a **LANGE** medical book

SMITH'S

General Urology

TWELFTH EDITION

Edited by

Emil A. Tanagho, MD
Professor and Chairman of Department of Urology
University of California School of Medicine
San Francisco

Jack W. McAninch, MD
Professor and Vice Chairman of Department of Urology
University of California School of Medicine
San Francisco
Chief of Urology, San Francisco General Hospital
San Francisco

APPLETON & LANGE
Norwalk, Connecticut/San Mateo, California

0-8385-8605-8

Notice: Our knowledge in clinical sciences is constantly changing. As new information becomes available, changes in treatment and in the use of drugs become necessary. The author(s) and the publisher of this volume have taken care to make certain that the doses of drugs and schedules of treatment are correct and compatible with the standards generally accepted at the time of publication. The reader is advised to consult carefully the instruction and information material included in the package insert of each drug or therapeutic agent before administration. This advice is especially important when using new or infrequently used drugs.

Copyright © 1988 by Appleton & Lange
A Publishing Division of Prentice Hall
Copyright © 1957, 1959, 1961, 1963, 1966, 1969, 1972, 1975, 1978, 1981, 1984 by Lange Medical Publications

Spanish Edition: Editorial El Manual Moderno, S.A. de C.V., Av. Sonora 206, Col. Hipodromo, 06100-Mexico, D.F.
Polish Edition: Panstwowy Zaklad Wydawnictw Lekarskich, P.O. Box 379, 00-950 Warsaw 1, Poland
Japanese Edition: Hirokawa Publishing Company, 27-14, Hongo 3, Bunkyo-ku, Tokyo 113, Japan
Portuguese Edition: Editora Guanabara Koogan S.A., Travessa do Ouvidor, 11, 20,040 Rio de Janeiro-RJ, Brazil

All rights reserved. This book, or any parts thereof, may not be used or reproduced in any manner without written permission. For information, address Appleton & Lange, 25 Van Zant Street, East Norwalk, Connecticut 06855.

88 89 90 91 / 5 4 3 2 1

Prentice-Hall International (UK) Limited, *London*
Prentice-Hall of Australia Pty. Limited, *Sydney*
Prentice-Hall Canada Inc., *Toronto*
Prentice-Hall Hispanoamericana, S.A., *Mexico*
Prentice-Hall of India Private Limited, *New Delhi*
Prentice-Hall of Japan, Inc., *Tokyo*
Simon & Schuster Asia Pte. Ltd., *Singapore*
Editora Prentice-Hall do Brasil, Ltda., *Rio de Janeiro*
Prentice-Hall, *Englewood Cliffs, New Jersey*

ISBN: 0-8385-8605-8
ISSN: 0892-1245

Cover: M. Chandler Martylewski

PRINTED IN THE UNITED STATES OF AMERICA

Table of Contents

Preface

Since 1957, when Donald Smith conceived and wrote the first edition of GENERAL UROLOGY, it has become the standard text for medical students and urology residents. With our assumption of the editorship of this, the 12th edition, it is our pleasure to honor Dr. Smith's contribution by renaming the text SMITH'S GENERAL UROLOGY.

The current edition is a very thorough revision and updating of the book, incorporating the following new or completely rewritten chapters:

Percutaneous Antegrade Endourology
Retrograde Instrumentation of the Urinary Tract (including laser and lithotripsy)
Sexually Transmitted Diseases in Men
Immunology of Genitourinary Tumors
Skin Diseases of the External Genitalia
Male Infertility
Sexual Dysfunction
Radionuclide Imaging (with all new illustrations showing the latest techniques)
Neuropathic Bladder Disorders

In addition to the above chapters, the rest of the book has been reviewed and updated. Particular emphasis has been placed on making the references current in all chapters, and the several hundred illustrations have been further modernized and improved, including many fine anatomic drawings and examples of the latest imaging techniques.

Students will find this book useful because of its concise, easy-to-follow format and organization and its mass of information. Interns and residents, as well as practicing physicians in urology or general medicine, will find it an efficient and current reference especially because of its stress on diagnosis and treatment.

As urologic subspecialties developed over the years, Dr. Smith invited the contributions of acknowledged experts. With the following new or greatly expanded chapters we continue this tradition: percutaneous and retrograde instrumentation, by Joachim Thüroff; radionuclide imaging, by Barry Kogan and Robert Hattner; sexually transmitted diseases in men, by Bruce Mayer and Richard Berger; immunology of genitourinary tumors, by Perinchery Narayan; skin diseases of the external genitalia, by Timothy Berger; male infertility, by Dale McClure; and sexual dysfunction, by Tom Lue.

General Urology is currently available in Japanese, Polish, Portuguese, and Spanish editions. The book has also been recorded in English on tape for use by the blind. The tape recording is available from Recording for the Blind, Inc., 20 Roszel Road, Princeton, NJ 08540.

It is our intent to provide in a concise format the information necessary for the understanding, diagnosis, and treatment of diseases managed by urologic surgeons. It has been our goal to keep the book current, to-the-point, and readable. Of incalculable assistance to us in this last respect has been the expertise of Jack Lange. For his skill and tact we are deeply appreciative.

Emil A. Tanagho
Jack W. McAninch

San Francisco
January, 1988

Authors

Mohamed M. Al Ghorab, MB, ChB, DS, MCh, FICS
Professor Emeritus of Urology, Faculty of Medicine, Alexandria University (Alexandria, Egypt).

William J.C. Amend, Jr., MD
Clinical Professor of Medicine, University of California School of Medicine (San Francisco).

Richard E. Berger, MD
Associate Professor of Urology, University of Washington School of Medicine, Seattle, and Chief of Urology, Harborview Medical Center (Seattle).

Timothy G. Berger, MD
Assistant Clinical Professor of Dermatology, University of California School of Medicine (San Francisco).

Felix A. Conte, MD
Professor of Pediatrics, University of California School of Medicine (San Francisco).

Nicholas J. Feduska, MD
Professor of Surgery, Transplant Service, University of California School of Medicine (San Francisco).

Peter H. Forsham, MD
Professor of Medicine and Pediatrics Emeritus, Former Chief of Endocrinology, and Former Director of Metabolic Research Unit, University of California School of Medicine (San Francisco).

Melvin M. Grumbach, MD
Edward B. Shaw Professor of Pediatrics and Chairman Emeritus, Department of Pediatrics, University of California School of Medicine (San Francisco).

Robert S. Hattner, MD
Associate Professor of Radiology, Chief of Nuclear Medicine Section, and Vice Chairman of Department of Radiology, University of California School of Medicine (San Francisco).

Douglas E. Johnson, MD
Professor of Urology, University of Texas M.D. Anderson Hospital & Tumor Institute (Houston).

Barry A. Kogan, MD
Assistant Professor of Urology and Chief of Pediatric Urology Service, University of California School of Medicine (San Francisco).

Marcus A. Krupp, MD
Clinical Professor of Medicine Emeritus, Stanford University School of Medicine (Stanford); Director Emeritus of Research Institute, Palo Alto Medical Foundation (Palo Alto, California).

Erich K. Lang, MD
Professor of Radiology, Louisiana State University Medical Center and Tulane School of Medicine (New Orleans); Chairman of Department of Radiology, Louisiana State Medical Center (New Orleans); Director of Department of Radiology, Charity Hospital (New Orleans).

Tom F. Lue, MD
Associate Professor of Urology, University of California School of Medicine (San Francisco).

Bruce M. Mayer, MD
Resident in Urology, University of Washington School of Medicine (Seattle).

Jack W. McAninch, MD
Professor and Vice Chairman of Department of Urology, University of California School of Medicine (San Francisco); Chief of Urology, San Francisco General Hospital (San Francisco).

R. Dale McClure, MD, FRCS(C)
Assistant Professor of Urology, University of California School of Medicine (San Francisco); Assistant Chief of Urology, Veterans Administration Hospital (San Francisco).

Edwin M. Meares, Jr., MD, FACS, FIDSA
Charles M. Whitney Professor and Chairman of Division of Urology, Tufts University School of Medicine (Medford, Massachusetts); Chairman of Department of Urology, New England Medical Center (Boston).

Perinchery Narayan, MD
Assistant Professor of Urology, University of California School of Medicine (San Francisco); Chief of Division of Urology, Veterans Administration Medical Center (San Francisco).

Alphonse J. Palubinskas, MD
Professor of Radiology and Urology and Chief of Section of Uroradiology, University of California School of Medicine (San Francisco).

Martin I. Resnick, MD
Professor and Chairman of Division of Urology, Case Western Reserve University School of Medicine (Cleveland).

Oscar Salvatierra, Jr., MD
Professor of Surgery and Urology and Chief of Transplant Service, University of California School of Medicine (San Francisco).

Richard A. Schmidt, MD, FACS
Associate Professor of Urology, University of California School of Medicine (San Francisco).

R. Ernest Sosa, MD
Assistant Professor of Surgery and Urology, The New York Hospital-Cornell Medical Center (New York).

J. Patrick Spirnak, MD
Assistant Professor of Urology, Case Western Reserve University School of Medicine (Cleveland); Director of Division of Urology, Cleveland Metropolitan General Hospital.

Samuel D. Spivack, MD
Clinical Professor of Medicine and Radiology, University of California School of Medicine (San Francisco).

David A. Swanson, MD
Associate Professor of Urology, University of Texas M.D. Anderson Hospital & Tumor Institute (Houston).

Emil A. Tanagho, MD
Professor and Chairman of Department of Urology, University of California School of Medicine (San Francisco).

Joachim W. Thüroff, MD
Associate Professor of Urology and Director of Urinary Stone Center, University of California School of Medicine (San Francisco); Associate Professor of Urology, Johannes Gutenberg University Medical School (Mainz, Federal Republic of Germany).

E. Darracott Vaughan, Jr., MD
James J. Colt Professor of Urology and Chairman of Division of Urology, Cornell University Medical College (New York); Attending Urologist-in-Chief, The New York Hospital.

Flavio G. Vincenti, MD
Clinical Professor of Medicine, University of California School of Medicine (San Francisco).

Andrew C. von Eschenbach, MD
Professor of Urology, University of Texas M.D. Anderson Hospital & Tumor Institute (Houston).

Richard D. Williams, MD
Professor of Urology and Chairman of Department of Urology, University of Iowa Hospitals and Clinics (Iowa City, Iowa); Chief of Urology, Veterans Administration Medical Center (Iowa City, Iowa).

Anatomy of the Genitourinary Tract

1

Emil A. Tanagho, MD

Urology deals with diseases and disorders of the male genitourinary tract and the female urinary tract. Surgical diseases of the adrenal gland are also included. These systems are illustrated in Figs 1–1 and 1–2.

ADRENALS

Gross Appearance

A. Anatomy: Each kidney is capped by an adrenal gland, and both organs are enclosed within Gerota's (perirenal) fascia. Each adrenal weighs about 5 g. The right adrenal is triangular in shape; the left is more rounded and crescentic. Each gland is composed of a cortex, chiefly influenced by the pituitary gland, and a medulla derived from chromaffin tissue.

B. Relations: Fig 1–2 shows the relation of the adrenals to other organs. The right adrenal lies between the liver and the vena cava. The left adrenal lies close to the aorta and is covered on its lower surface by the pancreas; superiorly and laterally, it is related to the spleen.

Histology

The adrenal cortex is composed of 3 distinct layers: the outer zona glomerulosa, the middle zona fasciculata, and the inner zona reticularis. The medulla lies centrally and is made up of polyhedral cells containing eosinophilic granular cytoplasm. These chromaffin cells are accompanied by ganglion and small round cells.

Blood Supply

A. Arterial: Each adrenal receives 3 arteries: one from the inferior phrenic artery, one from the aorta, and one from the renal artery.

B. Venous: Blood from the right adrenal is drained by a very short vein that empties into the vena cava; the left adrenal vein terminates in the left renal vein.

Lymphatics

The lymphatic vessels accompany the suprarenal vein and drain into the lumbar lymph nodes.

KIDNEYS

Gross Appearance

A. Anatomy: The kidneys lie along the borders of the psoas muscles and are therefore obliquely placed. The position of the liver causes the right kidney to be lower than the left (Figs 1–2 and 1–3). The adult kidney weighs about 150 g.

The kidneys are supported by the perirenal fat (which is enclosed in the perirenal fascia), the renal vascular pedicle, abdominal muscle tone, and the general bulk of the abdominal viscera. Variations in these factors permit variations in the degree of renal mobility. The average descent on inspiration or on assuming the upright position is 4–5 cm. Lack of mobility suggests abnormal fixation (eg, perinephritis), but extreme mobility is not necessarily pathologic.

On longitudinal section (Fig 1–4), the kidney is seen to be made up of an outer cortex, a central medulla, and the internal calices and pelvis. The cortex is homogeneous in appearance. Portions of it project toward the pelvis between the papillae and fornices and are called the columns of Bertin. The medulla consists of numerous pyramids formed by the converging collecting renal tubules, which drain into the minor calices.

B. Relations: Figs 1–2 and 1–3 show the relations of the kidneys to adjacent organs and structures. Their intimacy with intraperitoneal organs and the autonomic innervation they share with these organs explain, in part, some of the gastrointestinal symptoms that accompany genitourinary disease.

Histology

A. Nephron: The functioning unit of the kidney is the nephron, which is composed of a tubule that has both secretory and excretory functions (Fig 1–4). The secretory portion is contained largely within the cortex and consists of a renal corpuscle and the secretory part of the renal tubule. The excretory portion of this duct lies in the medulla. The renal corpuscle is composed of the vascular glomerulus, which projects into Bowman's capsule, which, in turn, is continuous with the epithelium of the proximal convoluted tubule. The secretory portion of the renal tubule is made up of the proximal convoluted tubule, the loop of Henle, and the distal convoluted tubule.

The excretory portion of the nephron is the collecting tubule, which is continuous with the distal end of the ascending limb of the convoluted tubule. It empties its contents through the tip (papilla) of a pyramid into a minor calix.

B. Supporting Tissue: The renal stroma is composed of loose connective tissue and contains blood vessels, capillaries, nerves, and lymphatics.

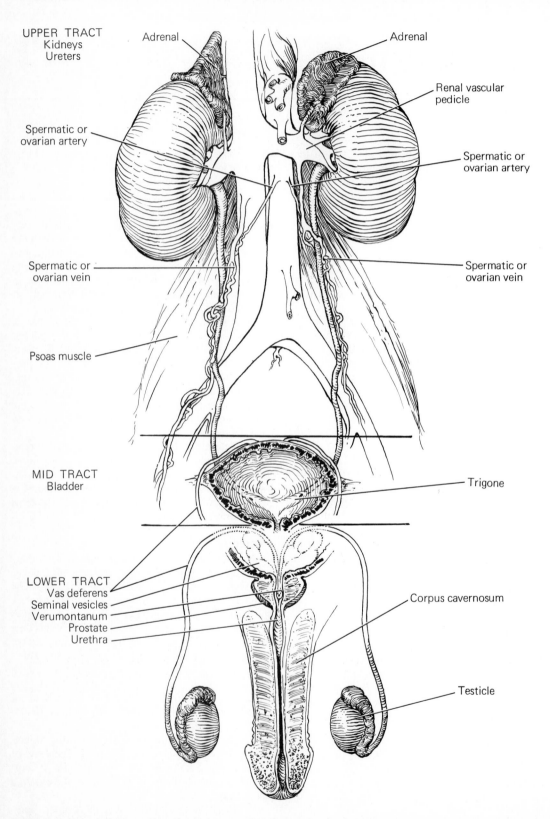

UPPER TRACT
Kidneys
Ureters

Adrenal

Adrenal

Renal vascular
pedicle

Spermatic or
ovarian artery

Spermatic or
ovarian artery

Spermatic or
ovarian vein

Spermatic or
ovarian vein

Psoas muscle

MID TRACT
Bladder

Trigone

LOWER TRACT
Vas deferens
Seminal vesicles
Verumontanum
Prostate
Urethra

Corpus cavernosum

Testicle

Figure 1–1. Anatomy of the male genitourinary tract. The upper and mid tracts have urologic function only. The lower tract has both genital and urinary functions.

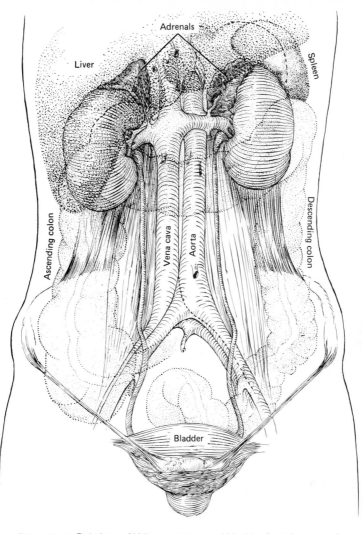

Figure 1–2. Relations of kidney, ureters, and bladder (anterior aspect).

Blood Supply
(Figs 1–2, 1–4, and 1–5)

A. Arterial: Usually there is one renal artery, a branch of the aorta, that enters the hilum of the kidney between the pelvis, which normally lies posteriorly, and the renal vein. It may branch before it reaches the kidney, and 2 or more separate arteries may be noted. In duplication of the pelvis and ureter, it is usual for each renal segment to have its own arterial supply.

The renal artery divides into anterior and posterior branches. The posterior branch supplies the mid segment of the posterior surface. The anterior branch supplies both upper and lower poles as well as the entire anterior surface. The renal arteries are all end arteries.

The renal artery further divides into interlobar arteries, which ascend in the columns of Bertin (between the pyramids) and then arch along the base of the pyramids (arcuate arteries). The renal artery then ascends as interlobular arteries. From these vessels, smaller (afferent) branches pass to the glomeruli. From the

glomerular tuft, efferent arterioles pass to the tubules in the stroma.

B. Venous: The renal veins are paired with the arteries, but any of them will drain the entire kidney if the others are tied off.

Although the renal artery and vein are usually the sole blood vessels of the kidney, accessory renal vessels are common and may be of clinical importance if they are so placed as to compress the ureter, in which case hydronephrosis may result.

Nerve Supply

The renal nerves derived from the renal plexus accompany the renal vessels throughout the renal parenchyma.

Lymphatics

The lymphatics of the kidney drain into the lumbar lymph nodes (Figs 19–1 and 19–2).

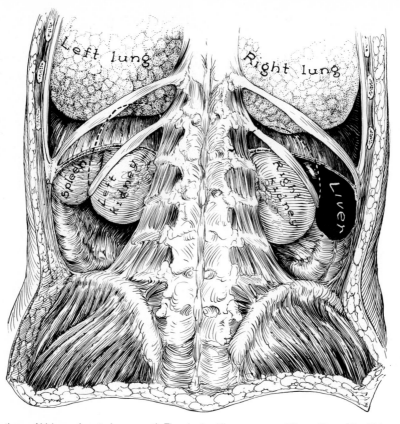

Figure 1–3. Relations of kidneys (posterior aspect). The dashed lines represent the outline of the kidneys where they are obscured by overlying structures.

CALICES, RENAL PELVIS, & URETER

Gross Appearance

A. Anatomy:

1. Calices–The tips of the minor calices (8–12 in number) are indented by the projecting pyramids (Fig 1–4). These calices unite to form 2 or 3 major calices, which join the renal pelvis.

2. Renal pelvis–The pelvis may be entirely intrarenal or partly intrarenal and partly extrarenal. Inferomedially, it tapers to form the ureter.

3. Ureter–The adult ureter is about 30 cm long, varying in direct relation to the height of the individual. It follows a rather smooth S curve. Areas of relative narrowing are found (1) at the ureteropelvic junction, (2) where the ureter crosses over the iliac vessels, and (3) where it courses through the bladder wall.

B. Relations:

1. Calices–The calices are intrarenal and are intimately related to the renal parenchyma.

2. Renal pelvis–If the pelvis is partly extrarenal, it lies along the lateral border of the psoas muscle and on the quadratus lumborum muscle; the renal vascular pedicle is placed just anterior to it. The left renal pelvis lies at the level of the first or second lumbar vertebra; the right pelvis is a little lower.

3. Ureter–As followed from above downward, the ureters lie on the psoas muscles, pass medially to the sacroiliac joints, and then swing laterally near the ischial spines before passing medially to penetrate the base of the bladder (Fig 1–2). In the female, the uterine arteries are closely related to the juxtavesical portion of the ureters. The ureters are covered by the posterior peritoneum; their lowermost portions are closely attached to it, while the juxtavesical portions are embedded in vascular retroperitoneal fat.

The vasa deferentia, as they leave the internal inguinal rings, sweep over the lateral pelvic walls anterior to the ureters (Fig 1–6). They lie medial to the latter before joining the seminal vesicle and penetrating the base of the prostate to become the ejaculatory ducts.

Histology
(Fig 1–4)

The walls of the calices, pelvis, and ureters are

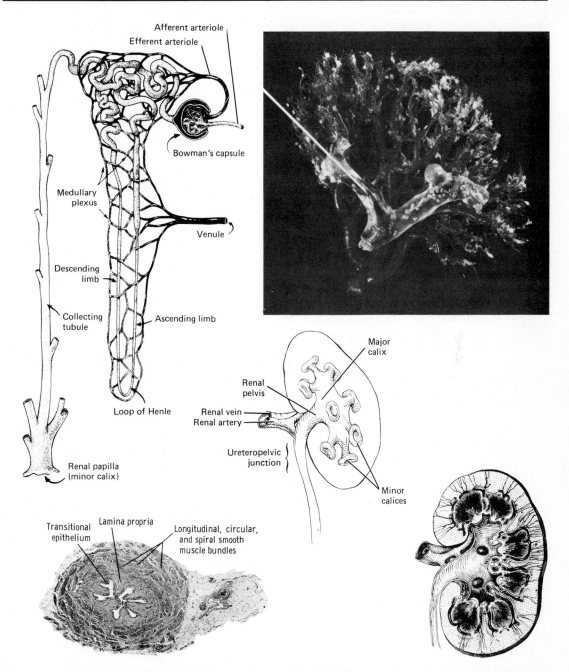

Figure 1–4. Anatomy and histology of the kidney and ureter. *Upper left:* Diagram of the nephron and its blood supply. (Courtesy of Merck, Sharp, & Dohme: Seminar: 1947;9[3].) *Upper right:* Cast of the pelvic caliceal system and the arterial supply of the kidney. *Middle:* Renal calices, pelvis, and ureter (posterior aspect). *Lower left:* Histology of the ureter. The smooth muscle bundles are arranged in both a spiral and longitudinal manner. *Lower right:* Longitudinal section of kidney showing calices, pelvis, ureter, and renal blood supply (posterior aspect).

composed of transitional cell epithelium under which lies loose connective and elastic tissue (lamina propria). External to these are a mixture of spiral and longitudinal smooth muscle fibers. They are not arranged in definite layers. The outermost adventitial coat is composed of fibrous connective tissue.

Blood Supply

A. Arterial: The renal calices, pelvis, and upper ureters derive their blood supply from the renal arteries; the mid ureter is fed by the internal spermatic (or ovarian) arteries. The lowermost portion of the ureter is served by branches from the common iliac, internal iliac (hypogastric), and vesical arteries.

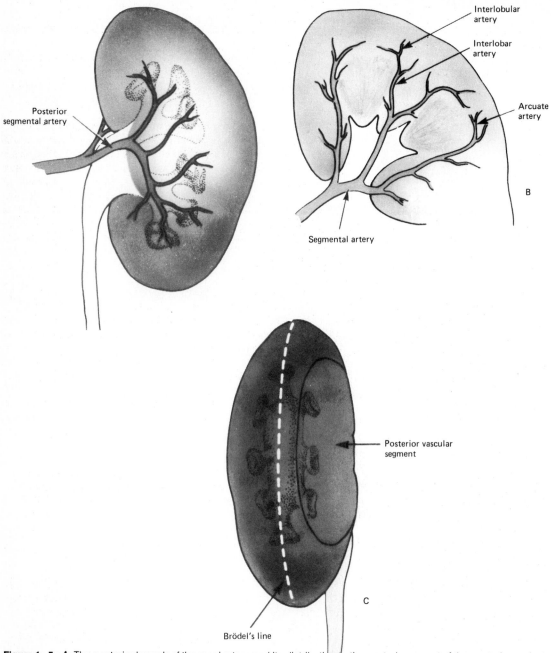

Figure 1–5. *A:* The posterior branch of the renal artery and its distribution to the central segment of the posterior surface of the kidney. *B:* Branches of the anterior division of the renal artery supplying the entire anterior surface of the kidney as well as the upper and lower poles at both surfaces. The segmental branches lead to interlobar, arcuate, and interlobular arteries. *C:* The lateral convex margin of the kidney. Brödel's line, which is 1 cm from the convex margin, is the bloodless plane demarcated by the distribution of the posterior branch of the renal artery.

B. Venous: The veins of the renal calices, pelvis, and ureters are paired with the arteries.

Lymphatics

The lymphatics of the upper portions of the ureters as well as those from the pelvis and calices enter the lumbar lymph nodes. The lymphatics of the mid ureter pass to the internal iliac (hypogastric) and common iliac lymph nodes; the lower ureteral lymphatics empty into the vesical and hypogastric lymph nodes (Figs 19–1 and 19–2).

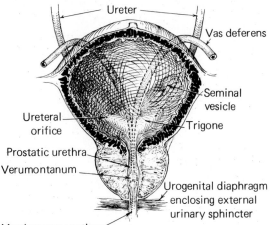

Figure 1–6. Anatomy and relations of the ureters, bladder, prostate, seminal vesicles, and vasa deferentia (anterior view).

BLADDER

Gross Appearance

The bladder is a hollow muscular organ that serves as a reservoir for urine. In women, its posterior wall and dome are invaginated by the uterus. The adult bladder normally has a capacity of 350–450 mL.

A. Anatomy: When empty, the adult bladder lies behind the pubic symphysis and is largely a pelvic organ. In infants and children, it is situated higher. When it is full, it rises well above the symphysis and can readily be palpated or percussed. When overdistended, as in acute or chronic urinary retention, it may cause the lower abdomen to bulge visibly.

Extending from the dome of the bladder to the umbilicus is a fibrous cord, the medial umbilical ligament, which represents the obliterated urachus. The ureters enter the bladder posteroinferiorly in an oblique manner and at these points are about 5 cm apart (Fig 1–6). The orifices, situated at the extremities of the crescent-shaped interureteric ridge that forms the proximal border of the trigone, are about 2.5 cm apart. The trigone occupies the area between the ridge and the bladder neck.

The internal sphincter, or bladder neck, is not a true circular sphincter but a thickening formed by interlaced and converging muscle fibers of the detrusor as they pass distally to become the smooth musculature of the urethra.

B. Relations: In males, the bladder is related posteriorly to the seminal vesicles, vasa deferentia, ureters, and rectum (Figs 1–8 and 1–9). In females, the uterus and vagina are interposed between the bladder and rectum (Fig 1–10). The dome and posterior surfaces are covered by peritoneum; hence, in this area the bladder is closely related to the small intestine and sigmoid colon. In both males and females, the bladder is related to the posterior surface of the pubic symphysis, and, when distended, it is in contact with the lower abdominal wall.

Histology
(Fig 1–7)

The mucosa of the bladder is composed of transitional epithelium. Beneath it is a well-developed submucosal layer formed largely of connective and elastic tissues. External to the submucosa is the detrusor muscle, which is made up of a mixture of smooth muscle fibers arranged at random in a longitudinal, circular, and spiral manner without any layer formation or specific orientation except close to the internal meatus, where the detrusor muscle assumes 3 definite layers: inner longitudinal, middle circular, and outer longitudinal.

Blood Supply

A. Arterial: The bladder is supplied with blood by the superior, middle, and inferior vesical arteries, which arise from the anterior trunk of the internal iliac (hypogastric) artery, and by smaller branches from the obturator and inferior gluteal arteries. In the female, the uterine and vaginal arteries also send branches to the bladder.

B. Venous: Surrounding the bladder is a rich plexus of veins that ultimately empties into the internal iliac (hypogastric) veins.

Lymphatics

The lymphatics of the bladder drain into the vesical, external iliac, internal iliac (hypogastric), and common iliac lymph nodes (Figs 19–1 and 19–2).

PROSTATE GLAND

Gross Appearance

A. Anatomy: The prostate is a fibromuscular and glandular organ lying just inferior to the bladder (Figs 1–6 and 1–8). The normal prostate weighs about 20 g and contains the posterior urethra, which is about 2.5 cm in length. It is supported anteriorly by the puboprostatic ligaments and inferiorly by the urogenital diaphragm (Fig 1–6). The prostate is perforated posteriorly by the ejaculatory ducts, which pass obliquely to empty through the verumontanum on the floor of the prostatic urethra just proximal to the striated external urinary sphincter (Fig 1–11).

According to the classification of Lowsley, the prostate consists of 5 lobes: anterior, posterior, median, right lateral, and left lateral. According to McNeal (1972), the prostate has a peripheral zone, a central zone, and transitional zone, an anterior segment, and a preprostatic sphincteric zone (Fig 1–12). The segment of urethra that traverses the prostate gland is the prostatic urethra. It is lined by an inner longitudinal layer of muscle (continuous with a similar layer of

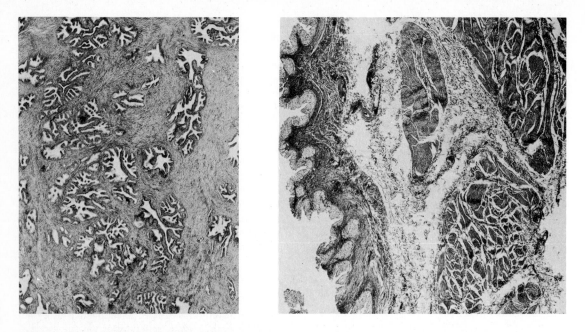

Figure 1–7. *Left:* Histology of the prostate. Epithelial glands embedded in a mixture of connective and elastic tissue and smooth muscle. *Right:* Histology of the bladder. The mucosa is transitional cell in type and lies upon a well-developed submucosal layer of connective tissue. The detrusor muscle is composed of interlacing longitudinal, circular, and spiral smooth muscle bundles.

the vesical wall). Incorporated within the prostate gland is an abundant amount of smooth musculature derived primarily from the external longitudinal bladder musculature. This musculature represents the true smooth involuntary sphincter of the posterior urethra in males.

Prostatic adenoma develops from the periurethral glands at the site of the median or lateral lobes. The posterior lobe, however, is prone to cancerous degeneration.

B. Relations: The prostate gland lies behind the pubic symphysis. Closely applied to the posterosuperior surface are the vasa deferentia and seminal vesicles (Fig 1–8). Posteriorly, it is separated from the rectum by the 2 layers of Denonvilliers' fascia, serosal rudiments of the pouch of Douglas, which once extended to the urogenital diaphragm (Fig 1–9).

Histology
(Fig 1–7)

The prostate consists of a thin fibrous capsule under which are circularly oriented smooth muscle fibers and collagenous tissue that surrounds the urethra (involuntary sphincter). Deep to this layer lies the prostatic stroma, composed of connective and elastic tissues and smooth muscle fibers in which are embedded the epithelial glands. These glands drain into the major excretory ducts (about 25 in number), which open chiefly on the floor of the urethra between the veru-

montanum and the vesical neck. Just beneath the transitional epithelium of the prostatic urethra lie the periurethral glands.

Blood Supply

A. Arterial: The arterial supply to the prostate is derived from the inferior vesical, internal pudendal, and middle rectal (hemorrhoidal) arteries.

B. Venous: The veins from the prostate drain into the periprostatic plexus, which has connections with the deep dorsal vein of the penis and the internal iliac (hypogastric) veins.

Nerve Supply

The prostate gland receives a rich nerve supply from the sympathetic and parasympathetic nerve plexuses.

Lymphatics

The lymphatics from the prostate drain into the internal iliac (hypogastric), sacral, vesical, and external iliac lymph nodes (Figs 19–1 and 19–2).

SEMINAL VESICLES

Gross Appearance

The seminal vesicles lie just cephalad to the prostate under the base of the bladder (Figs 1–6 and

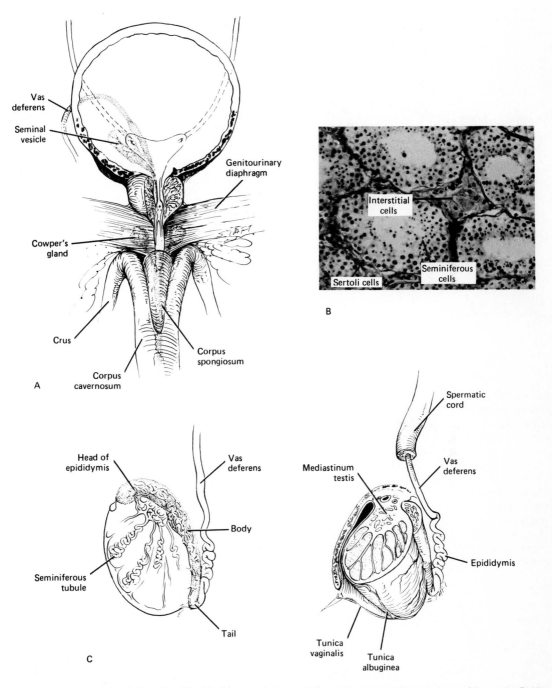

Figure 1–8. *A:* Anatomic relationship of the bladder, prostate, prostatomembranous urethra, and root of the penis. *B:* Histology of the testis. Seminiferous tubules lined by supporting basement membrane for the Sertoli and spermatogenic cells. The latter are in various stages of development. *C:* Cross sections of the testis and epididymis. (*A* and *C* are reproduced, with permission, from Tanagho EA: Anatomy of the lower urinary tract. Chap 1, pp. 46–74, in: *Campbell's Urology,* 5th ed. Vol 1. Walsh PC et al [editors]. Saunders, 1986.)

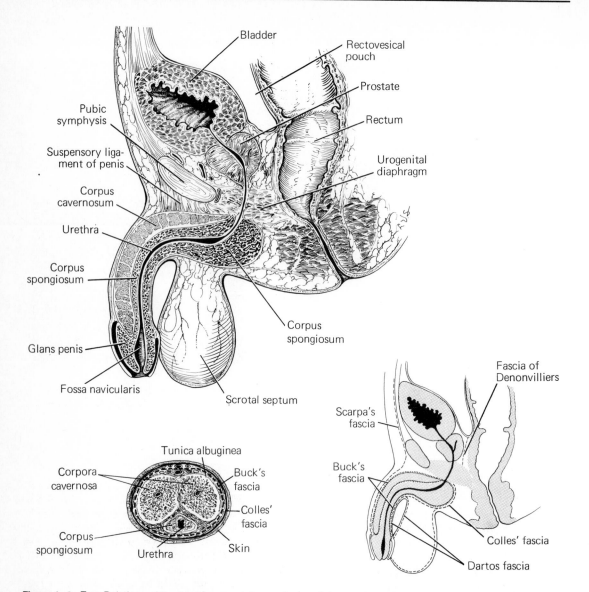

Figure 1-9. *Top:* Relations of the bladder, prostate, seminal vesicles, penis, urethra, and scrotal contents. *Lower left:* Transverse section through the penis. The paired upper structures are the corpora cavernosa. The single lower body surrounding the urethra is the corpus spongiosum. *Lower right:* Fascial planes of the lower genitourinary tract. (After Wesson.)

1-8). They are about 6 cm long and quite soft. Each vesicle joins its corresponding vas deferens to form the ejaculatory duct. The ureters lie medial to each, and the rectum is contiguous with their posterior surfaces.

Histology

The mucous membrane is pseudostratified. The submucosa consists of dense connective tissue covered by a thin layer of muscle that in turn is encapsulated by connective tissue.

Blood Supply

The blood supply is similar to that of the prostate gland.

Nerve Supply

The nerve supply is mainly from the sympathetic nerve plexus.

Lymphatics

The lymphatics of the seminal vesicles are those that serve the prostate (Figs 19-1 and 19-2).

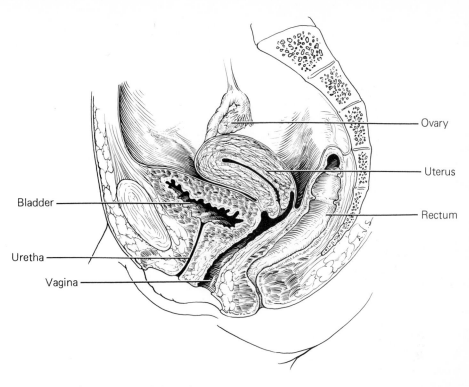

Figure 1–10. Anatomy and relations of the bladder, urethra, uterus and ovary, vagina, and rectum.

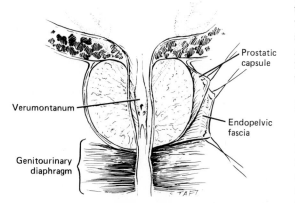

Figure 1–11. Section of the prostate gland shows the prostatic urethra, verumontanum, and crista urethralis, in addition to the opening of the prostatic utricle and the 2 ejaculatory ducts in the midline. Note that the prostate is surrounded by the prostatic capsule, which is covered by another prostatic sheath derived from the endopelvic fascia. The prostate is resting on the genitourinary diaphragm. (Reproduced, with permission, from Tanagho EA: Anatomy of the lower urinary tract. Chap 1, pp 46–74, in: *Campbell's Urology*, 5th ed. Vol 1. Walsh PC et al [editors]. Saunders, 1986.)

SPERMATIC CORD

Gross Appearance

The 2 spermatic cords extend from the internal inguinal rings through the inguinal canals to the testicles (Fig 1–8). Each cord contains the vas deferens, the internal and external spermatic arteries, the artery of the vas, the venous pampiniform plexus (which forms the spermatic vein superiorly), lymph vessels, and nerves. All of the above are enclosed in investing layers of thin fascia. A few fibers of the cremaster muscle insert on the cords in the inguinal canal.

Histology

The fascia covering the cord is formed of loose connective tissue that supports arteries, veins, and lymphatics. The vas deferens is a small, thick-walled tube consisting of an internal mucosa and submucosa surrounded by 3 well-defined layers of smooth muscle encased in a covering of fibrous tissue. Above the testes, this tube is straight. Its proximal 4 cm tends to be convoluted.

Blood Supply

A. Arterial: The external spermatic artery, a branch of the inferior epigastric, supplies the fascial coverings of the cord. The internal spermatic artery passes through the cord on its way to the testis. The deferential artery is close to the vas.

B. Venous: The veins from the testis and the coverings of the spermatic cord form the pampiniform

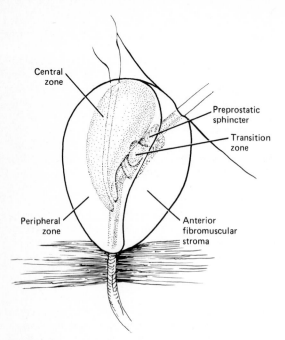

Figure 1–12. Anatomy of the prostate gland (adapted from McNeal). (Reproduced, with permission, from Tanagho EA: Anatomy of the lower urinary tract. Chap 1, pp 46–74, in: *Campbell's Urology*, 5th ed. Vol 1. Walsh PC et al [editors]. Saunders, 1986.)

plexus, which, at the internal inguinal ring, unites to form the spermatic vein.

Lymphatics

The lymphatics from the spermatic cord empty into the external iliac lymph nodes (Figs 19–1 and 19–2).

EPIDIDYMIS

Gross Appearance

A. Anatomy: The upper portion of the epididymis (globus major) is connected to the testis by numerous efferent ducts from the testis (Fig 1–8). The epididymis consists of a markedly coiled duct that, at its lower pole (globus minor), is continuous with the vas deferens. An appendix of the epididymis is often seen on its upper pole; this is a cystic body that in some cases is pedunculated but in others is sessile.

B. Relations: The epididymis lies posterolateral to the testis and is nearest to the testis at its upper pole. Its lower pole is connected to the testis by fibrous tissue. The vas lies posteromedial to the epididymis.

Histology

The epididymis is covered by serosa. The ductus epididymidis is lined by pseudostratified columnar epithelium throughout its length.

Blood Supply

A. Arterial: The arterial supply to the epididymis comes from the internal spermatic artery and the artery of the vas (deferential artery).

B. Venous: The venous blood drains into the pampiniform plexus, which becomes the spermatic vein.

Lymphatics

The lymphatics drain into the external iliac and internal iliac (hypogastric) lymph nodes (Figs 19–1 and 19–2).

TESTIS

Gross Appearance

A. Anatomy: The average testicle measures about $4 \times 3 \times 2.5$ cm (Fig 1–8). It has a dense fascial covering called the tunica albuginea testis, which, posteriorly, is invaginated somewhat into the body of the testis to form the mediastinum testis. This fibrous mediastinum sends fibrous septa into the testis, thus separating it into about 250 lobules.

The testis is covered anteriorly and laterally by the visceral layer of the serous tunica vaginalis, which is continuous with the parietal layer that separates the testis from the scrotal wall.

At the upper pole of the testis is the appendix testis, a small pedunculated or sessile body similar in appearance to the appendix of the epididymis.

B. Relations: The testis is closely attached posterolaterally to the epididymis, particularly at its upper and lower poles.

Histology
(Fig 1–8)

Each lobule contains 1–4 markedly convoluted seminiferous tubules, each of which is about 60 cm long. These ducts converge at the mediastinum testis, where they connect with the efferent ducts that drain into the epididymis.

The seminiferous tubule has a basement membrane containing connective and elastic tissue. This supports the seminiferous cells, which are of 2 types: (1) Sertoli (supporting) cells and (2) spermatogenic cells. The stroma between the seminiferous tubules contains connective tissue in which the interstitial Leydig cells are located.

Blood Supply

The blood supply to the testes is closely associated with that to the kidneys because of the common embryologic origin of the 2 organs.

A. Arterial: The arteries to the testes (internal spermatics) arise from the aorta just below the renal arteries and course through the spermatic cords to the testes, where they anastomose with the arteries of the vasa deferentia that branch off from the internal iliac (hypogastric) artery.

B. Venous: The blood from the testis returns in

the pampiniform plexus of the spermatic cord. At the internal inguinal ring, the pampiniform plexus forms the spermatic vein.

The right spermatic vein enters the vena cava just below the right renal vein; the left spermatic vein empties into the left renal vein.

Lymphatics

The lymphatic vessels from the testes pass to the lumbar lymph nodes, which in turn are connected to the mediastinal nodes (Figs 19–1 and 19–2).

SCROTUM

Gross Appearance

Beneath the corrugated skin of the scrotum lies the dartos muscle. Deep to this are the 3 fascial layers derived from the abdominal wall at the time of testicular descent. Beneath these is the parietal layer of the tunica vaginalis.

The scrotum is divided into 2 sacs by a septum of connective tissue. The scrotum not only supports the testes but, by relaxation or contraction of its muscular layer, helps to regulate their environmental temperature.

Histology

The dartos muscle, under the skin of the scrotum, is unstriated. The deeper layer is made up of connective tissue.

Blood Supply

A. Arterial: The arteries to the scrotum arise from the femoral, internal pudendal, and inferior epigastric arteries.

B. Venous: The veins are paired with the arteries.

Lymphatics

The lymphatics drain into the superficial inguinal and subinguinal lymph nodes (Figs 19–1 and 19–2).

PENIS & MALE URETHRA

Gross Appearance

The penis is composed of 2 corpora cavernosa and the corpus spongiosum, which contains the urethra, whose diameter is 8–9 mm. These corpora are capped distally by the glans. Each corpus is enclosed in a fascial sheath (tunica albuginea), and all are surrounded by a thick fibrous envelope known as Buck's fascia. A covering of skin, devoid of fat, is loosely applied about these bodies. The prepuce forms a hood over the glans.

Beneath the skin of the penis (and scrotum) and extending from the base of the glans to the urogenital diaphragm is Colles' fascia, which is continuous with Scarpa's fascia of the lower abdominal wall (Fig 1–9).

The proximal ends of the corpora cavernosa are attached to the pelvic bones just anterior to the ischial tuberosities. Occupying a depression on their ventral surface in the midline is the corpus spongiosum, which is connected proximally to the undersurface of the urogenital diaphragm, through which emerges the membranous urethra. This portion of the corpus spongiosum is surrounded by the bulbospongiosus muscle. Its distal end expands to form the glans penis.

The suspensory ligament of the penis arises from the linea alba and pubic symphysis and inserts into the fascial covering of the corpora cavernosa.

Histology

A. Corpora and Glans Penis: The corpora cavernosa, the corpus spongiosum, and the glans penis are composed of septa of smooth muscle and erectile tissue that enclose vascular cavities.

B. Urethra: The urethral mucosa that traverses the glans penis is formed of squamous epithelium. Proximal to this, the mucosa is transitional in type. Underneath the mucosa is the submucosa, which contains connective and elastic tissue and smooth muscle. In the submucosa are the numerous glands of Littre, whose ducts connect with the urethral lumen.

The urethra is surrounded by the vascular corpus spongiosum and the glans penis.

Blood Supply

A. Arterial: The penis and urethra are supplied by the internal pudendal arteries. Each artery divides into a deep artery of the penis (which supplies the corpora cavernosa), a dorsal artery of the penis, and the bulbourethral artery. These branches supply the corpus spongiosum, the glans penis, and the urethra.

B. Venous: The superficial dorsal vein lies external to Buck's fascia. The deep dorsal vein is placed beneath Buck's fascia and lies between the dorsal arteries. These veins connect with the pudendal plexus, which drains into the internal pudendal vein.

Lymphatics

Lymphatic drainage from the skin of the penis is to the superficial inguinal and subinguinal lymph nodes. The lymphatics from the glans penis pass to the subinguinal and external iliac nodes. The lymphatics from the deep urethra drain into the internal iliac (hypogastric) and common iliac lymph nodes (Figs 19–1 and 19–2).

FEMALE URETHRA

The adult female urethra is about 4 cm long and 8 mm in diameter. It is slightly curved and lies beneath the pubic symphysis just anterior to the vagina.

The epithelial lining of the female urethra is squamous in its distal portion and pseudostratified or transitional in the remainder. The submucosa is made up of connective and elastic tissues and spongy venous spaces. Embedded in it are many periurethral glands, which are most numerous distally; the largest of these are the periurethral glands of Skene, which open on the floor of the urethra just inside the meatus.

External to the submucosa is a longitudinal layer of smooth muscle continuous with the inner longitudinal layer of the bladder wall. Surrounding this is a heavy layer of circular smooth muscle fibers extending from the external vesical muscular layer. They constitute the true involuntary urethral sphincter. External to this is the circular striated (voluntary) sphincter surrounding the middle third of the urethra; this constitutes an intrusive element in the musculature of the urethra.

The arterial supply to the female urethra is derived from the inferior vesical, vaginal, and internal pudendal arteries. Blood from the urethra drains into the internal pudendal veins.

Lymphatic drainage from the external portion of the urethra is to the inguinal and subinguinal lymph nodes. Drainage from the deep urethra is into the internal iliac (hypogastric) lymph nodes (Figs 19–1 and 19–2).

Nerve Supply to the Genitourinary Organs

See Figs 3–2, 3–3, and 20–1.

REFERENCES

Adrenals

Ivemark B, Ekström T, Lagergren C: The vasculature of the developing and mature human adrenal gland. *Acta Paediatr Scand* 1967;**56:**601.

Johnstone FRC: The surgical anatomy of the adrenal glands with particular reference to the suprarenal vein. *Surg Clin North Am* 1964;**44:**1315.

Kidneys

Barger AC, Herd JA: The renal circulation. *N Engl J Med* 1971;**284:**482.

Cockett ATK: Lymphatic network of kidney. 1. Anatomic and physiologic considerations. *Urology* 1977;**9:**125.

Fetterman GH et al: The growth and maturation of human glomeruli and proximal convolutions from term to adulthood. *Pediatrics* 1965;**35:**601.

Fine H, Keen EN: Some observations on the medulla of the kidney. *Br J Urol* 1976;**48:**161.

Graves FT: The arterial anatomy of the congenitally abnormal kidney. *Br J Surg* 1969;**56:**533.

Hegedüs V: Arterial anatomy of the kidney: A three-dimensional angiographic investigation. *Acta Radiol [Diagn] (Stockh)* 1972;**12:** 604.

Hodson J: The lobar structure of the kidney. *Br J Urol* 1972;**44:**246.

Layton JM: The structure of the kidney from the gross to the molecular. *J Urol* 1963;**90:**502.

Mayerson HS: The lymphatic system with particular reference to the kidney. *Surg Gynecol Obstet* 1963;**116:**259.

Meyers MA: The reno-alimentary relationships. Anatomic-roentgen study of their clinical significance. *Am J Roentgenol* 1975;**123:**386.

Potter EL: Development of the human glomerulus. *Arch Pathol* 1965;**80:**241.

Resnick MI, Pounds DM, Boyce WH: Surgical anatomy of the human kidney and its applications. *Urology* 1981;**17:**367.

Roddie IC: Modern views of physiology. 20. The kidney. *Practitioner* 1970;**205:**242.

Vordermark JS II: Segmental anatomy of the kidney. *Urology* 1981;**17:**521.

Zamboni L, DeMartino C: Embryogenesis of the human renal glomerulus. 1. A histologic study. *Arch Panthol* 1968;**86:**279.

Calices, Renal Pelvis, & Ureters

Cussen LJ: The structure of the normal human ureter in infancy and childhood. *Invest Urol* 1967;**5:**179.

Elbadawi A, Amaku EO, Frank IN: Trilaminar musculature of submucosal ureter: Anatomy and functional implications. *Urology* 1973;**2:**409.

Hanna MK Et al: Ureteral structure and ultrastructure. 1. Normal human ureter. *J Urol* 1976;**116:**718.

Osathanondh V, Potter EL: Development of human kidney shown by microdissection. 2. Renal pelvis, calyces, and papillae. 3. Formation and interrelationships of collecting tubules and nephrons. 4. Formation of tubular portions of nephrons. 5. Development of vascular pattern of glomerulus. *Arch Pathol* 1963;**76:**277, 290 and 1966; **82:**391, 403.

Rizzo M et al: Ultrastructure of the urinary tract muscle coat in man: Calices, renal pelvis, pelviureteric junction and ureter. *Eur Urol* 1981;**7:**171.

Sykes D: The morphology of renal lobulations and calyces, and their relationship to partial nephrectomy. *Br J Surg* 1964;**51:**294.

Tanagho EA: The ureterovesical junction: Anatomy and physiology. Pages 394–404 in: *Scientific Foundations of Urology.* Chisholm GD, Williams DI (editors). Heinemann, 1982.

Weiss RM, Bassett AL, Hoffman BF: Adrenergic innervation of the ureter. *Invest Urol* 1978;**16:**123.

Bladder & Urethra

Elbadawi A: Ultrastructure of vesicourethral innervation. 1. Neuroeffector and cell junctions in male internal sphincter. *J Urol* 1982;**128:**180.

Elbadawi A, Schenk EA: A new theory of the innervation of bladder musculature. 2. Innervation of the vesicourethral junction and external urethral sphincter. *J Urol* 1974; **111:**613.

Fletcher TF, Bradley WE: Neuroanatomy of the bladder-urethra. *J Urol* 1978;**119:**153.

Gosling JA, Dixon DS: The structure and innervation of smooth muscle in the wall of the bladder neck and proximal urethra. *Br J Urol* 1975;**47:**549.

Hakky SI: Ultrastructure of the normal human urethra. *Br J Urol* 1979;**51:**304.

Hodges CV: Surgical anatomy of the urinary bladder and pelvic ureter. *Surg Clin North Am* 1964;**44:**1327.

Hutch JA: *Anatomy and Physiology of the Bladder, Trigone and Urethra.* Appleton-Century-Crofts, 1972.

Hutch JA: The internal urinary sphincter: A double loop system. *J Urol* 1971;**105**:375.

Olesen KP, Grau V: The suspensory apparatus of the female bladder neck. *Urol Int* 1976;**31**:33.

Tanagho EA: Anatomy of the lower urinary tract. Chap 1, pp 46–74, in: *Campbell's Urology,* 5th ed. Vol 1. Walsh PC et al (editors). Saunders, 1986.

Tanagho EA, Miller ER: Functional considerations of urethral sphincteric dynamics. *J Urol* 1973;**109**:273.

Tanagho EA, Pugh RCB: The anatomy and function of the ureterovesical junction. *Br J Urol* 1963;**35**:151.

Tanagho EA, Schmidt RA, de Araujo CG: Urinary striated sphincter: What is its nerve supply? *Urology* 1982; **20**:415.

Tanagho EA, Smith DR: The anatomy and function of the bladder neck. *Br J Urol* 1966;**38**:54.

Tanagho EA et al: Observations in the dynamics of the bladder neck. *Br J Urol* 1966;**38**:72.

Prostate Gland

Bruschini H, Schmidt RA, Tanagho EA: The male genitourinary sphincter mechanism in the dog. *Invest Urol* 1978;**15**:284.

Hutch JA, Rambo ON Jr: A study of the anatomy of the prostate, prostatic urethra and the urinary sphincter system. *J Urol* 1970;**104**:443.

McNeal JE: The prostate and prostatic urethra: A morphologic study. *J Urol.* 1972;**107**:1008.

Vaalsti A, Hervonen A: Autonomic innervation of the human prostate. *Invest Urol* 1980;**17**:293.

Wein AJ, Benson GS, Jacobowitz D: Lack of evidence for adrenergic innervation of external urethral sphincter. *J Urol* 1979;**121**:324.

Spermatic Cord

Ahlberg NE, Bartley O, Chidekel N: Right and left gonadal veins: An anatomical and statistical study. *Acta Radiol [Diagn] (Stockh)* 1966;**4**:593.

Bergman LL: The regional anatomy of the inguinal canal. *GP* (Oct) 1962;**26**:114.

Testis

Busch FM, Sayegh ES: Roentgenographic visualization of human testicular lymphatics: A preliminary report. *J Urol* 1963;**89**:106.

Female Urethra

Lindner HH, Feldman SE: Surgical anatomy of the perineum. *Surg Clin North Am* 1962;**42**:877.

Zacharin RF: The anatomic supports of the female urethra. *Obstet Gynecol* 1968;**32**:754.

2

Embryology of the Genitourinary System

Emil A. Tanagho, MD

At birth, the genital and urinary systems are related only in the sense that they share certain common passages. Embryologically, however, they are intimately related. Because of the complex interrelationships of the embryonic phases of the 2 systems, they will be discussed here as 5 subdivisions; the nephric system, the vesicourethral unit, the gonads, the genital duct system, and the external genitalia.

NEPHRIC SYSTEM

The nephric system develops progressively as 3 distinct entities: pronephros, mesonephros, and metanephros.

Pronephros

This is the earliest nephric stage in humans, and it corresponds to the mature structure of the most primitive vertebrate. It extends from the fourth to the fourteenth somites and consists of 6–10 pairs of tubules. These open into a pair of primary ducts that are also formed at the same level, extend caudally, and eventually reach and open into the cloaca. The pronephros is a vestigial structure that disappears completely by the fourth week of embryonic life (Fig 2–1).

Mesonephros

The mature excretory organ of the higher fish and amphibians corresponds to the embryonic mesonephros. It is the principal excretory organ during early embryonic life (4–8 weeks). It, too, gradually degenerates, although parts of its duct system become associated with the male reproductive organs. The mesonephric tubules develop from the intermediate mesoderm caudad to the pronephros shortly before pronephric degeneration. The mesonephric tubules differ from those of the pronephros in that they develop a cuplike outgrowth into which a knot of capillaries is pushed. This is called Bowman's capsule, and the tuft of capillaries is called a glomerulus. In their growth, the mesonephric tubules extend toward and establish a connection with the nearby primary nephric duct as it grows caudally to join the cloaca (Fig 2–1).

This primary nephric duct is now called the mesonephric duct. After establishing their connection with the nephric duct, the primordial tubules elongate and become S-shaped. As the tubules elongate, a series of secondary branchings increases their surface exposure, thereby enhancing their capacity for interchanging material with the blood in adjacent capillaries. Leaving the glomerulus, the blood is carried by one or more efferent vessels that soon break up into a rich capillary plexus closely related to the mesonephric tubules. The mesonephros, which forms early in the fourth week, reaches its maximum size by the end of the second month.

Metanephros

The metanephros, the final phase of development of the nephric system, originates from both the intermediate mesoderm and the mesonephric duct. Development begins in the 5- to 6-mm embryo with a budlike outgrowth from the mesonephric duct as it bends to join the cloaca. This ureteral bud grows cephalad and collects mesoderm from the nephrogenic cord of the intermediate mesoderm around its tip. This mesoderm with the metanephric cap moves, with the growing ureteral bud, more and more cephalad from its point of origin. During this cephalad migration, the metanephric cap becomes progressively larger, and rapid internal differentiation takes place. Meanwhile, the cephalad end of the ureteral bud expands within the growing mass of metanephrogenic tissue to form the renal pelvis (Fig 2–1). Numerous outgrowths from the renal pelvic dilatation push radially into this growing mass and form hollow ducts that branch and rebranch as they push toward the periphery. These form the primary collecting ducts of the kidney. Mesodermal cells become arranged in small vesicular masses that lie close to the blind end of the collecting ducts. Each of these vesicular masses will form a uriniferous tubule draining into the duct nearest to its point of origin. As the kidney grows, increasing numbers of tubules are formed in its peripheral zone. These vesicular masses develop a central cavity and become S-shaped. One end of the S coalesces with the terminal portion of the collecting tubules, resulting in a continuous canal. The proximal portion of the S develops into the distal and proximal convoluted tubules and into Henle's loop; the distal end becomes the glomerulus and Bowman's capsule. At this stage, the undif-

16

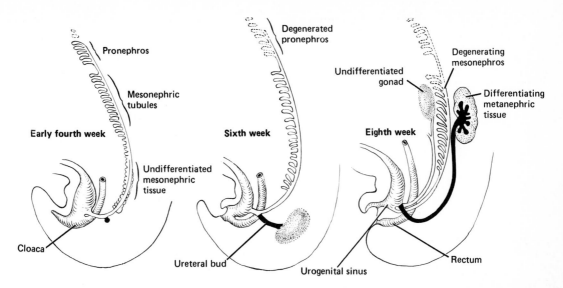

Figure 2–1. Schematic representation of the development of the nephric system. Only a few of the tubules of the pronephros are seen early in the fourth week, while the mesonephric tissue differentiates into mesonephric tubules that progressively join the mesonephric duct. The first sign of the ureteral bud from the mesonephric duct is seen. At 6 weeks, the pronephros has completely degenerated and the mesonephric tubules start to do so. The ureteral bud grows dorsocranially and has met the metanephrogenic cap. At the eighth week, there is cranial migration of the differentiating metanephros. The cranial end of the ureteric bud expands and starts to show multiple successive outgrowths. (Adapted from several sources.)

ferentiated mesoderm and the immature glomeruli are readily visible on microscopic examination (Fig 2–2). The glomeruli are fully developed by the 36th week or when the fetus weighs 2500 g (Osathanondh and Potter, *Arch Pathol* 1964;**77**:510). The metanephros arises opposite the 28th somite (fourth lumbar segment). At term, it has ascended to the level of the first lumbar or even the 12th thoracic vertebra. This ascent of the kidney is due not only to actual cephalad migration but also to differential growth in the caudal part of the body. During the early period of ascent (seventh to ninth weeks), the kidney slides above the arterial bifurcation and rotates 90 degrees. Its convex border is now directed laterally, not dorsally. Ascent proceeds more slowly until the kidney reaches its final position.

Certain features of these 3 phases of development must be emphasized: (1) The 3 successive units of the system develop from the intermediate mesoderm. (2) The tubules at all levels appear as independent primordia and only secondarily unite with the duct system. (3) The nephric duct is laid down as the duct of the pronephros and develops from the union of the ends of the anterior pronephric tubules. (4) This pronephric duct serves subsequently as the mesonephric duct and as such gives rise to the ureter. (5) The nephric duct reaches the cloaca by independent caudal growth. (6) The embryonic ureter is an outgrowth of the nephric duct, yet the kidney tubules differentiate from adjacent metanephric blastema.

ANOMALIES OF THE NEPHRIC SYSTEM

Failure of the metanephros to ascend leads to **ectopic kidney.** An ectopic kidney may be on the proper side but low (simple ectopy) or on the opposite side (crossed ectopy) with or without fusion. Failure to rotate during ascent causes a **malrotated kidney.**

Fusion of the paired metanephric masses leads to various anomalies—most commonly **horseshoe kidney.**

The ureteral bud from the mesonephric duct may bifurcate, causing a **bifid ureter** at varying levels depending on the time of the bud's subdivision. An accessory ureteral bud may develop from the mesonephric duct, thereby forming a **duplicated ureter,** usually meeting the same metanephric mass. Rarely, each bud has a separate metanephric mass, resulting in **supernumerary kidneys.**

If the double ureteral buds are close together on the mesonephric duct, they will open near each other in the bladder. In this case, the main ureteral bud, which is the first to appear and the most caudal on the mesonephric ducts, will reach the bladder first. It will then start to move upward and laterally and will be followed later by the second accessory bud as it reaches the urogenital sinus. The main ureteral bud (now more cranial on the urogenital sinus) will drain the lower portion of the kidney. The 2 ureteral buds have reversed their relationship as they moved from the mesonephric duct to the urogenital sinus. This is why

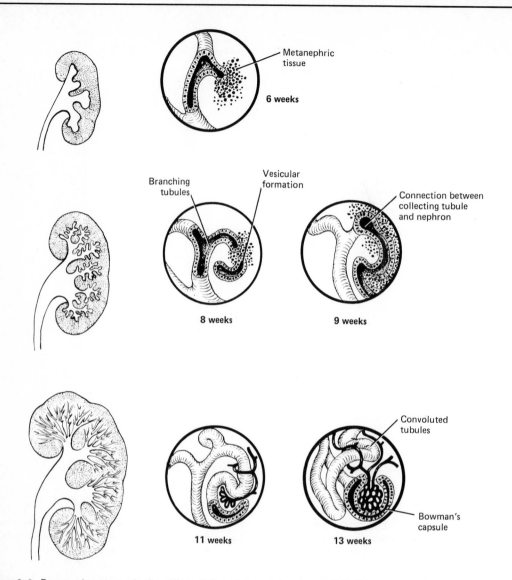

Figure 2–2. Progressive stages in the differentiation of the nephrons and their linkage with the branching collecting tubules. A small lump of metanephric tissue is associated with each terminal collecting tubule. These are then arranged in vesicular masses that later differentiate into a uriniferous tubule draining into the duct near which it arises. At one end, Bowman's capsule and the glomerulus differentiate; the other end establishes communication with the nearby collecting tubules.

double ureters always cross (Weigert-Meyer law). If the 2 ureteral buds are widely separated on the mesonephric duct, the accessory bud appears more proximal and will end in the bladder with an ectopic orifice lower than the normal one. This ectopic orifice could still be in the bladder close to its outlet, in the urethra, or even in the genital duct system (Fig 2–3). A single ureteral bud that arises higher than normal on the mesonephric duct can also end in a similar ectopic location.

Lack of development of a ureteral bud will result in **a solitary kidney** and a hemitrigone.

VESICOURETHRAL UNIT

The blind end of the hindgut caudad to the point of origin of the allantois expands to form the cloaca, which is separated from the outside by a thin plate of tissue (the cloacal membrane) lying in an ectodermal depression (the proctodeum) under the root of the tail. At the 4-mm stage, starting at the cephalad portion of the cloaca where the allantois and gut meet, the cloaca progressively divides into 2 compartments by the cau-

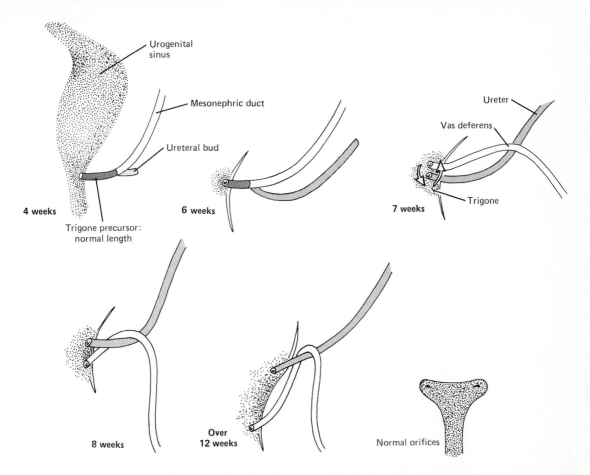

Figure 2–3. The development of the ureteral bud from the mesonephric duct and the relationship of both to the urogenital sinus. The ureteral bud appears at the fourth week. The mesonephric duct distal to this ureteral bud will be gradually absorbed into the urogenital sinus, resulting in separate endings for the ureter and the mesonephric duct. The mesonephric tissue that is incorporated into the urogenital sinus will expand and form the trigonal tissue.

dad growth of a crescentic fold, the urorectal fold. The 2 limbs of the fold bulge into the lumen of the cloaca from either side, eventually meeting and fusing. The division of the cloaca into a ventral portion (urogenital sinus) and a dorsal portion (rectum) is completed during the seventh week. During the development of the urorectal septum, the cloacal membrane undergoes a reverse rotation, so that the ectodermal surface is no longer directed toward the developing anterior abdominal wall but gradually is turned to face caudally and slightly posteriorly. This change facilitates the subdivision of the cloaca and is brought about mainly by development of the infraumbilical portion of the anterior abdominal wall and regression of the tail. The mesoderm that passes around the cloacal membrane to the caudal attachment of the umbilical cord proliferates and grows, forming a surface elevation, the genital tubercle. Further growth of the infraumbilical part of the abdominal wall progressively separates the umbilical cord from the genital tubercle. The division of the cloaca is completed before the cloacal membrane rup-

tures, and its 2 parts therefore have separate openings. The ventral part is the primitive urogenital sinus, which has the shape of an elongated cylinder and is continuous cranially with the allantois; its external opening is the urogenital ostium. The dorsal part is the rectum, and its external opening is the anus.

The urogenital sinus receives the mesonephric ducts. The caudad end of the mesonephric duct distal to the ureteral bud is progressively absorbed into the urogenital sinus. By the seventh week, the mesonephric duct and the ureteral bud have independent opening sites. This introduces an island of mesodermal tissue amid the surrounding endoderm of the urogenital sinus. As development progresses, the opening of the mesonephric duct (which will become the ejaculatory duct) migrates downward and medially. The opening of the ureteral bud (which will become the ureteral orifice) migrates upward and laterally. The absorbed mesoderm of the mesonephric duct expands with this migration to occupy the area limited by the final position of these tubes (Fig 2–3). This will later be differentiated as the trigonal structure, which is the only mesodermal inclusion in the endodermal vesicourethral unit.

The urogenital sinus can be divided into 2 main segments; the dividing line, the junction of the combined müllerian ducts with the dorsal wall of the urogenital sinus, is an elevation called Müller's tubercle, which is the most fixed reference point in the whole structure and which will be discussed below. The segments are as follows:

(1) The ventral and pelvic portion will form the bladder, part of the urethra in the male, and the whole urethra in the female. This portion receives the ureter.

(2) The urethral or phallic portion receives the mesonephric and the fused müllerian ducts. This will be part of the urethra in the male and forms the lower fifth of the vagina and the vaginal vestibule in the female.

During the third month, the ventral part of the urogenital sinus starts to expand and forms an epithelial sac whose apex tapers into an elongated, narrowed urachus. The pelvic portion remains narrow and tubular, and this will form the whole urethra in the female and the supramontanal portion of the prostatic urethra in the male. The splanchnic mesoderm surrounding the ventral and pelvic portion of the urogenital sinus begins to differentiate into interlacing bands of smooth muscle fibers and an outer fibrous connective tissue coat. By the 12th week, the layers characteristic of the adult urethra and bladder are recognizable (Fig 2–4).

The part of the urogenital sinus caudad to the opening of the müllerian duct will form the vaginal vestibule and contribute to the lower fifth of the vagina in the female (Fig 2–5). In the male, it forms the inframontanal part of the prostatic urethra and the membranous urethra. The penile urethra is formed by the fusion of the urethral folds on the ventral surface of the genital tubercle. In the female, the urethral folds remain separate and form the labia minora. The glandular urethra in the male is formed by canalization of the urethral plate. The bladder originally extends up to the umbilicus, where it is connected to the allantois that extends into the umbilical cord. The allantois usually is obliterated at the level of the umbilicus by the 15th week. The bladder then starts to descend by the 18th week. As it descends, its apex becomes stretched and narrowed, and it pulls on the already obliterated allantois, now called the urachus. By the 20th week, the bladder is well separated from the umbilicus and the stretched urachus will become the middle umbilical ligament.

PROSTATE

The prostate develops as multiple solid outgrowths of the urethral epithelium both above and below the entrance of the mesonephric duct. These simple, tubular outgrowths begin to develop in 5 distinct groups at the end of the 11th week and are complete by the 16th week (112-mm stage). They branch and rebranch, ending in a complex duct system that encounters the differentiating mesenchymal cells around this segment of the urogenital sinus. These mesenchymal cells start to develop around the tubules by the 16th week and become denser at the periphery to form the prostatic capsule. By the 22nd week, the muscular stroma is considerably developed, and it continues to increase progressively until birth.

From the 5 groups of epithelial buds, 5 lobes are eventually formed: anterior, posterior, median, and 2 lateral lobes. Initially, these lobes are widely separated, but later they meet, with no definite septums dividing them. Tubules of each lobe do not intermingle with each other but simply lie side by side.

The anterior lobe tubules begin to develop simultaneously with those of the other lobes. Although in the early stages the anterior lobe tubules are large and show multiple branches, gradually they contact and lose most of the branches. They continue to shrink, so that at birth they show no lumen and appear as small, solid embryonic epithelial outgrowths. In contrast, the tubules of the posterior lobe are fewer in number yet relatively larger, with extensive branching. These tubules, as they grow, extend posterior to the developing median and lateral lobes and form the posterior aspect of the gland, which may be felt rectally.

ANOMALIES OF THE VESICOURETHRAL UNIT

Failure of the cloaca to subdivide is rare and results in a **persistent cloaca.** Incomplete subdivision is more frequent, ending with **rectovesical, rectourethral,** or **rectovestibular fistulas** (usually with **imperforate anus** or **anal atresia**).

Failure of descent or incomplete descent of the bladder leads to a **urinary umbilical fistula (urethral fistula), urachal cyst,** or **urachal diverticulum** depending on the stage and degree of maldescent.

Development of the genital primordia in an area more caudal than normal can result in formation of the corpora cavernosa just caudad to the urogenital sinus outlet, with the urethral groove on its dorsal surface. This defect results in complete or incomplete **epispadias** depending on its degree. A more extensive defect results in **vesical exstrophy.** Failure of fusion of urethral folds leads to various grades of **hypospadias.** This defect, because of its mechanism, never extends proximal to the bulbous urethra. This is in contrast to epispadias, which usually involves the entire urethra up to the internal meatus.

GONADS

Most of the structures that make up the embryonic genital system have been taken over from other sys-

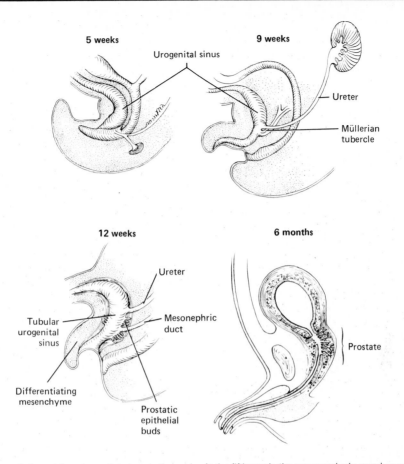

Figure 2–4. Differentiation of the urogenital sinus in the male. At the fifth week, the progressively growing urorectal septum is separating the urogenital sinus from the rectum. The former receives the mesonephric duct and the ureteral bud. It retains its tubular structure until the 12th week, when the surrounding mesenchyme starts to differentiate into the muscle fibers around the whole structure. The prostate gland develops as multiple epithelial outgrowths just above and below the mesonephric duct. During the third month, the ventral part of the urogenital sinus expands to form the bladder proper; the pelvic part remains narrow and tubular, forming part of the urethra. (Reproduced, with permission, from Tanagho EA, Smith DR: Mechanisms of urinary continence. 1. Embryologic, anatomic, and pathologic considerations. *J Urol* 1969; **100:**640.)

tems, and their readaptation to genital function is a secondary and relatively late phase in their development. The early differentiation of such structures is therefore independent of sexuality. Furthermore, each embryo is at first morphologically bisexual, possessing all the necessary structures for either sex. The development of one set of sex primordia and the gradual involution of the other is determined by the sex of the gonad.

The sexually undifferentiated gonad is a composite structure. Male and female potentials are represented by specific histologic elements (medulla and cortex) that have alternative roles in gonadogenesis. Normal differentiation involves the gradual predominance of one component.

The primitive sex glands make their appearance during the fifth and sixth weeks within a localized region of the thickening known as the urogenital ridge (this contains both the nephric and genital primordia). At the sixth week, the gonad consists of a superficial germinal epithelium and an internal blastema. The blastemal mass is derived mainly from proliferative ingrowth from the superficial epithelium that comes loose from its basement membrane.

During the seventh week, the gonad begins to assume the characteristics of a testis or ovary. Differentiation of the ovary usually occurs somewhat later than differentiation of the testis.

If the gonad develops into a testis, the gland increases in size and shortens into a more compact organ while achieving a more caudal location. Its broad attachment to the mesonephros is converted into a gonadal mesentery known as the mesorchium. The cells of the germinal epithelium grow into the underlying mesenchyme and form cordlike masses. These are radially arranged and converge toward the mesorchium, where a dense portion of the blastemal mass is also emerging as the primordium of the rete testis. A network of strands soon forms that is continuous with the testis cords. The latter also split into 3–4 daughter

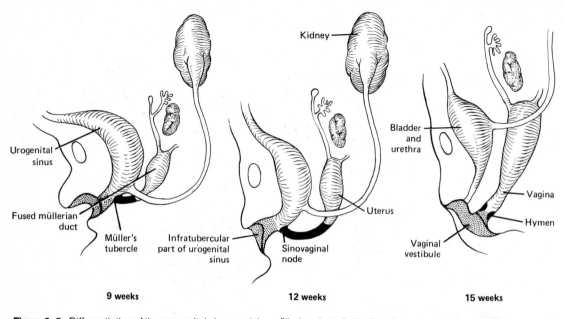

Figure 2–5. Differentiation of the urogenital sinus and the müllerian ducts in the female embryo. At 9 weeks, the urogenital sinus receives the fused müllerian ducts at Müller's tubercle (sinovaginal node; see p 25), which is solidly packed with cells. As the urogenital sinus distal to Müller's tubercle becomes wider and shallower (15 weeks), the urethra and fused müllerian duct will have separate openings. The distal part of the urogenital sinus will form the vaginal vestibule and the lower fifth of the vagina (*shaded area*), and that part above Müller's tubercle will form the urinary bladder and the entire female urethra. The fused müllerian ducts will form the uterus and the upper four-fifths of the vagina. The hymen is formed at the junction of the sinovaginal node and the urogenital sinus.

cords. These eventually become differentiated into the seminiferous tubules by which the spermatozoa are produced. The rete testis unites with the mesonephric components that will form the male genital ducts, as discussed below (Fig 2–6).

If the gonad develops into an ovary, it (like the testis) gains a mesentery (mesovarium) and settles in a more caudal position. The internal blastema differentiates in the ninth week into a primary cortex beneath the germinal epithelium and a loose primary medulla. A compact cellular mass bulges from the medulla into the mesovarium and establishes the primitive rete ovarii. At 3–4 months of age, the internal cell mass becomes young ova. A new definitive cortex is formed from the germinal epithelium as well as from the blastema in the form of distinct cellular cords (Pflüger's tubes), and a permanent medulla is formed. The cortex differentiates into ovarian follicles containing ova.

Descent of the Gonads

A. Testis: In addition to its early caudal migration, the testis later leaves the abdominal cavity and descends into the scrotum. By the third month of fetal life, the testis is located retroperitoneally in the false pelvis. A fibromuscular band (the gubernaculum) extends from the lower pole of the testis through the developing muscular layers of the anterior abdominal wall to terminate in the subcutaneous tissue of the

scrotal swelling. The gubernaculum also has several other subsidiary strands that extend to adjacent regions. Just below the lower pole of the testis, the peritoneum herniates as a diverticulum along the anterior aspect of the gubernaculum, eventually reaching the scrotal sac through the anterior abdominal muscles (the processus vaginalis). The testis remains at the abdominal end of the inguinal canal until the seventh month. It then passes through the inguinal canal behind (but invaginating) the processus vaginalis. Normally, it reaches the scrotal sac by the end of the eighth month.

B. Ovary: In addition to undergoing an early internal descent, the ovary becomes attached through the gubernaculum to the tissues of the genital fold and then attaches itself to the developing uterovaginal canal at its junction with the uterine (fallopian) tubes. This part of the gubernaculum between the ovary and uterus becomes the ovarian ligament; the part between the uterus and the labia majora becomes the round ligament of the uterus. These ligaments prevent extra-abdominal descent, and the ovary enters the true pelvis. It eventually lies posterior to the uterine tubes on the superior surface of the urogenital mesentery, which has descended with the ovary and now forms the broad ligament. A small processus vaginalis forms and passes toward the labial swelling, but it is usually obliterated at full term.

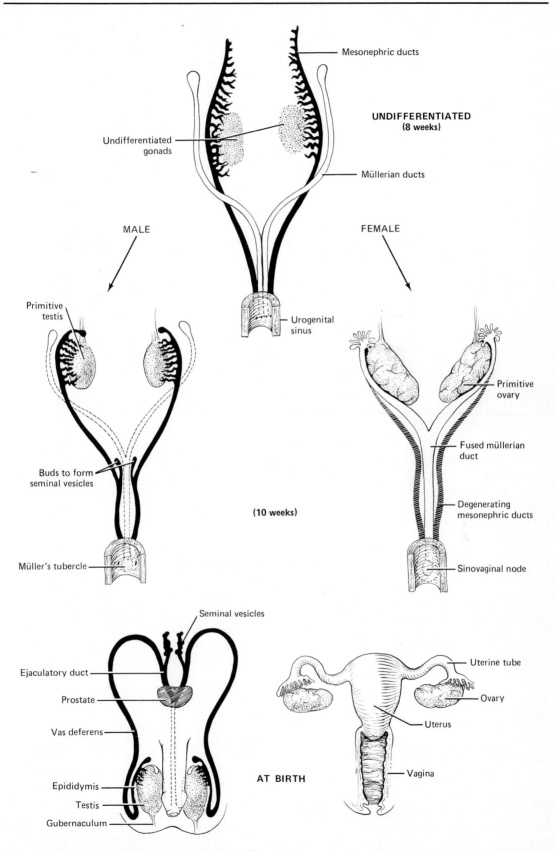

Figure 2–6. Transformation of the undifferentiated genital system into the definitive male and female systems.

GONADAL ANOMALIES

Lack of development of the gonads is called **gonadal agenesis.** Incomplete development with arrest at a certain phase is called **hypogenesis. Supernumerary gonads** are rare. The commonest anomaly involves descent of the gonads, especially the testis. Retention of the testis in the abdomen or arrest of its descent at any point along its natural pathway is called **cryptorchidism,** which may be either unilateral or bilateral. If the testis does not follow the main gubernaculum structure but follows one of its subsidiary strands, it will end in an abnormal position, resulting in **ectopic testis.**

Failure of union between the rete testis and mesonephros results in a testis separate from the male genital ducts (the epididymis) and azoospermia.

GENITAL DUCT SYSTEM

Alongside the indifferent gonads, there are, early in embryonic life, 2 different yet closely related ducts. One is primarily a nephric duct (wolffian duct), yet it will also serve as a genital duct if the embryo develops into a male. The other (müllerian duct) is primarily a genital structure from the start.

Both ducts grow caudally to join the primitive urogenital sinus. The wolffian duct (known as the pronephric duct at the 4-mm stage) joins the ventral part of the cloaca, which will be the urogenital sinus. This duct gives rise to the ureteral bud close to its caudal end. The ureteral bud will grow cranially and meet metanephrogenic tissue. That part of each mesonephric duct caudad to the origin of the ureteric bud becomes absorbed into the wall of the primitive urogenital sinus, so that the mesonephric duct and ureter open independently. This is achieved at the 15-mm stage (seventh week). During this period, starting at the 10-mm stage, the müllerian ducts start to develop. They reach the urogenital sinus relatively late—at the 30-mm stage (ninth week)—their partially fused blind ends producing the elevation called Müller's tubercle. Müller's tubercle is the most constant and reliable point of reference in the whole system.

If the gonad starts to develop into a testis (17-mm stage, seventh week), the wolffian duct will start to differentiate into the male duct system, forming the epididymis, vas deferens, seminal vesicles, and ejaculatory ducts. At this time, the müllerian duct proceeds toward its junction with urogenital sinus and immediately starts to degenerate. Only its upper and lower ends persist, the former as the appendix testis and the latter as part of the prostatic utricle.

If the gonad starts to differentiate into an ovary (22-mm stage, eighth week), the müllerian duct system forms the uterine (fallopian) tubes, uterus, and most of the vagina. The wolffian ducts, aside from their contribution to the urogenital sinus, remain rudimentary.

MALE DUCT SYSTEM

Epididymis

Because of the proximity of the differentiating gonads and the nephric duct, some of the mesonephric tubules are retained as the efferent ductules, and their lumens become continuous with those of the rete testis. These tubules, together with that part of the mesonephric duct into which they empty, will form the epididymis. Each coiled ductule makes a conical mass known as the lobule of the epididymis. The cranial end of the mesonephric duct becomes highly convoluted, completing the formation of the epididymis. This is an example of direct inclusion of a nephric structure into the genital system. Additional mesonephric tubules, both cephalad and caudad to those that were included in the formation of the epididymis, will remain as rudimentary structures, ie, the appendix of the epididymis and the paradidymis.

Vas Deferens, Seminal Vesicles, & Ejaculatory Ducts

The mesonephric duct caudad to that portion forming the epididymis will form the vas deferens. Shortly before this duct joins the urethra (urogenital sinus), a localized dilatation (ampulla) develops and the saccular convoluted structure that will form the seminal vesicle is evaginated from its wall. The mesonephric duct between the origin of the seminal vesicle and the urethra will form the ejaculatory duct. The whole mesonephric duct now achieves its characteristic thick investment of smooth muscle, with a narrow lumen along most of its length.

Both above and below the point of entrance of the mesonephric duct into the urethra, multiple outgrowths of urethral epithelium mark the beginning of the development of the prostate. As these epithelial buds grow, they meet the developing muscular fibers around the urogenital sinus, and some of these fibers become entangled in the branching tubules of the growing prostate and become incorporated into it, forming its muscular stroma (Fig 2–4).

FEMALE DUCT SYSTEM

The müllerian ducts, which are a paired system, are seen alongside the mesonephric duct. It is not known whether they arise directly from the mesonephric ducts or separately as an invagination of the celomic epithelium into the parenchyma lateral to the cranial extremity of the mesonephric duct, but the latter theory is favored. The müllerian duct develops and runs lateral to the mesonephric duct. Its opening into the celomic cavity persists as the peritoneal ostium of the uterine tube (later it develops fimbriae). The other end grows caudally as a solid tip and then crosses in front

Table 2–1. Male and female homologous structures.

Embryonic Structure	Male	Female
Mesonephric duct	Epididymis Vas deferens and seminal vesicles Ejaculatory ducts Appendix epididymidis Ureter, renal pelvis, etc Trigonal structure	Duct of epoophoron Gartner's duct Vesicular appendage Ureter, renal pelvis, etc Trigonal structure
Müllerian duct	Appendix testis Prostatic utricle	Uterine tubes Uterus Vagina (upper four-fifths)
Müller's tubercle	Verumontanum	Site of hymen
Sinovaginal bulb from urogenital sinus	Part of prostatic utricle	Lower one-fifth of vagina
Junction of sinovaginal bulb and urogenital sinus	Disappears normally (remnants probably form posterior urethral valves)	Hymen
Urogenital sinus Ventral and pelvic part	Urinary bladder (except the trigone) Supramontanal part of prostatic urethra	Urinary bladder (except the trigone) Whole urethra
Phallic or urethral portion	Inframontanal part of prostatic urethra Membranous urethra	Vaginal vestibule
Genital tubercle	Penis	Clitoris
Urethral folds	Penile urethra	Labia minora
Genital swellings	Scrotum	Labia majora
Gubernaculum	Gubernaculum testis	Ligament of ovary Round ligament of uterus
Genital glands	Testis	Ovary
Germinal cords	Seminiferous tubules	Pflüger's tube

of the mesonephric duct at the caudad extremity of the mesonephros. It continues its growth in a caudomedial direction until it meets and fuses with the müllerian duct of the opposite side. The fusion is partial at first, so there is a temporary septum between the 2 lumens. This later disappears, leaving one cavity that will form the uterovaginal canal. The potential lumen of the vaginal canal is completely packed with cells. The solid tip of this cord pushes the epithelium of the urogenital sinus outward, where it becomes Müller's tubercle (33-mm stage, ninth week). The müllerian ducts actually fuse at the 63-mm stage (13th week), forming the sinovaginal node, which receives a limited contribution from the urogenital sinus. (This contribution will form the lower fifth of the vagina.)

The urogenital sinus distal to Müller's tubercle, originally narrow and deep, shortens, widens, and opens to form the floor of the pudendal or vulval cleft. This results in separate openings for the vagina and urethra and also brings the vaginal orifice to its final position nearer the surface. At the same time, the vaginal segment increases appreciably in length. The vaginal vestibule is derived from the infratubercular segment of the urogenital sinus (in the male, the same segment will form the inframontanal part of the prostatic urethra and the membranous urethra). The labia minora are formed from the urethral folds (in the male they will form the pendulous urethra). The hymen is the remnant of the müllerian tubercle. The lower fifth of the vagina is derived from the portion of the urogenital sinus that combines with the sinovaginal node.

The remainder of the vagina and the uterus are formed from the lower (fused) third of the müllerian ducts. The uterine tubes (fallopian tubes, oviducts) are the cephalad two-thirds of the müllerian ducts (Fig 2–6).

ANOMALIES OF THE GONADAL DUCT SYSTEM

Nonunion of the rete testis and the efferent ductules can occur and, if bilateral, cause **azoospermia and sterility.** Failure of the müllerian ducts to approximate or to fuse completely can lead to various degrees of **duplication** in the genital ducts. **Congenital absence** of one or both uterine tubes or of the uterus or vagina occurs rarely.

Arrested development of the infratubercular segment of the urogenital sinus leads to its persistence, with the urethra and vagina having a common duct to the outside (**urogenital sinus).**

EXTERNAL GENITALIA

During the eighth week, external sexual differentiation begins to occur. Not until 3 months, however, do the progressively developing external genitalia attain characteristics that can be recognized as distinctively male or female. During the indifferent stage of sexual development, 3 small protuberances appear on the external aspect of the cloacal membrane. In front is the genital tubercle, and on either side of the membrane are the genital swellings.

With the breakdown of the urogenital membrane (17-mm stage, seventh week), the primitive urogenital sinus achieves a separate opening on the undersurface of the genital tubercle.

MALE EXTERNAL GENITALIA

The urogenital sinus opening extends on the ventral aspect of the genital tubercle as the urethral groove. The primitive urogenital orifice and the urethral groove are bounded on either side by the urethral folds. The genital tubercle becomes elongated to form the phallus. The corpora cavernosa are indicated in the seventh week as paired mesenchymal columns within the shaft of the penis. By the tenth week, the urethral folds start to fuse from the urogenital sinus orifice toward the tip of the phallus. At the 14th week, the fusion is complete and results in the formation of the penile urethra. The corpus spongiosum results from the differentiation of the mesenchymal masses around the formed penile urethra.

The glans penis becomes defined by the development of a circular coronary sulcus around the distal part of the phallus. The urethral groove and the fusing folds do not extend beyond the coronary sulcus. The glandular urethra develops as a result of canalization of an ectodermal epithelial cord that has grown through the glans. This canalization reaches and communicates with the distal end of the previously formed penile urethra. During the third month, a fold of skin at the base of the glans begins growing distally and, 2 months later, surrounds the glans. This forms the prepuce. Meanwhile, the genital swellings shift caudally

and are recognizable as scrotal swellings. They meet and fuse, resulting in the formation of the scrotum, with 2 compartments partially separated by a median septum and a median raphe, indicating their line of fusion.

FEMALE EXTERNAL GENITALIA

Until the eighth week, the appearance of the female external genitalia closely resembles that of the male except that the urethral groove is shorter. The genital tubercle, which becomes bent caudally and lags in development, becomes the clitoris. As in the male (though on a minor scale), mesenchymal columns differentiate into corpora cavernosa and a coronary sulcus identifies the glans clitoridis. The most caudal part of the urogenital sinus shortens and widens, forming the vaginal vestibule. The urethral folds do not fuse but remain separate as the labia minora. The genital swellings meet in front of the anus, forming the posterior commissure, while the swellings as a whole enlarge and remain separated on either side of the vestibule and form the labia majora.

ANOMALIES OF THE EXTERNAL GENITALIA

Absence or duplication of the penis or clitoris is very rare. More commonly, the penis remains rudimentary or the clitoris may show hypertrophy. These may be seen alone or, more frequently, in association with **pseudohermaphroditism.** Concealed penis and transposition of penis and scrotum are relatively rare anomalies.

Failure or incomplete fusion of the urethral folds results in **hypospadias** (see above). Penile development is also anomalous in cases of **epispadias** and **exstrophy** (see above).

REFERENCES

General

Allan FD: *Essentials of Human Embryology.* Oxford Univ Press, 1960.

Arey LB: *Developmental Anatomy: A Textbook and Laboratory Manual of Embryology,* 6th ed. Saunders, 1954.

Blechschmidt E: *The Stages of Human Development Before Birth: An Introduction to Human Embryology.* Saunders, 1961.

Corliss CE: *Patten's Human Embryology,* 4th ed. McGraw-Hill, 1976.

D'Albertson A et al: Prevalence of urinary tract abnormalities in large series of patients with uterovaginal atresia. *J Urol* 1981;**126:**623.

Frazer JES, Baxter JS: *Manual of Embryology: The Development of the Human Body,* 3rd ed. Williams & Wilkins, 1953.

Keith A: *Human Embryology and Morphology,* 6th ed. Williams & Wilkins, 1948.

Kjellberg SR, Ericsson NO, Rudhe U: *The Lower Urinary Tract in Childhood: Some Correlated Clinical and Roentgenologic Observations.* Year Book, 1957.

Marshall FF: Embryology of the lower genitourinary tract. *Urol Clin North Am* 1978;**5:**3.

Stephens FD: *Congenital Malformations of the Urinary Tract.* Praeger, 1983.

Stephens FD: Embryopathy of malformations. *J Urol* 1982;**127:**13.

Tanagho EA: Developmental anatomy and urogenital abnormalities. Pages 3–11 in: *Female Urology.* Raz S (editor). Saunders, 1983.

Tanagho EA: Embryologic development of the urinary tract. Pages 1–8 in: *AUA Update Series.* Ball TP (editor). American Urological Association, 1982.

Vaughan ED Jr, Middleton GW: Pertinent genitourinary embryology: Review for practicing urologist. *Urology* 1975;**6:**139.

Anomalies of the Nephric System

Akhtar M, Valencia M: Horseshoe kidney with unilateral renal dysplasia. *Urology* 1979;**13**:284.

Ayalon A et al: Ureterocele: A familial congenital anaomaly. *Urology* 1979;**13**:551.

Carrion H et al: Retrocaval ureter: Report of 8 cases and surgical management. *J Urol* 1979;**121**:514.

Correa RJ Jr, Paton RR: Polycystic horseshoe kidney. *J Urol* 1976;**116**:802.

Cowinn JL, Landry BW: Cystic diseases of the kidney in infants and children. *Radiol Clin North Am* 1968;**6**:191.

Douglas LL, Pott GA: Congenital ureteral diverticulum and solitary kidney. *J Urol* 1979;**122**:401.

Evans WP et al: Association of crossed fused renal ectopia and multicystic kidney. *J Urol* 1979;**122**:821.

Feldman SL, Lome LG: Renal dysplasia in horseshoe kidney. *Urology* 1982;**20**:74.

Gribetz ME, Leiter E: Ectopic ureterocele, hydroureter, and renal dysplasia: An embryogenic triad. *Urology* 1978; **11**:131.

Johnson DK, Perlmutter AD: Single system ectopic ureteroceles with anomalies of heart, testis and vas deferens. *J Urol* 1980;**123**:81.

Koyanagi T et al: Everting ureteroceles: Radiographic and endoscopic observation, and surgical management. *J Urol* 1980;**123**:538.

Leiter E: Persistent fetal ureter. *J Urol* 1979;**122**:251.

Lockhard JL, Singer AM, Glenn JF: Congenital megaureter. *J Urol* 1979;**122**:310.

Maatman TJ, DeOreo GA Jr, Kay R: Solitary pseudo-crossed renal ectopia. *J Urol* 1983;**129**:128.

Magee MC: Ureteroceles and duplicated systems: Embryologic hypothesis. *J Urol* 1980;**123**:605.

Magee MC: Ureteroceles in single versus duplicated systems: An embryologic hypothesis. *Urology* 1981;**18**:365.

Maizels M, Simpson SB Jr: Primitive ducts of renal dysplasia induced by culturing ureteral buds denuded of condensed renal mesenchyme. *Science* 1983;**219**:509.

Mandell J et al: Ureteral ectopia in infants and children. *J Urol* 1981;**126**:219.

Murphy WK, Palubinskas AJ, Smith DR: Sponge kidney: Report of 7 cases. *J Urol* 1961;**85**:866.

Osathanondh V, Potter EL: Pathogenesis of polycystic kidneys: Survey of results of microdissection. *Arch Pathol* 1964;**77**:510.

Osathanondh V, Potter EL: Pathogenesis of polycystic kidneys: Type 4 due to urethral obstruction. *Arch Pathol* 1964;**77**:502.

Scott JES: The single ectopic ureter and the dysplastic kidney. *Br J Urol* 1981;**53**:300.

Soderdahl DW, Shiraki IW, Schamber DT: Bilateral ureteral quadruplication. *J Urol* 1976;**116**:255.

Tanagho EA: Development of the ureter. Pages 1–12 in: *The Ureter,* 2nd ed. Bergman H (editor). Springer-Verlag, 1981.

Tanagho EA: Ureteroceles: Embryogenesis, pathogenesis and management. *J Cont Educ Urol* (Feb) 1979;**18**:13.

Tokunaka S et al: Morphological study of ureterocele: Possible clue to its embryogenesis as evidenced by locally arrested myogenesis. *J Urol* 1981;**126**:726.

Traut HF: The structural unit of the human kidney. *Contribution to Embryology,* No. 76, Carnegie Inst Pub No. 332. 1923;**15**:103.

Anomalies of the Vesicourethral Unit

Amar AD, Hutch JA: Anomalies of the ureter. Page 98 in: *Malformations.* Vol 7 of: *Encyclopedia of Urology.* Springer, 1968.

Ansell JS: Surgical treatment of exstrophy of bladder with emphasis on neonatal primary closure: Personal experience with 28 consecutive cases treated at University of Washington Hospitals from 1962 to 1977. Techniques and results. *J Urol* 1979;**121**:650.

Begg RC: The urachus, its anatomy, histology and development. *J Anat* 1930;**64**:170.

Browne D: Some congenital deformities of the rectum, anus, vagina and urethra. (Hunterian Lecture.) *Ann R Coll Surg Engl* 1951;**8**:173.

Chwalle R: The process of formation of cystic dilatations of the vesical end of the ureter and of diverticula at the ureteral ostium. *Urol Cutan Rev* 1927;**31**:499.

Crooks KK: Protean aspects of posterior urethral valves. *J Urol* 1981;**126**:763.

Cullen TS: *Embryology, Anatomy and Diseases of the Umbilicus Together With Diseases of the Urachus.* Saunders, 1916.

Das S, Amar AD: Extravesical ureteral ectopia in male patients. *J Urol* 1981;**125**:842.

Das S, Brosman SA: Duplication of male urethra. *J Urol* 1977;**117**:452.

Eagle JR Jr, Barrett GS: Congenital deficiency of abdominal musculature with associated genitourinary abnormalities: A syndrome. Report of nine cases. *Pediatrics* 1950; **6**:721.

Ericsson NO: Ectopic ureterocele in infants and children: A clinical study. *Acta Chir Scand [Suppl]* 1954;**197**:1. [Entire issue.]

Escham W, Holt HA: Complete duplication of bladder and urethra. *J Urol* 1980;**123**:773.

Haralson IP: Double bladder and urethra with imperforate anus and ureterorenal reflux: Case presentation with review of literature. *J Urol* 1980;**123**:776.

Hinman F Jr: Microphallus: Distinction between anomalous and endocrine types. *J Urol* 1980;**123**:412.

Hinman F Jr: Microphallus: Distinction between anomalous and endocrine types. *Trans Am Assoc Genitourin Surg* 1979;**71**:159.

Hinman F Jr: Surgical disorders of the bladder and umbilicus or urachal origin. *Surg Gynecol Obstet* 1961;**113**:605.

Kroovand RL, Al-Ansari RM, Perlmutter AD: Urethral and genital malformations in prune belly syndrome. *J Urol* 1982;**127**:94.

Landes RR, Melnick I, Klein R: Vesical exstrophy with epispadias: Twenty-year follow-up. *Urology* 1977;**9**:53.

Lattimer JK: Congenital deficiency of the abdominal musculature and associated genitourinary anomalies: A report of 22 cases. *J Urol* 1958;**79**:343.

Lattimer JK et al: Delayed development of scrotum in exstrophy. *J Urol* 1979;**121**:339.

Lattimer JK et al: Long-term follow-up after exstrophy closure: Late improvement and good quality of life. *J Urol* 1978;**119**:664.

Lenaghan D: Bifid ureters in children: An anatomical, physiological and clinical study. *J Urol* 1962;**87**:808.

Lowe FC, Jeffs RD: Wound dehiscence in bladder exstrophy: An examination of the etiologies and factors for initial failure and subsequent success. *J Urol* 1983;**130**:312.

Lowsley OO: Persistent cloaca in the female: Report of two cases corrected by operation. *J Urol* 1948;**59**:692.

Mackie GG: Abnormalities of the ureteral bud. *Urol Clin North Am* 1978;**5**:161.

Meyer R: Normal and abnormal development of the ureter in

the human embryo: A mechanistic consideration. *Anat Rec* 1946;**96**:355.

Morgan RJ, Williams DI, Pryor JP: Müllerian duct remnants in the male. *Br J Urol* 1979;**51**:481.

Randall A, Campbell EW: Anomalous relationship of the right ureter to the vena cava. *J Urol* 1935;**34**:565.

Sellers BB et al: Congenital megalourethra associated with prune belly syndrome. *J Urol* 1976;**116**:814.

Shima H et al: Developmental anomalies associated with hypospadias. *J Urol* 1979;**122**:619.

Sohrabi A et al: Duplication of male urethra. *Urology* 1978;**12**:704.

Stephens FD: *Congenital Malformations of the Rectum, Anus and Genitourinary Tracts*. Livingstone, 1963.

Stephens FD: The female anus, perineum and vestibule: Embryogenesis and deformities. *J Obstet Gynaecol Br Commonw* 1968;**8**:55.

Tanagho EA: Embryologic basis for lower ureteral anomalies: A hypothesis. *Urology* 1976;**7**:451.

Uehling DT: Posterior urethral valves: Functional classification. *Urology* 1980;**15**:27.

Wainstein ML, Persky L: Superior vesical fistula: An unusual form of exstrophy of the urinary bladder. *Am J Surg* 1968;**115**:397.

Wespes E et al: Blind ending bifid and double ureters. *Urology* 1983;**21**:586.

Gonadal Anomalies

Bartone FF, Schmidt MA: Cryptorchidism: Incidence of chromosomal anomalies in 50 cases. *J Urol* 1982;**127**:1105.

Brosman SA: Mixed gonadal dysgenesis. *J Urol* 1979;**121**:344.

Elder JS, Isaacs JT, Walsh PC: Androgenic sensitivity of gubernaculum testis: Evidence for hormonal/mechanical interactions in testicular descent. *J Urol* 1982;**127**:170.

Fallon B, Welton M, Hawtrey C: Congenital anomalies associated with cryptorchidism. *J Urol* 1982;**127**:91.

Honoré LH: Unilateral anorchism: Report of 11 cases with discussion of etiology and pathogenesis. *Urology* 1978; **11**:251.

Job J-C et al: Hormonal therapy of cryptorchidism with human chorionic gonadotrophin (HCG). *Urol Clin North Am* 1982;**9**:405.

Jones IRG, Young ID: Familial incidence of cryptorchidism. *J Urol* 1982;**127**:508.

Marshall FF, Shermeta DW: Epididymal abnormalities associated with undescended testis. *J Urol* 1979;**121**:341.

Marshall FF, Weissman RM, Jeffs RD: Cryptorchidism: Surgical implications of nonunion of epididymis and testis. *J Urol* 1980;**124**:560.

Pujol A et al: The value of bilateral biopsy in unilateral cryptorchidism. *Eur Urol* 1978;**4**:85.

Raiffer J, Walsh PC: Testicular descent: Normal and abnormal. *Urol Clin North Am* 1978;**5**:22.

Walsh PC: The differential diagnosis of ambiguous genitalia in the newborn. *Urol Clin North Am* 1978;**5**:213.

Symptoms of Disorders of the Genitourinary Tract

3

Jack W. McAninch, MD

In the workup of any patient, the history is of paramount importance; this is particularly true in urology. It will be necessary to discuss here only those urologic symptoms that are apt to be brought to the physician's attention by the patient. It is important to know not only whether the disease is acute or chronic but also whether it is recurrent, since recurring symptoms may represent acute exacerbations of chronic disease.

Obtaining the history is an art that depends upon the skill and methods used to elicit information. The history is only as accurate as the patient's ability to describe the symptoms. This subjective information is important in establishing an accurate diagnosis.

SYSTEMIC MANIFESTATIONS

Symptoms of fever and weight loss should be sought. The presence of fever associated with other symptoms of urinary tract infection may be helpful in evaluating the site of the infection. Simple acute cystitis is essentially an afebrile disease. Acute pyelonephritis or prostatitis is apt to cause high temperatures (to 40 °C [104 °F]), often accompanied by violent chills. Infants and children suffering from acute pyelonephritis may have high temperatures without other localizing symptoms or signs. Such a clinical picture, therefore, *invariably* requires bacteriologic study of the urine.

A history of unexplained attacks of fever occurring even years before may have been due to an otherwise asymptomatic pyelonephritis. Renal carcinoma sometimes causes fever that may reach 39 °C (102.2 °F) or more. The absence of fever does not by any means rule out renal infection, for it is the rule that chronic pyelonephritis does not cause fever.

Weight loss is to be expected in the advanced stages of cancer, but it may also be noticed when renal insufficiency due to obstruction or infection supervenes. In children who have "failure to thrive" (low weight and less than average height for age), chronic obstruction, urinary tract infection, or both should be suspected.

General malaise may be noted with tumors, chronic pyelonephritis, or renal failure.

The presence of many of these symptoms may be compatible with acquired immunodeficiency syndrome (AIDS; see Chapter 15).

LOCAL & REFERRED PAIN

Two types of pain have their origins in the genitourinary organs: local and referred. The latter is especially common.

Local pain is felt in or near the involved organ. Thus, the pain from a diseased kidney (T10–12, L1) is felt in the costovertebral angle and in the flank in the region of and below the 12th rib. Pain from an inflamed testicle is felt in the gonad itself.

Referred pain originates in a diseased organ but is felt at some distance from that organ. The ureteral colic (Fig 3–1) caused by a stone in the upper ureter may be associated with severe pain in the ipsilateral testicle; this is explained by the common innervation of these 2 structures (T11–12). A stone in the lower ureter may cause pain referred to the scrotal wall; in this instance, the testis itself is not hyperesthetic. The burning pain with voiding that accompanies acute cystitis is felt in the distal urethra in the female or in the glandular urethra in the male (S2–3).

Abnormalities of a urologic organ can also cause pain in any other organ (eg, gastrointestinal, gynecologic) that has a sensory nerve supply common to both (Figs 3–2 and 3–3).

Kidney Pain
(Fig 3–1)

Typical renal pain is usually felt as a dull and constant ache in the costovertebral angle just lateral to the sacrospinalis muscle and just below the 12th rib. This pain often spreads along the subcostal area toward the umbilicus or lower abdominal quadrant. It may be expected in those renal diseases that cause sudden distention of the renal capsule. Acute pyelonephritis (with its sudden edema) and acute ureteral obstruction (with its sudden renal back pressure) both cause this typical pain. It should be pointed out, however, that many urologic renal diseases are painless because their progression is so slow that sudden capsular distention does not occur. Such diseases include cancer, chronic pyelonephritis, staghorn calculus, tuberculosis, polycystic kidney, and hydronephrosis due to chronic ureteral obstruction.

Pseudorenal Pain
(Radiculitis)

Mechanical derangements of the costovertebral or costotransverse joints can cause irritation or pressure

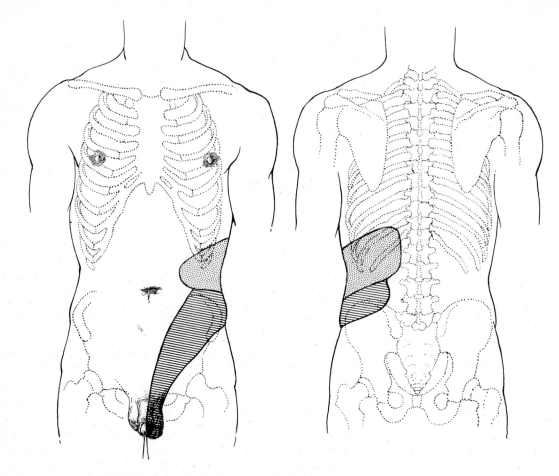

Figure 3–1. Referred pain from kidney (*dotted areas*) and ureter (*shaded areas*).

on the costal nerves. Disorders of this sort are common in the cervical and thoracic areas, but the most common sites are T10–12 (Smith and Raney, 1976). Irritation of these nerves causes costovertebral pain, often with radiation into the ipsilateral lower abdominal quadrant. The pain is positional in nature. Its first onset is usually quite acute, following the lifting of a heavy object, a blow to the costovertebral area, or a fall on the buttocks from a height. The pain is usually absent on arising from bed but is apt to increase as the day wears on. It is exacerbated by heavy physical work and is usually increased during an automobile trip over a rough road. It is apt to awaken the patient when a certain position is assumed (eg, lying on the right side) and is relieved by a change of position. Radiculitis may mimic ureteral colic or renal pain. True renal pain is seldom affected by movements of the spine.

Ureteral Pain
(Fig 3–1)

Ureteral pain is typically stimulated by acute obstruction (passage of a stone or a blood clot). In this instance, there is back pain from renal capsular distention combined with severe colicky pain (due to renal pelvic and ureteral muscle spasm) that radiates from the costovertebral angle down toward the lower anterior abdominal quadrant, along the course of the ureter. In men, it may also be felt in the bladder, scrotum, or testicle. In women, it may radiate into the vulva. The severity and colicky nature of this pain are caused by the hyperperistalsis and spasm of this smooth muscle organ as it attempts to rid itself of a foreign body or to overcome obstruction. It should be remembered that radiculitis may mimic ureteral pain.

The physician may be able to judge the position of a ureteral stone by the history of pain and the site of referral. If the stone is lodged in the upper ureter, the pain radiates to the testicle, since the nerve supply of this organ is similar to that of the kidney and upper ureter (T11–12). With stones in the mid portion of the ureter on the right side, the pain is referred to McBurney's point and may therefore simulate appendicitis; on the left side, it may resemble diverticulitis or other diseases of the descending or sigmoid colon (T12, L1). As the stone approaches the bladder, inflammation and edema of the ureteral orifice ensue, and symptoms of vesical irritability such as urinary frequency and urgency may occur. It is important to realize, however, that in mild ureteral obstruction, as seen in the congenital stenoses, there is usually no pain, either renal or ureteral.

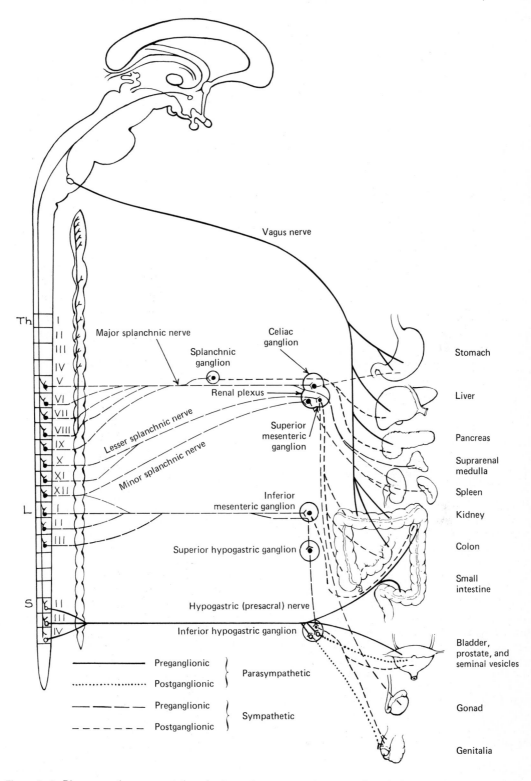

Figure 3–2. Diagrammatic representation of autonomic nerve supply to gastrointestinal and genitourinary tracts.

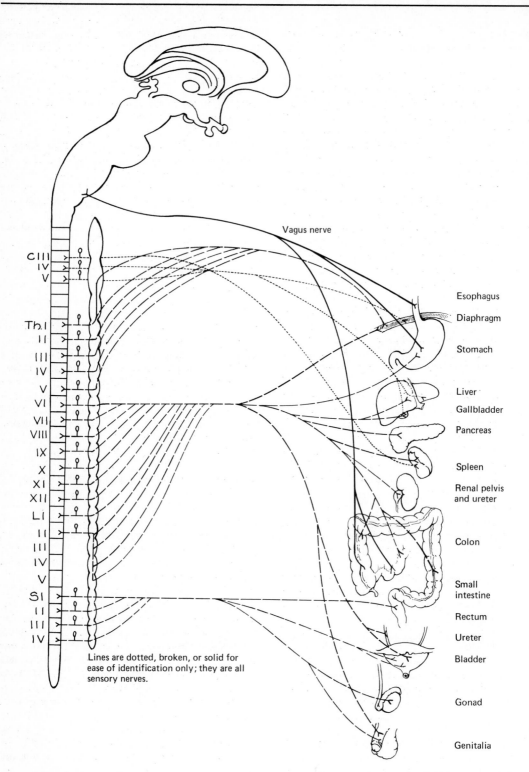

Figure 3–3. Diagrammatic representation of the sensory nerves of the gastrointestinal and genitourinary tracts.

Vesical Pain

The overdistended bladder of the patient in acute urinary retention will cause agonizing pain in the suprapubic area. Other than this, however, constant suprapubic pain not related to the act of urination is usually not of urologic origin. The relatively uncommon interstitial cystitis and vesical ulceration caused by tuberculosis or schistosomiasis may cause suprapubic discomfort (usually relieved by urination) when the bladder becomes full.

The patient in chronic urinary retention due to bladder neck obstruction or neurogenic bladder may experience little or no suprapubic discomfort even though the bladder reaches the level of the umbilicus.

The most common cause of bladder pain is infection; the pain is usually not felt over the bladder but is referred to the distal urethra and is related to the act of urination. Terminal dysuria may be a major complaint in severe cystitis.

Prostatic Pain

Direct pain from the prostate gland is not common. Occasionally, when the prostate is acutely inflamed, the patient may feel a vague discomfort or fullness in the perineal or rectal area (S2–4). Lumbosacral backache is occasionally experienced as referred pain from the prostate but is not a common symptom of prostatitis. Inflammation of the gland may cause dysuria, frequency, and urgency.

Testicular Pain

Testicular pain due to trauma, infection, or torsion of the spermatic cord is very severe and is felt locally, although there may be some radiation of the discomfort along the spermatic cord into the lower abdomen. It may involve the costovertebral area as well. Uninfected hydrocele, spermatocele, and tumor of the testis do not commonly cause pain. A varicocele may cause a dull ache in the testicle that is increased after heavy exercise. At times, the first symptom of an early indirect inguinal hernia may be testicular pain (referred). Pain from a stone in the upper ureter may be referred to the testicle.

Epididymal Pain

Acute infection of the epididymis is the only painful disease of this organ and is quite common. The pain begins in the scrotum, and some degree of neighborhood inflammatory reaction involves the adjacent testis as well, further aggravating the discomfort. In the early stages of epididymitis, pain may first be felt in the groin or lower abdominal quadrant. (If on the right side, it may simulate appendicitis.) This may be a referred type of pain but can be secondary to associated inflammation of the vas deferens. The discomfort associated with epididymitis may reach the costal angle and mimic ureteral stone on rare occasions.

Back & Leg Pain

Pain low in the back and radiating down one or both legs, especially when associated with symptoms of vesical neck obstruction in an older man, suggests metastases to the pelvic bones from cancer of the prostate.

GASTROINTESTINAL SYMPTOMS OF UROLOGIC DISEASES

Whether renal or ureteral disease is painful or not, gastrointestinal symptoms are often present. The patient with acute pyelonephritis will suffer not only from localized back pain, symptoms of vesical irritability, chills, and fever but also from generalized abdominal pain and distention. The patient who is passing a stone down the ureter will have typical renal and ureteral colic and, usually, hematuria and may experience severe nausea and vomiting as well as abdominal distention. However, the urinary symptoms so far overshadow the gastrointestinal symptoms that the latter are usually ignored. Inadvertent overdistention of the renal pelvis (eg, with opaque material in order to obtain adequate retrograde urograms) may cause the patient to become nauseated, to vomit, and to complain of cramplike pain in the abdomen. This clinical experiment demonstrates the renointestinal reflex, which may lead to confusing symptoms. In the vary common "silent" urologic deseases, some degree of gastrointestinal symptomatology may be present that could mislead the clinician into seeking the diagnosis in the intraperitoneal zone.

Cause of the Mimicry

A. Renointestinal Reflexes: These account for most of the confusion. They arise because of the common autonomic and sensory innervations of the 2 systems (Figs 3–2 and 3–3). Afferent stimuli from the renal capsule or musculature of the pelvis may, by reflex action, cause pylorospasm (symptoms of peptic ulcer) or other changes in tone of the smooth muscles of the enteric tract and its adnexa.

B. Organ Relationships: The right kidney is closely related to the hepatic flexure of the colon, the duodenum, the head of the pancreas, the common bile duct, the liver, and the gallbladder (Fig 1–3). The left kidney lies just behind the splenic flexure of the colon and is closely related to the stomach, pancreas, and spleen. Inflammations or tumors in the retroperitoneum thus may extend into or displace intraperitoneal organs, causing them to produce symptoms.

C. Peritoneal Irritation: The anterior surfaces of the kidneys are covered by peritoneum. Renal inflammation, therefore, will cause peritoneal irritation, which can lead to muscle rigidity and rebound tenderness.

The symptoms arising from chronic renal disease (eg, uninfected hydronephrosis, staghorn calculus, cancer, chronic pyelonephritis) may be entirely gastrointestinal and may simulate in every way the syndromes of peptic ulcer, gallbladder disease, appendicitis, or other less specific gastrointestinal complaints. If a thorough survey of the gastrointestinal tract fails to demonstrate suspected disease processes, the physician should give every consideration to study of the urinary tract.

SYMPTOMS RELATED TO THE ACT OF URINATION

Many conditions cause symptoms of "cystitis." These include infections of the bladder, vesical inflammation due to chemical or x-ray radiation reactions, interstitial cystitis, prostatitis, psychoneurosis, torsion or rupture of an ovarian cyst, and foreign bodies in the bladder. Often, however, the patient with chronic cystitis notices no symptoms of vesical irritability. Irritating chemicals or soap on the urethral meatus may cause cystitislike symptoms of dysuria, frequency, and urgency. This has been specifically noted in little girls taking frequent bubble baths.

Frequency, Nocturia, & Urgency

The normal capacity of the bladder is about 400 mL. Frequency may be caused by residual urine, which decreases the functional capacity of the organ. When the mucosa, submucosa, and even the muscularis become inflamed (eg, infection, foreign body, stones, tumor), the capacity of the bladder decreases sharply. This decrease is due to 2 factors: the pain resulting from even mild stretching of the bladder and the loss of bladder compliance resulting from inflammatory edema. When the bladder is normal, urination can be delayed if circumstances require it, but this is not so in acute cystitis. Once the diminished bladder capacity is reached, any further distention may be agonizing, and the patient may actually urinate involuntarily if voiding does not occur immediately. During very severe acute infections, the desire to urinate may be constant, and each voiding may produce only a few milliliters of urine. Day frequency without nocturia and acute or chronic frequency lasting only a few hours suggest nervous tension.

Diseases that cause fibrosis of the bladder are accompanied by frequency of urination. Examples of such diseases are tuberculosis, radiation cystitis, interstitial cystitis, and schistosomiasis. The presence of stones or foreign bodies causes vesical irritability, but secondary infection is almost always present.

Nocturia may be a symptom of renal disease related to a decrease in the functioning renal parenchyma with loss of concentrating power. Nocturia can occur in the absence of disease in persons who drink excessive amounts of fluids in the late evening. Coffee and alcoholic beverages, because of their specific diuretic effect, often produce nocturia if consumed just before bedtime. In older people who are ambulatory, some fluid retention may develop secondary to mild heart failure or varicose veins. With recumbency at night, this fluid is mobilized, leading to nocturia in these patients.

A very low or very high urine pH can irritate the bladder and cause frequency of urination. In chronic obstructive pulmonary disease, the Pa_{CO_2} is elevated. Compensation requires increased urinary excretion of chloride, leading to a low pH (Farcon and Morales, 1972). With hyperventilation, the urine becomes strongly alkaline.

Dysuria

Painful urination is usually related to acute inflammation of the bladder, urethra, or prostate. At times, the pain is described as "burning" on urination and is usually located in the distal urethra in men. Women usually localize the pain to the urethra. The pain is present only with voiding and disappears soon after micturition is completed. More severe pain sometimes occurs in the bladder just at the end of voiding, suggesting that inflammation of the bladder is the likely cause. Pain also may be more marked at the beginning of or throughout the act of urination. Dysuria often is the first symptom suggesting urinary infection and is often associated with urinary frequency and urgency.

Enuresis

Strictly speaking, enuresis means bedwetting at night. It is physiologic during the first 2 or 3 years of life but becomes troublesome, particularly to parents, after that age. It may be functional or secondary to delayed neuromuscular maturation of the urethrovesical component, but it may present as a symptom of organic disease (eg, infection, distal urethral stenosis in girls, posterior urethral valves in boys, neurogenic bladder). If, however, wetting occurs also during the daytime or if there are other urinary symptoms—or if the enuresis persists beyond age 5 or 6—urologic investigation is essential. In adult life, enuresis may be replaced by nocturia for which no organic basis can be found.

Symptoms of Bladder Outlet Obstruction
(See also Chapters 11 and 19.)

A. Hesitancy: Hesitancy in initiating the urinary stream is one of the early symptoms of bladder outlet obstruction. As the degree of obstruction increases, hesitancy is prolonged and the patient often strains to force urine through the obstruction. Prostate obstruction and urethral stricture are common causes of this symptom.

B. Loss of Force and Decrease of Caliber of the Stream: Progressive loss of force and caliber of the urinary stream is noted as urethral resistance increases despite the generation of increased intravesical pressure. This can be evaluated by measuring urinary flow rates, which in normal circumstances with a full bladder should approximate 20 mL/sec.

C. Terminal Dribbling: This becomes more and more noticeable as obstruction progresses and is a most distressing symptom.

D. Urgency: A strong, sudden desire to urinate is caused by hyperactivity and irritability of the bladder, resulting from obstruction, inflammation, or neuropathic bladder disease. In most circumstances, the patient is able to temporarily control the sudden need to void, but loss of small amounts of urine may occur (urgency incontinence).

E. Acute Urinary Retention: Sudden inability to urinate may supervene. The patient experiences increasingly agonizing suprapubic pain associated with severe urgency and may dribble only small amounts of urine.

F. Chronic Urinary Retention: This may cause little discomfort to the patient even though there is great hesitancy in starting the stream and marked reduction of its force and caliber. Constant dribbling of urine (paradoxic incontinence) may be experienced. It may be likened to water pouring over a dam.

G. Interruption of the Urinary Stream: Interruption may be abrupt and accompanied by severe pain radiating down the urethra. This type of reaction strongly suggests the complication of vesical calculus.

H. Sense of Residual Urine: The patient often feels that urine is still in the bladder even after urination has been completed.

I. Cystitis: Recurring episodes of acute cystitis suggest the presence of residual urine.

Incontinence
(See also Chapter 21.)

There are many reasons for incontinence. The history often gives a clue to its cause.

A. True Incontinence: The patient may lose urine without warning; this may be a constant or periodic symptom. The more obvious causes include exstrophy of the bladder, epispadias, vesicovaginal fistula, and ectopic ureteral orifice. Injury to the urethral smooth muscle sphincters may occur during prostatectomy or childbirth. Congenital or acquired neurogenic diseases may lead to dysfunction of the bladder and incontinence.

B. Stress Incontinence: When slight weakness of the sphincteric mechanisms is present, urine may be lost in association with physical strain (eg, coughing, laughing, rising from a chair) This is common in multiparous women who have weakened muscle support of the bladder neck and urethra. Occasionally, neuropathic bladder dysfunction can cause stress incontinence. The patient stays dry while lying in bed.

C. Urge Incontinence: This type of urgency may be so precipitate and severe that there is involuntary loss of urine. Urge incontinence not infrequently occurs with acute cystitis, particularly in women, since they seem to have relatively poor anatomic sphincters. Urge incontinence is a common symptom of an upper motor neuron lesion. It is often seen also in tense, anxious women even in the absence of infection.

D. Paradoxic (Overflow or False) Incontinence: This is loss of urine due to chronic urinary retention or secondary to a flaccid bladder. The intravesical pressure finally equals the urethral resistance; urine then constantly dribbles forth.

Oliguria & Anuria

Oliguria and anuria may be caused by acute renal failure (due to shock or dehydration), fluid-ion imbalance, or bilateral ureteral obstruction.

Pneumaturia

The passage of gas in the urine almost always means that there is a fistula between the urinary tract and the bowel. This occurs most commonly in the bladder or urethra but may be seen also in the ureter or renal pelvis. Carcinoma of the sigmoid colon, diverticulitis with abscess formation, regional enteritis, and trauma cause most vesical fistulas. Congenital anomalies account for most urethroenteric fistulas. Certain bacteria, by the process of fermentation, may rarely liberate gas.

Cloudy Urine

Patients often complain of cloudy urine, but it is most often cloudy merely because it is alkaline; this causes precipitation of phosphate. Infection can also cause urine to be cloudy and malodorous. A properly performed urinalysis will reveal the cause of cloudiness.

Chyluria

The passage of lymphatic fluid or chyle is noted by the patient as passage of milky white urine. This represents a lymphatic urinary system fistula. Most often, this is from obstruction of the renal lymphatics, which causes forniceal rupture and leakage. Filariasis, trauma, tuberculosis, and retroperitoneal tumors have caused the problem.

Bloody Urine

Hematuria is a danger signal that cannot be ignored. It is important to know whether urination is painful or not, whether the hematuria is associated with symptoms of vesical irritability, and whether blood is seen in all or only a portion of the urinary stream. Some individuals (particularly if they are anemic) will pass red urine after eating beets or taking laxatives containing phenolphthalein, in which case the urine is translucent rather than opaque and contains no red cells. Because of the wide use of rhodamine B as a coloring agent in cookies, cakes, cold drinks, and fruit juices, children commonly pass red urine after ingestion of these foods. This is the so-called Monday morning disorder. The hemoglobinuria that occurs as a feature of the hemolytic syndromes may also cause the urine to be red.

A. Bloody Urine in Relation to Symptoms and Diseases: Hematuria associated with renal colic suggests ureteral stone, although a clot from a bleeding renal tumor can cause the same type of pain.

Hematuria is not uncommonly associated with nonspecific, tuberculous, or schistosomal infection of the bladder. The bleeding is often terminal (bladder neck or prostate), although it may be present throughout urination (vesical or upper tract). Stone in the bladder often causes hematuria, but infection is usually present, and there are symptoms of bladder neck obstruction, neurogenic bladder, or cystocele. When a tumor of the bladder ulcerates, it is often complicated by infection and bleeding. Thus, symptoms of cystitis and hematuria are also compatible with tumors.

Dilated veins may develop at the bladder neck secondary to enlargement of the prostate. These may rupture when the patient strains to urinate.

Hematuria without other symptoms ("silent") must be regarded as a symptom of tumor of the bladder or kidney until proved otherwise. It is usually intermittent; bleeding may not recur for months. Complacency because the bleeding stops spontaneously must be condemned. Less common causes of silent hematuria are staghorn calculus, polycystic kidneys, solitary renal cyst, sickle cell disease, and hydronephrosis. Painless bleeding is common with acute glomerulonephritis. Recurrent bleeding is occasionally seen in children suffering from focal glomerulitis.

Richie and Kerr (1979) remind us that white patients can have sickle cell trait. Joggers frequently develop transient proteinuria and gross or microscopic hematuria (Boileau et al, 1980).

B. Time of Hematuria: Learning whether the hematuria is partial (initial, terminal) or total (present throughout urination) is often of help in identifying the site of bleeding. Initial hematuria suggests an anterior urethral lesion (eg, urethritis, stricture, meatal stenosis in young boys). Terminal hematuria usually arises from the posterior urethra, bladder neck, or trigone. Among the common causes are posterior urethritis and polyps and tumors of the vesical neck.

Total hematuria has its source at or above the level of the bladder (eg, stone, tumor, tuberculosis, nephritis).

OTHER OBJECTIVE MANIFESTATIONS

Urethral Discharge

Urethral discharge in men is one of the most common complaints in urology. The causative organism is usually *N gonorrhoeae* or *C trachomatis*. The discharge is often accompanied by local burning on urination or an itching sensation in the urethra (see Chapter 15).

Skin Lesions of the External Genitalia
(See Chapters 15 and 33.)

An ulceration of the glans penis or its shaft may represent syphilitic chancre, chancroid, herpes simplex, or squamous cell carcinoma. Venereal warts of the penis are common.

Visible or Palpable Masses

The patient may notice a visible or palpable mass in the upper abdomen that may represent renal tumor, hydronephrosis, or polycystic kidney. Enlarged lymph nodes in the neck may contain metastatic tumor from the prostate or testis. Lumps in the groin may represent

spread of tumor of the penis or lymphadenitis from chancroid, syphilis, or lymphogranuloma venereum. Painless masses in the scrotal contents are common and include hydrocele, varicocele, spermatocele, chronic epididymitis, hernia, and testicular tumor.

Edema

Edema of the legs may result from compression of the iliac veins by lymphatic metastases from prostatic cancer. Edema of the genitalia suggest filariasis or chronic ascites.

Bloody Ejaculation

Inflammation of the prostate or seminal vesicles can cause hematospermia.

Gynecomastia

This is often idiopathic. It is common in elderly men, particularly those taking estrogens for control of prostatic cancer. It is also seen in association with choriocarcinoma and interstitial cell and Sertoli cell tumors of the testis. Certain endocrinologic diseases, eg, Klinefelter's syndrome, may also cause gynecomastia.

Size of Penis in Infant or Child

Micropenis is probably due to fetal testosterone deficiency (see p 623). Megalopenis is caused by overactivity of the adrenal cortex (see Chapter 22) and is seen in association with interstitial cell tumor of the testis (see p 393).

Infertility
(See Chapter 36.)

Many men are referred to the urologist for fertility studies. The urologist should explore the patient's sexual habits and investigate diseases and disorders that have affected the scrotal contents (ie, mumps, torsion of the spermatic cord, epididymitis) and exposure to testicular toxins (eg, x-ray radiation).

COMPLAINTS RELATED TO SEXUAL PROBLEMS

Many people suffer from genitourinary complaints on a purely psychologic or emotional basis. In others, organic symptoms may be increased in severity because of tension states. It is therefore important to seek clues that might give evidence of emotional stress.

In women, the relationship of the menses to ureteral pain or vesical complaints should be determined, although menstruation may exacerbate both organic and functional vesical and renal difficulties.

Many patients, particularly women, recognize that the state of their "nerves" has a direct effect on their symptoms. They often realize that their "cystitis" develops following a tension-producing or anxiety-producing episode in their personal or occupational environment.

A. Sexual Difficulties in Men: Men may complain directly of sexual difficulty. However, they are often so ashamed of loss of sexual power that they cannot admit it even to a physician. In such cases they may ask for "prostate treatment" and hope that the physician will understand that they have sexual complaints and that they will be treated accordingly. The main sexual symptoms include impaired quality of erection, premature loss of erection, absence of ejaculate with orgasm, premature ejaculation, and even loss of desire.

B. Sexual Difficulties in Women: Women suffering from the psychosomatic cystitis syndrome almost always admit to an unhappy sex life. They notice that frequency or vaginal-urethral pain often occurs on the day following the incomplete sexual act. Many of them recognize the inadequacy of their sexual experiences as one of the underlying causes of urologic complaints; too frequently, however, the physician either does not ask them pertinent questions or, if patients volunteer this information, ignores it.

C. Sexual Difficulties of Suspected Psychosomatic Origin: In treating sexual difficulties of suspected psychosomatic origin, the physician should explore pertinent facts concerning childhood, adolescence (sex education and experiences), marriage problems, and relationships with relatives, business associates, etc. Even when psychosomatic disease is strongly suspected before history-taking has been completed, a thorough examination and laboratory survey must be done. Both psyche and soma may be involved, and the patient must be assured that there is no serious organic disease. Although sexual interest and activity decline with advancing years, physically healthy men and women may continue to be sexually active into their eighth or ninth decades.

REFERENCES

Local & Referred Pain

Delaere KP, Debruyne FM, Moonen WA: Extended bladder neck incision for outflow obstruction in male patients. *Br J Urol* 1983;**55**:225.

DeWolf WC, Fraley EE: Renal pain. *Urology* 1975;**6**:403.

Dowd JB: Flank pain in nonurologic disease. *Med Clin North Am* 1963;**47**:437.

Eisenberg RL et al: Evaluation of plain abdominal radiographs in the diagnosis of abdominal pain. *Ann Intern Med* 1982;**97**:257.

Nicholls AJ et al: Loin pain and haematuria in young women: Diagnostic pitfalls. *Br J Urol* 1982;**54**:209.

Smith DR, Raney FL Jr: Radiculitis distress as a mimic of renal pain. *J Urol* 1976;**116**:269.

Symptoms Related to the Act of Urination

Abuelo JG: Evaluation of hematuria. *Urology* 1983;**21**:215.

Bartholomew TH: Neurogenic voiding: Function and dysfunction. *Urol Clin North Am* 1985;**12**:67.

Boileau M et al: Stress hematuria: Athletic pseudonephritis in marathoners. *Urology* 1980;**15**:471.

Copley JB: Isolated asymptomatic hematuria in the adult. *Am J Med Sci* 1986;**291**:101.

Elzouki AY, Mir NA, Jeswal OP: Symptomatic urinary tract infection in pediatric patients: A developmental aspect. *Int J Pediatr Nephrol* 1985;**6**:267.

Fritz GK, Armbrust J: Enuresis and encopresis. *Psychiatr Clin North Am* 1982;**5**:283.

Jensen KM et al: Abdominal straining in benign prostatic hyperplasia. *J Urol* 1983;**129**:44.

Jensen KM et al: Uroflowmetry in neurologically normal children with voiding disorders. *Scand J Urol Nephrol* 1985;**19**:81.

Jones KW, Schoenberg HW: Comparison of the incidence of bladder hyperreflexia in patients with benign prostatic hypertrophy and age-matched female controls. *J Urol* 1985;**133**:425.

Koehler PR, Kyaw MM: Hematuria. *Med Clin North Am* 1975;**59**:201.

Kunin CM: Genitourinary infections in the patient at risk: Extrinsic risk factors. *Am J Med* 1984;**76**:131.

Levin S: Red urine: The Monday morning disorder of children. *Pediatrics* 1965;**36**:134.

Manoliu RA: Urethral calibre measurements on micturition cystourethrograms in adult males. 2. Subvesical obstruction. *Eur J Radiol* 1982;**2**:293.

Millard RJ: The clinical significance of bladder speed. *Br J Urol* 1984;**56**:165.

Resnick NM, Yalla SV: Management of urinary incontinence in the elderly. *N Engl J Med* 1985;**313**:800.

Richie JP, Kerr WS Jr: Sickle cell trait: Forgotten cause of hematuria in white patients. *J Urol* 1979;**122**:134.

Seeds JW, Mandell J: Congenital obstructive uropathies: Pre- and postnatal treatment. *Urol Clin North Am* 1986; **13**:155.

Shenoy UA: Current assessment of microhematuria and leukocyturia. *Clin Lab Med* 1985;**5**:317.

Tapp AJ, Cardozo L: The postmenopausal bladder. *Br J Hosp Med* 1986;**35**:20.

Thon W, Altwein JE: Voiding dysfunctions. *Urology* 1984;**23**:323.

Warshaw BL, Hymes LC, Woodard JR: Long-term outcome of patients with obstructive uropathy. *Pediatr Clin North Am* 1982;**29**:815.

Wiggelinkhuizen J, Landman C, Greenberg E: Chyluria. *Am J Dis Child* 1972;**124**:99.

4

Physical Examination of the Genitourinary Tract

Emil A. Tanagho, MD

The history will suggest whether a complete or partial examination is indicated. The symptom of urethral discharge probably does not require a thorough physical examination; on the other hand, painless hematuria certainly requires a careful examination of the genitourinary tract. In this chapter are discussed the urologic aspects of the physical examination.

Unusual Findings on General Examination

A. Gynecomastia: Gynecomastia is common and usually of no consequence. Williams (1963) found gynecomastia in 40% of a series of 447 autopsies. Its causes included prostatic carcinoma (treated with estrogen), testicular abnormalities, adrenocortical hyperplasia, adrenocortical tumors, interstitial cell tumors of the testis, certain diseases of the liver and thyroid, cirrhosis, and diabetes. Gynecomastia in a young man suggests to the urologist the presence of a choriocarcinomatous testicular tumor or Klinefelter's syndrome.

B. Hemihypertrophy: Hennessy, Cromie, and Duckett (1981) noted abdominal masses associated with this rare phenomenon. The masses were on the side of the hemihypertrophy and, in 7 patients, included 3 Wilms' tumors, 2 adrenal tumors, and a neuroblastoma. Saypol and Laudone (1983) have reviewed the literature on this subject.

C. Clues to Renal Anomalies: A child with gross deformity of an external ear and ipsilateral maldevelopment of the facial bones is likely to have a congenital abnormality of the kidney on the same side. Lateral displacement of the nipples has been associated with bilateral renal hypoplasia. Renal abnormalities have also been observed with congenital scoliosis and kyphosis as well as with prelevator imperforate anus.

D. Other Findings: Evidence of endocrinologic changes should be noted, eg, hypertrophy of the external genitalia, hirsutism, etc. The finding of hypertension suggests the possibility of pheochromocytoma or renovascular hypertension.

EXAMINATION OF THE KIDNEYS

Inspection

On occasion, a mass that is visible in the upper ab-

dominal area may, if soft (eg, as in hydronephrosis), be difficult to palpate. Fullness in the costovertebral angle may be consistent with cancer (eg, neuroblastoma in children) or perinephric infection. The presence and persistence of indentations in the skin from lying on wrinkled sheets suggest edema of the skin secondary to perinephric abscess. If this disease is suspected, have the patient lie on a rough towel and observe for indentations.

Palpation

The kidneys lie rather high under the diaphragm and lower ribs and are therefore well protected from injury. Because of the position of the liver, the right kidney is lower than the left. The kidneys are difficult to palpate in men because of the resistance of abdominal muscle tone and because the kidneys in men are more fixed than those in women and move only slightly with change of posture or respiration. The lower part of the right kidney can sometimes be felt, especially in thin patients, but the left kidney cannot usually be felt unless it is enlarged or displaced.

The most successful method of renal palpation is carried out with the patient lying supine on a hard surface (Fig 4–1). The kidney is lifted by one hand in the costovertebral angle. On deep inspiration, the kidney moves downward; when it is lowest, the other hand is pushed firmly and deeply beneath the costal margin in an effort to trap the kidney below that point. If this is successful, the anterior hand can palpate the size, shape, and consistency of the organ as it slips back into its normal position.

The kidney can sometimes best be palpated with the examiner standing behind the seated patient. At other times, if the patient is lying on one side, the uppermost kidney drops downward and medially, thereby making it more accessible to palpation.

Perlman and Williams (1976) have described a very effective method of identifying renal anomalies in the newborn. The fingers are placed in the costovertebral angle, with the thumb anterior. The thumb does the feeling. With this technique, the kidneys can be palpated 95% of the time. Anomalies were found in 0.5% of 11,000 newborns.

An enlarged renal mass suggests compensatory hypertrophy (if the other kidney is absent or atrophic), hydronephrosis, tumor, cyst, or polycystic disease. A

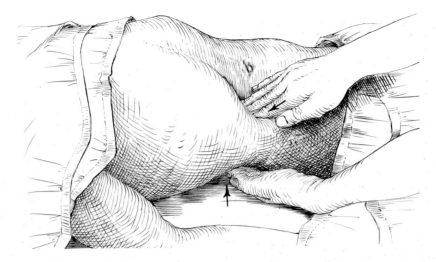

Figure 4–1. Method of palpation of the kidney. The posterior hand lifts the kidney upward. The anterior hand feels for the kidney. The patient then takes a deep breath; this causes the kidney to descend. As the patient inhales, the fingers of the anterior hand are plunged inward at the costal margin. If the kidney is mobile or enlarged, it can be felt between the 2 hands.

mass in this area, however, may be a retroperitoneal tumor, the spleen, a lesion of the bowel (eg, tumor, abscess), a lesion of the gallbladder, or a pancreatic cyst. Tumors may have the consistency of normal tissue; they may also be nodular. Hydronephroses may be firm or soft. Polycystic kidneys are usually nodular and firm.

An acutely infected kidney is tender, but this is difficult to elicit, since marked muscle spasm is usually present. Since normal kidneys are often tender also, this sign is not always helpful.

Although renal pain may be diffusely felt in the back, tenderness is usually well localized just lateral to the sacrospinalis muscle and just below the 12th rib (costovertebral angle [CVA]). This may be elicited by palpation or, more sharply, by first percussion over that area.

Percussion

At times, a greatly enlarged kidney cannot be felt on palpation, particularly if it is soft. This can be true of hydronephrosis. Such masses, however, may be readily outlined by percussion, both anteriorly and posteriorly; this part of the examination should never be omitted. Percussion is of particular value in outlining an enlarging mass in the flank following renal trauma (progressive hemorrhage), where tenderness and muscle spasm prevent proper palpation.

Transillumination

This maneuver may prove quite helpful in the child under age 1 year who presents with a suprapubic or flank mass. A 2- or 3-cell flashlight with an opaque flange protruding beyond the lens is an adequate instrument. The flashlight is applied at right angles to the

abdomen. The fiberoptic light cord, used to illuminate various optical instruments, is an excellent source of cold light. A dark room is required. A distended bladder or cystic mass will transilluminate; a solid mass will not. Flank masses may also be tested by applying the light posteriorly.

Differentiation of Renal & Radicular Pain

Radicular pain (see p 29) is commonly felt in the costovertebral and subcostal areas. It may spread along the course of the ureter as well and is the most common cause of so-called kidney pain. Every patient who complains of flank pain should be examined for evidence of nerve root irritation. Frequent causes are poor posture (scoliosis, kyphosis), arthritic changes in the costovertebral or costotransverse joints, impingement of a rib spur on a subcostal nerve, hypertrophy of costovertebral ligaments pressing on a nerve, and intervertebral disk disease (Smith and Raney, 1976). Radicular pain may be noted as an aftermath of a flank incision wherein a rib may become dislocated, causing the costal nerve to impinge on the edge of a ligament (Krauss, Khonsari, and Lilien, 1977). Pain experienced during the preeruptive phase of herpes zoster involving any of the segments between T11 and L2 may also simulate pain of renal origin.

Radiculitis usually causes hyperesthesia of the area of skin served by the irritated peripheral nerve. This hypersensitivity can be elicited by means of the pinwheel or by grasping and pinching both skin and fat of the abdomen and flanks. Pressure exerted by the thumb over the costovertebral joints will reveal local tenderness at the point of emergence of the involved peripheral nerve.

Auscultation

Auscultation of the costovertebral areas and upper abdominal quadrants may reveal a systolic bruit, which is often associated with stenosis or aneurysm of the renal artery. Bruits over the femoral arteries may be found in association with Leriche syndrome, which may be a cause of impotence.

EXAMINATION OF THE BLADDER

The bladder cannot be felt unless it is moderately distended. In the adult, if it is percussible, it contains at least 150 mL of urine. In acute or (more commonly) in chronic urinary retention, the bladder may reach or even rise above the umbilicus, in which case its outline may be seen and usually felt. (In chronic retention, where the bladder wall is flabby, the bladder may be difficult to palpate. In this instance, percussion is of great value.)

In the male infant or little boy, palpation of a hard mass deep in the center of the pelvis is compatible with a thickened hypertrophied bladder secondary to obstruction caused by posterior urethral valves.

A sliding inguinal hernia containing some bladder wall can be diagnosed (when the bladder is full) by compressing the scrotal mass. The bladder will be found to further distend.

A few instances have been reported wherein marked edema of the legs has developed secondary to compression of the iliac vessels by a distended bladder. Bimanual (abdominorectal or abdominovaginal) palpation may reveal the extent of a vesical tumor. To be successful, it must be done under anesthesia.

EXAMINATION OF THE EXTERNAL MALE GENITALIA

PENIS

Inspection

If the patient has not been circumcised, the foreskin should be retracted. This may reveal tumor or balanitis as the cause of a foul discharge. If retraction is not possible (ie, phimosis), surgical correction (dorsal slit or circumcision) is indicated.

The observation of a poor urinary stream is significant. In the newborn, neurogenic (neuropathic) bladder or the presence of posterior urethral valves should be considered. In men, such a finding suggests urethral stricture or prostatic obstruction.

The scars of healed syphilis may be an important clue. An active ulcer requires bacteriologic or pathologic study (eg, syphilitic chancre, epithelioma). Superficial ulcers or vesicles are compatible with herpes simplex; they are often interpreted by the patient as a serious sexually transmitted disease, possibly syphilis. Venereal warts may be observed.

Meatal stenosis is a common cause of bloody spotting in the male infant. On rare occasions, it may be of such degree as to cause advanced bilateral hydronephrosis. It is easily corrected by meatotomy.

The position of the meatus should be noted. It may be located proximal to the tip of the glans on either the dorsum (epispadias) or the ventral surface (hypospadias). In either instance, there is apt to be abnormal curvature of the penis—dorsally with epispadias, ventrally with hypospadias. The urethral orifice is often stenotic in the latter.

Micropenis or macropenis may be observed.

Palpation

Palpation of the dorsal surface of the shaft may reveal a fibrous plaque involving the fascial covering of the corpora cavernosa. This is typical of Peyronie's disease. Tender areas of induration felt along the urethra may signify periurethritis secondary to urethral stricture.

Urethral Discharge

Urethral discharge is the most common complaint referable to the male sex organ. Gonococcal pus is usually profuse, thick, and yellow or gray-brown. Nongonorrheal discharges may be similar in appearance but are often thin, mucoid, and scanty. Although gonorrhea must be ruled out as the cause of a urethral discharge, a high percentage of such cases will be found to be caused by chlamydiae. Patients with urethral discharge should also be examined for other sexually transmitted diseases; multiple infection is not uncommon.

Bloody discharge should suggest the possibility of a foreign body in the urethra (male or female), urethral stricture, or tumor.

Urethral discharge must always be sought before the patient is asked to void.

SCROTUM

Infections and inflammations of the skin of the scrotum are not common. Small sebaceous cysts are occasionally seen. Malignant tumors are rare. The scrotum is bifid when midscrotal or perineal hypospadias is present.

Elephantiasis of the scrotum is caused by obstruction to lymphatic drainage. It is endemic in the tropics and is due to filariasis. Elephantiasis may result from radical resection of the lymph nodes of the inguinal and femoral areas, in which case the skin of the penis is also involved. Small hemangiomas of the skin are common and may bleed spontaneously.

TESTIS

The testes should be carefully palpated with the fingers of both hands. A hard area in the testis proper must be regarded as a malignant tumor until proved otherwise. Transillumination of all scrotal masses should be done routinely. With the patient in a dark room, a strong flashlight or fiberoptic light is placed against the scrotal sac posteriorly. A hydrocele will cause the intrascrotal mass to glow red. Light will not be transmitted through a solid tumor. Tumors are often smooth but may be nodular. They seem abnormally heavy. A testis replaced by tumor or damaged by gumma is insensitive to pressure, and the usual sickening sensation is absent. About 10% of tumors are associated with a secondary hydrocele that may have to be aspirated before definitive palpation can be done.

The testis may be absent from the scrotum. This may represent transient (physiologic retractile testis) or true cryptorchidism. Palpation of the groins may reveal the presence of the organ.

The atrophic testis (following postoperative orchiopexy, mumps orchitis, or torsion of the spermatic cord) may be flabby and at times hypersensitive but is usually firm and hyposensitive. Although spermatogenesis may be lost, androgen function is occasionally maintained.

EPIDIDYMIS

The epididymis is sometimes rather closely attached to the posterior surface of the testis, and at other times it is quite free of it. The epididymis should be carefully palpated for size and induration. Induration means infection (primary tumors are exceedingly rare).

In the acute stage of epididymitis, the testis and epididymis are indistinguishable by palpation; the testicle and epididymis may be adherent to the scrotum, which is usually quite red. Tenderness is exquisite. With few exceptions, the infecting organism is either *Neisseria gonorrhoeae, Chlamydia trachomatis,* or *Escherichia coli.*

Chronic painless induration should suggest tuberculosis or schistosomiasis, although nonspecific chronic epididymitis is also a possibility. Other signs of tuberculosis of the genitourinary tract usually present include "sterile" pyuria, a thickened seminal vesicle, a nodular prostate, and "beading" of the vas deferens.

SPERMATIC CORD & VAS DEFERENS

A swelling in the spermatic cord may be cystic (eg, hydrocele or hernia) or solid (eg, connective tissue tumor). The latter is rare. Lipoma in the investing fascia of the cord may simulate hernia. Diffuse swelling and induration of the cord are seen with filarial funiculitis.

Careful palpation of the vas deferens may reveal thickening (eg, chronic infection), fusiform enlargements (the "beading" caused by tuberculosis), or even its absence. The latter finding is of importance in the infertile male; it is rare.

In the standing male, a mass of dilated veins (varicocele) may be noted behind and above the testis. The degree of dilatation decreases with recumbency and can be increased by the Valsalva maneuver. The major sequel of varicocele is infertility (see Chapter 36).

TESTICULAR TUNICS & ADNEXA

Hydroceles are usually cystic but on occasion are so tense that they simulate solid tumors. Transillumination makes the differential diagnosis. They may develop secondary to nonspecific acute or tuberculous epididymitis, trauma, or tumor of the testis. The latter is a distinct possibility if hydrocele appears "spontaneously" between the ages of 18 and 35. It should be aspirated to permit careful palpation of underlying structures.

Hydrocele usually surrounds the testis completely. Cystic masses that are separate from but in the region of the upper pole of the testis are probably spermatoceles. Aspiration reveals the typical thin, milky fluid, which contains sperms.

VAGINAL EXAMINATION

Diseases of the female genital tract may secondarily involve the urinary organs, thereby making a thorough gynecologic examination essential. Commonly associated are urethrocystitis secondary to urethral diverticulitis or cervicitis, pyelonephritis during pregnancy, and ureteral obstruction from metastatic nodes or direct extension in cancer of the cervix.

Inspection

In newborns and children especially, the vaginal vestibule should be inspected for a single opening (common urogenital sinus), labial fusion, split clitoris and lack of fusion of the anterior forchette (epispadias), or hypertrophied clitoris and scrotalization of the labia majora (adrenogenital syndrome).

The urinary meatus may reveal a reddened, tender, friable lesion (urethral caruncle) or a reddened, everted posterior lip, which is often seen with senile urethritis and vaginitis. Biopsy is indicated if a malignant tumor cannot be ruled out. The diagnosis of senile vaginitis (and urethritis) is established by staining a smear of the vaginal epithelium with Lugol's solution. It should be examined immediately after rinsing, because the brown dye in the cells fades quickly. Cells lacking glycogen (hypoestrogenism) do not take up the stain, whereas normal cells do.

Multiple painful small ulcers or blisterlike lesions may be noted; these probably represent herpesvirus type 2 infection, which may have serious sequels.

Smears and cultures of urethral or vaginal discharge should be made. Gonococci are relatively easy to identify; culture of chlamydiae requires techniques seldom available to the physician.

Evidence of skenitis and bartholinitis may reveal the source of persistent urethritis or cystitis. The condition of the vaginal wall should be observed. Bacteriologic study of the secretions may be helpful. Urethrocele and cystocele may cause residual urine and lead to persistent infection of the bladder. They are often found in association with stress incontinence. A bulge in the anterior vaginal wall may represent a urethral diverticulum. The cervix should be inspected to detect cancer or infection. Taking biopsy specimens or making Papanicolaou smears may be indicated.

Palpation

At times, the urethra, the base of the bladder, and the lower ureters may be tender on palpation, but little can be deduced from this. Induration of the urethra or trigonal area or a mass involving either may be a clue to an existing tumor. A soft mass found in this area could be a urethral diverticulum. Pressure on such a lesion may cause pus to extrude from the urethra. A stone in the lower ureter may be palpable. Evidence of enlargement of the uterus (eg, pregnancy, myomas) or diseases or inflammations of the colon or adnexa may afford a clue to the cause of urinary symptoms (eg, compression of a ureter by a malignant ovarian tumor, endometriosis, or diverticulitis of the sigmoid colon adherent to the bladder).

Carcinoma of the cervix may invade the base of the bladder, causing vesical irritability or hematuria; or its metastases to iliac lymph nodes may compress the ureters.

Rectal examination may afford further information and is the obvious route of examination in children and virgins.

RECTAL EXAMINATION OF THE MALE

SPHINCTER & LOWER RECTUM

The estimation of sphincter tone is of great importance. Laxity of the muscle strongly suggests similar changes in the urinary sphincters and detrusor and may be a clue to the diagnosis of neurogenic disease. The same is true for a spastic anal sphincter. In addition to the digital prostatic examination, the examiner should palpate the entire lower rectum to rule out stenosis, internal hemorrhoids, cryptitis, rectal fistulas, mucosal polyps, and rectal cancer and should use bidigital palpation for Cowper's glands. Testing perianal sensation is mandatory.

PROSTATE

A specimen of urine for routine analysis should be collected before the rectal examination is made. This is of the utmost importance, since prostatic massage (or even palpation at times) will force prostatic secretion into the posterior urethra. If this secretion contains pus, a specimen of urine voided after the rectal examination will be contaminated by it.

Size

The average prostate is about 4 cm in length and width. It is widest superiorly at the bladder neck. As the gland enlarges, the lateral sulci becomes relatively deeper and the median furrow becomes obliterated. The prostate may also elongate. The clinical importance of prostatic hyperplasia is measured by the severity of symptoms and the amount of residual urine and not by the size of the gland. On rectal examination, the prostate may be of normal size and consistency in a patient with acute urinary retention.

Consistency

Normally, the consistency of the gland is similar to that of the contracted thenar eminence of the thumb (with the thumb completely opposed to the little finger). It is rather rubbery. It may be mushy if congested (due to lack of intercourse or to chronic infection with impaired drainage), indurated (due to chronic infection with or without calculi), or stony-hard (due to advanced carcinoma).

The difficulty lies in differentiating firm areas in the prostate: fibrosis from nonspecific infection, granulomatous prostatitis, nodulation from tuberculosis, or firm areas due to prostatic calculi or early cancer. Generally speaking, nodules caused by infection are raised above the surface of the gland. At their edges, the induration gradually fades to the normal softness of surrounding tissue. In cancer, conversely, the suspicious lesion is usually not raised; it is hard and has a sharp edge, ie, there is an abrupt change in consistency on the same plane. It tends to arise in the lateral sulcus (Fig 4–2).

Even the most experienced clinicians sometimes have trouble making this differentiation. In the absence of other signs of tuberculosis and in the absence of pus in the prostatic secretion, cancer is likely, particularly if an x-ray fails to show prostatic calculi (which are seen just behind or above the symphysis). Serum acid phosphatase determinations and radiograms of bones are of no help in diagnosing early carcinoma of the prostate.

Mobility

The mobility of the gland varies. Occasionally, it has great mobility; at other times, very little. With advanced carcinoma, it is fixed because of local extension through the capsule. The prostate should be routinely massaged in the adult and its secretion examined microscopically. It should not be massaged, however, in the presence of an acute urethral discharge, acute

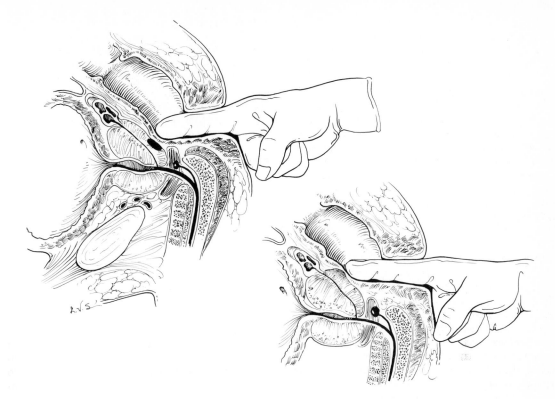

Figure 4–2. Differential diagnosis of prostatic nodules. *A:* Inflammatory area is raised above the surface of the gland; induration decreases gradually at its periphery. *B:* Cancerous nodule is not raised; there is an abrupt change in consistency at its edges.

prostatitis, or acute prostatocystitis; in men near the stage of complete urinary retention (because it may precipitate complete retention); or in men suffering from obvious cancer of the gland. Even without symptoms, massage is necessary, for prostatitis is commonly asymptomatic. Diagnosis and treatment of such silent disease is important in preventing cystitis and epididymitis.

Techniques of Massage

The patient should lean over the examining table so that his body is horizontal. His legs should be straight and his feet somewhat apart.

Methods of massage vary, but the basic maneuver is to press the gland substance firmly with the pad of the index finger in order to express secretion into the prostatic urethra. Start laterally and superiorly, and massage toward the midline. A rolling motion of the finger is less traumatic to the rectal mucosa and prostate gland and is better tolerated by the patient. Finally, the seminal vesicles should be stripped from above downward and medially (Fig 4–3).

Copious amounts of secretion may be obtained from some prostate glands and little or none from others. This of course depends to some extent upon the

vigor with which the massage is carried out. If no secretion is obtained, have the patient void even a few drops of urine; this will contain adequate secretion for examination. Microscopic examination of the secretion is done under low-power magnification. Normal secretion contains numerous lecithin bodies, which are refractile, like red cells, but much smaller than red cells. Only an occasional white cell is present. A few epithelial cells and, rarely, corpora amylacea are seen. Sperms may be present, but their absence is of no significance.

The presence of large numbers of pus cells is pathologic and suggests the diagnosis of prostatitis. Stained smears are usually impractical. It is difficult to fix this material on the slide, and even when this is successful, pyogenic bacteria are usually not found. Acid-fast organisms can often be found by appropriate staining methods.

On occasion, it may be necessary to obtain cultures of prostatic secretion in order to demonstrate nonspecific organisms, tubercle bacilli, gonococci, or chlamydiae. After thorough cleansing of the glans and emptying of the bladder (to mechanically cleanse the urethra), massage is done. Drops of secretion are collected in a sterile tube of appropriate culture medium.

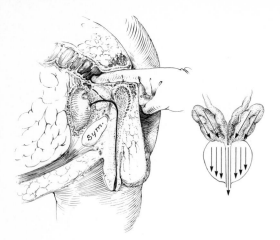

Figure 4–3. Technique of prostatic massage. The glandular substance is compressed from its lateral edges to the urethra, which lies in the center. (Drawing at right shows direction of pressure.) The seminal vesicles are then stripped from above downward.

SEMINAL VESICLES

Palpation of the seminal vesicles should be attempted. The vesicles are situated under the base of the bladder and diverge from below upward (Figs 1–8 and 4–3). Normal seminal vesicles are usually not palpable, but when they are overdistended they may feel quite cystic. In the presence of chronic infection (particularly tuberculosis or schistosomiasis) or in association with advanced carcinoma of the prostate, they may be markedly indurated. Stripping of the seminal vesicles should be done in association with prostatic massage, for the vesicles are usually infected when prostatitis is present. Primary tumors of the vesicles are very rare. A cystic mass may rarely be felt over the prostate or just above it. This probably represents a cyst of the müllerian duct or the utricle. The latter is occasionally associated with severe hypospadias.

LYMPH NODES
(See Figs 19–1 and 19–2)

It should be remembered that generalized lymphadenopathy usually occurs early in acquired immunodeficiency syndrome (AIDS) (see Chapter 15).

Inguinal & Subinguinal Lymph Nodes

With inflammatory lesions of the skin of the penis and scrotum or vulva, the inguinal and subinguinal lymph nodes may be involved. Such diseases include chancroid, syphilitic chancre, lymphogranuloma venereum, and, on occasion, gonorrhea.

Malignant tumors (squamous cell carcinoma) involving the penis, glans, scrotal skin, or distal urethra in women metastasize to the inguinal and subinguinal nodes. Testicular tumors do not spread to these nodes unless they have invaded the scrotal skin or the patient has previously undergone orchiopexy.

Other Lymph Nodes

Tumors of the testis and prostate may involve the left supraclavicular nodes. Tumors of the bladder and prostate typically metastasize to the internal iliac, external iliac, and preaortic nodes, although only occasionally are they so large as to be palpable. Upper abdominal masses near the midline in a young man should suggest metastases from cancer of the testis; the primary growth may be minute and completely hidden in the substance of what appears to be a normal testicle.

NEUROLOGIC EXAMINATION

A careful neurologic survey may uncover sensory or motor impairment that will account for residual urine (neuropathic bladder) or incontinence. Since the bladder and its sphincter are innervated by the second to fourth sacral segments, much information can be gained by testing anal sphincter tone and the sensation of the perianal skin and by eliciting the Achilles tendon and bulbocavernosus reflexes. The bulbocavernosus reflex is elicited by placing a finger in the patient's rectum and squeezing the glans penis or clitoris or by jerking on an indwelling Foley catheter. The normal reflex is contraction of the anal sphincter and bulbocavernosus muscles in response to these maneuvers. Blaivas, Zayed, and Labib (1981) performed cystometrograms in addition to eliciting the bulbocavernosus reflex. They found that cystometrograms allowed greater accuracy in judging the state of the sacral nerves: when the nerves were normal, the cystometrogram was normal and the reflex was almost always present; with complete sacral cord damage, the cystometrogram was abnormal and the reflex absent; but with incomplete sacral cord damage, the cystometrogram was abnormal and the reflex absent; but with incomplete sacral cord damage, although the cystometrograms were usually abnormal, about half of these patients had a normal bulbocavernosus reflex.

It is wise, particularly in children, to seek a dimple over the lumbosacral area. Palpate the sacrum to be sure it is present and normally formed. Sacral agenesis or partial development is compatible with deficits of S2–4. If findings seem abnormal, x-ray examination is indicated.

REFERENCES

Examination of the Kidneys

Hennessy WT, Cromie WJ, Duckett JW: Congenital hemihypertrophy and associated abdominal lesions. *Urology* 1981;**18:**576.

Hodges CV, Barry JM: Non-urologic flank pain: A diagnostic approach. *J Urol* 1975;**113:**644.

Koop CE: Abdominal mass in the newborn infant. *N Engl J Med* 1973;**289:**569.

Krauss DJ, Khonsari F, Lilien OM: Incapacitating flank pain of questionable origin. *Urology* 1977;**9:**51.

Marshall S, Lapp M, Schulte JW: Lesions of the pancreas mimicking renal disease. *J Urol* 1965;**93:**41.

Mofenson HC, Greensher J: Transillumination of the abdomen in infants. *Am J Dis Child* 1968;**115:**428.

Perlman M, Williams J: Detection of renal anomalies by abdominal palpation in newborn infants. *Br Med J* 1976;**3:**347.

Saypol DC, Laudone VP: Congenital hemihypertrophy with adrenal carcinoma and medullary sponge kidney. *Urology* 1983;**21:**510.

Smith DR, Raney FL Jr: Radiculitis distress as a mimic of renal pain. *J Urol* 1976;**116;**269.

Williams MJ: Gynecomastia: Its incidence, recognition and host characterization in 447 autopsy cases. *Am J Med* 1963;**34:**103.

Examination of the Bladder

Boyarsky S, Goldenberg J: Detection of bladder distention by suprapubic percussion. *NY State J Med* 1962;**62:**1804.

Carlsson E, Garsten P: Compression of the common iliac vessels by dilatation of the bladder. *Acta Radiol* 1960;**53:**449.

Patil UB: Estimation of residual urine in bladder: Use of vesical "thrill" test. *Urology* 1974;**4:**737.

External Genitalia in the Female

Redman JF, Bissada NK: How to make a good examination of the genitalia of young girls. *Clin Pediatr* 1976;**15:**907.

Neurologic Examination

Blaivas JG, Zayed AAH, Labib KB: The bulbocavernosus reflex in urology: A prospective study of 299 patients. *J Urol* 1981;**126;**197.

Bors E, Blenn KA: Bulbocavernosus reflex. *J Urol* 1959; **82:**128.

5

Urologic Laboratory Examination

Richard D. Williams, MD

Examination of specimens of urine, blood, and genitourinary secretions or exudates commonly directs the subsequent urologic workup and frequently establishes a diagnosis. Since approximately 20% of patients who visit a primary physician's office have urologic problems, it is important for the physician to have a broad knowledge of the laboratory methods available to test appropriate specimens. Judicious use of such tests will permit accurate, rapid, and cost-effective determination of the probable diagnosis and the treatment needs of patients with urologic disease.

EXAMINATION OF URINE

Urinalysis is unquestionably one of the most important and useful screening tests available, yet all too often the necessary details are neglected and significant information is overlooked or misinterpreted. Reasons for inadequate urinalyses include: (1) improper collection, (2) failure to examine the specimen immediately, (3) incomplete examination (eg, many hospital laboratories do not perform a microscopic analysis unless it is specifically requested), (4) inexperience of the examiner, and (5) inadequate appreciation of the significance of the findings.

Urine Collection

A. Timing of Collection: It is best to examine urine that has been properly obtained in the office. First-voided morning specimens are helpful for qualitative protein testing in patients with possible orthostatic proteinuria and for specific gravity assessment as a presumptive test of renal function in patients with minimal renal disease due to diabetes mellitus or sickle cell anemia or in those with suspected diabetes insipidus. Urine specimens that are obtained immediately after the patient has eaten or that have been left standing for a few hours become alkaline and thus may contain lysed red cells, disintegrated casts, or rapidly multiplying bacteria; therefore, a freshly voided specimen obtained a few hours after the patient has eaten is most reliable. The patient's state of hydration may alter the concentration of urinary constituents. Timed urine collections may be required for definitive assessment of renal function or proteinuria.

B. Method of Collection: The importance of the method of urine collection cannot be overstated.

Proper collection of the specimen is particularly important when patients have hematuria or proteinuria or are being evaluated for urinary tract infection. Examination of a urine specimen collected sequentially in several containers may help to identify the site of origin of hematuria or urinary tract infection (see pp 50 and 53). Because urine specimens obtained at home are usually improperly collected and examination is delayed while they are delivered to the office or laboratory, such specimens are usually useless. To gather consistent and meaningful urinalysis data, urine must be collected by a strictly uniform method in the physician's office or laboratory. The specimen should be obtained before a genital or rectal examination in order to prevent contamination from the introitus or expressed prostatic secretions. Urine obtained from a collecting device, eg, a condom or drainage bag, is not a proper specimen for urinalysis.

1. Men—It is usually simple to collect a clean-voided midstream urine sample from most men. Routine instructions may be printed on a sheet given to the patient or placed on the lavatory wall. The procedure should include (1) retraction of the foreskin (a common source of contamination of the specimen) and cleansing of the meatus with benzalkonium chloride or hexachlorophene; (2) passing the first part of the stream (15–30 mL) without collection; (3) collecting the next portion (approximately 50–100 mL) in a sterile specimen container, which is capped immediately afterward; and (4) complete emptying of the bladder into the toilet. A portion of the specimen is then immediately prepared for both macroscopic and microscopic examination, and the rest is saved in the sterile container for subsequent culture if this proves necessary.

With this midstream clean-catch method, the likelihood that the specimen will be contaminated by meatal or urethral secretions is markedly decreased, although not completely eliminated. In adult males, it is rarely necessary to collect urine by catheterization unless urinary retention is present or assessment of residual urine is required.

2. Women—It is virtually impossible for a woman to obtain a satisfactory clean-voided midstream specimen without help. A voided specimen from an unprepped patient is not useful unless it is completely normal. The best method for collecting a clean-voided midstream specimen from a woman is as follows: (1) The patient is placed on the examining table in the lithotomy position. (2) The vulva and urethral meatus are cleansed with benzalkonium chloride or hexachlorophene. (3) The labia are separated. (4) The patient is then instructed to initiate voiding into a container held close to the vulva. After she has passed the first 10–20 mL of urine, the next 50–100 mL is collected in a sterile container that is immediately capped. (5) The patient is then allowed to complete emptying of the bladder. Because this technique requires considerable effort, it is acceptable to have the patient obtain an initial specimen in a nonsterile container in the lavatory. If results of urinalysis are normal, no further study is indicated; if abnormal, a urine specimen must be obtained by the more exacting technique. In either case, the specimen should be prepared for immediate examination.

If a satisfactory specimen cannot be obtained by the above method, one should not hesitate to obtain a specimen by catheterization, although suprapubic needle aspiration is the only sure way to obtain urine uncontaminated by urethrovaginal secretions or perineal organisms. Catheterization may be necessary to determine whether residual urine is present or to eliminate nonvaginal sources of hematuria. The possibility of introducing bladder infection by catheter is minimal when catheterization is performed carefully and should not prevent one from obtaining essential information. A satisfactory device with an 8F catheter attached to a centrifuge tube is available commercially.

3. Children–Obtaining satisfactory urine specimens from young children can be particularly challenging. Urine for analyses other than bacterial cultures can be obtained by covering the cleansed urethral meatus with a plastic bag; urine specimens for cultures may require catheterization or suprapubic needle aspiration. In girls, catheterization with a small catheter attached to a centrifuge tube is appropriate, but boys should not be routinely catheterized. It is often preferable in either sex to proceed with suprapubic needle aspiration. This is easier if the patient has been previously hydrated, so that the bladder is full. Suprapubic needle aspiration is performed as follows: (1) Cleanse the suprapubic area by sponging with alcohol. (2) With a small amount of local anesthetic, raise an intradermal wheal on the midline 1–2 cm above the pubis (the bladder lies just above the pubis in young children). (3) Attach a 10-mL syringe to a 22-gauge needle. Insert the needle perpendicularly through the abdominal wheal into the bladder wall, maintaining gentle suction with the syringe so that urine will be aspirated as soon as the bladder is entered.

Macroscopic Examination

Macroscopic examination of urine can often provide a clue when diagnosis is difficult.

A. Color and Appearance: Urine is often colored owing to drugs: phenazopyridine will turn the urine orange; nitrofurantoin will turn it brown; and L-dopa, α-methyldopa, and metronidazole will turn it reddish-brown. Red urine does not always signify hematuria. A red discoloration unassociated with red blood cells in the urine can result from betacyanin excretion after beet ingestion, myoglobinuria due to significant muscle trauma, or hemoglobinuria following hemolysis. However, whenever red urine is seen, hematuria must be ruled out by microscopic analysis. Cloudy urine is commonly thought to represent pyuria, but more often the cloudiness is due to large amounts of amorphous phosphates and can be made to disappear with the addition of acid. The odor of urine is rarely clinically significant, except that a pungent odor may indicate that the specimen has been standing too long to be diagnostically useful.

B. Specific Gravity: The specific gravity of urine (normal, 1.003–1.030) is often important for diagnostic purposes: that of patients with significant intracranial trauma may be low due to a lack of antidiuretic hormone (ADH, vasopressin); that of patients with primary diabetes insipidus will be less than 1.010 even after overnight dehydration; that of patients with extensive acute renal tubular damage will consistently be 1.010; and a low specific gravity can be an early sign of renal damage from conditions such as sickle cell anemia. Urine specific gravity is the simplest time-honored test for evaluating hydration in postoperative patients. The specific gravity of the urine may affect the results of other urine tests: in dilute urine, a pregnancy test may be falsely negative; in concentrated urine, protein that is detected by dip-strips may be found on confirmatory quantitative tests to be present in insignificant amounts. The specific gravity of urine may be falsely elevated by the presence of glucose, protein, artificial plasma expanders, or intravenous contrast agents.

The specific gravity of urine can easily be tested in the physician's office by a hydrometer or a refractometer. Both devices require occasional monitoring for precise calibration, and the specific gravity must be corrected to a standard temperature. Occasionally, a urine osmolality determination will be required to confirm specific gravity findings. Recent studies of specific-gravity reagent drips have shown inferior results compared to those with a refractometer, and the reagent drip is therefore not recommended.

C. Chemical Tests: Within the last few years, chemically impregnated reagent strips that permit simultaneous rapid performance of a battery of chemical tests have become available and have replaced the more specific individual tests. In general, these strips are accurate and have simplified routine urinalysis greatly. However, they must be monitored routinely by appropriate controls (Bradley, Schumann, Ward, 1984), and more sophisticated chemical tests are occasionally required to confirm results. The dip-strips are reliable only when not outdated and when used with room-temperature urine.

1. pH–The pH of urine is important in only a few specific clinical situations. Patients with uric acid stones rarely have a urinary pH over 6.5 (uric acid is soluble in alkaline urine). Patients with calcium stones, nephrocalcinosis, or both may have renal tubular acidosis and will be unable to acidify urine below pH 6.0. With urinary tract infections caused by urea-splitting organisms (most commonly *Proteus* species), the urinary pH tends to be over 7.0. It should be reemphasized that urine obtained within 2 hours of a large meal or left standing at room temperature for several hours tends to be alkaline. The indicator paper in most dip-strips is quite accurate; however, confirmation by a pH meter may occasionally be required.

2. Protein—Dip-strips containing bromphenol blue can be used to determine the presence of protein in urine, but persistent abnormalities will require quantitative protein testing. Concentrated urine may give a false-positive result, as will urine containing numerous white blood cells or vaginal secretions. Occasional patients will have orthostatic proteinuria, which can be demonstrated by finding elevated protein levels in a specimen obtained after the patient has been in the upright position for several hours but normal levels in an early-morning specimen obtained before ambulation. Prolonged fever and excessive physical exertion are also common causes of transient proteinuria.

Persistently elevated protein levels in the urine may indicate significant disease, eg, glomerulopathy or cancer; therefore, specific quantitative protein tests on a timed urine collection, electrophoretic studies of the urine, or both are required to determine the specific type of protein that is present. Ginsberg et al (1983) found that they could accurately assess proteinuria by determining the protein:creatinine ratio in an early-morning or late-afternoon single-voided urine specimen. They found that the normal ratio is 0.2 mg or less of protein per milligram of creatinine and that a ratio of 3.5 or more represents significant proteinuria (more than 1 g of protein excreted every 24 hours). Results obtained by this method had an excellent correlation with the results of quantitative protein tests on 24-hour urine specimens. This new method of assessing proteinuria may obviate the need for the time-consuming and often inaccurate (due to incomplete collection) protein tests on 24-hour urine collections.

3. Glucose—The glucose oxidase-peroxidase tests utilized in dip-strips are quite accurate and specific for urinary glucose. False-positive results may be obtained when patients have ingested large doses of aspirin, ascorbic acid, or cephalosporins. An occasional patient will have a blood glucose level below 180 mg/dL and yet have significant glucosuria; this indicates a low renal threshold of glucose excretion. Most patients with a positive reading, however, have diabetes mellitus, which may result in specific urinary tract manifestations such as renal papillary necrosis, recurrent urinary tract infections, neurovesical dysfunction, or impotence.

4. Hemoglobin—The dip-strip test for hemoglobin is not specific for red cells and should be used only to screen for hematuria, with microscopic analysis of the urinary sediment for confirmation. Free hemoglobin or myoglobin in the urine may give a positive reading; ascorbic acid in the urine can inhibit the dip-strip reaction and give a false-negative result.

Microscopic Examination

Microscopic examination of the urinary sediment is an essential part of all urinalyses. To be most accurate, it should be done personally by an experienced physician. Early-morning urine is the best specimen if it can be examined within a few minutes of collection; however, this is rarely possible when the specimen is obtained at home, and for this reason, collection of a specimen for immediate examination in the office or hospital is the most useful method. In most cases, the sediment can be prepared as follows: (1) Centrifuge a 10-mL specimen at 2000 rpm for 5 minutes. (2) Decant the supernatant. (3) Suspend the sediment in the remaining 1 mL of urine by tapping the tube gently against a counter top. (4) Place 1 drop of the mixture on a microscope slide, cover with a coverslip, and examine first under a low-power (10×) and then under a high-power (40×) lens. For maximal contrast of the elements in the sediment, the microscope diaphragm should be nearly closed in order to prevent overillumination. Significant elements (particularly bacteria) are more easily seen if the slide is stained with methylene blue, but staining is not essential. Fig 5–1 shows typical findings in the urinary sediment.

A. Staining: Staining with methylene blue (available commercially) may be helpful in microscopic examination of urinary sediment.

The urinary sediment is prepared as follows: (1) Place a drop of the centrifuged sediment on a glass slide and fix it slowly with heat from a laboratory burner. (2) Cool the slide and cover it with methylene blue for 10–20 seconds. (3) Rinse with tap water and dry with mild heat. Do not blot. (4) Examine the slide under oil immersion (with 100× lens) without a coverslip.

The slide can be stained with Gram's stain (Table 5–1) instead of methylene blue, but this is more complex and time-consuming to perform and its only advantage over staining with methylene blue is that *Neisseria gonorrhoeae* (gram-negative intracellular diplococci) can be identified.

B. Interpretation:

1. Bacteria—The significance of bacteria in the urinary sediment is discussed in the section on bacteriuria (see below).

2. Leukocytes—Just as the presence of bacteria in the sediment is not an absolute indication of infection, neither is the finding of pyuria. The method used to collect the specimen and the hydration status of the patient can alter the significance of the findings. In the sediment from clean-voided midstream specimens from men and those obtained by suprapubic aspiration or catheterization in women, more than 5–8 white blood cells per high-power field is generally considered abnormal (pyuria). If the patient has symptoms of a urinary tract infection, pyuria, and bacteriuria, one is justified in making a diagnosis of infection and initiating empirical therapy. However, in a study of female patients with symptoms of urinary tract infection (Komaroff, 1984), 61% of those with pyuria had no bacterial growth from bladder urine obtained by catheter-

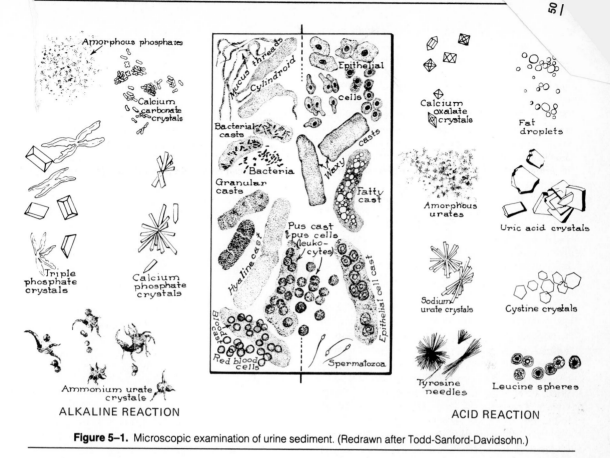

Figure 5–1. Microscopic examination of urine sediment. (Redrawn after Todd-Sanford-Davidsohn.)

ization or suprapubic aspiration. This underscores the unreliability of urinalysis *alone* for diagnosing urinary tract infections and further emphasizes the need for confirmation by bacterial cultures.

Renal tuberculosis can cause "sterile" acid-pyuria and should be considered in any patient with persistent pyuria and negative results on routine bacterial cultures. Specific staining of the urinary sediment for acid-fast bacteria (Ziehl-Neelsen stain) can be diagnostic; however, results will be positive from the sediment of spot specimens in only approximately 50% of patients with renal tuberculosis, whereas they are positive in the sediment of 24-hour specimens in 70–80% of such cases. *Mycobacterium smegmatis,* a commensal organism, may be present in the urine (particularly

in uncircumcised men) and can give false-positive results on acid-fast stains.

Urolithiasis can also cause pyuria. In patients with persistent pyuria, the physician should consider obtaining at least a plain x-ray of the abdomen and possibly an intravenous urogram to determine whether urolithiasis is present.

Previous studies have suggested that "glitter cells" (leukocytes with visible brownian movement of cytoplasmic granules) in the urinary sediment are pathognomonic of pyelonephritis; however, more recent evidence has shown that these cells are not limited to patients with pyelonephritis.

3. Red blood cells–The presence of even a few red blood cells in the urine (hematuria) is abnormal and requires further investigation. Although gross hematuria is more alarming to the patient, microscopic hematuria is no less significant. Causes of hematuria include strenuous exercise (long-distance running), vaginal bleeding, and inflammation of organs near or directly adjoining the urinary tract, eg, diverticulitis, appendicitis. Hematuria associated with cystitis or urethritis will generally clear after treatment. Persistent hematuria in an otherwise asymptomatic patient of either sex and any age signifies disease and is an indication for further testing.

In patients with microscopic hematuria, a 3-glass method for collection of urine can provide information

Table 5–1. Gram staining method (Hucker modification).

(1) Fix smear by heat.
(2) Cover with crystal violet for 1 minute.
(3) Wash with water. Do not blot.
(4) Cover with Gram's iodine for 1 minute.
(5) Wash with water. Do not blot.
(6) Decolorize for 10–30 seconds with gentle agitation in acetone (30 mL) and alcohol (70 mL).
(7) Wash with water. Do not blot.
(8) Cover for 10–30 seconds with safranin (2.5% solution in 95% alcohol).
(9) Wash with water and let dry.

on the site of origin of red blood cells. The method is as follows: (1) Give the patient 3 containers, labeled 1, 2, and 3 (or initial, mid, and terminal). (2) Instruct the patient to urinate and to collect the initial portion of urine (10–15 mL) in the first container, the middle portion (30–40 mL) in the second, and the final portion (5–10 mL) in the third. (3) Using the methods described above, centrifuge the 3 specimens individually, prepare slides of the urinary sediment (with or without staining), and examine them microscopically. If red blood cells predominate in the initial portion of the specimen, they are usually from the anterior urethra; those in the terminal portion are generally from the bladder neck or posterior urethra; and the presence of equal numbers of red blood cells in all 3 containers usually indicates a source above the bladder neck (bladder, ureters, or kidneys). It is important to collect the urine before physical examination (particularly before rectal examination in men) in order to avoid misleading results.

The 3-container test may not be necessary in patients with gross hematuria, since they can usually tell the physician which portion of the stream contains the darkest urine (ie, the most red blood cells).

A specific dysmorphic red blood cell configuration that can be seen with phase contrast microscopy of the urinary sediment and is highly indicative of active glomerular disease (Fig 5–2) has been described by Fairley and Birch (1982) and by Stamey and Kindrachuk (1984). This dysmorphism is thought to be a result of extreme changes in osmolality and the high concentration of urinary chemical constituents affecting red blood cells during passage through the kidney tubules. An examiner experienced in viewing red blood cell morphology can also detect these dysmorphic cells on routine microscopy if the light is diffracted appropriately. This finding represents a significant advance in routine urinalysis and should help define the origin of hematuria in patients with an elusive cause of bleeding.

Red cell casts are discussed below.

4. Epithelial cells–Squamous epithelial cells in the urinary sediment indicate contamination of the specimen from the distal urethra in males and the introitus in females; no other significance should be placed on them. It is not uncommon to find transitional epithelial cells in the normal urinary sediment; however, if they are present in large numbers or clumps and exhibit abnormal histology (including large nuclei, multiple nucleoli, and an increased ratio of nucleus to cytoplasm), they are indicative of a malignant process affecting the urothelium (Fig 5–3). Although staining the sediment with methylene blue may aid in visualizing the cells, the findings must be confirmed by an experienced cytopathologist.

5. Casts–Casts are formed in the distal tubules and collecting ducts and, for the most part, are not seen in normal urinary sediment; therefore, they commonly signify intrinsic renal disease.

Although **leukocyte casts** have been considered suggestive of pyelonephritis, they are not an absolute

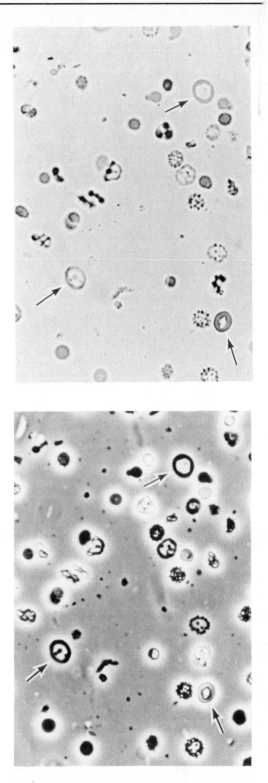

Figure 5–2. *Top:* Dysmorphic red cells in urine **(arrows)**, viewed under light microscopy (magnification 400×). *Bottom:* Dysmorphic red cells in urine (identical field), viewed under phase contrast microscopy. (Reproduced, with permission, from Stamey TA, Kindrachuk RW: *Urinary Sediment and Urinalysis: A Practical Guide for the Health Professional.* Saunders, 1984.)

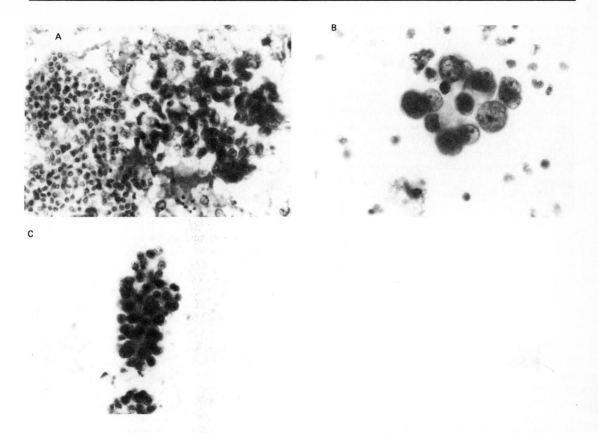

Figure 5–3. Papanicolaou-stained bladder cytology specimens. *A:* Normal cells (*left*) and malignant cells (*right*). *B:* High-power view of malignant cells. *C:* Papillary cluster of malignant cells. (Courtesy of Larry Kluskens, MD, Cytopathology Laboratory, University of Iowa.)

indicator and should not be used as the sole criterion for diagnosis. Leukocyte casts must be distinguished from **epithelial cell casts,** because the latter have little significance when present in small numbers. The distinction can be made easily if a small amount of acetic acid is added under the coverslip to enhance nuclear detail. Epithelial cell or leukocyte casts in large numbers signify underlying intrinsic renal disease requiring further diagnostic workup. In renal transplant recipients, an increase in the number of epithelial cells or casts from the renal tubules may be an early indication of acute graft rejection.

Red blood cell casts are pathognomonic of underlying glomerulitis or vasculitis.

Hyaline casts probably represent a mixture of mucus and globulin congealed in the tubules; in small numbers, they are not significant. Hyaline casts are commonly seen in urine specimens taken after exercise and in concentrated or highly acidic urine specimens. As mentioned above, casts are rarely seen in alkaline urine and are therefore not usually present in urine specimens that have been left standing or in specimens from patients unable to acidify urine (eg, those with advanced stages of chronic renal failure).

Granular casts most commonly represent disintegrated epithelial cells, leukocytes, or protein and indicate intrinsic renal tubular disease.

6. Other findings—The finding of crystals in urine can be helpful in some instances, but the mere presence of crystals does not indicate disease. Crystals form in normal urine below room temperature. Cystine, leucine, tyrosine, cholesterin, bilirubin, hematoidin, and sulfonamide crystals are abnormal findings of varying importance. Several types of crystals that may be found on microscopic examination of urinary sediment are shown in Fig 5–1.

The presence of trichomonads or yeast cells in the stained or unstained smear of sediment from a properly obtained urine specimen establishes both the diagnosis and the need for treatment.

Artifacts present in the urine sediment can be difficult to differentiate from real abnormalities. Dirt and small pieces of vegetable fiber or hair are frequently found, but the most common artifacts are starch granules from examination gloves.

Bacteriuria

A. Microscopic Examination: A presumptive diagnosis of bacterial infection may be made on the basis of results of microscopic examination of the urinary sediment. The significance of bacteria in the urinary sediment depends in part on the method used to collect the specimen, the specific gravity of the specimen, and whether the slide was stained. If several bacteria per high-power field are found in a urine specimen obtained by suprapubic aspiration or catheterization in a woman or in a properly obtained clean-voided midstream specimen from a man, a provisional diagnosis of bacterial infection can be made and empirical treatment started. The findings should be confirmed by bacterial culture. Finding several bacteria per high-power field in a voided specimen from a woman is of little significance. If the specific gravity of the urine specimen is low, the bacterial count may be low due to dilution; if the specific gravity is high, the converse is true. It is easier to distinguish and count bacteria and to differentiate leukocytes from transitional epithelial cells when slides are stained with methylene blue (see above).

B. Determining the Site of Origin of Infection: If the patient has a urinary tract infection but the site of the infection is not known, tests for antibody-coated bacteria may be performed. Although past studies indicated that the presence of antibody-coated bacteria in the urine pointed to the kidney as the site of infection, antibody-coated bacteria may also be found in the urine of patients with neurogenic bladder, prostatitis, and chronic or recurrent cystitis. The test may be useful, however, in locating the site of origin of recurrent bacteriuria (particularly in women) if specimens are collected separately from the bladder and both ureters.

Another method for determining the site of origin of bacteriuria and pyuria is discussed below in the section on examination of urethral discharge.

C. Bacterial Cultures: The presumptive diagnosis of bacterial infection based on microscopic examination of the urinary sediment should be confirmed by culture.

1. Indications and interpretation–Cultures can be used to estimate the number of bacteria in the urine (quantitative cultures), to identify the exact organism present, and to predict which drugs will be effective in treating the infection. Cultures are particularly important in patients with recurrent or persistent infections, renal insufficiency, or drug allergies.

The number of bacteria present in the urine (colony count) is influenced by the method used to collect the urine specimen, the patient's hydration status, and whether the patient has been taking antimicrobial drugs. These factors and the patient's symptoms must be considered in determining whether a urinary tract infection is present. The concept that urinary tract infection is present only when the urine specimen contains 10^5 or more bacteria per milliliter is not an absolute rule; a lower count does not exclude the possibility of an infection, particularly in a symptomatic patient. For example, a symptomatic patient with a urine specific gravity of 1.015 and a colony count of less than 10^5/mL in a clean-voided specimen may have a significant infection; a count of more than 10^3/mL in a specimen obtained by catheterization or an even lower count in a specimen obtained by suprapubic aspiration may also indicate significant bacteriuria. Cultures with growth of multiple organisms usually signify contamination, which may be due to an improper collection method or improper laboratory technique. The presence of a few organisms in a specimen with a low specific gravity is more significant than the same finding in a specimen with a high specific gravity, because the latter is more-dilute. The physician must take into account all of these factors when interpreting the results of bacterial cultures.

It is not always necessary to identify the specific organism causing the infection, particularly in "routine" lower urinary tract infections; however, identification of the causative organism may be important in patients with recurrent or persistent symptoms and signs of urinary tract infection. Some bacteria (eg, neisseriae, brucellae, mycobacteria, anaerobes), fungi, and yeasts will not grow with common culture methods, and thus special culture techniques are required.

Identifying the drugs to which the bacteria are sensitive may or may not be necessary. *Escherichia coli,* which causes 85% of "routine" urinary tract infections, is known to be sensitive to numerous oral antimicrobial drugs. However, in patients with septicemia, renal insufficiency, diabetes mellitus, or suspected enterococcal, *Proteus,* or *Pseudomonas* infections, it is important to determine the antibiotic sensitivity of the organism and the drug concentration necessary for efficacious treatment. Monitoring antibiotic levels in blood and urine during treatment may be indicated, especially in severely ill patients and those receiving highly toxic drugs. These measurements can be done by most hospital laboratories.

2. Rapid tests for bacteriuria–In general, seriously ill or hospitalized patients with urinary tract infections should have cultures processed by an accredited bacteriology laboratory. However, for "routine" infections encountered in office practice, there are many satisfactory, cost-effective testing methods.

Many rapid methods to screen for the presence of significant bacteriuria are available. They commonly utilize small strips impregnated with substances such as triphenyltetrazolium chloride; bacteria in the urine turn the reagent strips red. Although these tests and others like them are rapid and inexpensive, not all bacteria will react. Results may be equivocal in patients who are already being treated or whose urine is discolored. More recently, a filter mechanism for detecting bacteria and white cells in urine has been shown to be 96% accurate in predicting positive cultures and 98% sensitive to significant pyuria.

More reliable methods involve use of small strips or glass slides coated with eosin-methylene blue agar on one side and nutrient agar on the other. The strips or slides are dipped in the urine specimen and then incubated for 24 hours. Although these methods are easy to use, their disadvantages are (1) not all bacteria will grow under these conditions and (2) the accuracy of colony counts is debatable.

Perhaps preferable (but still subject to some of the same limitations) is use of a divided plastic culture plate with blood agar on one side and deoxycholate agar on the other. A known amount of urine is inoculated onto the agar on each side of the plate, and colony counts are determined at 24–48 hours. The numbers of bacteria in 1 mL of the original urine specimen can be determined by multiplying the number of colonies by the volume (in milliliters) and dilution (if any) of the inoculum. If antibiotic sensitivity testing is also desired, an additional culture plate can be inoculated and small antibiotic-impregnated disks placed on the agar. Zones of growth inhibition seen around the disks at 12–24 hours indicate sensitivity. These methods are satisfactory for most office situations, although some organisms (see above) may require specific media or conditions for growth.

3. Cultures for tuberculosis–Urine smears stained for acid-fast bacilli (Ziehl-Neelsen stain performed by the laboratory) may provide evidence to support the diagnosis of renal tuberculosis. However, regardless of the result of the smear, multiple urine cultures should be performed if renal tuberculosis is suspected, both to confirm the presence of *Mycobacterium* and to determine its species. Recently, numerous atypical mycobacteria have been found to cause renal tuberculosis. Since they are not always sensitive to the commonly used antituberculous drugs, sensitivity testing may also be indicated. Because the procedures for urine culture for mycobacteria vary from one laboratory to another, the physician should consult the laboratory beforehand. Mycobacteria grow slowly; thus, culture results may require 6–8 weeks or longer.

Other Urine Tests

Many other tests of urine can be helpful in determining the presence of urologic disease. The following tests are not routine and can rarely be performed in the physician's office.

A. Hormone Studies: Tests for abnormalities in adrenal hormone secretion are important in the workup of patients with suspected adrenal tumors. Pheochromocytoma and neuroblastoma can be detected by measuring the excretion of vanilmandelic acid (VMA). However, urinary levels of metanephrine, epinephrine, and norepinephrine are more sensitive indicators, particularly in cases of pheochromocytoma. While high levels of aldosterone in urine usually indicate an aldosterone-secreting tumor, drug interference may cause false-positive or false-negative results. Other adrenocortical tumors may be detected by their production of elevated levels of urinary 17-ketosteroids, although more specific urinary steroid tests are now available. In the past, determinations of urinary gonadotropin levels were helpful in the staging and follow-up of patients with testicular tumors or gestational trophoblastic tumors, but studies of the serum markers alpha-fetoprotein and the beta-subunit of hCG (human chorionic gonadotropin) have supplanted urinary studies in most of these patients (see Examination of Blood, Serum, & Plasma, below).

B. Studies of Stone Constituents: Patients with recurrent urolithiasis may have an underlying abnormality of excretion of calcium, uric acid, oxalate, magnesium, or citrate. Samples of 24-hour urine collections can be tested to determine abnormally high levels of each. A few patients may have elevated cystine levels in urine. The nitroprusside test, a simple qualitative screening test for cystine, may indicate the need for quantifying cystine levels in timed urine collections. Whenever a stone is recovered, a formal stone analysis is recommended.

C. Miscellaneous Studies: Tests of urinary levels of lactate dehydrogenase (LDH), carcinoembryonic antigen (CEA), and other tumor markers (see Chapters 18 and 19) are not specific and thus are not generally helpful. The measurement of urinary levels of hydroxyproline has recently been described as a useful test for determining both the presence of bone metastases and the efficacy of treatment in patients with advanced prostatic adenocarcinoma. In patients with suspected fistula of the urinary tract and bowel (eg, cancer of the colon, diverticulitis, regional ileitis), discoloration of the urine after ingestion of a poorly absorbed dye such as phenol red will confirm the diagnosis. In an equally satisfactory test for fistulas, the patient is instructed to ingest gelatin capsules filled with granulated charcoal and to submit a urine sample several days later; examination of the centrifuged urinary sediment will reveal the typical black granules if a fistula is present.

EXAMINATION OF URETHRAL DISCHARGE & VAGINAL EXUDATE

Urethral Discharge

Examination of urethral discharge in males can be particularly helpful in establishing a diagnosis. The following procedure (as outlined by Stamey and others; see Stamey, 1980), although exacting, provides proper specimens for determining the site of origin of bacteriuria or pyuria. Four sterile containers are labeled VB_1, VB_2, EPS, and VB_3 (VB = voided bladder urine; EPS = expressed prostatic secretions). The patient is instructed to retract the foreskin and cleanse the meatus with benzalkonium chloride or hexachlorophene and to collect the urine specimens, capping the containers immediately afterward. The initial 10–15 mL of urine is collected in container VB_1 and the subsequent 15–30 mL in container VB_2. The prostate is then massaged, and secretions are collected in container EPS. The patient then voids a final time, collecting the specimen in container VB_3. An aliquot of each specimen is centrifuged and the sediment prepared for microscopic examination as described above. A separate aliquot of each VB specimen and the EPS specimen is saved for subsequent culture if necessary. The presence of leukocytes or bacteria (or both) only in VB_1 indicates anterior urethritis; if present in all 3 VB specimens, they may indicate cystitis or upper urinary tract infection; if present in EPS or VB_3 only, they indicate a prostatic source of infection. Quantitative cultures can be similarly interpreted. Patients with positive results should be treated with appropriate antimicrobial drugs.

If the patient presents with the thick yellowish discharge typical of *N gonorrhoeae* infection, the discharge should be stained with Gram's stain and examined for gram-negative intracellular diplococci. It is important to remember that commensal bacteria in smegma may produce false-positive results. Nevertheless, treatment of patients with positive results should be started immediately and not delayed until the results of confirmatory cultures are available. A spot test for *N gonorrhoeae* (Gonodecten) appears to be useful (Fellman and William, 1982), but its accuracy is not completely defined; therefore, confirmation of results by conventional culture of the exudate is still recommended.

If the patient presents with clear or whitish urethral discharge, a smear of the discharge obtained by milking the urethra or from VB_1 should be stained with methylene blue or Gram's stain and examined microscopically. The presence of trichomonads, yeast cells, or bacteria in properly collected specimens indicates disease requiring appropriate treatment.

In cases of acute epididymitis, urinalysis and urine culture are often helpful in establishing the cause. Berger et al (1978) demonstrated that epididymitis is most commonly caused by *Chlamydia* species in young men and by *E coli* in men over 35 years of age. Since culturing chlamydiae is time-consuming and expensive, it is usually best to proceed with therapy based on the age of the patient and guided by clinical results.

Vaginal Exudate

Examination of the vaginal introitus is mandatory in evaluating symptoms involving the lower urinary tract in females. The underlying cause of vaginitis is often a viral, yeast, or protozoal infection or the presence of a foreign body (eg, retained tampon), and a simple physical examination may be all that is required for diagnosis.

Vaginal secretions obtained by use of a swab can be examined either stained or unstained. A drop of saline is added to a drop of the specimen on a glass slide, mixed thoroughly, and covered with a coverslip. Examination under a low- or high-power lens may reveal yeast cells or trichomonads, thus suggesting appropriate therapy. Since bacteria are always present in the vagina, they generally are not significant findings in a wet smear. Culture of vaginal secretions may, however, help to establish the cause of recurrent bacteriuria.

RENAL FUNCTION TESTS

If urologic disease is suspected, results of renal function tests may provide clues to the diagnosis, aid in determining which diagnostic studies should be performed or avoided, and assist in the choice of therapeutic alternatives.

Urine Specific Gravity

As noted above, specific gravity is a simple and reproducible test of renal function. With diminished renal function, the ability of the kidneys to concentrate urine lessens progressively until the specific gravity of urine reaches 1.006–1.010. However, the ability to dilute urine tends to be maintained until renal damage is extreme. Even in uremia, although the concentrating power of the kidneys is limited to a specific gravity of 1.010, dilution power in the specific gravity range of 1.002–1.004 may still be found. Determination of urine osmolality is undoubtedly a more meaningful measurement of renal function, but determination of specific gravity lends itself to office diagnosis.

Serum Creatinine

Creatinine, the end product of the metabolism of creatine in skeletal muscle, is normally excreted by the kidneys. Because daily creatinine production is amazingly constant, the serum level is a direct reflection of renal function. Serum creatinine levels will remain within the normal range (0.8–1.2 mg/dL in adults; 0.4–0.8 mg/dL in young children) until approximately 50% of renal function has been lost. Unlike most other excretory products, the serum creatinine level is not generally influenced by dietary intake or hydration status.

Endogenous Creatinine Clearance

Because creatinine production is stable and creatinine is filtered through the glomerulus (although a small amount is probably secreted), its renal clearance is essentially equal to the glomerular filtration rate. The endogenous creatinine clearance test has thus become the most accurate and reliable measure of renal function available without resorting to infusion of exogenous substances such as inulin or radionuclides. Determination of creatinine clearance requires only the collection of a timed (usually 24-hour) urine specimen and a serum specimen. The clearance can then be calculated as follows:

$$\text{Clearance} = \frac{UV}{P} \text{ where:}$$

U = creatinine in urine (in mg/dL)

P = creatinine in plasma (in mg/dL)

V = mL of urine excreted per minute or per 24 hours

The resulting clearance is expressed in milliliters per minute, with 90–110 mL/min considered normal.

Because muscle mass differs among individuals, further standardization has been achieved by using the following formula:

$$\frac{UV}{P} \times \frac{1.73 \text{ m}^2}{\text{Estimated surface area}} = \frac{\text{Corrected}}{\text{clearance}}$$

A corrected clearance level of 70–140 mL/min is considered normal.

Although creatinine is highly reliable as an estimate of renal function, values may be falsely low, particularly if only part of the urine is collected over the timed period or if the serum specimen is not collected at the same time.

Blood Urea Nitrogen

Urea is the primary metabolite of protein catabolism and is excreted entirely by the kidneys. The blood urea nitrogen level is therefore related to the glomerular filtration rate. Unlike creatinine, however, blood urea nitrogen is influenced by dietary protein intake, hydration status, gastrointestinal bleeding, and urinary obstruction. Approximately two-thirds of renal function must be lost before a significant rise in blood urea nitrogen level will be evident. For these reasons, an elevated blood urea nitrogen level is less specific for renal insufficiency than an elevated serum creatinine level. However, the blood urea nitrogen:creatinine ratio can provide specific diagnostic information—it is normally 10:1; in dehydrated patients and those with bilateral urinary obstruction or urinary extravasation, the ratio may range from 20:1 to 40:1; and patients with advanced hepatic insufficiency and overhydrated patients may exhibit a lower than normal blood urea nitrogen level and blood urea nitrogen:creatinine ratio. Patients with renal insufficiency may develop extremely high blood urea nitrogen levels that can be partially controlled by a decrease in dietary protein.

EXAMINATION OF BLOOD, SERUM, & PLASMA

Some of the serum and blood tests of diagnostic usefulness in urology are discussed above. The following are also applicable to urologic disease.

Complete Blood Count

Normochromic normocytic anemia is often seen with chronic renal insufficiency. Chronic blood loss from microscopic hematuria is usually not sufficient to cause anemia, although gross hematuria certainly can be. A specific increase in the number of red blood cells, as manifested by elevated hemoglobin and hematocrit levels (erythrocytosis, not polycythemia), may be indicative of a paraneoplastic syndrome associated with renal cell cancer. The white blood cell count is usually nonspecific, although marked elevations may indicate an underlying leukemia that may be the cause of urologic symptoms; in such cases, further testing is indicated to determine the specific diagnosis prior to any urologic surgery.

Blood Clotting Studies

Clotting studies are generally not necessary, unless insidious disorders such as von Willebrand's disease, hepatic disease, or a sensitivity to ingested salicylates are suspected in patients with unexplained hematuria. The determination of prothrombin time and bleeding time (and perhaps partial thromboplastin time) is usually sufficient. A platelet count is important in patients receiving chemotherapy and those who have received extensive radiation therapy.

Electrolyte Studies

Serum sodium and potassium determinations may be indicated in patients taking diuretics or digitalis preparations and in patients who have just undergone transurethral prostatectomy. Serum calcium determinations are useful in patients with calcium urolithiasis. Elevated calcium levels are occasionally indicative of a paraneoplastic syndrome in patients with renal cell cancer. Serum albumin levels should be measured simultaneously with calcium levels in order to assess adequately the significance of the latter.

Enzyme Studies

Serum acid phosphatase is still a useful marker of prostatic cancer, usually signifying metastatic disease when levels are consistently and significantly elevated. The enzymatic tests (particularly the thymolphthalein monophosphate method) are quite reliable, although prostatic infarction, recent prostatic massage, or hemolysis may cause false-positive results. Radioimmunoassays are more sensitive but have not been shown to have substantial advantage over the enzymatic methods. Recently, prostate-specific antigen (PSA) has been shown to be elevated in approximately 60% of patients with prostate cancer, falling precipitously with effective treatment and rising early with recurrences. Alkaline phosphatase is useful as a marker of bone metastasis in prostatic cancer.

Hormone Studies

Serum parathyroid hormone studies are useful in determining the presence of a parathyroid adenoma in patients with urolithiasis and an elevated serum calcium level. Measurement of parathyroid hormone is not reliable, however, as a sole screening test for parathyroid adenoma and should not be used routinely in all patients with urolithiasis. Serum renin levels may be elevated in patients with renal hypertension, although many conditions can cause false-positive results. Studies of adrenal steroid hormones (eg, aldosterone, cortisol, epinephrine, norepinephrine) are useful in determining adrenal function or the presence of adrenal tumors. Determinations of serum levels of the beta-subunit of hCG and of alpha-fetoprotein are indispensable in staging and in treatment follow-up for testicular tumors. One of these tumor markers is usually elevated in up to 85% of patients with non-seminomatous testicular tumors and can predict the recrudescence of tumor several months before disease is clinically evident. Serum testosterone studies can help to establish the cause of impotence or infertility.

Other Studies

The finding of elevated fasting plasma glucose levels in patients with urologic disease can establish the diagnosis of diabetes mellitus and thus indicate a possible cause of renal insufficiency, neurovesical dysfunction, impotence, or recurrent urinary tract infection. Serum uric acid levels are often elevated in patients with uric acid stones. Elevated serum complement levels may be diagnostic of underlying glomerulopathies.

Urologic diseases are rarely confined solely to urologic organs and may cause or result from diseases in other organ systems.

REFERENCES

Abuelo JG: Proteinuria: Diagnostic principles and procedures. *Ann Intern Med* 1983;**98:**186.

Adams LJ: Evaluation of Ames Multistix-SG for urine specific gravity versus refractometer specific gravity. *Am J Clin Pathol* 1983;**80:**871.

Baum N, Dichoso CC, Carlton CE Jr: Blood urea nitrogen and serum creatinine: Physiology and interpretations. *Urology* 1975;**5:**583.

Berger RE et al: *Chlamydia trachomatis* as a cause of acute "idiopathic" epididymitis. *N Engl J Med* 1978;**298:**301.

Bradley M, Schumann GB, Ward PCJ: Examination of urine. Chap 18, pp 380–458, in: *Todd-Sanford-Davidsohn's Clinical Diagnosis and Management by Laboratory Methods,* 17th ed. Henry JB (editor). Saunders, 1984.

Brody LH, Salladay JR, Armbruster K: Urinalysis and the urinary sediment. *Med Clin North Am* 1971;**55:**243.

Carlton CE Jr, Scardino PT: Initial evaluation. Chap 6, pp 276–285, in: *Campbell's Urology,* 5th ed. Vol 1. Harrison JH et al (editors). Saunders, 1986.

Emanuel B, Aronson N: Neonatal hematuria. *Am J Dis Child* 1974;**128:**204.

Fairley KF, Birch DF: Hematuria: A simple method for identifying glomerular bleeding. *Kidney Int* 1982;**21:**105.

Felman YM, William DC: New 3-minute in vitro diagnostic test for gonorrhea in the male without use of conventional culture or gram stain. *Urology* 1982;**19:**252.

Friedman SA, Gladstone JL: The effects of hydration and bladder incubation time on urine colony counts. *J Urol* 1971; **105:**428.

Galambos JT, Herndon EG Jr, Reynolds GH: Specific gravity determination: Fact or fancy. *N Engl J Med* 1964;**270:**506.

Gavan TL: In vitro antimicrobial susceptibility testing: Clinical implications and limitations. *Med Clin North Am* 1974; **58:**493.

Gillenwater JY et al: Home urine cultures by the dip-strip method: Results in 289 cultures. *Pediatrics* 1976;**58:**508.

Ginsberg JM et al: Use of single voided urine samples to estimate quantitative proteinuria. *N Engl J Med* 1983;**309:**1543.

Gleckman R: A critical review of the antibody-coated bacteria test. *J Urol* 1979;**122:**770.

Gleckman R, Crowley M: Epididymitis as cause of antibody-coated bacteria in urine. *Urology* 1979;**14:**241.

Greenhill A, Gruskin AB: Laboratory evaluation of renal function. *Pediatr Clin North Am* 1976;**23:**661.

Hardy JD, Furnell PM, Brumfitt W: Comparison of sterile bag, clean catch and suprapubic aspiration in the diagnosis of urinary infection in early childhood. *Br J Urol* 1976;**48:**279.

Hendler ED, Kashgarian M, Hayslett JP: Clinicopathological correlations of primary haematuria. *Lancet* 1972;**1:**458.

Kampmann J et al: Rapid evaluation of creatinine clearance. *Acta Med Scand* 1974;**196:**517.

Kass EH: Asymptomatic infections of the urinary tract. *Trans Assoc Am Phys* 1956;**69:**56.

Kassirer JP, Gennou FJ: Laboratory evaluation of renal function. Pages 41–91 in: *Diseases of the Kidney,* 3rd ed. Strauss MB, Welt LG (editors). Little, Brown, 1979.

Khanna OP, Son DL: Screening for urinary tract infection using Bac-T-Screen bacteriuria device. *Urology* 1986;**27:**424.

Komaroff AL: Acute dysuria in women. *N Engl J Med* 1984; **310:**368.

Kunin CM, DeGroot JE: Self-screening for significant bacteriuria: Evaluation of dip-strip combination nitrite/culture test. *JAMA* 1975;**231:**1349.

Kunin CM, DeGroot JE: Sensitivity of a nitrite indicator strip method in detecting bacteriuria in preschool girls. *Pediatrics* 1977;**60:**244.

Labovits ED et al: "Benign" hematuria with focal glomerulitis in adults. *Ann Intern Med* 1972;**77:**723.

Littlewood JM, Jacobs SI, Ramsden CH: Comparison between microscopical examination of unstained deposits of urine and quantitative culture. *Arch Dis Child* 1977;**52:**894.

Madaio MP, Harrington JT: The diagnosis of acute glomerulonephritis. *N Engl J Med* 1983;**309:**1299.

McLin PH, Tavel FR: Urine culture and direct drug disc sensitivity testing: A rapid simple method for use in the office. *Clin Med* (Dec) 1971;**78:**16.

Merritt JL, Keys TF: Limitations of the antibody-coated bacteria test in patients with neurogenic bladder. *JAMA* 1982; **247:**1723.

Nanji AA, Adam W, Campbell DJ: Routine microscopic examination of the urine sediment: Should we continue? *Arch Pathol Lab Med* 1984;**108:**399.

Nettleman MD et al: Cost-effectiveness of culturing for *Chlamydia trachomatis:* A study in a clinic for sexually transmitted diseases. *Ann Intern Med* 1986;**105:**189.

Pontes JE et al: Serum prostatic antigen measurement in localized prostatic cancer: Correlation with clinical course. *J Urol* 1982;**128:**1216.

Sanford JP et al: Evaluation of the "positive" urine culture: An approach to the differentiation of significant bacteria from contaminants. *Am J Med* 1956;**20:**88.

Stamey TA: Chap 1, pp 1–51, in: *Pathogenesis and Treatment of Urinary Tract Infections.* Williams & Wilkins, 1980.

Stamey TA, Kindrachuk RW: *Urinary Sediment and Urinalysis: A Practical Guide for the Health Professional.* Saunders, 1984.

Stamm WE et al: Diagnosis of coliform infection in acutely dysuric women. *N Engl J Med* 1982;**307:**463.

Unni Mooppan MM et al: Use of urinary hydroxyproline excretion as a tumor marker in diagnosis and follow-up of prostatic carcinoma. *The Prostate* 1983;**4:**397.

Wright DN, Saxon B, Matsen JM: Use of the Bac-T-Screen to predict bacteriuria from urine specimens held at room temperature. *J Clin Microb* 1986;**24:**214.

Wyatt RJ, McRoberts JW, Holland NH: Hematuria in childhood: Significance and management. *J Urol* 1977;**117:**366.

Imaging of the Urinary Tract

6

A. J. Palubinskas, MD

Diagnostic imaging is a dynamic recent development in medical practice with great potential for benefiting patient care. Nothing has contributed more to the improvement of existing anatomic imaging devices and the development of new ones than digital computers and their related electronics. With computers, the vast numbers of data collected in analog fashion by the basic imaging mechanics of radiography, ultrasonography, computerized tomography (CT scanning), and magnetic resonance (MR; nuclear magnetic resonance, NMR) tomography are converted electronically into digits corresponding to the different intensities of the original bits of information. These digits are stored in the computer and can be recalled, combined, and manipulated in various ways to achieve reconverted analog images. Hard copies of selected images can be made at the time of the study, or the information can be stored permanently in digital form for subsequent retrieval and conversion to analog images.

Radiography (roentgenography) is the oldest method of urologic imaging, having been used to demonstrate radiopaque urinary calculi shortly after the discovery of x-rays by Wilhelm Röntgen in 1895. Since then, it has continued to be used for diagnosis in every branch of medicine, and it is currently the most widely available method of medical imaging. Newer imaging methods (eg, scintigraphy, sonography, CT scan, and magnetic resonance tomography) are competing with, complementing, and, increasingly, replacing long-established uroradiographic techniques.

URORADIOGRAPHY

X-rays are electromagnetic waves with photon energies that fall between those of gamma rays and ultraviolet radiations in the electromagnetic spectrum. Radiography makes use of the fact that all substances and tissues differ in their ability to absorb x-rays passing through them. A radiopaque contrast medium is frequently employed to help distinguish separate structures and thus make radiograms easier to "read."

It is well known that improperly used x-rays can have harmful effects, particularly on the gonads and on fetuses early in gestation, but roentgenography is safe when properly used by trained personnel.

Although newer imaging techniques are replacing radiography for diagnosis of some urologic problems, radiography remains the backbone of urologic practice. It is often the first and sometimes the single most effective examination. Therefore, the urologist should be familiar with current x-ray equipment and uroradiologic techniques. The basic types of commonly used uroradiologic studies are plain abdominal films, urograms, cystourethrograms, urethrograms, and angiograms. These studies and enhancement by radiographic subtraction are described separately below. Some uroradiologic studies widely used in the past, eg, retroperitoneal gas insufflation (for visualization of the adrenals and kidneys) and pelvic pneumography (for visualization of pelvic organs), have become obsolete.

Basic Equipment & Techniques

A. Equipment:

1. Radiography–The basic requirements for radiography are a high-voltage electrical source, an x-ray tube, x-ray film, and some type of film holder. In practice, film holders are built into a variety of upright stands, tables, and rapid film changers.

2. Fluoroscopy–Shortly after the discovery of x-rays, real-time radiographic imaging (fluoroscopy) was accomplished by direct viewing in a darkened room of the images produced by x-rays passing through the subject and striking radiosensitive fluorescent screens.

3. Radiography-fluoroscopy (RF)–Modern x-ray units are vastly improved and much safer than the old ones and contain both radiographic and fluoroscopic capabilities. RF units combined with an electronic image intensifier and a television system are the mainstays of any diagnostic radiology department.

4. Image intensification–Radiographic image intensifiers came into use about 30 years ago and are now standard components of RF systems. Image intensifiers electronically augment the ordinary dim fluoroscopic image so that it may be viewed in daylight. Most modern RF units with image intensifiers also have television cameras tied into the system so that the intensified picture can be recorded and relayed to a television monitor conveniently placed for viewing, either in the x-ray room or elsewhere.

5. Real-time radiographic image recording–Any single frame of the real-time electronically intensified fluoroscopic image can be recorded on "spot" x-ray film, or the continuing real-time image can be recorded on videotape to allow real-time replay or study of single frames.

6. Data transmission systems—Increasingly, radiographic and other anatomic images are being transmitted from the examination site to stations in the same building or through standard telephone lines or via microwave or cable facilities to distant receivers, permitting clinicians to examine the studies at locations quite distant from the imaging site.

B. Patient Preparation: It is no longer considered necessary that patients be dehydrated in preparation for urography. Indeed, dehydration is to be avoided in infants, debilitated and aged patients, and patients with diabetes mellitus, renal failure, multiple myeloma, or hyperuricemic states.

On the other hand, preliminary bowel cleansing is very desirable, although children under age 10 years usually need no bowel preparation for urography. Bowel preparation for a urogram should be no less conscientious than that required for a barium enema examination of the colon. There are many ways to obtain good bowel preparation, and the choice may be made according to individual preference.

C. Radiopaque Urographic Contrast Media: An important concept extensively exploited in diagnostic radiology is that sharply contrasting and easily separable x-ray images can be produced by interfacing body tissues and structures with substances that are significantly different in radio-absorptivity. Such radiographic contrast media include liquids (almost all of which contain iodine), gels, solids (eg, barium preparations), and gases (most commonly air, nitrous oxide, and carbon dioxide).

Some contrast media can only be administered by one route, which limits their usefulness for multisystem anatomic imaging. For example, barium is used almost exclusively for gastrointestinal x-ray studies. Others, eg, some water-soluble iodine-containing preparations, can be administered by several routes, including intravascularly, and can be used to study many organ systems. The latter type of medium is especially useful in urographic and angiographic x-ray studies.

D. Adverse Reactions to Urographic Contrast Media: All procedures utilizing intravascular contrast media carry a small but definite risk of adverse reactions. The overall incidence of adverse reactions is about 5%.

Most reactions are minor, eg, nausea, vomiting, hives, rash, or flushing, and usually require no treatment other than reassurance. However, cardiopulmonary and anaphylactic reactions can occur with little or no warning and can be life-threatening or fatal. According to various reports, the incidence of death due to intravascular injection of contrast media ranges from 1 per 10,000 to 1 per 70,000, with most recent reports indicating a mortality rate of about 1 per 40,000.

Subjects with a history of allergies have a somewhat higher incidence of reactions to intravenous contrast media. There are no reliable methods for pretesting patients for possible adverse reactions. Therefore, the risks and benefits of using intravascular urographic contrast media should be carefully evaluated beforehand for each patient.

Recently developed nonionic contrast media have produced fewer adverse reactions than the higher-osmolarity ionic intravascular contrast agents now in general use. Although considerably more expensive than ionic agents, these new nonionic agents are being used increasingly, particularly in patients with previous significant reactions to conventional ionic contrast agents or in patients with a strong history of allergies.

Treatment of adverse reactions involves the use of antihistamines, epinephrine, vascular volume expanders, and cardiopulmonary drugs as well as ancillary treatment procedures indicated by the nature and severity of the reaction.

In some cases, imaging techniques not requiring contrast media are inadequate and examination using intravascular contrast media is absolutely critical even though the patient has a history of severe reaction to such media. Such patients have been given corticosteroids in an effort to prevent recurrence of the untoward response. This preventive treatment is not always successful, however.

Advantages & Disadvantages

Radiography produces excellent anatomic images of almost any body part. Costs of equipment and ex-

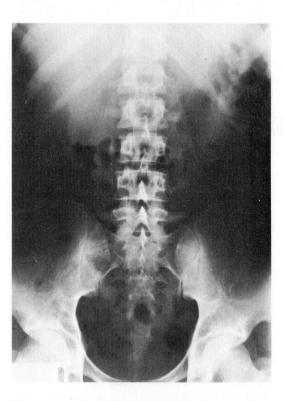

Figure 6–1. Normal plain film of the abdomen (KUB). Representative film, ordinary technical quality, and average patient bowel preparation. The kidneys are poorly outlined because of the small amount of perinephric fat. Healthy, lean 22-year-old man with back pain.

aminations are moderate compared to those of some other imaging systems. Space requirements for ordinary radiographic equipment are not excessive, and sophisticated portable equipment is available for use in hospital wards, operating rooms, and intensive care units. Because there are a great many specialists exclusively trained in radiography, its use is not confined to large medical centers. The major disadvantage of radiographic imaging is its fundamental basis in ionizing radiation.

1. PLAIN FILM OF THE ABDOMEN
(Figs 6–1 through 6–4.)

A plain film of the abdomen, frequently called a KUB (kidney-ureter-bladder) film, is the simplest uroradiologic study and the first performed in any radiographic examination of the abdomen or urinary tract. It is usually the preliminary radiogram in more extended radiologic examinations of the urinary tract, such as urography. It is usually taken with the patient supine, but when indicated, it may be taken with the patient in other positions. It may demonstrate abnormalities in bones, adrenals, and other structures as well as giving information about the state of the kidneys and extrarenal urinary tract.

Because kidney outlines can usually be seen on the plain film of the abdomen (although they may be obscured if there is very little perirenal fat), the size, number, shape, and position of the kidneys can be determined. This contributes useful urologic information. For example, finding on a plain film symmetrically shrunken rather than enlarged kidneys in a patient with unexplained uremia would be useful in excluding surgically remediable bilateral urinary tract obstruction as the cause of the renal failure.

The size of normal kidneys varies widely, not only between like individuals but also with age, sex, and body stature. The long diameter of the kidney is the most widely used and most convenient radiographic measurement. The average adult kidney is about 12–14 cm long, and the left kidney is ordinarily slightly longer than the right one. In children over 2 years of age, the length of a normal kidney is approximately equal to the distance from the top of the first to the bottom of the fourth lumbar vertebral body. In adults, the length of a normal kidney is approximately 3–4.5 times the height of the second lumbar vertebra.

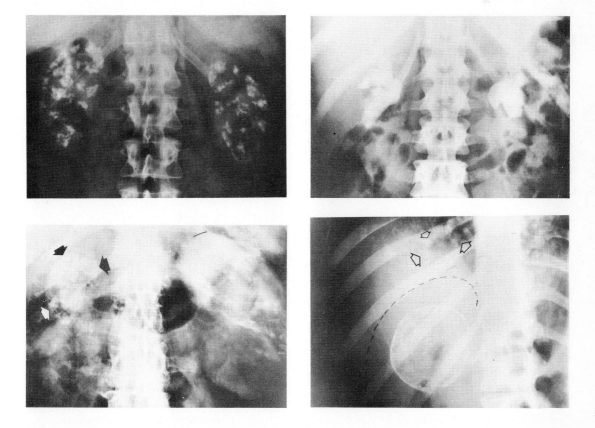

Figure 6–2. Plain films of the abdomen with abnormal radiopacities. *Upper left:* Bilateral nephrocalcinosis. Young adult male with renal tubular acidosis. *Upper right:* Bilateral staghorn calculi. 37-year-old woman with chronic pyelonephritis and history of previous right staghorn pyelolithotomy. *Lower left:* Renal tuberculosis. Shrunken, autonephrectomized and calcified right tuberculous kidney (*arrows*). 74-year-old man with history of renal and thoracolumbar spinal tuberculosis. *Lower right:* Papillary adenocarcinoma of right kidney. Remarkable tumor surface calcifications. Multiple pulmonary metastases (*arrows*) from the renal cancer. 22-year-old woman with painless soft tissue mass in the neck.

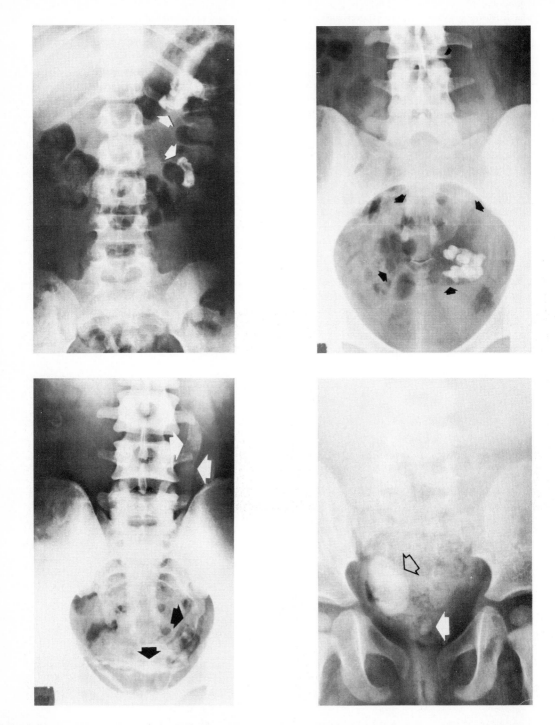

Figure 6–3. Plain films of the abdomen with abnormal radiopacities. *Upper left:* Benign retroperitoneal teratoma with bone formations. 9-year-old asthmatic girl with asymptomatic infradiaphragmatic calcifications (*arrows*) noted on routine chest film. *Upper right:* Benign ovarian cystic teratoma with teeth. Rounded cyst contains radiolucent fat (*arrows*) and a nest of well-formed teeth. 22-year-old woman with left pelvic mass. *Lower left:* Schistosomiasis calcification (*arrows*) in bladder and left ureter. 19-year-old male native of Aden with weight loss and hematuria. *Lower right:* Large vaginolith (*open arrow*) and small, barely visible bladder calculus (*solid arrow*). 4-year-old girl with common urogenital sinus.

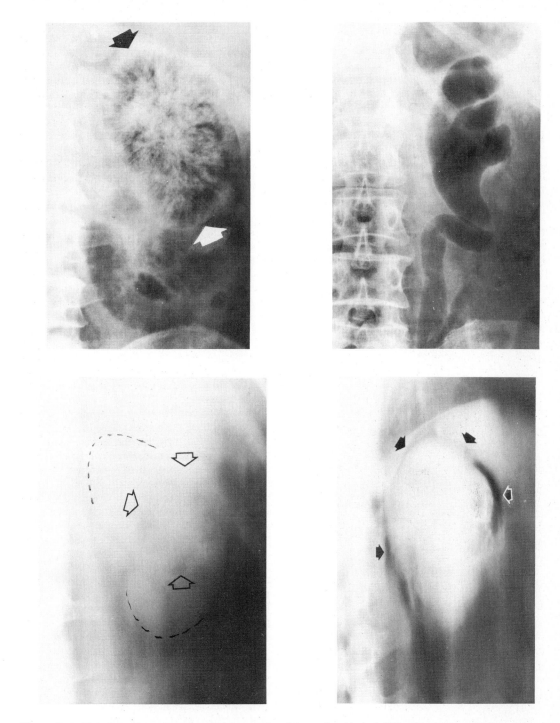

Figure 6–4. Plain films of the abdomen with abnormal radiolucencies. *Upper left:* Emphysematous pyelonephritis. Interstitial striated pattern of radiolucent gas throughout the entire left kidney. Similar changes were present in the right kidney. 58-year-old diabetic man with pyuria and septic shock. *Upper right:* Gas pyelogram. No interstitial gas, but gas fills dilated left kidney calices, pelvis, and ureter. 50-year-old diabetic woman with sepsis and left upper urinary tract infection due to gas-forming microorganisms. *Lower left:* Renal angiomyolipoma. Plain film tomogram shows left kidney mass containing radiolucent fat (*arrows*). 69-year-old woman with weight loss and left flank pain. *Lower right:* Calcified renal *Echinococcus* cysts. Retroperitoneal gas insufflation study, tomogram, adult male. Note how radiolucent gas (*arrows*) has dissected in the retroperitoneum about the minimally calcified cysts in the upper pole of the kidney.

Identification on the plain film of calcification or calculi anywhere in the urinary tract (Figs 6–2 and 6–3) may help to identify specific kidney diseases (eg, the calcifications occasionally seen in a kidney cancer) or may suggest primary disease elsewhere (eg, the occasional patient with nephrocalcinosis whose underlying primary disease is hyperparathyroidism).

2. UROGRAPHY
(Figs 6–5 through 6–11.)

The collecting structures of the kidneys, ureters, and bladder can be demonstrated radiologically by the following methods.

Excretory Urograms

The excretory urogram (Fig 6–5), formerly called an intravenous pyelogram (IVP), is most commonly used. Excretory urograms can demonstrate a wide variety of urinary tract lesions (Figs 6–6 and 6–7), are simple to perform, and are well tolerated by most patients. Occasionally, however, retrograde urograms (see below) may be required if the excretory urogram is unsatisfactory or the patient has a history of significant adverse reaction to intravascular contrast

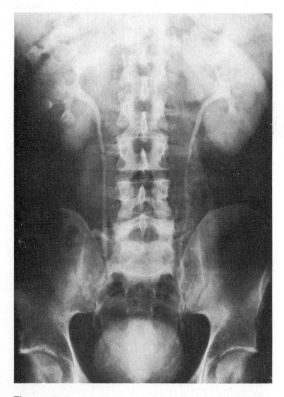

Figure 6–5. Normal excretory urogram. High-volume contrast medium study. The kidneys are normal in shape, size, and position; the calices and pelves are normal. The ureters are well shown because of the diuresis effect of the high volume of contrast medium. The bladder is normal. Healthy young adult male potential kidney donor.

media. The advent of excretory urography using high volumes of radiopaque contrast media and ureteral compression (see below) has decreased the need for the more invasive retrograde urograms.

Sonography and CT scan are now used instead of urography in many cases, and as magnetic resonance imaging is used more frequently, urography will probably be used even less. Nevertheless, urography remains the best, if not the only, imaging study capable of demonstrating small lesions in the urinary tract (eg, papillary necrosis, medullary sponge kidney, small uroepithelial tumors, pyeloureteritis cystica). These lesions cannot be seen with nonurographic techniques.

A. Standard Technique: Following a preliminary plain film of the abdomen, radiograms of the abdomen are taken at timed intervals after the intravenous injection of a suitable iodine-containing radiopaque contrast medium. Such substances are promptly excreted by normal kidneys, almost entirely by glomerular filtration.

The volume and speed of injection of the radiographic contrast medium (rapid bolus, slow infusion, etc), as well as the number and type of films taken following injection, vary depending upon the institution at which the studies are performed and the patient's age, physical condition, and clinical problem. Several modifications of the standard technique have improved the study generally or increased its value in particular diseases.

B. High-Volume Technique: In most patients, use of standard intravenous radiopaque medium in the amount recommended by the manufacturer will usually result in satisfactory diagnostic urograms. The amount of iodine commonly used in patients with normal renal function is approximately 300 mg/kg body weight. The use of greater than average amounts of standard contrast medium—and thus greater amounts of iodine per kilogram of body weight—may be indicated in selected patients. The high volumes may be injected either rapidly as a bolus or more slowly as an infusion; the bolus method produces better visualization and a better urographic nephrogram than the infusion method.

C. Rapid-Sequence ("Hypertensive") Technique: This modification of the standard excretory urogram was devised to make the study more useful in the diagnosis of renovascular hypertension. In this method, the procedure for the standard intravenous urogram is altered to include several radiograms taken at intervals during the first few minutes after bolus injection of the contrast medium. This technique has increased somewhat the diagnostic value of the ordinary urogram in patients suspected of having renal artery occlusive disease without prolonging the study or adding appreciably to its cost.

The rapid-sequence radiograms are examined for findings that could indicate renal artery stenosis, eg, significant decrease in the size of the affected kidney or delayed appearance of the contrast medium, with later hyperconcentration in that kidney.

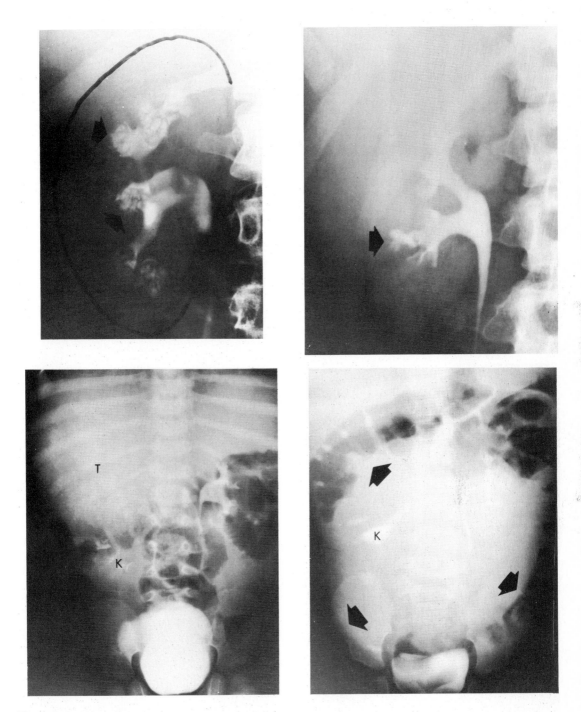

Figure 6–6. Abnormal excretory urograms. *Upper left:* Medullary sponge kidney. Pronounced medullary tubular ectasia (*arrows*) of entire right kidney. Similar findings in upper pole pyramids of left kidney. Small medullary calculi were present in some areas of tubular ectasia in both kidneys. 34-year-old female with repeated bouts of chills, fever, and left flank pain. *Upper right:* Renal tuberculosis. Irregular cavitation of lower pole pyramid (*arrow*). 22-year-old woman with positive urine culture for tuberculosis. *Lower left:* Adrenal neuroblastoma. Diffuse small calcifications in a large right upper quadrant mass (T) depressing the right kidney (K). 12-year-old girl with proptosis of the right eye and an abdominal tumor. *Lower right:* Wilms' tumor. Huge tumor of right kidney filling the entire abdomen (*arrows*), displacing bowel, and deforming collecting structures of the right kidney (K). Left kidney normal. 21-month-old girl with large abdominal mass.

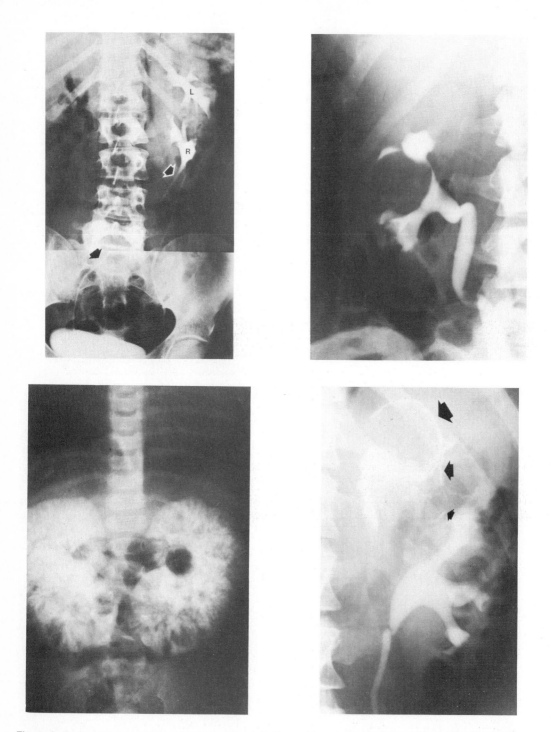

Figure 6–7. Abnormal excretory urograms. *Upper left:* Crossed fused ectopia. Composite of 2 films from an excretory urogram shows ectopic right kidney (R) fused to left kidney (L). Right ureter (*arrows*) crosses midline and enters normally into right side of bladder. Healthy 31-year-old female potential kidney donor. *Upper right:* Renal artery aneurysm. Right kidney collecting structures draped around a central mass. See corresponding arteriogram (Fig 6–22, upper right). 41-year-old woman with hypertension and right abdominal bruit. *Lower left:* Infantile polycystic kidney disease. Very large kidneys with radiopaque spoke pattern radiating out to cortex, 26 hours after administration of intravenous contrast medium. 4-month-old girl with bilateral abdominal masses. *Lower right:* Renal cell carcinoma. Unusual circular and curvilinear eggshell calcifications (*arrows*) in the tumor, which is compressing the infundibulum to deform upper pole calices. 39-year-old man with history of "unroofing of left kidney cyst" 3 years earlier.

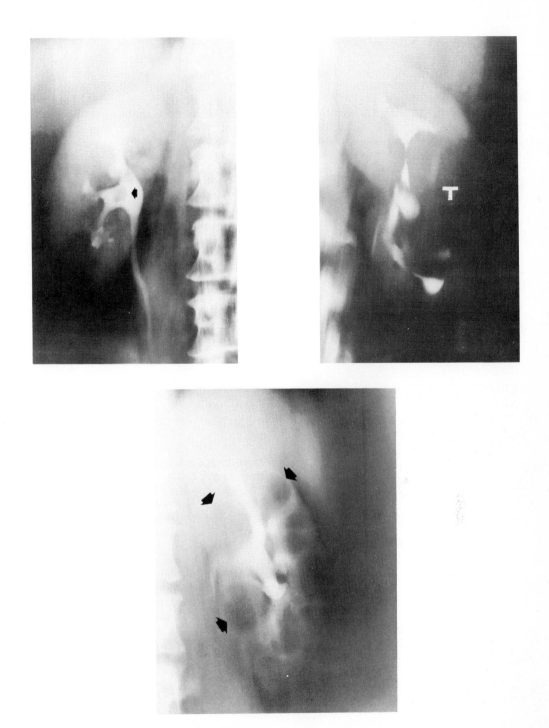

Figure 6–8. Radiographic tomography. Tomography is used to image a plane in the body. The technique is particularly useful in uroradiology, often permitting demonstration of lesions otherwise hidden by overlying soft tissues or obscuring bowel shadows. *Upper left:* Transitional cell carcinoma. The tumor in the pelvis (*arrow*) is clearly shown free of obscuring gas shadows present on the nontomographic films. 56-year-old man with history of renal calculi. *Upper right:* Renal cell carcinoma (T). Displacement of mid-kidney collecting structures and a nephrogram defect are seen free of obscuring splenic flexure fecal shadows that were present on the nontomographic films. 44-year-old woman with fever, weight loss, anemia, and history of contralateral nephrectomy for carcinoma 15 years earlier. *Bottom:* Adult polycystic kidney disease. The tomographic plane of the left kidney is outside the level of the bowel and shows to more advantage the numerous radiolucent cysts (*arrows*). Similar appearance in right kidney. 29-year-old man with family history of "cysts in the kidneys."

This rapid-sequence study was popular for years, but it is now agreed that it is at best only minimally effective as a screening study for suspected renovascular hypertension.

D. Other Techniques: Additional modifications of the standard excretory urogram can be used. **Radiographic tomography,** x-ray imaging of a selected plane in the body, permits recognition of kidney structures that otherwise are obscured on standard radiograms by extrarenal shadows, eg, those due to bone or feces (Fig 6–8). **Image-intensified fluoroscopy** permits real-time study of urinary tract dynamics. **"Immediate" films,** which are taken directly after the rapid (bolus) injection of contrast medium, almost al-

ways show a dense nephrogram and permit better visualization of renal outlines. **Abdominal (ureteral) compression devices** that temporarily obstruct the upper urinary tracts during excretory urograms dramatically improve the filling of renal collecting structures. **"Delayed" films,** which are taken later on the same day or on the day after the contrast medium is administered, often contribute useful urologic information. **"Upright" films,** taken with the patient standing or partially erect, reveal the degree of mobility and drainage of the kidneys and, if taken immediately after the patient has voided **("postvoiding" film),** show any residual urine in the bladder.

Retrograde Urograms

Retrograde urography is a moderately invasive procedure that requires cystoscopy and the placement of catheters in the ureters. A radiopaque contrast medium is introduced into the ureters or renal collecting structures through the ureteral catheters (Figs 6–9 through 6–11), and radiograms of the abdomen are then taken. The study, which is more difficult than an excretory urogram, must be performed by a urologist. Some type of local or general anesthesia must be used, and the procedure can occasionally cause later morbidity or urinary tract infection.

Retrograde urograms may be necessary if excretory urograms are unsatisfactory, if the patient has a history of adverse reaction to intravenous contrast media, or if other methods of imaging are unavailable or inappropriate.

Percutaneous Antegrade Urograms

This method of outlining the renal collecting structures and ureters is occasionally used when urinary tract imaging is necessary but excretory or retrograde urography has failed or is contraindicated or when there is a nephrostomy tube in place and delineation of the collecting system of the upper urinary tract is desired. The contrast medium is introduced either through nephrostomy tubes, if these are present (nephrostogram), or by direct injection into the renal collecting structures via a percutaneous puncture through the patient's back.

Percutaneous Retrograde Urograms

These studies of the upper urinary tract are made by retrograde injection of contrast medium through the opening of a skin ureterostomy or pyelostomy (skin ureterogram, skin urogram) or through the ostium of an interposed conduit, usually a segment of small bowel ("loopogram").

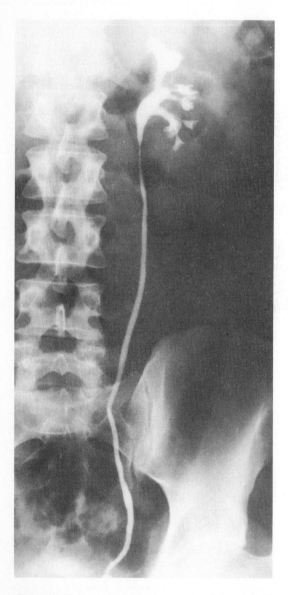

Figure 6–9. Normal retrograde urogram. Intrarenal collecting structures, pelvis, and ureter are normal. Adult male with microscopic hematuria and previous technically unsatisfactory excretory urogram.

3. CYSTOGRAPHY & VOIDING CYSTOURETHROGRAPHY (Figs 6–12 through 6–15.)

A cystogram is a radiogram showing radiopaque

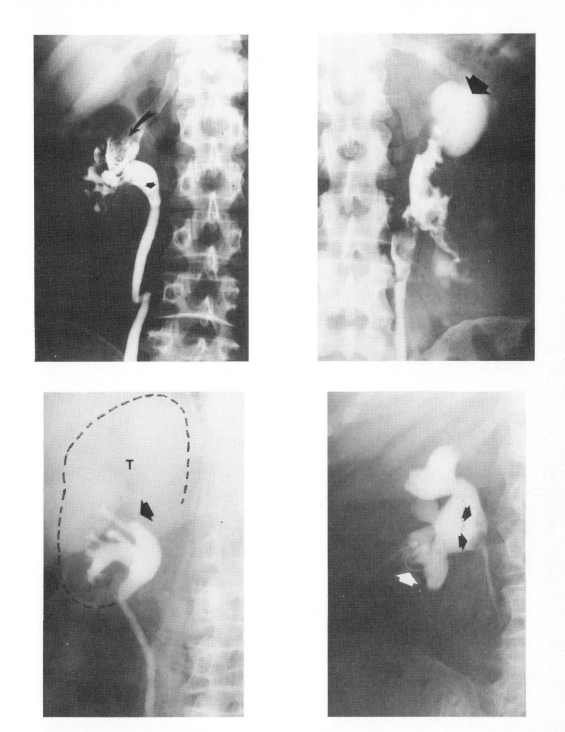

Figure 6–10. Abnormal retrograde urograms and nephrostograms; lower ureters not shown. *Upper left:* Transitional cell carcinoma. Severe deformity with filling defects in right upper pole calices (*curved arrow*) and blood clots in lower calices and at ureteropelvic junction (*straight arrow*). 65-year-old man with gross hematuria and right flank pain. *Upper right:* Squamous cell carcinoma. Marked irregular filling defects involving calices, pelvis, and proximal ureter, with communicating abscess cavity in upper pole (*arrow*). Kidney also showed squamous metaplasia and contained calculi. 51-year-old woman with 2-week history of left flank cellulitis and tenderness. *Lower left:* Renal cell carcinoma. Right upper pole mass (T) with amputation of superior calices and infundibulum (*arrow*). 76-year-old man with pulmonary metastases. *Lower right:* Fungus balls. Nephrostogram revealing 2 filling defects (*arrows*) in renal pelvis. Copious fungal matter aspirated through nephrostomy catheter. 65-year-old diabetic woman who had undergone left nephrectomy, with percutaneous nephrostomy catheter (*white arrow*) for obstruction of right kidney.

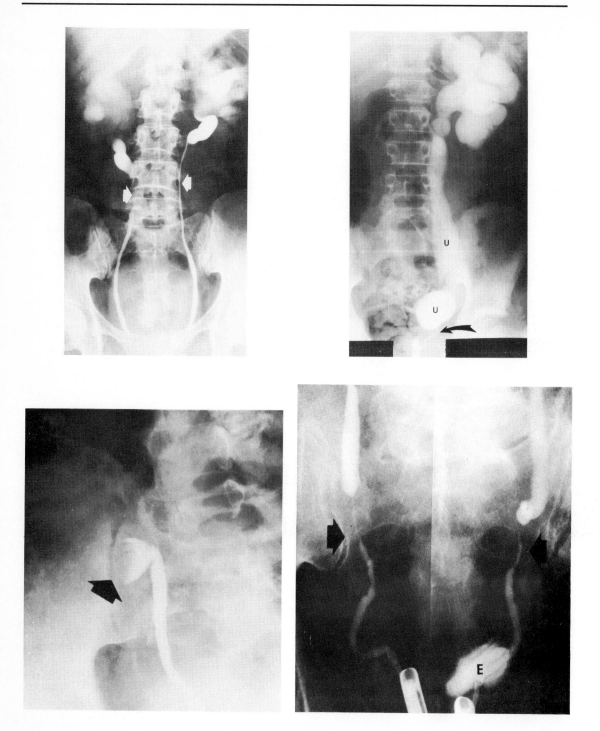

Figure 6–11. Abnormal retrograde urograms. *Upper left:* Idiopathic retroperitoneal fibrosis. Smooth narrowing of both mid ureters (*arrows*), with bilateral proximal ureterectasis and hydronephrosis. 51-year-old woman with no urinary tract symptoms. *Upper right:* Functional ureteral obstruction. Obstruction was due to congenitally abnormal muscle arrangements in the affected very distal ureter (*curved arrow*). Pronounced hydronephrosis and dilatation of ureter (U) proximal to the short segment of abnormal ureter. 13-year-old boy with repeated urinary tract infections. *Lower left:* Transitional cell carcinoma of the ureter. No contrast medium has passed beyond the large, bulky, right ureteral tumor (*arrow*). The ureteral widening below the tumor is distinctive and is sometimes referred to as the "champagne glass" sign (in this instance, the glass is tipped on its side). 76-year-old man with nonfunctioning right kidney. *Lower right:* Ureteral constrictions secondary to extension of carcinoma of the colon. Bilateral distal ureteral narrowings (*arrows*) with upper tract obstruction. Composite of separate retrograde urograms. E = unintended extravasation about tip of left ureteral catheter. 76-year-old man with cancer of the sigmoid colon.

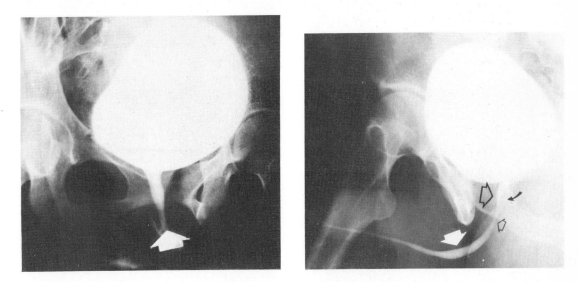

Figure 6–12. Normal voiding cystourethrograms. *Left:* Normal female bladder and urethra. Arrow indicates urethral meatus. 22-year-old woman with voiding symptoms. *Right:* Normal male bladder and urethra. Large open arrow = prostatic urethra; small open arrow = membranous urethra; closed arrow = cavernous urethra; curved arrow = veramontanum. 27-year-old man with vague right lower abdominal and testicular pain.

outlining of the bladder cavity. Cystograms are seen as part of ordinary excretory urograms, but direct radiographic cystograms can be obtained by instilling a radiopaque fluid directly into the bladder. The contrast medium is usually instilled via a transurethral catheter, but when necessary, it can be administered via percutaneous suprapubic bladder puncture. Radiograms of the filled bladder are taken using standard overhead x-ray tube equipment, or less frequently, "spot" films are taken during real-time, direct, image-intensified fluoroscopy.

Voiding cystourethrograms are radiograms of the bladder and urethra obtained during micturition.

In addition to their use in imaging the bladder and urethra, cystography and cystourethrography are important radiologic techniques for detecting vesicoureteral reflux and are the bases of several radiographic methods used in the workup of patients with urinary stress incontinence.

4. URETHROGRAPHY
(Figs 6–15 through 6–18.)

The urethra can be imaged radiographically by retrograde injection of radiopaque fluid or in antegrade fashion with voiding cystourethrography. The antegrade technique is required when lesions of the posterior urethra, eg, posterior urethral valves, are suspected; the retrograde technique is more useful for examining the anterior urethra. An antegrade urethrogram can also be obtained by taking radiograms as the patient voids at the termination of an excretory urogram, when the bladder is filled with contrast medium.

5. VASOGRAPHY
(Fig 6–19.)

Vasoseminal vesiculography is most often used in the investigation of male sterility. The radiopaque contrast medium is introduced into the sex duct system by direct injection into an ejaculatory duct following panendoscopy or, more commonly, by injection into the vas deferens after it has been surgically exposed through a small incision in the scrotum.

6. LYMPHANGIOGRAPHY
(Fig 6–20.)

Injection of an oily contrast medium through a cannula into a lymphatic vessel in the foot produces radiopacification of the inguinal, pelvic, and retroperitoneal lymphatic system. The main value of this procedure is in demonstrating metastatic infiltration of regional lymph nodes; thus, it is useful in the study of patients with cancers of the testis, penis, bladder, and prostate.

Considerable manual dexterity is required to cannulate lymphatic vessels in the feet, and lymphangiography can be a tedious procedure. Although CT scans are being used with increasing frequency to search for pelvic and abdominal lymphadenopathy, some physicians believe that lymphangiograms can show tumor infiltration not visible on CT scans, particularly lymph nodes involved with disease but not yet enlarged. Enlargement is the primary diagnostic feature recognized on CT scans.

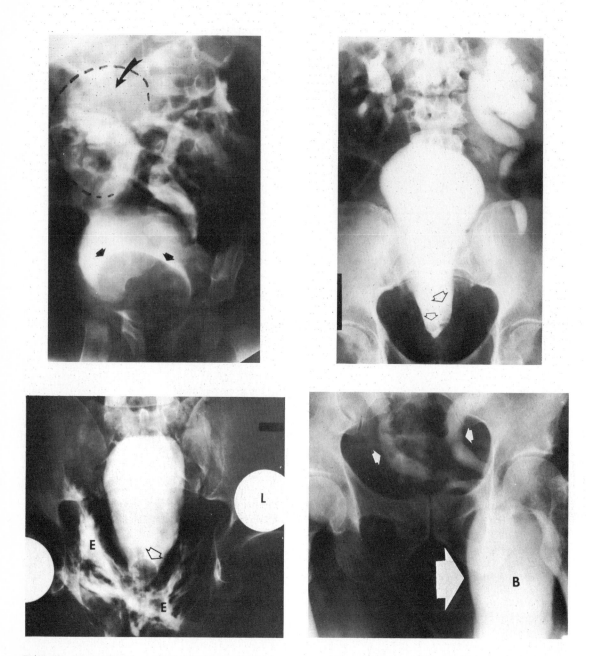

Figure 6-13. Abnormal cystograms: retrograde cystograms or "cystograms" as part of excretory urogram studies. *Upper left:* Ectopic ureterocele. Giant ureterocele (*straight arrows*) to hydronephrotic, nonfunctioning upper portion (*curved arrow*) of duplex right kidney. 9-month-old-girl with urinary tract infections. *Upper right:* Pelvic lipomatosis. Pear-shaped bladder and increased radiolucency of the pelvic soft tissues secondary to pelvic lipomatosis of severity sufficient to produce obstructive dilatation of the upper urinary tracts. Filling defects (*arrows*) at bladder base due to cystitis glandularis. 62-year-old man with intermittent left flank pain. *Lower left:* Rupture of the membranous urethra. Pear-shaped bladder secondary to extraperitoneal extravasation (E) and perivesical hematoma. Arrow = inflated balloon of Foley catheter. 41-year-old man with renal transplant, after a motor vehicle accident that resulted in pelvic bone fractures, separation of the sacroiliac joints, and dislocation of the left (L) but not the right hip prosthesis (patient has bilateral hip prostheses). *Lower right:* Bladder hernia. Bilateral obstructive ureterectasis (*small arrows*) secondary to remarkable herniation of the entire bladder (*large arrow*, B) into the inguinal region, 5'5", 225-pound, 53-year-old man with panniculus reaching to mid thigh, complaining of difficulty voiding.

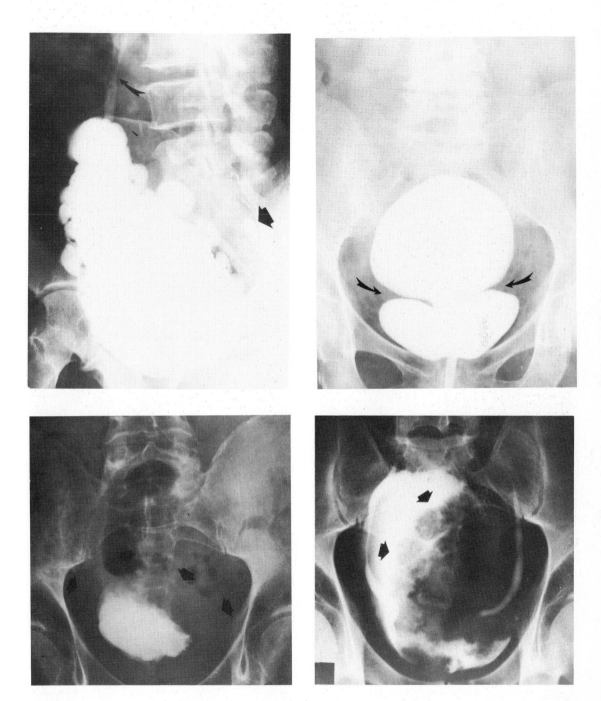

Figure 6–14. Abnormal cystograms: retrograde cystograms or "cystograms" as part of excretory urogram studies. *Upper left:* Neurogenic bladder. This neurogenic bladder has a "Christmas-tree" shape, with gross trabeculation and many diverticula. Residual myelographic contrast medium in spinal canal (*straight arrow*). Right vesicoureteral reflux (*curved arrow*). 70-year-old man with urinary incontinence. *Upper right:* Congenital "hourglass" bladder. Transverse concentric muscular band (*arrows*) separates upper and lower bladder segments, both of which contracted and emptied simultaneously and completely with voiding. 66-year-old woman with urinary stress incontinence. *Lower left:* Hodgkin's disease of bladder. Global thickening of the bladder (*arrows*), more apparent on the left. 54-year-old man with generalized Hodgkin's disease. *Lower right:* Papillary transitional cell bladder carcinoma. Huge (12 cm) cauliflowerlike bladder mass (*arrows*) filling almost the entire bladder. "Cystogram" film of an excretory urogram in a 40-year-old man with recurrent bladder tumor.

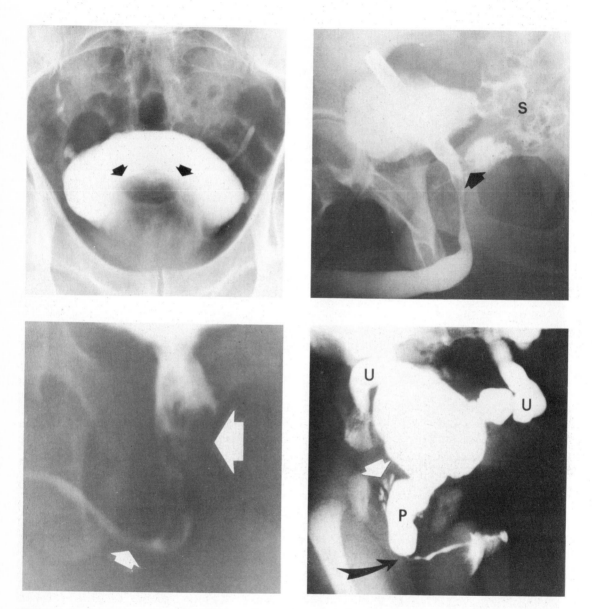

Figure 6–15. Abnormal prostate and posterior urethra: cystograms and urethrograms. *Upper left:* Benign prostatic hyperplasia. Gross enlargement of prostate gland producing marked elevation (*arrows*) of the bladder base. The bladder shows small diverticula and slight trabeculation. Excretory urogram (cystogram) in a 65-year-old man with history of obstructive voiding symptoms. *Upper right:* Foreign body (eyeliner pencil cover) lodged in bladder and prostatic urethra, with urethrorectal fistula. Radiopaque medium enters rectum and sigmoid colon (S) through fistula (*arrow*) from prostatic urethra. Retrograde urethrogram in a 43-year-old transsexual man. *Lower left:* Rhabdomyosarcoma of prostate. Lobulated filling defects (*large arrow*) encroaching on widened prostatic urethra. Voiding cystourethrogram in a 5-year-old boy with voiding difficulties. Small arrow = cavernous urethra. *Lower right:* Posterior urethral valves. Marked dilatation and elongation of prostatic urethra (P), with reflux into prostatic ducts (*straight arrow*) secondary to posterior urethral valves (*curved arrow*) with bilateral vesicoureteral reflux into dilated ureters (U). Voiding cystourethrogram in a 10-day-old boy.

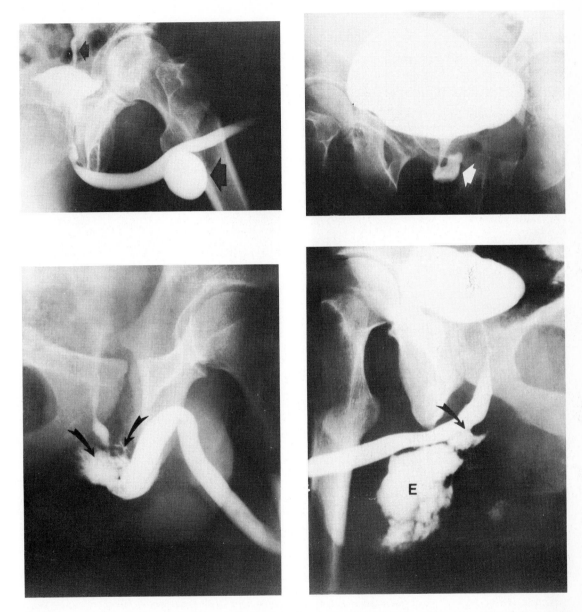

Figure 6–16. Abnormal anterior urethras: voiding cystourethrograms and retrograde urethrograms. *Upper left:* Urethral diverticulum in a male. 4-cm anterior urethral diverticulum (*large arrow*) and left vesicoureteral reflux (*small arrow*). Voiding cystourethrogram in a 78-year-old man with history of urethral diverticulum of unknown etiology. *Upper right:* Urethral diverticulum in a female. Large irregular diverticulum (*arrow*). Voiding cystourethrogram in a 51-year-old woman with voiding difficulties and suspected urethral stricture. *Lower left:* Ruptured urethra. Extravasation of contrast medium around the bulbous urethra (*arrows*). Retrograde urethrogram in a 16-year-old boy in whom blunt perineal trauma was followed by bloody urethral discharge and inability to void. *Lower right:* Urethroscrotal fistula. Extravasation (E) into extraurethral tissues from fistula in bulbous urethra (*arrow*). Retrograde urethrogram in a 26-year-old man after end-to-end urethroplasty for stricture.

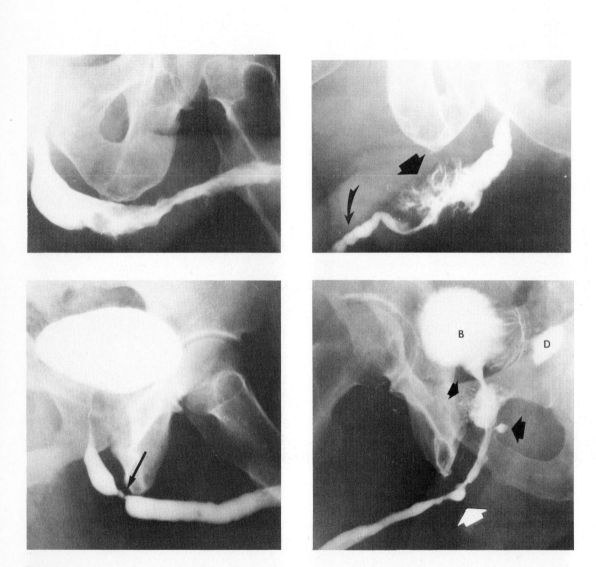

Figure 6–17. Abnormal anterior urethras: retrograde urethrograms. *Upper left:* Urethral carcinoma. Gross irregularities with filling defects involving most of penile urethra. Poorly differentiated carcinoma of anterior urethra in a 59-year-old man with obstructive voiding symptoms and inguinal adenopathy. *Upper right:* Urethral carcinoma. Filling of irregular sinus tracts and channels in a large epidermoid carcinoma of the bulbocavernous urethra (*straight arrow*). There are multiple thin transverse strictures of the penile urethra (*curved arrow*). 75-year-old man with obstructive voiding symptoms and 30-year history of urethral strictures requiring dilatations. *Lower left:* Focal urethral stricture (*arrow*). Middle-aged man with obstructive voiding symptoms who denied any previous urethritis. *Lower right:* Urethral strictures. Multiple strictures in the bulbocavernous urethra (*lower arrow*) with reflux into Cowper's gland (*middle arrow*) and prostatic ducts (*upper arrow*). B = bladder; D = bladder diverticulum. 62-year-old man with 25-year history of urethral strictures requiring frequent dilatations.

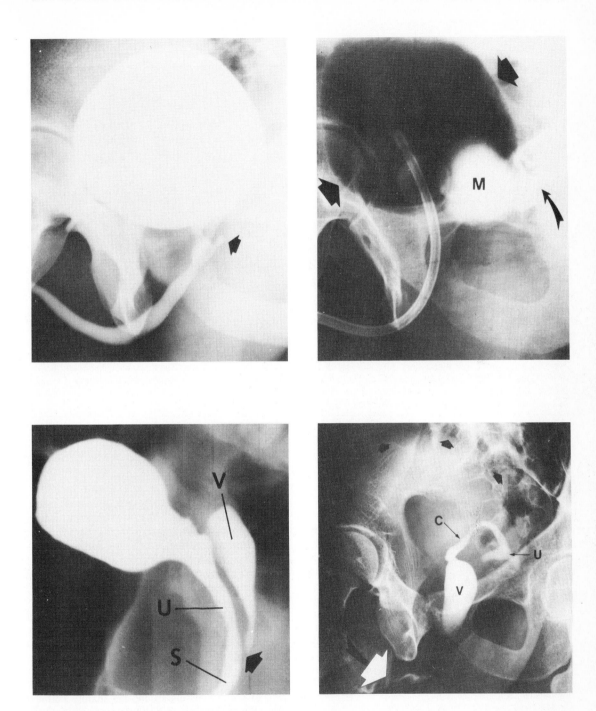

Figure 6–18. Congenital genitourinary anomalies: voiding cystograms and retrograde urethrograms. *Upper left:* Utricle. Midline outpouching (*arrow*) from verumontanum between orifices of ejaculatory ducts, representing müllerian duct remnant. Voiding cystourethrogram in a 25-year-old man with dysuria and urinary tract infections. *Upper right:* Müllerian duct cyst. Gas cystogram combined with injection of utricle, oblique view. M = grossly dilated utricle (müllerian duct cyst); straight arrows = bladder distended with air; curved arrow = coincident partial filling of left seminal vesicle and vas deferens. 34-year-old man with urgency, frequency, and suspected retrograde ejaculation. *Lower left:* Common urogenital sinus. Vagina (V) and urethra (U) join (*at arrow*) into a common urogenital sinus (S). Voiding cystourethrogram in a 3-week-old female pseudohermaphrodite with ambiguous genitalia and congenital adrenal hyperplasia. *Lower right:* Male pseudohermaphrodite. Bladder is distended with urine (*black arrows*). Retrograde urethrogram via hypospadiac meatus has fortuitously and selectively filled with contrast medium an extensive müllerian duct remnant consisting of vagina (V), cervix and cervical canal (C), and retroverted uterus (U). Residual contrast medium in hypoplastic anterior urethra (*white arrow*). 27-year-old man with small external genitalia, hypospadias, and perineal pain.

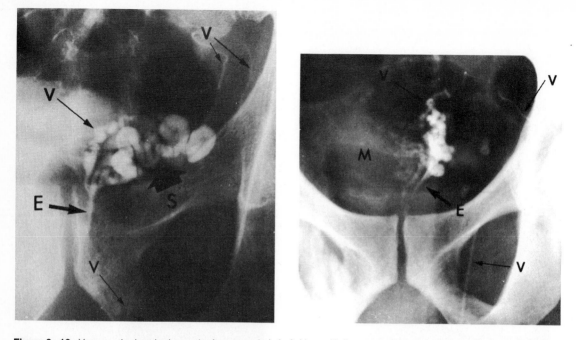

Figure 6–19. Vasoseminal vesiculography (vasography). *Left:* Normal left vasoseminal vesiculogram. V = vas deferens; S = seminal vesicle; E = ejaculatory duct. 40-year-old man with hypospermia. *Right:* Seminal vesiculitis. Bilateral vasogram. Mass (M) produced by the swollen, nonfilling right seminal vesicle has displaced both ejaculatory ducts (E) toward the left and indented the medial aspect of the proximal left seminal vesicle and vas deferens (V). 33-year-old man with painful ejaculations after repair of right varicocele.

7. ANGIOGRAPHY
(Figs 6–21 through 6–27.)

Angiography is visualization of blood vessels by use of radiopaque contrast media. Angiographic study of the urinary tract is almost exclusively used to visualize renal structures. Vesical angiography and penile angiography are seldom performed and of limited value. Although angiography is an established imaging technique with proved value and an acceptable incidence of complications and morbidity, it is moderately invasive and relatively expensive and usually requires a hospital stay. Increasing use of sonography, CT scanning, and digital angiography (see below) has resulted in a decrease in the use of angiography for diagnosis of urologic problems.

Aortorenal & Selective Renal Arteriography
(Figs 6–21 through 6–23.)

Arteriographic study of the kidneys is performed almost exclusively by percutaneous needle puncture and catheterization of the common femoral arteries or, much less often, the axillary arteries. Rapid serial radiograms are obtained during and after bolus injection of suitable radiopaque contrast medium into the aorta at the level of the renal arteries (aortorenal arteriogram, "flush" abdominal aortogram) or into one of the renal arteries (selective renal arteriogram).

In urologic practice, aortograms and renal arteriograms are most often performed to investigate renal tumors or renovascular lesions, to obtain vascular maps before surgery is performed, or to evaluate the suitability of potential kidney donors.

Adenocarcinomas of the kidney usually have obvious abnormal vessels and are generally hypervascular, whereas transitional cell carcinomas are notoriously poorly vascularized and difficult to identify by angiography. Renal hamartomas are often indistinguishable from adenocarcinomas on angiography, but their fat content readily distinguishes them from adenocarcinomas on CT scans.

Benign renal cysts are avascular, with displacement of normal vessels around the sharply outlined cysts. Renal abscesses can mimic renal cysts on angiography, although hyperemic inflammatory vessels may be visible around an abscess.

Although sonograms and CT scans readily demonstrate the nature and extent of most renal tumors, many surgeons obtain abdominal and renal angiograms as vascular maps in order to determine the vascular limits of tumors, their degree of hypervascularity, whether they have other blood supplies in addition to the renal arteries (see figure 6–21, lower right), and whether renal vein tumor thrombi are present.

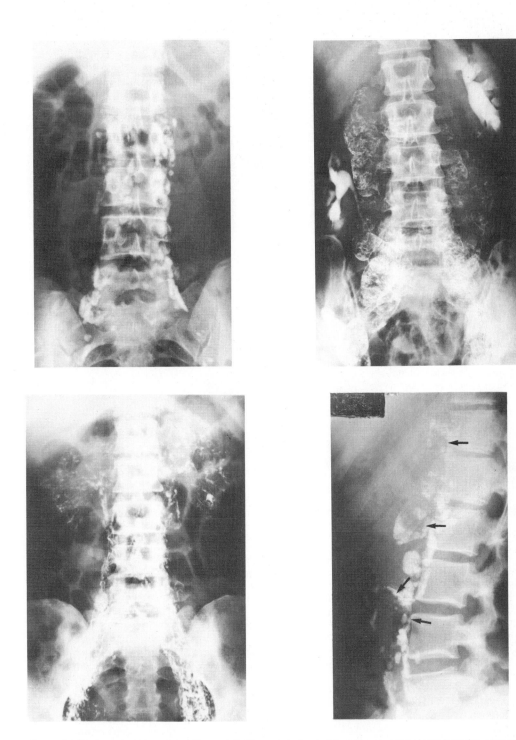

Figure 6–20. Lymphangiography. *Upper left:* Normal abdominal lymphangiogram. Lymph nodes appear normal. 15-year-old girl with fevers of unknown etiology. *Upper right:* Hodgkin's disease. Kidneys and ureters displaced by grossly involved abdominal and pelvic lymph nodes. 52-year-old woman with stage IV Hodgkin's disease. *Lower left:* Filariasis. Remarkable pattern of dilated, tortuous pelvic, abdominal, and renal lymphatics representing development of an extensive network of collateral channels secondary to obstruction of normal pathways. 42-year-old native of Okinawa with 12-year history of chyluria. *Lower right:* Metastatic testicular choriocarcinoma. Enlarged thoracolumbar lymph nodes partially replaced by metastatic tumor (*arrows*). 26-year-old man with enlarged left supraclavicular node, after orchiectomy for choriocarcinoma.

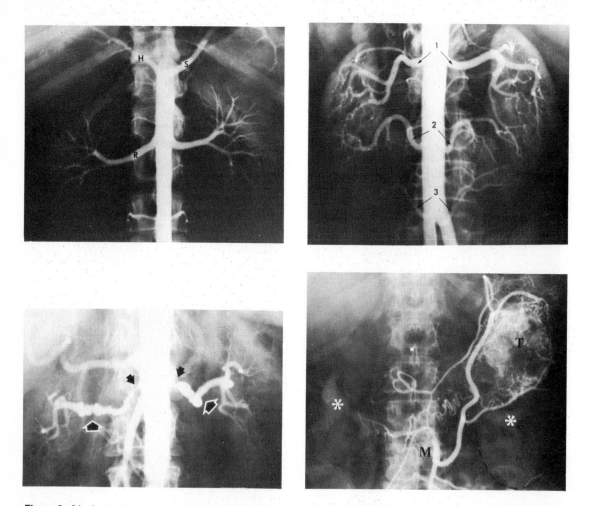

Figure 6–21. Angiography: aortorenal arteriography. *Upper left:* Normal abdominal aortogram. The aortic catheter is hidden by the opacified normal aorta. Right (R) and left renal arteries and branches are well shown, as are the splenic (S) and hepatic (H) arteries arising from the celiac axis. The superior mesenteric artery is superimposed over the aortic silhouette and is not visible on this study. 28-year-old healthy female potential kidney donor. *Upper right:* Multiple renal arteries. Horseshoe kidney with 3 renal arteries on each side, the 2 lowermost (3) supplying the renal isthmus. 42-year-old man with recurrent calculous disease, after left pyelolithotomy. *Lower left:* Bilateral renal artery stenoses. Typical angiographic appearance and location of stenoses caused by atherosclerosis (*small arrows*) and fibromuscular dysplasia (*large arrows*). 58-year-old woman with abdominal bruits and a 16-year history of hypertension. *Lower right:* Vascular parasitism by kidney cancer. Selective inferior mesenteric arteriogram (M) demonstrating large blood supply to a hypervascular adenocarcinoma (T) of the upper pole. * = renal pelvis. 69-year-old woman with polycythemia.

Inferior Venacavography & Selective Renal Venography (Figs 6–24 through 6–26.)

The common femoral veins are the usual site for catheterization and injection of contrast medium to visualize the inferior vena cava and renal veins.

Inferior venacavography (Figs 6–24 and 6–25) is ineffective for demonstration of small paracaval masses or minimally enlarged retroperitoneal lymph nodes, but it can show lesions large enough to obstruct, distort, or displace the vena cava. It is useful to demonstrate extension of thrombus or tumor from renal veins into the vena cava. Renal vein tumor or thrombus that does not extend into the vena cava will not be evident on inferior venacavograms but can be visualized by selective renal venography (Fig 6–26).

Sonography and CT scanning are being used increasingly for visualization of abnormalities in the inferior vena cava and main renal veins.

Adrenal Angiography (Fig 6–22.)

Adrenal angiograms are not often performed. They are technically difficult because the multiple arteries supplying the adrenals are small and the adrenal veins are difficult to catheterize selectively. In addition, selective adrenal venography is not without hazard; the veins in the glands are particularly susceptible to rupture, and serious injury to the gland has resulted from intravasation of contrast medium into the adrenal parenchyma.

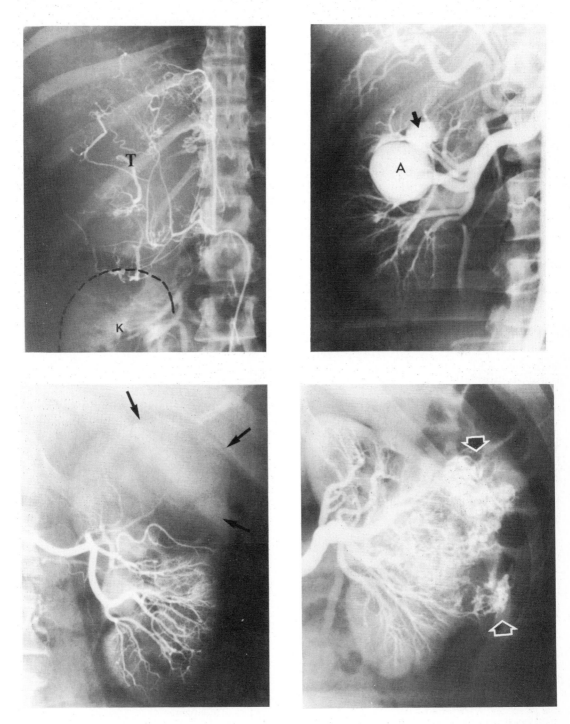

Figure 6–22. Angiography: selective adrenal and renal arteriography. *Upper left:* Adrenal carcinoma. Large, moderately vascular adrenal tumor (T) depressing right kidney (K). Selective adrenal arteriogram in a 24-year-old woman with weight gain and episodes of weakness, sweating, tachycardia, and hypoglycemia. *Upper right:* Renal artery aneurysm. The aneurysm (A) is producing some obstruction to an upper pole calix (*arrow*). See corresponding excretory urogram (Fig 6–7, upper right). Aortorenal arteriogram in a 41-year-old woman with hypertension and an abdominal bruit. *Lower left:* Simple renal cyst. The angiographic appearance of the totally avascular upper pole mass (*arrow*) is not diagnostic and is indistinguishable from some other lesions, including avascular cancer. 73-year-old man with left renal mass on excretory urogram and sonographic diagnosis of probable simple cyst. *Lower right:* Renal cell carcinoma. Large hypervascular mass with pathologic vessels extending outside kidney (*arrows*). 45-year-old man with left knee pain (due to lytic femur metastasis).

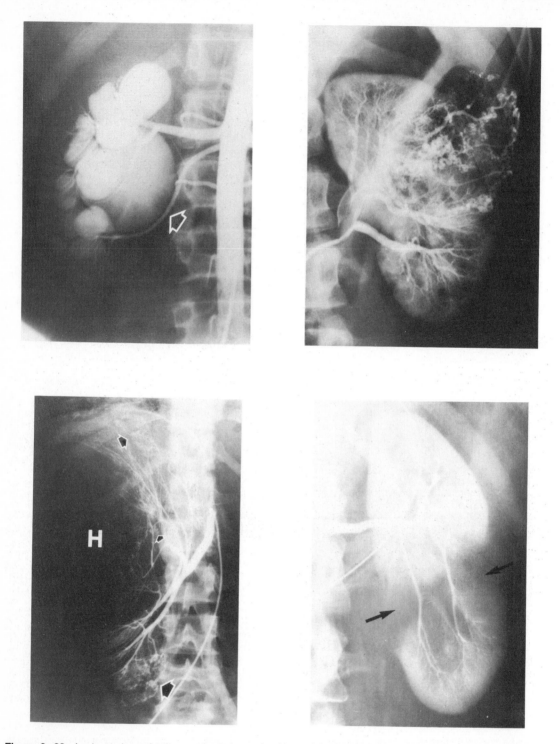

Figure 6–23. Angiography: selective renal arteriography. *Upper left:* Ureteropelvic junction obstruction. Obstruction caused by crossing renal artery (*arrow*). 12-year-old girl with right hydronephrosis. *Upper right:* Renal hamartoma (angiomyolipoma). Hypervascular mass with abnormal vasculature. Hamartomas are usually indistinguishable angiographically from renal cell carcinomas. 13-year-old boy with tuberous sclerosis and bilateral renal masses. *Lower left:* Intrarenal hematoma. Renal artery branches are draped about a large intrarenal hematoma (H) secondary to hemorrhage from one or more renal angiomyolipomas (*arrows*). 28-year-old woman with tuberous sclerosis, right flank pain, gross hematuria, and falling hematocrit. *Lower right:* Transverse kidney fracture (*arrows*). Two arteries to the lower pole are still patent and supply blood to some of the separated lower fragment. 47-year-old man with gross hematuria following motor vehicle accident.

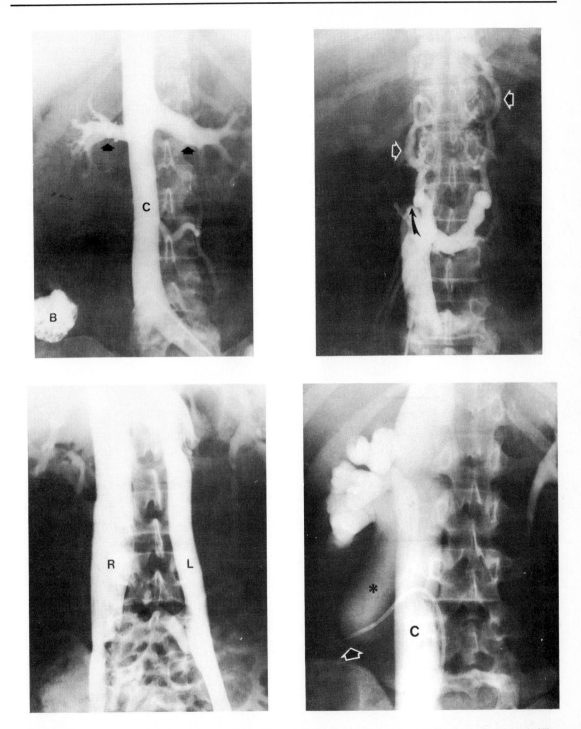

Figure 6–24. Angiography: inferior venacavography. *Upper left:* Normal inferior vena cava (C). Unusual retrograde filling of morphologically normal renal veins (*arrows*) from antegrade injection into the inferior vena cava is probably due to reduced venous outflow from the kidneys with the patient in Valsalva maneuver. B = retained contrast material in the cecum from previous barium enema examination. Woman with arteriolar nephrosclerosis and renal failure. *Upper right:* Inferior vena cava obstruction. Complete block of the vena cava (*curved arrow*) by extension from right renal vein of tumor thrombus from a right renal carcinoma. Note cephalad blood return via the paralumbar veins (*straight arrows*). 60-year-old man with gross hematuria. *Lower left:* Double inferior vena cava (R, L). Persistent left supracardinal vein anomaly. 23-year-old man after orchiectomy for testicular teratocarcinoma. *Lower right:* Retrocaval ureter. Hydronephrosis and proximal ureterectasis secondary to congenitally abnormal course of the right ureter behind the inferior vena cava (C). Catheter is in the right ureter, with its tip (*arrow*) at the lower curve of the redundant, dilated proximal ureter (*). 17-year-old girl with history of pyelonephritis.

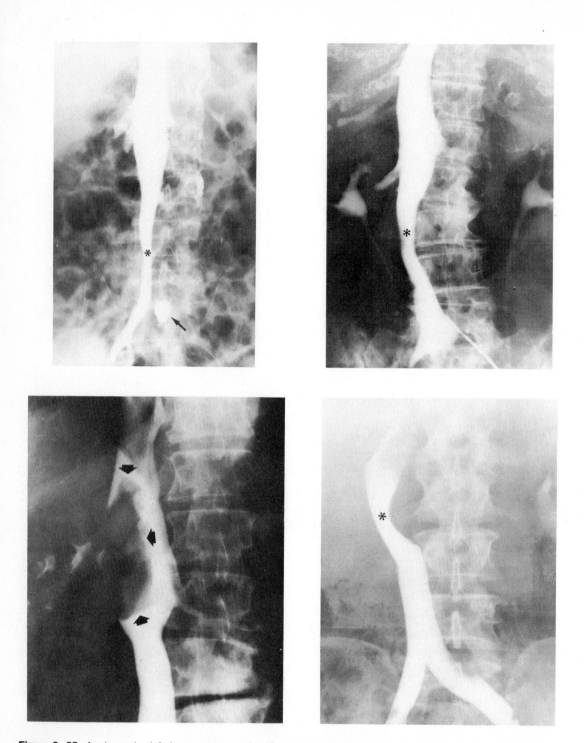

Figure 6–25. Angiography: inferior venacavography. *Upper left:* Idiopathic retroperitoneal fibrosis. Circumferential narrowing (*) of the infrarenal vena cava. Arrow = residual contrast medium in the spinal canal from previous myelogram. 47-year-old man with proteinuria and rapidly progressive renal failure. *Upper right:* Adenopathy due to metastatic bladder carcinoma. Metastatic lymph node masses displacing and narrowing the midlumbar inferior vena cava (*) from the left. 81-year-old man with edema of the left leg after carcinoma of the bladder and urethra. *Lower left:* Tumor thrombus. Renal cell carcinoma of the right kidney with filling defect of tumor thrombus extending from the renal vein into the vena cava (*arrows*). 62-year-old man with hematuria. *Lower right:* Lymphoma. Large lymphomatous nodes deforming and narrowing the inferior vena cava from the left (*) at the level of the kidneys. 58-year-old man with splenomegaly.

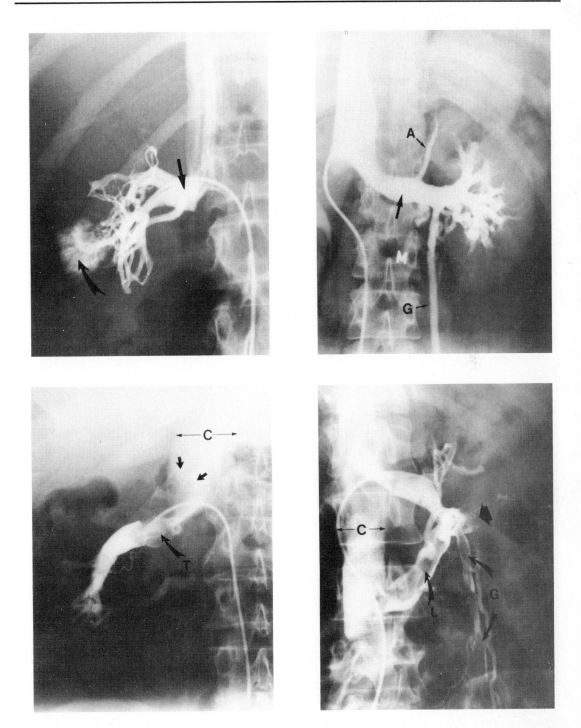

Figure 6–26. Angiography: renal venography. *Upper left:* Normal right renal vein. The right renal vein (*straight arrow*) is short and, unlike the left renal vein, does not receive the adrenal or gonadal vein; these veins empty directly into the inferior vena cava. Curved arrow = segmental intravasation of contrast medium from inadvertent wedging of the catheter tip in a small vein during injection. 19-year-old man with glomerulonephritis and nephrotic syndrome. *Upper right:* Normal left renal vein. On the left side, the adrenal (A) and gonadal (G) veins enter the renal vein (*arrow*). M = radiographic localization marker. Young woman with proteinuria. *Lower left:* Tumor thrombus. Straight arrow = upper margin of filling defect of the renal vein tumor thrombus (T) that extends into the vena cava (C). 68-year-old man with gross hematuria from adenocarcinoma of the right kidney. *Lower right:* Circumaortic left renal vein thrombosis. The catheter is in the patent upper limb of the venous anomaly. There is thrombosis of the intrarenal vein (*straight arrow*), with extension of thrombus into the lower limb (L) of the circumaortic renal vein and into the gonadal vein (G). C = inferior vena cava. 54-year-old man with nephrotic syndrome and edema of the legs and scrotum.

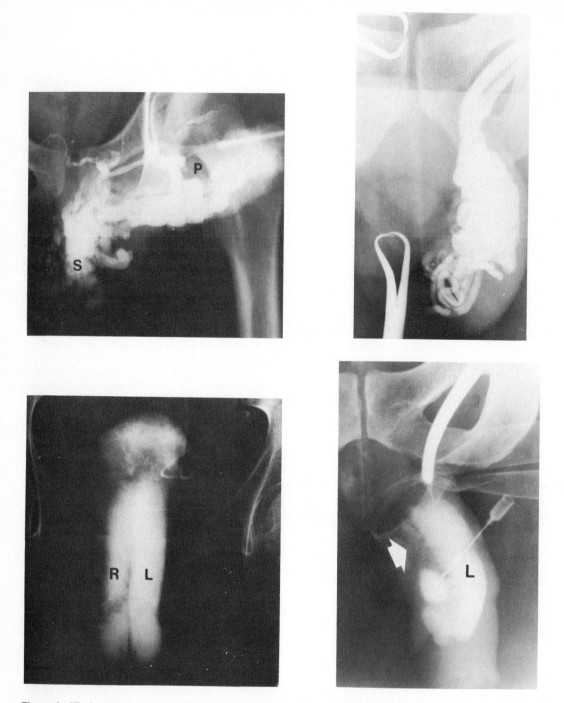

Figure 6–27. Angiography: miscellaneous urovenography. *Upper left:* Penoscrotal varices. Penile venography. Many tortuous veins in the penis (P) and scrotum (S). 14-year-old boy with long-standing penile and scrotal varicosities and numerous scrotal phleboliths. *Upper right:* Varicocele. Gonadal venography. Dilated, tortuous varicosities of the pampiniform plexus in the left scrotum. 31-year-old man with recurrence of scrotal pain after varicocele ligation. *Lower left:* Normal corpora cavernosogram. Injection of contrast medium into the left corpus (L), with normal (albeit slightly less) filling of the right corpus (R). 57-year-old man with impotence. *Lower right:* Penile fibrosis. Corpora cavernosogram. Injection of right corpus produces no filling of the proximal right corpus (*arrow*); there is normal filling of the left corpus (L). 33-year-old man with "crooked penis" following unsuccessful penile prosthesis operation.

The need for adrenal angiography has been reduced because sonography, CT scanning, and magnetic resonance tomography are increasingly effective for adrenal imaging.

Miscellaneous Urologic Angiography (Fig 6–27)

Although angiography has little or no value in examination of the ureter, bladder, and prostate, angiograms of these structures may be indicated in particular clinical situations, in which case the studies are usually "tailored" to the clinical problem.

Corpus cavernosograms are made by direct injection of suitable contrast material into the corpora cavernosa of the penis. They can be useful in examining for Peyronie's disease, impotence, priapism, and traumatic penile lesions but are not commonly performed.

8. RADIOGRAPHIC SUBTRACTION

Images of all body structures through which x-rays have passed are included in conventional radiograms, with the result that images of structures of little or no interest are invariably superimposed on and obscuring those of clinical importance. Radiographic subtraction is a technique for removing (subtracting) unwanted shadows on the radiogram, leaving only the images of pertinent structures.

Until recently, radiographic subtraction has been a time-consuming manual process (Fig 6–28). Computerized image subtraction has now been incorporated into radiographic systems. Such systems include image intensifiers and digital computers that electronically convert the information in the intensified images into digits which are automatically compared, subtracted, and reformatted to display a subtracted image for immediate inspection.

At present, computerized radiographic subtraction is used almost exclusively in angiographic studies **(digital angiography).** With computerized radiographic subtraction equipment, it is possible to obtain satisfactory arteriograms of larger vessels, eg, the aorta, extracranial carotid arteries, and main renal arteries, with intravenous injection of radiopaque contrast medium and thus avoid the more invasive procedures involving arterial punctures and catheterization.

Other radiographic subtraction systems now being developed (energy-selective radiography) have the potential to make radiographic subtraction possible in all radiographic studies. For example, use of dual-energy radiographic systems will permit selective subtraction of obscuring shadows due to bowel gas or bone from excretory urograms, leaving only unobscured urographic images.

SONOGRAPHY

Basic Principles

Sound is the propagation of a cyclic vibratory motion through a deformable medium. Sound is not an electromagnetic wave and, unlike x-rays, radiowaves, or visible light, cannot travel through a vacuum. A wave frequency of one cycle per second (cps) is called a hertz (Hz). Sound frequencies greater than 20 kHz are beyond the range of human hearing and are called ultrasound. Medical sonography uses ultrasound apparatuses to produce body images. The frequencies commonly used in medical sonography are 2.25, 3.5, and 5 MHz.

Ultrasound waves for imaging are generated by transducers, devices that convert electrical energy to sound energy and vice versa. These transducers are special piezoelectric crystals that emit ultrasound waves when they are deformed as an electrical voltage is applied and, conversely, generate an electrical potential when struck by reflected sound waves. Thus, they act as both sound transmitters and sound detectors. In imaging, repeated bursts of ultrasound from the transducer are transmitted through tissues. Between transmissions, the transducer acts as a sound receiver.

Ultrasound imaging is based on the principle that acoustic energy is differentially attenuated by tissues of varying density, in somewhat the same way as x-rays are. But unlike radiograms, ultrasound images are *reflection* images formed when part of the sound that was emitted by the transducer bounces back from tissue interfaces to the transducer. These reflected sounds vary in intensity and time according to the nature and location of the tissues from which they are reflected. In general concept, medical sonography resembles sonar.

The reflected sound energies are received by the transducer and converted into electrical signals that are amplified and stored in a computer. The information is converted by the computer into analog echo images of the acoustical profile of the tissues being examined. The images can be viewed directly in real time; permanently recorded on hard copy, film, or videotape; or both.

Clinical Sonographic Imaging

Sonography produces good images of the urinary tract (Figs 6–29 through 6–33) and is being used increasingly as the initial screening procedure in suspected urinary tract disease, particularly when exposure to x-rays is undesirable or intravenous contrast medium is contraindicated.

The renal calices and central sinus tissues produce strong sonographic echoes; echoes from the renal pyramid are less intense; and those from the renal cortex are of intermediate strength—slightly less intense than those from the liver. Uncomplicated cysts and ordinary fluid-filled structures (eg, a distended bladder,

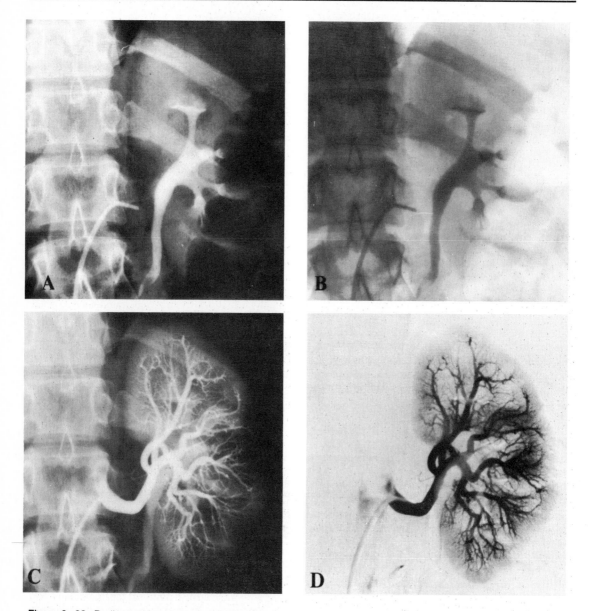

Figure 6–28. Radiographic subtraction. Radiograms A–D illustrate the theory and the steps taken to obtain subtraction radiograms manually. Computerized digital subtraction has replaced this laborious manual process. *A:* Left kidney urogram with angiographic catheter in left renal artery. The kidney is excreting contrast medium from an earlier aortorenal arteriogram. *B:* "Mask" made by exposing radiogram *A* on subtraction "masking" film. *C:* Renal arteriogram taken immediately after film *A. D:* Final subtraction film, made by exposing carefully superimposed "mask" (*B*) and arteriogram (*C*) on subtraction "print" film. Obscuring images of bones, bowel gas, and renal collecting structures have been removed (subtracted) almost completely.

a dilated ureter, or hydronephrosis) are anechoic, whereas renal tumors, complicated cysts, and abscesses produce echoes to varying degrees ranging from minimal to intense. Renal hamartomas are usually hyperechoic.

Sonography is the primary method of examining a fetus suspected of having major urinary tract disease, particularly obstructive disease. It is the method of choice in some cases and is excellent for examination of many types of urinary tract abnormalities, including congenital, acquired, obstructive, and nonobstructive

lesions. It is useful in examination of kidneys not visualized by excretory urography, in renal transplant problems, and in testicular and scrotal diseases. It is very useful to determine localization for percutaneous aspiration and for biopsy.

Advantages & Disadvantages

The advantages of sonography are its safety, noninvasiveness, excellent spatial and temporal resolution, relative speed of performing tests, inexpensiveness, and flexibility for imaging in many planes. The equip-

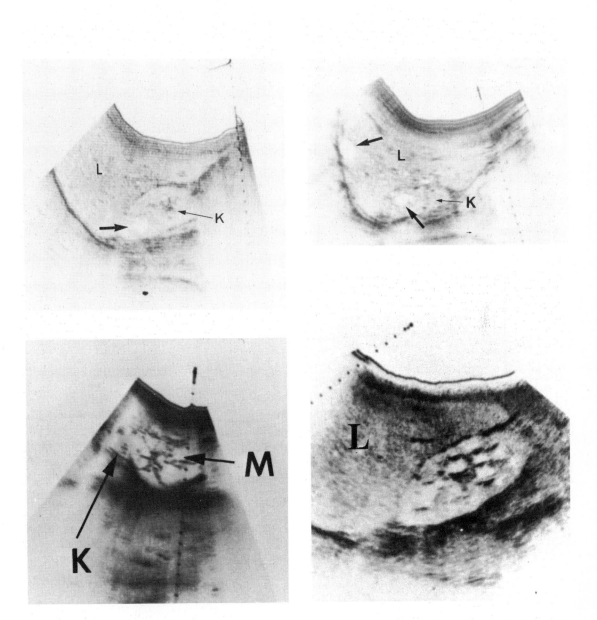

Figure 6–29. Sonography: kidney sonograms. *Upper left:* Simple renal cyst. Anechoic right renal defect (*arrow*). K = kidney; L = liver. *Upper right:* Cysts (*arrows*) in dome of liver (L) and in kidney (K). Young adult with polycystic kidney disease. *Lower left:* Multilocular cyst. Longitudinal scan shows hyperechoic strands and septums in an otherwise hypoechoic mass (M) in the lower pole of the left kidney (K). 16-month-old girl with left flank mass. *Lower right:* Hydronephrosis. Dilated hypoechoic calices are well seen. L = liver. Adult with right flank pain.

ment is relatively small in comparison with other imaging equipment and is mobile.

The major disadvantages of sonography are that structures behind bones or bowel gas cannot be imaged, there is a low signal-to-noise ratio, special training is necessary for proper interpretation of sonograms, and a skilled operator is required.

CT SCANNING
(Computed Body Tomography)

Basic Principles

In radiography, a broad beam of x-rays passes through the subject to produce an image on a detector, the x-ray film. In CT scanning, a thin, collimated

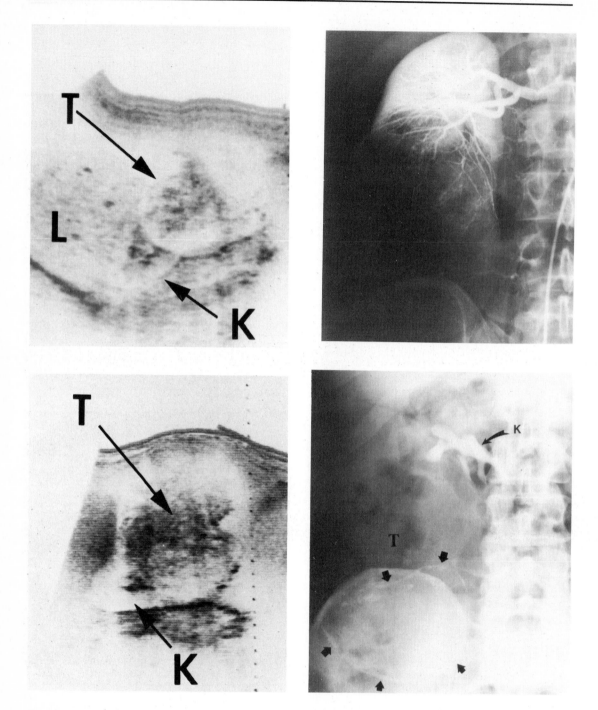

Figure 6–30. Sonography: kidney sonograms with other imaging studies for comparison. *Upper left:* Renal cell carcinoma. Longitudinal scan through liver (L), right kidney (K), and kidney tumor (T). The tumor has irregular central hyperechoic tissue. 60-year-old man with right flank pain and hematuria. See comparative arteriogram at right. *Upper right:* Selective right renal arteriogram, same patient. The tumor mass is almost avascular, with equivocal appearance of arterial vessels at the tumor-kidney interface. The sonogram and the arteriogram were complementary, but the sonogram was more definitive. *Lower left:* Benign hemorrhagic cyst with cyst wall calcification. Appearance similar to that of sonogram above, with large hyperechoic mass (T) of lower pole of right kidney (K). Old blood products in the cyst produced the hyperechogenicity. Sonographic diagnosis: malignant renal tumor. 59-year-old diabetic with gout, hypertension, and right abdominal mass. See comparative excretory urogram at right. *Lower right:* Excretory urogram, same patient. Right kidney (K) displaced and collecting structures indented by a huge mass (T) with curvilinear calcifications (*arrows*) in its lowest half. Excretory urographic diagnosis: renal mass with curvilinear calcification, cyst versus tumor. The sonogram and the excretory urogram were complementary studies, but neither gave the correct diagnosis.

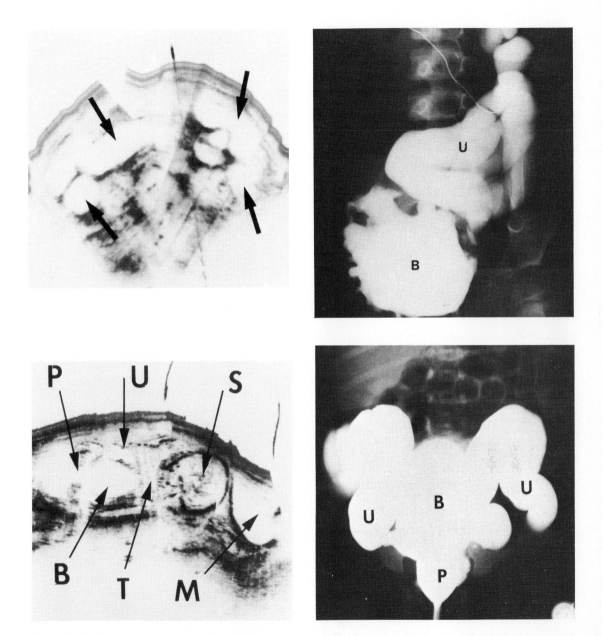

Figure 6–31. Sonography: urinary tract sonograms with other imaging studies for comparison. *Upper left:* Hydroureterectasis. Transverse abdominal scan demonstrating large, bilateral, redundant, anechoic structures (*arrows*). 9-year-old boy with prune belly syndrome and renal failure. *Upper right:* Same patient, cystourethrogram. Bladder (B) diverticulosis and trabeculation with vesicoureteral reflux into dilated, redundant left ureter (U). No right vesicoureteral reflux. The sonogram had demonstrated the bilateral ureterectasis. *Lower left:* Posterior urethral valves. Longitudinal in utero (fetal) sonogram. The fetal bladder (B) is grossly distended, and the posterior urethra (P) and one ureter (U) of the fetus are dilated. M = maternal bladder; S = fetal skull; T = fetal thorax. *Lower right:* Cystourethrogram, same patient as fetal sonogram. Newborn with bilateral vesicoureteral reflux. Dilated ureters (U) and prostatic urethra (P). B = bladder.

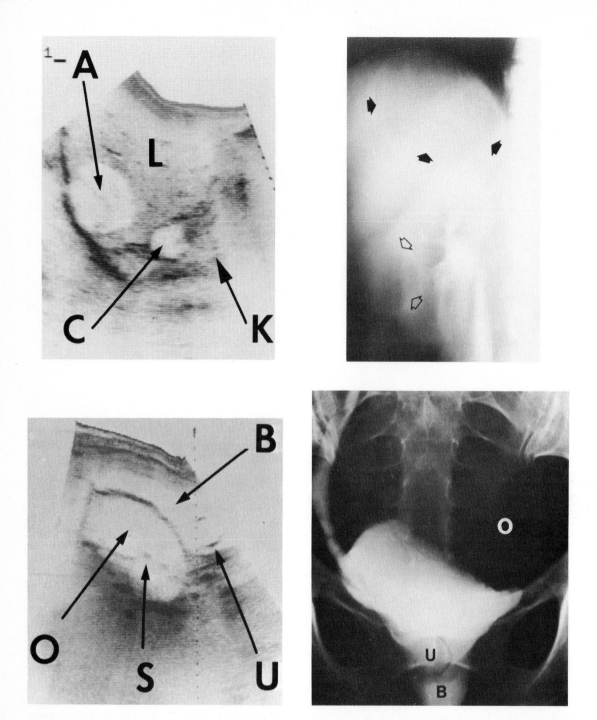

Figure 6–32. Sonography: kidney and bladder sonograms with other imaging studies for comparison. *Upper left:* Simple renal cyst and amebic liver abscess. Longitudinal scan through liver (L) and kidney (K) demonstrates an anechoic simple renal cyst (C) and an amebic liver abscess with some internal echoes (A). 68-year-old man with prostatism and history of amebic liver abscess. *Upper right:* Simple renal cyst (*open arrows*) and amebic liver abscess (*solid arrows*). Excretory urogram (tomogram). Compare with sonogram of same patient (*at left*). *Lower left:* Bladder neck and ureterocele prolapse into vagina and septated ovarian cyst. Longitudinal scan shows bladder (B), ureterocele (U), and a cystic ovarian retro-vesical mass (O) containing hyperechoic septations (S). 68-year-old woman with history of hysterectomy for uterine pro-lapse. *Lower right:* Cystogram from excretory urogram, same patient. Compare with sonogram at left. The bladder pro-lapse (B) and ureterocele (U) are well shown, and a right ureterectasis is evident; the paravesical mass compressing the bladder is shown (O), but its cystic nature is not apparent.

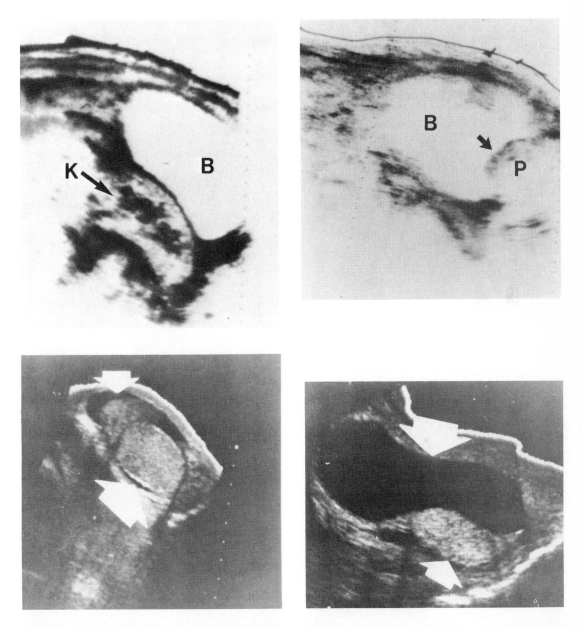

Figure 6–33. Sonography: pelvis and scrotum. *Upper left:* Pelvic kidney. Longitudinal scan shows ectopic hydronephrotic kidney (K) indenting the bladder (B). *Upper right:* Enlarged prostate. The hyperplastic prostate (P) indents the bladder (B). *Lower left:* Epididymitis and hydrocele. Normal testicle (*large arrow*), anechoic hydrocele, and swollen epididymis (*small arrow*). *Lower right:* Hydrocele. Longitudinal scan of normal testicle (*small arrow*) with large anechoic hydrocele (*large arrow*).

beam of x-rays is passed through the subject, and the detector is some type of phototube or ionization chamber rather than x-ray film. CT scans give remarkable definition of body anatomy (Figs 6–34 through 6–37).

When scanning, the interconnected x-ray source and detector system is rapidly rotated in the gantry around the recumbent patient, the detectors recording a number of transmitted x-rays during the very short scan period. Digital computers assemble and integrate the collected information as directed by the operator at the CT console. The information is finally reconstructed into a cross-sectional image (tomogram) that is displayed directly on a television screen. The image can be photographed, stored in digital form for later retrieval, or both. The newest CT scanners have scanning cycles of less than 2 seconds, and scanners with much shorter scanning times are being developed.

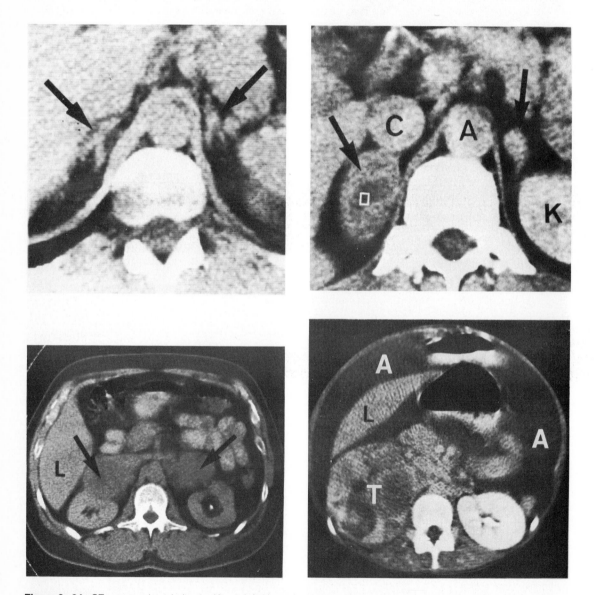

Figure 6–34. CT scans: adrenal glands. *Upper left:* Normal adrenals. At this level, in this patient, both adrenals (*arrows*) have an inverted Y shape. 34-year-old man with extra-adrenal pheochromocytoma. *Upper right:* Bilateral pheochromocytomas (*arrows*). Larger tumor on the right has a lower attenuation center (*cursor*). A = aorta; C = inferior vena cava; K = left kidney. 33-year-old man with multiple endocrine adenomatosis syndrome, after parathyroid adenoma and parathyroid carcinoma, with family history of medullary carcinoma. *Lower left:* Bilateral adrenal lymphoma. Enlarged adrenal glands (*arrows*) anterior to normal kidneys. L = liver. 53-year-old man with abdominal pain and histiocytic lymphoma of the central nervous system. *Lower right:* Carcinoma of the right adrenal. Scan through normal left kidney and large cystic and necrotic retrohepatic adrenal tumor (T). A = ascites; L = liver. 17-year-old girl with right abdominal mass and ascites.

Clinical CT Scanning

Because collapsed or fluid-filled loops of bowel can mimic soft tissue masses on CT images, radiopaque contrast medium is administered orally or rectally at the time of the CT study to identify gastrointestinal structures. Radiopaque contrast medium may also be injected intravascularly at the time of the scan to produce contrast delineation of the urinary tract and vascular structures (the so-called enhanced CT scan).

Radiograms and CT scans are reflections of the amount of x-rays reaching the respective detectors after passing through body tissues. Tissues that absorb much of the x-ray beam, eg, bone, will appear as white (radiopaque) shadows on the CT scan, just as they do on conventional radiograms; tissues that absorb little photon energy, eg, fat and gas, record as black (radiolucent) shadows. Body tissues have their own individual radioattenuating values, denoted by CT numbers. Water has been assigned a CT number of 0; fat and gas have negative CT numbers; bone and metal have positive CT numbers; and soft tissues have various positive CT numbers greater than 0 (the CT number of water) but less than the CT number of bone. The value at any point on the CT scan can easily be determined by the CT apparatus.

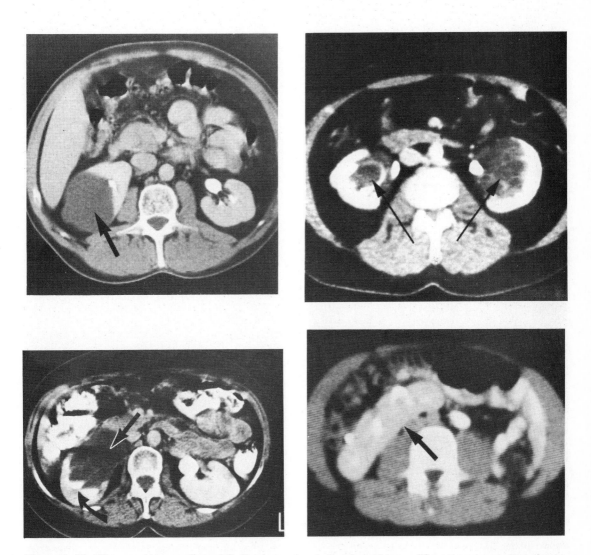

Figure 6–35. CT scans: kidneys. *Upper left:* Simple renal cyst. Cyst (*arrow*) has a CT number close to that of water. 49-year-old man with flank pain. *Upper right:* Bilateral peripelvic cysts (*arrows*). 52-year-old man with right flank mass found on routine physical examination. *Lower left:* Hydronephrosis. Dilated right renal pelvis (*straight arrow*) with layering of excreted contrast medium in distended calices (*curved arrow*). 54-year-old woman with obstructed distal right ureter from ovarian carcinoma. *Lower right:* Crossed fused renal ectopia (*arrow*). 14-year-old asymptomatic boy with abdominal mass palpated on school medical examination.

The most eye-pleasing CT scans are in patients with large amounts of body fat, because the black CT image of fat throws the tissues and organs with higher CT numbers into sharp relief. Renal cysts have CT numbers close to that of water and lower than those of tumors, complicated cysts, and abscesses. Angiomyolipomas have negative CT numbers corresponding to their fat content.

Although CT scanning can be used to image all parts of the urinary tract, it is used almost exclusively for examination of the abdominal and pelvic urinary tract. CT scanning is effective for staging and following urologic tumors and for determining localization for percutaneous aspiration and biopsy. With the increasing use of CT scanning alone or combined with sonography, there has been a sharp decrease in the use of conventional and invasive radiographic studies of the urinary tract.

Advantages & Disadvantages

The advantages of CT scanning of the urinary tract are that it demonstrates organ morphology, particularly of retroperitoneal structures, exceptionally well; is relatively easy to interpret without special training; and can be done on an outpatient basis.

Its disadvantages are its basis in ionizing radiation; the cost, size, and immobility of the equipment; and the cost of the studies, which are more expensive than sonography and most radiographic examinations.

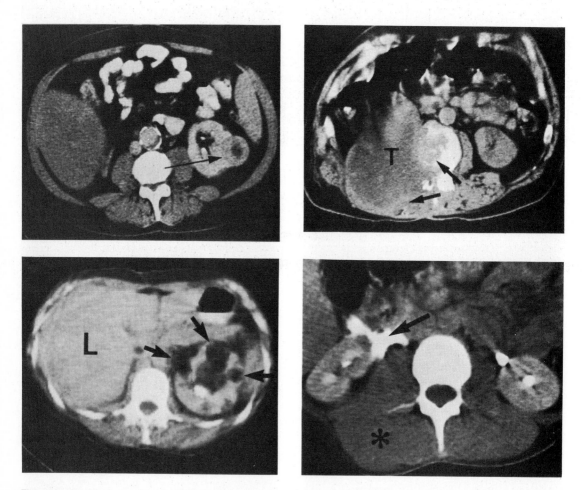

Figure 6–36. CT scans: kidneys. *Upper left:* Renal cell carcinoma. The left renal tumor (*arrow*) shows central necrosis. Note calcification in the arteriosclerotic abdominal aorta. 61-year-old man with previous right nephrectomy for renal carcinoma. *Upper right:* Recurrent renal adenocarcinoma. Massive recurrence in right renal fossa (T), with extensive invasion of posterior soft tissues and destruction of vertebral bodies (*arrows*). 51-year-old man after right nephrectomy for carcinoma. *Lower left:* Renal angiomyolipomas. Multiple low-attenuation mass lesions in the left kidney (*arrows*) with negative CT numbers compatible with fat. L = liver. 35-year-old woman with multiple bilateral renal hamartomas. *Lower right:* Right renal pelvic laceration. Enhanced CT scan through the kidneys showing extravasation of radiopaque material (*arrow*). Hemorrhage into the psoas and back muscles has enlarged their image (*). 22-year-old man with laceration of the right renal pelvis due to a stab wound.

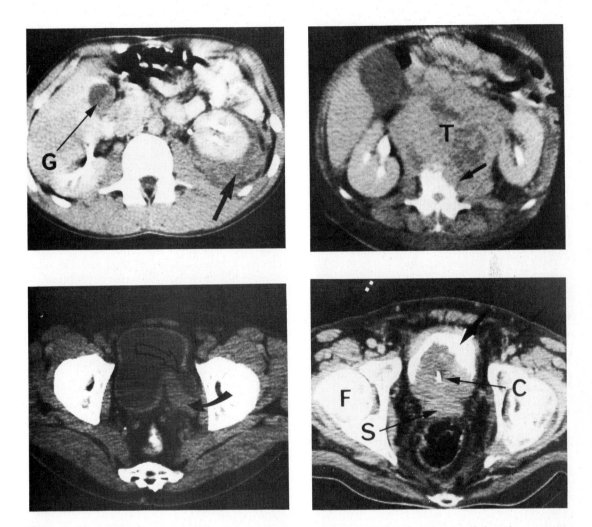

Figure 6–37. CT scans: retroperitoneum, bladder, prostate. *Upper left:* Perirenal hematoma. Hematoma (*arrow*) displaces the left kidney anteriorly. G = gallbladder. 16-year-old boy with acute glomerulonephritis; low-grade fever and left flank pain following left renal biopsy. *Upper right:* Retroperitoneal metastatic seminoma. Huge retroperitoneal mass of metastatic nodes (T) destroying vertebral body (*arrow*), obliterating outlines of central abdominal and retroperitoneal structures, and displacing kidneys laterally and bowel anteriorly. 46-year-old man with metastatic anaplastic testicular seminoma. *Lower left:* Transitional cell carcinoma in a bladder diverticulum. Open arrow points to mouth of diverticulum; solid arrow points to tumor of posterior wall of diverticulum. 65-year-old man with microhematuria. *Lower right:* Prostatic carcinoma. Irregular margin of enlarged prostate indenting posterior bladder (*arrow*). C = transurethral catheter; S = seminal vesicles; F = head of femur, 65-year-old man with prostatic carcinoma invading the bladder, seminal vesicles, and perirectal tissues.

MAGNETIC RESONANCE (MR) IMAGING (Nuclear Magnetic Resonance [NMR] Tomography)

Basic Principles

Clinical MR anatomic imaging has its basis in the nuclear properties of the hydrogen atoms in the body. The nucleus of a hydrogen atom consists of a single proton. Any atom containing an odd total number of protons and neutrons has the nuclear property of spin, with the result that the nucleus behaves like a tiny magnet.

Ordinarily, the axes of spin of the hydrogen nuclei in the body are randomly oriented. However, if the whole body or part of it is placed in a strong magnetic field (like that produced in MR imagers by large magnets housed in suitable gantries), the hydrogen nuclei of the body part within the magnetic field precess (wobble like a top) around the lines of magnetic force.

If these hydrogen nuclei in the magnetic field are then additionally stimulated by very short pulses of radiowaves of appropriate frequency, they absorb energy and invert their orientation with respect to the magnetic field, ie, they are elevated to a state of higher energy. Once the short radiofrequency pulse terminates, the hydrogen nuclei return at various speeds to their original (low-energy) orientation in the magnetic field, emitting energy in the form of radiowaves in the process. This phenomenon is called nuclear magnetic resonance. The hydrogen nuclei continue to resonate as long as the radiowave pulses continue. The emitted energies from the resonating hydrogen nuclei are collected and form the basis of the final MR scan.

MR tomographic images are reflections of the hydrogen densities in the various body tissues, modified importantly by the differing physical, cellular, and chemical microenvironments and any flow (fluid) characteristics of the tissues. Whereas x-rays have a directional element the point of origin and direction of which can be controlled, the energy signals emitted from nuclei under MR investigation contain no innate information defining their origin. In MR imaging, that information is obtained by the use of added gradient magnetic coils which vary the magnetic field in space, thereby changing the nature of the emitted MR signals from the different body regions to permit exact localization of the hydrogen nuclei emitting the signals.

There are biologically important nuclei other than hydrogen that are MR-sensitive, including those of phosphorus, sodium, and potassium, but these more complex nuclei have lower inherent sensitivities to MR and occur in lower physiologic concentrations than hydrogen. The present lesser capacity of these nuclei to be imaged by MR notwithstanding, the potential use of imaging these nuclei for tissue typing and mapping and as biologic tracers (MR spectroscopy) is under intense research and development. Although the principles of MR have been applied in chemistry for many years, the first MR image (of water in thin-walled glass capillaries) was produced only a little more than a decade ago. In the short time since this first crude MR image was made, the development of appropriate magnets, computers, related electronic equipment, and imaging technology has resulted in the availability of MR units capable of collecting the re-emitted radiowave signals, converting them to digits, coding them spatially, and reconstructing the information into tomographic body images that resemble CT scans (Figs 6–38 through 6–41).

Although there are still only a relatively small number of MR systems currently in operation, it is agreed that MR is potentially the most powerful and versatile imaging technique in medicine.

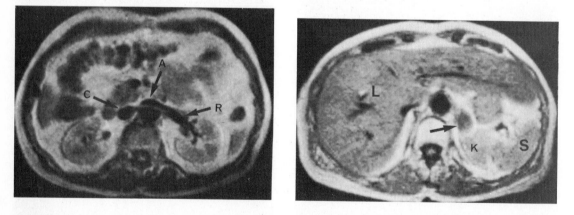

Figure 6–38. MR imaging: transverse scan of kidneys and adrenals. *Left:* Normal kidneys. Perinephric fat registers an intense (white) MR signal, the opposite of the black image of fat on CT scans. Moving blood in the renal vessels (R), aorta (A), and inferior vena cava (C) is MR-silent, rendering black images. *Right:* Carcinoid tumor metastatic to left adrenal (arrow). High-intensity (white) images of fat separate the enlarged adrenal silhouette from the left kidney (K). L = liver; S = spleen.

Clinical MR Imaging
(Figs 6–38 through 6–41)

In MR imaging, rigidly bound hydrogen nuclei, eg, those in compact bone and other calcified structures (like arteriosclerotic plaques), register as black zones on the MR image, ie, they are MR-silent.

Hydrogen nuclei that move through the plane of imaging too rapidly to register an MR signal are also MR-silent, ie, they register as black zones on the image. Approximately 50 milliseconds are required to register the MR signal from protons in a field. Thus, moving blood, for example, is imaged in various shades of black depending on the rate of blood flow.

Fat is registered by MR as a bright, intense white image, the opposite of the black image it gives on radiograms and CT scans.

Tissues of the brain, spinal cord, viscera, and muscles produce MR signals of intensities between the brightest white images of fat and the black images of cortical bone. Bone marrow, because of its fat content, has a high-intensity (white) image.

Advantages & Disadvantages

There are many advantages to MR imaging. It uses no ionizing radiation, and no harmful genetic or somatic effects have been attributed to the energy ranges used for clinical imaging. No bowel preparation or fluid and food restrictions are necessary, and contrast media are not required to distinguish the gastrointestinal tract or vascular structures. Paramagnetic contrast agents are now being developed that should further enhance the advantages of MR in the near future. MR offers great flexibility for imaging in many planes—axial, sagittal, and coronal planes being the most useful clinically. The images produced by MR give spatial resolution superior to that obtained with ultrasound, with more specific tissue characterization. Indeed, MR gives better information about soft tissues than any other method of imaging.

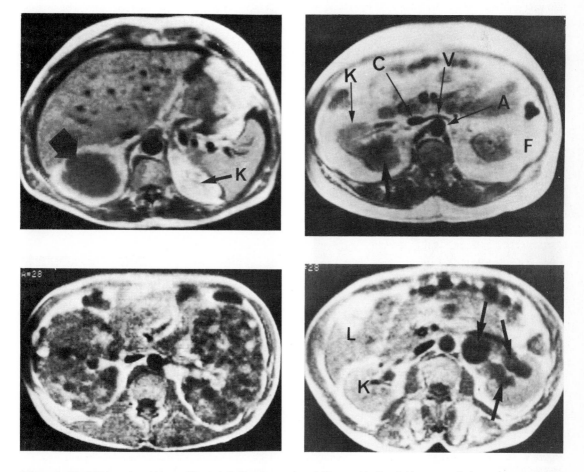

Figure 6–39. MR imaging: kidney. *Upper left:* Simple renal cyst. The cyst in the right upper pole (*arrow*) appears as a low-intensity structure. K = left kidney. *Upper right:* Renal cell carcinoma. The tumor (*arrow*) bulges from the posteromedial aspect of the right kidney (K). Retroperitoneal fat (F) surrounds the kidneys and has an intense MR image. V = left renal vein crossing anterior to aorta (A) to enter the inferior vena cava (C). Note the MR silence (black) of moving blood in these vessels. *Lower left:* Polycystic kidney disease. Huge kidneys with numerous cysts of differing MR image intensities. *Lower right:* Hydroureteronephrosis. Arrows = low-intensity MR signal of urine in dilated calices and pelvis; K = normal right kidney; L = liver.

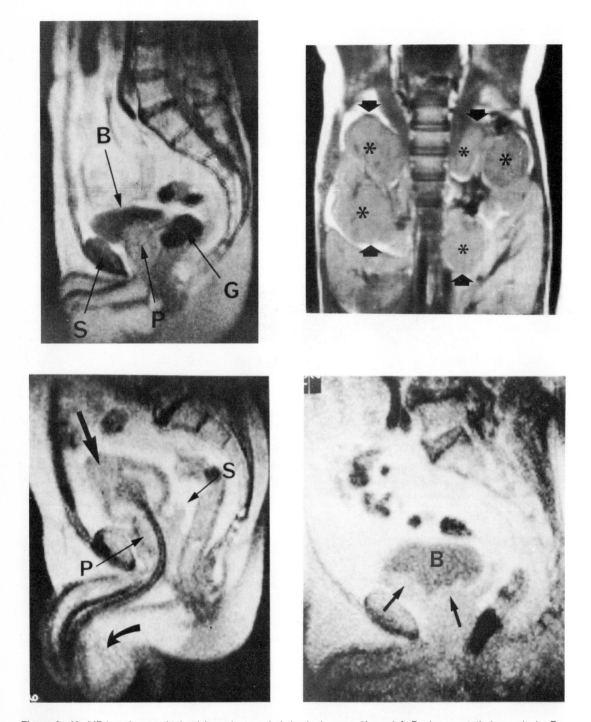

Figure 6–40. MR imaging: sagittal pelvic and coronal abdominal scans. *Upper left:* Benign prostatic hyperplasia. Enlarged prostate (P) indents the base of the bladder (B). G = gas in rectum; S = pubic symphysis. *Upper right:* Enlarged kidneys (*arrows*) from bilateral multifocal Wilms' tumors (asterisks). 3-year-old female with bilateral renal masses. *Lower left:* Bladder carcinoma. There is a transurethral Foley catheter in the bladder. P = prostate; S = seminal vesicle; curved arrow = scrotum; straight arrow = extensive bladder tumor. *Lower right:* Bladder carcinoma. Extensive tumor (*arrows*) irregularly indents the base of the bladder (B).

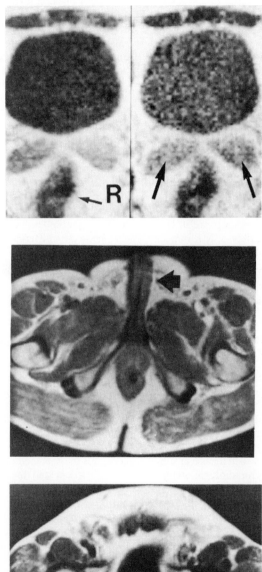

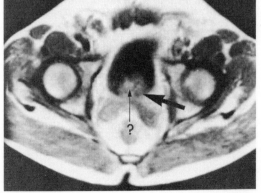

Figure 6–41. MR imaging: transverse pelvic scans. *Top:* Normal bladder and seminal vesicles (*arrows*). Two different imaging modes are shown. R = rectum. *Center:* Normal penis (*arrow*) and pelvic structures. MR imaging provides excellent soft tissue differentiation. Note the intense (white) MR imaging of the perirectal and subcutaneous fat. *Bottom:* Enlarged prostate. The hyperplastic gland (*large arrow*) indents the bladder. The prostate also contained a focus of carcinoma, possibly the small area of more intense MR signal (?) indicated by the small arrow.

The disadvantages of MR imaging are as follows: MR has a low sensitivity for calcification and calcified lesions. Image acquisition takes longer than with CT scanning and much longer than the patient can halt respiration; consequently, some blurring of images occurs during breathing, especially in the upper abdomen. The equipment is large and expensive, and preparing a site for it is also expensive. The studies are expected to cost more than most other imaging procedures. Because a strong magnetic field is used, strict security measures are needed to prevent injury due to loose metallic objects being drawn into the magnetic field. Ferromagnetic surgical clips, especially on vessels in the brain, represent a potential hazard, and patients with metal joint replacements or pacemakers cannot be exposed to the powerful magnetic field used in MR imaging. The magnetic field and the radiofrequency pulses affect the functioning of nearby electronic equipment.

There are at present only a limited number of MR facilities in clinical operation, and most are in large medical centers. However, a number of MR imaging units are commercially available, and it is expected that many more MR facilities will soon exist.

COMPARISON OF IMAGING METHODS
(Figs 6–42 through 6–46.)

Radiography, sonography, CT scanning, and magnetic resonance tomography all have individual advantages and disadvantages. As new imaging methods have been developed, changes have occurred in both the amount each type of imaging is used and the purposes for which it is used. For example, increased familiarity with and confidence in sonography and CT scanning have resulted in a decrease in the use of some long-established conventional uroradiologic studies, eg, excretory urography, retrograde urography, and lymphography; and fewer adrenal and renal angiograms are being performed for strictly diagnostic purposes. MR imaging promises to produce another dramatic change in medical and urologic diagnosis once MR imaging equipment and trained personnel become more widely available.

Several factors are involved in these changes: (1) the increased effectiveness of newer imaging methods over older ones for some aspects of urodiagnosis; (2) the availability of equipment, trained technical personnel to operate it, and physicians to interpret the results; (3) increased awareness of the hazards of ionizing radiation, and (4) the desire to avoid using invasive diagnostic procedures if possible.

Because so many different types of imaging are available, each with different costs, risks, and areas of effectiveness, it may be difficult for the clinician to decide which method will yield the most information with the least cost and risk. A particular study may be critical in one specific diagnostic situation but useless in another. For example, sonography, CT scanning, and MR tomography are usually ineffective in demonstrating small uroepithelial tumors, and an excretory urogram is the study of choice for such lesions. Sonography is an excellent noninvasive, relatively inexpensive method for differentiating simple cysts from other mass lesions in the kidney but is much less effective in imaging the retroperitoneum than CT scanning. Sonography also relies considerably on the skill of the operator. Angiography can delineate the source and extent of vessels supplying blood to renal tumors, but the examination uses ionizing radiation and is moderately invasive and relatively expensive, commonly requiring a hospital stay. CT scanning produces excellent images and is currently the best available way to image the retroperitoneum and the method of choice for imaging the adrenal glands, but it is more expensive than other imaging studies. MR tomography, still in its early development and available in relatively few facilities, already rivals CT scanning in imaging capability; for certain structures, eg, the brain and spinal cord, it is the best method for anatomic imaging.

The patient and the clinician both benefit from careful consultation designed to ensure that the methods of imaging chosen are of value in diagnosis or treatment planning and do not duplicate or merely confirm established findings with loss of time and additional expense.

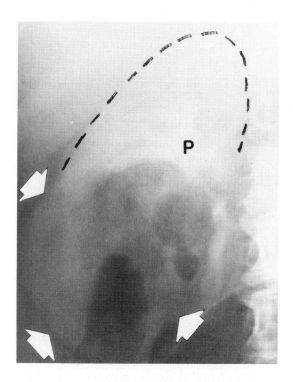

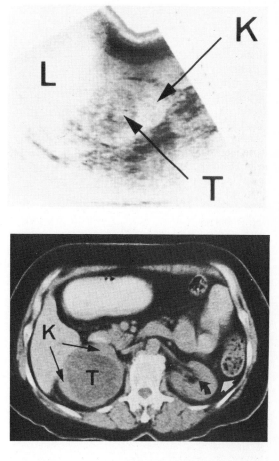

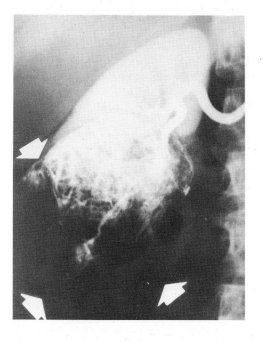

Figure 6–42. Comparison of imaging methods: adeno-carcinoma of the right kidney. 73-year-old woman with right flank pain and hematuria. *Upper left:* Excretory uro-gram. Renal pelvis (P) and lower calices displaced by a large, poorly outlined mass (*arrows*). Urographic diagno-sis: renal mass; question simple cyst versus tumor. *Upper right:* Sonogram. Longitudinal scan through liver (L), lat-eral portion of hyperechoic tumor (T), and lower pole of kidney (K). Sonographic diagnosis: probable angiomyo-lipoma. *Lower left:* Selective arteriogram of upper of 2 right renal arteries. Pathologic hypervascularity to upper part of tumor. The lower artery provided an equally hypervascular blood supply to lower portion of tumor between arrows. Angiographic diagnosis: renal carcinoma rather than an-giomyolipoma. *Lower right:* CT scan. The CT number of the tumor (T) is less than that of adjacent kidney pa-renchyma (K) enhanced by contrast medium and much greater than low-attenuation fat as seen in the left renal si-nus (*curved arrow*) and adjacent perinephric space (*straight arrow*). CT diagnosis: renal carcinoma.

In this patient, the CT examination was specific and ex-cluded the possibility of angiomyolipoma that was raised by the sonographic study.

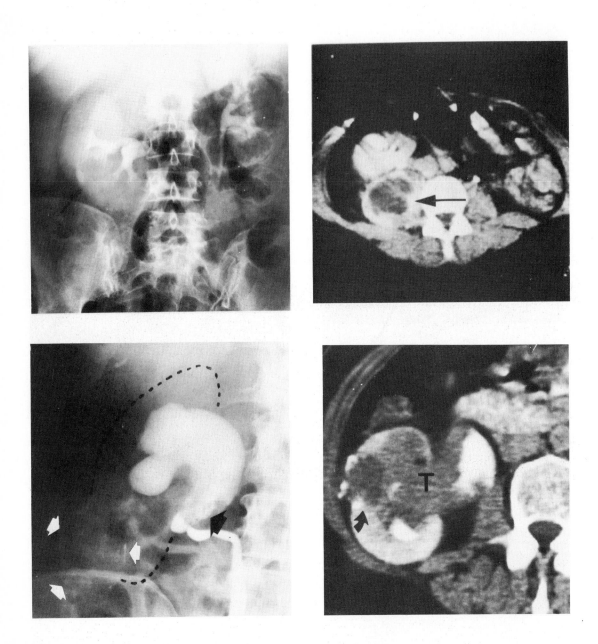

Figure 6–43. Comparison of imaging methods. *Upper left:* Psoas abscess. Excretory urogram reveals abnormal orientation of the right kidney and an enlarged right psoas muscle. *Upper right:* CT scan, same patient. CT imaging clearly identifies the psoas abscess (*arrow*). CT scanning is exceptionally helpful for imaging retroperitoneal structures. The abscess was drained percutaneously under CT control. *Lower left:* Transitional cell carcinoma and a calcified renal cyst. Retrograde urogram shows filling defects due to tumor in renal pelvis (*black arrow*) at ureteropelvic junction and eggshell calcification in a lower pole mass (*white arrows*). Note that the infundibulum and calices of the lower pole failed to opacify. 45-year-old woman with hematuria. *Lower right:* CT scan, same patient. The cystic nature of the calcified renal mass (*curved arrow*) is evident, and the CT scan shows better the considerable extent of the tumor (T), which involves most of the lower pole of the kidney and extends into the dilated renal pelvis.

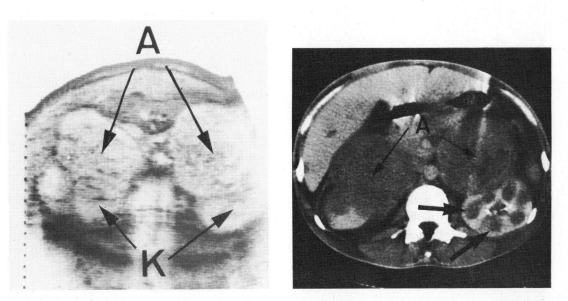

Figure 6–43 (cont'd) *Left:* Adrenal and renal lymphoma. Transverse sonographic scan through the kidneys (K). The adrenals (A) are greatly enlarged. The sonographic appearance of the kidneys is not diagnostic on this particular scan cut. 26-year-old man with fever, weight loss, adrenal insufficiency, and diffuse histiocytic lymphoma. *Right:* CT scan, same patient. Radiopaque contrast medium-enhanced study opacifies the renal parenchyma and highlights the lower-attenuation lymphomatous areas (*large arrows*). The massive adrenal enlargement (A) is well shown. Both sonography and CT scanning demonstrated the pathologic changes well.

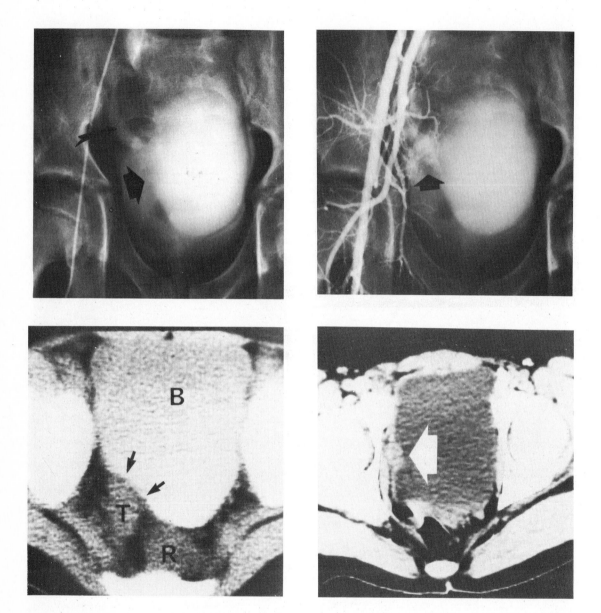

Figure 6–44. Comparison of imaging methods: metastatic extra-adrenal familial pheochromocytoma. 10-year-old boy with hypertension and seizures precipitated by abdominal palpation. Family history of multiple extra-adrenal pheochromocytomas in the mother. *Upper left:* Excretory urogram. The right ureter is dilated and elevated (*curved arrow*), with the right posterior portion of the bladder disposed toward the left (*straight arrow*). Urographic diagnosis: question extra-adrenal paravesical pheochromocytoma. *Upper right:* Right femoral arteriogram. Tumor stain (*arrow*) in right paravesical location. Angiographic diagnosis: extra-adrenal paravesical pheochromocytoma. *Lower left:* CT scan. Transverse tomogram through bladder (B) shows the tumor (T) indenting the bladder (*arrows*). R = rectum. *Lower right:* CT scan. Transverse tomogram through bladder. Recurrence of symptoms following removal of the right paravesical pheochromocytoma prompted another CT study, which shows recurrent tumor (*arrow*) in the bladder wall.

Each imaging study complemented or supplemented the previous one. None, however, diagnosed the small liver metastases discovered at surgery.

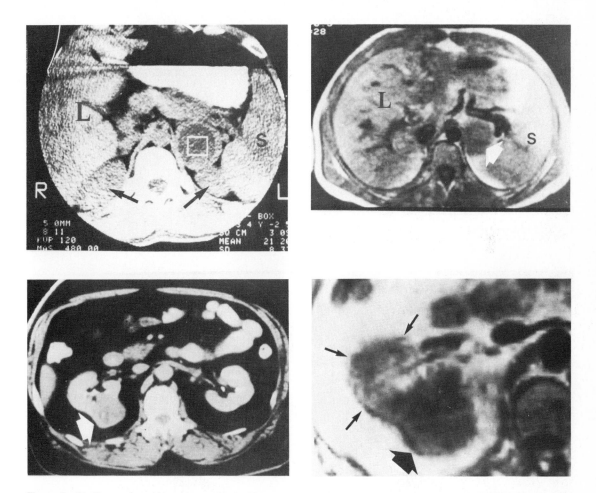

Figure 6–45. Comparison of imaging methods. *Upper left:* Adrenal pheochromocytoma. CT scan. The CT cursor is over a central cystic core of the left adrenal tumor. L = liver; S = spleen; arrows = upper poles of kidneys. 25-year-old man with 5-year history of paresthesias, palpitations, and sweating. *Upper right:* MR imaging, same patient. This MR tomogram was taken at a slightly higher level than the CT scan. The tomogram passes through the adrenal tumor (*arrow*) but is above the upper poles of kidneys. The cystic character of the tumor is not as evident as it was on the CT scan. *Lower left:* Renal cell carcinoma. CT scan. The tumor bulging from the posteromedial aspect of the right kidney (*arrow*) has irregular atten-uation areas representing necrotic zones within the cancer. The left kidney is normal. Note the low-attenuation CT image (black) of perirenal fat. Adult male with renal mass found on excretory urogram. *Lower right:* MR tomogram of right kidney, same patient. With the particular method used for this scan, the carcinoma (*large arrow*) has a less intense (blacker) MR image than the normal kidney (*small arrows*). Note the intense white MR image of retroperitoneal and perirenal fat.

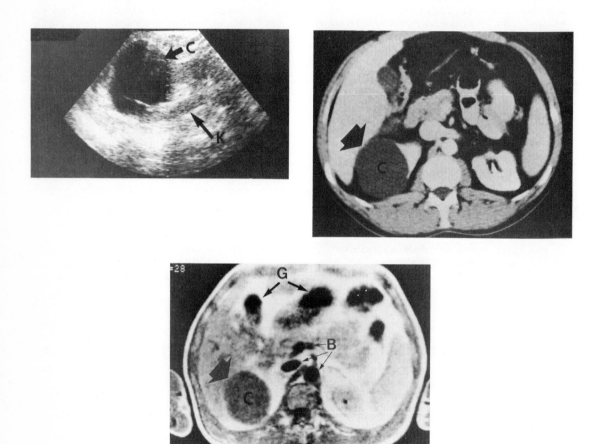

Figure 6–46. Comparison of imaging methods: simple cyst, left kidney. 49-year-old man with bilateral flank pain. *Upper left:* Sonogram. An anechoic right renal mass (C) is demonstrated, with a well-defined back wall and acoustic enhancement deep to the mass, findings diagnostic of a simple cyst of the kidney (K). *Upper right:* CT scan. This CT image adds no information about the right kidney and cyst that was not obtained from the sonogram. Note the low-attenuation CT image of the cyst (*C, arrow*), with a CT number about that of water. *Bottom:* MR tomogram. This study, made at a slightly higher level than the CT scan, also adds no information to that obtained from the sonogram. Compare the low-intensity MR image of the cyst fluid (C) with the MR silence of bowel gas (G) and moving blood (B) in the aorta, vena cava, and other vessels. The sonogram was a definitive diagnostic study in this patient, and the CT and MR examinations were unnecessary.

REFERENCES

Radiography

Abrams HL (editor): *Abrams Angiography: Vascular and Interventional Radiology,* 3rd ed. Little, Brown, 1983.

Alvarez RE, Cassel D: Film-based digital x-rays: Using energy-selective processing to subtract unwanted materials. *Diagn Imaging* (May) 1983;**52**:36.

Anton PA, Abramowsky CR: Adult polycystic renal disease presenting in infancy: A report emphasizing the bilateral involvement. *J Urol* 1982;**128**:1290.

Baker SR, Elkin M: *Plain Film Approach to Abdominal Calcifications.* Vol 21 of: *Monographs in Clinical Radiology.* Saunders, 1983.

Blickman JG, Taylor GA, Lebowitz RL: Voiding cystourethrography: The initial radiologic study in children with urinary tract infection. *Radiology* 1985;**156**:659.

Bolz KD, Skalpe IO, Gutteberg TJ: Iohexol and metrizoate in urography in children: Comparison between a nonionic and an ionic contrast medium. *Acta Radiol [Diagn]* 1984;**25**:155.

Choi SH, Anllo V: Left renal vein "nutcracker" phenomenon. *Urology* 1982;**20**:549.

Clark RA, Alexander ES: Digital subtraction angiography of the renal arteries: Prospective comparison with conventional arteriography. *Invest Radiol* 1983;**18**:6.

Davidson AJ (editor): *Radiology of the Kidney.* Saunders, 1985.

Doubilet P et al: Excretory urography in current practice: Evidence against overutilization. *Radiology* 1985;**154**:607.

Dyer R et al: The segmental nephrogram. *AJR* 1985;**145**:321.

Fanous H et al: Renal cell carcinoma extending into vena cava and right atrium. *Urology* 1983;**22**:215.

Ford K et al: Seminal vesiculography in evaluation of the infertile male. *Fertil Steril* 1982;**37**:552.

Friedland GW et al (editors): *Uroradiology: An Integrated Approach.* Churchill Livingstone, 1983.

Greenberger PA, Patterson R, Tapio CM: Prophylaxis against repeated radiocontrast media reactions in 857 cases: Adverse experience with cimetidine and safety of beta-adrenergic antagonists. *Arch Intern Med* 1985;**145**:2197.

Hartman GW et al: Mortality during excretory urography. *AJR* 1982;**139**:919.

Hatch TR, Barry JM: The value of excretory urography in staging bladder cancer. *J Urol* 1986;**135**:49.

Hendee WR: Real and perceived risks of medical radiation exposure. *West J Med* 1983;**138**:380.

Hoffer FA, Lebowitz RL: Intermittent hydronephrosis: A unique feature of ureteropelvic junction obstruction caused by a crossing renal vessel. *Radiology* 1985;**156**:655.

Kaude JV et al: Renal morphology and function immediately after extracorporeal shockwave lithotripsy. *AJR* 1985;**145**:305.

Kruger RA, Riederer SA: *Basic Concepts of Digital Subtraction Angiography.* Hall, 1984.

Kuchta SG, Manco LG, Evans JA: Prominent iliopsoas muscles producing a gourd-shaped deformity of the bladder. *J Urol* 1982;**127**:1188.

Kumar D et al: Case profile: Bilateral emphysematous pyelonephritis. *Urology* 1982;**20**:96.

Lang EK (editor): *Current Concepts of Uroradiology.* Williams & Wilkins, 1984.

Lebowitz RL et al: International system of radiographic grading of vesicoureteric reflux: International Reflux Study in Children. *Pediatr Radiol* 1985;**15**:105.

Leiberman E, Macchia RJ: Excretory urography in women with urinary tract infection. *J Urol* 1982;**127**:263.

Leiter E, Whitehead ED, Desai SB: Fungus balls in renal pelvis. *NY State J Med* 1982;**82**:64.

Leonidas JC et al: The one-film urogram in urinary tract infection in children. *AJR* 1983;**141**:61.

Lue TF et al: Functional evaluation of penile veins by cavernosography in papaverine-induced erection. *J Urol* 1986;**135**:479.

Michel JR: Radiological examination of the male urethra. *Medicamundi* 1982;**27**:77.

Moreau J-F, Mazzara L: *Intravenous Urography.* Wiley, 1983.

Nabizadeh I, Morehouse HT, Freed SZ: Hydatid disease of kidney. *Urology* 1983;**22**:176.

Nocks BN et al: Transitional cell carcinoma of renal pelvis. *Urology* 1982;**19**:472.

Panto PN, Davies P: Delayed reactions to urographic contrast media. *Br J Radiol* 1986;**59**:41.

Patriquin HB, O'Regan S: Medullary sponge kidney in childhood. *AJR* 1985;**145**:315.

Siminovitch JMP, Montie JE, Straffon RA: Inferior venacavography in the preoperative assessment of renal adenocarcinoma. *J Urol* 1982;**128**:908.

Smith SEW: Unexpected anterior urethral diverticula. *Clin Radiol* 1986;**37**:55.

Sommer FG et al: Renal imaging with dual energy projection radiography. *AJR* 1982;**138**:317.

Spring DB: Urinary tract fungal disease. Pages 105–113 in: *Diagnostic Radiology.* Margulis AR, Gooding CA (editors). Mosby, 1985.

Spring DB et al: Radiologists and informed-consent lawsuits. *Radiology* 1985;**156**:245.

Steinhardt GF, Slovis TL, Perlmutter AD: Simple renal cysts in infants. *Radiology* 1985;**155**:349.

Stephens FD: *Congenital Malformations of the Urinary Tract.* Praeger, 1983.

Strijk SP, Debruyne FMJ, Herman CJ: Lymphography in the management of urologic tumors. *Radiology* 1982;**146**:39.

Templeton PA, Pais SO: Renal artery occlusion in PAN. *Radiology* 1985;**156**:308.

Thomsen HS, Rygaard H, Strandberg C: Micturating cystourethrography and vesicoureteral reflux. *Eur J Radiol* 1985;**5**:318.

Thornbury JR, Stanley JC, Fryback DG: Hypertensive urogram: A nondiscriminatory test for renal vascular hypertension. *AJR* 1982;**138**:43.

Wasserman NF, La Pointe S, Posalaky IP: Ureteral pseudodiverticulosis. *Radiology* 1985;**155**:561.

Wechsler RJ, Brennan RE: Teardrop bladder: Additional considerations. *Radiology* 1982;**144**:281.

Weiner SN et al: Hematuria secondary to left peripelvic and gonadal vein varices. *Urology* 1983;**22**:81.

Weiss RM, Glickman MG: Venography of the undescended testis. *Urol Clin North Am* 1982;**9**:387.

Sonography

Chan JCM, Brewer WH, Still WJ: Renal biopsies under ultrasound guidance: 100 consecutive biopsies in children. *J Urol* 1983;**129**:103.

Charboneau JW et al: Spectrum of sonographic findings in 125 renal masses other than benign simple cyst. *AJR* 1983;**140**:87.

Dunne MG, Cunat JS: Sonographic determination of fetal gender before 25 weeks gestation. *AJR* 1983;**140**:741.

Fong KW et al: Fetal renal cystic disease: Sonographic-pathologic correlation. *AJR* 1986;**146**:767.

Gooding AW: High-resolution sonography of the scrotum. Pages 49–56 in: *Diagnostic Radiology*. Margulis AR, Gooding CA (editors). Mosby, 1985.

Grantham JG et al: Testicular neoplasms: 29 tumors studied by high-resolution US. *Radiology* 1985;**157**:775.

Grossman H et al: Sonographic diagnosis of renal cystic diseases. *AJR* 1983;**140**:81.

Hadlock FP, Deter RL, Carpenter RJ: Sonography of the fetal genitourinary tract. *Semin Ultrasound* 1984;**5**:213.

Han BK, Babcock DS: Sonographic measurements and appearance of normal kidneys in children. *AJR* 1985;**145**:611.

Hennigan HW Jr, DuBose TH: Sonography of the normal female urethra. *AJR* 1985;**145**:839.

Hricak H (editor): *Genitourinary Ultrasound*. Churchill Livingstone, 1986.

Jeffrey RB et al: Sensitivity of sonography in pyonephrosis: A reevaluation. *AJR* 1985;**144**:71.

Kangarloo H et al: Urinary tract infection in infants and children evaluated by ultrasound. *Radiology* 1985;**154**:367.

Kink W 3rd, Kimme-Smith C, Winter J: Renal stone shadowing: An investigation of contributing factors. *Radiology* 1985;**154**:191.

Kuligowska E et al: Interventional ultrasound in detection and treatment of renal inflammatory disease. *Radiology* 1983;**147**:521.

Lue TF et al: Vasculogenic impotence evaluated by high-resolution ultrasonography and pulsed Doppler spectrum analysis. *Radiology* 1985;**155**:777.

Lupetin AR et al: The traumatized scrotum: Ultrasound evaluation. *Radiology* 1983;**148**:203.

Mahony BS et al: Fetal renal dysplasia: Sonographic evaluation. *Radiology* 1984;**152**:143.

Montana MA et al: Sonographic detection of fetal ureteral obstruction. *AJR* 1985;**145**:595.

Nussbaum AR et al: Ectopic ureter and ureterocele: Their varied sonographic manifestations. *Radiology* 1986;**159**:227.

Oppenheimer DA, Carrol BA, Yousem S: Sonography of the normal neonatal adrenal gland. *Radiology* 1983;**146**:157.

Resnick MI, Kursh ED: Transurethral ultrasonography in bladder cancer. *J Urol* 1986;**135**:253.

Resnick MI, Sanders RC: *Ultrasound in Urology*. Williams & Wilkins, 1984.

Rifkin MD, Kurtz AB, Goldbert BB: Sonographically guided transperineal prostatic biopsy: Preliminary experience with a longitudinal linear-array transducer. *AJR* 1983;**140**:745.

Rifkin MD et al: Endoscopic ultrasonic evaluation of the prostate using a transrectal probe: Prospective evaluation and acoustic characterization. *Radiology* 1983;**149**:265.

Sanders RC: Ultrasonic assessment of genitourinary anomalies in utero. In: *Ultrasonography in Obstetrics and Gynecology*. Sanders RC, James AE Jr (editors). Appleton-Century-Crofts, 1985.

Schwerk WB, Schwerk WN, Rodeck G: Venous renal tumor extension: A prospective US evaluation. *Radiology* 1985;**156**:491.

Taylor KJW (editor): *Atlas of Ultrasonography*. Churchill Livingstone, 1985.

Weinreb JC et al: Cystic renal mass evaluation: Real-time versus static imaging. *J Clin Ultrasound* 1986;**14**:29.

White SJ et al: Sonography of neuroblastoma. *AJR* 1983. **141**:465.

Wood BP et al: Ureterovesical obstruction and megaloureter: Diagnosis by real-time US. *Radiology* 1985;**156**:79.

Zafaranloo S, Gerard PS, Wise G: Bilateral neonatal testicular torsion: Ultrasonographic evaluation. *J Urol* 1986;**135**:589.

CT Scanning

Baert AF et al: Dynamic CT of the urogenital tract. *Urol Radiol* 1982;**4**:69.

Balfe DM et al: Evaluation of renal masses considered indeterminate on computed tomography. *Radiology* 1982;**142**:421.

Baron RL et al: Computed tomography of transitional-cell carcinoma of the renal pelvis and ureter. *Radiology* 1982;**144**:125.

Bosniak MA et al: computed tomography of ureteral obstruction. *AJR* 1982;**138**:1107.

Degesys GE et al: Retroperitoneal fibrosis: Use of CT in distinguishing among possible causes. *AJR* 1986;**146**:57.

Gatewood OMB et al: computerized tomography in the diagnosis of transitional cell carcinoma of the kidney. *J Urol* 1982;**127**:876.

Gatewood OMB et al: Renal vein thrombosis in patients with nephrotic syndrome: CT diagnosis. *Radiology* 1986;**159**:117.

Glasser J et al: Localization of impalpable testis by computed tomography. *Urology* 1983;**22**:206.

Goldman SM, Siegelman SS: Computerized tomography in the scheme of things. (Editorial.) *J Urol* 1982;**127**:724.

Greenberg M et al: Use of computerized tomography in the evaluation of filling defects of the renal pelvis. *J Urol* 1982;**127**:1172.

Hedgcock MW: CT Evaluation of the adrenal glands. Pages 65–81 in: *Diagnostic Radiology*. Margulis AR, Gooding CA (editors). Mosby, 1985.

Kenney PJ et al: Adrenal glands in patients with congenital renal anomalies: CT appearance. *Radiology* 1985;**155**:181.

Lang EK, Sullivan J: Categorization of traumatic injury to the upper urinary tract by dynamic CT. Pages 83–90 in: *Diagnostic Radiology*. Margulis AR, Gooding CA (editors). Mosby, 1985.

Lee JKT, Sagel SS, Stanley RJ (editors): *Computed Body Tomography*. Raven, 1983.

Levine E, Grantham JJ: High-density renal cysts in autosomal dominant polycystic kidney disease demonstrated by CT. *Radiology* 1985;**154**:477.

McAninch JW, Federle MP: Evaluation of renal injuries with computerized tomography. *J Urol* 1982;**128**:456.

Moss AA: Computed tomography of the adrenal glands. Chap 16, pp 837–876, in: *Computed Tomography of the Body*. Moss AA, Gamsu G, Genant HK (editors). Saunders, 1983.

Moss AA: Computed tomography of the kidneys. Chap 15, pp 763–836, in: *Computed Tomography of the Body*. Moss AA, Gamsu G, Genant HK (editors). Saunders, 1983.

Moss AA, Gamsu G, Genant HK (editors): *Computed Tomography of the Body*. Saunders, 1983.

Parienty RA, Pradel J, Parienty I: Cystic renal cancers: CT characteristics. *Radiology* 1985;**157:**741.

Rajfer J et al: The use of computerized tomography scanning to localize the impalpable testis. *J Urol* 1983;**129:**942.

Rauschkolb EN et al: Computed tomography of renal inflammatory disease. *J Comput Assist Tomogr* 1982;**6:** 502.

Richie JP, Garnic MB, Finberg H: Computerized tomography: How accurate for abdominal staging of testis tumors? *J Urol* 1982;**127:**715.

Sawczuk IS et al: Sensitivity of computed tomography in evaluation of pelvic lymph node metastases from carcinoma of bladder and prostate. *Urology* 1983;**21:**81.

Stanley RJ: Computed tomography of neoplastic renal lesions. Pages 181–189 in: *NMR, Interventional Radiology, and Diagnostic Imaging Modalities.* Moss AA (editor). Department of Radiology, University of California, San Francisco, 1983.

Thoeni RF: Computed tomography of the pelvis. Chap 20, pp 987–1053, in: *Computed Tomography of the Body.* Moss AA, Gamsu G, Genant HK (editors). Saunders, 1983.

van Waes PF, Ruijs SH, Feldberg MA: Computed tomographic techniques in urogenital malignancies. Pages 191–198 in: *NMR, Interventional Radiology, and Diagnostic Imaging Modalities.* Moss AA (editor). Department of Radiology, University of California, San Francisco, 1983.

van Waes PFGM et al: Direct coronal and direct sagittal CT of abdomen and pelvis: An approach to staging malignancies. *RadioGraphics* 1986;**6:**213.

Weyman PJ, McClennan BL, Lee JKT: Computed tomography of calcified renal masses. *AJR* 1982;**138:**1095.

Zeman RK et al: Computed tomography of renal masses: Pitfalls and anatomic variants. *RadioGraphics* 1986;**6:**351.

Magnetic Resonance Tomography

Alfidi RJ et al: Preliminary experimental results in humans and animals with a superconducting, whole-body, nuclear magnetic resonance scanner. *Radiology* 1982;**143:**175.

Bradbury EM, Radda GK, Allen PS: Nuclear magnetic resonance techniques in medicine. *Ann Intern Med* 1983;**98:** 514.

Brasch RC, Ogan MD, Englestad BL: Magnetic resonance pharmaceutical contrast enhancement. Pages 15–22 in: *Diagnostic Radiology.* Margulis AR, Gooding CA (editors). Mosby, 1985.

Bryan PJ et al: Magnetic resonance imaging of the prostate. *AJR* 1986;**146:**543.

Butler H et al: Magnetic resonance imaging of the abnormal female pelvis. *AJR* 1984;**143:**1259.

Cohen MD: *Pediatric Magnetic Resonance Imaging.* Saunders, 1986.

Crooks LE, Kaufman L: Basic physical principles. Pages 13–39 in: *Clinical Magnetic Resonance Imaging.* Margulis AA et al (editors). Radiological Research and Education Foundation, 1983.

Crooks LE, Kaufman L: Physical principles of nuclear magnetic resonance imaging. Pages 1–4 in: *NMR, Interventional Radiology, and Diagnostic Imaging Modalities.* Moss AA (editor). Department of Radiology, University of California, San Francisco, 1983.

Crooks LE et al: Clinical efficiency of nuclear magnetic resonance imaging. *Radiology* 1983;**146:**123.

Dietrich RB, Kangarloo H: Kidneys in infants and children: Evaluation with MR. *Radiology* 1986;**159:**215.

Fisher M et al: Female urethral carcinoma: MRI staging. *AJR* 1985;**144:**603.

Fisher MR, Hricak H, Crooks LE: Urinary bladder MR imaging. 1. Normal and benign conditions. *Radiology* 1985; **157:**467.

Fisher MR, Hricak H, Tanagho EA: Urinary bladder MR imaging. 2. Neoplasm. *Radiology* 1985;**157:**471.

Glazer GM et al: Adrenal tissue characterization using MR imaging. *Radiology* 1986;**158:**73.

Hricak H et al: Magnetic resonance imaging in the diagnosis and staging of renal and perirenal neoplasms. *Radiology* 1985;**154:**709.

Lasser EC: New developments in contrast media. *West J Med* 1985;**143:**372.

LiPuma JP: Magnetic resonance imaging of the kidney. *Radiol Clin North Am* 1984;**22:**925.

Lueng AWL et al: Magnetic resonance imaging of the kidneys. *AJR* 1984;**143:**1215.

Margulis AR et al (editors): *Clinical Nuclear Magentic Resonance Imaging.* Radiological Research and Education Foundation, 1983.

Moon KL et al: Nuclear magnetic resonance imaging of the adrenal gland: A preliminary report. *Radiology* 1983;**147:** 155.

Moss AA (editor): *NMR, Interventional Radiology, and Diagnostic Imaging Modalities.* Department of Radiology, University of California, San Francisco, 1983.

Mulopulos GP, Patel SK, Pessis D: MR imaging of xanthogranulomatous pyelonephritis. *J Comput Assist Tomogr* 1986;**10:**154.

New PFJ et al: Potential hazards and artifacts of ferromagnetic and nonferromagnetic surgical and dental materials and devices in nuclear magnetic resonance imaging. *Radiology* 1983;**147:**139.

Pavlicek W et al: The effects of nuclear magnetic resonance on patients with cardiac pacemakers. *Radiology* 1983; **147:**149.

Poon PY et al: Magnetic resonance imaging of the prostate. *Radiology* 1985;**154:**143.

Pykett IL et al: Principles of nuclear magnetic resonance imaging. *Radiology* 1982;**143:**157.

Schwartz JL, Crooks LE: NMR imaging produces no observable mutations or cytotoxicity in mammalian cells. *AJR* 1982;**139:**583.

Smith FW: Two years' clinical experience with NMR imaging. *Appl Radiol* 1983;**12(3):**29.

Smolin MF: Magnetic resonance imaging and other radiology advances in urology. *West J Med* 1985;**142:**821.

Williams RD, Hricak H: Magnetic resonance imaging in urology. *J Urol* 1984;**132:**641.

Comparison of Various Imaging Modalities

Auh YH et al: Extraperitoneal paravesical spaces: CT delineation with US correlation. *Radiology* 1986;**159:**319.

Auh YH et al: Intraperitoneal paravesical spaces: CT delineation with US correlation. *Radiology* 1986;**159:**311.

Bloomfield JA: *Introduction to Organ Imaging.* Medical Examination Publishing Co., 1984.

Cronan JJ, Zeman RK, Rosenfield AT: Comparison of computerized tomography, ultrasound and angiography in staging renal cell carcinoma. *J Urol* 1982;**127:**712.

Denkhaus H et al: Comparative study of suprapubic sonography and computed tomography for staging of prostatic carcinoma. *Urol Radiol* 1983;**5:**1.

Dietrich RB, Kangarloo H: Kidneys in infants and children: Evaluation with MR. *Radiology* 1986;**159**:215.

Falke THM et al: MR imaging of the adrenals: Correlation with computed tomography. *J Comput Assist Tomogr* 1986;**10**:242.

Hidalgo H et al: Parapelvic cysts: Appearance on CT and sonography. *AJR* 1982;**138**:667.

Hoddick W et al: CT and sonography of severe renal and perirenal infections. *AJR* 1983;**140**:517.

Jeffrey RB, Federle MP: CT and ultrasonography of acute renal abnormalities. *Radiol Clin North Am* 1983;**21**:515.

Laing FC, Jeffrey RB Jr, Wing VW: Ultrasound versus excretory urography in evaluating acute flank pain. *Radiology* 1985;**154**:613.

Lang EK: Comparison of dynamic and conventional computed tomography, angiography, and ultrasonography in the staging of renal cell carcinoma. *Cancer* 1984; **54**:2205.

Lang EK, Sullivan J, Frentz G: Renal trauma: Radiological studies. Comparison of urography, computed tomography, angiography, and radionuclide studies. *Radiology* 1985;**154**:1.

Lien HH et al: Comparison of computed tomography, lymphography, and phlebography in 200 consecutive patients with regard to retroperitoneal metastases from testicular tumor. *Radiology* 1983;**146**:129.

Moss AA, Goldberg HI: Correlations between nuclear magnetic resonance and computed tomography in body imaging. Pages 27–36 in: *NMR, Interventional Radiology, and Diagnostic Imaging Modalities*. Moss AA (editor). Department of Radiology, University of California, San Francisco, 1983.

Newhouse JH (editor): Symposium on imaging and intervention in the renal fossa. *Radiol Clin North Am* 1984; **22**:285. [Entire issue.]

Rifkin MD: *Diagnostic Imaging of the Lower Genitourinary Tract*. Raven, 1984.

Rumack CM: Evaluation of abdominal masses in children. Pages 135–138 in: *Diagnostic Radiology*. Margulis AR, Gooding CA (editors). Mosby, 1985.

Staub WH (editor): *Manual of Diagnostic Imaging: A Clinician's Guide to Clinical Problem Solving*. Little, Brown, 1985.

Subramanyam BR et al: Diffuse xanthogranulomatous pyelonephritis: Analysis by computed tomography and sonography. *Urol Radiol* 1982;**4**:5.

Subramanyam BR et al: Replacement lipomatosis of the kidney: Diagnosis by computed tomography and sonography. *Radiology* 1983;**148**:791.

Troupin RH: *Diagnostic Imaging in Clinical Medicine*. Year Book, 1985.

Weigert F, Schulz U, Kromer HD: Renal abscess: Report of a case with sonographic, urographic and CT evaluation. *Eur J Radiol* 1985;**5**:224.

Wolverson MK et al: Comparison of computed tomography with high-resolution real-time ultrasound in the localization of the impalpable undescended testis. *Radiology* 1983;**146**:133.

Interventional Uroradiology*

7

Erich K. Lang, MD

Interventional uroradiologic procedures can be divided into 2 major groups: (1) those performed via a percutaneous route and (2) those performed via an intravascular route (interventional arteriography).

Percutaneous diagnostic procedures include puncture and aspiration of renal cysts, guided thin needle biopsy, antegrade urography, the Whitaker test, and percutaneous cystourethrography. Although the use of invasive diagnostic procedures has declined as improved noninvasive imaging methods have become available (see Chapter 6), there still remain situations in which diagnosis can only be made by means of invasive imaging techniques. The percutaneous route is also used to dissolve or break up stones and remove them, to place ureteral catheters, and to dilate ureteral strictures.

Intravascular methods are used for embolization of renal cell carcinomas, arteriovenous fistulas and malformations, and bleeding sites—including intractable hemorrhage of the bladder or pelvic organs—and for dilation of stenotic arteries.

GUIDED PUNCTURE & ASPIRATION OF RENAL CYSTS

Because most asymptomatic space-occupying lesions in the kidneys occur in older patients, it is important that diagnostic procedures be as noninvasive as possible while giving acceptably accurate results. Although most renal cysts are benign and imaging methods for diagnosing both benign renal cysts and solid renal tumors are highly sensitive and specific, a substantial group of space-occupying lesions in the kidneys (inflammatory mass lesions, infected cysts, and hematomas) cannot be diagnosed with acceptable specificity or accuracy by imaging techniques alone. Guided puncture and aspiration of renal cysts has proved highly effective in increasing the specificity and accuracy of diagnosis in this group of indeterminate lesions (Lang, 1980).

About 94% of all benign renal cysts can be diagnosed by ultrasonography or CT scanning (Lang, 1980). However, the remainder cannot be diagnosed with certainty by these methods, and therefore it is necessary to confirm the diagnosis by puncture and as-

piration of the cyst followed by histochemical and cytologic assessment of the aspirate and a double-contrast study of the cyst to determine whether it is benign (Lang, 1980). Fluoroscopic, CT, or ultrasonographic guidance greatly facilitates the puncture of space-occupying lesions (Lang, 1980) and is necessary to confirm the site of aspiration.

The double-contrast study of the cyst is performed by instilling contrast medium and air into the cyst and then obtaining anterior, posterior, upright, decubitus, and oblique radiograms. This study should visualize all inner surfaces of the cyst and identify any protruding nodules or masses (Fig 7–1).

The aspirated fluid must be assessed visually for color, turbidity, and the presence of blood; histochemically for its content of fat, protein, amylase, and lactate dehydrogenase; and cytologically for the presence of malignant or inflammatory cells. If infection is suspected, the fluid should be cultured for bacteria (Lang, 1977).

Benign renal cysts contain clear, straw-colored fluid with low levels of fat, protein, lactate dehydrogenase, and amylase.

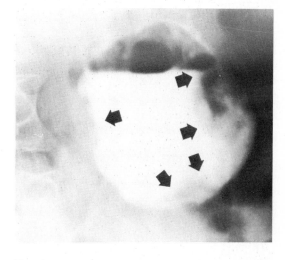

Figure 7–1. A double-contrast study showing multiple filling defects (*arrows*) protruding into the lumen of a renal cyst. The aspirate was murky; had high levels of fat, protein, and lactate dehydrogenase; and contained neoplastic cells that were readily identified on cytologic examination. An unequivocal diagnosis of renal cell carcinoma in the renal cyst was established.

---

*For a more detailed discussion of interventional uroradiology in the treatment of calculi, see Chapter 16.

Cystic or necrotic tumors or tumors within cysts generally yield a murky aspirate with high concentrations of fat, protein, and lactate dehydrogenase. Neoplastic cells are usually identifiable on cytologic examination; for best results, the aspirate should be filtered through a micropore filter and the residue on the filter examined cytologically (Lang, 1971). Double-contrast studies often show tumor nodules protruding into the lumen of the cyst in such cases (Fig 7–1).

Inflammatory cysts tend to yield murky aspirates with moderately elevated fat and protein levels and significantly elevated amylase and lactate dehydrogenase levels. Inflammatory cells may be seen on cytologic examination. Cultures of the aspirate usually identify the organism causing the infection.

GUIDED THIN NEEDLE BIOPSY

Guided thin needle biopsy is used to obtain specimens from an indeterminate lesion for histopathologic and bacteriologic diagnosis. Usually, the lesion is found by imaging but insufficient information is available for diagnosis. In most such cases, it is necessary to determine whether the lesion is a tumor or an inflammatory mass. A definitive diagnosis can usually be made on the basis of histopathologic examination of the biopsy specimen.

CT scanning, ultrasonography, or fluoroscopy should be used to guide thin needle biopsies. It is essential to obtain permanent records (eg, photographs of CT scans) showing the site from which the biopsy specimen was taken (Fig 7–2). If the results of histopathologic examination are negative, ie, normal, it is particularly important to prove that the specimen came from the suspect area.

If cytologic examination indicates that the lesion is an inflammatory mass, cultures and antimicrobial sensitivity studies should be performed. Not infrequently, the bacteria thought on the basis of urine cultures and antibody-coated bacteria tests (see p 52) to cause an upper urinary tract infection are different from those cultured from the specimen obtained by thin needle biopsy (Lang and Price, 1983).

Thin needle biopsy is also of value in determining whether tumors of the genitourinary tract have metastasized to lymph nodes or spread by extension to adjacent tissues or organs (Fig 7–3). This method may be used either for diagnosis or for confirmation of a diagnosis made by other means. The information thus obtained is useful in staging and managing tumors of the genitourinary tract.

ANTEGRADE UROGRAPHY

Antegrade urography is a diagnostic tool that demonstrates morphologic details in the upper urinary tract which may not be visible on retrograde urograms or intravenous contrast films. Although computerized radionuclide urography allows differentiation of pre-renal and postrenal obstructive disease, antergrade urography is more informative: the exact site—and often the cause (calculus, iatrogenic stricture, stricture due to inflammation or tumor)—of obstruction can be determined and the extent of damage assessed (Fig 7–4). It has also been found useful to identify the site of obstruction in patients with ureteroileotomies who fail to opacify the upper collecting system by reflux on the loopogram. Antegrade urograms are also most useful in identifying leakage or dehiscence of ureteroileostomy (Lang and Glorioso, 1986) (Fig

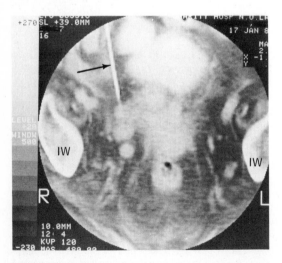

Figure 7–2. Thin needle biopsy of enlarged internal iliac nodes carried out with CT scan guidance. The site of the biopsy is documented by the pertinent CT scans. Arrow indicates biopsy needle. IW = iliac wings.

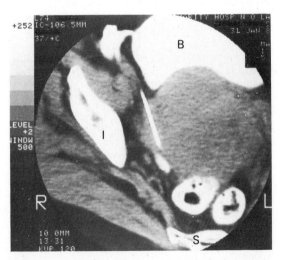

Figure 7–3. A CT-guided thin needle biopsy of a superolateral extension of a mass originating from the prostate proves the mass to be a prostatic carcinoma. B = bladder, I = iliac wing, S = sacrum.

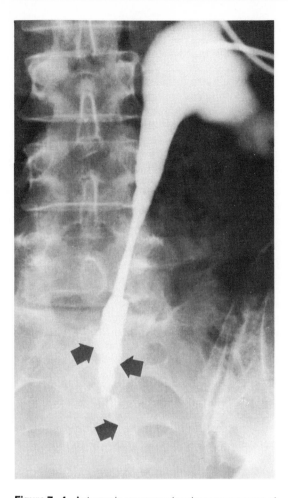

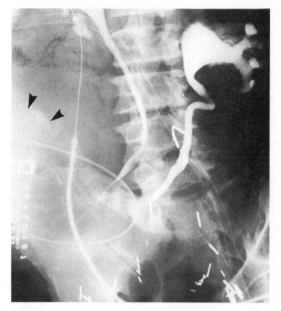

Figure 7–5. Antegrade percutaneous ureterogram demonstrates patency of the ureters but extravasation of contrast medium into a large urinoma (*arrowheads*). A partial dehiscence at the ureteroileostomy site exists.

Figure 7–4. Antegrade urogram showing encasement of the right mid ureter (*top arrows*) and finally complete obstruction (*bottom arrow*) by what proved to be recurrent carcinoma of the cervix extending along the ureteral lymphatics.

7–5). The study can be expanded to include a brush biopsy or a Whitaker test (see below) if this is desired. On the basis of the information obtained, the physician can plan definitive treatment.

Antegrade urography is performed as follows: The collecting system is punctured percutaneously via an oblique translumbar approach. This is done using CT scans, fluoroscopy, or ultrasonography for guidance; and a 22-gauge Shiba needle is generally employed. Once the collecting system is entered, the system is decompressed by aspiration of urine. The aspirated urine should be cultured for bacteria (Pfister and Newhouse, 1979). The system must be decompressed before contrast medium is instilled. If the collecting system is overdistended, bacteria may be forced through the fornices into the bloodstream, and septicemia can result (Lang and Price, 1983). For best demonstration of intraluminal lesions, the contrast medium should be diluted.

This study can easily be expanded to include a brush biopsy of the suspect lesion. If a brush biopsy is desired, an 18-gauge thin-walled needle is introduced in tandem with the Shiba needle. After the urogram is obtained, a deflectable brush (Wilson-Eskridge) can be introduced through the 18-gauge needle and biopsies of exfoliated tissue from any suspect lesion can be obtained under fluoroscopic guidance (Lang et al, 1978) (Fig 7–6). Radiographs should be taken as a permanent record of the site of biopsies.

WHITAKER TEST

The Whitaker test can also be performed in conjunction with percutaneous antegrade urography. This test assesses the clinical significance of obstruction by determining the effects of various filling rates on the pressure within the renal pelvis and on renal blood flow. Clinically significant obstruction also causes a reduction in the rate of renal blood flow that can be documented by computed radionuclide urography. Although computerized radionuclide urography appears to have replaced the Whitaker test in screeening patients with possible obstructive lesions, the latter is still considered the definitive test for determining the need for surgical correction of an obstruction of the ureteropelvic junction or the ureter.

The test is performed as follows: After the antegrade urogram is obtained, the 18-gauge thin-walled needle in the renal pelvis is connected via flexible tubing to a manometer so that intrapelvic pressures can be measured. By means of a 3-way stopcock, saline can

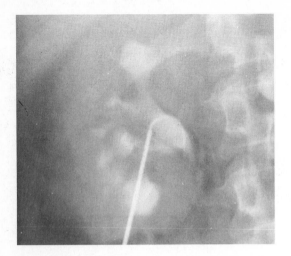

Figure 7–6. Brush biopsy of a suspect mass with a Wilson-Eskridge deflectable brush introduced under fluoroscopic guidance through an 18-gauge thin-walled needle that has been advanced into the pelvis of the right kidney. (Reproduced, with permission, from Lang EK et al: Brush biopsy of pyelocalyceal lesions via a percutaneous translumbar approach. *Radiology* 1978;**129**:623.)

be infused into the renal pelvis at flow rates of 5, 10, or 20 mL/min. After several minutes of perfusion at a given rate, during which time equilibrium will be reached, the intrapelvic pressure is recorded on a strip recording. Because the intrapelvic pressure is affected by changes in intra-abdominal pressure, the intravesical pressure (which is a function of both detrusor pressure and intra-abdominal pressure) is recorded simultaneously; the recorded intrapelvic pressure is later corrected for any change that occurred simultaneously in the bladder and renal pelvis (Pfister and Newhouse, 1979). This procedure is repeated with the other flow rates. After nonstress pressures are recorded, furosemide can be administered intravenously; it causes an increase in the flow rate (filling rate) that simulates the reaction to stress.

If the intrapelvic pressure reaches 160–200 mm of water when the filling rate is 10–20 mL/min, the obstruction is considered clinically significant.

PERCUTANEOUS CYSTOURETHROGRAPHY

Cystourethrography combines cystography and urethrography. It is used to demonstrate abnormalities of the bladder and urethra. Radiopaque contrast medium can be instilled via a transurethral catheter or a percutaneous suprapubic bladder puncture. The latter is the procedure of choice in patients with urethral valves, meatal stenosis, or lower urinary tract anomalies; in those who have recently undergone urethral surgery; and sometimes in those with urethral strictures.

A. Suprapubic Bladder Puncture: Bladder puncture is easier if the patient has been previously hydrated, so that the bladder is full. Ultrasound guidance can be used but is usually not necessary. The puncture may be performed under a local anesthetic, but a quick, direct puncture is quite painless. The fully distended bladder is easily entered via a puncture in the midline about 1–2 cm above the pubis. An Intercath system, if available, is a good means of introducing a flexible catheter into the bladder.

B. Tests:

1. Bacteriologic examination of urine– When urine is flowing freely from the catheter, a small specimen should be aspirated for microscopic examination and culture.

2. Cystourethrography– Only a small amount of contrast medium need be instilled into the bladder. After the contrast medium is instilled through the catheter, an anteroposterior film and oblique views should be obtained. Then voiding cystourethrograms should be obtained—in male patients, an oblique projection; in females, an anteroposterior projection and, if possible, a simultaneous lateral projection (biplane fluoroscopy). The image from the image intensifier should be split to allow simultaneous fluoroscopic observation and permanent documentation on film.

C. Complications: The incidence of complications from suprapubic bladder puncture is exceedingly low; in fact, in patients with anomalies of the lower urinary tract, cystourethrography performed using suprapubic bladder puncture is considered safer than cystourethrography performed using transurethral catheterization (Goldberg and Meyer, 1973).

PERCUTANEOUS STONE DISSOLUTION

Dissolution of renal calculi was first attempted using irrigation via retrograde ureteral catheters (Suby and Albright, 1943). Although this method was sound in principle, difficulties in maintaining effective drainage during perfusion resulted in a high rate of complications. Thus, the technique had limited acceptance.

With the advent of percutaneous nephrostomy, large-bore nephrostomy tubes that could effectively perfuse and drain the pyelocaliceal system became available (Newhouse and Pfister, 1982). With this technology, it is easy to maintain high perfusion rates, eg, 200–300 mL/h, and dissolve calculi in a reasonable length of time. A large number of calculi previously thought refractory to dissolution can be treated by this method.

A. Indications: Patients with uric acid, cystine, or struvite stones who are poor candidates for surgery or in whom the urine pH cannot be manipulated by parenteral administration of sodium bicarbonate may be treated by percutaneous stone dissolution (Spataro, Linke, and Barbaric, 1978; Smith, 1979).

B. Technique: It is best to use 2 catheters for perfusion: a percutaneous nephrostomy tube and a retrograde catheter, or 2 percutaneous nephrostomy tubes. Use of 2 catheters ensures drainage of the perfuseate and safeguards against sudden large increases in intrapelvic pressure that could result in rupture of the fornices and entry of potentially toxic solutions into the venous system. Usually one catheter is inserted in a cephalad calix and the other in the renal pelvis near the ureteropelvic junction. This arrangement ensures that the perfuseate will circulate around the stone.

Before solvent is used, a trial irrigation with sterile saline should be performed to ascertain that the system is patent and operates properly. The maximal perfusion rate should be maintained for at least 5 minutes, during which time the intrapelvic pressure should be monitored; the pressure must not exceed 150 mm of water.

Sodium bicarbonate solution is used to dissolve uric acid stones, acetylcysteine for cystine stones, and Suby's solution G (Newhouse and Pfister, 1982) or hemiacidrin (see p 266) for struvite stones. With this method, uric acid stones dissolve most rapidly—often within 24 hours—particularly if a high perfusion rate is maintained. Dissolution of cystine and struvite stones usually requires prolonged perfusion (up to 7 days).

It is sometimes possible to combine perfusion and extraction, first dissolving as much stone as possible and then removing small residual calculi with a Dormier basket through the nephrostomy tract.

Perfusion therapy should be temporarily discontinued if the patient becomes febrile but may be resumed when the febrile reaction subsides.

LITHOTRIPSY & PERCUTANEOUS STONE EXTRACTION

Lithotripsy and percutaneous extraction of renal and ureteral stones are performed via either an existing percutaneous nephrostomy tract or one that is specially developed to allow the most direct access to the calculus (Dunnick et al, 1985). Stones may be either removed intact or—particularly when they are large—broken up (lithotripsy) and then removed. The advantages of percutaneous lithotripsy and extraction are that the procedure does not require prolonged hospitalization and, therefore, is relatively inexpensive. Its disadvantages are that it is a long and technically complex operation (Lang, 1987).

A. Technique: Under fluoroscopic guidance, a percutaneous nephrostomy tract is developed through renal parenchyma along the straightest line to the stones. The tract is then dilated so that it is large enough for removal of the largest stone. With the patient heavily sedated and under local anesthesia, a Grüntzig balloon catheter 10 cm long and 10 mm in diameter can be used to dilate the tract to 26F in a single procedure.

Following balloon dilation, an Amplatz sheath is introduced over polyurethane dilators. Thereafter, all manipulations are performed through this sheath.

Before extraction is begun, a safety guide wire is advanced into the ureter and a working guide wire is advanced into the area of interest (Castaneda-Zuniga et al, 1982) (Fig 7–7).

Extraction can be carried out under fluoroscopic guidance or under direct vision with a nephroscope or ureteroscope. Stones up to 9 mm in size can be readily extracted through a 26F sheath with a Dormier basket or any of a variety of other extraction devices. If the renal pelvis is ample, most stones up to 9 mm in size can be extracted with a basket under fluoroscopic guidance. Direct visualization with a nephroscope is necessary if the pelvis is small or if stones are lodged in infundibula or calices. Stones lodged in the upper ureters are best teased back into the renal pelvis with a steerable guide wire and then extracted from the pelvis. If this maneuver fails, a flexible ureteroscope may be advanced to the stone and the stone extracted under direct vision (Banner and Pollack, 1982) (Fig 7–8).

B. Nephrolithotripsy: Large calculi can be broken up by electrohydraulic or ultrasonic nephrolithotripsy and the fragments extracted as described above. The lithotripsy probe passes readily through a 26F nephroscope (Marberger, Stackl, and Gruby, 1982). When the probe is in direct contact with the stone, electrical or sonic energy is transmitted through the probe to break up the stone. Small fragments are removed by continuous suction through the nephroscope and larger fragments by use of a stone basket or forceps (Fig 7–9).

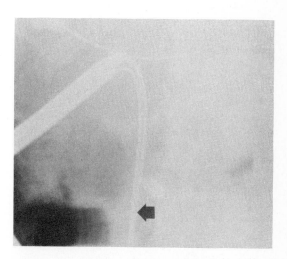

Figure 7–7. The percutaneous nephrostomy tract has been dilated by balloon catheters or bougie catheters, an Amplatz sheath has been introduced, and working and safety guide wires have been advanced into the ureter.

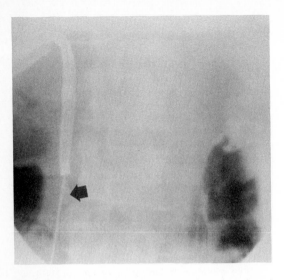

Figure 7–8. A flexible ureteroscope has been introduced into the renal pelvis through an Amplatz sheath and advanced along the guide wire to the stone (*arrow*) lodged in the upper right ureter.

C. Follow-Up Measures: Complete removal of the stone or stones should be verified by both direct observation through a nephroscope and radiographic studies.

A large nephrostomy catheter is then placed in the kidney to provide drainage and tamponade and to allow ready access for follow-up studies, for repeat extraction procedures if small fragments have been retained, or for both purposes.

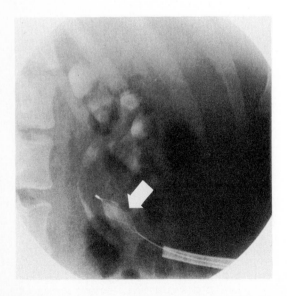

Figure 7–9. Retrieval of fragment of stone retained in the inferior calix using a Dormier basket (*arrow*).

EXTRACORPOREAL SHOCK-WAVE LITHOTRIPSY

Extracorporeal shock-wave lithotripsy (ESWL) is rapidly becoming the method of choice for management of calculi in the upper tract collecting system (Chaussy et al, 1985). The method allows for nonoperative and relatively noninvasive pulverization and subsequent elimination of calculi. The patient is submerged in a water bath, and under biplane fluoroscopic control, the calculus is centered in a shock-wave field. The shock waves are transmitted through the water bath and the body of the patient and are centered in the calculus, which is fragmented. Although fragments of different sizes result, they tend to be small enough to pass relatively easily through the ureter. Thus, calculi can be eliminated by a relatively noninvasive approach. A patent passageway, infundibula, and ureter are prerequisites for use of this technique.

PERCUTANEOUS PROCEDURES ON THE URETER

Placement of a Ureteral Stent Catheter

Percutaneous placement of a ureteral stent catheter is advocated in all conditions involving ureteral injury that would benefit from conservative management. Extravasation of urine from a dehiscence of the ureter must be stopped and the urinoma drained. The flow of urine must be temporarily rerouted. This was formerly accomplished by means of surgical nephrostomy, but percutaneous nephrostomy is now the procedure of choice. Prompt institution of drainage by percutaneous placement of a ureteral stent catheter will usually preserve renal function, prevent formation of urinomas, and encourage healing. This method of treatment is particularly valuable in patients in whom vascular embarrassment of long segments of the ureter due to trauma, iatrogenic injury, or radiation injury is suspected, because surgical correction of the problem entails extensive interposition procedures and thus is much more difficult.

A. Classification of Ureteral Fistulas: The site of the ureteral fistula and the extent of dehiscence must be ascertained by antegrade and retrograde ureterograms.

Anatomically, ureteral fistulas are grouped as follows: ureterovaginal, ureteroenteric, ureterocutaneous, ureteroretroperitoneal (urinoma), and lymphaticoureteral. Ureterovaginal fistulas are the most common type and tend to occur as complications of radical pelvic surgery, radiation treatment of advanced carcinoma of the cervix, or both (Wrigley, Prem, and Fraley, 1976). Ureteroenteric fistulas are most commonly complications of inflammatory disease, eg, Crohn's disease, diverticulitis, or regional enterocolitis. Ureterocutaneous and ureteroretroperitoneal fistulas occur as complications of penetrating trauma or calculous disease.

If the ureter is partially dehiscent, conservative management by long-term drainage via an indwelling ureteral catheter will usually result in satisfactory healing of the dehiscence (Lang, *Radiology* 1981;**138**:311). However, if the ureter is distorted or almost completely severed, retrograde catheterization and placement of a ureteral stent catheter may be impossible (Gibbons et al, 1976). In such cases, it is often possible to place an antegrade ureteral stent catheter through the area of dehiscence via a percutaneous nephrostomy (Lang, *Radiology* 1981;**138**:311).

If a large segment of ureter is missing owing to trauma or devitalization, the defect must be bridged and effective drainage into the bladder reconstructed by means of Boari flaps, transureteroureterostomies, ureteral reimplantation, or isolated bowel loop interposition (Konigsberg, Blunt, and Muecke, 1975; Lang, 1984).

B. Technique: Although a guide wire usually can be advanced into the ureter through an existing percutaneous nephrostomy, manipulation of the guide wire may be facilitated if the renal pelvis is repunctured in a straight line with the ureter. A guide wire deflector is useful for negotiating acute angles in the path of the ureter. Even when the ureter is almost completely severed, the guide wire may follow existing tissue bridges into the distal ureteral segment and thence into the bladder (Fig 7–10). Biplane fluoroscopy is very helpful in passing the guide wire (Lang, *Radiology* 1981;**138**:311).

Once the guide wire has been passed into the bladder, the distance from the renal pelvis to the bladder is measured so that multiple vents can be placed in a stent catheter at the correct level for drainage of the renal pelvis. The stent catheter is then introduced over the guide wire. This permits urine to drain into the bladder (Fig 7–11). The external end of the stent catheter serves as a safety valve, permitting drainage of urine to the outside if the distal end of the catheter becomes obstructed for any reason, and makes it easy to exchange one stent catheter for another.

An antegrade stent catheter is usually kept in place for 6–12 weeks. During this period, the catheter is exchanged several times to increase the catheter bore in order to prevent formation of tight strictures at the site of injury (Lang, *Radiology* 1981;**138**:311).

It is customary to continue using percutaneous stent catheters, since they are easily exchanged. However, it is possible to replace the percutaneous stent catheter with an indwelling internal stent catheter (Cook double pigtail catheter) (Fig 7–12). For this purpose, the distance from the renal pelvis to the bladder is measured and a double-J catheter of appropriate length selected. The double-J catheter is then advanced into position over a guide wire with a "pusher." Once the distal coil is properly positioned in the bladder and the proximal coil in the renal pelvis, the guide wire is withdrawn while the double-J catheter is held in position by the pusher. If it is later necessary to exchange this catheter for another double-J catheter, this can be

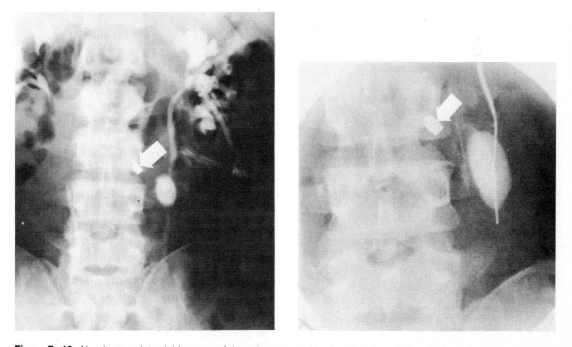

Figure 7–10. Nearly complete dehiscence of the ureter caused by gunshot wound. *Left:* Antegrade urogram showing extravasation of contrast medium from the dehiscence. *Right:* Despite the dehiscence, a guide wire has been passed along existing tissue bridges into the distal ureteral segment and a stent catheter subsequently placed in position. Arrows indicate projectile.

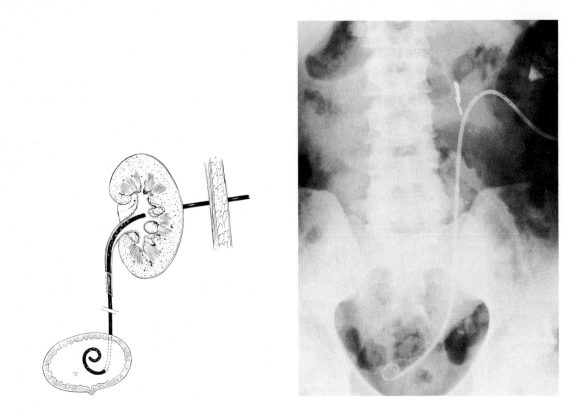

Figure 7–11. Multiple vents have been cut into a pigtail catheter, which was then inserted into the renal pelvis to allow urine to drain from the renal pelvis into the bladder or an external receptacle. (Reproduced, with permission, from Lang EK: Diagnosis and management of ureteral fistulas by percutaneous nephrostomy and antegrade stent catheter. *Radiology* 1981;**138**:311.)

done by retrieving the distal end of the original J catheter cystoscopically and reinserting a guide wire to the level of the renal pelvis, then inserting the new catheter.

C. Results: Conservative management of ureteral injury by means of percutaneous ureteral stent catheters eliminates the need for complex surgery, requires less hospitalization time, and usually produces good results. Although strictures may develop in the area of vascular impairment, these can be corrected later by transluminal dilation. If the segment of ureter that was injured is large, surgical correction may be required.

Balloon Dilation of Ureteral Strictures

Certain benign ureteral strictures, particularly fresh postoperative strictures, appear to be amenable to dilation by balloon catheter (Banner et al, 1983). In many cases, balloon dilation obviates the need for chronic indwelling ureteral stent catheters, additional surgery, or both.

Although Grüntzig balloons can sometimes be introduced in a retrograde fashion and positioned across the stricture, this approach is often impossible because of difficulty in negotiating the ureterovesical angle and

tortuous segments of the distal ureter. Therefore, an antegrade percutaneous approach is usually preferred (Lang, 1984).

A. Technique: A guide wire is introduced via an antegrade percutaneous nephrostomy and threaded across the stenosis. A balloon (usually 7F, 6 mm in diameter and 2 cm long) is introduced, centered over the stricture, and gradually inflated to its maximal diameter. Inflation is maintained for about 2 minutes, until the deformity imparted by the stricture upon the normally sausage-shaped balloon has disappeared. It may be necessary to repeat this procedure 3–4 times. Symmetric inflation of the balloon indicates successful dilation of the stricture (Fig 7–13).

Following successful dilation, an 8–10F ureteral stent catheter is placed in position and left in place for 7–14 days.

B. Results: Antegrade percutaneous transluminal balloon dilation produces the best results in fresh postoperative strictures after ureterolithotomies and in strictures that develop when ureteral injuries are managed by internal stenting.

Strictures that develop at ureteroileostomy sites usually show a similar favorable response, but longstanding and densely fibrotic strictures are often refractory to balloon dilation. Strictures due to cancer or

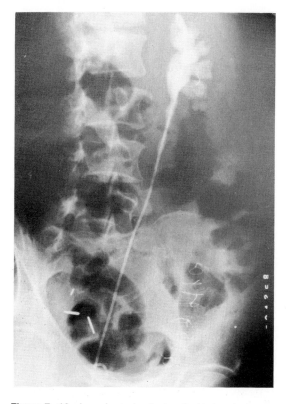

Figure 7–12. An antegrade stent catheter has been replaced by a Cook double-J catheter. This exchange can be readily carried out over a guide wire advanced into the bladder through the antegrade stent catheter.

to avascular necrosis complicating radical pelvic surgery, radiation therapy, or both usually show only a limited response to balloon dilation and recur after a short time.

Long strictures, which are often caused by avascu-

lar necrosis, are not amenable to dilation by balloon catheters. Occasionally, bougie dilation with a tapered VanAndel catheter may be successful in these patients. Strictures that develop in the ureter of a transplanted kidney—probably owing to small juxta-ureteral urinomas, chronic rejection, or both—respond particularly well to bougienage with a VanAndel catheter (Lang and Price, 1983).

TRANSCATHETER EMBOLIZATION OF RENAL CELL CARCINOMA

Surgical treatment of renal tumors is facilitated by preliminary transcatheter embolization of tumors and their host kidneys. Surgical treatment of renal cell carcinoma is no longer limited to carcinomas confined to the kidney. Advances in surgical techniques make it possible to attack lesions extending into the perinephric space, involving Gerota's fascia, and invading adjacent organs (Skinner et al, 1971). Even extensions of tumor thrombi into the renal vein, inferior vena cava, and right atrium are no longer absolute contraindications to surgical intervention (Bissada, Abdel-sayed, and Holder, 1977).

With renal tumors, arteriography was formerly used only for detailed preoperative assessment of tumor extension and for planning the surgical approach; more recently, it has also been used for treatment (Lang, Sullivan, and deKernion, 1983). Both the renal tumor and the host kidney can be treated by transcatheter embolization with inert embolic material or sclerosing material in preparation for "bloodless surgery" (Wallace et al, 1981). Occlusion of the vascular supply of the kidney makes possible early ligation of the renal vein. Since the renal vein is encountered first when exposing the kidney via a transabdominal approach, its ligation theoretically may

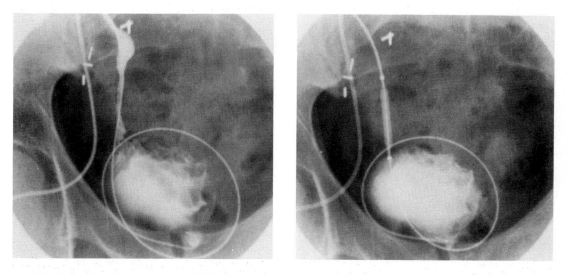

Figure 7–13. *Left:* Significant stricture of the distal portion of the right ureter. The stricture is 10 cm long and is probably a consequence of a radical Wertheim hysterectomy. *Right:* A 7F Grüntzig balloon catheter with a balloon 5 mm in diameter and 5 cm in length has been appropriately placed across the stricture to dilate it.

prevent dissemination of tumor cells when the kidney and the tumor are subsequently mobilized. Transcatheter embolization of the vascular bed of the kidney and its tumor also causes accentuation of cleavage planes 24–48 hours later, and this is said to facilitate surgical resection. Recently, the improved host immune response in patients after transcatheter embolization of renal tumors has been credited with disappearance of pulmonary metastases (Wallace et al, 1981). This is thought to be due to stimulation of the host's immune system by antigens released from the necrotic tumor.

A. General Considerations: To ensure total embolization of the kidney and its tumor, the embolic or sclerosing material must be distributed throughout both. Superselective engagement of branch vessels or use of an occlusive balloon catheter is an important precaution necessary to prevent inadvertent embolization of distant organs due to regurgitation of embolic material into the aorta.

B. Simple Embolization: Initially, $2 \times 2 \times 2$ mm Gelfoam or Ivalon particles were usually used for transcatheter embolization of renal tumors. Currently, 100% ethanol is usually used (Klatte, 1981) because it produces more permanent obliteration of the vascular bed (Fig 7–14). Renal tumors embolized with Gelfoam or Ivalon tend to regain a blood supply either by retrograde collateral filling from extrarenal sources or by re-establishment of blood flow in the occluded segments (Lang, Sullivan, and deKernion, 1983).

C. Embolization for Radiation Therapy: Transcatheter embolization with radioactive particles can create an interstitial infarct implant capable of delivering high-dose radiation to the tumor (Lang, Sullivan, and deKernion, 1983). This method can be used both for definitive treatment of inoperable tumors and for reducing tumor mass in the hope of rendering inoperable tumors operable.

By using radiopharmaceuticals with appropriate half-lives and radiation characteristics, it is possible to limit radiation almost exclusively to the tumor-bearing area and thus minimize the dose to the host (Lang, Sullivan, and deKernion, 1983). Use of a radiopharmaceutical with a long half-life prolongs irradiation and increases the probability of damage to tumor cells during their mitotic phase. [125]I is the preferred radiopharmaceutical. It is commercially available in preparations that fit the lumen of catheters customarily used for selective catheterization of renal tumors.

Superselective engagement of as many tumor branch arteries as possible and release of as many infarct particles as possible ensure the best geometric distribution of radioactive sources throughout the tumor (Fig 7–15). This in turn ensures homogeneous irradiation of the entire tumor. The distribution of radioactive particles is governed in part by variations in blood flow to different regions of the tumor. Since irradiation of a tumor produces fibrosis and reduced perfusion, performing transcatheter embolization with serial fractional introduction of the radiopharmaceutical tends to improve the distribution of radioactive parti-

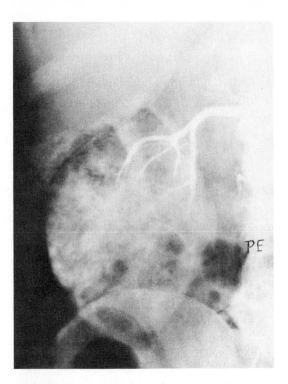

Figure 7–14. Transcatheter embolization of renal tumor. Follow-up arteriogram after intra-arterial administration of 12 mL of 96% ethanol shows a stationary column of contrast medium in the main renal artery and its main branches. There is no flow into peripheral blood vessels or into the rich vascular system of the tumor, which has been totally obliterated by the administration of ethanol. PE = postembolization.

cles. Areas that received a lower dose from the first fractional implant will retain better perfusion; thus, radioactive particles from subsequent fractions will tend to flow into these areas rather than into areas with decreased vascular perfusion due to radiation fibrosis.

D. Results: Transcatheter embolization with inert embolic material or ethanol has been very helpful in facilitating subsequent surgical resection of tumors. If properly performed (ie, using superselective catheterization or balloon catheters), the procedure is safe and has no serious complications. Nearly all patients thus treated have transient pain and elevations in temperature; appropriate analgesics should be used. Surgery need not be delayed because the patient's temperature is elevated owing to necrosis of the devascularized tumor.

Transcatheter embolization with radioactive particles has significantly increased the survival of patients with advanced stages of renal tumors (Lang and deKernion, 1981). Although cures have not been reported with this method, it has produced relief of pain, cessation of hematuria, and long-term remissions in patients with advanced stage renal cell carcinoma not amenable to surgical resection.

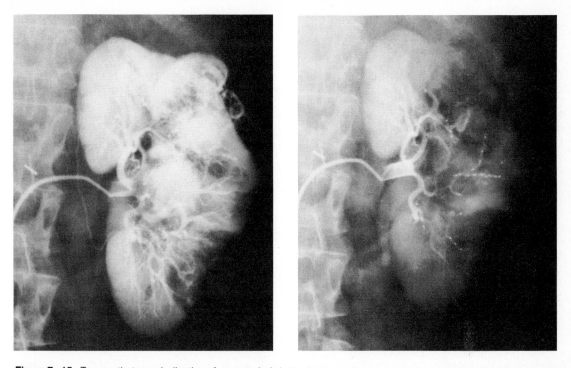

Figure 7–15. Transcatheter embolization of a tumor. *Left:* Late phase arteriogram showing a densely stained tumor in the mid pole of the left kidney. *Right:* Following transcatheter embolization with radioiodine (^{125}I seeds), distribution of the radioactive particles throughout the tumor-bearing area is satisfactory.

TRANSCATHETER EMBOLIZATION OF BLEEDING SITES & ARTERIOVENOUS MALFORMATIONS & FISTULAS OF THE KIDNEY

Transcatheter embolization offers an attractive alternative to surgical intervention in the management of bleeding sites, arteriovenous malformations, and arteriovenous fistulas of the kidney. This method is particularly effective in the management of traumatic arteriovenous fistulas (Fig 7–16).

A. Arteriovenous Fistulas: Because blood is siphoned from other segments of the kidney and shunted through an arteriovenous fistula, renin release is often activated from ischemic renal parenchyma; this causes hypertension. Occlusion of the arterial supply of an arteriovenous fistula will normalize perfusion of the remainder of the kidney and thereby correct the condition.

The size of the vessel feeding the arteriovenous fistula determines the choice of the occlusive device to be used. Detachable balloons can be placed in position via a catheter and then released. Gianturco coils are also useful to obliterate medium or large vessels feeding arteriovenous fistulas. Small vascular umbrellas appear to produce the most complete occlusion.

B. Bleeding Sites: Transcatheter embolization can be used to occlude actively bleeding vessels permanently or temporarily. Embolization of the bleeding sites with autologous blood clot alone or reinforced

with ϵ-aminocaproic acid (Amicar) is preferred if they appear to be supplied from lobar or smaller renal branch arteries. Although such blood clots eventually lyse, fibroblasts seal the defect within 24 hours, and this seal should prevent further hemorrhage.

Placement of a balloon catheter may be considered in the presence of life-threatening hemorrhage from major vessels. The balloon can be inflated in the main artery or in the branch that is hemorrhaging in order to curtail further hemorrhage, and the lumen of the catheter can be used to gain access to the renal parenchyma. Thus, the balloon catheter can provide temporary hemostasis and can also be used to perfuse the organ with iced saline solution in preparation for "bench surgery."

C. Results: Both of the above techniques have been credited with saving kidneys, and in many cases they have made surgical intervention unnecessary.

TRANSCATHETER EMBOLIZATION IN THE MANAGEMENT OF INTRACTABLE HEMORRHAGE FROM THE PELVIS & BLADDER

Intractable hemorrhage from the bladder or pelvic organs may occur as a complication of surgical procedures (eg, transurethral resection of the prostate) or may be caused by pelvic tumors or traumatic injuries. If hemorrhage cannot be controlled by conserva-

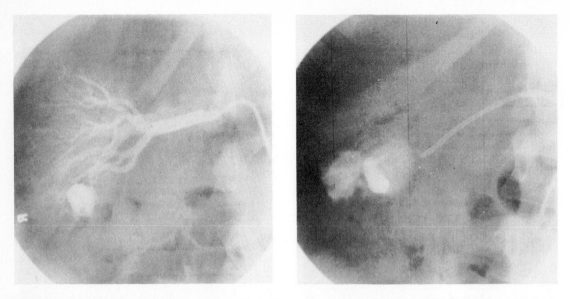

Figure 7–16. *Left:* Traumatic pseudoaneurysm and small traumatic arteriovenous fistula. *Right:* The feeding artery is selectively catheterized and will be occluded with 2-mm Ivalon cubes.

tive measures, eg, irrigation, administration of ϵ-aminocaproic acid (Amicar), and fulguration, transcatheter embolization should be considered as an alternative to surgical intervention. Transcatheter embolization has been effectively used for definitive treatment of hemorrhages caused by trauma and by pelvic tumors.

The aim is to control the hemorrhage and stabilize the patient without permanently disrupting the blood supply of the affected tissues. To achieve this, blood flow must be restricted at the level of the smallest branch vessel that will curtail the hemorrhage. Before embolization is undertaken, careful arteriographic assessment is necessary to determine which blood vessel should be occluded and whether other organs depend on blood supplied by that vessel. Particularly in older patients, some major vessels (eg, the inferior mesenteric artery) may have arteriosclerotic occlusions, and organs ordinarily supplied by these vessels may depend entirely on collateral flow. Obviously, vessels that provide the sole blood supply to organs cannot be embolized, since this would jeopardize the dependent organs. Once the offending vessel is identified and it is determined that embolization is possible, superselective catheterization of the vessel is attempted, and then embolization is performed.

In patients with bleeding due to trauma, autologous blood clot alone or reinforced with ϵ-aminocaproic acid is the embolic material of choice. Because such clots eventually lyse, restitution of flow in the affected vessel ensures a safeguard against tissue necrosis (Lang and deKernion, 1981).

If the hemorrhage is due to tumor, it may be desirable to occlude the vessel more permanently. Ivalon particles $1 \times 1 \times 1$ mm in size are best for this purpose, since they tend to lodge in small muscular arteries. Oc-

clusion at this level ensures collateral flow via the precapillary plexus and therefore safeguards against total deprivation of tissue perfusion, which could cause avascular necrosis of the bladder (Hietala, 1978). Occlusion of the small muscular arteries results in a substantial drop in pulse pressure, which fosters thrombosis of the bleeding terminal branch vessels and thereby controls hemorrhage (Fig 7–17).

TRANSLUMINAL ANGIOPLASTY

Transluminal angioplasty has become the procedure of choice for the management of fibromuscular hyperplasia and arteriosclerotic lesions of the renal arteries causing hypertension (Sos et al, 1984). An intraluminal balloon catheter is used to dilate the stenotic area of the artery and thereby increase flow to the kidney.

A. Indications: Both lesions involving the main renal artery and those involving major branch vessels can be dilated transluminally. Arteriosclerotic plaques that extend contiguously from the renal artery onto the aorta are more difficult to treat by this technique, because placing the balloon across the orifice of the renal artery with a portion of the balloon protruding into the aorta predisposes to intimal flap formation and its attendant complications.

B. Technique: After the lesion has been located and assessed by angiography or digital subtraction angiography, a balloon catheter is advanced to the lesion by the Seldinger technique. Depending upon the precise location of the lesion, a transfemoral or transaxillary approach may be favored. A guide wire is advanced into the distal branches of the renal artery to ensure that the balloon remains in a stable position.

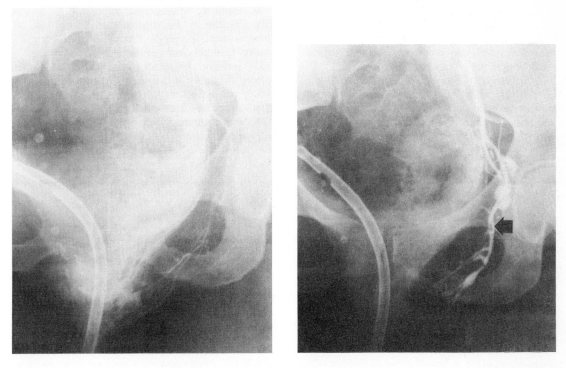

Figure 7–17. Transcatheter embolization to control intractable hemorrhage due to tumor. *Left:* Arteriogram showing densely stained mass in left fornix of vagina and parametrium. *Right:* Marked reduction in staining of tumor in the fornix of the vagina, vaginal vault, and left parametrium after transcatheter embolization of the anterior division of the left internal iliac artery with Ivalon (*arrow*). Life-threatening hemorrhage was successfully controlled by occluding the blood supply of the tumor.

The balloon is then placed across the lesion and inflation is begun. The balloon can be inflated using either hand pressure on a 2- to 5-mm syringe or equipment monitored by a pressure gauge.

Initially, the lesion imposes a deformity on the inflated balloon. When the lesion "gives," ie, when dilation is successful, there is no longer a deformity of the balloon (Fig 7–18).

Small intimal tears and flaps may occur as a consequence of the dilation and predispose to thrombosis of

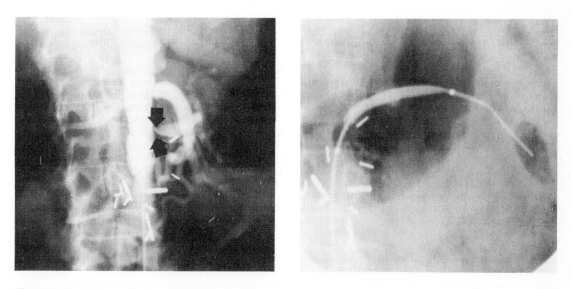

Figure 7–18. *Left:* Aortogram showing a tight arteriosclerotic stenosis of the left renal artery (*arrows*). *Right:* A Grüntzig balloon catheter has been advanced across the stenosis and inflated. Satisfactory dilatation of the stenotic lesion is indicated by the normal shape of the balloon.

the vessel. To prevent thrombosis, the patient's blood should be heparinized so that the partial thromboplastin time is 1 1/2–2 times normal for at least 3 days. Thereafter, aspirin may be given as an anticoagulant for a prolonged period of time.

C. Follow-Up: Intravenous digital angiography is a relatively noninvasive method for follow-up examination of an angioplasty site. Computed radionuclide urography can be used to monitor the renal plasma flow rate (RPF) (Schwarten, 1984).

D. Results: Transluminal angioplasty is particularly effective in the treatment of lesions due to fibromuscular hyperplasia. Up to 95% of such lesions respond favorably and permanently (Colapinto et al, 1982). Initially, about 85% of arteriosclerotic lesions respond favorably to this treatment; however, about 50% of such lesions recur 6 months to 2 years after the initial procedure. Although a recurrent lesion can be treated by transluminal angioplasty, the success rate of repeat dilation is only about 50%.

REFERENCES

Banner MP, Pollack HM: Percutaneous extraction of renal and ureteral calculi. *Radiology* 1982;**144**:7.

Banner MP et al: Catheter dilatation of benign ureteral strictures. *Radiology* 1983;**147**:427.

Bissada NK, Abdelsayed M, Holder JC: Renal carcinoma: Diagnostic and therapeutic aspects. *Am Fam Physician* (Aug) 1977;**16**:100.

Castaneda-Zuniga WR et al: Nephrostolithotomy: Percutaneous technique for urinary calculus removal. *AJR* 1982;**139**:7.

Chaussy C et al: Extracorporeal shock wave lithotripsy (ESWL) for treatment of urolithiasis. *Radiology* 1985;**154**:273.

Colapinto RF et al: Percutaneous transluminal dilatation of the renal artery: Follow-up studies on renovascular hypertension. *AJR* 1982;**139**:727.

Dunnick NR et al: Percutaneous approach to nephrolithiasis. *AJR* 1985;**144**:451.

Gibbons RP et al: Experience with indwelling ureteral stent catheters. *J Urol* 1976;**155**:22.

Goldberg BB, Meyer H: Ultrasonically guided suprapubic urinary bladder aspiration. *Pediatrics* 1973;**51**:70.

Hietala SO: Urinary bladder necroses following selective embolization of the internal iliac artery. *Acta Radiol* [*Diagn*] 1978;**19**:316.

Klatte E: Effective occlusion of the renovascular bed by selective catheter infusion of 100% ethyl alcohol in patients with renal cell carcinoma. [Paper presented to the Association of University Radiologists, New Orleans, April, 1981.]

Konigsberg H, Blunt KJ, Muecke EC: Use of Boari flap in lower ureteral injuries. *Urology* 1975;**5**:751.

Lang EK: Antegrade ureteral stenting for dehiscence, strictures and fistulae. *AJR* 1984;**143**:795.

Lang EK: Asymptomatic space-occupying lesions of the kidney: A programmed sequential approach and its impact on quality and cost of health care. *South Med J* 1977;**70**:277.

Lang EK: Co-existence of cyst and tumor in the same kidney. *Radiology* 1971;**101**:7.

Lang EK: Diagnosis and management of ureteral fistulas by percutaneous nephrostomy and antegrade stent catheter. *Radiology* 1981;**138**:311.

Lang EK: Percutaneous nephrostolithotomy and lithotripsy: A multi-institutional survey of complications. *Radiology* 1987;**162**:25.

Lang EK: Roentgenologic approach to the diagnosis and management of cystic lesions of the kidney: Is cyst exploration mandatory? *Urol Clin North Am* 1980;**7**:677.

Lang EK: Transcatheter embolization of pelvic vessels for control of intractable hemorrhage. *Radiology* 1981;**140**:331.

Lang EK, deKernion JB: Transcatheter embolization of advanced renal cell carcinoma with radioactive seeds. *J Urol* 1981;**126**:581.

Lang EK, Glorioso L III: Management of urinomas by percutaneous drainage procedures. *Radiol Clin North Am* 1986;**24**:551.

Lang EK, Price ET: Redefinitions of indications for percutaneous nephrostomy. *Radiology* 1983;**147**:419.

Lang EK, Sullivan J, deKernion JB: Work in progress: Transcatheter embolization of renal cell carcinoma with radioactive infarct particles. *Radiology* 1983;**147**:413.

Lang EK et al: Brush biopsy of pyelocalyceal lesions via a percutaneous translumbar approach. *Radiology* 1978;**129**:623.

Marberger M, Stackl W, Gruby W: Percutaneous litholapaxy of renal calculi with ultrasound. *Eur Urol* 1982;**8**:236.

Newhouse JH, Pfister RC: Percutaneous dissolution of renal stones. Chapter 40 in: *Interventional Radiology*. Athanasoulis CA et al (editors). Saunders, 1982.

Pfister RC, Newhouse JH: Interventional percutaneous pyeloureteral techniques. 1. Antegrade pyelography and ureteral perfusion. 2. Percutaneous nephrostomy and other procedures. (2 parts.) *Radiol Clin North Am* 1979;**17**:344, 351.

Schwarten DE: Percutaneous transluminal angioplasty of the renal arteries: Intravenous digital subtraction angiography for follow-up. *Radiology* 1984;**150**:369.

Skinner DJ et al: Diagnosis and management of renal cell carcinoma. *Cancer* 1971;**28**:1165.

Smith AD et al: Dissolution of cystine calculi by irrigation with acetylcysteine through percutaneous nephrostomy. *Urology* 1979;**13**:422.

Sos TA et al: Percutaneous transluminal renal angioplasty and renovascular hypertension due to atheroma or fibromuscular dysplasia. *Radiology* 1984;**151**:547.

Spataro RF, Linke CA, Barbaric ZL: The use of percutaneous nephrostomy and urinary alkalinization in the dissolution of obstructing uric acid stones. *Radiology* 1978;**129**:629.

Suby HI, Albright F: Dissolution of phosphatic urinary calculi by the retrograde introduction of citrate solution containing magnesium. *N Engl J Med* 1943;**228**:81.

Wallace S et al: Embolization of renal cell carcinoma: Experience with 100 patients. *Radiology* 1981;**138**:563.

Whitaker RH: Equivocal pelvi-ureteric obstruction. *Br J Urol* 1976;**47**:771.

Whitaker RH, Buxton-Thomas M: A comparison of pressure flow studies and renography in equivocal upper urinary tract obstruction. *J Urol* 1984;**131**:446.

Wrigley JV, Prem KA, Fraley EE: Pelvic exenteration: Complications of urinary diversion. *J Urol* 1976;**116**:428.

Percutaneous Antegrade Endourology

8

Joachim W. Thüroff, MD

In contrast to techniques of retrograde instrumentation, which invade the urinary tract via the urethra, techniques of antegrade instrumentation involve access via percutaneous puncture. This approach must respect the intrarenal anatomy just as in open surgical nephrotomy, and imaging techniques are essential to guide the procedure.

First, and most importantly, a puncture route must be established that will provide straightforward access to the target and safe, bloodless instrumentation. Thus, the location and direction of the puncture tract and the site of entry into the renal collecting system determine the success of all subsequent steps of radiologically and endoscopically controlled instrumentation. Visualization of the puncture needle and target and precise guidance to the target require the use of imaging techniques such as ultrasound, fluoroscopy, or, in selected cases, CT scanning.

For percutaneous puncture, ultrasound is the technique of choice. For subsequent procedures (eg, tract dilation, nephrostomy catheter placement), fluoroscopy is required. For intrarenal surgical procedures, endoscopy provides a comprehensive view.

Contraindications to percutaneous kidney puncture are blood clotting anomalies due to coagulopathies or anticoagulant medical therapy. Preparation and draping of the surgical field are required as for open surgery, and the same standards of asepsis must be followed. Local anesthesia only is sufficient for puncture of the kidney and small-bore tract dilation (6–12F) for antegrade insertion of a ureteral stent or nephrostomy catheter. Lidocaine hydrochloride 1% USP, 10 mL, can be given for infiltration of the skin and tissue along the intended route of puncture down to the renal capsule. During dilation of the tract, administration of a local anesthetic in lubricant (eg, lidocaine hydrochloride jelly 2%) serves the dual purpose of anesthetization and lubrication. Dilation of nephrostomy tracts up to 30F and extraction of small renal stones can be done under local anesthesia. However, extracorporeal shock-wave lithotripsy (ESWL) is now the treatment of choice for most of these small stones.

Percutaneous nephrolithotomy (PNL) is still indicated for treatment of staghorn calculi and stones in caliceal diverticula, but the extent of intrarenal instrumentation for stone disintegration and extraction usually requires epidural or general anesthesia. Because puncture, tract dilation, and stone disintegration and removal are preferably performed as a one-stage procedure, the use of local anesthesia in PNL is limited.

IMAGING & PUNCTURE TECHNIQUES

Percutaneous puncture of the renal collecting system may be performed for diagnostic procedures (eg, antegrade pyelography, pressure/perfusion studies) or to establish an access route for therapeutic interventions such as percutaneous catheter placement or endoscopic procedures (Table 8–1). Regardless of indication, techniques for imaging and percutaneous puncture of the kidneys and retroperitoneum are identical.

Both ultrasonic scanning and fluoroscopy provide visualization and guidance for safe, accurate percutaneous puncture, but ultrasound has definite advantages:

(1) Intravenous or retrograde administration of contrast dye is unnecessary.

(2) Continuous on-line control of needle advancement is possible without exposure to radiation.

(3) Radiolucent, non-contrast-enhancing renal and extrarenal structures (eg, renal cysts, retroperitoneal tumors) can be visualized and punctured accurately.

(4) All underlying tissue along an intended percutaneous nephrostomy tract can be seen (eg, bowel or lung).

(5) Imaging in all 3 dimensions is easily obtainable simply by tilting and rotating the scanning head.

(6) The 2-dimensional image of the scanning plane

Table 8–1. Indications for percutaneous puncture of the renal collecting system.

Diagnostic indications
Antegrade pyelography
Pressure/perfusion study (Whitaker test)
Therapeutic indications
Nephrostomy catheter drainage
Antegrade ureteral stenting
Dilation of ureteral strictures
Perfusion chemolysis of renal stones
Percutaneous nephrolithotomy (PNL)
Percutaneous endopyeloplasty
Percutaneous resection and coagulation of urothelial tumors

can actually provide 3-dimensional information. If both the puncture needle and the target are visualized and the needle is directed and aligned accordingly, it will travel exactly within the scanning plane and will not deviate laterally into the third dimension.

Once the puncture needle has entered the renal collecting system, fluoroscopy is required for control and guidance of subsequent steps (eg, guide wire insertion, tract dilation, catheter insertion). In selected cases, insertion and placement of a nephrostomy catheter in a dilated renal system may be possible with ultrasonic control only. However, while the rigid puncture needle can be readily visualized and directed within the 2-dimensional ultrasonic scanning plane, flexible instruments such as guide wires and catheters follow the anatomy of the renal collecting system and may therefore deviate from the scanning plane. Fluoroscopy provides a 2-dimensional image with complete integration of all information from the third (anterior-posterior) dimension, so that the entire length of radiopaque catheters, wires, etc, can be visualized.

For percutaneous puncture of the renal collecting system, the patient should be placed on the fluoroscopy table in the prone position. Radiolucent bolsters may be placed under the abdomen to correct for lumbar lordosis and to support the kidney. A standard puncture site is in the posterior axillary line midway between the 12th rib and the ileal crest; this site ensures that the patient will not later lie on the nephrostomy catheter as long as it is left in place. Ultrasonic scanning is performed below the 12th rib to obtain a median longitudinal scan through the kidney. For optimal coupling of the ultrasonic beam to the skin, sterile gel (eg, K-Y jelly) is applied to the skin at the scanning site. The position, rotation, and tilt of the scanning head, which determine the plane of ultrasonic scanning, must be oriented along the normal topography of the kidney. In the frontal view of an intravenous pyelogram (IVP), the longitudinal axis of the kidney usually follows the psoas muscle, its cranial extension meeting the midline at about a 30-degree angle (Fig 8–1A). In the transverse view of a CT scan, the transverse axis of the kidney forms about a 45-degree angle with both a horizontal and a sagittal line (Fig 8–1B). The position and direction of the transducer should be roughly oriented to the following marks: below the 12th rib (if possible), cranial to the puncture site, with a 30-degree caudal-lateral rotation and a 45-degree lateral tilt of the scanning head. Fine adjustment of the position and direction of the scanning head must be made during imaging.

Factors that may influence the choice of scanning technique and puncture site include patient size; position and rotation of the kidney; anomalies of bony structures; positions of the colon, spleen, liver, and lung relative to the kidney; and the target of puncture (upper, middle, or lower calix; caliceal diverticulum). Ultrasound can image all these structures, and the scanning head can be positioned to provide the best visualization and optimal puncture site for each patient.

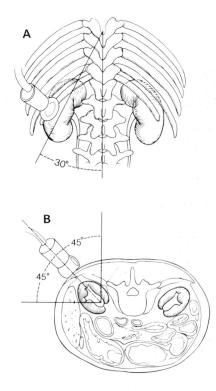

Figure 8–1. Renal ultrasound. *A:* The longitudinal axis of the kidney forms a 30-degree angle with the midline. *B:* The transverse axis of the kidney forms a 45-degree angle with both a horizontal and a vertical line.

Thus, a puncture site as high as above the 11th rib may be chosen if the lung is not visualized in the puncture route. A different puncture site must be chosen if bowel gas or the liver or spleen is visualized within the intended nephrostomy route.

If puncture is performed for nephrostomy drainage of a dilated system or antegrade stent placement only, the site of entry into the collecting system is not as critical as for endoscopic stone manipulation or other procedures. However, on principle, the route of puncture should always aim through a pyramid into a dorsal calix; puncture into an infundibulum may result in bleeding from segmental and interlobar vessels in the renal sinus, and direct puncture of the renal pelvis renders dilation of the nephrostomy tract and insertion of catheters and instruments difficult, with increased risk of accidental catheter dislodgment after successful entry. Performance of PNL for complicated stones such as staghorn calculi or stones in caliceal diverticula requires careful planning and precise entry into the target area of the renal collecting system. In large, complete staghorn calculi, where PNL is to be performed for debulking the stone volume (followed by ESWL for disintegrating retained caliceal stones), puncture is usually performed through a lower dorsal calix, a position from which the lower caliceal group, the renal pelvis, and part of the upper caliceal group can be easily reached with rigid instruments. How-ever, for staghorn stones that can be completely re-moved by PNL alone (without ESWL), another route (eg, middle or upper calix puncture) may be chosen. Stones in caliceal diverticula are better approached by direct puncture of the diverticulum than by puncture of the collecting system with endoscopic access to the di-verticulum. In every case, peripheral puncture of the collecting system through a papilla allows maximal utilization of available space.

Once chosen, the target for access to the renal col-lecting system must be visualized ultrasonically. The cutaneous puncture site should be caudad to the trans-ducer head in extension of the transverse axis (width) of the scanning plane (most transducers have a mark indicating the axis of the scanning plane relative to the transducer head, or an attachment for a needle guide at this site). Skin and fascia are incised with a No. 11 blade. At this time, the scanning head may be shifted over the incision to measure the exact distance be-tween the incision and the target. A 16- to 18-gauge puncture needle (Fig 8–2) may then be inserted blindly through the incision and aimed in the direction previously determined by ultrasound. However, the needle should never be advanced blindly farther than through the abdominal fascia.

The scanning head is now placed in such a way that both the target and the puncture needle are visualized in the same scanning plane, and the needle is aligned so that its tip can be clearly seen. Time and patience may be necessary to align the direction of the needle and the position of the scanning head so that both the needle and the target can be seen simultaneously on the monitor. Vibrating the needle will make the tip more visible while the position of the scanning head is being adjusted. If the angle of puncture is too steep or too flat, the needle can be withdrawn into the subcuta-

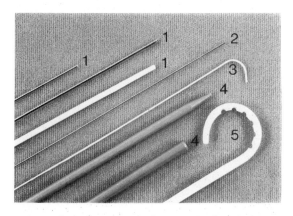

Figure 8–2. Universal nephrostomy set (Angiomed, USA), containing (1) coaxial 17.5-gauge needle/6F catheter system with obturator; (2) fine needle (22 gauge); (3) 0.035-in stiff guide wire with floppy J-tip; (4) coaxial 10F dilator/12F introducer catheter system; and (5) 10F pigtail nephrostomy catheter.

neous fat and reinserted through the abdominal wall. The needle can be safely moved back and forth down to the renal capsule as often as necessary, but the renal parenchyma should ideally be punctured only once.

A needle guide can be used to direct the needle ex-actly within the ultrasonic scanning plane. This device usually has a slot or duct configuration and must be sterilized and attached to the transducer head. With some needle guides, the angle of puncture relative to the median long axis of the scanning plane (depth) is also fixed and may be indicated on the monitor by an electronically generated beam. If a steeper or flatter angle of puncture is desired, the entire scanning head and attached needle guide must be tilted, and the choice of puncture site is therefore limited. Another drawback of this device is that it does not allow for in-dependent adjustment of the puncture and scanning di-rection if the needle deviates from its intended direc-tion after being advanced through the skin. This frequently occurs in patients with scars from previous operations and becomes more of a problem the farther the target is from the cutaneous puncture site. Free-hand puncture with individual adjustment of puncture and scanning direction is preferable in these cases.

Movement of the kidney during respiration may complicate puncture if the target is small and is visible on the monitor only during a specific respiratory phase. If the direction of the needle and the position of the target are aligned and both are clearly seen on the monitor, the needle is advanced through the renal cap-sule during the appropriate phase of respiration (Fig 8–3). In this phase, the kidney is usually moved to some extent by the puncture needle so that visualiza-tion of needle and target may be momentarily blurred. However, as soon as the tip of the needle has pene-trated the fibrous renal capsule, it is seen even more clearly as it is advanced through the renal paren-chyma, which is only slightly echogenic, and into a di-lated calix, the renal pelvis, or a renal cyst, all of which are free of internal echoes. If both the tip of the needle and the target are visualized clearly at the same spot on the scanning plane, the needle will be in the de-sired space.

A stone may actually be felt by the needle tip, or its movement may be observed on the monitor. Ante-grade injection of a small amount of contrast dye will fluoroscopically outline the renal collecting system af-ter successful puncture. However, if the collecting system has not first been successfully punctured, con-trast dye may fill the interlobar veins, which form a basketlike structure around the calices, or may ex-travasate. In rare cases in which contrast dye is in-jected into the adventitia of the renal collecting sys-tem, extravasation may assume the configuration of the collecting system, mimicking successful puncture. Care must be taken to inject the least amount of dye necessary so that further fluoroscopic and ultrasonic orientation will not be hindered. A larger amount of dye injected outside the collecting system may com-press the calix to be entered and render puncture more difficult. At this stage, the position of the needle tip

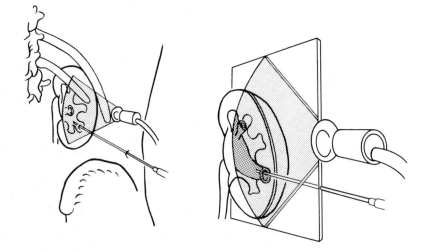

Figure 8–3. Ultrasonically guided puncture of a dorsal lower calix. Needle must be in the scanning plane to be visualized.

should be checked by repeated ultrasonic viewings and the findings compared with the fluoroscopic appearance. If the position of the needle tip on ultrasound is close to its destination (as ascertained by a small vibratory movement), the needle should be retracted a few millimeters only and then readvanced at the appropriate angle and tilt. Once the collecting system is entered (Fig 8–4A), fluoroscopy alone is used to guide procedures.

If fluoroscopy is used instead of ultrasound for guiding renal puncture, a fine-needle (20–22 gauge) puncture technique may be used. Intravenous or retrograde administration of contrast dye is needed. With retrograde injection, a ureteral balloon occlusion catheter can be inserted into the ureteropelvic junction to cause slight distention of the renal collecting system; this will facilitate puncture of a nondilated system. First, a 16- to 18-gauge needle is inserted through the abdominal wall only, and a longer fine needle is then inserted coaxially through the larger needle (Fig 8–4B). This technique increases control of the fine needle. As soon as the fine needle has entered the collecting system, the larger needle can be advanced over the fine needle serving as a guide. A regular guide wire can then be inserted after withdrawal of the fine needle through the large needle into the collecting system.

Urine aspirated from the collecting system should be cultured, especially if there is suspicion of a urinary tract infection from the history or the appearance of the aspirated urine.

ANTEGRADE PYELOGRAPHY & PRESSURE/PERFUSION STUDIES

Renal puncture is rarely indicated for diagnostic antegrade pyelography only, because less invasive radiographic techniques are available (eg, intravenous pyelography with tomograms, ultrasound, CT scan-

ning, magnetic resonance imaging, retrograde pyelography). However, obtaining a radiograph after antegrade injection of contrast dye should be an integral part of every percutaneous puncture for any indication. Before contrast dye is injected, urine must be aspirated to decompress an obstructed collecting system. The contrast dye should be diluted to 20–30% for better visualization of details; antegrade pyelography will then provide images of the collecting system with about the same resolution of detail as retrograde pyelography.

Antegrade pyelography is also performed in con-

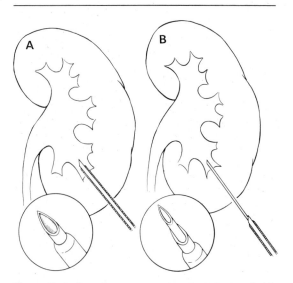

Figure 8–4. Percutaneous puncture techniques. *A:* Ultrasonically guided technique: puncture with a 16- to 18-gauge coaxial needle/catheter system. *B:* Fluoroscopically guided technique: coaxial fine-needle puncture through a larger needle/catheter system.

junction with a percutaneous pressure/perfusion study (Whitaker test) to assess pyeloureteral resistance. Percutaneous urodynamic studies of the dilated upper urinary tract are indicated only in the 10–30% of cases in which noninvasive radioisotope studies (diuresis renogram; see Chapter 9) fail to differentiate an obstructed from a nonobstructed dilated system (more likely in distal ureteral obstruction than in pelvic-ureteral obstruction, in which diuresis renograms are reliable).

The Whitaker test provides simultaneous measurements of intrapelvic and intravesical pressures during antegrade perfusion, with flow rates of 5, 10, 15, and 20 mL/min. Puncture of the renal collecting system is performed with a coaxial needle/catheter system with an outer 6F catheter for the renal pressure/perfusion study; thus, puncture and catheter insertion can be done as a one-step procedure. Perfusion is started with flow rates of 5–10 mL/min until a steady-state equilibrium of pressure readings is reached and the entire upper urinary tract is opacified (Fig 8–5). Pressure readings may be obtained intermittently from the perfusion catheter via a 3-way stopcock or continuously, if a double-lumen nephrostomy catheter or 2 separate catheters for perfusion and pressure measurement are used. Continuous recordings during perfusion from a single perfusion catheter via a T connection yield erroneous pressure readings (the smaller the lumen of the nephrostomy catheter and the higher the perfusion rate, the higher the pressure reading), unless the resistance of the entire system was previously calibrated for each rate of perfusion. In order to obtain accurate pressure readings, the positions of the intrapelvic and intravesical pressure manometers must be adjusted to the level of the renal pelvis and bladder, respectively. At a flow rate of 10 mL/min, differential pressures (renal pelvic pressure minus bladder pressure) below 13 cm of water are normal, between 14 and 22 cm of water suggest mild obstruction, and above 22 cm of water suggest moderate to severe obstruction. At flow rates of 15 mL/min and 20 mL/min, upper limits of normal pressure are 18 cm and 21 cm of water, respectively.

PERCUTANEOUS CATHETER PLACEMENT

Percutaneous nephrostomy catheter placement for drainage and decompression of the upper urinary tract is indicated if retrograde ureteral catheterization is not advisable (eg, in sepsis secondary to ureteral obstruction) or proves to be impossible (eg, impassable ureteral obstruction due to stone, tumor, or stricture). Nephrostomy catheters may also be used for diagnostic purposes (Whitaker test) or therapeutic procedures (chemolysis of stones). After percutaneous endourologic procedures, a nephrostomy catheter is usually left indwelling for a few days. To convert a nephrostomy catheter diversion into an internal stent drainage, antegrade ureteral stenting through the nephrostomy tract may be attempted even in cases in which previous attempts at retrograde stenting have failed. The antegrade approach to stenting can be expected to be successful if failure of retrograde stenting was not related to mere mechanical ureteral obstruction but rather to ureteral tortuosity, false passage (ureterovaginal fistula, urinoma after open surgery), or inability to identify the orifice endoscopically (ureteroileal anastomosis).

In percutaneous puncture for catheter placement, the diameter of the tract will depend on the size of the catheter to be inserted. For diagnostic procedures such as pressure/perfusion studies (Whitaker test), a 6F catheter is sufficient. Catheters of this size can be placed in a one-step procedure of puncture if coaxial needle/catheter systems are used (Fig 8–2). For therapeutic interventions such as nephrostomy drainage or antegrade ureteral stenting, softer, larger catheters must be inserted, and puncture tract dilation is necessary before catheter insertion. For dilation of a puncture tract, a 0.035- or 0.038-inch guide wire must be inserted into the collecting system, either directly through the puncture needle or through the outer catheter of a coaxial needle/catheter system. Curved-

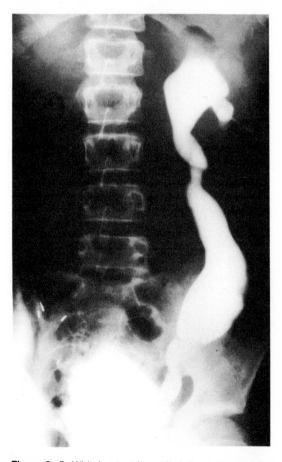

Figure 8–5. Whitaker test in a dilated upper tract after vesicoureteral reimplantation (prune belly syndrome). Antegrade perfusion with 10 mL/min results in a vesicopelvic pressure gradient of 10 cm of water, with unobstructed flow.

tip (J) guide wires are less likely to cause damage to the mucosa of the renal pelvis than are straight guide wires. One of the most common problems of tract dilation is kinking of the guide wire during insertion of fascial dilators; therefore, guide wires with a floppy tip and a stiff proximal section are preferable over floppy guide wires. If the tip of the guide wire cannot be advanced into the renal pelvis because it is trapped in a dilated calix with a narrow infundibulum or because an obstructing stone hinders passage, the outer catheter of a coaxial needle/catheter system can be used to manipulate the guide wire into the collecting system (Fig 8–6A), or angiographic catheters with different curved-tip configurations may be inserted over the guide wire for this purpose. Once the guide wire is in the correct position (upper calix, renal pelvis, upper ureter), radiopaque fascial dilators can be inserted under fluoroscopic control with rapid forth-and-back rotating movements. If flexible plastic fascial dilators are used, sequential insertion of dilators of progressively increasing size (usually in 2F steps) is necessary. If stiff metal or Kevlar dilators are used, dilation from 6F to 10–12F is possible in a one-step procedure.

After tract dilation, relatively stiff nephrostomy catheters (eg, polyethylene catheters) can be introduced easily over the guide wire. However, if softer catheters (eg, silicone or polyurethane catheters) are to be inserted, use of an introducer catheter is helpful. An introducer catheter is also helpful for antegrade ureteral stenting and for insertion of nephrostomy catheters with various self-retaining configurations of the tip (eg, pigtail). These catheters can be stretched into a straight configuration while being inserted through the introducer catheter and over a guide wire; the tip will resume its original configuration due to memory function of the material once the guide wire is withdrawn. The introducer catheter can be inserted with the last fascial dilator in a one-step procedure if a coaxial dilator/introducer catheter system is used (Figs 8–6B and C). The use of an introducer catheter provides universal access to the renal collecting system for placement of all types of catheters (nephrostomy catheters [Fig 8–6D], ureteral stents, balloon dilation catheters) and safety and working wires for different systems of large-bore nephrostomy tract dilation required for insertion of endoscopic instruments.

Nephrostomy catheters should be soft to avoid discomfort and irritation of the renal pelvis and should have a self-retaining mechanism or should be placed

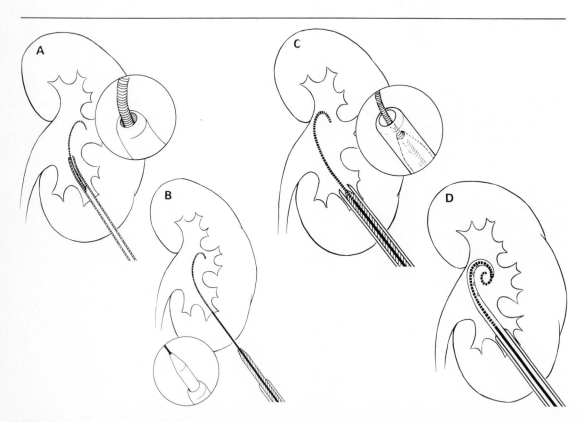

Figure 8–6. Small-bore tract dilation and nephrostomy catheter insertion. *A:* J-guide wire inserted through the needle/catheter system and advanced with assistance of the catheter into the renal pelvis. *B:* Insertion of a coaxial dilator/introducer catheter system over the guide wire. Stiff proximal section of the guide wire prevents extrarenal kinking. *C:* After the dilator has entered the collecting system, the introducer catheter is advanced over its tip. *D:* Pigtail nephrostomy catheter is inserted into the renal pelvis over the guide wire and through the introducer catheter.

with enough slack to prevent dislodgment from the collecting system if pulled inadvertently. The most commonly used nephrostomy catheters are Malecot catheters with or without a ureteral catheter extension distal to the retaining mechanism, pigtail catheters, and loop catheters. Loop catheters have the best self-retaining mechanism, but this may cause serious complications if the catheter is accidentally pulled out of the kidney.

Antegrade ureteral stenting can be done through an introducer catheter using either open- or closed-tip stents. Catheters with open-tip configuration are advanced with a pusher catheter over a guide wire, which must be inserted through the introducer sheath down the ureter and into the bladder as a first step. Catheters with closed-tip configuration are advanced by pushing the indwelling wire. In either technique, a thread should be pulled through one of the proximal side holes of the catheter so that the catheter can be pulled back into the renal pelvis if it is advanced too far. The thread must be pulled out before the guide wire is withdrawn so that the pusher catheter can hold the double-J stent in place.

An introducer catheter may also be used for insertion of a 7F balloon dilation catheter over a guide wire into the ureter to dilate ureteral strictures to 12–18F with balloon pressures of up to 15 atm. After successful dilation, an 8–10F stent is usually left indwelling for several weeks. This technique is most successful in ureteral strictures as a complication of recent surgery for benign disorders, except ureteropelvic obstruction. Long-standing strictures or strictures due to tumor compression of the ureter, radiation damage, or ischemic ureteral necrosis after radical pelvic surgery are not likely to respond favorably to balloon dilation. Long-term results with this technique cannot be determined from most published data, either because the period of follow-up was short or because periodically repeated balloon dilations were used.

PERFUSION-CHEMOLYSIS OF RENAL STONES

Nephrostomy catheters may be used for perfusion of the renal collecting system with chemolytic agents for renal stone dissolution. Stones composed of uric acid, cystine, struvite, or apatite are amenable to chemolysis. However, the success of oral chemolysis (for uric acid stones) and ESWL has limited the use of percutaneous chemolysis to adjunctive treatment of residual stones after open surgery, PNL, or ESWL. Primary percutaneous chemolysis may still be indicated in patients who are poor anesthetic risks, since anesthesia is required for several alternative procedures. Benefits of percutaneous chemolysis must be weighed against disadvantages and possible risks, eg, prolonged hospitalization for dissolution of large stones (cystine, struvite, or apatite stones) and possible complications of treating infection stones (sepsis, hypermagnesemia).

To limit risks, perfusion chemolysis should always be performed with a double-catheter system for irrigation and simultaneous continuous drainage. This is achieved by using either 2 separately or coaxially inserted nephrostomy catheters (Fig 8–7A) or a ureteral catheter in conjunction with a nephrostomy catheter (Fig 8–7B). To ensure effective flow around the stone, the irrigation catheter must be placed close to the stone. Lack of continuous, complete drainage of the perfusate with increased intrapelvic pressures above 30 cm of water may lead to pyelotubular and pyelovenous reflux of chemolytic agents and, possibly, infected urine, resulting in hypermagnesemia (perfusion with hemiacidrin or Suby's solution G or M) and sepsis. Irrigation should be started only in the absence of urinary tract infection or if infection is under control. Irrigation must first be tested with saline at the lowest possible height above kidney level to achieve a flow rate of 100–120 mL/h. Discomfort, pain, or leakage of perfusate may indicate inappropriate drainage of the irrigant, and patients should be instructed to interrupt the irrigation themselves in such instances.

Uric acid stones can be dissolved by sodium or potassium bicarbonate solution; cystine stones with D-penicillamine, acetylcysteine, or tromethamine-E solution; and struvite and apatite stones with Suby's solution G or M or hemiacidrin (renacidin; not FDA-approved for renal irrigation). Patients must be monitored for developing urinary tract infection or fever, and serum creatinine, phosphorus (hemiacidrin-perfusion), and serum magnesium studies (perfusion with hemiacidrin, Suby's solution G or M) must be obtained every other day.

The time necessary for complete stone dissolution depends on the composition and size of the stone and may vary from a few days (uric acid stones) to several weeks (cystine or struvite stones).

ENDOSCOPIC INTRARENAL INSTRUMENTATION

Nephroscopes are endoscopic instruments with sheaths of 15–26F that are inserted percutaneously through a nephrostomy tract. Standard rigid instruments are available in sizes 24–26F; these have fiberoptic telescopes with offset eyepieces (Fig 8–8A). Rigid instruments such as graspers and ultrasound probes can be inserted through a central working channel (Fig 8–8B). Flexible nephroscopes may be used as well. These have a deflecting mechanism for the tip that allows inspection of otherwise difficult-to-reach calices. A smaller working channel allows insertion of flexible instruments such as stone baskets, wire graspers, and electrohydraulic probes. Fewer types of instrumentation can be performed with flexible nephroscopes, and optical quality and durability are less than with the rigid nephroscopes.

Nephroscopy is rarely indicated for diagnostic purposes only; in most cases, it is performed for percuta-

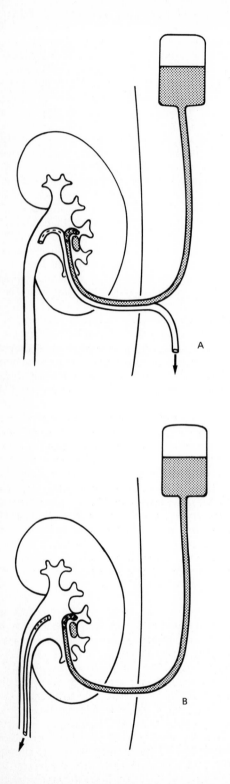

Figure 8–7. Catheter placement for perfusion chemolysis of renal stones. *A:* Perfusion and drainage of the irrigating fluid through 2 nephrostomy catheters. *B:* Perfusion through nephrostomy catheter, and drainage of the irrigant through ureteral catheter.

neous lithotripsy and extraction of renal stones (PNL). PNL had gradually replaced open surgery for removal of renal stones, but ESWL is now used in more than 80% of cases. PNL is still indicated in the 10–15% of cases for which ESWL is not the primary choice of treatment. Such cases include obstruction not caused by stones, large-volume stones, and stones that cannot be positioned within the focus of the shock waves. Nephroscopy may also be used for direct-vision internal incision of ureteropelvic strictures and for palliative treatment of urothelial cancer of the upper urinary tract.

Insertion of a nephroscope into the renal collecting system requires dilation of the puncture tract to 24–30F. Different systems of dilators can be employed, all of which are introduced over a working wire. A safety wire should be inserted parallel to the working wire and advanced into an upper calix or upper ureter to guide the way back into the collecting system in case the dilator and working wire become dislodged accidentally. Use of an introducer catheter during the small-bore tract dilation to 10–12F facilitates parallel insertion of safety and working wires. The central metal catheter of a coaxial metal dilator system (Fig 8–9A), the central plastic catheter for insertion of sequential plastic dilators, or a balloon dilator catheter can be inserted over the working wire. Balloon dilator catheters of 9F size can dilate a nephrostomy tract to a diameter of 30F under pressure up to 15 atm in a one-step procedure. This may prove difficult or impossible if perirenal scar tissue from previous operation does not allow complete expansion of the balloon over its entire length. Sequential plastic dilators allow stepwise dilation of the tract under fluoroscopic control; however, upon withdrawal for insertion of the next larger sized dilator, compression of the tract is lost intermittently and bleeding occurs into the collecting system, sometimes hindering endoscopy. Coaxial metal dilators (Fig 8–9B) (each dilator slides over the next smaller one) allow stepwise tract dilation even in the presence of severe scarring without intermittent loss of nephrostomy tract compression. With any dilation technique, the last step is insertion of a working sheath, which may be either the 24–26F metal working sheath of the nephroscope or a larger plastic sheath. With the balloon dilation technique, the working sheath must be introduced over a plastic dilator; with use of serial plastic or coaxial metal dilators, the working sheath will slide over the next smaller dilator. A 28–30F plastic working sheath is preferable to a metal nephroscope sheath in all cases in which extensive, prolonged instrumentation is anticipated (eg, staghorn stones). Larger plastic sheaths not only provide better irrigation with lower intrapelvic pressures than do continuous-flow nephroscope sheaths but also allow easier extraction of large stone fragments.

Renal Stones

In the era of ESWL, use of PNL is limited to 3 types of cases:

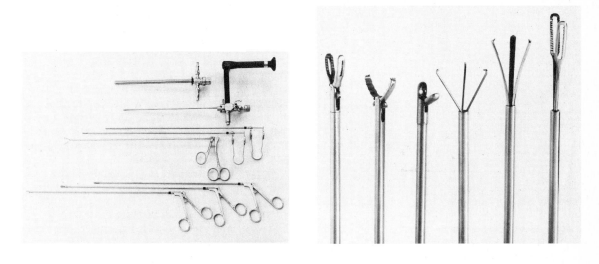

Figure 8–8. Rigid nephroscope. *Left:* A continuous-flow sheath, telescope with offset eyepiece for central access to a straight working channel, and rigid forceps and graspers. *Right:* Graspers and forceps for percutaneous endoscopic stone extraction.

(1) Obstruction not caused by stones (eg, stones in a caliceal diverticulum [Figs 8–10A and B], stones in association with ureteropelvic stenosis). These stones could be broken up by ESWL, but gravel would not pass spontaneously.

(2) Large-volume stones (Figs 8–11A and B) (eg, staghorn stones). These stones can be treated by several sessions of ESWL. However, problems associated with passing large quantities of gravel (eg, ureteral obstruction, pain, fever, and sepsis) can be prevented by first percutaneously debulking the stone and then performing ESWL for endoscopically inaccessible stones.

(3) Stones that cannot be positioned within the focus of the shock wave (eg, stones in kidneys with abnormal position due to congenital anomalies of the urinary tract or skeleton, stones in transplanted kidneys).

Of these cases, large-volume staghorn stones are a much more common indication for PNL than stones that can be extracted in toto. Small stones can be extracted with a variety of rigid forceps and graspers (Fig 8–8B). Stones may be retrieved from difficult-to-reach calices with flexible wire baskets and graspers inserted through flexible nephroscopes. Large stones must be disintegrated using mechanical, ultrasonic, or

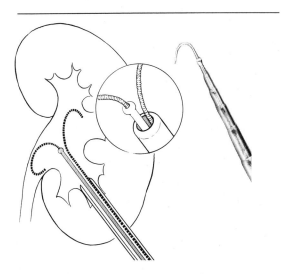

Figure 8–9. Large-bore tract dilation for nephroscopy. *Left:* Insertion of the central catheter of the Alken dilator system over a working wire through an introducer catheter (see also Fig 8–7). An introducer catheter allows parallel insertion of a safety wire into the collecting system. *Right:* Alken coaxial metal dilators for sequential tract dilation without loss of tract compression. Final step is coaxial insertion of a plastic working sheath or the metal nephroscope sheath.

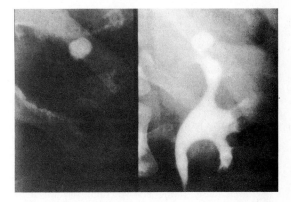

Figure 8–10. Stone in upper caliceal diverticulum requiring PNL. *Left:* KUB. *Right:* IVP.

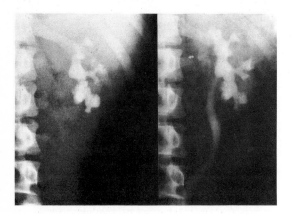

Figure 8–11. Staghorn stone requiring combined PNL and ESWL. *Left:* KUB. *Right:* IVP.

electrohydraulic energy. Strong nutcracker-type forceps (visual lithotrite, stone punch; derived from instruments for transurethral bladder stone disintegration) can be used only in a spacious renal pelvis. Hollow ultrasonic probes allow for controllable, systematic stone disintegration under continuous suction for removal of sand and smaller fragments. Electrohydraulic probes are more powerful than ultrasonic probes and may also be used through flexible nephroscopes but do not provide continuous suction and are associated with a higher risk of scattering stone fragments into inaccessible calices and of damaging the mucosa of the renal pelvis. However, with electrohydraulic probes, disintegration of especially hard or large stones is faster.

For relatively soft stones, continuous disintegration and evacuation of fragments with ultrasound probes is most time-efficient. Hard stones are preferably broken up into the largest possible fragments that can still be extracted through the working sheath. The ureteropelvic portion of a staghorn stone should be left in place until the procedure is nearly completed, as it will act like a plug in a drain to prevent the loss of fragments into the ureter. An antegradely or retrogradely positioned ureteral balloon occlusion catheter might serve the same purpose; however, the extra procedure of retrograde ureteral catheterization is rarely indicated.

Normal saline should be used as the irrigation fluid except in the case of electrohydraulic lithotripsy, in which 1/6 normal saline is more appropriate. However, even with the low-pressure system provided by the large plastic working sheath, considerable amounts of irrigation fluid may be absorbed if small veins are opened and intrarenal manipulation is prolonged. This may cause TUR syndrome with use of hypotonic fluids. Intraoperative administration of diuretics (eg, mannitol, 12.5 g) is advisable and also has proved effective in preventing intrarenal reflux. If there is suspicion of extravasation, contrast dye must

be injected and a diagnostic radiograph obtained. Upon completion of the procedure, a plain film should be obtained and a nephrostomy catheter placed. A Foley catheter with a 5-mL balloon may be inserted through a fenestrated trocar or the plastic working sheath, which then is withdrawn and cut lengthwise for removal from the Foley catheter. Malecot catheters or straight polyethylene catheters (eg, chest tubes) may be used as well and should be secured to the skin with 2 sutures. A final nephrostogram documents appropriate position of the catheter.

Nephrostomy catheters may be removed after 1–4 days, the interval depending on the amount and duration of instrumentation and related persistence of hematuria. If ESWL is to be performed, it can be done 1–4 days after the percutaneous procedure. The nephrostomy catheter should be left in place during and after ESWL to provide drainage for urine and stone gravel and to allow for a second endoscopic procedure if some of the stone fragments do not pass spontaneously after ESWL.

Ureteropelvic Stenoses

With the advent of PNL, other endosurgical techniques have been developed that are similar to procedures used in the lower urinary tract. Direct-vision internal incision of ureteropelvic stenoses seems to be a natural outgrowth of endoscopic techniques in the upper urinary tract. Compared to fluoroscopy-guided balloon dilation, which tears the stricture by exerting radial forces, this technique offers the advantage of a narrow incision of definable length and depth. This incision must be extended into the perirenal fat and is stented for 4–6 weeks to allow for healing, according to the principle of Davis' intubated ureterotomy. The procedure seems to work best in patients in whom open surgical pyeloplasty has failed (the latter is still the method of choice for congenital ureteropelvic obstruction). Long-term follow-up data are too incomplete to suggest that endopyeloplasty should be a standard form of treatment.

Urothelial Tumors

Another new technique of endoscopic surgery in the upper urinary tract is use of electroresection, electrocoagulation, and neodymium:YAG laser coagulation for treatment of urothelial tumors. However, with the limited experience in treating upper urinary tract urothelial cancer endoscopically, these techniques must still be considered experimental and limited to palliative surgery.

PERCUTANEOUS ASPIRATION & BIOPSY

Percutaneous puncture of cystic or solid lesions of the kidney and the adjacent retroperitoneum is usually performed for diagnostic purposes, in some cases combined with therapeutic drainage and obliteration of fluid-filled spaces (Tables 8–2 and 8–3). Because

Table 8–2. Indications for puncture of renal and retroperitoneal lesions.

Diagnostic indications
  Fluid aspiration and serum chemistry
  Bacterial culture and sensitivity testing
  Cytologic studies
  Contrast dye injection and radiography
  Histologic studies (renal biopsies)
Therapeutic indications
  Catheter drainage (urinoma, abscess, hematoma, lymphocele)
  Fluid evacuation and injection of sclerosing agents (simple renal graft)

most of these lesions are not radiopaque and will not concentrate intravenously administered contrast dye, they cannot be easily visualized with fluoroscopy. Thus, ultrasound or CT scanning is the imaging technique of choice to depict these lesions and guide percutaneous puncture. The technique of ultrasonically guided puncture is the same whether the target is the renal collecting system or a cystic or solid renal or extrarenal lesion. Depending on the purpose of the puncture, the size and configuration of puncture needles may vary. For cytologic aspiration, a fine-needle (20–22 gauge) aspiration technique is used that is comparable to fine-needle aspiration biopsy of the prostate. There is no evidence that one type of needle is preferable to the others. For aspiration and evacuation of renal cysts or extrarenal fluid collections (urinoma, lymphocele), the same coaxial needle/catheter system can be used as for percutaneous puncture of the renal collecting system. A small catheter is left in place to ensure complete drainage of fluid. When fluids of high viscosity (abscess, hematoma) are to be drained, larger-bore catheters (12–20F) must be inserted, necessitating dilation of the percutaneous tract. Percutaneous renal biopsy for histologic diagnosis and classification of renal disease is performed with 14- to 16-gauge needles (eg, Franklin-Silverman, Tru-cut) at the lower pole of the kidney.

Table 8–3. Differential diagnosis of renal and retroperitoneal lesions.

Renal cystic lesion
  Benign cyst
  Hydrocalix
  Abscess
  Hematoma
  Cystic tumor
  Tumor in cyst
Retroperitoneal fluid collection
  Urinoma
  Lymphocele
  Hematoma
  Cystic tumor
Solid renal and retroperitoneal lesions
  Benign tumor
  Malignant primary tumor
  Metastatic tumor

Renal Cysts

Renal cysts are found in about 50% of autopsy specimens in persons over age 50 years and are a frequent accidental finding on ultrasound or CT studies. On ultrasound examination, a simple benign cyst will appear as a smooth-walled, echo-free spherical lesion that may protrude exophytically from the kidney, cause indentation of the renal parenchyma, or compress the renal collecting system. Septations in a cyst and multilocular cysts may be difficult to differentiate from tumors on ultrasound, and CT scanning may become necessary; however, only a few cases require diagnostic percutaneous puncture. Indications for puncture are an irregular, thick wall and internal echoes on ultrasound examination, density numbers on CT scanning higher than those of serous fluid, and hematuria. Puncture for therapeutic procedures (evacuation of fluid and instillation of a sclerosing agent) is indicated only if, due to its size or location, the cyst causes compression and obstruction of an infundibulum or the ureter, or discomfort and pain.

Various tests may be performed on aspirated fluid. No one test is pathognomonic except cytologic findings of malignant cells. However, neoplasms within a cyst are exceedingly rare, and cystic degeneration of a renal neoplasm can usually be easily identified by ultrasound and CT scanning. Benign cysts contain clear, straw-colored fluid with low fat and protein content and lactic acid dehydrogenase (LDH) levels of less than 250 IMU/mL. Cancer is suspected if the fluid is bloody or murky and has a high content of fat, protein, and lactic acid dehydrogenase. After aspiration of 20–30% of the cystic fluid, the same amount of 60% contrast dye is injected, and diagnostic radiographs are obtained in the prone, supine, upright, decubitus, and Trendelenburg positions. If necessary, another 20–30% of the cystic fluid may be replaced by air for obtaining double-contrast radiographs.

For therapeutic obliteration of cysts, sclerosing agents such as Pantopaque or 95% ethanol can be injected after complete evacuation of the cystic fluid through the catheter. A volume of 10–100 mL of 95% ethanol, approximating 10–20% of the original volume of cystic fluid, is injected into the cyst and should be drained after 30 minutes.

Retroperitoneal Fluid Collections

Low-viscosity retroperitoneal fluid collections (urinoma, lymphocele) are usually a complication of surgical procedures. However, urinoma may also be caused by exogenous trauma or by forniceal rupture due to acute ureteral obstruction. Percutaneous techniques of catheter drainage eliminate the need for open surgical revision in most cases. Insertion of a small (6–10F) catheter (with numerous side holes) is usually sufficient. Adjunctive procedures are performed to ensure sealing of the fluid leak and obliteration of the cystic lesion. With urinoma, the upper urinary tract must also be drained by a ureteral catheter or percutaneous nephrostomy catheter until drainage from the urinoma stops. Lymphoceles that develop following pelvic or retroperitoneal lymphadenectomy or renal transplantation often undergo spontaneous regression and usually do not require puncture and drainage. However, large lymphoceles developing after retroperitoneal lymphadenectomy may cause pain and even ureteral obstruction (Fig 8–12). Patients should be treated with parenteral nutrition and abdominal compression by bandaging, but if lymph drainage after percutaneous puncture and catheter placement persists for more than 1 week, surgical intervention with intraperitoneal marsupialization of the lymphocele and ligation or electrocoagulation of lymphatic vessels is indicated.

High-viscosity fluid collections (hematoma, abscess) usually require large-bore (12–20F) percutaneous catheters for sufficient drainage. Perirenal hematomas are most frequently caused by surgical or exogenous trauma and rarely develop spontaneously in the presence of a bleeding diathesis or owing to rupture of a renal tumor. Indications for percutaneous drainage are rare, as most small hematomas (which should be followed with ultrasound and CT scanning)

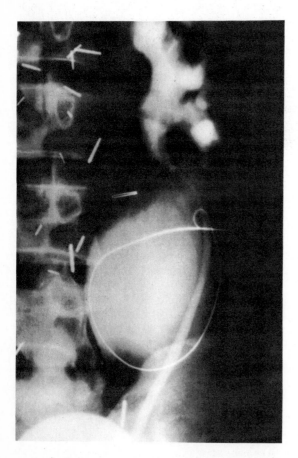

Figure 8–12. Percutaneous drainage of a lymphocele causing ureteral displacement and compression.

resolve spontaneously. Hematomas that increase in size require surgical intervention rather than percutaneous drainage. Secondary infection of a hematoma can be an indication for percutaneous drainage. Most perirenal abscesses are a complication of open surgery; hematogenic renal abscess (renal carbuncle) is less frequent. Indications for puncture and drainage should be based on findings on CT scan of a unifocal process that can be effectively and safely drained percutaneously. Multifocal renal abscesses are not amenable to percutaneous drainage.

Renal & Retroperitoneal Tumors

Percutaneous aspiration biopsy of renal and retroperitoneal tumors is indicated if less invasive radiologic studies are inconclusive and if cytologic studies may have an important impact on further medical or surgical therapy (Fig 8–13). If curative treatment by open surgery seems to be feasible, aspiration biopsy is generally not indicated. If malignancy of a renal lesion is uncertain and if conservative, organ-sparing operation is technically feasible, renal-sparing surgery plus performance of intraoperative frozen section might be preferable over percutaneous aspiration biopsy. However, rather than performing radical nephrectomy for a possibly benign lesion, aspiration biopsy should be performed first. In multifocal or possibly metastatic lesions, cytologic evaluation can be crucial for planning surgical or medical therapy, and in these cases, aspiration biopsy is usually indicated. There is a 10–25% incidence of false-negative findings on cytologic examination. As a rare complication, tumor seeding in the puncture tract has been described. The aspirate is immediately spread on glass slides. For standard Papanicolaou stains, alcohol fixation must be used.

Renal Biopsy

Renal biopsy for diagnosis and classification of medical renal diseases can be performed percutaneously as opposed to open surgical biopsy. Because specimens, rather than aspirates, are needed for diagnostic histologic study, large-bore (14–16 gauge) Franklin-Silverman or Tru-cut needles are used. Ultrasonic or fluoroscopic guidance is preferable over blind renal puncture. However, even with puncture aimed precisely at the dorsal lower pole of the kidney, where accidental injury to large vessels is less likely, bleeding is to be expected because of the vascularity of the parenchyma and is the major complication of this procedure (about 5% of cases, with a mortality rate of 0.1%). Hematoma can usually be followed conservatively by ultrasound and CT scanning, but transvascular embolization, open surgical revision, and even nephrectomy have been required following diagnostic renal biopsy. Therefore, open surgical biopsy rather than percutaneous biopsy is indicated in patients with solitary kidneys or uncontrolled hypertension.

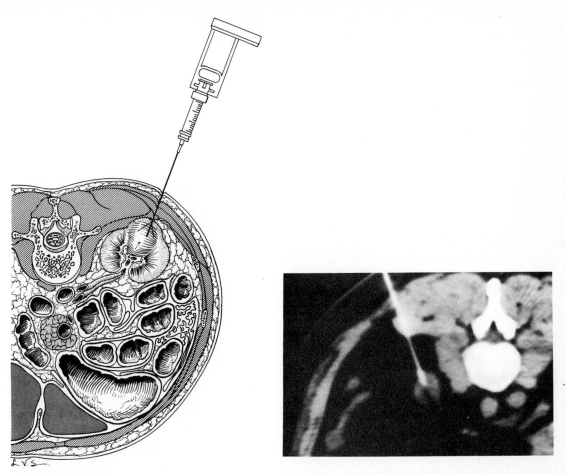

Figure 8–13. Percutaneous fine-needle biopsy. *Left:* Aspiration biopsy of a renal lesion. *Right:* Guidance with CT scanning for fine-needle aspiration biopsy of an exophytic renal cell carcinoma.

REFERENCES

Percutaneous Puncture & Catheter Placement

Alken P: Teleskopbougierset zur perkutanen Nephrostomie. *Aktuel Urol* 1981;**12**:216.

Babcock JR, Shkolnik A, Cook WA: Ultrasound-guided percutaneous nephrostomy in the pediatric patient. *J Urol* 1979;**121**:327.

Banner MP et al: Catheter dilatation of benign ureteral strictures. *Radiology* 1983;**147**:427.

Bartley O, Chidekel N, Redberg C: Percutaneous drainage of the renal pelvis for uremia due to obstructed urinary outflow. *Acta Chir Scand* 1965;**129**:443.

Bigongiari LR: The Seldinger approach to percutaneous nephrostomy and ureteral stent placement. *Urol Radiol* 1981;**2**:141.

Bigongiari LR: Transluminal dilatation of ureteral strictures. Chap 6, pp 113–118, in: *Percutaneous and Interventional Urology and Radiology*. Lang EK (editor). Springer-Verlag, 1986.

Burnett KR et al: Percutaneous nephrostomy utilizing B-mode and real-time ultrasound guidance: The lateral approach and puncture facilitation with furosemide. *J Clin Ultrasound* 1982;**10**:252.

Clayman RV et al: Rapid balloon dilatation of the nephrostomy tract for nephrostolithotomy. *Radiology* 1983;**147**:884.

Druy EM, Gharib M, Finder CA: Percutaneous nephroureteral drainage and stenting for postsurgical ureteral leaks. *AJR* 1983;**141**:389.

Elyaderani MK, Kandzari SJ: Percutaneous nephrostomy. Chap 2, pp 23–54, in: *Invasive Uroradiology: A Manual of Diagnostic and Therapeutic Techniques*. Elyaderani MK et al (editors). Heath, 1984.

Finney RP: Double-J and diversion stents. *Urol Clin North Am* 1982;**9**:89.

Fowler JE Jr, Meares EM Jr, Goldin AR: Percutaneous nephrostomy: Techniques, indications, and results. *Urology* 1975;**6**:428.

Fritzsche PJ: Antegrade and retrograde ureteral stenting. Chap 5, pp 91–111, in: *Percutaneous and Interventional Urology and Radiology*. Lang EK (editor). Springer-Verlag, 1986.

Glanz S et al: Percutaneous transrenal balloon dilatation of the ureter. *Radiology* 1983;**149**:101.

Goldin AR: Percutaneous ureteral splinting. *Urology* 1977; **10**:165.

Goodwin WE, Casey WC, Woolf W: Percutaneous trocar (needle) nephrostomy in hydronephrosis. *JAMA* 1955; **157**:891.

Gordon RL et al: Replacing the "fallen out" catheter. *Radiology* 1980;**134**:537.

Günther R, Alken P, Altwein JE: Percutaneous nephropyelostomy using a fine-needle puncture set. *Radiology* 1979;**132**:228.

Günther R, Alken P, Altwein JE: Ureterobstruktion: Perkutane transrenale Uretersplintung. *Aktuel Urol* 1978;**4**:195.

Günther R, Altwein JE, Alken P: Internal urinary diversion by a percutaneous ureteric splint. *Br J Urol* 1980;**52**:165.

Günther R, Altwein JE, Georgi M: Feinnadelpunktion zur antegraden Pyelographie und perkutanen Nephropyelostomie. *ROFO* 1977;**127**:439.

Günther R, Marberger M, Klose K: Transrenal ureteral embolization. *Radiology* 1979;**132**:317.

Harris RD, McCullough DL, Talner LB: Percutaneous nephrostomy. *J Urol* 1976;**115**:628.

Heckemann R et al: Percutaneous nephropyelostomy under continuous real-time ultrasound guidance. *Urol Radiol* 1981;**3**:171.

Hutschenreiter G, Alken P, Klippel KF: Ultraschallgesteuerte perkutane Nephrostomie. *Urologe [A]* 1979; **18**:157.

Jeffrey RB Jr, Kuligowska E: Interventional ultrasound. Chap 5, pp 113–134, in: *Genitourinary Ultrasound*. Hricak H (editor). Churchill Livingstone, 1986.

Johnson M, Lindberg B, Risholm L: Percutaneous nephropyelosotomy in cases of ureteral obstruction. *Scand J Urol Nephrol* 1972;**6**:51.

Kadir S, White RI Jr, Engel R: Balloon dilatation of a ureteropelvic junction obstruction. *Radiology* 1982; **143**:263.

Kaplan JO et al: Dilatation of a surgically ligated ureter through a percutaneous nephrostomy. *AJR* 1982;**139**:188.

Kaye KW, Goldberg ME: Applied anatomy of the kidney and ureter. *Urol Clin North Am* 1982;**9**:3.

Lang EK: Diagnosis and management of ureteral fistulas by percutaneous nephrostomy and antegrade stent catheter. *Radiology* 1981;**138**:311.

Lang EK, Price ET: Redefinitions of indications for percutaneous nephrostomy. *Radiology* 1983;**147**:419.

Lang EK et al: The management of urinary fistulas and strictures with percutaneous ureteral stent catheters. *J Urol* 1979;**122**:736.

Lange PH: Diagnostic and therapeutic urologic instrumentation. Chap 8, pp 510–540, in: *Campbell's Urology*, 5th ed. Walsh PC et al (editors). Saunders, 1986.

Lieberman SF et al: Percutaneous antegrade transluminal ureteroplasty for renal allograft ureteral stenosis. *J Urol* 1982;**128**:122.

Miller RP et al: Percutaneous approach to the ureter. *Urol Clin North Am* 1982;**9**:31.

Oosterlinck W, De Sy WA: A new percutaneous nephrostomy set. *J Urol* 1983;**129**:466.

Pedersen JF: Percutaneous nephrostomy guided by ultrasound. *J Urol* 1974;**112**:157.

Pedersen JF et al: Ultrasonically-guided percutaneous nephrostomy: Report of 24 cases. *Radiology* 1976; **119**:429.

Pfister RC: Percutaneous nephrostomy. Chap 1, pp 1–27, in: *Percutaneous and Interventional Urology and Radiology*. Lang EK (editor). Springer-Verlag, 1986.

Pollack HM, Banner MP: Replacing blocked or dislodged percutaneous nephrostomy and ureteral stent catheters. *Radiology* 1982;**145**:203.

Reimer DE, Oswalt GC Jr: Iatrogenic ureteral obstruction treated with balloon dilation. *J Urol* 1981;**126**:689.

Ring EJ, McLean GK: Pages 379–410 in: *Interventional Radiology: Principles and Techniques*. Little, Brown, 1981.

Rosen RJ et al: Obstructed ureteroileal conduits: Antegrade catheter drainage. *AJR* 1980;**135**:1201.

Saitoh M, Watanabe H: Ultrasonically guided percutaneous pyeloscopy. *Urology* 1981;**17**:457.

Sanders RC: Renal puncture techniques. Chap 16, pp 353–372, in: *Ultrasound in Urology*, 2nd ed. Resnick MI, Sanders RC (editors). Williams & Wilkins, 1984.

Seldinger SI: Catheter replacement of the needle in percutaneous arteriography. *Acta Radiol* 1953;**39**:368.

Singh B, Kim H, Wax SH: Stent versus nephrostomy: Is there a choice? *J Urol* 1979;**121**:268.

Smith AD et al: A modified Stamey catheter kit for long-term percutaneous nephrostomy drainage. *Radiology* 1981; **139**:230.

Stables DP: Percutaneous nephrostomy: Techniques, indications, and results. *Urol Clin North Am* 1982;**9**:15.

Thüroff JW, Alken P: Ultrasound for renal puncture and fluoroscopy for tract dilatation and catheter placement: A combined approach. *Endourology* 1987;**2**:1.

Turner AG et al: The role of anterograde pyelography in the transplant kidney. *J Urol* 1980;**123**:812.

Walz PH et al: Technik und Fehlermöglichkeiten der perkutanen Nephrostomie unter sonographischer Kontrolle. *Aktuel Urol* 1981;**12**:232.

Antegrade Pressure/Perfusion Studies

Amis ES Jr, Pfister RC, Newhouse JH: Resistances of various renal instruments used in ureteral perfusion. *Radiology* 1982;**143**:267.

Coolsaet BLRA et al: Urodynamic investigation of the wide ureter. *J Urol* 1980;**124**:666.

Djurhuus JC, Nerstrom B, Rask-Andersen H: Dynamics of upper urinary tract in man: Peroperative electrophysiological findings in patients with manifest or suspected hydronephrosis. *Acta Chir Scand [Suppl]* 1976;**472**:49.

Djurhuus JC, Stage P: Percutaneous intrapelvic pressure registration in hydronephrosis during diuresis. *Acta Chir Scand [Suppl]* 1976;**472**:43.

Elyaderani MK, Kandzari SJ: Antegrade pyelography and the ureteral perfusion test. Chap 1, pp 9–22, in: *Invasive Uroradiology: A Manual of Diagnostic and Therapeutic Techniques*. Elyaderani MK et al (editors). Heath, 1984.

Jaffe RB, Middleton AW Jr: Whitaker test: Differentiation of obstructive from nonobstructive uropathy. *AJR* 1980; **134**:9.

King LR: Megaloureter: Definition, diagnosis and management. (Editorial.) *J Urol* 1980;**123**:222.

Mortensen J et al: The relationship between pressure and flow in the normal pig renal pelvis: An experimental study of the range of normal pressures. *Scand J Urol Nephrol* 1983;**17**:369.

Newhouse JH, Pfister RC: Percutaneous upper urinary tract dynamics in equivocal obstruction (Whitaker). *Urol Radiol* 1981;**2**:191.

Newhouse JH et al: Whitaker test after pyeloplasty: Establishment of normal ureteral perfusion pressures. *AJR* 1981;**137**:223.

Pfister RC: Obstruction and percutaneous ureteral urodynamics: The Whitaker Test. Chap 2, pp 29–54, in: *Percutaneous and Interventional Urology and Radiology*. Lang EK (editor). Springer-Verlag, 1986.

Toguri AG, Fournier G: Factors influencing the pressure-flow-perfusion system. *J Urol* 1982;**127**:1021.

Weinstein BJ, Skolnick ML: Ultrasonically guided antegrade pyelography. *J Urol* 1978;**120**:319.

Whitaker RH: Clinical application of upper urinary tract dynamics. *Urol Clin North Am* 1979;**6**:137.

Whitaker RH: Equivocal pelvic-ureteric obstruction. *Br J Urol* 1975;**47**:771.

Whitaker RH: An evaluation of 170 diagnostic pressure flow studies in the upper urinary tract. *J Urol* 1979;**121**:602.

Whitaker RH: Investigating wide ureters with ureteral pressure flow studies. *J Urol* 1976;**116**:81.

Whitaker RH: Methods of assessing obstruction in dilated ureters. *Br J Urol* 1973;**45**:15.

Whitaker RH: Percutaneous upper urinary tract dynamics in equivocal obstruction. *Urol Radiol* 1981;**2**:187.

Whitaker RH: Some observations and theories on the wide ureter and hydronephrosis. *Br J Urol* 1975;**47**:377.

Whitaker RH, Buxton-Thomas MS: A comparison of pressure flow studies and renography in equivocal upper urinary tract obstruction. *J Urol* 1984;**131**:446.

Percutaneous Renal Stone Treatment

Alken P, Altwein JE: Die perkutane Nephrolitholapaxie. *Verh Dtsch Ges Urol* 1980;**31**:109.

Alken P, Günther R, Thüroff J: Percutaneous nephrolithotomy: A routine procedure? *Br J Urol [Suppl]* 1983;**51**:1.

Alken P, Huschenreiter G, Günther R: Percutaneous kidney stone removal. *Eur Urol* 1982;**8**:304.

Alken P et al: Extracorporeal shock wave lithotripsy (ESWL): Alternatives and adjuvant procedures. *World J Urol* 1985;**3**:48.

Alken P et al: Percutaneous stone manipulation. *J Urol* 1981;**125**:463.

Bissada NK, Meacham KR, Redman JF: Nephrostoscopy with removal of renal pelvic calculi. *J Urol* 1974;**112**:414.

Blaivas JG, Pais VM, Spellman RM: Chemolysis of residual stone fragments after extensive surgery for staghorn calculi. *Urology* 1975;**6**:680.

Cato AR, Tulloch AGS: Hypermagnesemia in a uremic patient during renal pelvis irrigation with renacidin. *J Urol* 1974;**111**:313.

Chaussey C, Schmiedt E: Shock wave treatment for stones in the upper urinary tract. *Urol Clin North Am* 1983;**10**:743.

Clayman RV et al: Nephrostolithotomy: Percutaneous removal of renal and ureteric calculi. *Br J Urol [Suppl]* 1983;**51**:6.

Clayman RV et al: Percutaneous nephrolithotomy: An approach to branched and staghorn renal calculi. *JAMA* 1983;**250**:73.

Clayman RV et al: Percutaneous nephrolithotomy: Extraction of renal and ureteral calculi from 100 patients. *J Urol* 1984;**131**:868.

Crissey MM, Gittes RF: Dissolution of cystine ureteral calculus by irrigation with tromethamine. *J Urol* 1979;**121**:811.

Dretler SP, Pfister RC, Newhouse JH: Renal-stone dissolution via percutaneous nephrostomy. *N Engl J Med* 1979;**300**:341.

Dunnick NR: Percutaneous approach to urinary tract calculi. Chap 4, pp 75–89, in: *Percutaneous and Interventional Urology and Radiology*. Lang EK (editor). Springer-Verlag, 1986.

Fernström I: Percutaneous extraction of renal calculi: Technique and results. *Br J Urol [Suppl]* 1983;**51**:25.

Fernström I, Johansson B: Percutaneous pyelolithotomy: A new extraction technique. *Scand J Urol Nephrol* 1976;**10**:257.

Fostvedt GA, Barnes RW: Complications during lavage therapy for renal calculi. *J Urol* 1963;**89**:329.

Freiha FS, Hemady K: Dissolution of uric acid stones: Alternative to surgery. *Urology* 1976;**8**:334.

Günther RW, Alken P: Percutaneous litholapaxy and extrac-

tion of renal calculi. Chap 3, pp 55–74, in: *Percutaneous and Interventional Urology and Radiology*. Lang EK (editor). Springer-Verlag, 1986.

Jacobs SC, Gittes RF: Dissolution of residual renal calculi with hemiacidrin. *J Urol* 1976;**115**:2.

Kandzari SJ, Elyaderani MK: Retrograde extraction, chemolysis, and intraoperative ultrasonographic localization of urinary calculi. Chap 5, pp 133–153, in: *Invasive Uroradiology: A Manual of Diagnostic and Therapeutic Techniques*. Elyaderani MK et al (editors). Heath, 1984.

Kurth KH, Hohenfellner R, Altwein JE: Ultrasound litholapaxy of a staghorn calculus. *J Urol* 1977;**117**:242.

Lange PH et al: Percutaneous removal of caliceal and other "inaccessible" stones: Instruments and techniques. *J Urol* 1984;**132**:439.

LeRoy AJ, Segura JW: Percutaneous ultrasonic lithotripsy. *Urol Radiol* 1984;**6**:88.

Letourneau J et al: Nephrostolithotomy: The percutaneous approach to kidney stones. Chap 4, pp 97–132, in: *Invasive Uroradiology: A Manual of Diagnostic and Therapeutic Techniques*. Elyaderani MK et al (editors). Heath, 1984.

Marberger M: Disintegration of renal and ureteral calculi with ultrasound. *Urol Clin North Am* 1983;**10**:729.

Marberger M: Ultrasonic lithotripsy of renal calculi: A 3-year experience. *Br J Urol [Suppl]* 1983;**51**:41.

Marberger M, Stackl W, Hruby W: Percutaneous litholapaxy of renal calculi with ultrasound. *Eur Urol* 1982;**8**:236.

Marberger M et al: Late sequelae of ultrasonic lithotripsy of renal calculi. *J Urol* 1985;**133**:170.

Miller RA, Wickham JEA, Kellett MJ: Percutaneous destruction of renal calculi: Clinical and laboratory experience. *Br J Urol [Suppl]* 1983;**51**:51.

Mulvaney WP: The hydrodynamics of renal irrigations: With reference to calculus solvents. *J Urol* 1963;**89**:765.

Rathert P et al: Ultraschall-Lithotripsie von Ureter- und Nierensteinen: Experimentelle und erste klinische Untersuchungen. *Verh Dtsch Ges Urol* 1977;**28**:365.

Reddy PK et al: Percutaneous removal of caliceal and other "inaccessible" stones: Results. *J Urol* 1984;**132**:443.

Sachse H: Erfahrungen mit der Elektrolithotripsie. *Verh Dtsch Ges Urol* 1970;**23**:171.

Segura JW, LeRoy AJ: Percutaneous ultrasonic lithotripsy. *Urology* 1984;**23**(5 Spec No):7.

Segura JW et al: Percutaneous lithotripsy. *J Urol* 1983;**130**:1051.

Segura JW et al: Percutaneous removal of kidney stones: Preliminary report. *Mayo Clin Proc* 1982;**57**:615.

Segura JW et al: Percutaneous removal of kidney stones: Review of 1000 cases. *J Urol* 1985;**134**:1077.

Sheldon CA, Smith AD: Chemolysis of calculi. *Urol Clin North Am* 1982;**9**:121.

Smith AD, Clayman RV, Castaneda-Zuniga WR: Use of Mauermeyer stone punch via percutaneous nephrostomy. *J Urol* 1982;**128**:1285.

Smith AD, Lee WJ: Percutaneous stone extraction. *Br J Urol [Suppl]* 1983;**51**:84.

Smith AD et al: Dissolution of cystine calculi by irrigation with acetylcysteine through percutaneous nephrostomy. *Urology* 1979;**13**:422.

Smith AD et al: Percutaneous nephrostomy in the management of ureteral and renal calculi. *Radiology* 1979;**133**:49.

Stark H, Savir A: Dissolution of cystine calculi by pelviocaliceal irrigation with D-penicillamine. *J Urol* 1980;**124**:895.

Suby HI, Albright F: Dissolution of phosphatic urinary calculi by the retrograde introduction of citrate solution containing magnesium. *N Engl J Med* 1943;**228**:81.

Thüroff JW, Alken P: Stones in caliceal diverticula: Removal by percutaneous nephrolithotomy. In: *Endo-Urology: New and Approved Techniques*. Jonas U (editor). Springer-Verlag, 1987.

Thüroff JW, Hutschenreiter G: Case report: Percutaneous nephrostomy and instrumental extraction of a blocking renal calculus under local anesthesia. *Urol Int* 1980;**35**:375.

Tseng CH et al: Dissolution of cystine calculi by pelviocaliceal irrigation with tromethamine-E. *J Urol* 1982; **128**:1281.

Wickham JEA, Kellett MJ: Percutaneous nephrolithotomy. *Br Med J* 1981;**283**:1571.

Wickham JEA, Kellett MJ, Miller RA: Elective percutaneous nephrolithotomy in 50 patients: An analysis of the technique, results and complications. *J Urol* 1983; **129**:904.

Percutaneous Endoscopic Surgery

Badlani G, Eshghi M, Smith AD: Percutaneous surgery for ureteropelvic junction obstruction (endopyelotomy): Technique and early results. *J Urol* 1986;**135**:26.

Clayman RV: Percutaneous nephroscopy: A nonoperative approach to the diagnosis and treatment of renal disease. *Br J Urol* [Suppl] 1983;**51**:18.

Clayman RV et al: Percutaneous intrarenal electrosurgery. *J Urol* 1984;**131**:864.

Davis DM: Intubated ureterotomy: A new operation for ureteral and ureteropelvic strictures. *Surg Gynecol Obstet* 1943;**76**:513.

Malloy TR: Laser treatment of ureter and upper collecting system. In: *Lasers in Urologic Surgery*. Smith JA Jr (editor). Year Book, 1985.

Wickham JEA: Percutaneous pyelolysis. Chap 8, p 150, in: *Percutaneous Renal Surgery*. Wickham JEA, Miller RA (editors). Churchill Livingstone, 1983.

Percutaneous Aspiration & Biopsy

Almkuist RD, Buckalew VM Jr: Techniques of renal biopsy. *Urol Clin North Am* 1979;**6**:503.

Banner MP et al: Multilocular renal cysts: Radiologic-pathologic correlation. *AJR* 1981;**136**:239.

Barth KH: Fine needle aspiration biopsy for metastatic tumors of the kidneys and urogenital tract. Chap 8, pp 137–146, in: *Percutaneous and Interventional Urology and Radiology*. Lang EK (editor). Springer-Verlag, 1986.

Baumgartner BR, Bernardino ME: Percutaneous drainage of abscesses, urinomas, and hematomas of the genitourinary tract and retroperitoneum. Chap 7, pp 119–135, in: *Percutaneous and Interventional Urology and Radiology*. Lang EK (editor). Springer-Verlag, 1986.

Bean WJ: Renal cysts: Treatment with alcohol. *Radiology* 1981;**138**:329.

Bolton WK, Vaughan ED: A comparative study of open surgical and percutaneous renal biopsies. *J Urol* 1977; **117**:696.

Brun C, Raaschou F: The results of 500 percutaneous renal biopsies. *Arch Intern Med* 1958;**102**:716.

Buonocore E, Skipper GJ: Steerable real-time sonographically guided needle biopsy. *AJR* 1981;**136**:387.

Burnstein J, Woodside JR: Malignant hemorrhagic renal cyst with occult neoplasm. *Radiology* 1977;**123**:599.

Bush WH Jr, Burnett LL, Gibbons RP: Needle tract seeding of renal cell carcinoma. *AJR* 1977;**129**:725.

Caldamone AA, Frank IN: Percutaneous aspiration in the treatment of renal abscess. *J Urol* 1980;**123**:92.

Coleman BG et al: Hyperdense renal masses: A computed tomographic dilemma. *AJR* 1984;**143**:291.

Corad MR, Sanders RC, Mascardo AD: Perinephric abscess aspiration using ultrasound guidance. *AJR* 1977;**128**:459.

Diaz-Buxo JA, Donadio JV Jr: Complications of percutaneous renal biopsy: An analysis of 1,000 consecutive biopsies. *Clin Nephrol* 1975;**4**:223.

Elyaderani MK, Kandzari SJ: Percutaneous aspiration and biopsy procedures. Chap 6, pp 155–190, in: *Invasive Uroradiology: A Manual of Diagnostic and Therapeutic Techniques*. Elyaderani MK et al (editors). Heath, 1984.

Elyaderani Mk, Subramanian VP, Burgess JE: Diagnosis and percutaneous drainage of a perinephric abscess by ultrasound and fluoroscopy. *J Urol* 1981;**125**:405.

Ferrucci JT et al: Malignant seeding of the tract after thin-needle aspiration biopsy. *Radiology* 1979;**130**:345.

Gerzof SG: Percutaneous drainage of renal and perinephric abscess. *Urol Radiol* 1981;**2**:171.

Gerzof SG, Gale ME: Computed tomography and ultrasonography for diagnosis and treatment of renal and retroperitoneal abscesses. *Urol Clin North Am* 1982;**9**:185.

Gibbons RP, Bush WH Jr, Burnett LL: Needle tract seeding following aspiration of renal cell carcinoma. *J Urol* 1977; **118**:865.

Goldman SM et al: Renal carbuncle: The use of ultrasound in its diagnosis and treatment. *J Urol* 1977;**118**:525.

Heaston DK et al: Narrow gauge needle aspiration of solid adrenal masses. *AJR* 1982;**138**:1143.

Johnson WC et al: Treatment of abdominal abscesses: Comparative evaluation of operative drainage versus percutaneous catheter drainage guided by computed tomography or ultrasound. *Ann Surg* 1981;**194**:510.

Kark RM et al: An analysis of 500 percutaneous renal biopsies. *Arch Intern Med* 1958;**101**:439.

Kressel HY, Filly RA: Ultrasonographic appearance of gas-containing abscesses in the abdomen. *AJR* 1978;**130**:71.

Kuligowska E et al: Interventional ultrasound in detection and treatment of renal inflammatory disease. *Radiology* 1983;**147**:521.

Lang EK: Coexistence of cyst and tumor in the same kidney. *Radiology* 1971;**101**:7.

Lang EK: Diagnosis and management of renal cysts. Chap 9, pp 147–175, in: *Percutaneous and Interventional Urology and Radiology*. Lang EK (editor). Springer-Verlag, 1986.

Lee DA et al: Late complications of percutaneous renal biopsy. *J Urol* 1967;**97**:793.

Lee JKT et al: Acute focal bacterial nephritis: Emphasis on gray scale sonography and computed tomography. *AJR* 1980;**134**:87.

Lundström B: Angiographic abnormalities following percutaneous needle biopsy of the kidney. *Acta Radiol* [Suppl] 1972;**321**:1.

Madewell JE et al: Multilocular cystic nephroma: A radiologic pathologic correlation of 58 patients. *Radiology* 1983;**146**:309.

McClennan BL et al: CT of the renal cyst: Is cyst aspiration necessary? *AJR* 1979;**133**:671.

Mindell HJ: On the use of Pantopaque in renal cysts. *Radiology* 1976;**119**:747.

Muth RG: The safety of percutaneous renal biopsy: An analysis of 500 consecutive cases. *J Urol* 1965;**94**:1.

Parienty RA et al: Diagnostic value of CT numbers in pelvocalyceal filling defects. *Radiology* 1982;**145**:743.

Parker RA et al: Percutaneous aspiration biopsy of renal allografts using ultrasound localization. *Urology* 1980; **15**:534.

Pedersen JF: Percutaneous puncture guided by ultrasonic multitransducer scanning. *J Clin Ultrasound* 1977;**5:**175.

Raskin MM, Roen SA, Viamonte M Jr: Effect of intracystic pantopaque on renal cysts. *J Urol* 1975;**114:**678.

Raskin MM et al: Percutaneous management of renal cysts: Results of a four-year study. *Radiology* 1975;**115:**551.

River GL et al: Unusual complications of kidney biopsy. *J Urol* 1970;**103:**15.

Samellas W: Death due to septicemia following percutaneous needle biopsy of the kidney. *J Urol* 1964;**91:**317.

Schmidt A, Baker R: Renal biopsy in children: Analysis of 61 cases of open wedge biopsy and comparison with percutaneous biopsy. *J Urol* 1976;**116:**79.

Sibler SJ, Clark RE: Treatment of massive hemorrhage after renal biopsy with angiographic injection of clot. *N Engl J Med* 1975;**292:**1387.

Spigos D, Capek V, Jonasson O: Percutaneous biopsy of renal transplants using ultrasonographic guidance. *J Urol* 1977;**117:**699.

Sussman S et al: Hyperdense renal masses: A CT manifestation of hemorrhagic renal cysts. *Radiology* 1984;**150:**207.

Tao LC et al: Percutaneous fine-needle aspiration biopsy. 1. Its value to clinical practice. *Cancer* 1980;**45:**1480.

vanSonnenberg E et al: Percutaneous drainage of abscesses and fluid collections: Technique, results, and applications. *Radiology* 1982;**142:**1.

von Schreeb T et al: Renal adenocarcinoma: Is there a risk of spreading tumor cells in diagnostic puncture? *Scand J Urol Nephrol* 1967;**1:**270.

Wajsman Z et al: Transabdominal fine needle aspiration of retroperitoneal lymph nodes in staging of genitourinary tract cancer (correlation with lymphography and lymph node dissection findings). *J Urol* 1982;**128:**1238.

Wehle MJ, Grabstald H: Contraindications to needle aspiration of a solid renal mass: Tumor dissemination by renal needle aspiration. *J Urol* 1986;**136:**446.

Wein AJ et al: Applications of thin needle aspiration biopsy in urology. *J Urol* 1979;**121:**626.

Zornoza J et al: Transperitoneal percutaneous retroperitoneal lymph node aspiration biopsy. *Radiology* 1977;**122:**111.

9

Radionuclide Imaging

Barry A. Kogan, MD, & Robert S. Hattner, MD

Radioisotopic imaging of the genitourinary tract permits anatomic and functional evaluations without disturbance of physiologic processes. These studies have benefited from numerous technical advances in radiopharmaceuticals, scintillation cameras, and computer processing. Currently, the most common studies emphasize the physiologic properties of radiopharmaceuticals and, consequently, allow for dynamic, functional evaluations of the organ system.

Radiopharmaceuticals

Imaging radiopharmaceuticals are moieties with specific physiologic properties allowing them to trace normal and abnormal processes. They are labeled with a readily available radionuclide that can be easily imaged, most commonly technetium-99m (^{99m}Tc) or iodine-131 (^{131}I). Because extremely small molar quantities of radionuclide can provide a photon flux adequate for imaging, radiopharmaceuticals rarely disturb the physiologic processes of the organs being investigated. These radioisotopes are safe and noninvasive, with radiation exposure being in most instances considerably less than in standard radiographic or fluoroscopic procedures. Owing to the tiny quantities used, allergic reactions are virtually unknown and the potential toxicity of contrast media is avoided. In most instances, the radiopharmaceutical is delivered intravenously and the agent enters the target organ physiologically. Thus, nuclear medicine images are not as much anatomic as they are functional—the concentration of the pharmaceutical being proportionate to the amount of function as much as to the anatomy of the organ being investigated.

Scintillation Camera

The amount of radiopharmaceutical present within a given organ is monitored externally by a scintillation camera. The camera has a central crystal, a collimator, and a photomultiplier. The crystal, made of thallium-drifted sodium iodide, is generally circular and optically clear. It is 20–50 cm in diameter and 6–12 mm thick. A photon interacting in the crystal causes a quantitative release of visible light photons proportionate to the energy of the incident photon. The collimator usually has parallel channels of dense radiation-absorbing material, usually lead, which are applied to the crystal in such a way that only photons with a path parallel to the long axis of the channel are permitted to reach the crystal and react with it. By doing this, the 3-dimensional distribution of radiopharmaceutical is converted into a 2-dimensional projection of the activity. The photomultiplier is attached to the back of the crystal on the side opposite the collimator. This device detects visible light photons released from the crystal and uses an electronic algebraic scheme to determine the spatial location of the incident photon. As each incident photon is examined independently, the scintillation camera samples the source distribution at random and can be used to sample the distribution of radioactivity over short time intervals. This produces a quantitative cinematic data set that can then be subjected to computer analysis. The data are also mapped onto film by converting the electron pulses to light flashes for subsequent photography.

Computer Analysis

The analog signals from the scintillation camera are digitized and stored in the computer memory. In most instances, they are subsequently transferred to a peripheral storage device, for example, a magnetic disk. A standard mini- or microcomputer is then programmed to direct the acquisition, analysis, and display of data. The acquisition program is flexible and allows for specification of the precision of spatial sampling, the temporal resolution, the study length, and the total amount of data to be collected. In renal cortical imaging, for instance, the data are collected based on the total number of counts for each image. In contrast, for diuretic renography, the data are collected in a series of images each of the same duration, independent of the number of counts per image. Analysis programs allow study of a particular region of interest and will also compute and display activity in a quantitative manner (eg, as a function of time). This is used extensively for diuretic renography. Finally, the display program can provide graphs, images, and tables that can be photographed for the clinician's use. Other analysis programs use the linear systems theory to solve multiple differential equations and analyze raw data to look at the rate of disappearance of radioisotopes from various body pools. This type of computer analysis is used for calculations of the glomerular filtration rate (GFR) with Tc-99m diethylenetriamine-pentaacetic acid (^{99m}Tc-DTPA).

As in most investigations, communication between clinician and nuclear medicine specialist is essential, as the choice of radioisotope, imaging technique, and computer analysis should be adapted and adjusted to the particular problem.

KIDNEY

Nuclear medicine studies of the kidney remain extremely valuable for noninvasive evaluation of renal function and anatomy. In some instances, these are the only studies capable of delineating the anatomy.

Function

When quantifying renal function, either glomerular or tubular function can be measured. Glomerular function has traditionally been assessed by the GFR and tubular function by renal blood flow (RBF). Any substance that is freely filtered by the glomerulus but is not reabsorbed or secreted by the tubular or collecting duct cells can be used to quantify the GFR. The polysaccharide inulin meets these criteria and has been the classic agent used for this purpose. It remains the "gold standard" by which other agents are judged. GFR can be expressed in the following equation:

$$\text{Urinary concentration of inulin} \times \frac{\text{Volume of urine}}{} = \text{Plasma concentration of inulin}$$

Unfortunately, accurate measurement of inulin clearance is complex, time-consuming, and expensive, making it impractical for clinical use. Labeling inulin with a radioisotope allows for easier quantification of concentrations. ^{14}C-inulin is available for these purposes, but it requires special handling and is also not useful in the clinical setting. The most commonly used alternatives are iothalamate, chromium-51 ethylenediaminetetraacetic acid (^{51}Cr-EDTA), or ^{99m}Tc-DTPA. All are excreted in a manner similar to that of inulin and are easier to handle and measure. ^{51}Cr-EDTA and iothalamate are stable, and assessment of GFR with them correlates well with inulin clearance, but accurate measurements depend on collection of multiple serum and urine samples. ^{99m}Tc-DTPA has the advantage of providing excellent renal images as well, allowing simultaneous imaging and clearance measurements. Clearances can be measured in the same way as with ^{51}Cr-EDTA, or a close estimate can be obtained by quantitative analysis of scintillation counts obtained on gamma camera imaging (Gates, 1982, 1983). An important advantage of this technique is the ease with which simultaneous split renal function studies can be obtained. This is of considerable practical benefit.

RBF is measured by determining the clearance of a substance that is completely eliminated from blood in one pass through the kidney. Para-aminohippuric acid (PAH) meets this criterion, and its clearance has been the traditional reference standard for measurement of RBF. As with inulin, it is not easy to measure PAH clearance, nor is it easy to radiolabel PAH. However, ^{131}I-hippuran is widely available and is almost completely extracted from renal blood in one pass; hence, it provides accurate measurements of RBF. It is also used for renal imaging; however, ^{123}I-hippuran, although considerably more expensive, has better imaging qualities and is used more commonly in Europe (O'Reilly et al, 1977). Its clearance also correlates well with PAH clearances. The absolute uptake of technetium-99m dimercaptosuccinic acid (^{99m}Tc-DMSA) can also be used for this purpose, but, again, its measurement is not straightforward (Daly et al, 1979).

The easy assessment of renal function is invaluable in urology. Further, the ability to quantify individual renal function noninvasively allows for comparison of renal health before, during, and after treatment for a number of urologic diseases (eg, vesicoureteral reflux or ureteropelvic junction obstruction). This is perhaps the principal advantage of nuclear medicine techniques over all other imaging modalities. In fact, they constitute the only noninvasive method of determining individual renal function.

Imaging

Two basic types of renal imaging are possible: (1) cortical imaging, with agents that are bound to renal parenchymal cells, and (2) imaging of the collecting system, with agents that are excreted in the urine. Some agents are known to do both (eg, technetium-99m glucoheptonate).

^{99m}Tc-DMSA is most commonly used for cortical imaging. A dose of 71 μCi/kg, but not less than 0.3 mCi, is given intravenously. Although a small amount is excreted in the urine, at least 50% is bound to renal proximal tubular cells within 4 hours. Images taken thereafter show detail of the renal parenchyma. This is particularly useful when looking for segmental abnormalities of the kidney (eg, renal scarring, tumors, or evidence of trauma).

^{99m}Tc-DTPA (171 μCi/kg, but not less than 2 mCi) and ^{131}I-hippuran (1 μCi/kg, but not less than 20 μCi) are the agents most often used for "excretory" imaging, since large amounts of these are rapidly excreted in the urine. Image resolution is much less satisfactory than with traditional uroradiographic studies (eg, excretory urograms), and these agents are therefore not used for examining details of the collecting system. Although nuclear medicine techniques provide crude anatomic information (enough, for instance, to delineate the level of upper tract obstruction) (Koff et al, 1984), their principal advantage is quantification of amounts of radioisotope entering and leaving the collecting system, allowing for dynamic, functional, and anatomic imaging simultaneously.

As noted above, each agent has somewhat different physiologic properties, causing their functional and anatomic capabilities to vary. The choice of agent can greatly affect the information obtained, and it is therefore preferable to tailor the study to the clinical problem under evaluation. This will be demonstrated by looking more closely at the clinical applications in which radioisotopes are most helpful.

UPPER URINARY TRACT OBSTRUCTION

Traditionally, a dilated upper urinary tract has been assumed to be obstructed, but this is not always the case (eg, following pyeloplasty, the collecting system may remain dilated but may not be obstructed). Sonography or excretory urography can delineate the anatomy but in many cases will not determine the degree of obstruction. Nuclear medicine studies are helpful, as they quantify the amount of radioisotope entering and leaving the collecting system. These studies are dynamic in that quantification is done sequentially and, when indicated, after diuresis (O'Reilly et al, 1978; Koff, Thrall, and Keyes, 1979).

In evaluating obstruction, radionuclide renography is performed with an agent that is excreted in the urine, in most instances ^{99m}Tc-DTPA. ^{131}I-hippuran can be used, but the image quality is not as good, and ^{123}I-hippuran is not readily available in the USA because of cost. After injection of the radioisotope, a series of images is obtained, usually one every 5 minutes, with the duration of imaging held constant. The amount of emptying of the system can be visually determined by observing the decrease in activity in the kidney over time. With computerized techniques, a region of interest is selected over the kidney (or in the case of ureteral dilation, over the distal ureter) and the number of counts at any given time quantified. The number of counts can be expressed as a function of time and a time-activity curve generated (see Fig 28–12). In the dilated system, which does not readily drain, a diuretic (usually furosemide, 0.5–1 mg/kg) is given when the collecting system is full of radioisotope. After administration of the diuretic, the unobstructed system will drain and the number of counts over the kidney will decrease. In the obstructed system, however, the amount of radioisotope will stay constant or even increase (Fig 9–1).

In some instances, diagnosis of obstruction is clearcut. However, in most cases, the obstruction is partial, and the surgeon must determine when operative intervention is appropriate. A number of investigators have documented the usefulness of diuretic renography in these circumstances (Kass, Majd, and Belman, 1985). However, there is no definitive criterion, and the final decision remains a clinical one. The shape of the time-activity curve is a measure of the severity of the obstruction, and a number of authors have attempted to use the slope of the curve or the time until 50% of the isotope has drained to judge this. A problem with this technique is that each case must be individualized, as the rapidity of drainage is determined not only by the degree of obstruction but also by the size and compliance of the collecting system, as well as by the amount of urinary output provoked by the diuretic. In fact, when a kidney has been significantly damaged by ob-

struction, it may respond poorly to the diuretic; the dilated system may not fill sufficiently to induce drainage. The time-activity curve must be interpreted cautiously in these patients, as limited or delayed "washout" of radioisotope may be falsely interpreted as an indication of obstruction. Modifications are being developed to make the scan more sensitive and specific (English et al, 1987). However, because of individual variations, the clinician must be actively involved in interpretation of these studies (Maizels et al, 1986). When properly performed and interpreted, these studies are the only noninvasive technique available for documenting the degree of obstruction. In cases where function is too poor, diagnosis of obstruction is better made by other means, usually pressure-flow studies.

In practice, these studies are useful in following patients with long-term hydronephrosis. Examples are newborns with antenatally diagnosed hydronephrosis, children with posterior urethral valves, and patients after surgery for a ureteropelvic junction obstruction or vesicoureteral reflux (Koff et al, 1981; Bayne and Shapiro, 1985).

CHRONIC PYELONEPHRITIS

Evaluation of renal damage from urinary infections has traditionally been done with excretory urography. The classic abnormalities include small kidneys, thinned parenchyma, and blunted calices, with thinning of the parenchyma primarily overlying the calices. These changes, although pathognomonic, are not always seen, partly because it is difficult to obtain a high-quality excretory urogram during childhood when careful follow-up of renal growth is most important, since vesicoureteral reflux with associated pyelonephritis is a major cause of renal damage. The difficulties with excretory urography are multifactorial. (1) Young children have diminished renal function, even when compared on a per kilogram basis with adults. (2) Bowel preparation is not used, as it may cause excessive dehydration. (3) Crying causes swallowing of air and markedly increases bowel gas. (4) Abnormally positioned kidneys may be hidden by bony structures. (5) The use of oblique films and tomography is limited by attempts to keep exposure to radiation to a minimum.

Nuclear medicine obviates many of these problems. ^{99m}Tc-DTPA scans can be used, but only the images obtained in the first several minutes are valuable because thereafter the radioisotope is excreted in the urine and the images are primarily of the collecting system. A better alternative is an agent that images the renal cortex primarily, the optimal one being ^{99m}Tc-DMSA (Kogan et al, 1983). By binding directly to renal proximal tubular cells, these agents provide excellent delineation of parenchymal anatomy. Because the binding is permanent and the half-life of the radiolabeled DMSA is 6 hours, images can be obtained in different positions to visualize specific lesions more com-

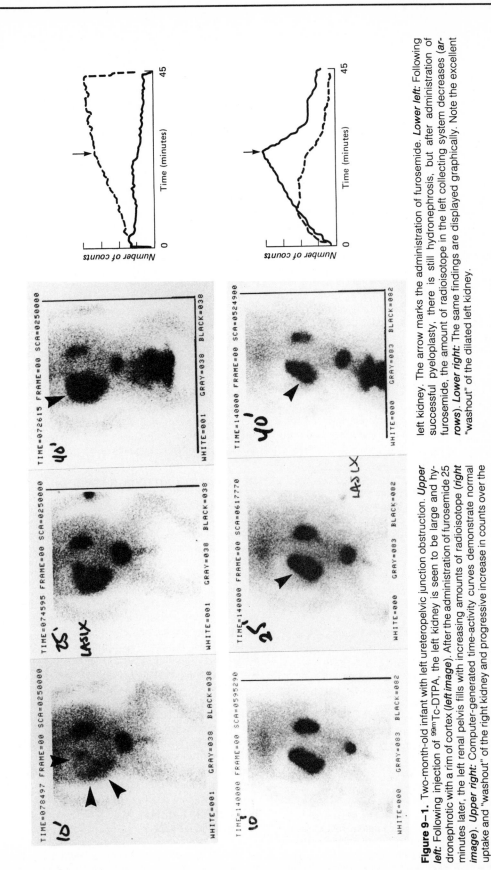

Figure 9–1. Two-month-old infant with left ureteropelvic junction obstruction. *Upper left:* Following injection of ⁹⁹ᵐTc-DTPA, the left kidney is seen to be large and hydronephrotic with a rim of cortex (*left image*). After the administration of furosemide 25 minutes later, the left renal pelvis fills with increasing amounts of radioisotope (*right image*). *Upper right:* Computer-generated time-activity curves demonstrate normal uptake and "washout" of the right kidney and progressive increase in counts over the left kidney. The arrow marks the administration of furosemide. *Lower left:* Following successful pyeloplasty, there is still hydronephrosis, but after administration of furosemide, the amount of radioisotope in the left collecting system decreases (*arrows*). *Lower right:* The same findings are displayed graphically. Note the excellent "washout" of the dilated left kidney.

pletely. Where necessary, 24-hour images can be obtained to reduce the background further and to allow any radioisotope in the urine to be excreted, giving further definition to the renal parenchymal images.

These studies are particularly beneficial in chronic pyelonephritis (Fig 9–2). First, they are not affected by bowel gas, bony structures, or any of the other problems associated with excretory urography. Further, they appear to be more sensitive than excretory urography, even when a high-quality study is available. This is probably due to the fact that the injured renal parenchyma will not bind the radiopharmaceutical immediately after being damaged, whereas on excretory urography, the size and shape of the kidney do not change until the injured area is replaced by collagen and the collagen contracts, distorting the calices and thinning the cortex.

Clinically, renal cortical scans are invaluable shortly after an episode of pyelonephritis in order to document the amount of renal damage. This is important in planning therapy and particularly useful in evaluating the results of treatment (eg, in determining the progression of scarring in children followed medically for vesicoureteral reflux; Stoller and Kogan, 1986).

RENAL TRANSPLANTATION

After renal transplantation, the kidney must be continously monitored. Numerous disease processes can

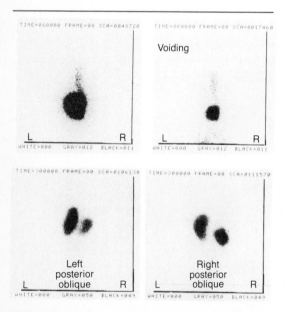

Figure 9–2. Six-month-old girl with recurrent urinary tract infection. *Top:* Posterior images from a nuclear cystogram, performed by injecting ^{99m}Tc-DTPA into a urethral catheter and filling the bladder with saline. Images are also obtained during voiding. Right vesicoureteral reflux is demonstrated during both filling and voiding. *Bottom:* Left posterior oblique and right posterior oblique images from a ^{99m}Tc-DMSA scan clearly delineate right renal scarring.

lead to graft dysfunction (eg, acute tubular necrosis, acute rejection, cytomegalovirus infection, acute pyelonephritis, cyclosporine toxicity, aminoglycoside toxicity, and recurrence of the original renal disease). Measurement of serum creatinine is the most common clinical determination of renal function, but changes are slow and this measurement is relatively insensitive to small changes in function. Nuclear medicine studies are highly sensitive and provide quantitative information with low risk (Hattner and Engelstad, 1984). Many different techniques have been investigated and a number of good results published, but no single radionuclide has emerged as universal. Perhaps the most common protocol involves a combination of quantitative analysis and qualitative evaluation of ^{131}I-hippuran kinetics. Although nonspecific, this study permits repeated evaluations and comparison even during acute tubular necrosis. This capability is particularly beneficial in following patients after cadaveric transplants, in which there is a higher incidence of acute tubular necrosis. Urinary extravasation or obstruction can be identified on the hippuran images, and major vascular abnormalities can be identified on a ^{99m}Tc-DTPA flow study (ie, monitoring the radionuclide on its first transit through the bloodstream and kidney).

Although hippuran kinetics are extremely sensitive in detecting subtle changes in renal function, the clinician must be aware that they are nonspecific. Determining the cause of diminished function requires correlation with other clinical data.

RENOVASCULAR HYPERTENSION

In typical renovascular hypertension, there is decreased blood flow and diminished uptake and delayed excretion of radioisotope over the involved area, the renal mass is smaller, and there is compensatory hypertrophy of uninvolved areas (Fig 9–3). This is best demonstrated by agents that correlate with RBF (eg, ^{131}I-hippuran). In recent years, ^{99m}Tc-DMSA has been shown to be particularly valuable, especially in delineating segmental vascular disease (Stringer et al, 1984; Rosen, Treves, and Ingelfinger, 1985).

Unfortunately, the classic findings are not often seen; hence, traditional nuclear scans are not very sensitive or specific. Recently, captopril has been used to exaggerate the differences between perfused and nonperfused areas of the kidneys (Geyskes et al, 1986). Although this may ultimately prove useful, it is likely that nuclear medicine techniques will remain too nonspecific to be useful for screening purposes. Currently, radioisotopes are primarily beneficial in localizing segmental disease and as a noninvasive means of evaluating kidneys after revascularization.

FUNCTIONAL RENAL MASS QUANTIFICATION

One of the most important problems in clinical urology and nephrology is the quantification of renal

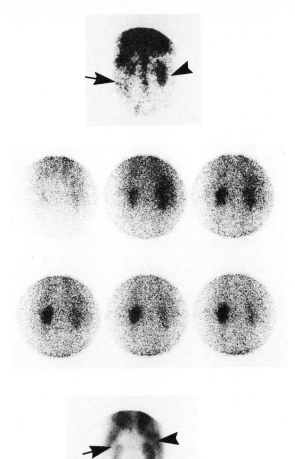

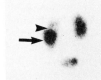

Figure 9–4. DMSA renal cortical scans. *Left:* Posterior images from a 3-month-old girl with left duplication and ureterocele. The dilated upper pole (*arrowhead*) has 12% of the total renal function compared with the lower pole (*arrow*), which has 32%. Enough function remained so that heminephroureterectomy was deemed unnecessary. *Right:* Posterior images from a 1-week-old female with a horseshoe kidney, right duplication, and ureterocele arising from the upper pole segment. This scan delineates the renal anatomy better than any other study.

Figure 9–3. Images of a 65-year-old man with severe hypertension. *Top:* Posterior image from a ⁹⁹ᵐTc-DTPA blood flow study. The aorta is clearly seen, as is the right kidney (*arrowhead*). The blood flow to the left kidney is delayed (*arrow*). *Middle:* On a ¹³¹I-hippuran study done immediately following, there is not only slow uptake but delayed excretion. Images were obtained at 4-minute intervals. *Bottom:* A delayed ⁹⁹ᵐTc-DTPA image shows the small left kidney (*arrow*) and the larger, possibly hypertrophied, right kidney (*arrowhead*).

mass. Excretory urography provides some information on renal size and amount of contrast excretion, but this only loosely correlates with function. Similarly, sonography can evaluate renal size and character (ie, echogenicity) but, again, is not functional. On the other hand, radioisotopes, by virtue of their physiology, provide functional information; the amount of uptake of radioisotope is proportionate to the amount of function. Excretory agents can be used for this purpose but are not optimal because many kidneys being evaluated are abnormal in shape and position and have dilated collecting systems or vesicoureteral reflux.

Cortical agents (eg, ⁹⁹ᵐTC-DMSA) are superior in these instances (Gordon, 1987) (Fig 9–4).

In practice, these studies are useful in evaluating unilateral renal pathology. In order to decide whether a significantly damaged kidney should be removed, it is crucial to know what percentage of renal function the kidney contributes. Radioisotopic imaging is the only currently available study that can provide this information noninvasively.

SPACE-OCCUPYING RENAL LESIONS

Renal cortical agents are capable of delineating mass lesions within the kidney, particularly those larger than 1–2 cm. Because of numerous technologic advances in recent years, ultrasonography, CT scanning, and MRI can provide similar information while also evaluating associated renal and extrarenal findings. Hence, nuclear medicine studies are not the investigation of choice in patients with renal infarctions, tumors, or lesions due to trauma. However, in unusual circumstances or when some of the above studies are unavailable, renal cortical agents can provide extremely useful information (eg, delineating the degree of segmental renal damage from trauma or differentiating a hypertrophied column of Bertin from a renal tumor). A high-quality ⁹⁹ᵐTC-DMSA scan can clearly differentiate functional from nonfunctional renal tissue.

BLADDER

Radioisotopic imaging of the bladder is useful primarily for detecting vesicoureteral reflux. This was first discussed in 1959 by Winter (Winter, 1959).

Refinements in widefield gamma camera imaging and new radioisotopes have made this technique highly sensitive and useful, especially in children (Conway et al, 1972; Merick, Uttley, and Wild, 1977).

A catheter is placed in the bladder, and the bladder is filled with normal saline to which 1 mCi of ^{99m}Tc-DTPA has been added. The cooperative child is placed upright on a portable toilet or bedpan. Once the bladder is distended, the catheter is removed and the child voids. Gamma camera imaging is performed from behind and is continuous during both filling and voiding. The images obtained will often demonstrate reflux (Fig 9-2). Very mild degrees of reflux can also be identified by computer analysis of radioactivity over the kidneys. The test can be combined with a simple cystometrogram to obtain more information and to increase accuracy (Nasrallah et al, 1978). A variation of this technique (indirect radionuclide cystography) avoids catheterization (Conway and Kruglik, 1976). A standard renogram is performed, and time-activity curves are obtained for regions of interest over the kidneys. The bladder fills with radioisotope as the radionuclide is excreted by the kidneys. The amount of radioactivity over the kidneys and ureters is monitored and quantified before, during, and after voiding. An increase in radioactivity in the kidney or ureter is indicative of vesicoureteral reflux. The indirect radionuclide cystogram has the major advantage of avoiding urethral catheterization. However, it is unreliable if the patient moves during the study (common in children) or has associated hydronephrosis or poor renal function (also common). Hence, for practical purposes, this technique is not nearly as useful as the former procedure.

The major advantage of radioisotopic cystography is its high sensitivity with relatively limited radiation exposure, approximately 1/100th that obtained from conventional voiding cystourethrography. Because image resolution is relatively poor, fine anatomic detail is not as well seen as with traditional radiography, and this procedure is not useful as the initial study of the lower urinary tract in males, where visualization of the urethra is important. It is also of questionable usefulness as the first study in females with urinary tract infection because the spine is not visualized, a ureterocele may not be seen, and visualization of bladder wall thickening and trabeculation is not possible. It is, however, an ideal test for follow-up studies of children with vesicoureteral reflux either after ureteral reimplantation or during expectant management for spontaneous resolution. In these children, the quality of image resolution is not important but limited exposure to radiation is, particularly when many studies must be performed.

TESTIS

The primary benefit of radionuclide imaging of the testis is in differentiating degrees of testicular vascu-larity. Angiography is performed with a bolus injection of ^{99m}Tc sodium pertechnetate (0.21 mCi/kg, but not less than 2 mCi) and imaging at 5-second intervals during its first pass through the groin area. Approximately 10 minutes later, blood pool images are obtained, as concentration of this agent correlates reasonably well with vascularity. Areas of increased vascularity appear denser than normal, and avascular tissues appear as a filling defect.

This study is used primarily to differentiate testicular torsion from epididymitis. The latter classically appears as an area of hypervascularity and the former as avascular (Fig 9-5). A number of reports have suggested that this technique is both sensitive and specific (Falkowski and Firlit, 1980; Blacklock et al, 1983).

Unfortunately, there are some limitations. First, because torsion must be diagnosed and treated immediately, a nuclear medicine technician must be available on short notice 24 hours a day. Further, false-negative and false-positive results do occur (Stoller, Kogan, and Hricak, 1985). Late torsion may appear as a hypervascular area due to an inflammatory response, and intermittent torsion can also demonstrate hypervascularity and result in delayed diagnosis and correction. A large hydrocele and even gross purulence can result in a large defect, simulating torsion (Wilkins et al, 1985). In summary, radioisotopic studies of the scrotum can be helpful in the differential diagnosis of acute scrotal pain, but the diagnosis is primarily made on clinical grounds and the scan should be used only as an adjunct.

ADRENAL SCINTIGRAPHY

Adrenal Cortex

The adrenal cortex uses blood cholesterol as the primary substrate for steroid synthesis, in contrast to other organs, which synthesize cholesterol de novo from acetate. Hence, radiolabeled derivatives of cholesterol are taken up by the adrenal and can be imaged 3-5 days after injection (Lieberman et al, 1971). The best agent for this purpose is 7-iodomethy1-19-norcholesterol labeled with ^{131}I (NP59) (Sarkar et al, 1975). These scans are useful in both Cushing's syndrome and Conn's syndrome (Beierwaltes, 1984).

In Cushing's syndrome, it is important to distinguish between a primary adrenal source of corticosteroids and a paraneoplastic or pituitary source. Often biochemical and other radiographic tests can help, but NP59 can distinguish the origin when it is unclear (Fig 9-6). Either a pituitary or paraneoplastic source of ACTH will stimulate both adrenals, and both will be imaged. A primary adrenal adenoma will also be seen, but the increased corticosteroids suppress the pituitary, and the contralateral adrenal will therefore be suppressed and will not take up NP59. In contrast, a metabolically active adrenal cortical carcinoma will synthesize its own cholesterol and corticosteroids and consequently suppress both adrenals. In these cases,

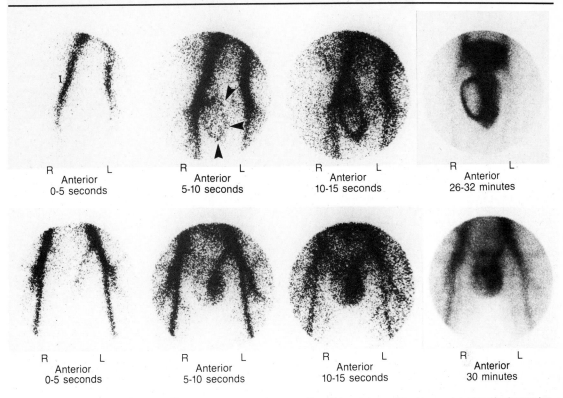

R Anterior L
0-5 seconds

R Anterior L
5-10 seconds

R Anterior L
10-15 seconds

R Anterior L
26-32 minutes

R Anterior L
0-5 seconds

R Anterior L
5-10 seconds

R Anterior L
10-15 seconds

R Anterior L
30 minutes

Figure 9–5. Scrotal scanning with ⁹⁹ᵐTc-sodium pertechnetate. *Top:* This adolescent had proved right testicular torsion. Early scans of the pelvis show both iliac arteries (I) and increased flow around the right testis (*arrowheads*). However, later pictures, especially the 30-minute delayed film, demonstrate a clear photogenic area involving the right testis. *Bottom:* In contrast, this young man with left epididymo-orchitis has obviously increased blood flow to the entire left scrotum. Again, the delayed film demonstrates the increased flow clearly. (Courtesy of M. C. C. Ling.)

neither adrenal will be visualized.

In Conn's syndrome, primary hyperaldosteronism is demonstrated by biochemical studies. It is then therapeutically important to distinguish between bilateral adrenal hyperplasia and a unilateral adenoma. This can be done by suppressing both adrenals with dexamethasone and then imaging with NP59. The scan will image any autonomously functioning tissue, either the

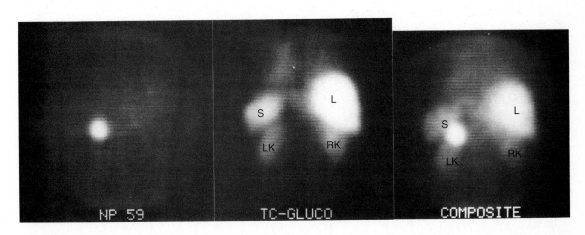

Figure 9–6. In this 45-year-old woman with Cushing's syndrome, CT scanning suggested a left adrenal mass, but biochemical studies were unclear as to the primary pathology. *Left:* An NP59 scan shows very strong uptake in the abdomen. *Center:* A ⁹⁹ᵐTc-glucoheptinate scan was performed to localize the uptake in relation to the liver (L), spleen (S), right kidney (RK), and left kidney (LK). *Right:* A composite of both scans shows that the uptake is clearly unilateral and in the left adrenal. A left adrenal adenoma was removed, and the patient was cured.

unilateral adenoma or the bilateral hyperplastic glands. The appropriate surgical approach can then be planned.

In the USA, high-resolution CT scanning has largely supplanted the adrenal cortical scan. However, when CT scanning is equivocal or unavailable (as it is in many parts of the world), cortical scanning with NP59 remains very useful.

Adrenal Medulla

In somewhat the same manner as cholesterol in the adrenal cortex, metaiodobenzylguanidine (MIBG) is taken up by adrenergic neurons. It can be radiolabeled with radioiodine and used to image the adrenal medulla and other endocrinologically active adrenergic tissues, in particular pheochromocytoma and neuroblastomas (Sisson et al, 1981; Munkner, 1985; Hattner et al, *AJR* 1984; Hattner et al, *Noninvasive Med Imaging* 1984).

^{123}I-MIBG is 85–90% sensitive and virtually 100% specific for localizing pheochromocytomas (Sisson et al, 1984) (Fig 9–7). This is particularly helpful in extra-adrenal pheochromocytomas when CT scanning is unrevealing or when symptoms and signs of pheochromocytoma persist after resection, indicating multiple neoplasms. Because the incidence of this may be as high as 10%, some surgeons perform routine preoperative MIBG scans. ^{123}I-MIBG is also helpful in screening the family members of patients with type 2 multiple endocrine neoplasia, in whom a high incidence of pheochromocytoma or adrenal medullary hyperplasia is seen. In a few cases, large doses of ^{131}I-MIBG have been used therapeutically in patients with otherwise untreatable metastatic malignant pheochromocytoma (Sisson et al, 1984).

In patients with neuroblastoma, ^{123}I-MIBG is almost 100% sensitive and specific. This is crucial for staging and subsequently defining the optimal therapy. Imaging with MIBG has uncovered numerous soft tissue and bony metastases not found by any other means. Consequently, it has considerable promise as a means of delivering high doses of radiation directly to metastatic neuroblastoma. Trials of ^{131}I-MIBG radiotherapy are now under way in patients with otherwise unresponsive stage IV tumors. Early results are encouraging (Hoefnagel et al, 1987).

SKELETAL SCINTIGRAPHY

Bone scans obtained with conventional bone-seeking radiopharmaceuticals such as [99m]TC-methylenediphosphonate (MDP) occupy a unique place in the staging of cancer patients. Nowhere is this more true than in urogenital cancers, particularly carcinoma of the prostate (McNeil, 1984) (Fig 9–8).

MDP and similar compounds are chemisorbed to the surface of bone crystals, intercollating into crystal imperfections. The relative localization of a radiopharmaceutical is equal to the product of its extraction efficiency, blood flow, and blood concentration. Since blood concentration after intravenous injection is equal throughout the body and since MDP has a very high extraction efficiency, it follows that the bone scan correlates mostly with the vascularity of the skeleton. The response of bone to a variety of insults is limited but nearly always includes increased blood flow; hence, bony lesions are seen as foci of increased radioisotope in scans. Overall, the sensitivity of bone scans in skeletal metastasis for prostate cancer exceeds 95%, making it particularly important in the evaluation and follow-up of patients with this disease. It should be remembered, however, that scans are nonspecific, and suspicious areas on radionuclide scanning should be evaluated by plain radiographs as well (eg, to differentiate between metastasis and osteoarthritis).

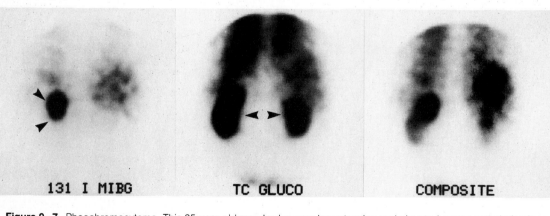

Figure 9–7. Pheochromocytoma. This 35-year-old man had severe hypertension and elevated serum catecholamines. *Left:* A ^{131}I-MIBG scan shows marked uptake in the left abdomen. *Center:* A ^{99m}Tc-glucoheptinate scan was done to help localize the lesion. The kidneys are clearly seen. *Right:* A composite view shows the lesion in the left adrenal. With surgical excision of a left adrenal pheochromocytoma, the patient was cured.

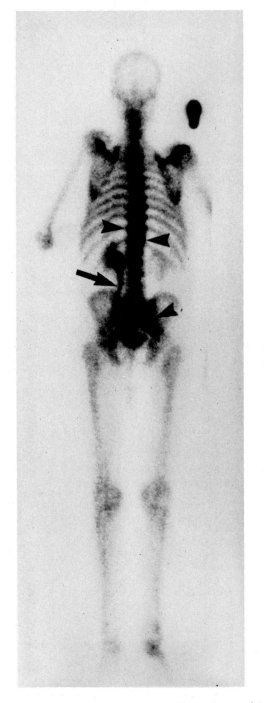

Figure 9–8. An 83-year-old man with carcinoma of the prostate. A ^{99m}Tc-MDP bone scan shows metastasis in the sacrum and at T10 and T11 (*arrowheads*). Since some radioisotope is excreted in the urine, the obstructed left ureter is also well delineated (*arrow*).

SCINTIGRAPHIC DETECTION OF OCCULT INFLAMMATION

Gallium-67 (^{67}Ga) was originally investigated as a tumor imaging agent but has been disappointing in this regard. It has found considerable use in detection of acute and chronic inflammation (Halpern and Hagan, 1980). The exact mechanism of localization of ^{67}Ga in inflammatory foci is disputed. Because it resembles ferric iron, it probably binds to iron-binding molecules of microorganisms (siderophores) and to lactoferrin, an iron-binding protein abundant in neutrophils. For unknown reasons, ^{67}Ga is also accumulated by macrophages. Since any or all of these cells are found at the site of inflammatory processes, ^{67}Ga is an excellent compound for finding inflammation.

Gallium scans are hampered by nonspecific colonic activity, which significantly reduces their imaging capabilities. Nonetheless, they can serve to direct further diagnostic workup in cases of occult inflammation (eg, suspected perinephric abscess, interstitial nephritis, or pelvic abscess). They can also be used to confirm suspicious or nondiagnostic findings seen on other studies.

Indium-111-labeled granulocytes are prepared by labeling the patient's own white blood cells with ^{111}In. These cells are then reinjected into the patient. Although the labeled granulocytes are distributed throughout the body, areas of high concentration are easily imaged with a gamma camera. In contrast to ^{67}Ga, there is minimal colonic binding. These scans are therefore very sensitive and specific for acute suppurative infections (Coleman, 1982). Unfortunately, these labeled granulocytes are not as accurate for finding chronic inflammatory conditions. Because the radiolabeling is generally performed out of hospital by a community radiopharmacy, these scans are relatively expensive and usually available only during regular working hours, a distinct disadvantage, since this particular study is often needed urgently. Nonetheless, in selected cases these scans can be extremely useful.

FUTURE CONSIDERATIONS

Monoclonal Antibodies

In the early 1970s, it became possible to create large quantities of pure antibodies in a relatively inexpensive way. Monoclonal antibodies are made by immunizing a mouse, then hybridizing the mouse's spleen cells with murine myeloma cells and subsequently growing these hybridomas within other mice. A continuous supply of pure antibodies can be created. These antibodies can be developed against a variety of antigens and are used primarily for in vitro immunoassays.

By choosing a tumor-specific antigen, it is theoretically possible to radiolabel the monoclonal antibodies to the tumor in question. In practice, monoclonal antibodies highly specific for prostatic and renal cell carcinoma have been produced. Cancer-specific radiopharmaceuticals have been used to image these neoplasms with moderate success, and it is hoped that in the future this technique will permit radioimmunotherapy, so that radioisotopes can be directed only against the neoplasm, allowing for high-dose radiation therapy to the tumor yet limiting toxicity to normal tissues (Larson, Carrasquillo, and Reynolds, 1984).

New Radioisotopes

^{123}I-hippuran and ^{131}I-hippuran have been 2 of the principal radiopharmaceuticals used for renal imaging. They are especially valued because their excretion correlates with RBF. However, ^{99m}Tc is preferred to most other radionuclides because it is readily available, inexpensive, and ideally suited to the scintillation cameras currently used for imaging and quantification.

Mercaptoacetyltriglycine (MAG3) is a compound that is excreted in a manner similar to that of hippuran and PAH but is easily labeled with ^{99m}Tc (Taylor et al, 1987). Although only now in clinical trials, ^{99m}Tc-MAG3 may well replace other more commonly used radioisotopes due to its easy availability, relatively low cost, good imaging qualities, and improved radiation dosimetry.

REFERENCES

Bayne DP, Shapiro CE: Diuretic radionuclide urography: Functional assessment following pyeloplasty. *J Urol* 1985;**134**:344.

Beierwaltes WH: The adrenals. Pages 56–69 in: *Textbook of Nuclear Medicine*. Vol 2: *Clinical Applications*, 2nd ed. Harbert J, DaRocha AFG (editors). Lea & Febiger, 1984.

Blacklock ARE et al: Radionuclide imaging in scrotal swellings. *Br J Urol* 1983;**55**:749.

Coleman RE: Radiolabeled leukocytes. Pages 119–141 in: *Nuclear Medicine Annual 1982*. Freeman LM, Weissman H (editors). Raven Press, 1982.

Conway JJ, Kruglik GD: Effectiveness of direct and indirect radionuclide cystography in detecting vesicoureteral reflux. *J Nucl Med* 1976;**17**:81.

Conway JJ et al: Detection of vesicoureteral reflux with radionuclide cystography: A comparison study with roentgenographic cystography. *Am J Roentgenol Rad Ther Nucl Med* 1972;**115**:720.

Daly MJ et al: Differential renal function using technetium-99m dimercaptosuccinic acid (DMSA): In vitro correlation. *J Nucl Med* 1979;**20**:63.

English PJ et al: Modified method of diuresis renography for the assessment of equivocal pelviureteric junction obstruction. *Br J Urol* 1987;**59**:10.

Falkowski WS, Firlit CF: Testicular torsion: The role of radioisotopic scanning. *J Urol* 1980;**124**:886.

Gates GF: Glomerular filtration rate: Estimation from fractional renal accumulation of ^{99m}Tc-DTPA (stannous). *AJR* 1982;**138**:565.

Gates GF: Split renal function testing using Tc-99m DTPA: A rapid technique for determining differential glomerular filtration. *Clin Nucl Med* 1982;**8**:400.

Geyskes GG et al: Renography with captopril: Changes in a patient with hypertension and unilateral renal artery stenosis. *Arch Intern Med* 1986;**146**:1705.

Gordon I: Indications for ^{99m}technetium dimercapto-succinic acid scan in children. *J Urol* 1987;**137**:464.

Halpern S, Hagan P: Gallium-67 citrate imaging in neoplastic and inflammatory disease. In: *Nuclear Medicine Annual 1980*. Freeman LM, Weissman H (editors). Raven Press, 1980.

Hattner RS, Engelstad BE: Radionuclide evaluation of renal transplants. Pages 319–342 in: *Nuclear Medicine Annual 1984*. Freeman LM, Weissmann HS (editors). Raven Press, 1984.

Hattner RS et al: Localization of m-iodo (^{131}I) benzylguanidine in neuroblastoma. *AJR* 1984;**143**:373.

Hattner RS et al: Scintigraphic detection of pheochromocytomas using m-iodo (^{131}I) benzylguanidine. *Noninvasive Med Imaging* 1984;**1**:105.

Hoefnagel CA et al: Radionuclide diagnosis and therapy of neural crest tumors using iodine-131 metaiodobenzylguanidine. *J Nucl Med* 1987;**28**:308.

Kass EJ, Majd M, Belman AB: Comparison of the diuretic renogram and the pressure perfusion study in children. *J Urol* 1985;**134**:92.

Koff SA, Thrall JH, Keyes JW Jr: Diuretic radionuclide urography: A noninvasive method for evaluating nephroureteral dilatation. *J Urol* 1979;**122**:451.

Koff SA et al: Diuretic radionuclide localization of upper urinary tract obstruction. *J Urol* 1984;**132**:513.

Koff SA et al: Early postoperative assessment of the functional patency of ureterovesical junction following ureteroneocystostomy. *J Urol* 1981;**125**:554.

Kogan BA et al: ^{99m}Tc-DMSA scanning of diagnose pyelonephritic scarring in children. *Urology* 1983;**21**:641.

Larson SM, Carrasquillo JA, Reynolds JC: Radioimmunodetection and radioimmunotherapy. *Cancer Invest* 1984;**2**:363.

Lieberman LM et al: Diagnosis of adrenal disease by visualization of human adrenal glands with ^{131}I-19-iodocholesterol. *N Engl J Med* 1971;**285**:1387.

Maizels M et al: Troubleshooting the diuretic renogram. *Urology* 1986;**28**:355.

McNeil BJ: Value of bone scanning in neoplastic disease. *Semin Nucl Med* 1984;**14**:277.

Merrick MV, Uttley WS, Wild R: A comparison of two techniques of detecting vesicoureteric reflux. *Br J Radiol* 1977;**50**:792.

Munkner T: ^{131}I-meta-iodobenzylguanidine scintigraphy of neuroblastomas. *Semin Nucl Med* 1985;**15**:154.

Nasrallah PF et al: Quantitative nuclear cystogram: Aid in determining spontaneous resolution of vesicoureteral reflux. *Urology* 1978;**12**:654.

O'Reilly PH et al: Diuresis renography in equivocal urinary tract obstruction. *Br J Urol* 1978;**50**:76.

O'Reilly PH et al: 123-Iodine: A new isotope for functional renal scanning. *Br J Urol* 1977;**49**:15.

Rosen PR, Treves S, Ingelfinger J: Hypertension in children: Increased efficacy of technetium Tc 99m succimer in screening for renal disease. *Am J Dis Child* 1985;**139**:173.

Sarkar JD et al: A new and superior adrenal scanning agent: Np-59. *J Nucl Med* 1975;**16**:1038.

Sisson JC et al: Radiopharmaceutical treatment of malignant pheochromocytoma. *J Nucl Med* 1984;**25**:197.

Sisson JC et al: Scintigraphic localization of pheochromocytoma. *N Engl J Med* 1981;**305**:12.

Stoller ML, Kogan BA: Sensitivity of ^{99m}technetium-dimercaptosuccinic acid for diagnosis of chronic pyelonephritis: Clinical and theoretical considerations. *J Urol* 1986;**135**:977.

Stoller, ML, Kogan BA, Hricak H: Spermatic cord torsion: Diagnostic limitations. *Pediatrics* 1985;**76**:929.

Stringer DA et al: Comparison of aortography, renal vein renin sampling, radionuclide scans, ultrasound and IVU in the investigation of childhood renovascular hypertension. *Br J Radiol* 1984;**57**:111.

Taylor A Jr et al: Evaluation of Tc-99m mercaptoacetyltriglycine in patients with impaired renal function. *Radiology* 1987;**162**:365.

Wilkins SA Jr et al: Acute appendicitis presenting as acute left scrotal pain: Diagnostic considerations. *Urology* 1985;**25**:634.

Winter CC: A new test for vesicoureteral reflux: An external technique using radioisotopes. *J Urol* 1959;**81**:105.

10 | Retrograde Instrumentation of the Urinary Tract

Joachim W. Thüroff, MD

Instrumentation of the urinary tract is performed for diagnostic or therapeutic indications through different routes of access using a variety of techniques for orientation, most of which are imaging techniques (Table 10–1). Urethral catheterization is a typical retrograde instrumentation of the urinary bladder that is usually performed "blindly" (ie, without obtaining specific information regarding the individual anatomy of the access route). If there is suspicion of deviation in anatomy along the route of access to the urinary tract, diagnostic information must be obtained to allow safe instrumentation. For retrograde transurethral and transureteral access to various segments of the urinary tract, endoscopy is usually the most reliable guide for safe instrumentation. However, a diagnostic radiograph obtained prior to endoscopic instrumentation, using retrograde or intravenous injection of contrast dye, is helpful in predicting the difficulty and extent of an endosurgical procedure (eg, incision of urethral stricture).

In planning percutaneous access (eg, cystostomy), ultrasonic imaging is usually more useful than fluoroscopy, as it does not rely on the use of contrast dye and provides imaging of all underlying tissues along the intended route of access (eg, bowel in relation to an intended percutaneous cystostomy tract). This technique can be helpful for safe percutaneous placement of a cystostomy catheter but is even more important for precise placement of a percutaneous nephrostomy tract (see Chapter 8).

All these techniques of instrumentation invade a basically sterile urinary tract. The surgical field must be prepped and draped as for open surgery, and the same standards of asepsis must be followed.

For atraumatic, confortable transurethral instrumentation, generous use of a water-soluble lubricant is essential. The lubricant should be injected retrogradely into the urethra rather than applied to the outside of a catheter or instrument, since most of it would be stripped off upon insertion into the external meatus. Transurethral instrumentation using catheters or other flexible instruments (eg, flexible cystoscopes) requires topical anesthesia only. Retrograde injection of a solution of local anesthetic in lubricant (eg, 10 mL of lidocaine hydrochloride jelly USP, 2%) will serve both as an anesthetic and a lubricant. In males, a penile clamp should be placed for 5–10 minutes to allow sufficient time for the anesthetic to numb the urethral mucosa.

Table 10–1. Instrumentation of the lower urinary tract.

Indications
Diagnostic
Therapeutic
Access
Transrectal
Transurethral
Percutaneous
Orientation
Blind
Palpation
Fluoroscopy
Ultrasound
Endoscopy

Instrumentation of the male urethra with rigid instruments may be too uncomfortable in some patients to be done under anesthesia only. Additional sedation with barbiturates, tranquilizing agents, or narcotics may be necessary even if the procedure is being performed only for diagnostic purposes. If therapeutic interventions such as lithotripsy, fulguration, or electroresection are intended, regional (spinal, epidural) or general anesthesia is required.

URETHRAL CATHETERIZATION

Urethral catheterization is rarely indicated for diagnostic purposes only, except in females for obtaining urine specimens for culture. In males, midstream specimens are usually adequate for diagnosing urinary tract infection because contamination of urine is less likely than in females. Residual urine is easily checked noninvasively by ultrasound rather than by urethral catherization. Nevertheless, transurethral catheters are routinely used for vesical and urethral pressure measurements in urodynamic studies and for retrograde instillation of contrast dye in radiographic studies (eg, cystograms and voiding cystourethrograms in combined radiographic-urodynamic studies, detection of vesicoureteral reflux). For all other cases, voiding cystourethrograms may be obtained without urethral catheterization if they are scheduled in connection with an intravenous pyelogram so that the intravenously administered contrast dye can also be used for the voiding study.

Urethral catheters are used with therapeutic intention for relief of urinary retention, for drainage of

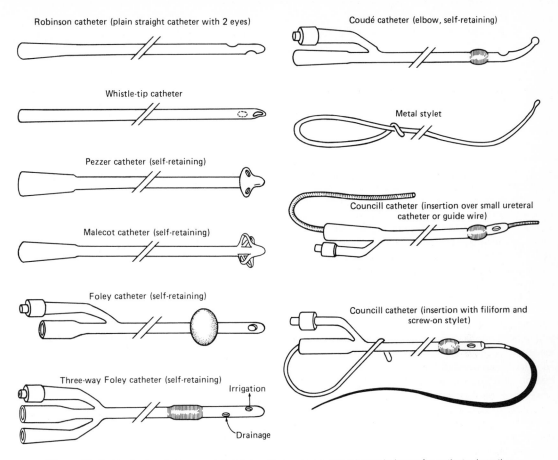

Figure 10–1. Urethral catheters, metal stylet, catheter and guide wire techniques for catheter insertion.

urine and monitoring of urinary output perioperatively and postoperatively, and for urethral stenting after urethroplasty or urethral trauma.

Catheter Design

Catheters differ in size and shape, type of material, number of lumens, and type of retaining mechanism (Fig 10–1). Standard sizes of external diameters of catheters and most endoscopic instruments are given according to Charriére's French scale in units of 0.33 mm (=1 French [F] or 1 Charriére [Charr]). Thus, 3F equals 1 mm in diameter and 30F equals 10 mm in diameter. Choice of size and design of catheter for transurethral catheterization depends on the purpose of instrumentation. For one-time intermittent catheterization of the urethra, plain straight catheters (Robinson) of 16–18F size are appropriate; the same sizes are used in self-retaining indwelling Foley catheters. In men, larger sizes of indwelling catheters tend to cause retention of urethral secretions and, subsequently, urethritis and possible urethral stricture; epididymitis may occur if large catheters are used over prolonged periods. Nevertheless, after transurethral endoscopic surgery of the prostate or the bladder, catheters with a larger diameter (20–24F) may be necessary to prevent retention of blood clots (especially if

3-lumen Foley catheters are used for continuous simultaneous bladder drainage and irrigation). After open or endoscopic urethroplasty, catheters may have multiple functions (ie, a stent for healing, an indwelling drain for urethral secretions and blood, and bladder drainage). The standard indwelling Foley catheter may not be appropriate for all these purposes; therefore, a suprapubic cystostomy catheter may be used for bladder drainage and a fenestrated catheter (with the proximal end not inserted into the bladder) as a urethral stent and drain.

For most cases, straight urethral catheters are adequate; however, if negotiation of the male urethra is difficult, curved-tip catheters (coudé catheter) should be used (Fig 10–1), as they are more easily engaged in the infrapubic angulation between the bulbous and membranous urethra. The most commonly used indwelling transurethral catheter is the Foley catheter with an inflatable balloon as a retaining mechanism. This is a double-lumen catheter (one lumen is used for activation of the balloon), and this means that the lumen available for urinary drainage is smaller than in a single-lumen catheter with the same external diameter. Because these catheters have a valve mechanism for inflation and deflation of the balloon (which is usually not detachable), a special fenestrated cannula must be used for percutaneous insertion if these catheters are to be used as cystostomy or nephrostomy catheters. The Councill catheter has a hole at its tip that can be passed coaxially over a guide wire, a thin ureteral catheter, or a filiform, which can be attached to a catheter stylet (Fig 10–1). This design allows safe transurethral placement of the catheter in difficult cases as well as guided percutaneous catheter placement without use of a fenestrated cannula. Self-retaining catheters without a ballon-and-valve mechanism (Pezzer catheter, Malecot catheter) must be inserted with a stylet to stretch the self-retaining mechanism of the tip, which will resume its original configuration after being inserted because of the memory function of the catheter material. If pulled inadvertently, these catheters are more easily dislodged than Foley catheters; however the absence of a balloon and second lumen-and-valve mechanism and the comparatively small space required for good drainage at the tip are advantages of these designs for use as cystostomy and nephrostomy catheters.

The rigidity of the catheter, the ratio between internal and external diameters, and the biocompatibility will depend on the material of which it is made. The tendency for encrustation and mucosal irritation is related to the structure of the catheter material, surface tension, smoothness, and hydrophilia. Silicone catheters are the most biocompatible and should be chosen if long-term use is anticipated, as the risk of urethritis and urethral stricture is reduced even if catheters are only changed every 4–6 weeks. However, silicone catheters are less rigid and have a smaller lumen-to-external-diameter ratio than catheters made of other materials.

Latex is the standard material used for urethral catheters. It is soft but is more likely to become encrusted than silicone if used in long-term indwelling catheters. Polyethylene and polyvinyl chloride catheters are more rigid and have a better lumen-to-external-diameter ratio, but they are not as biocompatible as silicone catheters for long-term use; these materials are therefore best used for one-time catheters and for small catheters (eg, ureteral catheters).

Technique of Catheterization

A. In Men: Prepping, draping, urethral lubrication, and anesthetization (see above) should be completed. The catheter is grasped near its tip with sterile gloves or by sterile forceps and is inserted into the external meatus while the penis is stretched with the other hand. The penis must be grasped laterally at the corpora cavernosa to avoid squeezing the urethra against the corpora. The catheter must be advanced gently, and if there is resistance to further advancement, the site of resistance should be determined by palpation of the catheter tip. The male urethra normally offers resistance at the membranous urethra; this is either due to involuntary constriction of the external sphincter because of discomfort or anxiety or due to resistance at the infrapubic angulation between the bulbous and the membranous urethra. In the latter

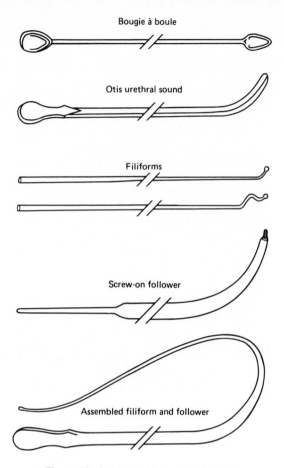

Bougie à boule

Otis urethral sound

Filiforms

Screw-on follower

Assembled filiform and follower

Figure 10–2. Urethral probes and sounds.

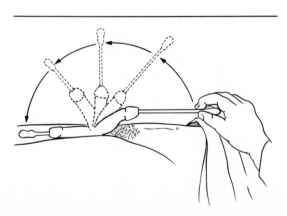

Figure 10–3. Insertion of a curved sound into the male urethra.

case, the tip of the catheter can be guided by a finger inserted into the rectum or a curved-tip catheter might be tried because it will follow the angulation of the urethra more easily. Once the resistance of the external sphincter has been overcome, the catheter can usually be easily advanced into the bladder, even in the presence of an obstructing prostatic adenoma. Bladder neck stricture may be a barrier that cannot be bypassed with a soft catheter. If the catheter is not rigid enough to follow the angulations of the male urethra, a metal stylet can be used to advance the catheter into the bladder (Fig 10–1). Care must be taken not to injure the urethra by overly forceful manipulation or by passing the tip of the stylet through a side hole of the catheter. For insertion of a catheter on a stylet or other rigid, curved instruments such as metal sounds, the penis must be stretched nearly horizontally cephalad; during insertion, the handle of the instrument must be moved in a half circle in the sagittal plane and will be nearly vertical if the tip of the instrument passes through the external sphincter region. The handle will be horizontal and pointing caudad if the instrument is in the bladder (Fig 10–3). This maneuver should be done only if it can be performed without undue force. If there is suspicion of a stricture, filiforms might be used to guide the route into the bladder for screw-on followers (Fig 10–2) or for a screw-on stylet to insert a Councill-tip catheter (Fig 10–1). However, because blind manipulation in the presence of a stricture may create a false passage, a percutaneous cystostomy tube should be placed for urinary drainage (see below) if the patient is in urinary retention. Definitive treatment (endoscopic or open urethroplasty) can then be planned after radiographic evaluation of the extent of the stricture (see Chapter 30).

B. In Women: Short, straight catheters are best, especially for self-catheterization. For self-catheterization, which is indicated for neurogenic and other voiding disorders, a mirror can be used to visualize the external meatus after spreading the labia. In female hypospadias, the meatus may be difficult to visualize, and self-catheterization may be impossible. Insertion of a vaginal speculum helps to engage a urethral catheter in those cases. If transurethral catheter insertion is difficult because of an anatomic or topographic anomaly such as a urethral diverticulum or urethrocystocele, the tip of the catheter can be guided by a finger inserted into the vagina. For obtaining urine specimens for culture, short catheters with sterile urine collection bags firmly attached can be used.

URETHRAL CALIBRATION & DILATION

Technique

A. In Men: Calibration of the male urethra can be performed by sequentially engaging catheters of increasing size or by use of bougie à boules (Fig 10–2), judging resistance, or "jump and hang," during the passage. In the presence of a stricture, a filiform may

be passed into the bladder, and screw-on followers can be used for calibration as well as for dilation of the stricture. However, sequential dilation of urethral strictures by insertion of catheters of increasing size exerts shear and tear forces to the mucosa and is likely to produce extended scarring. Thus, recurrence of stricture is common if periodic urethral dilation is terminated. Balloon dilation of a stricture with 7–9F balloon dilators (which can be passed over a guide wire and inflated up to 30F under a pressure of up to 15 atm) does not exert shear forces. The long-term efficiency of this technique as compared to endoscopic or open urethroplasty is unknown as yet.

Before insertion of a resectoscope sheath into the bladder for electroresection or other endoscopic procedures (see below), a strictured or narrow pendulous urethra may be dilated with the Otis urethrotome up to 30F and longitudinally incised at the 12 o'clock position. However, modern resectoscope sheaths of 20–24F size make this maneuver rarely necessary.

B. In Women: In females, bougie à boules of progressively larger diameter are used for calibration of the urethra. These olive-tip plastic or metal sounds are introduced into the bladder and then withdrawn. If, upon withdrawal, resistance is felt or the distal urethra reveals a "white ring," a urethral obstruction may be present. However, correlation between findings on calibration and on objective urodynamic assessment of urethral obstruction is poor unless there is an obvious high-grade stenosis. Dilation of the female urethra is commonly performed using the Otis urethrotome in the same manner as described above. However, there is a risk of overstretching the urethra, which may result in urinary incontinence.

URETHROSCOPY & DIRECT-VISION INTERNAL URETHROTOMY

In urethral lesions, endoscopy can identify the lesion, and appropriate diagnostic procedures (eg, biopsy) or therapeutic interventions (eg, internal urethrotomy) can be performed under direct vision. For retrograde urethroscopy, a cystoscope sheath or a special urethroscope sheath may be used with a fiberoptic 0-degree telescope lens. If a high-grade urethral stricture is encountered, a 5F ureteral catheter may be introduced under vision to serve as a guide for direct-vision internal urethrotomy. The direct-vision internal urethrotome allows longitudinal incision of the stricture with a cold knife (not using cutting or fulgurating electrical current); this is usually performed at the 12 o'clock position through the full thickness of the stricture. A silicone Foley catheter (18–24F) is used for stenting and bladder drainage for a period lasting from a few days to 6 weeks, depending on the extent of stricture as well as on individual stenting protocols.

CYSTOURETHROSCOPY

Cystourethroscopy is the standard endoscopic procedure for diagnostic evaluation of the lower urinary tract. This is the diagnostic procedure of choice for evaluation of most disorders of the urethra, prostate, and bladder. Endoscopic macroscopic evaluation of tumors, ulcers, and chronic inflammation of the bladder wall must be complemented in most cases by microscopic studies of biopsies, which can usually be obtained under topical anesthesia only if a "cold" biopsy forceps (without cutting or fulgurating electrical current) is used.

During endoscopic evaluation of the lower urinary tract, the anatomy must be examined systematically in a standardized fashion for urethral lesions (eg, strictures, diverticula, verrucae, tumors); size and configuration of the prostate and bladder neck; and tumors, stones, diverticula, trabeculation, ulcers, and other inflammatory changes of the bladder. However, while cystourethroscopy provides an excellent means of evaluating the anatomy of the lower urinary tract and the pathologic changes thereof, only a few endoscopic findings will suggest compromised function of the lower urinary tract. Indirect signs of abnormal function are hypertrophy of the bladder neck, bladder diverticula, and bladder wall hypertrophy and trabeculation. Bladder trabeculation is suggestive of an abnormal work load of the detrusor, either due to mechanical or functional infravesical obstruction (eg, prostate adenoma or sphincter spasticity) or to bladder hyperactivity (eg, hyperreflexia, unstable bladder). For detection and classification of these and other functional disorders of the bladder and urethra, urodynamic studies are more appropriate than endoscopy (see Chapter 21).

Cystourethroscopy may be performed with rigid or flexible instruments. While standard rigid instruments provide clearer visualization and a larger working channel that will accommodate a greater variety of instruments, flexible instruments have some definitive advantages: endoscopy of the male urethra can be done with minimal discomfort in the supine position and under topical anesthesia only, and "invisible" areas of the bladder such as the immediate vicinity of the bladder neck can be visualized because of the deflecting capabilities of the instruments. However, rigid instruments always provide better optical quality and durability than flexible ones. Thus, flexible cystoscopes are used mainly in males for the sake of comfort.

Rigid cystoscopes have sheaths of 8–24F and fiberoptic telescopes with an angle of view of 0–170 degrees. Lenses of 0 degrees are the best for visualizing the urethra, 30-degree lenses for inspection of the bladder in women, and 30- or 70-degree lenses for visualizing the bladder in men (the choice of lens depending on the size of the prostate). The bladder neck might be visualized by using a lens with a view of 120–170 degrees. Cystoscopy can be performed as retrograde urethrocystoscopy, with insertion of the viewing instrument through the entire urethra, or the cystoscope sheath may be inserted blindly into the bladder with an obturator in place of the telescope. After completion of cystoscopy, the urethra can be visualized during withdrawal of the instrument. However, whenever a urethral anomaly is suspected (eg, urethral stricture), the first technique is preferable in order to avoid damage and loss of information.

Inspection of the entire bladder wall must be done at different stages of filling; with minimal filling, an overview of all areas may be obtained, and with further filling, more details may be seen as the bladder wall unfolds. To visualize the bladder dome completely, it may be necessary to place the patient in the Trendelenburg position and exert manual sugrapubic pressure.

The bladder should be only half-filled for classification of the configuration and position of ureteral orifices in the evaluation of vesicoureteral reflux. For endoscopic diagnosis of interstitial cystitis, the bladder must be filled to capacity in order for the

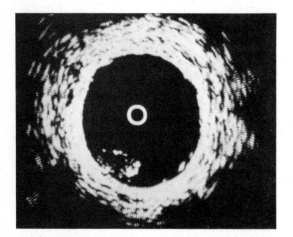 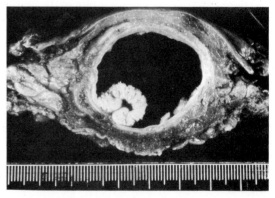

Figure 10–4. Multifocal bladder cancer. *Left:* Transurethral ultrasound. *Right:* Cystectomy specimen.

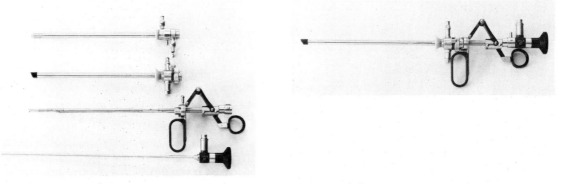

Figure 10–5. Transurethral resectoscope. *Left:* Continuous-flow sheath, standard sheath, working element with cutting loop, telescope. *Right:* Instrument assembled.

characteristic glomerulations and ecchymoses to be seen. When specimens are collected for cytologic examination, normal saline must be used for bladder irrigation.

TRANSURETHRAL & TRANSRECTAL ULTRASOUND

Miniature ultrasound probes may be used through cystoscopy sheaths or in the rectum for imaging of the prostate, bladder, and seminal vesicles. Transrectal ultrasound provides imaging of the seminal vesicles and the prostate showing size, shape, and echogenic areas within the prostate suggesting inflammatory changes or cancer. Transurethral ultrasound easily depicts bladder tumors (Fig 10–4) and gross transmural extensions thereof but is not reliable in differentiating between mucosal lesions and infiltration of tumors into the detrusor muscle. Further investigation is necessary to determine the value of ultrasound for diagnosing and staging tumors of the prostate and bladder and to define the indications for these studies.

TRANSURETHRAL SURGERY: ELECTRORESECTION, LASER, LITHOTRIPSY

Resectoscopes are endoscopes with sheaths of 10–30F (Fig 10–5) for transurethral surgery of the urethra, prostate, and bladder. If electrical current is applied to a wire loop while the loop is being retracted, strips, or "chips," of tissue can be cut. The chips must be evacuated from the bladder through the resectoscope sheath. This endosurgical technique can be used for resection of the prostate as well as for resection of bladder tumors. The loop acts as a monopolar electrode, with the indifferent electrode fixed at the patient's thigh. Two different modes of high-frequency current are available for cutting and fulguration and combinations thereof; a variety of probes such as hooks for bladder neck incision and balls for coagulation of larger areas are interchangeable with the loop. During electrosurgery, the bladder must be irrigated with nonhemolytic and near-isotonic solution (eg, 1.5% glycine solution).

The telescope and working element must be removed periodically from the resectoscope sheath to evacuate the bladder contents. A continuous-flow resectoscope design allows for simultaneous irrigation and drainage; this is particularly helpful in resecting large adenomas of the prostate. The continuous-flow technique can also be achieved using standard instruments and a suprapubic cystostomy catheter for drainage of the irrigating solution.

A new approach for treatment of bladder tumors is transurethral application of laser beams. Lasers generate electromagnetic waves of visible or invisible light, which consist of one wavelength (or color) only (monochromatic). They are emitted in synchronized phases, forming a strictly parallel beam with minimal divergence (coherence). The laser energy is absorbed by tissue, creating heat and causing local coagulation or vaporization of tissue. Owing to coherence of the beam, the laser light seems to be highly focused, allowing precise endoscopic application of energy. Lasers differ according to the medium used to generate energy and by the wavelengths of the emitted energy. The neodymium:YAG laser is most commonly used in urology; this emits invisible light at a wavelength of 1060 nm, which passes easily through water and coagulates tissue to a depth of 5 mm. CO_2 lasers emit invisible light at a wavelength of 10,600 nm, which is absorbed by water and readily vaporizes tissue but does not penetrate deeper than 0.03 mm. Argon lasers emit green light at a wavelength of 488–514 nm, which is preferably absorbed by melanin and hemoglobin and penetrates tissue to a depth of 1 mm.

In the treatment of bladder tumors, the neodymium:YAG laser allows for sealing of lymphatic channels and denaturation of tissue throughout the full thickness of the bladder wall, thus enabling the surgeon to treat even deep infiltrating tumors transurethrally (this is not possible by electroresection, because of the risk of bladder perforation and spreading of tumor cells). Urethral strictures, verrucae of the urethra and penis, and cancer of the penis have been treated successfully by neodymium:YAG laser coagulation.

The argon laser is used in the treatment of multifocal superficial tumors and carcinoma in situ of the bladder after photosensitizers (hematoporphyrin derivatives) have been administered systemically. These photosensitizers are absorbed by all cells but cleared more slowly from malignant cells, rendering them specifically susceptible to laser energy. Intravesically dispersed argon lasers will be specifically absorbed by these photosensitizers, acting on tumor cells to release singlet oxygen, superoxides, and hydroxyl radicals, and eventually causing cell death. Normal cells will not be harmed. CO_2 lasers have not yet been used endoscopically on a large scale, as appropriate fiber delivery systems for endoscopic application are still under investigation. CO_2 laser energy is readily absorbed by water, necessitating the use of gas (eg, CO_2) instead of irrigation fluid in endoscopy; low tissue penetration limits potential use to treatment of superficial bladder tumors and urethral strictures.

Transurethral laser treatment of bladder tumors, as well as use of lasers for ureterorenoscopic and percutaneous nephroscopic destruction of urothelial tumors of the upper urinary tract, is still in the phase of clinical experimentation, and further work is required to demonstrate its benefit over conventional treatment modalities and to clearly delineate indications.

Stones in the urinary bladder may be extracted through the resectoscope sheath or—if too large—must be first disintegrated by mechanical, ultrasonic, or electrohydraulic energy. A strong nutcracker-type forceps (visual lithotrite, stone punch) can be used to crush smaller stones under endoscopic vision. For large stones, electrohydraulic or ultrasonic probes are preferable. Ultrasonic probes allow controllable systematic stone disintegration with continuous suction applied through the hollow probe to evacuate sand and smaller fragments. This is useful for disintegration of stones in the renal pelvis during percutaneous nephrolithotomy (PNL) (see Chapter 8) to prevent scattering of fragments into inaccessible calices or the ureter. However, dispersal of fragments is not so much a concern in the bladder, because of its large capacity and simple structure. For bladder stones, electrohydraulic disintegration is preferable, because electrohydraulic probes are more powerful and stone disintegration is therefore more rapid. Fragments are readily evacuated from the bladder with a syringe or an Ellik evacuator.

URETERAL CATHETERIZATION

Indications for retrograde pyelography have declined steadily due to the availability of noninvasive,

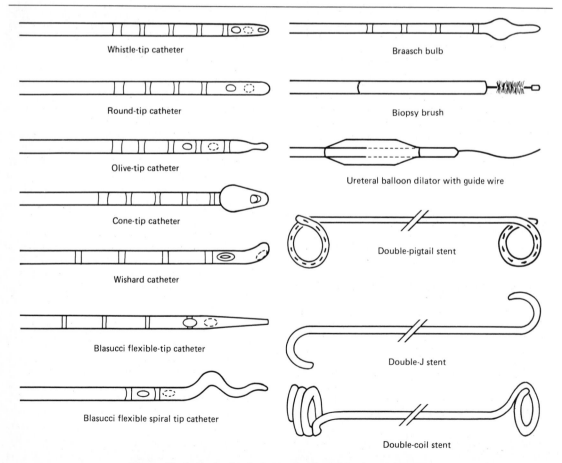

Figure 10–6. Ureteral catheters and self-retaining internal stents.

Whistle-tip catheter

Round-tip catheter

Olive-tip catheter

Cone-tip catheter

Wishard catheter

Blasucci flexible-tip catheter

Blasucci flexible spiral tip catheter

Braasch bulb

Biopsy brush

Ureteral balloon dilator with guide wire

Double-pigtail stent

Double-J stent

Double-coil stent

highly diagnostic radiographic techniques (eg, intravenous pyelography with tomography, renal ultrasound, CT scanning, and magnetic resonance imaging [MRI]). For diagnosis of filling defects of the upper urinary tract, ultrasound and CT studies readily differentiate between radiolucent stones and other filling defects. However, small lesions in the collecting system may still be better imaged by retrograde pyelography, and during the same study, selective urine specimens can be obtained for cytologic examination or tissue specimens can be obtained by ureteral brushing to verify a malignant lesion.

Evaluation of ureteral strictures or ureterovaginal fistulas often requires retrograde radiography supplementary to intravenous pyelography to exactly determine the distal extent of a lesion for planning of surgical repair. Retrograde pyelography may be performed in patients with allergic reactions to contrast dye, in whom standard intravenous pyelography would carry an undue risk.

Indications for stenting the ureter became more frequent with extracorporeal shock-wave lithotripsy (ESWL), (PNL), and ureterorenoscopy for treatment of upper urinary tract stones. Indwelling ureteral stents are further indicated perioperatively after reimplantation of ureters into the bladder or into segments of bowel and may be used to bridge a ureteral obstruction that is not amenable to surgical repair.

Ureteral catheters, which can be inserted through working channels of cystoscopes and ureterorenoscopes, are available in sizes 3–10F. They are made of the more rigid materials such as polyvinyl chloride or polyethylene, which provide sufficient rigidity in small-sized catheters with a reasonable lumen-to-external-diameter ratio. Some ureteral catheters are available with wire mandrels to provide even greater rigidity for ease of insertion and advancement.

There are many configurations of catheter tips (Fig 10–6). The cone-tip catheter is designed specifically for retrograde ureteropyelography. A catheter with a 6–10F cone is injected with contrast dye before engagement into the ureteral orifice to remove all air bubbles. The cone tip must be attached to the orifice only, and the contrast dye to be injected should be diluted to about 20–30% for better outlining of details. Antibiotics such as neomycin may be added, or commercially available solutions of contrast dye and antibiotics may be used (eg, 30% Renografin and 2.5% neomycin). If available, fluoroscopy should be used during injection of contrast dye to determine the exact amount of dye needed, and radiographs may be taken at appropriate intervals in different positions. If contrast dye is injected blindly, great care must be taken not to overdistend the renal collecting system and cause pyelotubular or pyelovenous backflow or extravasation, which eventually may lead to sepsis. If the catheter tip seals tightly at the orifice and prevents leakage of contrast dye, a nondilated upper urinary tract might accept as little as 0.5–1.5 mL of contrast dye. However, if the upper urinary tract is dilated or if there is leakage around the catheter tip, more contrast

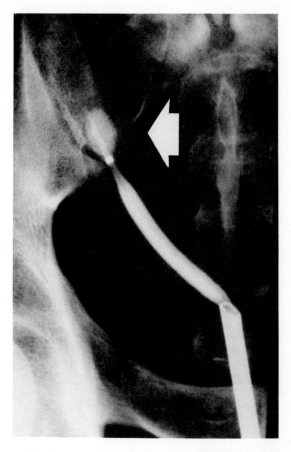

Figure 10–7. Ureteral dilation with balloon catheter before ureterorenoscopic removal of a distal ureteral stone (*arrow*).

dye may be needed. One radiograph should be taken during injection of contrast dye, a second immediately after injection, and a third after 5 minutes, when the dye has been allowed to mix with the urine while the ureteral catheter remains plugged. A final drainage film taken 10 minutes after removal of the catheter helps to determine the degree and localization of urinary stasis.

A round tip is safest for catheter advancement through the ureter into the renal pelvis or for retrograde manipulation of ureteral stones for subsequent treatment by ESWL. Olive-tip, filiform-tip (Blasucci), and curved-tip (Wishard and Blasucci) catheters may be used to negotiate ureteral strictures or bypass a ureteral stone. Open-tip catheters can be advanced over previously inserted guide wires, and if balloon dilator catheters are used, ureteral strictures may be dilated or the intramural segment of the ureter may be dilated prior to insertion of a ureterorenoscope (Fig 10–7). For dilation of ureteral strictures, 7F catheters with balloons 2.5–4 cm in length (which expand to 12–18F under pressures of up to 15 atm) are commonly used. After successful dilation, an 8–10F stent is usually left indwelling for several weeks. This technique seems to yield the best results in ureteral

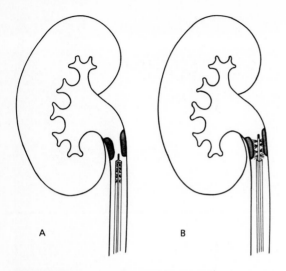

Figure 10–8. Brushing of a proximal ureteral lesion. *A:* Insertion of the brush covered by a catheter. *B:* Advancement of the brush through the lesion.

strictures as a complication of recent surgery for benign disorders, except for ureteropelvic junction obstruction. Long-standing strictures or strictures due to tumor compression of the ureter, radiation damage, or ischemic ureteral necrosis after radical pelvic surgery are not expected to respond favorably to balloon dilation. However, the long-term efficacy of this technique as compared to that of open surgical repair is yet to be determined.

To obtain more detailed information regarding lesions of the ureter or renal pelvis than that available from selective urinary cytology, a ureteral brush encased in a protective sheath may be advanced to the lesion under fluoroscopic control; at this point, the protective sheath is pulled back and the brush is advanced to gather sufficient tissue from the lesion for cytologic and histologic examination (Fig 10–8). After brushing, an additional sample of urine should be obtained from the ureter for cytologic studies.

Ureteral catheters, which may be left indwelling for a longer period of time for stenting after operation or for drainage of the upper urinary tract, are made from soft materials such as silicone or polyurethane. These catheters have a self-retaining mechanism (pigtail or J configuration of the proximal end). After the catheter has been stretched and advanced through the ureter, this configuration will be resumed owing to memory function of the material. The same J configuration is present at the distal end of the stent (Fig 10–6). These catheters must be introduced with guide wires to stretch the loops and provide sufficent rigidity for advancement through the ureter. Catheters with open-tip configuration are advanced by a pusher catheter over a guide wire, which must be positioned as a first step. Closed-tip catheters are advanced by pushing the indwelling guide wire. After final positioning of the stent, the guide wire is withdrawn while a pusher catheter holds the stent in the desired posi-

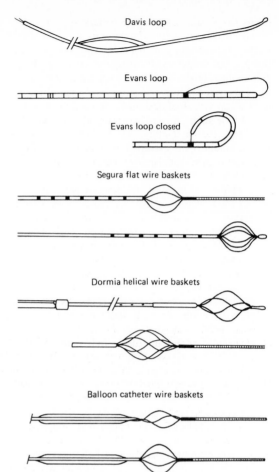

Figure 10–9. Loops, wire baskets, and wire baskets with balloon catheters for extraction of ureteral stones.

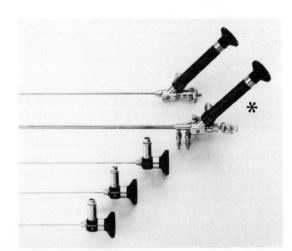

Figure 10–10. Ureterorenoscopes: Telescopes with center and offset eyepieces for use through a 12.5F working sheath. 10.5F ureterorenoscope with integrated sheath (*asterisk*).

tion. Indwelling ureteral stents can be removed without repeated cystoscopy by means of a thread pulled through a side hole at the distal end of the catheter and brought out through the urethra.

For retrieval of ureteral stones, a variety of baskets and loop catheters (Fig 10–9) is available for use through the cystoscope or ureterorenoscope. Techniques of application range from cystoscopic insertion and blind placement of the basket to fluoroscopically controlled catheter placement and endoscopically (ureterorenoscopy; see below) controlled stone extraction. Some catheters (eg, loop catheters) may be safely placed blindly or under fluoroscopic control, but most do not allow acute extraction of stones. Wire basket catheters (Dormia baskets) allow acute extraction of ureteral stones if the wires of the basket can be wrapped around the stone to hold it firmly. However, if this is done under fluoroscopic control only, possible perforation of the ureter with the basket may not be detected, and avulsion of the ureter with the basket may occur. The safest techniques of endoureteral stone manipulation are endoscopically controlled procedures, which are now being challenged by ESWL for noninvasive disintegration of ureteral stones.

URETERORENOSCOPY

Ureterorenoscopes are endoscopes for retrograde insertion into the ureter (Fig 10–10). They were developed from extended pediatric cystoscopes. Rigid ureterorenoscopes are available in sizes 9–13.5F. The choice of size depends on the diagnostic or therapeutic purpose. Flexible ureterorenoscopes as small as 7F in diameter are undergoing clinical trials as diagnostic instruments with theoretically the same low surgical risk as simple ureteral catheterization. Larger flexible ureterorenoscopes of 9–13.5F provide a limited irrigation and working channel for insertion of stone baskets, wire graspers, and electrohydraulic or laser probes for stone disintegration but do not offer the optical quality and durability of rigid instruments.

A rare indication for diagnostic ureterorenoscopy is lesions of the ureter and renal pelvis that cannot be identified or classified with any of the less invasive procedures such as retrograde pyelography, selective urinary cytology, CT scanning, or MRI. Indications for therapeutic ureterorenoscopy are disintegration and removal of ureteral stones. Direct-vision internal ureterotomy of ureteral strictures and endosurgical treatment of ureteral tumors by electroresection or laser coagulation are the subjects of promising ongoing clinical trials, but neither modality can be considered a standard treatment at this time.

Treatment of ureteral stones under direct vision is the main purpose of ureterorenoscopy, especially since most renal stones are amenable to ESWL but not all fragments and ureteral stones pass through the ureter spontaneously. A ureterorenoscope sheath for interchangeable telescopes with axial or offset eyepieces is most useful; the latter allows for insertion of

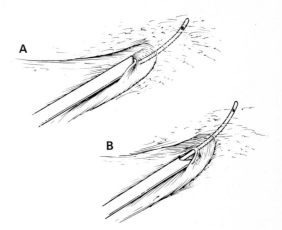

Figure 10–11. Ureterorenoscopy. *A:* Straightforward advancement of the instrument over a thin ureteral catheter can catch the mucosa of the orifice. *B:* With 180-degree upside-down rotation of the instrument, the ureteral catheter holds the orifice open like a tent.

rigid working instruments such as ultrasound probes through a central working channel. Insertion of the ureterorenoscope may be facilitated by dilation of the intramural ureter, either with plastic dilators of increasing size, which are slid over a guide wire, or with a balloon dilator catheter. Dilation of the ureter is often unnecessary if a small (3–5F) ureteral catheter is inserted through the ureterorenoscope into the ureter as a guide and the ureterorenoscope is then rotated 180 degrees and introduced in an upside-down orientation (Fig 10–11). In this position, the ureteral catheter will spread the roof of the intramural ureter like a tent and the nose of the instrument will slide flat on the trigone into the orifice. The orifice will be dilated only to the extent necessary for insertion of the instrument.

Stones may be retrieved by grasping forceps or by wire baskets under direct vision. However, if stones are too large to be extracted whole, intraureteral disintegration with ultrasonic or electrohydraulic probes is necessary. To prevent the flushing of fragments back into the renal pelvis, a 3F wire basket can be used to fix the position of the stone during disintegration or a 3F balloon catheter can be passed alongside the stone and inflated proximally. Ultrasonic probes allow controlled, safe disintegration of stones in the ureter but are not as effective as electrohydraulic probes, which have a slightly higher risk of damaging the ureter. If ureteral perforation occurs as a complication of intraureteral manipulation, ureteral stenting using a 7–8F double-J stent for 2–4 weeks usually allows healing without late sequalas. Stents should be used for a few days even after uncomplicated ureterorenoscopy to prevent pain from urinary stasis due to edema of the intramural ureter. Stents are easily introduced into the renal pelvis through the ureterorenoscope sheath after final inspection of the ureter to ensure that all stone fragments have been removed.

SUPRAPUBIC CYSTOSTOMY

Percutaneous placement of a suprapubic cystostomy catheter for bladder drainage is preferable to insertion of a transurethral catheter in several instances: (1) urinary retention due to urethral stricture, if the stricture is to be corrected by open or endoscopic surgery at a later time; (2) urethral trauma, with disruption of the urethra; (3) long-term catheter drainage of the bladder if intermittent urethral catheterization is not feasible; and (4) drainage of the bladder after plastic surgery of the urethra.

Use of a suprapubic cystostomy catheter is a simple, reliable measure to prevent some complications of long-term transurethral catheterization such as urethritis, urethral stricture, and epididymitis. Percutaneous placement of a suprapubic cystostomy catheter is safe and reliable if some precautions are observed: (1) the procedure should not be performed in patients with blood coagulation disorders due to coagulopathy or anticoagulant therapy; (2) the bladder must be filled to capacity; and (3) abnormalities of anatomy or topography of the bladder (eg, prolapse, previous surgery of the lower abdomen and pelvis) require diagnostic radiographic or ultrasonic evaluation before a cystostomy catheter may be placed safely.

Cystostomy catheters—like other indwelling catheters—must be biocompatible, with a low tendency for encrustation, and should have an intravesical self-retaining mechanism so that they are not dislodged during emptying of the bladder. For percutaneous placement of a cystostomy catheter, a trocar assembly must be used, the design of which depends on the type of catheter to be inserted. Foley catheters may be inserted through a fenestrated cannula, which is inserted into the bladder with a trocar; Malecot

catheters with a trocar needle (Stamey cystostomy); and pigtail catheters through a peel-away hollow needle (Braun-Melsungen design) or a fenestrated needle (Angiomed design) (Fig 10–12). The percutaneous tract must be anesthetized first. If a fine needle is used for this purpose, an initial test puncture of the bladder may be performed with the same needle to ensure proper aiming of puncture direction. The puncture must be performed with the patient in the supine position, the puncture site being located about 2 inches cranial of the pubic symphysis in the midline. The puncture needle should be held perpendicular to the skin.

If there is any doubt regarding the degree of bladder filling, anatomic abnormalities, or position of the bowel relative to the intended cystostomy tract, ultrasonic scanning should be performed and may also be used to guide the needle during puncture. Cystostomy catheters, even if equipped with self-retaining mechanisms, should be secured to the skin, either by taping or suturing.

PROSTATE BIOPSY

Biopsy of the prostate gland for diagnosis and grading of malignant tumors can be performed either transrectally or through the perineum. The transrectal route allows accurate puncture of suspicious areas, as the needle is guided by the palpating finger. However, transrectal ultrasound scanners with attached needle guides allow for puncture of small suspicious areas via a perineal route with about the same accuracy of puncture as the transrectal technique. Advantages of the perineal approach are lower risk of infection in the puncture site and no need for bowel preparation; dis-

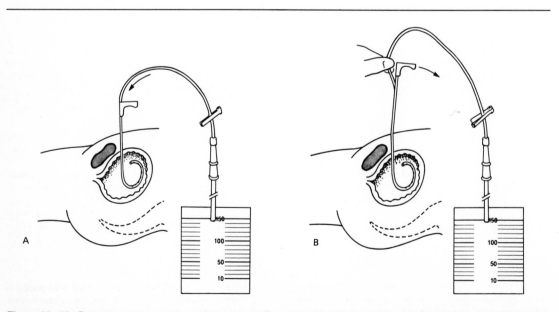

Figure 10–12. Percutaneous cystostomy placement. **A:** Puncture of the bladder with a fenestrated needle and insertion of a pigtail catheter. **B:** Withdrawal of the puncture needle and dislodgment of the cystostomy catheter from the needle.

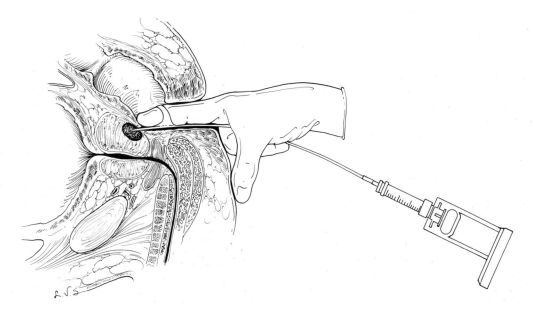

Figure 10–13. Transrectal aspiration biopsy. Advancement of a fine needle into the lesion under digital control. During forth-and-back movement of the needle in a fan-type motion, suction is applied with a plunger and syringe. A transrectal prostate biopsy is also obtained under digital control by inserting the trocar needle (Tru-cut needle) into the lesion and then advancing the outer cannula to cut off tissue extending into the recessed area of the trocar needle. Both trocar and cannula are removed, along with a cylinder of prostatic tissue.

advantages are the need for local anesthesia and the fact that the fine-needle technique (see below) is not applicable through this approach.

If a histologic diagnosis is to be made, a cylinder of tissue must be obtained with a specially designed biopsy needle (eg, Tru-cut needle) (Fig 10–13). For cytologic diagnosis, a transrectal fine-needle aspiration technique (Franzen needle) may be used. Advan-

tages of the fine-needle technique are lower risk of infection and bleeding, as well as including a larger volume of tissue, because the needle is moved back and forth in a fan-type motion through the prostate while suction is applied by an aspiration syringe. However, an experienced cytologist must be available to make the diagnosis with the same accuracy as with a histologic specimen.

REFERENCES

Urethral Catheterization Cystoscopy

Berci G: Instrumentation 1: Rigid endoscopes. Pages 74–112 in: *Endoscopy*. Berci G (editor). Appleton-Century-Crofts, 1976.

Berci G: Instrumentation 2: Flexible fiber endoscopes. Pages 113–132 in: *Endoscopy*. Berci G (editor). Appleton-Century-Crofts, 1976.

Berci G: Television. Pages 271–279 in: *Endoscopy*. Berci G (editor). Appleton-Century-Crofts, 1976.

Berci G et al: Permanent film records. Pages 242–270 in: *Endoscopy*. Berci G (editor). Appleton-Century-Crofts, 1976.

Brocklehurst JC: The management of indwelling catheters. *Br J Urol* 1978;**50**:102.

Burke JP et al: Prevention of catheter-associated urinary tract infections: Efficacy of daily meatal care regimens. *Am J Med* 1981;**70**:655.

Clayman RV, Reddy P, Lange PH: Flexible fiberoptic and rigid-rod lens endoscopy of the lower urinary tract: A prospective controlled comparison. *J Urol* 1984;**131**:715.

Cox CE, Hinman F Jr: Experiments with induced bacteriuria,

vesical emptying and bacterial growth on the mechanism of bladder defense to infection. *J Urol* 1961;**86**:739.

Desautels RE, Chibaro EA, Lang JR: Maintenance of sterility in urinary drainage bags. *Surg Gynecol Obstet* 1981;**154**:838.

Koss EH, Schneiderman JJ: Entry of bacteria in urinary tracts of patients with in-lying catheter. *N Engl J Med* 1957;**256**:556.

Lange PH: Diagnostic and therapeutic urologic instrumentation. Chap 8, pp 510–540, in: *Campbell's Urology,* 5th ed. Walsh PC et al (editors). Saunders, 1986.

Lapides J et al: Clean, intermittent self-catheterization in the treatment of urinary tract disease. *J Urol* 1972;**107**:458.

Nanninga JB: Care of the catheter-dependent patient. *Urol Clin North Am* 1980;**7**:41.

Transrectal & Transurethral Ultrasound

Carpentier PJ, Schröder FH: Transrectal ultrasonography in the follow-up of prostatic carcinoma patients: A new prognostic parameter? *J Urol* 1984;**131**:903.

Carpentier PJ, Schröder FH, Blom JHM: Transrectal ultrasonography in the follow-up of prostatic carcinoma patients. *J Urol* 1982;**128:**742.

Chodak GW et al: Comparison of digital examination and transrectal ultrasonography for the diagnosis of prostatic cancer. *J Urol* 1986;**135:**951.

Gammelgaard J, Holm HH: Transurethral and transrectal ultrasonic scanning in urology. *J Urol* 1980;**124:**863.

Harada K: Disorders of the prostate. Chap 11, pp 239–251, in: *Ultrasound in Urology,* 2nd ed. Resnick MI, Sanders RC (editors). Williams & Wilkins, 1984.

Holm HH, Gammelgaard J: Ultrasonically guided precise needle placement in the prostate and the seminal vesicles. *J Urol* 1981;**125:**385.

Itzchak Y, Singer D, Fischelovitch Y: Ultrasonographic assessment of bladder tumors: 1. Tumor detection. *J Urol* 1981;**126:**31.

Nakamura S, Niijima T: Staging of bladder cancer by ultrasonography: A new technique by transurethral intravesical scanning. *J Urol* 1980;**124:**341.

Nakamura S, Niijima T: Transurethral real-time scanner. *J Urol* 1981;**125:**781.

Peeling WB et al: Diagnosis and staging of prostatic cancer by transrectal ultrasonographic system. *Ultrasound Med Biol* 1979;**5:**129.

Resnick MI, Willard JW, Boyce WH: Transrectal ultrasonography in the evaluation of patients with prostatic carcinoma. *J Urol* 1980;**124:**482.

Rifkin MD: Ultrasonography of the lower genitourinary tract. *Urol Clin North Am* 1985;**12:**645.

Rifkin MD, Kurtz AB: Prostate ultrasound. Chap 9, pp 195–219, in: *Genitourinary Ultrasound.* Hricak H (editor). Churchill Livingstone, 1986.

Rifkin MD et al: Endoscopic ultrasonic evaluation of the prostate using a transrectal probe: Prospective evaluation and acoustic characterization. *Radiology* 1983;**149:**265.

Schüller J et al: Intravesical ultrasound tomography in staging bladder carcinoma. *J Urol* 1982;**128:**264.

Shapeero LG, Friedland GW, Perkash I: Transrectal sonographic voiding cystourethrography: Studies in neuromuscular bladder dysfunction. *AJR* 1983;**141:**83.

Singer D, Itzchak Y, Fischelovitch Y: Ultrasonographic assessment of bladder tumors. 2. Clinical staging. *J Urol* 1981;**126:**34.

Watanabe H et al: Mass screening program for prostatic diseases with transrectal ultrasonotomography. *J Urol* 1977;**117:**746.

Watanabe H et al: Transrectal ultrasonotomography of the prostate. *J Urol* 1975;**114:**734.

Laser

Beisland HO, Sander S, Fossberg E: Neodymium:YAG laser irradiation of urinary bladder tumors: Follow-up study of 100 consecutively treated patients. *Urology* 1985;**25:**559.

Benson RC Jr: Treatment of diffuse transitional cell carcinoma in situ by whole bladder hematoporphyrin derivative photodynamic therapy. *J Urol* 1985;**134:**675.

Benson RC Jr et al: Treatment of transitional cell carcinoma of the bladder with hematoporphyrin derivative phototherapy. *J Urol* 1983;**130:**1090.

Bülow H, Bülow U, Frohmüller HG: Transurethral laser urethrotomy in man: A preliminary report. *J Urol* 1979;**121:**286.

Hofstetter A, Frank F: Laser use in urology. Page 146 in: *Surgical Application of Lasers.* Dixon JA (editor). Year Book, 1983.

Hofstetter A, Frank F, Keiditsch E: Laser treatment of the bladder: Experimental and clinical results. In: *Lasers in Urologic Surgery.* Smith JA (editor). Year Book, 1985.

Jocham D: Photodynamic techniques in the treatment of bladder cancer. In: *Advances in Urologic Oncology.* Williams RD (editor). Macmillan, 1987.

Malloy TR: Laser treatment of ureter and upper collecting system. In: *Lasers in Urologic Surgery.* Smith JA (editor). Year Book, 1985.

Malloy TR, Wein AJ, Shanberg A: Superficial transitional cell carcinoma of the bladder treated with neodymium:YAG laser: A study of recurrence rate within the first year. *J Urol* 1984;**131:**251.

Rosemberg SK, Fuller T, Jacobs H: Continuous-wave carbon dioxide laser treatment of giant condylomata acuminata of the distal urethra and perineum: Technique. *J Urol* 1981;**126:**827.

Rosemberg SK, Jacobs H, Fuller T: Some guidelines in the treatment of urethral condylomata with carbon dioxide laser. *J Urol* 1982;**127:**906.

Rosenberg SJ, Williams RD: Photodynamic therapy of bladder carcinoma. *Urol Clin North Am* 1986;**13:**435.

Rothauge CF: Urethroscopic recanalization of urethral stenosis using an argon laser. *Urol* 1980;**16:**158.

Schaeffer AJ: Use of the CO_2 laser in urology. *Urol Clin North Am* 1986;**13:**393.

Smith JA Jr: Endoscopic applications of laser energy. *Urol Clin North Am* 1986;**13:**405.

Staehler G et al: Therapy of bladder tumors with the neodymium-YAG laser: A critical assessment. In: *Bladder Cancer.* Liss, 1984.

von Eschenbach AC: The neodymium-yttrium aluminum garnet (Nd:YAG) laser in urology. *Urol Clin North Am* 1986;**13:**381.

Vourc'h G et al: Two unusual cases of gas embolism following urethral surgery under laser. *Intensive Care Med* 1982;**8:**239.

Willscher MK: Endoscopic delivery of CO_2 laser energy. In: *Lasers in Urologic Surgery.* Smith JA (editor). Year Book, 1985.

Ureteral Catheterization

Bigongiari LR: Transluminal dilatation of ureteral strictures. Chap 6, pp 113–118, in: *Percutaneous and Interventional Urology and Radiology.* Lang EK (editor). Springer-Verlag, 1986.

Camacho MF et al: Double-ended pigtail ureteral stent: Useful modification to single end ureteral stent. *Urology* 1979;**13:**516.

Elyaderani MK, Kandzari SJ: Ureteral stent insertion and brush biopsy. Chap 3, pp 55–95, in: *Invasive Uroradiology: A Manual of Diagnostic and Therapeutic Techniques.* Elyaderani MK et al (editors). Heath, 1984.

Finney RP: Double-J and diversion stents. *Urol Clin North Am* 1982;**9:**89.

Finney RP: Experience with new double-J ureteral catheter stent. *J Urol* 1978;**120:**678.

Fritzche PJ: Antegrade and retrograde ureteral stenting. Chap 5, pp 91–111, in: *Percutaneous and Interventional Urology and Radiology.* Lang EK (editor). Springer-Verlag, 1986.

Mardis HK, Hepperlen TW, Kammandel H: Double pigtail ureteral stent. *Urology* 1979;**14:**23.

Oswalt GC Jr, Bueschen AJ, Lloyd IK: Upward migration of indwelling ureteral stents. *J Urol* 1979;**122:**249.

Ramsay JWA et al: The effects of double J stenting on unobstructed ureters: An experimental and clinical study. *Br J Urol* 1985;**57:**630.

Smith AD: The universal ureteral stent. *Urol Clin North Am* 1982;**9:**103.

Stone Basketing, Ureterorenoscopy

Abdelsayed M, Onal E, Wax SH: Avulsion of the ureter caused by stone basket manipulation. *J Urol* 1977; **118**:868.

Dourmashkin RL: Cystoscopic treatment of stones in the ureter with special reference to large calculi: Based on a study of 1550 cases. *J Urol* 1945;**54**:245.

Ford TF, Payne SR, Wickham JE: The impact of transurethral ureteroscopy on the management of ureteric calculi. *Br J Urol* 1984;**56**:602.

Ford TF, Watson GM, Wickham JE: Transurethral ureteroscopic retrieval of ureteric stones. *Br J Urol* 1983;**55**:626.

Harrison GSM, Davies GA, Holdsworth PJ: Twelve-year experience using the dormia basket for the extraction of ureteric stones. *Eur Urol* 1983;**9**:93.

Huffman JL, Bagley DH, Lyon ES: Treatment of distal ureteral calculi using rigid ureteroscope. *Urology* 1982; **20**:574.

Huffman JL et al: Endoscopic diagnosis and treatment of upper-tract urothelial tumors: A preliminary report. *Cancer* 1985;**55**:1422.

Huffman JL et al: Transurethral removal of large ureteral and renal pelvic calculi using ureteroscopic ultrasonic lithotripsy. *J Urol* 1983;**130**:31.

Kandzari SJ, Elyaderani MK: Retrograde extraction, chemolysis, and intraoperative ultrasonographic localization of urinary calculi. Chap 5, pp 113–153, in: *Invasive Uroradiology: A Manual of Diagnostic and Therapeutic Techniques*. Elyaderani MK et al (editors). Heath, 1984.

Lupu AN, Fuchs GJ, Chaussy CG: A new approach to ureteral-stone manipulation for ESWL. *Endourology* 1986;**1**:13.

Lyon ES, Banno JJ, Schoenberg HW: Transurethral ureteroscopy in men using juvenile cystoscopy equipment. *J Urol* 1979;**122**:152.

Lyon ES, Huffman JL, Bagley DH: Ureteroscopy and uretero-pyeloscopy. *Urology* 1984;**23(5 Spec No.)**:29.

Lyon ES, Kyker JS, Schoenberg HW: Transurethral ureteroscopy in women: A ready addition to the urological armamentarium. *J Urol* 1978;**119**:35.

Pérez-Castro Ellendt E, Martinez-Piñeiro JA: Ureteral and renal endoscopy: A new approach. *Eur Urol* 1982;**8**:117.

Pérez-Castro Ellendt E, Martinez-Piñeiro JA: La ureterorenoscopia transuretral: Un actual proceder urológico. *Arch Esp Urol* 1980;**33**:445.

Ruter AB: Ureteral balloon dilatation and stone basketing. *Urology* 1984;**23(5 Spec No.)**:44.

Rutner AB, Fucilla IS: An improved helical stone basket. *J Urol* 1976;**116**:784.

Schwartz BA, Wise HA II: Endourologic techniques for the bladder and urethra. *Urol Clin North Am* 1982;**9**:165.

Shihata AA, Greene JE: Ureteric stone extraction by a new double-balloon catheter: An experimental study. *J Urol* 1983;**129**:616.

Stackl W, Marberger M: Late sequelae of the management of ureteral calculi with the ureterorenoscope. *J Urol* 1986;**136**:386.

Suprapubic Cystostomy

Schmidt RA: Postoperative catheter drainage. Chap 19, pp 267–274, in: *Surgery of Female Incontinence*, 2nd ed. Stanton SS, Tanagho EA (editors). Springer-Verlag, 1986.

Shapiro J, Hoffmann J, Jersky J: A comparison of suprapubic and transurethral drainage for postoperative urinary retention in general surgical patients. *Acta Chir Scand* 1982;**148**:323.

Rasmussen OV et al: Suprapubic vs urethral bladder drainage following surgery for renal cancer. *Acta Chir Scand* 1977;**143**:371.

Wilson EA, Sprague AD, Van Nagell JR Jr: Suprapubic cystostomy in gynecologic surgery: A comparison of two methods. *Am J Obstet Gynecol* 1973;**115**:991.

Cytology, Biopsy Histology

Barry JM et al: The influence of retrograde contrast medium on urinary cytodiagnosis: A preliminary report. *J Urol* 1978;**119**:633.

Crawford ED et al: Prevention of urinary tract infection and sepsis following transrectal prostatic biopsy. *J Urol* 1982;**127**:449.

Epsoti PL: Cytologic malignancy grading for prostatic carcinoma for transurethral aspiration biopsy. *Scand J Urol Nephrol* 1971;**5**:199.

Epstein NA: Prostatic biopsy: A morphologic correlation of aspiration cytology with needle biopsy histology. *Cancer* 1976;**38**:2078.

Franzen S et al: Cytological diagnosis of prostatic tumors by transrectal aspiration biopsy: A preliminary report. *Br J Urol* 1960;**32**:193.

Gill WB, Lu C, Bibbo M: Retrograde brush biopsy of the ureter and renal pelvis. *Urol Clin North Am* 1979;**6**:573.

Lieberman RP, Cummings KB, Leslie SW: Sheathed catheter system for fluoroscopically guided retrograde catheterization, and brush and forceps biopsy of the upper urinary tract. *J Urol* 1984;**131**:450.

Rife CC, Farrow GM, Utz DC: Urine cytology of transitional cell neoplasms. *Urol Clin North Am* 1979;**6**:599.

Segura JW: Prostatic biopsy technique. Chap 90, pp 935–938, in: *Urologic Surgery*, 3rd ed. Glenn JF, Boyce WH (editors). Lippincott, 1983.

11 Urinary Obstruction & Stasis

Emil A. Tanagho, MD

Because of their damaging effect on renal function, obstruction and stasis of urinary flow are among the most important of urologic disorders. Either leads eventually to hydronephrosis, a peculiar type of atrophy of the kidney that may terminate in renal insufficiency or, if unilateral, complete destruction of the organ. Furthermore, obstruction leads to infection, which causes additional damage to the organs involved.

Classification

Obstruction may be classified according to etiology (congenital or acquired), duration (acute or chronic), degree (partial or complete), and level (upper or lower urinary tract).

Etiology

Congenital anomalies, more common in the urinary tract than in any other organ system, are generally obstructive. In adult life, many types of acquired obstruction can occur.

A. Congenital: The common sites of congenital narrowing are the external meatus in boys (meatal stenosis) or just inside the external urinary meatus in little girls, the distal urethra (stenosis), posterior urethral valves, ectopic ureters, ureteroceles, and the ureterovesical and ureteropelvic junctions. Another congenital cause of urinary stasis is damage to sacral roots 2–4 as seen in spina bifida and myelomeningocele. Vesicoureteral reflux causes both vesical and renal stasis (see Chapter 12).

B. Acquired: Acquired obstructions are numerous and may be primary in the urinary tract or secondary to retroperitoneal lesions that invade or compress the urinary passages. Among the common causes are (1) urethral stricture secondary to infection or injury; (2) benign prostatic hyperplasia or cancer of the prostate; (3) vesical tumor involving the bladder neck or one or both orifices; (4) local extension of cancer of the prostate or cervix into the base of the bladder, occluding the ureters; (5) compression of the ureters at the pelvic brim by metastatic nodes from cancer of the prostate or cervix; (6) ureteral stone; (7) retroperitoneal fibrosis or malignant tumor; and (8) pregnancy.

Neurogenic dysfunction affects principally the bladder. The upper tracts are damaged secondarily by ureterovesical obstruction or reflux and, often, complicating infection. Severe constipation, especially in children, can cause bilateral hydroureteronephrosis from compression of the lower ureters.

Elongation and kinking of the ureter secondary to vesicoureteral reflux commonly lead to ureteropelvic obstruction and hydronephrosis. Unless a voiding cystourethrogram is obtained in all children with this lesion, the primary cause may be missed and improper treatment given.

Pathogenesis & Pathology

Obstruction and neuropathic vesical dysfunction have the same effects on the urinary tract. These changes can best be understood by considering (1) the effects upon the lower tract (distal to the bladder neck) of severe external urinary meatal stricture and (2) the effects upon the mid tract (bladder) and upper tract (ureter and kidney) of benign prostatic hyperplasia.

A. Lower Tract: Hydrostatic pressure proximal to the obstruction causes dilation of the urethra. The wall of the urethra may become thin, and a diverticulum may form. If the urine becomes infected, spontaneous urethral rupture with urinary extravasation may occur. The prostatic ducts may become widely dilated.

B. Mid Tract: In the earlier stages (compensatory phase), the muscle wall of the bladder becomes hypertrophied and thickened. With decompensation, it becomes less contractile and, therefore, weakened.

1. Stage of compensation–In order to balance the increasing urethral resistance, the bladder musculature hypertrophies. Its thickness may double or triple. Complete emptying of the bladder is thus made possible.

Hypertrophied muscle may be seen microscopically. With secondary infection, the effects of infection are often superimposed. There may be edema of the submucosa, which may be infiltrated with plasma cells, lymphocytes, and polymorphonuclear cells.

At cystoscopy, surgery, or autopsy, the following evidence of this compensation may be visible (Fig 11–1):

a. Trabeculation of the bladder wall–The wall of the distended bladder is normally quite smooth. With hypertrophy, individual muscle bundles stand out taut and give a coarsely interwoven appearance to the mucosal surface. The trigonal muscle and the interureteric ridge, which normally are only slightly raised above the surrounding tissues, respond to obstruction by hypertrophy of their smooth musculature. The ridge then becomes prominent. This trigonal hypertrophy causes increased resistance to urine flow in the intravesical ureteral segments owing to accentu-

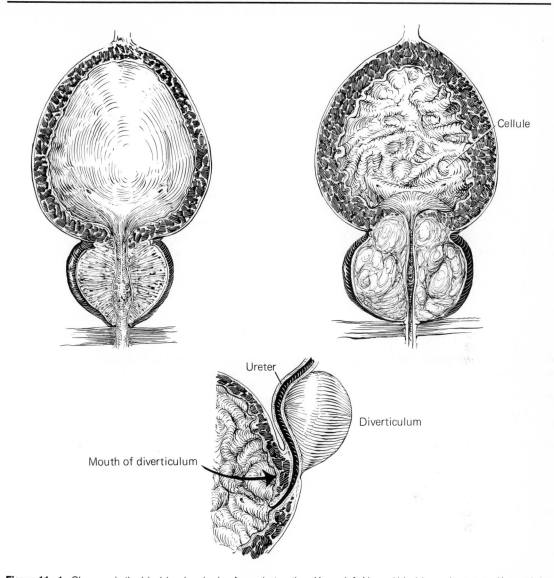

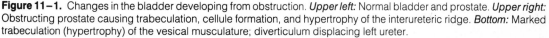

Figure 11–1. Changes in the bladder developing from obstruction. *Upper left:* Normal bladder and prostate. *Upper right:* Obstructing prostate causing trabeculation, cellule formation, and hypertrophy of the interureteric ridge. *Bottom:* Marked trabeculation (hypertrophy) of the vesical musculature; diverticulum displacing left ureter.

ated downward pull upon them. It is this mechanism that causes relative functional obstruction of the ureterovesical junctions, leading to back pressure on the kidney and hydroureteronephrosis. The obstruction increases in the presence of significant residual urine, which further stretches the ureterotrigonal complex. (A urethral catheter will relieve the obstruction somewhat by eliminating the trigonal stretch. Definitive prostatectomy leads to permanent release of stretch and gradual softening of trigonal hypertrophy with relief of the obstruction.)

b. Cellules–Normal intravesical pressure is about 30 cm of water at the beginning of micturition. Pressures 2–4 times as great may be reached by the trabeculated (hypertrophied) bladder in its attempt to force urine past the obstruction. This pressure tends to push mucosa between the superficial muscle bundles, causing the formation of small pockets, or cellules (Fig 11–1).

c. Diverticula–If cellules force their way entirely through the musculature of the bladder wall, they become saccules, then actual diverticula, which may be embedded in perivesical fat or covered by peritoneum, depending upon their location. Diverticula have no muscle wall and are therefore unable to expel their contents into the bladder efficiently even after the primary obstruction has been removed. When secondary infection occurs, it is difficult to eradicate; surgical removal of the diverticula may be required. If a diverticulum pushes through the bladder wall on the anterior surface of the ureter, the ureterovesical junction will become incompetent (see Chapter 12).

d. Mucosa–In the presence of acute infection, the mucosa may be reddened and edematous. This may lead to temporary vesicoureteral reflux in the presence of a "borderline" junction. The chronically inflamed membrane may be thinned and pale. In the absence of infection, the mucosa appears normal.

2. Stage of decompensation–The compensatory power of the bladder musculature varies greatly. One patient with prostatic enlargement may have only mild symptoms of prostatism but a large obstructing gland that can be palpated rectally and observed cystoscopically; another may suffer acute retention and yet have a gland of normal size on rectal palpation and what appears to be only a mild obstruction cystoscopically.

In the face of progressive urethral obstruction, possibly aggravated by prostatic infection with edema or by congestion from lack of intercourse, decompensation of the detrusor may occur, resulting in the presence of residual urine after voiding. The amount may range up to 500 mL or more.

C. Upper Tract:

1. Ureter–In the early stages of obstruction, intravesical pressure is normal while the bladder fills and is increased only during voiding. The pressure is not transmitted to the ureters and renal pelves because of the competence of the ureterovesical "valves." (A true valve is not present; the ureterotrigonal unit, by virtue of its intrinsic structure, resists the retrograde flow of urine.) However, owing to trigonal hypertrophy (see above) and to the resultant increase in resistance to urine flow across the terminal ureter, there is progressive back pressure on the ureter and kidney, resulting in ureteral dilatation and hydronephrosis. Later, with the phase of decompensation accompanied by residual urine, there is an added stretch effect on the already hypertrophied trigone that increases appreciably the resistance to flow at the lower end of the ureter and induces further hydroureteronephrosis. With decompensation of the ureterotrigonal complex, the valvelike action may be lost, vesicoureteral reflux occurs, and the increased intravesical pressure is then transmitted directly to the renal pelves, aggravating the degree of hydroureteronephrosis.

Secondary to the back pressure resulting from reflux or from obstruction by the hypertrophied and stretched trigone or by a ureteral stone, the ureteral musculature thickens in its attempt to push the urine downward by increased peristaltic activity (stage of compensation). This causes elongation and some tortuosity of the ureter (Fig 11–2). At times, this change becomes marked, and bands of fibrous tissue develop. On contraction, the bands further angulate the ureter, causing secondary ureteral obstruction. Under these circumstances, removal of the obstruction below may not prevent the kidney from undergoing complete destruction due to the secondary ureteral obstruction.

Finally, because of increasing pressure, the ureteral wall becomes attenuated and therefore loses all of its contractile power (stage of decompensation). Dilatation may be so extreme that the ureter resembles a loop of bowel (Figs 11–3 and 12–8, upper right).

2. Kidney–The pressure within the renal pelvis is normally close to zero. When this pressure increases because of obstruction or reflux, the pelvis and calices dilate. The degree of hydronephrosis that develops depends upon the duration, degree, and site of the obstruction (Fig 11–4). The higher the obstruction, the greater the effect upon the kidney. If the renal pelvis is entirely intrarenal and the obstruction is at the ureteropelvic junction, all the pressure will be exerted upon the parenchyma. If the renal pelvis is extrarenal, only part of the pressure produced by a ureteropelvic stenosis will be exerted on the parenchyma; this is because the extrarenal renal pelvis is embedded in fat and dilates more readily, thus "decompressing" the calices (Fig 11–2).

In the earlier stages, the pelvic musculature undergoes compensatory hypertrophy in its effort to force urine past the obstruction. Later, however, the muscle becomes stretched and atonic (and decompensated).

The progression of hydronephrotic atrophy is as follows:

(1) The earliest changes in the development of hydronephrosis are seen in the calices. The end of a normal calix (as seen on a urogram, Fig 6–5) is concave because of the papilla that projects into it; with increase in intrapelvic pressure, the fornices become blunt and rounded. With persistence of increased intrapelvic pressure, the papilla becomes flattened, then convex (clubbed) as a result of compression enhanced by ischemic atrophy (Fig 11–5). The parenchyma between the calices is affected to a lesser extent. The changes in the renal parenchyma are due to (1) compression atrophy from increase in intrapelvic pressure (more accentuated with intrarenal pelves) and (2) ischemic atrophy from hemodynamic changes, mainly manifested in arcuate vessels that run at the base of the pyramids parallel to the kidney outline and are more vulnerable to compression between the renal capsule and the centrally increasing intrapelvic pressure.

This spotty atrophy is caused by the nature of the blood supply of the kidney. The arterioles are "end arteries"; therefore, ischemia is most marked in the areas farthest from the interlobular arteries. As the back pressure increases, hydronephrosis progresses, with the cells nearest the main arteries exhibiting the greatest resistance.

This increased pressure is transmitted up the tubules. The tubules become dilated, and their cells atrophy from ischemia.

It should be pointed out that a few instances of dilated renal pelves and calices are not due to the presence of obstruction. Rarely, the renal cavities are congenitally capacious and thus simulate hydronephrosis. More commonly, hydronephrosis may occur in childhood due to the back pressure associated with vesicoureteral reflux. If the valvular incompetence resolves (and this is common), some degree of the hydronephrotic changes may persist. These persisting changes may cause the physician to suspect the presence of obstruction, which may lead to unnecessary

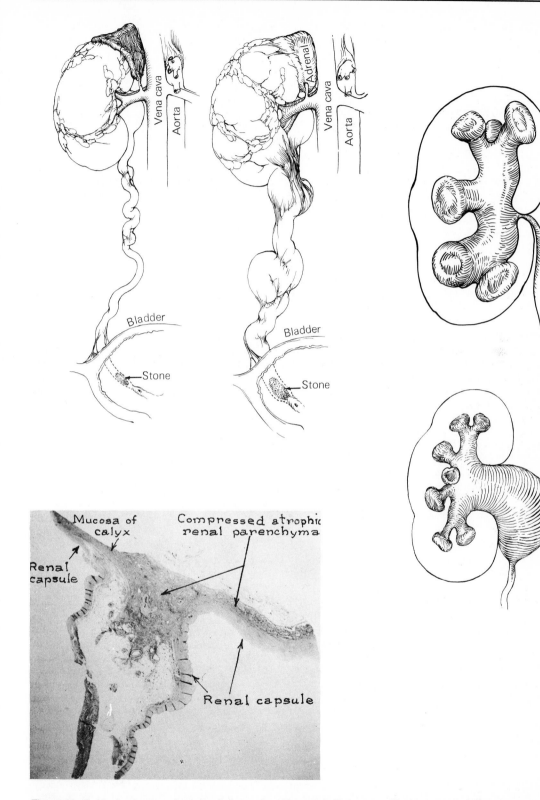

Figure 11–2. Mechanisms and results of obstruction. *Upper left:* Early stage. Elongation and dilatation of ureter due to mild obstruction. *Upper center:* Later stage. Further dilatation and elongation with kinking of the ureter; fibrous bands cause further kinking. *Lower left:* Photomicrograph of advanced hydronephrosis. Thin layer of renal parenchyma covered by fibrous capsule. *Upper right:* Intrarenal pelvis. Obstruction transmits all back pressure to parenchyma. *Lower right:* Extrarenal pelvis, when obstructed, allows some of the increased pressure to be dissipated by the pelvis.

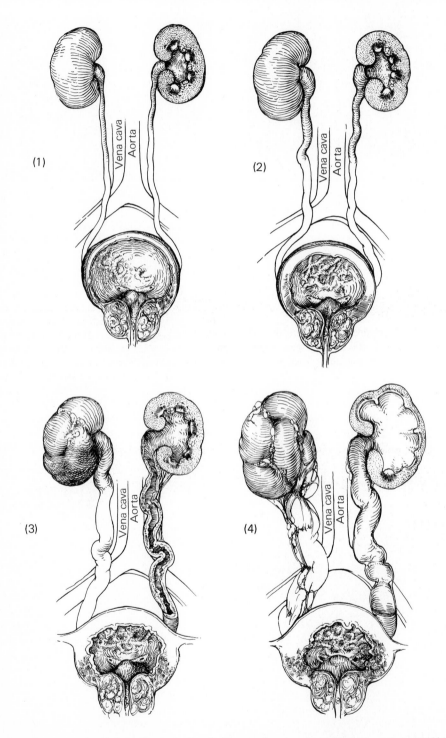

Figure 11–3. Pathogenesis of bilateral hydronephrosis. Progressive changes in bladder, ureters, and kidneys from obstruction of an enlarged prostate: thickening of bladder wall, dilatation and elongation of ureters, and hydronephrosis.

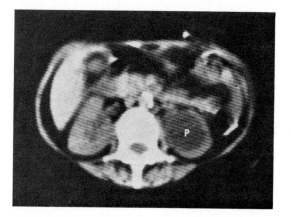

Figure 11–4. Hydronephrotic left renal pelvis. Low-density mass (P) in left renal sinus had attenuation value similar to that of water, suggesting the correct diagnosis. Unless intravenous contrast material is used, differentiation from peripelvic cyst may be difficult.

surgery. An isotope renogram or the Whitaker test (see p 113) can be performed to determine whether organic obstruction is present.

(2) Only in unilateral hydronephrosis are the advanced stages of hydronephrotic atrophy seen. Eventually the kidney is completely destroyed and appears

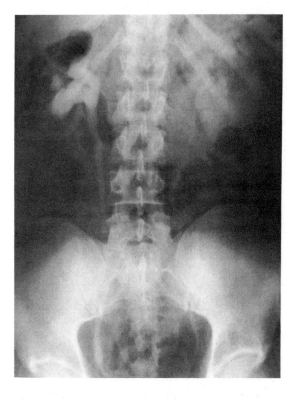

Figure 11–5. Lower right ureteral obstruction. Mild to moderate dilatation of the collecting system with rounded blunting of the calices.

as a thin-walled sac filled with clear fluid (water and electrolytes) or pus (Fig 11–6).

If obstruction is unilateral, the increased intrarenal pressure will cause some suppression of renal function on that side. The closer the intrapelvic pressure approaches the glomerular filtration pressure (6–12 mm Hg), the less urine can be secreted. Glomerular filtration rate and renal plasma flow are reduced, concentrating power is gradually lost, and the urea: creatinine concentration ratio of urine from the hydronephrotic kidney is lower than that of urine from the normal kidney.

Hydronephrotic atrophy is an unusual type of pathologic change. Other secretory organs (eg, the submaxillary gland) cease secreting when their ducts are obstructed. This causes primary (disuse) atrophy. The completely obstructed kidney, however, continues to secrete urine. (If this were not so, hydronephrosis could not occur, since it depends upon increased intrarenal pressure.) As urine is excreted into the renal pelvis, fluid and, particularly, soluble substances are reabsorbed, through either the tubules or the lymphatics. This has been demonstrated by injecting phenolsulfonphthalein (PSP) into the obstructed renal pelvis. It disappears (is reabsorbed) in a few hours and is excreted by the other kidney. If the intrapelvic pressure in the hydronephrotic kidney rapidly increases to a level approaching filtration pressure (resulting in cessation of filtration), a safety mechanism is activated that produces a break in the surface lining of the collecting structure at the weakest point—the fornices. This leads to escape and extravasation of urine from the renal pelvis into the parenchymal interstitium (pyelointerstitial backflow). The extravasated fluid will be absorbed by the renal lymphatics, and the pressure in the renal pelvis will drop, allowing further filtration of urine. This explains the process by which the markedly hydronephrotic kidney continues to function. Further evidence of the occurrence of extravasation and reabsorption is that the markedly hydronephrotic kidney does not contain urine in the true sense; only water and a few salts are present.

Functional impairment in unilateral hydronephrosis, as measured by PSP tests or excretory urograms, will be greater and will increase faster than that seen in bilateral hydronephrotic kidneys showing comparable damage on urography. As unilateral hydronephrosis progresses, the normal kidney undergoes compensatory hypertrophy (particularly in children) of its nephrons (renal counterbalance), thereby assuming the function of the diseased kidney in order to maintain normal total renal function. For this reason, successful anatomic repair of the ureteral obstruction of such a kidney may fail to improve its powers of waste elimination.

If both kidneys are equally hydronephrotic, a strong stimulus is continually being exerted on both to maintain maximum function. This is also true of a hydronephrotic solitary kidney. Consequently, the return of function in these kidneys after repair of their obstructions is at times remarkable.

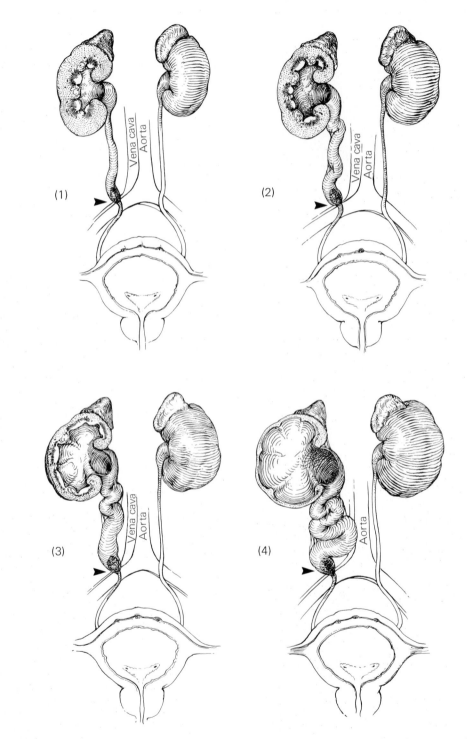

Figure 11–6. Pathogenesis of unilateral hydronephrosis. Progressive changes in ureter and kidney secondary to obstructing calculus (*arrows*). As the right kidney undergoes gradual destruction, the left kidney gradually enlarges (compensatory hypertrophy).

Experimental studies have shown recovery of function after release of complete obstruction of up to 4 weeks' duration. In 2 well-documented human cases, function was recovered after obstruction of 56 and 69 days. However, irreversible loss of function can begin as early as 7 days, as evidenced by dilatation and necrosis of the proximal tubules, which progressively increase with time.

The extent of recovery after partial obstruction is difficult to determine preoperatively. Renal scanning with DMSA (dimercaptosuccinic acid) is most helpful. Temporary drainage, especially by nephrostomy, followed by tests to assess renal function is the best measure.

Physiologic Explanation of Symptoms of Bladder Neck Obstruction

The following hypothesis has been proposed to explain the syndrome known as "prostatism," which occurs with progressive vesical obstruction:

The bladder, like the heart, is a hollow muscular organ that receives fluid and forcefully expels it. And, like the heart, it reacts to an increasing work load by going through the successive phases of compensation and finally decompensation.

Normally, contraction of the detrusor muscle and the trigone pulls the bladder neck open and forms a funnel through which the urine is expelled. The intravesical pressure generated in this instance varies between 20 and 40 cm of water; this force further widens the bladder neck.

With bladder neck obstruction, hypertrophy of the vesical musculature develops, allowing the intravesical voiding pressure to rise to 50–100 cm or more of water in order to overcome the increased outlet resistance. Despite this, the encroaching prostate appears to interfere with the mechanisms that ordinarily open the internal orifice. Also, the contraction phase may not last long enough for all of the urine to be expelled; "exhaustion" of the muscle occurs prematurely. The refractory phase then sets in, and the detrusor is temporarily unable to respond to further stimuli. A few minutes later, voiding may be initiated again and completed.

A. Compensation Phase:

1. Stage of irritability– In the earliest stages of obstruction of the bladder neck, the vesical musculature begins to hypertrophy. The force and size of the urinary stream remain normal because the balance is maintained between the expelling power of the bladder and urethral resistance. During this phase, however, the bladder appears to be hypersensitive. As the bladder is distended, the need to void is felt. In the individual with a normal bladder, these early urges can be inhibited, and the bladder relaxes and distends to receive more urine. However, in the patient with a hypertrophied detrusor, the contraction of the detrusor is so strong that it virtually goes into spasm, producing the symptoms of an irritable bladder. The earliest symptoms of bladder neck obstruction, therefore, are urgency (even to the point of incontinence) and frequency, both day and night.

2. Stage of compensation– As the obstruction increases, further hypertrophy of the muscle fibers of the bladder occurs, and the power to empty the bladder completely is thereby maintained. During this period, in addition to urgency and frequency, the patient notices hesitancy in initiating urination while the bladder develops contractions strong enough to overcome resistance at the bladder neck. The obstruction causes some loss in the force and size of the urinary stream, and the stream becomes slower as vesical emptying nears completion (exhaustion of the detrusor as it nears the end of the contraction phase).

B. Decompensation Phase: If vesical tone becomes impaired or if urethral resistance exceeds detrusor power, some degree of decompensation (imbalance) occurs. The contraction phase of the vesical muscle becomes too short to completely expel the contents of the bladder, and some urine remains in the bladder (residual urine).

1. Acute decompensation– The tone of the compensated vesical muscle can be temporarily embarrassed by rapid filling of the bladder (high fluid intake) or by overstretching of the detrusor (postponement of urination though the urge is felt). This may cause increased difficulty of urination, with marked hesitancy and the need for straining to initiate urination; a very weak and small stream; and termination of the stream before the bladder completely empties (residual urine). Acute and sudden complete urinary retention may also occur.

2. Chronic decompensation– As the degree of obstruction increases, a progressive imbalance between the power of the bladder musculature and urethral resistance develops. Therefore, it becomes increasingly difficult to expel all the urine during the contraction phase of the detrusor. The symptoms of obstruction become more marked. The amount of residual urine gradually increases, and this diminishes the functional capacity of the bladder. Progressive frequency of urination is noted. On occasion, as the bladder decompensates, it becomes overstretched and attenuated. It may contain 1000–3000 mL of urine. It loses its power of contraction, and overflow (paradoxic) incontinence results.

Clinical Findings

A. Symptoms:

1. Lower and mid tract (urethra and bladder)– Symptoms of obstruction of the lower and mid tract are typified by the symptoms of urethral stricture, benign prostatic hyperplasia, neurogenic bladder, and tumor of the bladder involving the vesical neck. The principal symptoms are hesitancy in starting urination, lessened force and size of the stream, and terminal dribbling; hematuria, which may be initial with stricture and total with prostatic obstruction or vesical tumor; and burning on urination, cloudy urine (due to complicating infection), and acute urinary retention.

2. Upper tract (ureter and kidney)– Symptoms

of obstruction of the upper tract are typified by the symptoms of congenital ureteral stenosis or ureteral or renal stone. The principal complaints are pain in the flank radiating along the course of the ureter, gross total hematuria (from stone), gastrointestinal symptoms, chills, fever, burning on urination, and cloudy urine with onset of infection, which is the common sequel to obstruction or vesicoureteral reflux. Nausea, vomiting, loss of weight and strength, and pallor are due to uremia secondary to bilateral hydronephrosis. A history of vesicoureteral reflux in childhood may be significant.

Obstruction of the upper tract may be silent even when uremia supervenes.

B. Signs:

1. Lower and mid tract—Palpation of the urethra may reveal induration about a stricture. Rectal examination may show atony of the anal sphincter (damage to the sacral nerve roots) or benign or malignant enlargement of the prostate. Vesical distention may be found.

Although observation of the force and caliber of the urinary stream affords a rough estimate of maximum flow rate, the rate can be measured accurately with a urine flowmeter or, even more simply, by the following technique: Have the patient begin to void. When observed maximum flow has been reached, interpose a container to collect the urine, and simultaneously start a stopwatch. After exactly 5 seconds, remove the container. The flow rate in milliliters per second can easily be calculated. The normal urine flow rate is 20–25 mL/s in males and 25–30 mL/s in females. Any flow rate under 15 mL/s should be regarded with suspicion. A flow rate under 10 mL/s is indicative of obstruction or weak detrusor function. Flow rates associated with an atonic neurogenic (neuropathic) bladder (diminished detrusor power), or with urethral stricture or prostatic obstruction (increased urethral resistance) may be as low as 3–5 mL/s. A cystometrogram will differentiate between these 2 causes of impaired flow rate. After definitive treatment of the cause, the flow rate should return to normal.

In the presence of a vesical diverticulum or vesicoureteral reflux, although detrusor power is normal, the urinary stream may be impaired because of the diffusion of intravesical pressure into the diverticulum and vesicoureteral junction as well as the urethra. Excision of the diverticulum or repair of the vesicoureteral junctions leads to efficient expulsion of urine via the urethra.

2. Upper tract—An enlarged kidney may be discovered by palpation or percussion. Renal tenderness may be elicited if infection is present. Cancer of the cervix may be noted; it may invade the base of the bladder and occlude one or both ureteral orifices, or its metastases to the iliac lymph nodes may compress the ureters. A large pelvic mass (tumor, pregnancy) can displace and compress the ureters. Children with advanced urinary tract obstruction (usually due to posterior urethral valves) may develop ascites. Rupture of the renal fornices allows leakage of urine, which

passes into the peritoneal cavity through a tear in the peritoneum.

C. Laboratory Findings: Anemia may be found secondary to chronic infection or in advanced bilateral hydronephrosis (stage of uremia). Leukocytosis is to be expected in the acute stage of infection. Little if any elevation of the white blood count accompanies the chronic stage.

Large amounts of protein are usually not found in the obstructive uropathies. Casts are not common from hydronephrotic kidneys. Microscopic hematuria may indicate renal or vesical infection, tumor, or stone. Pus cells and bacteria may or may not be present.

In the presence of unilateral hydronephrosis, results of the PSP test will be normal because of the contralateral renal hypertrophy. Suppression of PSP excretion indicates bilateral renal damage, residual urine (vesical or bilateral ureterorenal), or vesicoureteral reflux.

In the presence of significant bilateral hydronephrosis, urine flow through the renal tubules is slowed. Thus, urea is significantly reabsorbed but creatinine is not. Blood chemistry therefore reveals a urea:creatinine ratio well above the normal 10:1.

D. X-Ray Findings: (Fig 11–7.) A plain film of the abdomen may show enlargement of renal shadows, calcific bodies suggesting ureteral or renal stone, or tumor metastases to the bones of the spine or pelvis. Metastases in the spine may be the cause of spinal cord damage (neuropathic bladder); if they are osteoblastic, they are almost certainly from cancer of the prostate.

Excretory urograms will reveal almost the entire story unless renal function is severely impaired. They are more informative when obstruction is present because the radiopaque material is retained. These urograms will demonstrate the degree of dilatation of the pelves, calices, and ureters. The point of ureteral stenosis will be revealed. Segmental dilatation of the lower end of a ureter implies the possibility of vesicoureteral reflux (Fig 11–7), which can be revealed by cystography. The cystogram may show trabeculation as an irregularity of the vesical outline and may show diverticula. Vesical tumors, nonopaque stones, and large intravesical prostatic lobes may cause radiolucent shadows. A film taken immediately after voiding will show residual urine. Few tests that are as simple and inexpensive give the physician so much information.

Retrograde cystography shows changes of the bladder wall caused by distal obstruction (trabeculation, diverticula) or demonstrates the obstructive lesion itself (enlarged prostate, posterior urethral valves, cancer of the bladder). If the ureterovesical valves are incompetent, ureteropyelograms will be obtained by reflux.

Retrograde urograms may show better detail than the excretory type, but care must be taken not to overdistend the passages with too much opaque fluid; small hydronephroses can be made to look quite large. The degree of ureteral or ureterovesical obstruction

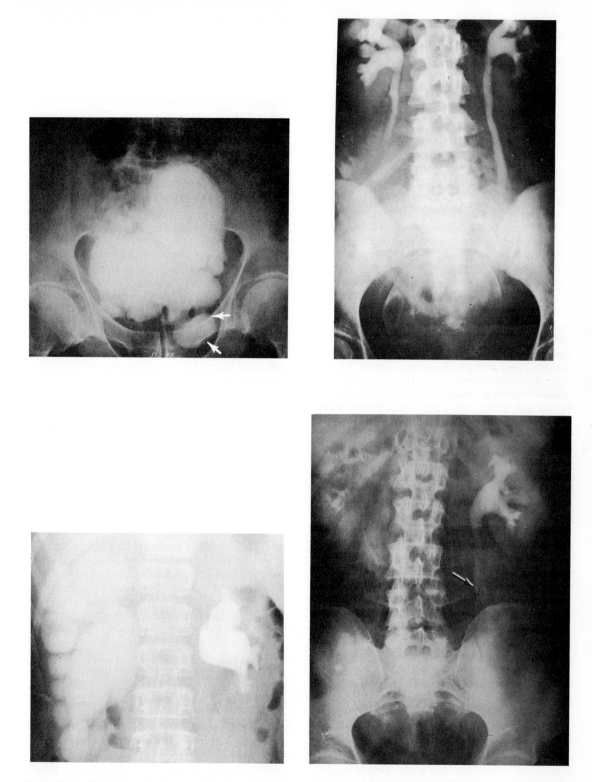

Figure 11–7. Changes in bladder, ureters, and kidneys caused by obstruction. *Upper left:* Cystogram showing benign prostatic enlargement and multiple diverticula. Arrows point to femoral hernia that probably developed as a result of straining to urinate. *Upper right:* Pregnancy. Significant dilatation and elongation of upper right ureter due to compression at the pelvic line. Left side normal. *Lower left:* Excretory urogram, 70 minutes after injection. Advanced right hydronephrosis secondary to ureteropelvic obstruction. Mild ureteropelvic obstruction on left. *Lower right:* Stone in left ureter (*at arrow*) with mild hydronephrosis.

can be judged by the degree of delay of drainage of the radiopaque fluid instilled.

CT scanning and sonography can also help determine the extent of dilatation and parenchymal atrophy.

E. Isotope Scanning: (See Chapter 9.) In the presence of obstruction, the radioisotope renogram may show depression of both the vascular and secretory phases and a rising rather than a falling excretory phase due to retention of the radiopaque urine in the renal pelvis.

The ^{131}I activity recorded on the gamma camera will show that the isotope is poorly taken up, slowly transported through the parenchyma, and accumulated in the renal pelvis.

F. Instrumental Examination: Exploration of the urethra with a catheter or other instrument is a valuable diagnostic measure. Passage may be blocked by a stricture or tumor. Spasm of the external sphincter may make passage difficult. Passage of the catheter immediately after voiding allows estimation of the amount of residual urine in the bladder. Residual urine is common in bladder neck obstruction (enlarged prostate), cystocele, and neurogenic (neuropathic) bladder. Residual urine is usually absent with urethral stricture, even though the urinary stream may be markedly impaired.

Measurement of vesical tone by means of cystometry is helpful in diagnosing neurogenic bladder and in differentiating between bladder neck obstruction and vesical atony.

Inspection of the urethra and bladder by means of cystoscopy and panendoscopy may reveal the primary obstructive agent. Catheters may be passed to the renal pelves and urine specimens obtained. The function of each kidney may be measured (PSP test), and retrograde ureteropyelograms can be made.

G. Interventional Uroradiology: If there is doubt about the presence of true obstruction, either the Whitaker test (see p 113) or an isotope renogram can be done. However, Whitaker and Buxton-Thomas (1984) have shown that neither test is without error.

Differential Diagnosis

A thorough examination usually leaves no doubt about the diagnosis. The differential diagnosis under these circumstances is rarely difficult. If seemingly simple infection does not respond to medical therapy or if infection recurs, obstruction or vesicoureteral reflux is the probable cause, and complete study of the urinary tract is indicated.

Complications

Stagnation of urine leads to infection, which then may spread throughout the entire urinary system. Once established, infection is difficult and at times impossible to eradicate even after the obstruction has been relieved.

Often the invading organisms are urea-splitting (*Proteus,* staphylococci), which causes the urine to become alkaline. Calcium salts precipitate and form bladder or kidney stones more easily in alkaline urine.

If both kidneys are affected, the result may be renal insufficiency. Secondary infection increases renal damage.

Pyonephrosis is the end stage of a severely infected and obstructed kidney. The kidney is functionless and filled with thick pus. At times, a plain film of the abdomen may show an air urogram caused by gas liberated by infecting organisms.

Treatment

A. Relief of Obstruction: Treatment of the main causes of obstruction and stasis (benign prostatic hyperplasia, cancer of the prostate, neurogenic bladder, ureteral stone, posterior urethral valves, and ureteral stenosis) is described in detail elsewhere in this book.

1. Lower tract obstruction (distal to the bladder)—With patients in whom secondary renal or ureterovesical damage (reflux in the latter) is minimal or nonexistent, correction of the obstruction is sufficient. If significant reflux is demonstrated and does not subside spontaneously after relief of obstruction, surgical repair may be needed. Repair becomes imperative if there is considerable hydronephrosis in addition to reflux. Preliminary drainage of the bladder by an indwelling catheter or other means of diversion (eg, loop ureterostomy) is indicated in order to preserve and improve renal function. If, after a few months of drainage, reflux persists, the incompetent ureterovesical junction should be surgically repaired.

2. Upper tract obstruction (above the bladder)—If tortuous, kinked, dilated, or atonic ureters have developed secondary to lower tract obstruction (so that they are themselves obstructive), vesical drainage will not protect the kidneys from further damage; the urine proximal to the obstruction must be diverted by nephrostomy or ureterostomy. The kidneys then may regain some function. Over a period of many months, the ureter may become less tortuous and less dilated; its obstructive areas may open up. If radiopaque material instilled into the nephrostomy tube passes readily to the bladder, it may be possible to remove the nephrostomy tube. If obstruction or reflux persists, surgical repair is indicated. Permanent urinary diversion (eg, ureteroileal conduit) may be necessary.

If one kidney has been irreversibly damaged, as measured by kidney function tests, urography, sonography, CT scan, or scintigraphy, nephrectomy may be necessary.

B. Eradication of Infection: Once the obstruction is removed, every effort should be made to eradicate infection. If the infection has been severe and prolonged, antibiotics may fail to sterilize the urinary tract.

Prognosis

No simple statement can be made about the prognosis in this group of patients. The outcome depends upon the cause, site, degree, and duration of the obstruction. The prognosis is also definitely influenced by complicating infection, particularly if it has been present for a long time.

If renal function is fair to good, if the obstruction or other causes of stasis can be corrected, and if complicating infection can then be eradicated, the prognosis is generally excellent.

REFERENCES

Aaronsen IA: Compensated obstruction of the renal pelvis. *Br J Urol* 1980;**52**:79.

Almgård LE, Fernström I: Percutaneous nephropyelostomy. *Acta Radiol [Diagn] (Stockh)* 1974;**15**:288.

Alton DJ, McDonald P: Urinary obstruction in the neonatal infant. *Radiol Clin North Am* 1975;**13**:343.

Amis ES et al: Ultrasonic inaccuracies in diagnosing renal obstruction. *Urology* 1982;**19**:101.

Aron B, Tessler A, Morales P: Angiography in hydronephrosis. *Urology* 1973;**2**:231.

Belis JA et al: Radionuclide determination of individual kidney function in treatment of chronic renal obstruction. *J Urol* 1982;**127**:636.

Belman AB, King LR: Vesicostomy: Useful means of reversible urinary diversion in selected infants. *Urology* 1973;**1**:208.

Berdon WE et al: Hydronephrosis in infants and children: Value of high dosage excretory urography in predicting renal salvageability. *Am J Roentgenol* 1970;**109**:380.

Bergstrom H: The diagnostic value of renography in suspected obstruction of the urinary tract during pregnancy. *Acta Obstet Gynecol Scand* 1975;**54**:65.

Bourne RB: Intermittent hydronephrosis as a cause of abdominal pain. *JAMA* 1966;**198**:1218.

Bratt C-G, Aurell M, Lindstedt G: Proximal tubular function in human hydronephrotic kidneys. *J Urol* 1981;**125**:9.

Bredin HC et al: The surgical correction of congenital ureteropelvic junction obstructions in normally rotated kidneys. *J Urol* 1974;**111**:460.

Bryan PJ, Azimi F: Ultrasound in diagnosis of congenital hydronephrosis due to obstruction of pelviureteric junction. *Urology* 1975;**5**:17.

Caine M, Perlberg S, Shapiro A: Phenoxybenzamine for benign prostatic obstruction: Review of 200 cases. *Urology* 1981;**17**:542.

Cherrie RJ, Kaufman JJ: Pyeloplasty for ureteropelvic junction obstruction in adults: Correlation of radiographic and clinical results. *J Urol* 1982;**129**:711.

Chibber PJ et al: ^{99m}Technetium DMSA and the prediction of recovery in obstructive uropathy. *Br J Urol* 1982;**53**:492.

Cohen B et al: Ureteropelvic junction obstruction: Its occurrence in 3 members of a single family. *J Urol* 1980;**120**:361.

Cremin BJ: Urinary ascites and obstructive uropathy. *Br J Urol* 1975;**48**:113.

DeMaeyer P et al: Clinical study of technetium dimercaptosuccinic acid uptake in obstructed kidneys: Comparison with creatinine clearance. *J Urol* 1982;**128**:8.

Devine CJ Jr, Devine PC: Urethral strictures. (Editorial.) *J Urol* 1980;**123**:506.

Edelmann CM Jr, Spitzer A: The maturing kidney: A modern view of well-balanced infants with imbalanced nephrons. *J Pediatr* 1969;**75**:509.

Emmott RC, Tanagho EA: Ureteral obstruction due to fecal impaction in patient with colonic loop urinary diversion. *Urology* 1980;**15**:496.

Engel RME: Permanent urinary diversion in childhood: Indications and types. *Urology* 1974;**3**:178.

Fanestil DD, Blackard CE: Etiology of postobstructive diuresis: Ouabain-sensitive adenosine triphosphate deficit and elevated solute excretion in the postobstructed dog kidney. *Invest Urol* 1976;**14**:148.

Fourcroy JL, Azoury B, Miller HC: Bilateral ureteral obstruction as a complication of vascular graft surgery. *Urology* 1980;**15**:556.

Fowler JE Jr, Meares EM Jr, Goldin AR: Percutaneous nephrostomy: Techniques, indications, and results. *Urology* 1975; **6**:428.

Fowler R, Jensen F: Percutaneous antegrade pyelography in small infants and neonates. *Br J Radiol* 1975;**48**:987.

Gill WB, Curtis GA: The influence of bladder fullness on upper urinary tract dimensions and renal excretory function. *J Urol* 1977;**117**:573.

Gillenwater JY et al: Renal function after release of chronic unilateral hydronephrosis in man. *Kidney Int* 1975;**7**:179.

Hanna MK, Jeffs RD: Primary obstructive megaureter in children. *Urology* 1975;**6**:419.

Hinman F Jr: Hydronephrosis. Pages 1–15 in: *Practice of Surgery.* Goldsmith HS (editor). Harper & Row, 1980.

Hinman F Jr, Oppenheimer RO, Katz IL: Accelerated obstruction at ureteropelvic junction in adults. *J Urol* 1983;**129**:812.

Hull JC, Kumar S, Pletka PG: Reflex anuria from unilateral ureteral obstruction. *J Urol* 1980;**123**:265.

Hutch JA, Tanagho EA: Etiology of non-occlusive ureteral dilatation. *J Urol* 1965;**93**:177.

Ibrahim A, Asha HA: Prediction of renal recovery in hydronephrotic kidneys. *Br J Urol* 1978;**50**:222.

Johnston JH: The presentation of management of neonatal obstructive uropathies. *Postgrad Med J* 1972;**48**:486.

Johnston JH et al: Pelvic hydronephrosis in children: A review of 219 personal cases. *J Urol* 1977;**117**:97.

Josephson S: Experimental obstructive hydronephrosis in newborn rats. 3. Long-term effect on renal function. *J Urol* 1983;**129**:396.

Kalika V et al: Prediction of renal functional recovery after relief of upper urinary tract obstruction. *J Urol* 1981;**126**:301.

Kelalis PP: Urinary diversion in children by the sigmoid conduit: Its advantages and limitations. *J Urol* 1974;**112**:666.

Kelalis PP et al: Ureteropelvic obstruction in children: Experiences with 109 cases. *J Urol* 1971;**106**:418.

Koff SA, Thrall JH, Keyes JW Jr: Diuretic radionuclide methods for investigating hydroureteronephrosis. *Eur Urol* 1982; **8**:82.

Krohn AG et al: Compensatory renal hypertrophy: The role of immediate vascular changes in its production. *J Urol* 1970; **103**:564.

Leff LO, Smith JP: Achalasia in children and adults. *Urology* 1973;**2**:139.

Lupton EW et al: Diuresis renography and morphology in upper urinary tract obstruction. *Br J Urol* 1979;**51**:10.

Lupton EW et al: Diuresis renography and the results of pyeloplasty for idiopathic hydronephrosis. *Br J Urol* 1979;**51**:449.

Maizels M, Stephens FD: Values of ureter as cause of primary obstruction of ureter: Anatomic, embryologic and clinical aspects. *J Urol* 1980;**123**:742.

Mayor G et al: Renal function in obstructive nephropathy: Long-term effects of reconstructive surgery. *Pediatrics* 1975; **56**:740.

Michaelson G: Percutaneous puncture of the renal pelvis, intrapelvic pressure and the concentrating capacity of the kidney in hydronephrosis. *Acta Med Scand [Suppl]* 1974;**559**:1. [Entire issue.]

Milewski PJ: Radiograph measurements and contralateral renal size in primary pelvic hydronephrosis. *Br J Urol* 1978; **50**:289.

Ossandon F, Androulakakis P, Ransley PG: Surgical problems in pelvioureteral junction obstruction of lower moiety in incomplete duplex systems. *J Urol* 1981;**125**:871.

Perlmutter AD, Kroovand RL, Lai Y-W: Management of ureteropelvic obstruction in first year of life. *J Urol* 1980; **123**:535.

Perlmutter AD, Patil J: Loop cutaneous ureterostomy in infants and young children: Late results in 32 cases. *J Urol* 1972; **107**:655.

Pope TL Jr et al: Nuclear scintigraphy and ultrasound in diagnosis of congenital ureteropelvic junction obstruction. *J Urol* 1980;**124**:917.

Reimer DE, Oswalt GC Jr: Iatrogenic ureteral obstruction treated with balloon dilation. *J Urol* 1981;**126**:689.

Remigailo RV et al: Ileal conduit urinary diversion: Ten-year review. *Urology* 1976;**7**:343.

Rose JS et al: B-mode sonographic evaluation of abdominal masses in the pediatric patient. *Am J Roentgenol* 1974;**120**:691.

Schmidt JD et al: Complications, results and problems of ileal conduit diversions. *J Urol* 1973;**109**:210.

Schulman A, Herlinger H: Urinary tract dilatation in pregnancy. *Br J Radiol* 1975;**48**:638.

Shapiro SR, Bennett AH: Recovery of renal function after prolonged unilateral ureteral obstruction. *J Urol* 1976;**115**:136.

Sharma D: Scrotal flap urethroplasty in the primary management of the "watering-can perineum." *Br J Urol* 1979;**51**:400.

Smart WR: Chapter 55 in: *Urology,* 3rd ed. Campbell MF, Harrison JH (editors). Saunders, 1970.

Stage KH, Lewis S: Use of radionuclide washout test in evaluation of suspected upper urinary tract obstruction. *J Urol* 1981;**125**:379.

Stephens FD: Idiopathic dilatations of the urinary tract. *J Urol* 1974;**112**:819.

Tanagho EA: Congenitally obstructed bladders: Fate after defunctionalization. *J Urol* 1974;**111**:102.

Tanagho EA: The pathogenesis and management of megaureter. Pages 85–116 in *Excerpta Medica in Paediatric Urology.* Johnson JH, Goodwin WF (editors). North Holland, 1974.

Tanagho EA, Meyers FH: Trigonal hypertrophy: A cause of ureteral obstruction. *J Urol* 1965;**93**:678.

Tanagho EA, Smith DR, Guthrie TH: Pathophysiology of functional ureteral obstruction. *J Urol* 1970;**104**:73.

Thompson IA, Bruns TNC: Neonatal ascites: A reflection of obstructive disease. *J Urol* 1972;**107**:509.

Walsh PC et al: Percutaneous antegrade pyelography in hydronephrosis: Preoperative assessment. *Urology* 1973; **1**:537.

Walther PC, Parsons CL, Schmidt JD: Direct vision internal urethrotomy in management of urethral strictures. *J Urol* 1980; **123**:497.

Walzer A, Loenigsberg M: Prenatal evaluation of partial obstruction of the urinary tract. *Radiology* 1980;**135**:93.

Waterhouse K, Laungani G, Patil U: Surgical repair of membranous urethral strictures: Experience with 105 consecutive cases. *J Urol* 1980;**123**:500.

Whitaker RH: Equivocal pelvi-ureteric obstruction. *Br J Urol* 1976;**47**:771.

Whitaker RH, Buxton-Thomas M: A comparison of pressure flow studies and renography in equivocal upper urinary tract obstruction. *J Urol* 1984;**131**:446.

Whitfield HN et al: Frusemide intravenous urography in the diagnosis of pelviureteric junction obstruction. *Br J Urol* 1979; **51**:445.

Whitfield HN et al: Renal transit time measurements in the diagnosis of ureteric obstruction. *Br J Urol* 1982;**53**:504.

Witherow RO, Whitaker RH: The predictive accuracy of antegrade pressure flow studies in equivocal upper tract obstruction. *Br J Urol* 1982;**53**:496.

Wolf FN, Whitaker RH: Late followup of dynamic evaluation of upper urinary tract obstruction. *J Urol* 1982;**128**:346.

Youssef AMR, Cockett ATK, Mee AD: Internal urethrotomy using Sachse knife for managing urethral strictures. *Urology* 1980;**15**:562.

Zincke H, Malek RS: Experience with cutaneous and transureteroureterostomy. *J Urol* 1974;**111**:760.

Vesicoureteral Reflux

12

Emil A. Tanagho, MD

Under normal circumstances, the ureterovesical junction allows urine to enter the bladder but prevents urine from regurgitating into the ureter, particularly at the time of voiding. In this way, the kidney is protected from high pressure in the bladder and from contamination by infected vesical urine. When this valve is incompetent, the chance for development of urinary infection is significantly enhanced, and pyelonephritis is then inevitable. With few exceptions, pyelonephritis—acute, chronic, or healed—is secondary to vesicoureteral reflux.

ANATOMY OF THE URETEROVESICAL JUNCTION

An understanding of the causes of vesicoureteral reflux requires a knowledge of the anatomy of the ureterovesical valve. Anatomic studies performed by Hutch (1972) and by Tanagho and Pugh (1963) (Fig 12–1) are incorporated into the following discussion.

Mesodermal Component

This structure, which arises from the wolffian duct, is made up of 2 parts that are innervated by the sympathetic nervous system:

A. The Ureter and the Superficial Trigone: The smooth musculature of the renal calices, pelvis, and extravesical ureter is composed of helically oriented fibers that allow for peristaltic activity. As these fibers approach the vesical wall, they are reoriented into the longitudinal plane. The ureter passes obliquely through the vesical wall; the intravesical ureteral segment is thus composed of longitudinal muscle fibers only and therefore cannot undergo peristalsis. As these smooth muscle fibers approach the ureteral orifice, those that form the roof of the ureter swing to either side to join those that form its floor. They then spread out and join equivalent muscle bundles from the other ureter and also continue caudally, thus forming the superficial trigone. The trigone passes over the neck of the bladder, ending at the verumontanum in the male and just inside the external urethral orifice in the female. Thus, the ureterotrigonal complex is one structure. Above the ureteral orifice, it is tubular; below that point, it is flat.

B. Waldeyer's Sheath and the Deep Trigone: Beginning at a point about 2–3 cm above the bladder, an external layer of longitudinal smooth muscle surrounds the ureter. This muscular sheath passes through the vesical wall, to which it is connected by a few detrusor fibers. As it enters the vesical lumen, its roof fibers diverge to join its floor fibers, which then spread out, joining muscle bundles from the contralateral ureter and forming the deep trigone, which ends at the bladder neck.

Endodermal Component

The vesical detrusor muscle bundles are intertwined and run in various directions. However, as they converge upon the internal orifice of the bladder, they tend to become oriented into 3 layers:

A. Internal Longitudinal Layer: This layer continues into the urethra submucosally and ends just inside the external meatus in the female and at the caudal end of the prostate in the male.

B. Middle Circular Layer: This layer is thickest anteriorly and stops at the vesical neck.

C. Outer Longitudinal Layer: These muscle bundles take a circular and spiral course about the external surface of the female urethra and are incorporated within the peripheral prostatic tissue in the male. They constitute the true vesicourethral sphincter.

The vesical detrusor muscle is innervated by the parasympathetic nerves (S2–4).

PHYSIOLOGY OF THE URETEROVESICAL JUNCTION

Although many investigators had suspected that normal trigonal tone tended to occlude the intravesical ureter, it remained for Tanagho et al (1965) to prove it. Using nonrefluxing dogs, they demonstrated the following:

(1) Interruption of the continuity of the trigone resulted in reflux. An incision was made in the trigone 3 mm below the ureteral orifice, resulting in an upward and lateral migration of the ureteral orifice with shortening of the intravesical ureter. Reflux was demonstrable. After the incision healed, reflux ceased.

(2) Unilateral lumbar sympathectomy resulted in paralysis of the ipsilateral trigone. This led to lateral and superior migration of the ureteral orifice and reflux.

(3) Electrical stimulation of the trigone caused the ureteral orifice to move caudally, thus lengthening the intravesical ureter. This maneuver caused a marked rise in resistance to flow through the ureterovesical junction. Ureteral efflux of urine ceased. Intravenous

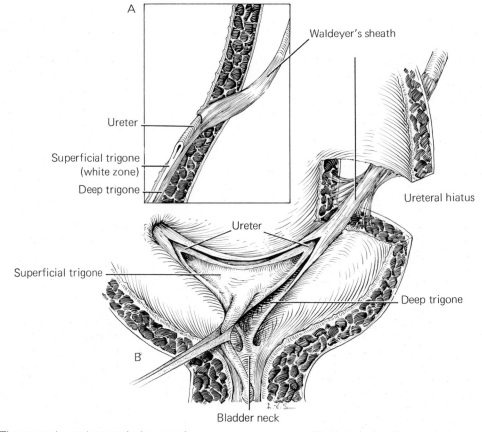

The ureteral muscle extends downward and becomes the superficial trigone.

Waldeyer's sheath extends downward and becomes the deep trigone.

Figure 12–1. Normal ureterotrigonal complex. *A:* Side view of ureterovesical junction. Waldeyer's muscular sheath invests the juxtavesical ureter and continues downward as the deep trigone, which extends to the bladder neck. The ureteral musculature becomes the superficial trigone, which extends to the verumontanum in the male and stops just short of the external meatus in the female. *B:* Waldeyer's sheath is connected by a few fibers to the detrusor muscle in the ureteral hiatus. This muscular sheath, inferior to the ureteral orifices, becomes the deep trigone. The musculature of the ureters continues downward as the superficial trigone. (Redrawn and modified, with permission, from Tanagho EA, Pugh RCB: The anatomy and function of the ureterovesical junction. *Br J Urol* 1963;**35**:151.)

injection of epinephrine caused the same reaction. On the other hand, isoproterenol caused the degree of occlusion to drop below normal. If, however, the trigone was incised, electrical stimulation of the trigone or the administration of epinephrine failed to increase ureteral occlusive pressure.

(4) During gradual filling of the bladder, intravesical pressure increased only slightly, whereas pressure within the intravesical ureter rose progressively—owing, apparently, to increasing trigonal stretch. A few seconds before the expected sharp rise in intravesical pressure generated for voiding, the closure pressure in the intravesical ureter rose sharply and was maintained for 20 seconds after detrusor contraction had ceased. This experiment demonstrated that ureterovesical competence is independent of detrusor action and is governed by the tone of the trigone, which contracts vigorously just before voiding, thus helping to open

and funnel the vesical neck. At the same time, significant pull is placed upon the intravesical ureter, so that it is occluded during the period when intravesical pressure is high. During the voiding phase, there is naturally no efflux of ureteral urine.

One may liken this function to the phenomenon of the Chinese thimble: The harder the finger (trigone) pulls, the tighter the thimble (intravesical ureter) becomes. Conversely, a deficient pull may lead to incomplete closure of the ureterovesical junction.

It was concluded from these experiments that normal ureterotrigonal tone prevents vesicoureteral reflux. Electrical or pharmacologic stimulation of the trigone caused increased occlusive pressure in the intravesical ureter and increased resistance to flow down the ureter, whereas incision or paralysis of the trigone led to reflux. The theory that ureterovesical competence was maintained by intravesical pressure com-

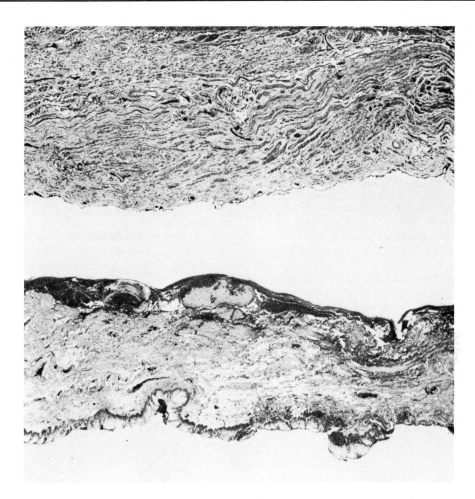

Figure 12–2. Histology of the trigone in primary reflux. *Top:* Normal trigone demonstrating wealth of closely packed smooth muscle fibers. *Bottom:* The congenitally attenuated trigonal muscle that accompanies vesicoureteral reflux. Note absence of inflammatory cells. (Reproduced, with permission, from Tanagho EA et al: Primary vesicoureteral reflux: Experimental studies of its etiology. *J Urol* 1965;**93**:165.)

pressing the intravesical ureter against its backing of detrusor muscle was thereby disproved.

Biopsy of the trigone (and the intravesical ureter) in patients with primary reflux revealed marked deficiency in the development of its smooth muscle (Fig 12–2). Electrical stimulation of such a trigone caused only a minor contraction of the ureterotrigonal complex. This work led to the conclusion that the common cause of reflux, particularly in children, is congenital attenuation of the ureterotrigonal musculature.

VESICOURETERAL REFLUX

CAUSES

The major cause of vesicoureteral reflux is attenuation of the trigone and its contiguous intravesical ureteral musculature. Any condition that shortens the intravesical ureter may also lead to reflux, but this is less common. Familial vesicoureteral reflux has been observed by a number of authors. It appears to be a genetic trait.

Congenital Causes

A. Trigonal Weakness ("Primary Reflux"): This is by far the most common cause of ureteral reflux. It is most often seen in little girls, though it occurs occasionally also in boys. Reflux in adults—usually women—probably represents the same congenital defect. Weakness of one side of the trigone leads to a decrease in the occlusive pressure in the ipsilateral intravesical ureter. Diffuse ureterotrigonal weakness causes bilateral reflux.

It is postulated that ureteral trigonal weakness is related to the development of the ureteral bud on the mesonephric duct. It is known that the ureter acquires its musculature from its cranial end caudally, so that if a segment is muscularly deficient, it is deficient in its most caudad part. It is also postulated that if the ureter is too close to the urogenital sinus on the mesonephric duct, it will join the latter relatively early in embryonic life, before acquiring adequate mesenchymal tissue around itself to be differentiated later into proper trigonal musculature as well as lower ureter. This embryologic hypothesis explains all the known features of refluxing ureters: their muscular weakness, their lateral placement on the bladder base with a very short submucosal segment, and their usual association with weak ureteral musculature and gaping ureteral orifices (which, in severe cases, will assume a golf-hole endoscopic appearance at their junction with the bladder wall). It also explains why, in duplicated systems, if there is only one refluxing unit, it is the upper orifice (which originated closer to the urogenital sinus on the mesonephric duct and thus has the least muscular development).

In the normal state, the intravesical ureterotrigonal muscle tone exerts a downward pull, whereas the extravesical ureter tends to pull cephalad (Fig 12–3). If trigonal development is deficient, not only is its occlusive power diminished but the ureteral orifice tends to migrate upward toward the ureteral hiatus. The degree of this retraction relates to the degree of incompetence

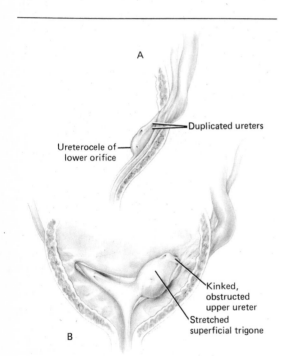

Figure 12–3. *A:* Small ureterocele developing in a duplicated system (where it always involves a lower ureteral orifice). *B:* Expansion of submucosal segment leads to lifting and angulation of ipsilateral lower pole ureteral orifice. Duplicated system ureteroceles are rarely so small. (Diagrammatic representation.) (Reproduced, with permission, from Tanagho EA: Ureteroceles: Embryogenesis, pathogenesis and management. *J Cont Educ Urol* [Feb] 1979;18:13.

of the junction (Fig 12–4). If the ureteral orifice lies over the ureteral hiatus in the bladder wall (so-called golf-hole orifice), it is completely incompetent. The degree of incompetence is judged by the findings on excretory urography and cystography and the cystoscopic appearance of the ureteral orifices.

B. Ureteral Abnormalities:

1. Complete ureteral duplication–(Fig 12–5.) The intravesical portion of the ureter to the upper renal segment is usually of normal length, whereas that of the ureter to the lower pole is abnormally short; this orifice is commonly incompetent. However, Stephens (1964) demonstrated that the musculature of the superiorly placed orifice is attenuated, which further contributes to its weakness.

2. Ectopic ureteral orifice–A single ureter or one of a pair may open well down on the trigone, at the vesical neck, or in the urethra. In this instance, vesicoureteral reflux is the rule. This observation makes it clear that the length of the intravesical ureter is not the sole factor in reflux. Stephens (1964) observed that such intravesical ureteral segments are usually devoid of smooth muscle. Thus, they have no occlusive force.

3. Ureterocele–A ureterocele involving a single ureter rarely allows reflux, but this lesion usually involves the ureter that drains the upper pole of a duplicated kidney. Because the ureteral orifice is obstructed, the intramural ureter becomes dilated. This increases the diameter of the ureteral hiatus, thus further shortening the intravesical segment of the other ureter, which therefore may become incompetent. Resection of the ureterocele usually causes its ureter to reflux freely as well.

Vesical Trabeculation

Occasionally, a heavily trabeculated bladder may be associated with reflux. The causes include spastic neurogenic bladder and severe obstruction distal to the bladder. These lesions, however, are associated with trigonal hypertrophy as well; the resultant extra pull on the ureterotrigonal muscle tends to protect the junction from incompetence. In a few such cases, however, the vesical mucosa may protrude through the ureteral hiatus just above the ureter to form a diverticulum, or saccule (Fig 12–6). The resulting dilatation of the hiatus shortens the intravesical segment; reflux may then occur.

Edema of the Vesical Wall Secondary to Cystitis

As noted above, valves vary in their degrees of incompetence. A "borderline" junction may not allow reflux when the urine is sterile, but valvular function may be impaired when cystitis causes associated edema involving the trigone and intravesical ureter. In addition, the abnormally high voiding pressure may lead to reflux, in which case secondary pyelonephritis may ensue. After cure of the infection, cystography again reveals no reflux. It is believed that a completely normal junction will not decompensate even under these circumstances.

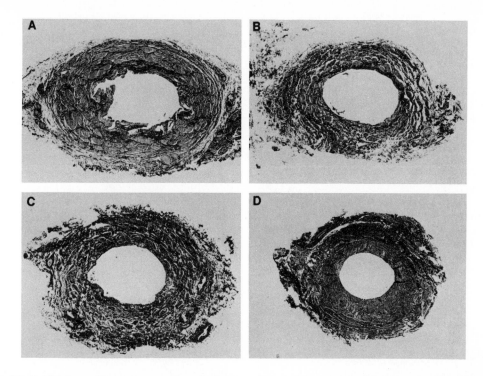

Figure 12–4. Histology of the various grades of submucosal muscular weakness of the ureteral orifice. (See also Fig 12–9.) *A:* Normal. Minimal deficiency. (Cone orifice.) *B:* More marked muscular weakness. (Stadium orifice.) *C:* Marked muscular deficiency. (Horseshoe orifice.) *D:* Extreme muscular deficiency. Only a few muscle fibers can be seen; the rest is collagen tissue.

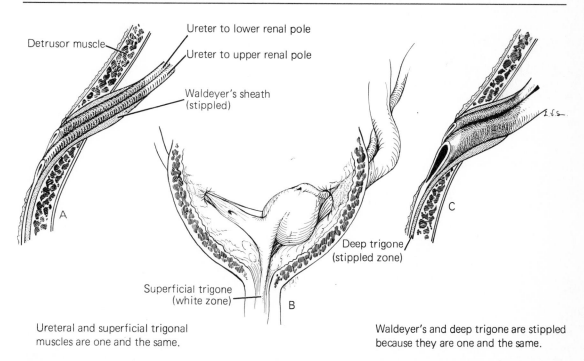

Figure 12–5. Ureteral duplication and ureterocele as causes of vesicoureteral reflux. *A:* Ureteral duplication showing juxtavesical and intravesical ureters encased in common sheath (Waldeyer's). The superior ureter, which always drains the lower renal pole, has a shorter intravesical segment; in addition, it is somewhat devoid of muscle. It therefore tends to allow reflux. *B:* Duplication with ureterocele that always involves caudal ureter, which drains upper renal pole. Pinpoint orifice is obstructive, causing hydroureteronephrosis. Resulting wide dilatation of ureter and ureteral hiatus shortens the intravesical segment of the other ureter, often causing it to reflux. *C:* Resection of ureterocele allows reflux into that ureter.

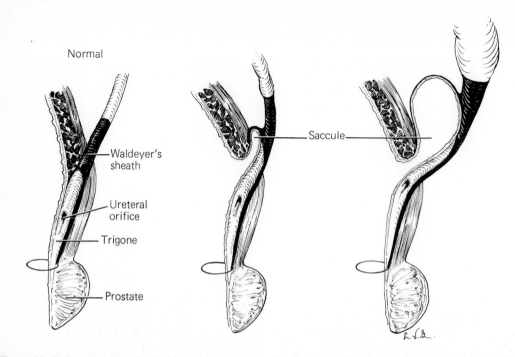

Figure 12–6. Development of ureteral saccule, seen occasionally in cases of primary reflux but more commonly in obstructed or neurogenic bladders with marked trabeculation. Note that the vesical mucosa herniates through the ureteral hiatus, pulling the ureteral orifice upward with it. The orifice may ultimately open in the saccule rather than in the bladder.

It has been shown that pyelonephritis of pregnancy is associated with vesicoureteral reflux. Many patients give a history of urinary tract infections during childhood. The implication is that they "outgrew" reflux at puberty, but if bacteriuria becomes established during pregnancy their "borderline" valves may become incompetent. This condition may be aggravated by the hormones of pregnancy, which may contribute to a further loss of tone of the ureterotrigonal complex. After delivery, reflux is usually no longer demonstrable (Hutch and Amar, 1972).

Eagle-Barrett (Prune Belly) Syndrome

This is a relatively rare condition in which there is failure of normal development of the abdominal muscles and the smooth muscle of the ureters and bladder. Bilateral cryptorchidism is the rule. At times, talipes equinovarus and hip dislocation are also noted. Because the smooth muscle of the ureterotrigonal complex is deficient, reflux is to be expected; advanced hydroureteronephrosis is therefore found.

Iatrogenic Causes

Certain operative procedures may lead to either temporary or permanent ureteral regurgitation.

A. Prostatectomy: With any type of prostatectomy, the continuity of the superficial trigone is interrupted at the vesical neck. If the proximal trigone moves upward, temporary reflux may occur. This mechanism may account for the high fever (and even bacteremia) that is sometimes observed when the

catheter is finally removed. Fortunately, in 2–3 weeks the trigone again becomes anchored and reflux ceases.

Preexisting trigonal hypertrophy (due to prostatic obstruction) helps to compensate for the effect of trigonal interruption; thus, reflux may never occur.

B. Wedge Resection of the Posterior Vesical Neck: This procedure, often ill-advisedly performed in conjunction with plastic revision of the vesical neck for supposed vesical neck stenosis or dysfunction, may also upset trigonal continuity and allow reflux.

C. Ureteral Meatotomy: Extensive ureteral meatotomy may be followed by reflux. Fortunately, however, limited incision of the roof of the intravesical ureter divides few muscle fibers, since they have left the roof to join muscle fibers on the floor. Wide resection for treatment of vesical cancer is often followed by ureteral reflux.

D. Resection of Ureterocele: If the ureteral hiatus is widely dilated, this procedure is often followed by reflux.

Contracted Bladder

A bladder that is contracted secondary to interstitial cystitis, tuberculosis, radiotherapy, carcinoma, or schistosomiasis may be associated with ureteral reflux.

COMPLICATIONS

Vesicoureteral reflux damages the kidney through one or both of 2 mechanisms: (1) pyelonephritis and (2) hydroureteronephrosis.

Pyelonephritis

Vesicoureteral reflux is one of the common contributing factors leading to the development of cystitis, particularly in females. When reflux is present, bacteria reach the kidney and the urinary tract cannot empty itself completely, so that infection is perpetuated. Pyelonephritis is discussed in more detail in Chapter 13.

Hydroureteronephrosis
(See also pp172–175.)

Dilatation of the ureter, renal pelvis, and calices is usually observed in association with reflux (Fig 12–7), sometimes to an extreme degree (Fig 12–8). In males, because they have a relatively long segment

of sterile urethra, such changes are often seen in the absence of infection. Sterile reflux is less damaging than infected reflux.

There are 3 reasons for the dilatation:

(1) Increased work load: The ureter is meant to transport the urine secreted by the kidney to the bladder only once. In the presence of reflux, variable amounts of urine go back and forth, and the work load may be doubled, quadrupled, or increased 10-fold or even more. Eventually, the ureter is not able to transport the increased volume of urine, and stasis and dilatation result.

(2) High hydrostatic pressure: The ureter is protected from the high pressures of the urinary bladder by a competent ureterovesical junction. If there is free

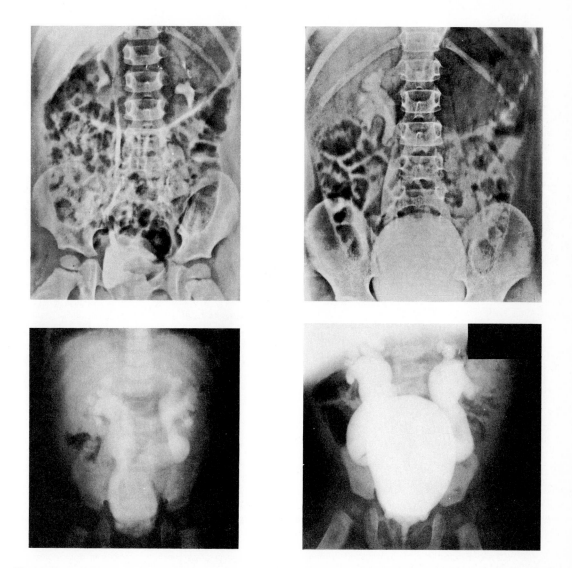

Figure 12–7. Excretory urogram with changes that imply right vesicoureteral reflux. *Upper left:* Excretory urogram showing normal right urogram and a ureter that is mildly dilated and remains full through its entire length. The ureteral change implies reflux. *Upper right:* Cystogram demonstrates the reflux. Note, now, the degree of dilatation of the ureter, pelvis, and calices. *Lower left:* Excretory urogram shows bilateral hydroureteronephrosis with pyelonephritic scarring. These findings imply the presence of reflux. *Lower right:* Voiding cystourethrogram. Free reflux bilaterally.

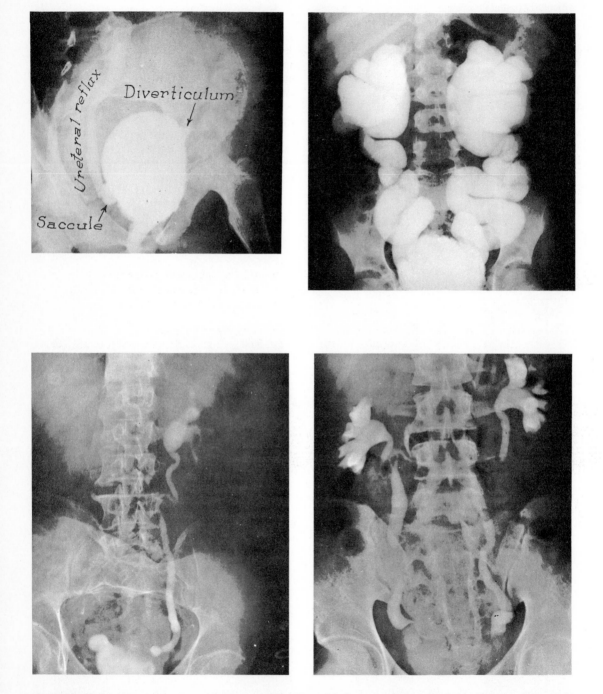

Figure 12–8. Cystograms revealing vesicoureteral reflux. *Upper left:* Saccule at right ureterovesical junction. *Upper right:* Meningomyelocele. Reflux with severe bilateral hydroureteronephrosis; serum creatinine, 0.6 mg/dL; PSP excretion, 5% in 1 hour. *Lower left:* Postprostatectomy patient with reflux on left and bilateral saccules. *Lower right:* Ten-year-old boy with meningomyelocele. Bladder has been emptied. Impairment of drainage at ureterovesical junctions is demonstrated. (Courtesy of JA Hutch.)

reflux, the high intravesical pressure will be directly transmitted to the ureteral and pelvic walls, which results in marked stretching and dilatation.

(3) Weak ureteral musculature: In reflux, the ureteral wall is invariably deficient in musculature to some degree. The more severe the reflux, the more apparent the muscular deficiency. Some cases show more massive dilatation than others. The properly muscularized ureter is better able to resist and compensate for overwork and hydrostatic pressure than the muscularly deficient ureter. The latter tends to undergo further dilatation once it is subjected to any increased intraluminal pressure.

Whether sterile reflux is harmful is the subject of controversy. We feel there is conclusive evidence that severe sterile reflux can lead to parenchymal damage. Pyelointerstitial backflow or pyelotubular backflow under the high pressures of reflux (not infrequently seen during cystographic studies) leads to extravasation of urine in the interstitium of the kidney. The presence of urine in any interstitium will result in a marked inflammatory response with cellular infiltration, resulting finally in fibrosis and scarring. On a long-term basis, this can lead to parenchymal changes indistinguishable from pyelonephritic scarring caused by inflammation due to bacterial infection. This damage may be termed reflux nephropathy. If severe, it will produce parenchymal damage serious enough to lead to end stage kidney disease.

Ransley's studies (1976) indicate that intrarenal reflux is more likely to occur in the presence of flat, concave, or compound papillae, as their collecting ducts tend to open with an increase in intrapelvic pressure and reflux. Papillae prone to reflux are more commonly seen in the polar segments of the kidney. Normal papillae might also permit intrarenal reflux if flattened as a result of the changes due to reflux.

Intravesical pressure is transmitted through the incompetent ureteral orifice. This back pressure is quite high at the time of voiding. Furthermore, the ureteropelvic and ureterovesical junctions are less distensible than the rest of the ureter. Either junction may have trouble passing the normal amount of secreted urine plus the refluxed urine; functional obstruction may result. A common cause of ureteropelvic and ureterovesical "obstruction" is vesicoureteral reflux. Such changes indicate the need for cystography.

INCIDENCE

Incompetence of the ureterovesical junction is an abnormal condition. Peters et al found no reflux in 66 premature infants; Lich et al found none in 26 infants studied during the first 2 days of life; and Leadbetter et al obtained normal cystograms in 50 adult males (see Smith, 1978).

Vesicoureteral reflux occurs in 50% of children with urinary tract infection but in only 8% of adults with bacteriuria. This discrepancy is explained by the fact that girls usually have pyelonephritis, whereas women usually have cystitis only. Bacteriuria does not always imply pyelonephritis.

The fairly competent ("borderline") valve refluxes only during an acute attack of cystitis. Since cystography is performed in such cases only after the infection has been eradicated, the incidence of reflux found on cystography is abnormally low. On the other hand, reflux is demonstrable in 85% of patients whose excretory urograms reveal significant changes typical of healed pyelonephritis.

When infection associated with reflux occurs during the first few weeks of life, many patients are septic and uremic. Most are boys with posterior urethral valves. After age 6 months, the female:male ratio of infection with reflux is 10:1.

CLINICAL FINDINGS

A history compatible with acute pyelonephritis implies the presence of vesicoureteral reflux. This is most commonly seen in females, particularly little girls. Persistence of recurrent "cystitis" should suggest the possibility of reflux. Such patients often have asymptomatic low-grade pyelonephritis.

Symptoms Related to Reflux

A. Symptomatic Pyelonephritis: The usual symptoms in adults are chills and high fever, renal pain, nausea and vomiting, and symptoms of cystitis. In children, only fever and vague abdominal pains and sometimes diarrhea are apt to occur.

B. Asymptomatic Pyelonephritis: The patient may have no symptoms whatsoever. The incidental findings of pyuria and bacteriuria may be the only clues. This points up the need for a proper urinalysis in all children.

C. Symptoms of Cystitis Only: In these cases, bacteriuria is resistant to antimicrobial drugs, or infection quickly recurs following treatment. These patients may have reflux with asymptomatic chronic pyelonephritis.

D. Renal Pain on Voiding: Surprisingly, this is a rare complaint in patients with vesicoureteral reflux.

E. Uremia: The last stage of bilateral reflux is uremia due to destruction of the renal parenchyma by hydronephrosis or pyelonephritis (or both). The patient often adjusts to renal insufficiency and may appear quite healthy. Many renal transplants are performed in patients whose kidneys have deteriorated secondarily to reflux and accompanying infection. Early diagnosis, based upon careful urinalysis, would have led to the proper diagnosis in childhood. Progressive pyelonephritis is, with few exceptions, preventable.

F. Hypertension: In the later stages of atrophic pyelonephritis, a significant incidence of hypertension is observed.

Symptoms Related to the Underlying Disease

The clinical picture is often dominated by the signs and symptoms of the primary disease.

A. Urinary Tract Obstruction: Little girls may have hesitancy in initiating the urinary stream and an impaired or intermittent stream secondary to spasm of the periurethral striated muscle (see Distal Urethral Stenosis in Chapter 31). In males, the urinary stream may be slow as a result of posterior urethral valves (infants) or prostatic enlargement (men over age 50).

B. Spinal Cord Disease: The patient may have a serious neurogenic disease such as paraplegia, quadriplegia, multiple sclerosis, or meningomyelocele. Symptoms may be limited to those of neurogenic bladder: incontinence of urine, urinary retention, and vesical urgency.

Physical Findings

During an attack of acute pyelonephritis, renal tenderness may be noted. Its absence, however, does not rule out chronic renal infection.

Palpation and percussion of the suprapubic area may reveal a distended bladder secondary to obstruction or neurogenic disease.

The finding of a hard midline mass deep in the pelvis in a male infant is apt to represent a markedly thickened bladder caused by posterior urethral valves.

Examination may reveal a neurologic deficit compatible with a paretic bladder.

Laboratory Findings

The most common complication of reflux, particularly in females, is infection. Bacteriuria without pyuria is not uncommon. In males, the urine may be sterile because of the long, sterile urethra.

PSP excretion will be diminished in uremia. The curve, even when renal function is normal, may be "flat" because some of the urine excreted in the first half-hour may be refluxed back up to the kidneys; with gross bilateral reflux, the total PSP excretion may be alarmingly low. The serum creatinine may be elevated in the advanced stage of renal damage, but it may be normal even when the degree of reflux and hydronephrosis is marked (Fig 12–8, upper right); the PSP test is the best screening test in this case.

X-Ray Findings

The plain film may reveal evidence of spina bifida, meningomyelocele, or absence of the sacrum and thus point to a neurologic deficit. Even in vesicoureteral reflux, excretory urograms may be normal, but usually one or more of the following clues to the presence of reflux is noted (Fig 12–7): (1) a persistently dilated lower ureter, (2) areas of dilatation in the ureter, (3) ureter visualized throughout its entire length, (4) presence of hydroureteronephrosis with a narrow juxtavesical ureteral segment, (5) changes of healed pyelonephritis (caliceal clubbing with narrowed infundibula or cortical thinning).

A normal intravenous urogram does not rule out reflux.

The presence of ureteral duplication suggests the possibility of reflux into the lower pole of the kidney. In this case, hydronephrosis or changes compatible with pyelonephritic scarring may be seen. Abnormality of the upper segment of a duplicated system can be caused by the presence of an ectopic ureteral orifice with reflux or by obstruction secondary to a ureterocele.

Reflux is diagnosed by demonstrating its existence with one of the following techniques: simple or delayed cystography, voiding cystourethrography, or voiding cinefluoroscopy. Radionuclide scanning can be used: 1 mCi of ^{99m}Tc is instilled into the bladder along with sterile saline solution, and the gamma camera will reveal ureteral reflux (see Chapter 9).

Reflux can be demonstrated by a technique using indigotindisulfonate sodium (indigo carmine), a blue dye. The bladder is filled with sterile water containing 5 mL of indigo carmine per 100 mL, after which the patient voids and the bladder is thoroughly flushed out with sterile water. The ureteral orifices are then viewed cystoscopically for blue-tinged efflux. This technique has the advantage that no ionizing radiation is used, and its efficiency is equal to that of voiding cystourethrography. In general, reflux demonstrable only with voiding implies a more competent valve than does reflux that occurs at low pressures. As has been pointed out, failure to demonstrate reflux on one study does not rule out intermittent reflux.

The voiding phase of the cystogram may reveal changes compatible with distal urethral stenosis with secondary spasm of the voluntary periurethral muscles in girls (Fig 31–1) or changes diagnostic of posterior urethral valves in young boys.

Instrumental Examination

A. Urethral Calibration: In females, urethral calibration using bougies à boule should be done. Distal urethral stenosis is almost routinely found in little girls suffering from urinary infection. Dilation of the ring of stenosis is an important step in improving the hydrodynamics of voiding: lowering intravesical voiding pressure and eliminating the presence of residual vesical urine (see Chapter 31). Less commonly, urethral stenosis is discovered in women and should be treated.

B. Cystoscopy: Most little girls with reflux have smooth-walled or only slightly trabeculated bladders. Chronic cystitis, ureteral duplication, or ureterocele may be evident. An orifice may be ectopic and be found at the bladder neck or even in the urethra. As the bladder is filled, a small diverticulum may form on the roof of the ureteral orifice (Fig 12–6). These findings imply the possibility of reflux. The major contribution of cystoscopy is to allow study of the morphology of the ureteral orifice and its position in relation to the vesical neck (Fig 12–9).

1. Morphology–The orifice of a normal ureter has the appearance of a volcanic cone. That of a

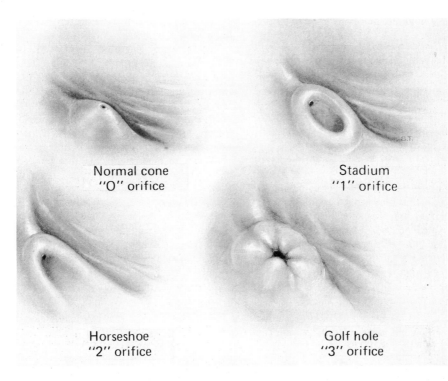

Normal cone
"0" orifice

Stadium
"1" orifice

Horseshoe
"2" orifice

Golf hole
"3" orifice

Figure 12–9. Cystoscopic appearance of the normal ureteral orifice and 3 degrees of incompetence of the ureterovesical junction. (See also Fig 12–4.) (Reproduced, with permission, from Lyon RP, Marshall SK, Tanagho EA: The ureteral orifice: Its configuration and competency. *J Urol* 1969;**102**:504.)

slightly weaker valve looks like a football stadium; an even weaker one has the appearance of a horseshoe with its open end pointing toward the vesical neck. The completely incompetent junction has a "golf-hole" orifice that lies over the ureteral hiatus.

2. Position—By and large, the more defective the appearance of the ureteral orifice, the farther from the vesical neck it lies. The degree of lateralization of the orifice reflects the degree of ureterotrigonal deficiency.

DIFFERENTIAL DIAGNOSIS

Functional (nonocclusive) vesicoureteral obstruction may cause changes similar to those suggesting the presence of reflux on excretory urography. Multiple cystograms fail to show reflux. Tanagho, Smith, and Guthrie (1970) showed that this congenital obstruction is due to an abundance of circularly oriented smooth muscle fibers in the ureteral musculature at this point. Its action is sphincteric.

Significant obstruction distal to the vesical neck leads to hypertrophy of both the detrusor and trigonal muscles. The latter exert an exaggerated pull upon the intravesical ureter and thus cause functional obstruction (Tanagho and Meyers, 1965). Hydroureteronephrosis is therefore to be expected; vesicoureteral reflux is uncommon.

Other lesions that may cause hydroureteronephrosis without reflux include low ureteral stone, occlusion

of the ureter by cervical or prostatic cancer, urinary tract tuberculosis, and schistosomiasis.

TREATMENT

It is impossible to give a concise and definitive discourse on the treatment of vesicoureteral reflux because of the many factors involved and because there is no unanimity of opinion among urologists on this subject. In general, probably more than half of the cases of primary reflux that occur in children can be controlled by nonsurgical means; the rest will require some form of operative procedure. Adults with reflux will usually require vesicoureteroplasty.

Medical Treatment

A. Indications: A child with primary reflux (attenuated trigone) who has fairly normal upper tracts on urographic study and whose ureterovesical valves appear fair to good on cystoscopy has an excellent chance of "outgrowing" the defect, particularly if cystograms show only transient or "high-pressure" reflux.

A boy with posterior urethral valves may cease to reflux once these valves are destroyed.

In a woman who occasionally develops acute pyelonephritis following intercourse but whose urine quickly clears on antimicrobial therapy, reflux will probably be controlled if she takes steps to prevent vesical infections (see treatment of acute cystitis, p 221). This is particularly true if reflux cannot be demonstrated cystographically when her urine is sterile. The maintenance of sterile urine will allow her "borderline" valve to remain competent.

B. Methods of Treatment: Dilation of the ring of distal urethral stenosis in little girls or of posterior urethral valves in boys usually gives excellent results, reducing intravesical voiding pressure and abolishing vesical residual urine and reflux.

Urinary infection should be definitively treated with antimicrobial drugs, after which chronic suppressive therapy should be continued for 6 months or more.

Triple voiding is the least effective method of treating reflux. Since vesicoureteral reflux prevents the urinary tract from emptying itself completely, thus destroying the vesical defense mechanism, triple voiding once a day is helpful if the child is old enough to be trained. When reflux is present, the bladder empties itself on voiding, but some urine ascends to the kidneys and then returns to the bladder. Voiding again a few minutes later will push less urine into the ureters. A third voiding will usually completely empty the urinary tract. This allows the patient's own natural resistance to operate to a maximum degree.

Children with reflux often have thin-walled bladders and do not perceive the normal urge to void when the bladder is full. Further detrusor tone is lost with overfilling, increasing the likelihood of residual urine. Such children should "void by the clock" every 3–4 hours whether they have the urge or not. Vesical residual urine may then be minimized.

Infant girls with markedly dilated upper urinary tracts may be tided over by means of an indwelling urethral catheter. Over a period of months, ureteral dilatation and elongation may regress; renal function is protected. At a convenient and strategic time, more definitive therapy can be accomplished.

C. Evaluation of Success of Medical Treatment: Urinalysis should be done at least once a month for a year or more. Maintenance of sterile urine is an encouraging sign. Cystograms should be repeated every 4–6 months. Excretory urography or nuclear renal scan should be performed at 6 and 12 months to be sure that renal deterioration does not occur.

About half of children with reflux are cured by medical treatment.

Surgical Treatment

A. Indications: Reflux caused by the following abnormalities will not disappear spontaneously: (1) ectopic ureteral orifice, (2) ureteral duplication, (3) ureterocele associated with ureteral duplication and reflux into the uninvolved ureter, (4) "golf-hole" ureteral orifice, and (5) low-pressure reflux with significant hydroureteronephrosis.

Surgery is indicated (1) if it is not possible to keep the urine sterile and reflux persists; (2) if acute pyelonephritis recurs despite a strict medical regimen and chronic suppressive antimicrobial therapy; (3) if increased renal damage is demonstrated by serial ex-

cretory urograms; or (4) if reflux persists for 1 year after institution of therapy.

B. Types of Surgical Treatment: In cases of markedly impaired kidney function and massively dilated ureters, preliminary urinary diversion may be required to improve renal function and to allow dilated ureters to regain tone, after which definitive relief of obstruction (eg, posterior urethral valves) and ureterovesicoplasty can be performed at the optimum time. Some patients with irreversible lesions causing reflux (eg, meningomyelocele) or badly damaged and atonic ureters may require permanent diversion of the urine (ie, ureteroileocutaneous anastomosis).

1. Temporary urinary diversion–If refluxed urine drains freely into the bladder, cystostomy (or an indwelling urethral catheter in girls) may prove helpful. If the ureters are dilated and kinked, a low redundant loop can be brought to the skin. The ureter is opened at this point and urine collected into an ileostomy bag. Later, the loop and the section of ureter distal to it can be resected and the ureter proximal to the loop reimplanted into the bladder. Nephrostomy may be necessary if there is no ureteral redundancy.

2. Permanent urinary diversion–If it is felt that successful ureterovesicoplasty cannot be accomplished, a Bricker type of diversion is indicated. If renal function is poor and the ureters are widely dilated and atonic, ureterocutaneous diversion may be the procedure of choice.

3. Other surgical procedures–

a. If reflux is unilateral, with the affected kidney badly damaged and the other kidney normal, nephrectomy is indicated.

b. If one renal pole of a duplicated system is essentially functionless, heminephrectomy with removal of its entire ureter should be done. If there is moderate hydronephrosis of one renal pole with duplication, an alternative is anastomosis of the dilated ureter or pelvis to the normal ureter or pelvis. The remainder of the dilated refluxing ureter should be removed.

c. In unilateral reflux, anastomosis of the lower end of the refluxing ureter into the side of its normal mate (transureteroureterostomy) has a few proponents.

4. Definitive repair.

Definitive Repair of Ureterovesical Junction (Ureterovesicoplasty)

A. Principles of Repair: (Tanagho, 1970.)

1. Resect the lower 2–3 cm of the ureter whose muscle is underdeveloped.

2. Free up enough extravesical ureter so that an intravesical segment 2.5 cm long can be formed.

3. Place the intravesical ureter in a submucosal position.

4. Suture the wall of the new ureteral orifice to the cut edge of the trigonal muscle.

B. Types of Operation: The following procedures satisfy the above principles and have been successful in a high percentage of cases: suprahiatal repair, increasing the length of intravesical ureter above the level of the ureteral hiatus (Paquin, 1959; Politano and Leadbetter, 1958); infrahiatal repair, the advancement procedures of Hutch (1963) and Glenn and Anderson (1967); combined supra- and infrahiatal repair, which is the most attractive; and transtrigonal repair (Cohen, 1975).

If the ureters are unduly tortuous, the redundant portions must be resected. If widely dilated, the lower ends must be tailored to a more normal size.

C. Results of Ureterovesicoplasty: About 93% of patients no longer show reflux after ureterovesicoplasty. About 3% develop ureterovesical stenosis that requires reoperation. At least 75% have and maintain sterile urine without antimicrobial drugs 3–6 months after surgery. Many patients in whom bacteriuria persists have cystitis only. This has been demonstrated by finding that renal urine specimens collected by ureteral catheters are sterile. Febrile attacks cease. Considering that only the most severe and advanced cases are submitted to surgical repair, these are impressive results, and they exceed by far the cure rates reported when only antimicrobial drugs are used (10–15%). This operation is rightly considered one of the most significant accomplishments of modern urology.

PROGNOSIS

In patients with reflux who are judged to have fairly competent valves, conservative therapy as outlined above is highly successful in the cure of the reflux and therefore infection.

Patients with very incompetent ureterovesical valves subjected to surgical repair also have an excellent prognosis. A few children, however, have such badly damaged urinary tracts when finally submitted to diagnostic procedures that little help other than permanent urinary diversion can be offered.

REFERENCES

Ahmed S, Tan H: Complications of transverse advancement ureteral reimplantation: Diverticulum formation. *J Urol* 1982;**127**:970.

Amar AD: Vesicoureteral reflux in adults: A 12-year study of 122 patients. *Urology* 1974;**3**:184.

Amar AD, Singer B, Chabra K: The practical management of vesicoureteral reflux in children: A review of 12 years' experience with 236 patients. *Clin Pediatr* 1976;**15**:562.

Ambrose SS et al: Observations on small kidney associated with vesicoureteral reflux. *J Urol* 1980;**123**:349.

Angel JR, Smith TW Jr, Roberts JA: Hydrodynamics of pyelorenal renal reflux. *J Urol* 1979;**122**:20.

Arap S, Abrao EG, Menezes de Goes G: Treatment and prevention of complications after extravesical antireflux technique. *Eur Urol* 1981;**7**:263.

Arap S et al: The extra-vesical antireflux plasty: Statistical analysis. *Urol Int* 1971;**26**:241.

Askari A, Belman AB: Vesicoureteral reflux in black girls. *J Urol* 1982;**127**:747.

Atwell JD, Allen NH: The interrelationship between paraureteric diverticula, vesicoureteric reflux and duplication of the pelvicaliceal collecting system: A family study. *Br J Urol* 1980;**52**:269.

Atwell JD, Cox PA: Growth of the kidney following unilateral antireflux surgery. *Eur Urol* 1981;**7**:257.

Badcock JR, Keats GK, King LR: Renal changes after uncomplicated antireflux operation. *J Urol* 1976;**115**:720.

Bakshandeh K, Lynne C, Carrion H: Vesicoureteral reflux and end stage renal disease. *J Urol* 1976;**116**:557.

Bauer SB, Colodny AH, Retik AB: The management of vesicoureteral reflux in children with myelodysplasia. *J Urol* 1982;**128**:102.

Bourne HH et al: Intrarenal reflux and renal damage. *J Urol* 1976;**115**:304.

Burkholder GV, Harper RC, Beach PD: Congenital absence of the abdominal muscles. *Am J Clin Pathol* 1970;**53**:602.

Carter TC, Tomskey GC, Ozog LS: Prune-belly syndrome: Review of 10 cases. *Urology* 1974;**3**:279.

Cattolica EV: Renal scarring and primary reflux in adults. *Urology* 1974;**4**:397.

Chisholm GD et al: DMSA scan and the prediction of recovery in obstructive uropathy. *Eur Urol* 1982;**8**:227.

Cohen SJ: Ureterozystoneostomie: Eine neue antireflux Technik. [Ureterocystoneostomy: A new technique for reflux prevention.] *Aktuelle Urologie* 1975;**6**:1.

Coleman JW, McGovern JH: Ureterovesical reimplantation in children: Surgical results in 491 children. *Urology* 1978;**12**:514.

DeKlerk DP, Reiner WG, Jeffs RD: Vesicoureteral reflux and ureteropelvic junction obstruction: Late occurrence of ureteropelvic obstruction after successful ureteroneocystostomy. *J Urol* 1979;**121**:816.

Devine PC et al: Vesicoureteral reflux in children: Indications for surgical and nonsurgical treatment. *Urology* 1974;**3**:315.

Duckett JW, Bellinger MF: A plea for standardized grading of vesicoureteral reflux. *Eur Urol* 1982;**8**:74.

Duckett JW Jr: Ureterovesical junction and acquired vesicoureteral reflux. *J Urol* 1982;**127**:249.

Elo J et al: Character of urinary tract infections and pyelonephritic renal scarring after antireflux surgery. *J Urol* 1982;**129**:343.

Fair WR et al: Urinary tract infections in children. 1. Young girls with non-refluxing ureters. *West J Med* 1974;**121**:366.

Garrett RA, Schlueter DP: Complications of antireflux operations: Causes and management. *J Urol* 1973;**109**:1002.

Geist RW, Antolak SJ Jr: The clinical problems of children with sterile ureteral reflux. *J Urol* 1972;**108**:343.

Glenn JF, Anderson EE: Distal tunnel ureteral reimplantation. *J Urol* 1967;**97**:623.

Gonzales ET, Leitner WA, Glenn JF: An analysis of various modes of therapy for vesicoureteral reflux. *Int Urol Nephrol* 1972;**4**:235.

Hawtry CE et al: Ureterovesical reflux in an adolescent and adult population. *J Urol* 1983;**130**:1067.

Hendren WH: Complications of megaureter repair in children. *J Urol* 1975;**113**:228.

Hendren WH: Reoperation for the failed ureteral reimplantation. *J Urol* 1974;**111**:403.

Hodson CJ: The radiological contribution toward the diagnosis of chronic pyelonephritis. *Radiology* 1967;**88**:857.

Huland H et al: Vesicoureteral reflux in end stage renal disease. *J Urol* 1979;**121**:10.

Hutch JA: The mesodermal component: Its embryology, anatomy, physiology and role in prevention of vesicoureteral reflux. *J Urol* 1972;**108**:406.

Hutch JA: Ureteric advancement operation: Anatomy, technique, and early results. *J Urol* 1963;**89**:180.

Hutch JA, Amar AD: *Vesicoureteral Reflux and Pyelonephritis.* Appleton-Century-Crofts, 1972.

Johnston JH: Vesicoureteric reflux with urethral valves. *Br J Urol* 1979;**51**:100.

Johnston JH, Farkas A: The congenital refluxing megaureter: Experiences with surgical reconstruction. *Br J Urol* 1976;**48**:153.

Kiesavan P, Fowler R: Vesicoureteric reflux and ureterovesical obstruction. *Urology* 1977;**10**:105.

Koff SA, Murtagh DS: The uninhibited bladder in children: Effect of treatment of recurrence of urinary infection and on vesicoureteral reflux resolution. *J Urol* 1983;**130**:1138.

Kogan SJ, Freed SZ: Postoperative course of vesicoureteral reflux associated with benign obstructive prostatic disease. *J Urol* 1974;**112**:322.

Leadbetter GW Jr: Skin ureterostomy with subsequent ureteral reconstruction. *J Urol* 1972;**107**;462.

Lenaghan D et al: The natural history of reflux and long-term effects of reflux on the kidney. *J Urol* 1976;**115**:728.

Lewy PR, Belman AB: Familial occurrence of nonobstructive, noninfectious vesicoureteral reflux with renal scarring. *J Pediatr* 1975;**86**:851.

Lue TF et al: Vesicoureteral reflux and staghorn calculi. *J Urol* 1982;**127**:247.

Lyon RP: Renal arrest, *J Urol* 1973;**109**:707.

Lyon RP: Treatment of vesicoureteral reflux: Point system based on 20 years of experience. *Urology* 1980;**16**:38.

Lyon RP, Marshall SK, Scott MP: Treatment of vesicoureteral reflux: Point system based on 20 years of experience. *Trans Am Assoc Genitourin Surg* 1979;**71**:146.

Lyon RP, Marshall SK, Tanagho EA: The ureteral orifice: Its configuration and competency. *J Urol* 1969;**102**:504.

MacGregor M: Pyelonephritis lenta: Consideration of childhood urinary infection as the forerunner of renal insufficiency in later life. *Arch Dis Child* 1970;**45**:159.

Majd M, Belman AB: Nuclear cystography in infants and children. *Urol Clin North Am* 1979;**6**:395.

Malek RS et al: Vesicoureteral reflux in the adult. 3. Surgical correction: Risks and benefits. *J Urol* 1983;**130**:882.

Marshall S et al: Ureterovesicoplasty: Selection of patients, incidence and avoidance of complications: A review of 3527 cases. *J Urol* 1977;**118**:829.

Middleton AW Jr, Nixon GW: Lack of correlation between upper tract changes on excretory urography and significant vesicoureteral reflux. *J Urol* 1980;**123**:227.

Miller HC, Caspari EW: Ureteral reflux as genetic trait. *JAMA* 1972;**220**:842.

Mulcahy JJ, Kelalis PP: Non-operative treatment of vesicoureteral reflux. *J Urol* 1978;**120**:336.

Mundy AR et al: Improvement in renal function following ureteric reimplantation for vesicoureteric reflux. *Br J Urol* 1982;**53**:542.

Nasrallah PF et al: Quantitative nuclear cystogram: Aid in determining spontaneous resolution of vesicoureteral reflux. *Urology* 1978;**12**:654.

Orikasa S et al: Effect of vesicoureteral reflux on renal growth. *J Urol* 1978;**119**:25.

Paquin AJ Jr: Ureterovesical anastomosis: The description and evaluation of a technique. *J Urol* 1959;**82**:573.

Parrott TS, Woodard JR: Reflux in opposite ureter after successful correction of unilateral vesicoureteral reflux. *Urology* 1976;**7**:276.

Politano VA, Leadbetter WF: An operative technique for correction of vesicoureteral reflux. *J Urol* 1958;**79**:932.

Rabinowitz R et al: Primary massive reflux in children. *Urology* 1979;**13**:248.

Rabinowitz R et al: Surgical treatment of the massively dilated ureter in children. 1. Management by cutaneous ureterostomy. *J Urol* 1977;**117**:658.

Randel DE: Surgical judgment in the management of vesicoureteral reflux. *J Urol* 1978;**119**:113.

Ransley PG: The renal papilla and intrarenal reflux. In: *Scientific Foundations of Urology.* Williams PI, Chisholm GD (editors). Year Book, 1976.

Ransley PG: Vesicoureteral reflux: Continuous surgical dilemma. *Urology* 1978;**12**:246.

Roberts JA: Experimental pyelonephritis in the monkey. 4. Vesicoureteral reflux and bacteria. *Invest Urol* 1976;**14**:198.

Rolleston GL, Maling TMJ, Hodson CJ: Intrarenal reflux and the scarred kidney. *Arch Dis Child* 1974;**49**:531.

Rose JS, Glassberg KI, Waterhouse K: Intrarenal reflux and its relationship to renal scarring. *J Urol* 1975;**113**:400.

Sala NL, Rubi RA: Ureteral function in pregnant women. 5. Incidence of vesicoureteral reflux and its effect upon ureteral contractility. *Am J Obstet Gynecol* 1972;**112**:871.

Salvatierra O Jr, Kountz SL, Belzer FO: Primary vesicoureteral reflux and end-stage renal disease. *JAMA* 1973;**226**:1454.

Salvatierra O Jr, Tanagho EA: Reflux as a cause of end stage kidney disease: Report of 32 cases. *J Urol* 1977;**117**:441.

Savage DCL et al: Covert bacteriuria of childhood: A clinical and epidemiological study. *Arch Dis Child* 1973;**43**:8.

Servadio C, Nissenkorn I, Baron J: Radioisotope cystography using ^{99m}Tc sulfur colloid for the detection and study of vesicoureteral reflux. *J Urol* 1974;**111**:750.

Siegel SR, Sokoloff B, Siegel B: Asymptomatic and symptomatic urinary tract infection in infancy. *Am J Dis Child* 1973;**125**:45.

Smith DR: Vesicoureteral reflux and other abnormalities of the ureterovesical junction. Chapter 10 in: *Urology,* 4th ed. Campbell MF, Harrison JH (editors). Saunders, 1978.

Stephens FD: Intramural ureter and ureterocele. *Postgrad Med J* 1964;**40**:179.

Stephens FD: Treatment of megaloureters by multiple micturition. *Aust NZ J Surg* 1957;**27**:130.

Stickler GB et al: Primary interstitial nephritis with reflux: A cause of hypertension. *Am J Dis Child* 1971;**122**:144.

Tanagho EA: The pathogenesis and management of megaureter. Pages 85–116 in: *Reviews in Paediatric Urology.* Johnston JH, Goodwin WE (editors). North-Holland, 1974.

Tanagho EA: Surgical revision of the incompetent ureterovesical junction: A critical analysis of techniques and requirements. *Br J Urol* 1970;**42**:410.

Tanagho EA: Ureteral tailoring. *J Urol* 1971;**106**:194.

Tanagho EA, Guthrie TH, Lyon RP: The intravesical ureter in primary reflux. *J Urol* 1969;**101**:824.

Tanagho EA, Jonas U: Reduced bladder capacity: Cause of ureterovesical reflux. *Urology* 1974;**4**:421.

Tanagho EA, Meyers FH: Trigonal hypertrophy: A cause of ureteral obstruction. *J Urol* 1965;**93**:678.

Tanagho EA, Pugh RCB: The anatomy and function of the ureterovesical junction. *Br J Urol* 1963;**35**:151.

Tanagho EA, Smith DR, Guthrie TH: Pathophysiology of function ureteral obstruction. *J Urol* 1970;**104**:73.

Tanagho EA et al: Primary vesicoureteral reflux: Experimental studies of its etiology. *J Urol* 1965;**93:**165.

Udall DA et al: Transureteroureterostomy. *Urology* 1973;**2:**401.

Uehling DT, Wear JB Jr: Concentrating ability after antireflux operation. *J Urol* 1976;**116:**1.

Vesicoureteral reflux and its familial distribution. (Editorial.) *Br Med J* 1975;**4:**726.

Wacksman J, Anderson EE, Glenn JF: Management of vesicoureteral reflux. *J Urol* 1978;**119:**814.

Walker RD III et al: Renal growth and scarring in kidneys with reflux and concentrating defect. *J Urol* 1983;**129:**784.

Warren MM, Kelalis PP, Stickler GB: Unilateral ureteroneocystostomy: The fate of the contralateral ureter. *J Urol* 1972;**107:**466.

Weiss RM, Biancani P: Characteristics of normal and refluxing ureterovesical junctions. *J Urol* 1983;**129:**858.

Welch KJ, Kearney GP: Abdominal muscular deficiency syndrome: Prune belly. *J Urol* 1974;**111:**693.

Whitaker RH: Reflux induced pelvi-ureteric obstruction. *Br J Urol* 1976;**48:**555.

Whitaker RH, Flower CDR: Ureters that show both reflux and obstruction. *Br J Urol* 1979;**51:**471.

Williams DI: The natural history of reflux. *Urol Int* 1971;**26:**350.

Williams GL: et al: Vesicoureteric reflux in patients with bacteriuria in pregnancy. *Lancet* 1968;**2:**1202.

Willscher MK et al: Infection of the urinary tract after antireflux surgery. *J Pediatr* 1967;**89:**743.

Woodard JR: Vesicoureteral reflux. *J Urol* 1981;**125:**79.

Zel G, Retik AB: Familial vesicoureteral reflux. *Urology* 1973;**2:**249.

13

Nonspecific Infections of the Genitourinary Tract

Edwin M. Meares, Jr., MD

The "nonspecific" infections of the genitourinary tract are a group of diseases with similar manifestations that are caused mainly by aerobic gram-negative rods (eg, *Escherichia coli, Proteus mirabilis*) and gram-positive cocci (eg, staphylococci, enterococci) and to a lesser extent by obligate anaerobic bacteria (eg, *Bacteroides fragilis,* peptostreptococci). In addition, "nonspecific" infections of the urethra frequently are caused by organisms that require special techniques of identification (eg, *Chlamydia trachomatis, Ureaplasma urealyticum, Gardnerella vaginalis*). These "nonspecific" infections are distinguished from infections caused by "specific" organisms, each of which causes a clinically unique disease (eg, tuberculosis, gonorrhea, actinomycosis).

In acute infections, a single infective pathogen usually is found; 2 or more pathogens often are seen in chronic infections, particularly those in patients with neuropathic bladders, vesicoenteric fistulas, or long-term urinary catheters. Various urinary pathogens are listed in Table 13–1.

Most uncomplicated urinary tract infections acquired outside the hospital environment (nonnosocomial) are caused by coliform bacteria, chiefly *E coli*. These pathogens tend to be susceptible to a variety of oral antimicrobial agents and respond quickly to short-term therapy. Hospital-acquired (nosocomial) infections often involve more resistant pathogens (eg, *Pseudomonas aeruginosa, Serratia marcescens*) and may require parenteral antimicrobial agents. Infections caused by urease-producing (urea-splitting) organisms (eg, *P mirabilis*) are associated with markedly alkaline urine and a tendency for phosphates to precipitate from the urine to form magnesium ammonium phosphate (struvite) and calcium phosphate (apatite) urinary stones.

These infections can involve any of the genital or urinary organs and eventually can spread from one site to any or all of the others (Fig 13–1). Renal infections are of the greatest importance because of the parenchymal destruction they cause. Since many noninfectious genitourinary conditions mimic the signs and symptoms of infectious genitourinary diseases, identification of the infectious agent by appropriate culture methods is important in diagnosis and management. Furthermore, antimicrobial sensitivity testing is often of paramount importance in clinical management.

Definitions of Common Infectious Syndromes

A. Acute Urethral Syndrome: (Women.) Dysuria and frequency with variable other bladder or urethral symptoms; characterized by "no growth" or low counts of bacteria on urine cultures. At times accompanied by vaginitis. May be caused by bacteria or *C trachomatis*.

B. Acute Urethritis: (Men.) Dysuria accompanied by urethral discharge without concomitant infection of the bladder. Most often represents a sexually transmitted disease caused by *Neisseria gonorrhoeae* (yellow discharge) or by nongonococcal agents, eg, *C trachomatis* or *U urealyticum* (white discharge).

C. Acute Cystitis: Painful urination with frequency, urgency, and a variable incidence of hematuria, suprapubic and low back discomfort, and malodorous urine. Fever is low-grade or absent. Pyuria and bacteriuria (generally $\geq$ 100,000 colonies/mL) are characteristic.

D. Acute Pyelonephritis: Chills and fever (often high), flank pain, and irritative voiding dysfunction. Usually unilateral; often accompanied by bac-

Table 13–1. Microorganisms commonly causing genitourinary tract infections.

Gram-positive cocci	Gram-negative rods	Other pathogens
Staphylococcus aureus	*Escherichia coli*	Chlamydiae (*Chlamydia trachomatis*)
Staphylococcus epidermidis	*Enterobacter* sp	Fungi *(Candida* sp)
Staphylococcus saprophyticus	*Gardnerella vaginalis (Haemophilus*	Mycoplasmas *(Ureaplasma urealyticum)*
Streptococcus, group D	*vaginalis)*	Obligate anaerobic bacteria
Streptococcus fecalis (enterococci)	*Klebsiella* sp	*Trichomonas vaginalis*
Streptococcus bovis	*Proteus mirabilis*	Viruses
Streptococcus, group B	*Proteus* sp (indole-positive)	
Gram-negative cocci	*Pseudomonas aeruginosa*	
Neisseria gonorrhoeae (non-β-	*Serratia* sp	
lactamase-producing)		
Neisseria gonorrhoeae (β-lactamase-		
producing)		

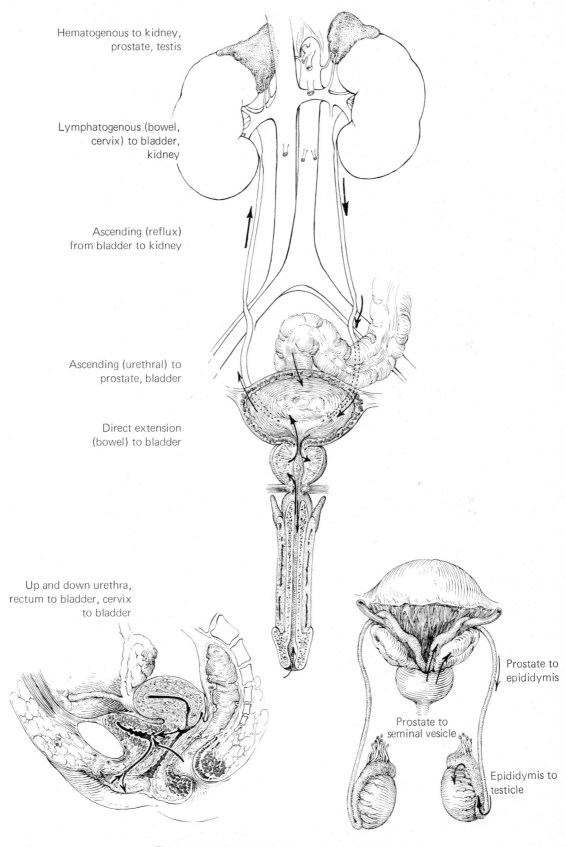

Hematogenous to kidney, prostate, testis

Lymphatogenous (bowel, cervix) to bladder, kidney

Ascending (reflux) from bladder to kidney

Ascending (urethral) to prostate, bladder

Direct extension (bowel) to bladder

Up and down urethra, rectum to bladder, cervix to bladder

Prostate to epididymis

Prostate to seminal vesicle

Epididymis to testicle

Figure 13–1. Routes of infection in the genitourinary tract.

teremia. Characterized by bacteriuria (generally ≥ 100,000 colonies/mL) and pyuria, often with white blood cell casts and glitter cells.

E. Acute Prostatitis: Chills and fever accompanied by severe irritative and variable degrees of obstructive voiding dysfunction; characterized by a tender, swollen, and indurated prostate. Purulent prostatic secretions, usually caused by infection with coliform bacilli. Often accompanied by bacteriuria; sometimes associated with bacteremia.

F. Acute Pelvic Inflammatory Disease: (Women.) Ascending infection from the vagina and endocervix to the intrapelvic genital organs (uterus, uterine tubes, ovaries); characterized by chills and fever, pelvic pain, and variable vaginal discharge; often confused with acute urinary tract infection. Mainly caused by *N gonorrhoeae* or nongonococcal infection (aerobic or anaerobic bacteria, *C trachomatis*).

G. Acute Epididymitis: Painful swelling of one or both epididymides with fever and a variable incidence of dysuria and pyuria. In young men, usually associated with sexually transmitted urethritis (*N gonorrhoeae* or *C trachomatis*); in older men, most often associated with prostatitis (infections with coliform bacilli).

H. Asymptomatic Bacteriuria: Significant bacteriuria (usually ≥ 100,000 colonies/mL) in bladder or renal urine, with or without pyuria, in a patient with no symptoms of urinary tract infection. Must be distinguished from contamination by urethral or vaginal organisms due to poor techniques of specimen collection.

I. Chronic Urinary Tract Infection: This confusing and imprecise term is best avoided; it implies persistent or recurrent urinary tract infection.

J. Chronic Prostatitis: An imprecise term that encompasses a variety of syndromes of variable cause and clinical sequelae: chronic bacterial prostatitis, chronic nonbacterial prostatitis, and prostatodynia.

K. Chronic Pyelonephritis: A confusing term, its exact meaning depending upon its usage. Primarily a radiologic diagnosis based upon urographic evidence of characteristic renal scarring and caliceal deformity. In patients with persistent renal bacterial infection, it may be associated with recurrent renal symptoms, bacteriuria, and pyuria; however, many patients with radiologic evidence of chronic pyelonephritis have negative urine cultures and no evidence of active infection.

L. Reinfecting Recurrent Urinary Tract Infection: New organisms ascend the urethra from outside the urinary tract and cause new urinary tract infections at variable intervals after a previous infection has been eradicated.

M. Relapsing Recurrent Urinary Tract Infection: An organism persists within the urinary tract during therapy and emerges in urine cultures after completion of therapy.

New Observations Concerning Urinary Tract Infections

During the past few years, research has clarified certain aspects of genitourinary tract infections and changed some of the traditional concepts about urinary tract infections.

(1) Urinary tract infection is the most common bacterial infection of humans of all ages.

(2) The incidence and sequelae of urinary tract infections and the considerations necessary in their diagnosis and treatment vary by sex and age (Table 13–2).

(3) Nearly 20% of women with sterile urine (obtained by suprapubic needle aspiration of the bladder) will produce a clean-voided midstream urine specimen that upon culture shows < 10,000 bacterial colonies/mL (Stamey, 1980).

(4) A recent study (Stamm et al, 1982) found that the bladder urine of acutely symptomatic women contained significantly fewer coliform bacteria than the traditional diagnostic criterion of ≥ 100,000 bacteria/mL of midstream urine. Indeed, these investigators found that only 51% of women with symptomatic urinary tract infections with coliform bacteria were identified by using the diagnostic criterion of ≥ 100,000 bacteria/mL.

(5) The presence of pyuria correlates poorly with the definitive diagnosis of urinary tract infection; pyuria may be present in the absence of urinary tract infection, and vice versa.

(6) The history and physical examination alone cannot reliably differentiate either renal infection from lower urinary tract infection or (in women) bladder infection from urethral syndrome.

(7) Deep tissue infection of the kidney and prostate and superficial infection of the bladder require different clinical management.

(8) Clinical differentiation between upper tract infection and lower tract infection by noninvasive tests is generally unreliable (Table 13–3).

(9) Conventional 7- to 14-day therapy is not ideal for most forms of urinary tract infection; deep tissue infection requires more intensive therapy and superficial mucosal infection less intensive therapy.

Table 13–2. Prevalence of urinary tract infections according to age and sex.

Age Group	Prevalence (1%)	Approximate Sex Ratio (Male : Female)
Neonatal	1	1.5:1
Preschool age	2–3	1:10
School age	1–2	1:30
Reproductive age	2.5	1:50
Elderly (65–70 years) living at home	20	1:10
Elderly (> 80 years) living at home	30	1:2
Elderly living in hospitals or chronic care facilities	30	1:1

Table 13–3. Studies to identify site of urinary tract infection (upper tract versus lower tract).

Invasive but accurate
Percutaneous aspiration of renal pelvis
Cystoscopy with ureteral catheterization
Bladder washout test of Fairley
Noninvasive but often inaccurate
Serum antibody studies
  Hemagglutination tests
  Direct bacterial agglutination tests
Urinary antibody (antibody-coated bacteria test)
Test for autoantibodies to Tamm-Horsfall protein
Level of C-reactive protein
Urinary level of lactate dehydrogenase
Urinary level of β_2-microglobulin
Maximal urinary concentrating ability

(10) For acute, uncomplicated urinary tract infections in women, single-dose therapy with various antimicrobial agents has proved as efficacious as traditional 10-day therapy and has fewer adverse reactions (see Antimicrobial Treatment of Urinary Tract Infections, p 233).

New Classification of Urinary Tract Infections

The use of terms such as "chronic" infection and "relapsing" infection has led to confusion. For this reason, Stamey (1980) has suggested a new classification that is gaining in popularity. This classification is especially useful in tracing the natural history of urinary tract infection for individual patients; it also enhances individual clinical management.

A. First Infection: For any individual, the first documented urinary tract infection. From a therapeutic standpoint, all infections thereafter fall within one of the other categories of this classification. First infections in young women tend to be uncomplicated; less than a third will recur in the ensuing 18 months.

B. Unresolved Bacteriuria: Those cases of urinary tract infection in which the urinary tract is not actually sterilized during therapy. Cultures obtained during therapy or immediately after therapy show that the infecting pathogen was not totally eliminated (even if the counts were reduced) by therapy. The main causes of unresolved bacteriuria are the following:

1. Bacterial resistance to the drug selected for treatment.
2. Patient noncompliance in taking medication.
3. Rapid development of resistance by initially sensitive bacteria.
4. Mixed infections with bacterial strains having different antimicrobial susceptibilities.
5. Rapid reinfection with a new, resistant species during initial therapy for the original (sensitive) organism.
6. Renal insufficiency (azotemia).
7. Giant staghorn calculi that are heavily infected.

C. Bacterial Persistence: Those cases of urinary tract infection in which the urine cultures become sterile during therapy but a persistent source of infection in contact with the urine and urinary tract is not sterilized, with resultant reinfection of the urine by the same organisms. Some causes of bacterial persistence are as follows:

1. Infected urinary calculi.
2. Chronic bacterial prostatitis.
3. Unilateral, atrophic infected kidney.
4. Vesicovaginal and vesicointestinal fistulas.
5. Obstructive nephropathy.
6. Infected pyelocaliceal diverticula.
7. Infected ureteral stumps following nephrectomy for pyelonephritis or pyonephrosis.
8. Infected necrotic papillae from papillary necrosis.
9. Infected urachal cysts.
10. Infected medullary sponge kidneys.
11. Urethral diverticula.
12. Foreign bodies.

D. Reinfections: Those cases of urinary tract infection in which a *new* infection occurs (generally by ascending the urethra from outside the urinary tract) with *new* pathogens at variable intervals after a previous infection has been eradicated. It is likely that at least 80% of all recurrent urinary tract infections are reinfections, probably secondary to altered host defenses. A better understanding of the biologic susceptibility to infection and reinfection is necessary for improved clinical management and prevention of urinary tract infections.

Pathogenesis of Urinary Tract Infection

The mode of entry of bacteria into the genitourinary tract cannot always be traced with certainty. There are 4 major pathways.

A. Ascending Infection: Ascending infection from the urethra clearly is the most common cause of genitourinary tract infections in men and urinary tract infections in girls and women. Because the female urethra is short and there is a tendency for rectal bacteria to colonize the perineum and vaginal vestibule, girls and women are especially susceptible to ascending urinary tract infection. Studies performed in nuns show a remarkably low incidence of urinary tract infection compared with that in age-matched sexually active women, which suggests that sexual intercourse and childbearing enhance the susceptibility of women to urinary tract infection (Kunin and McCormack, 1968).

B. Hematogenous Spread: Infection of the genitourinary tract by hematogenous spread is uncommon, notable exceptions being tuberculosis, renal abscesses, and perinephric abscesses. Conversely, bacteria often enter the bloodstream in the course of acute infections of the kidney and prostate. Bacteremia is more likely to complicate urinary tract infection when structural and functional abnormalities exist (eg, obstructive uropathy) than when the urinary tract is normal.

C. Lymphatogenous Spread: Infection of the genitourinary tract by means of lymphatic channels probably occurs, but this is rare. There is speculation but little proof that bacterial pathogens travel through the rectal and colonic lymphatics to the prostate and bladder and through the periuterine lymphatics to the female genitourinary tract.

D. Direct Extension From Another Organ: Intraperitoneal abscesses, especially those associated with inflammatory bowel disease, fulminant pelvic inflammatory disease in women, paravesical abscesses, and genitourinary tract fistulas (especially vesicovaginal and vesicointestinal fistulas), can infect the urinary tract by means of direct extension.

Susceptibility Factors & Defense Mechanisms in Urinary Tract Infections

Schaeffer (1983) reviewed the susceptibility factors and defense mechanisms known to influence the occurrence of urinary tract infection. Although it is known that the bacteria responsible for urinary tract infections reside primarily in the fecal flora, the factors that allow these bacteria to invade the genitourinary tract and produce infectious syndromes remain somewhat uncertain. Compelling evidence suggests, in female patients, that pathogenic bacteria from the rectum initially colonize the vaginal mucosa and spread by way of the urethra to enter the bladder. Sexual intercourse, urethral manipulation, and childbearing have been implicated as factors that enhance this ascent. Susceptibility factors and defense mechanisms may be considered in terms of those *extrinsic* to the bladder (those involving the urethra and vaginal introitus in females and the prostate and urethra in males) and those *intrinsic* to (ie, within) the bladder.

A. Bacterial Virulence Factors: Most urinary tract infections are caused by *E coli;* indeed, this organism accounts for about 90% of first occurrences of urinary tract infections among outpatients. Although more than 150 strains of *E coli* are recognized, most such infections are caused by serogroups O1, O2, O4, O6, O18, and O75. It is not known whether a given strain causes urinary tract infection because it is the predominant organism in the host's fecal flora or because it has special propensity to cause urinary tract infection.

Shortliffe and Stamey (1986) recently reviewed pertinent information about bacterial adherence as a virulence factor in the pathogenesis of urinary tract infection. It is known that *E coli* strains from children with acute pyelonephritis have a high propensity to adhere to vaginal and uroepithelial cells, whereas strains from girls with asymptomatic bacteriuria or strains from normal feces have low bacterial adherence. This adherence is mediated by bacterial fimbriae, or pili, which are nonflagellar, proteinaceous appendages that protrude from the bacterial cell surface like tiny hairs. These pili are classified on the basis of their ability to agglutinate erythrocytes of different animal species and by different sugars that are known to block this hemagglutination.

Certain pathogenic strains of *E coli* have type 1

pili, which agglutinate guinea pig erythrocytes, and this hemagglutination is inhibited by the sugar D-mannose. Strains with type 1 pili, which are characterized by mannose-sensitive hemagglutination (MSHA), react selectively to specific sugar sequences in the form of glycolipids or glycoproteins on the surfaces of host epithelial cells and cause the bacteria to adhere to the cell.

Other pathogenic strains of *E coli* have type 2 pili, which agglutinate human (not guinea pig) erythrocytes, and this hemagglutination is not inhibited by the sugar D-mannose. Strains with type 2 pili, which are characterized by mannose-resistant hemagglutination (MRHA), react specifically with uroepithelial cell receptors that are special forms of glycolipids. The most important specific adhesion involves certain pili interacting with uroepithelial cell receptors that are glycolipids of the globoseries identical to the glycosphingolipids of blood group P. Indeed, the terminal disaccharide of the P blood group, the P^k glycosphingolipid, is the receptor involved in MRHA that is caused by pyelonephritic strains of *E coli*. The bacterial pili that interact specifically with these receptors are called P pili, or P fimbriae. Receptors for P pili are present in the kidney, especially in the renal tubular cells, as well as on uroepithelial cells.

A striking relationship between P-fimbriated strains of *E coli* and the type of urinary tract infection present (pyelonephritis versus cystitis) has been observed in children. In one study of 35 patients with pyelonephritis, 94% had infection with P-fimbriated strains. In contrast, of 26 patients with cystitis, only 19% had P-fimbriated strains; of 36 patients with asymptomatic bacteriuria, only 14%; and of 82 healthy controls with fecal strains, only 7% (Kallenius et al, 1981). Similar findings have occurred in adult women with acute nonobstructive pyelonephritis (Jacobson et al, 1985). The presence or absence of vesicoureteral reflux apparently affects the type of adhesions that characterize the pathogens that cause pyelonephritis. Most girls with anatomically normal urinary tracts develop pyelonephritis caused by P-fimbriated bacterial strains. In contrast, most girls who have vesicoureteral reflux develop pyelonephritis caused by bacterial strains that are P-fimbriae negative (Lomberg et al, 1983).

Most *E coli* isolates causing urinary tract infection possess both type 1 (MSHA) and type 2 (MRHA) pili and binding properties. Urinary mucus, or slime, which in the bladder is identical to the Tamm-Horsfall protein elaborated by the renal tubules, contains mannose receptors. It is thought that mannose-sensitive adhesions are responsible for binding *E coli* strains to this urinary slime and that a 2-phase process is responsible for the attachment of uropathogenic strains. The *E coli* organisms first adhere to urinary slime by means of a mannose-sensitive attachment. If no other adhesive properties are present, the bacteria will be excreted with the mucus and infection does not occur. If, however, mannose-resistant properties are also present, such as those mediated by P pili, the bacteria will adhere to the uroepithelial cells and infection can ensue.

Although these recent discoveries are important, many questions remain unanswered concerning the pathogenesis of urinary tract infections.

B. Extrinsic Susceptibility Factors in Women:

1. Introital factors— The identification of factors regulating the receptivity of vaginal epithelial cells to colonization by bacteria, especially pathogenic bacteria, is currently the subject of intense investigation. Colonization of bacteria on mucosal surfaces seems to depend on the ability of the organism to adhere to surface epithelial cells. Shaeffer, Jones, and Dunn (1981) showed that *E coli* isolated from urine adhere in vitro more readily to vaginal cells from women with recurrent urinary tract infections than to similar cells from healthy controls. They also showed that such *E coli* adhere readily to the buccal mucosal cells of women with recurrent urinary tract infections—an observation suggesting that genetic factors may be involved. Stamey et al (1978), as well as other researchers, have observed an apparent direct relationship between the quantity and quality of local cervicovaginal antibody in the vaginal fluid and the likelihood of vaginal colonization by pathogens and recurrent urinary tract infection.

2. Urethral factors— Urethral factors are difficult to study. Bacterial adherence to the surface epithelium, bacterial infection of the periurethral glands, and the nature and turbulence of urinary flow bathing the urethral surface are probably important factors in susceptibility to urinary tract infection.

C. Extrinsic Susceptibility Factors in Men: The preponderance of evidence suggests that the main route of infection in men who experience urinary tract infection is ascent from urethral colonization. Contrary to the situation in girls and women, the male urethra is not near the anus, nor is there an adjacent mucosal surface (the vagina) that may be colonized by bacteria. Furthermore, the prostate normally secretes a potent antibacterial substance that probably serves as a natural defense mechanism against ascending urinary tract infection. Fair, Couch, and Wehner (1976) identified this substance as a zinc salt and observed that it was absent or present in reduced amounts in men with bacterial prostatitis. Chronic bacterial infection of the prostate appears to be the main cause of recurrent urinary tract infection in men (see Nonspecific Infections of the Prostate Gland, p 223).

D. Intrinsic Susceptibility Factors: Several factors intrinsic to the bladder have been shown to influence the susceptibility of both men and women to urinary tract infection. Cox and Hinman (1961) showed that bacteria placed in the bladders of human volunteers were promptly cleared by normal spontaneous voiding without treatment. Thus, efficient voiding itself may serve as a defense mechanism against bladder infection. Neurogenic bladder dysfunction, residual urine, and the presence of a foreign body increase susceptibility to bladder infection. Other fac-

tors that may prove important are under investigation. These concern the ease with which bacteria adhere to bladder surface cells: surface mucin, surface glycosaminoglycan, urinary antibody, and the antimicrobial properties of urine (especially high osmolality and extremes of pH) (Uehling and Iversen, 1982; Schaeffer, 1983). Genetic factors also may prove important.

E. Ureteral and Renal Factors: In addition to factors related to general host susceptibility to infection, there are several factors that relate specifically to ascending infection from the bladder to the upper urinary tracts: the presence or absence of vesicoureteral reflux, the quality of ureteral peristalsis, and the relative susceptibility of the renal medulla to infection. Obstructive uropathy, diminished renal blood flow, primary renal disease, and renal or ureteral foreign bodies have all been implicated as factors that increase the susceptibility of the kidney to infection.

NONSPECIFIC INFECTIONS OF THE KIDNEYS

ACUTE PYELONEPHRITIS

Etiology

Acute pyelonephritis is an infectious inflammatory disease that involves both the parenchyma and the pelvis of the kidney; it may affect one or, on occasion, both kidneys.

Aerobic gram-negative bacteria are the principal causative agents; common strains of *E coli* are the predominant pathogens. All species of *Proteus* are especially important because they are potent producers of urease, an enzyme that splits urea and produces highly alkaline urine that favors the precipitation of phosphates to form magnesium ammonium phosphate (struvite) and calcium phosphate (apatite) stones. *Klebsiella* species are less potent producers of urease but elaborate other substances that favor urinary stone formation.

Gram-positive bacteria, specifically coagulase-negative staphylococci (*S epidermidis* and *S saprophyticus*), *S aureus,* and streptococci group D (enterococci), occasionally cause pyelonephritis. Staphylococci may infect the kidney by the hematogenous route and cause bacteriuria and renal abscesses. Obligate anaerobic bacteria rarely cause pyelonephritis.

Pathology

A. Gross: The kidney usually is enlarged as a consequence of inflammatory edema. Small, raised, yellowish abscesses surrounded by a hemorrhagic rim typically are seen on the subcapsular surface. On cut section, the abscesses appear mainly in the cortex as small rounded areas with a wedge-shaped configuration in focal distribution. Straight yellowish streaks (pus-filled collecting tubules) spread from the cortex and course along the medulla to the papillae. The mucosal surfaces of the renal pelvis and calices are frequently congested, thickened, and covered by exudate.

B. Microscopic: Especially in the cortex, the parenchyma shows extensive tissue destruction by acute inflammation. Polymorphonuclear leukocytes tend to pervade the interstitium and tubules. In addition, infiltration by lymphocytes, plasma cells, and eosinophils is common. The renal medulla is similarly involved. Likewise, the epithelium of the renal pelvis and caliceal system shows acute inflammatory changes. Unless inflammation is severe, the glomeruli are much less involved. The focal nature of renal involvement with inflammation is most significant.

Pathogenesis
(Fig 13–2)

Renal infection usually ascends from the urethra and lower genitourinary tract. Hematogenous infection of the kidney occurs infrequently; lymphatic spread occurs rarely, if ever.

The short urethra in girls and women and its close proximity to the anus allow periurethral pathogenic bacteria easy access to the bladder during sexual intercourse or urethral manipulation. Girls and women with breached local defenses due to biologic, anatomic, or other abnormalities frequently experience introital and periurethral colonization by pathogenic enteric bacteria and are especially prone to infection that ascends from the urethra.

Males are less susceptible to ascending urethral infection because the male urethra is much longer than the female urethra and the meatus is not so near the anus and because the prostate normally secretes antibacterial factors that give some protection against invading pathogens.

Once pathogenic bacteria reach the bladder via the urethra, whether infection becomes established is influenced by the quality of the bladder defenses: the efficacy of voiding and muscle coordination, the antimicrobial properties of the urine, and factors that allow or inhibit bacterial adherence to surface cells.

Once bladder infection is established, whether infection ascends via the ureters and involves the kidneys is influenced by microbial virulence factors, the presence or absence of vesicoureteral reflux, the quality of ureteral peristalsis, and the susceptibility of the renal medulla to infection.

Clinical Findings

A. Symptoms: The usual symptoms of acute pyelonephritis include abrupt onset of shaking chills, moderate to high fever, a constant ache in the loin (unilateral or bilateral), and symptoms of cystitis: frequency, nocturia, urgency, and dysuria. Significant malaise and prostration are the rule; nausea, vomiting, and even diarrhea are common. Young children most often complain of poorly localized abdominal discomfort and seldom localize the discomfort specifically to the flank.

B. Signs: The patient generally appears quite ill. Intermittent chills are associated with fever ranging from 38.5 to 40 °C (101–104 °F) and tachycardia (the pulse rate may range from 90/min to 140/min or

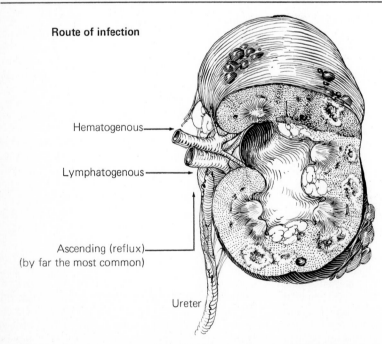

Route of infection

Hematogenous

Lymphatogenous

Ascending (reflux)
(by far the most common)

Ureter

Chief findings
Costovertebral angle pain
Tenderness
Chills and fever
Frequency and burning
Nausea and vomiting
Pus and bacteria in urine

Figure 13–2. Pathogenesis of acute pyelonephritis.

faster). Fist percussion over the costovertebral angle overlying the affected kidney usually causes pain. The kidney often cannot be palpated, because of tenderness and overlying muscle spasm. Abdominal distention may be marked, and rebound tenderness may suggest an intraperitoneal lesion. Auscultation usually reveals a quiet intestine.

C. Laboratory Findings: The hemogram typically shows significant leukocytosis (polymorphonuclear neutrophils and band cells); the erythrocyte sedimentation rate is increased. Urinalysis usually shows cloudy fluid with heavy pyuria, bacteriuria, mild proteinuria, and often microscopic or gross hematuria. Leukocyte casts and glitter cells (large polymorphonuclear neutrophils containing cytoplasmic particles that exhibit dramatic brownian movement) are occasionally seen. Quantitative urine culture generally grows the responsible pathogen in heavy density ($\geq$ 100,000 colonies/mL); sensitivity tests are helpful in therapy and of vital importance in the management of complicating bacteremia. Serial blood cultures are indicated, because bacteremia commonly accompanies acute pyelonephritis. In uncomplicated acute pyelonephritis, total renal function generally remains normal, and the serum creatinine level is not elevated.

D. X-Ray Findings: A plain film of the abdomen may show some degree of obliteration of the renal outline owing to edema of the kidney and perinephric fat. Suspicious calcifications must be carefully evaluated, because infected renal stones and calculous obstruction complicating pyelonephritis require special management.

Excretory urograms performed during the acute stage of uncomplicated pyelonephritis usually show few abnormalities but are important in surveying for possible complicating factors. The severely infected kidney may appear enlarged, show a decreased nephrogram effect on the initial film, and reveal little or no caliceal radiopaque material. Following appropriate therapy, the urograms return to normal (Davidson and Talner, 1973).

Voiding cystograms are best delayed until several weeks after the infection is cleared; otherwise, transient vesicoureteral reflux, often associated with the accompanying cystitis, may be confused with more serious permanent reflux.

E. Radionuclide Imaging: At times, imaging the kidneys with gallium-67 helps to determine the site of infection and distinguish between acute pyelonephritis and renal abscess. Despite some false-positive and false-negative images, Hurwitz et al (1976) claim 86% accuracy in confirming acute pyelonephritis by this method.

Differential Diagnosis

Because of the location and nature of the pain, pancreatitis at times may be confused with acute pyelonephritis. Elevated serum amylase and normal results of urinalysis help to confirm a diagnosis of pancreatitis and rule out pyelonephritis.

Basal pneumonia is a febrile illness that causes pain in the subcostal area. The pleuritic nature of the pain and the chest x-ray usually allow differentiation.

Acute intra-abdominal disease, including such conditions as acute appendicitis, cholecystitis, and diverticulitis, must at times be distinguished from acute pyelonephritis. Although the signs and symptoms may be confusing initially, the normal urinalysis associated with primary gastrointestinal disease and other laboratory tests should make the differential diagnosis uncomplicated.

In women, the onset of acute pelvic inflammatory disease (PID) at times must be distinguished from acute pyelonephritis. Characteristic physical findings and negative urine cultures should make differentiation fairly easy.

In male patients with febrile genitourinary tract infection, the main differential diagnosis consists of acute pyelonephritis, acute prostatitis, and acute epididymo-orchitis. Characteristic physical findings and symptoms in prostatitis and epididymitis should make this differentiation easy.

Acute pyelonephritis must be distinguished from renal abscess and perinephric abscess. Radiographic studies often are necessary to confirm the specific diagnosis.

Complications

When acute pyelonephritis is recognized promptly and treated appropriately, complications are uncommon. The outlook for patients with acute pyelonephritis complicated by underlying renal disease or urologic abnormalities is considerably worse. In such cases, the bacterial pathogens often are abnormally resistant to antimicrobial agents. Kidney stones, especially infected calculi, may preclude effective control and cure unless they are removed. Infections associated with obstructive uropathy are difficult to cure, often become chronic, and frequently lead to bacteremia.

The most serious complication of acute pyelonephritis is septicemia complicated by shock. An unusual but often fatal type of pyelonephritis is emphysematous pyelonephritis—a condition usually seen in diabetics, wherein the pathogen (usually a strain of *E coli*) liberates gas into the infected tissues (Ahlering et al, 1985).

With adequate treatment, acute pyelonephritis in adults without renal disease or complicating urologic abnormalities usually heals without producing renal scars or permanent damage. On the other hand, acute pyelonephritis in infants and children whose renal development is not complete, especially when complicated by renal disease or urologic abnormalities, most often produces permanent renal damage and scarring.

Prevention

Because the immature, developing kidney is at great risk of permanent scarring, atrophy, and functional loss due to attacks of acute pyelonephritis, all urinary tract infections in infants and children must be thoroughly evaluated and vigorously treated. Complete urologic evaluation is mandatory to identify and treat underlying abnormalities that predispose to and complicate urinary tract infections in these children. Children who tend to develop reinfections must be followed carefully; they often require long-term prophylactic administration of antimicrobial drugs.

Although adults with no underlying renal disease or urologic abnormalities seldom develop permanent renal damage as a consequence of acute pyelonephritis, the disease can cause considerable morbidity and possibly death. Predisposing or complicating factors must be carefully evaluated and treated. Patients prone to persistent infection or rapid reinfection also may require long-term preventive antimicrobial therapy.

Treatment

A. Specific Measures: When the infection is severe or complicating factors are present, hospitalization may be required. Urine and blood specimens must be obtained immediately for culture; recognized pathogens must be tested for antimicrobial sensitivity. Until the results of these tests are known, antimicrobial drugs should be given empirically. Although clinicians differ in their choice of antimicrobial agents, our preference is to administer an aminoglycoside (amikacin, gentamicin, or tobramycin) plus ampicillin intravenously in full dosage (see Antimicrobial Treatment of Urinary Tract Infections, p 233). If the pathogen is sensitive and the clinical response is favorable, this treatment is continued for about 1 week and then replaced with an appropriate oral antimicrobial drug for an additional 2 weeks. Complicating factors, eg, obstructive uropathy or infected stones, must be recognized early and dealt with effectively if complications are to be avoided.

B. General Measures: Complete bed rest is advised until symptoms subside. Medication should be given for pain, fever, and nausea. It is important to give fluids intravenously and orally to ensure adequate hydration and maintenance of adequate urinary output.

C. Failure of Response: If the clinical response remains poor after 48–72 hours of therapy, reevaluation is necessary to assess for possible complicating factors (eg, obstructive uropathy) or the use of inappropriate drugs. Excretory urography is required; if this is contraindicated, retrograde urography must be done. Unless treated quickly and effectively, obstructive uropathy complicating acute pyelonephritis can lead to bacteremia and irreversible renal damage.

D. Follow-Up Care: Clinical improvement does not always imply cure of the infection. In about one-third of patients, symptoms improve despite persistence of the bacterial pathogen. Therefore, repeat urine cultures are important during and after therapy for a follow-up period of at least 6 months.

Prognosis

When identified promptly and treated appropriately in a patient who has no underlying complicating factors, acute pyelonephritis carries a good prognosis for cure without sequels. The likelihood of serious sequels and a less favorable prognosis varies with the severity of complicating factors and the patient's age at the onset.

CHRONIC PYELONEPHRITIS

Etiology & Pathogenesis

The exact meaning of the term chronic pyelonephritis is controversial because the radiologic findings are similar whether or not there is persistent renal bacterial infection. Therefore, some clinicians prefer the term chronic tubulointerstitial renal disease due to bacterial infection.

Acute uncomplicated urinary tract infections do not, as previously thought, commonly lead to renal scarring and progressive renal disease. This is especially true in adults; indeed, chronic pyelonephritis appears to be a disease that usually originates in childhood and is carried into adulthood. Prospective studies of the natural history of urinary tract infection have shown that, in the absence of complicating factors such as diabetes, calculi, analgesic nephropathy, or obstructive uropathy, urinary tract infection is a relatively benign condition that seldom leads to renal damage or functional loss. The results of these studies and their clinical implications were carefully documented in a review by Asscher (1980).

The renal scars typical of chronic bacterial pyelonephritis characteristically occur in immature, developing kidneys as a consequence of urinary tract infections in infancy and childhood. The coarse renal scarring noted mainly in the polar regions in these children is known as chronic childhood pyelonephritis or chronic atrophic pyelonephritis. A dilated calix is found beneath each of the scars, because the calices are pulled out by the cicatrization of the renal parenchyma (Asscher, 1980). Current evidence suggests that the most important interrelationship in the pathogenesis of the renal scarring is that between urinary tract infection and vesicoureteral reflux. The severity of renal scarring seems to vary directly with the severity and grade of vesicoureteral reflux in infected children; the most pronounced scarring appears to occur in those who manifest intrarenal reflux (Rolleston, Mailing, and Hodson, 1974). Furthermore, new kidney scars seldom develop after age 4 years. Indeed, the Cardiff-Oxford Bacteriuria Study Group (1978) followed 208 girls between the ages of 5 and 12 years for 4 years and found that none with normal kidneys at initial study developed renal scars, even in the presence of vesicoureteral reflux and persistent infection. However, scars progressed or new scars were observed in 12 girls in whom initial study showed renal scarring and who experienced vesicoureteral reflux and persistent urinary tract infection throughout follow-up.

Pathology

On gross inspection, the kidney shows atrophy of variable degree depending upon the severity and uniformity of involvement. The renal surface usually is pitted and depressed in areas of scarring, and the capsule is pale and strips poorly. In kidneys with minimal involvement, the cut surface shows good preservation of cortical and medullary zones in most areas; in those with advanced disease, extensive disruption of normal structures by inflammation and fibrosis is typical. The pelvic mucosa may appear pale and fibrotic (Fig 13–3).

Histologic examination shows diffuse infiltration of the parenchyma with plasma cells and lymphocytes in affected areas. The tubules show variable degeneration; some are dilated and contain proteinaceous material. Affected glomeruli are fibrotic or frankly hyalinized. Considerable thickening of arteries and arterioles is the rule. In addition to the areas of scarring and chronic inflammation, patchy areas of acute inflammation may be seen. Parenchymal scarring overlying dilated calices is most typical.

Because the pathologic changes in chronic bacterial pyelonephritis are quite similar to those in many types of noninfectious interstitial nephritis, histologic examination alone cannot confirm the bacterial origin of chronic pyelonephritis with certainty. Undoubtedly, the incidence of true chronic bacterial pyelonephritis is considerably lower than might be expected from the finding of changes of chronic pyelonephritis in 10–15% of routine autopsies.

Clinical Findings

A. Symptoms: Episodes of acute infection may occur in children (and occasionally adults) with chronic bacterial pyelonephritis. Typical symptoms (see p 202) are produced. Fever is usually present only during acute infection. In the absence of acute infection, patients with chronic pyelonephritis may be asymptomatic. When chronic pyelonephritis is advanced and bilateral, symptoms related to hypertension, anemia, and azotemia may be seen.

B. Signs: Unless an acute infection develops, no specific physical findings are typical of chronic pyelonephritis. Advanced cases of chronic pyelonephritis may be associated with hypertension.

C. Laboratory Findings: Unless chronic pyelonephritis is complicated by an acute infection or azotemia, the hemogram usually is normal. The findings on urinalysis vary with the severity of renal impairment and the presence of active infection. Significant pyuria and bacteriuria may or may not be found. Significant proteinuria implies advanced disease with glomerular involvement. If bacteriuria is present, urine cultures are positive. Depending upon the stage of the disease, the serum creatinine and blood urea nitrogen may be normal or elevated.

D. X-Ray Findings: A plain film of the abdomen may show that one or both kidneys are small and irregular; urolithiasis may be evident. Typically, the excretory urogram is abnormal and is characterized by pa-

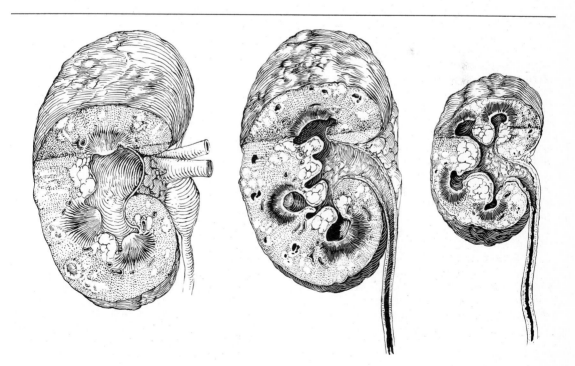

Figure 13–3. Progressive pathologic changes in kidney resulting from repeated attacks of acute pyelonephritis with progressive scarring. *Left:* Early stage of focal parenchymal scarring. *Center:* Progressive scarring with narrowing of the necks of the calices, which therefore become dilated (Fig 13–4). *Right:* End stage of recurrent pyelonephritis (stage of atrophy).

renchymal scarring and atrophy overlying dilated calices; parenchymal irregularity and delayed excretion with poor concentration of the medium also are characteristic (Figs 13–3 and 13–4). In unilateral atrophic pyelonephritis, compensatory hypertrophy of the contralateral kidney is often seen. Dilatation or fullness of the ureter of the affected kidney may signify vesicoureteral reflux (Fig 12–7). Retrograde urograms show similar changes. Voiding cystourethrography, especially in children, often demonstrates vesicoureteral reflux.

E. Instrumental Examination: When active infection is present, cystoscopy usually shows signs of cystitis. Abnormal configuration or position of a ureteral orifice suggests the possibility of valvular incompetence and vesicoureteral reflux. Following thorough washing of the bladder with sterile water, the passage of ureteral catheters to the upper tracts and collection of urine specimens for culture may localize the site of infection.

Differential Diagnosis

In the absence of symptoms suggesting acute pyelonephritis (significant fever and loin pain), the differentiation between infection of the upper and lower urinary tract is often difficult (Table 13–3). By definition, patients with chronic pyelonephritis show typical renal scarring on excretory urograms, whereas patients with only lower tract infection usually have normal kidneys. However, patients with renal scars often have sterile urine and may experience bouts of only lower tract infection; moreover, adults with uncomplicated urinary tract infection and normal urograms sometimes have upper tract infection without significant fever, loin pain, or other signs and symptoms of renal infection. Thus, the distinction between lower urinary tract infection (urethral syndrome and cystitis in women, chronic bacterial prostatitis and cystitis in men) and upper urinary tract infection often is difficult unless invasive procedures are used (Table 13–3).

Chronic pyelonephritis must be distinguished from other causes of chronic tubulointerstitial renal disease, especially analgesic nephropathy. Renal tuberculosis must be considered in the differential diagnosis. Urine smears and cultures positive for mycobacteria and urograms showing the changes typical of renal tuberculosis make this differentiation. At times, renal scans, angiograms, or CT scans are needed to differentiate renal tumors from the changes of chronic pyelonephritis noted on urograms.

Complications

In chronic bacterial pyelonephritis, most of the renal scarring and damage occurs during childhood; indeed, childhood pyelonephritis is responsible for the most severe sequels of urinary tract infection. Adults with normal kidneys and urinary tracts seldom have renal scarring or functional loss despite repeated bouts of pyelonephritis. However, adults with renal infec-

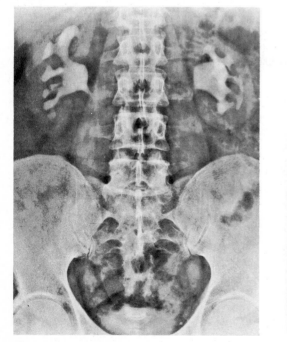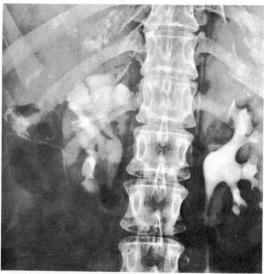

Figure 13–4. Healed pyelonephritis. *Left:* Excretory urogram showing flattening and clubbing of the calices; edge of renal shadow close to ends of the calices. These changes reflect numerous past episodes of acute pyelonephritis. *Right:* Excretory urogram showing marked atrophy of parenchyma of right kidney, with calices of upper pole extending to renal capsule. Left kidney normal.

tion complicated by conditions such as diabetes, underlying renal disease, urolithiasis, or obstructive uropathy are at risk of progressive renal damage and functional loss.

Patients with chronic pyelonephritis are apt to develop bacteremia, hypertension, and renal stones, particularly infected stones. Some mechanisms thought to be responsible for the progression of childhood bacterial pyelonephritis to chronic renal failure in adulthood are (1) inadequately treated recurrent or persistent infection, (2) failure of the kidney to grow, (3) development of progressive immunologic renal damage, (4) renal damage caused by complicating hypertension, (5) damage caused by the renal back pressure effect of severe vesicoureteral reflux, and (6) development of infected renal calculi, especially those caused by urea-splitting bacteria.

Prevention

Prevention of the renal scarring and progressive renal damage seen in chronic bacterial pyelonephritis requires early detection of childhood urinary tract infections, careful prevention and treatment of all urinary tract infections throughout childhood into adulthood, and prompt identification and repair of all surgically correctable conditions that adversely affect optimal medical management.

Treatment

A. Specific Measures:

1. Medical measures—Adults and (especially) children with evidence of chronic pyelonephritis require careful medical management. This entails prompt identification and eradication of established urinary tract infection and prevention of recurrent urinary tract infection. Pathogen-specific antimicrobial therapy is required to eradicate established urinary tract infection; the long-term use of continuous antimicrobial therapy often is required, especially in children, to prevent reinfection. The specific clinical situation determines the type and duration of such therapy.

2. Surgical measures—Contributing anatomic defects (particularly those causing obstructive uropathy) should be corrected and calculi (especially infected stones) removed by surgical means. High-grade vesicoureteral reflux or vesicoureteral reflux of lesser degree in patients who respond suboptimally to medical management requires surgical repair.

B. General Measures: If progressive renal damage and functional loss are to be minimized, the patient must be followed closely, urinary tract infections must be controlled tightly, and complications must be identified promptly and treated adequately. The hypertension associated with unilateral atrophic pyelonephritis may be renin-mediated; the patient should be evaluated for possible therapeutic nephrectomy.

Prognosis

The outlook for patients with chronic pyelo-

nephritis varies with the age of onset, the successful correction of contributing anatomic defects, the severity of complicating factors, and the successful control of urinary tract infections. Chronic pyelonephritis seldom progresses to chronic renal failure requiring dialysis and renal transplantation; when it does, this is usually a result of inadequately treated chronic pyelonephritis of childhood.

XANTHOGRANULOMATOUS PYELONEPHRITIS

Xanthogranulomatous pyelonephritis is an uncommon form of chronic bacterial infection of the kidney that may occur at any age but is most often seen in middle-aged or older women. The condition rarely is bilateral. Symptoms include loin pain, fever, vesical irritability, malaise, anorexia, and weight loss. Physical findings include flank tenderness in 55% of patients, a palpable flank mass in 52%, and hypertension in 20% (Elder, 1984). Most patients have a history of renal calculi, obstructive nephropathy, diabetes mellitus, or urologic surgery.

The affected kidney is usually enlarged, and its pyelocaliceal system is dilated by pus (pyonephrosis) or calculi or both. Grossly, the kidney typically shows orange-yellow nodules of inflamed parenchymal tissue adjacent to areas of tissue necrosis and suppuration; small, localized abscesses are commonly found. Histologically, the inflamed tissue consists of neutrophils, lymphocytes, plasma cells, necrotic debris, and giant cells; most characteristic are large macrophages with foamy cytoplasm containing much lipid material. At times, these cells may be mistaken for those seen in renal clear cell carcinoma.

Laboratory findings include an abnormal hemogram (67% of patients are anemic, and 46% show leukocytosis) and an abnormal urinalysis (pyuria is present in most patients, along with microhematuria and bacteriuria) (Elder, 1984). The urine culture usually is positive, and *P mirabilis* and *E coli* are most commonly recovered.

The x-ray findings vary with the severity of involvement of the affected kidney by obstruction, calculi, and parenchymal damage. Excretory urography often shows a nonfunctioning kidney with one or more renal calculi; parenchymal calcifications frequently are seen in advanced cases. Renal angiography generally depicts a relatively avascular mass or masses. CT scanning is particularly useful in diagnosis and in assessing the extent of disease.

It is difficult to differentiate xanthogranulomatous pyelonephritis from other causes of renal masses preoperatively. Nephrectomy usually is required but may be difficult owing to intense perinephritis.

BACTEREMIA & SEPTIC SHOCK

Gram-negative bacteremia is a serious, often life-threatening disease. Complicating shock occurs in approximately 40% of cases. Data indicate a progressive increase in the incidence of gram-negative bacteremia and septic shock, especially in large medical centers. Indeed, septic shock is one of the most frequent causes of shock seen in medical practice. The genitourinary tract is an important source of bacteremia, and the 4 most common organisms seen in gram-negative bacteremia are common genitourinary tract pathogens: *E coli*, *Proteus* sp, *Klebsiella* sp, and *P aeruginosa*. The mortality rate due to gram-negative bacteremia is estimated at 25%; however, that due to gram-negative bacteremia complicated by shock approaches 50%.

Predisposing Factors

Several factors are thought to predispose patients to the onset of bacteremia and septic shock; in general, however, septicemia occurs primarily in hosts with altered defense mechanisms or when the pathogen gains access to sites normally protected by host defenses.

In the USA, the incidence of gram-negative bacteremia is highest among hospitalized patients 60 years of age or older. Both the incidence and severity of outcome of bacteremia are influenced greatly by the severity of underlying disease. Unfavorable factors include debilitating diseases such as diabetes mellitus, azotemia, congestive heart disease, and cancer and states of malnutrition and starvation. Among those most susceptible to gram-negative bacteremia with shock are patients with severe granulocytopenia (< 500/μL) or those receiving immunosuppressive agents such as corticosteroids, antimetabolites, or various chemotherapeutic agents, especially when the drugs are combined with irradiation.

Three types of widely used medical devices—indwelling urethral catheters, intravenous catheters, and ventilatory equipment—are regarded as the most frequent sources of gram-negative bacteremia. Unless antimicrobial therapy and other preventive measures are employed, manipulation, instrumentation, and surgical procedures performed on the genitourinary tract are especially likely to cause gram-negative bacteremia.

Factors predisposing to septic shock are less clearly defined than are those predisposing to bacteremia. In general, shock occurs most frequently in patients who are over age 50 and have the most severe underlying diseases. The incidence of shock is definitely increased in patients who do not have a fever of greater than 37.6 °C (99.6 °F) during the first 24 hours after the onset of bacteremia. Surprisingly, the incidence of shock does not appear to be related to the type of gram-negative bacterial rod causing infection.

Among patients with septic shock, the highest mortality rates are associated with the use of inappropriate antibiotic therapy, delayed admission to an intensive care unit, and decreased cardiac output that fails to respond to therapy.

Pathophysiology & Pathology of Bacteremic Shock

It is commonly thought that bacterial endotoxins (lipopolysaccharides) are responsible for the early manifestations and onset of bacteremic shock. Several recent studies suggest that these endotoxins are not the true cause or the only mechanism involved. The pathophysiologic mechanism of gram-negative bacteremic shock is not fully understood; this type of shock can best be explained as a phenomenon resulting from a complex interaction between the fibrinolytic, coagulation, complement, and kinin systems and their effects upon the microcirculation and hemostasis.

Two relatively consistent patterns of hemodynamic change occur in bacteremic shock; the first phase is called "early" or "warm" shock, and the second "late" or "cold" shock. Early shock is typified by hyperdynamic circulation. Its characteristics are as follows: (1) increased or normal cardiac output, (2) decreased peripheral resistance, (3) high or normal central venous pressure, (4) hyperventilation with respiratory alkalosis, and (5) lactate accumulation. In late shock, the more classic clinical picture of shock (a cold, clammy patient with cyanosis and a weak, thready pulse) is typical. Late shock is characterized by (1) decreased cardiac output, (2) increased peripheral resistance (vasoconstriction), (3) decreased central venous pressure, (4) hyperventilation, (5) lactate accumulation, and (6) a shift from respiratory alkalosis to metabolic acidosis.

Early in the development of bacteremic shock, the decrease in peripheral resistance (vascular tone) is disproportionate to the increase in cardiac output; this leads to inadequate tissue and organ perfusion. Hyperventilation is common early in bacteremic shock, and the excessive blowing off of carbon dioxide results in respiratory alkalosis. Because tissue and organ perfusion remains inadequate, there is increasing anoxia and accumulation of lactate. Among other factors, bradykinin generation is thought to cause increased vascular permeability (with loss of intravascular fluid into the tissues) and marked systemic arteriolar dilatation, venoconstriction, and hypotension.

The hyperdynamic circulation of early shock eventually changes to the decreased cardiac output and increased peripheral resistance characteristic of late shock. Myocardial depression and a fall in tissue oxygen consumption have been implicated in this shift. Cerebral anoxia leads to confusion, stupor, and possibly coma. Diminished renal perfusion often leads to oliguria and salt and water retention and may result in acute tubular necrosis.

Disseminated intravascular coagulation (DIC) occurs occasionally in cases of bacteremia but is almost always associated with bacteremic shock. Activation of factor XII (Hageman factor) by gram-negative bacteria is thought to initiate the syndrome, with subsequent activation of the fibrinolytic and intrinsic clotting cascade producing concomitant intravascular coagulation and fibrinolysis. Bleeding from the skin, subcutaneous tissues, or mucous membranes of the mouth, nose, or gastrointestinal tract may ensue.

The most serious abnormalities due to bacteremic shock occur in the lung; indeed, the development of "shock" lung (adult respiratory distress syndrome) and resultant pulmonary failure is a common cause of death in cases of septic shock. The alveoli thicken owing to marked tissue anoxia, accumulation of intraalveolar fluid and sludged material associated with disseminated intravascular coagulation, hemorrhagic atelectasis, and round cell infiltration; lung compliance decreases markedly, and the ventilation-perfusion ratio is impaired. Eventually, the resulting hypoxia is unresponsive to the administration of 100% oxygen alone, and mechanical positive pressure ventilation is required for improvement.

Clinical Findings

A. Symptoms: The patient develops a fever that typically ranges from 38.5 to 40 °C (101–104 °F), with or without associated chills. Initial anxiety soon may be followed by confusion, stupor, or coma. Symptoms of an associated genitourinary tract infection may be present, or urethral instrumentation may have been performed a few hours previously.

B. Signs: The patient's initial anxiety and agitation usually change to confusion and stupor. Early in septic shock, the skin seems warm and the pulse bounding despite hypotension. The late phase of septic shock is characterized by cyanosis; cold, pale, moist skin; and a weak, thready pulse associated with hypotension. Respirations are shallow and rapid; capillary refilling in the nail beds is prolonged; and oliguria usually develops. Other physical findings may be present depending upon the underlying cause of the sepsis.

C. Laboratory Findings: Leukopenia usually is observed in infants; in adults, the leukocyte count generally is elevated with a shift to the left. Disseminated intravascular coagulation is characterized by thrombocytopenia, the presence of circulating fibrin split products, and decreased levels of coagulation factors II, V, and VII. Initially, the hematocrit may be increased as a result of loss of plasma into the interstitial tissues. Because renal blood flow is diminished, the specific gravity of the urine is increased, and the ratio of serum urea nitrogen to serum creatinine may exceed the normal 10:1. Diminished coronary artery blood flow and the presence of circulating substances that depress myocardial function cause ischemia; the appearance of the ECG may lead to the erroneous conclusion that myocardial infarction has occurred. An increase in the blood levels of fatty acids and glucose is common.

Since the source of the bacteremia often is the urinary tract, pyuria and bacteriuria may be found. It is essential to obtain urine specimens for Gram staining and culture and serial blood specimens for culture and sensitivity testing. Aerobic gram-negative bacilli, predominantly *E coli,* are the usual pathogens.

Since pulmonary insufficiency usually develops in

septic shock, frequent estimates of arterial blood gases and serum electrolytes are necessary. Initially, there are marked reductions in arterial P_{O_2} and P_{CO_2}, and respiratory alkalosis prevails; ultimately, metabolic acidosis develops. The serum lactate level (normal, 0.44–1.8 mmol/L) is important in estimating prognosis. Values of 5 mmol/L or more are associated with a high mortality rate and reflect severe tissue anoxia. Conversely, a progressive decrease in the serum lactate level during therapy is an encouraging sign.

D. X-Ray Findings: Chest roentgenograms demonstrate diffuse alveolar infiltrates that may progress to homogenous pulmonary consolidation as part of "shock lung."

Differential Diagnosis

Bacteremia alone is accompanied by chills, fever, and positive results of blood cultures, but hypotension and oliguria do not occur. Elderly patients referred from chronic care facilities often present clinical pictures that may be confused with a diagnosis of bacteremia with shock. These patients often are dehydrated and hypovolemic and have low-grade fevers associated with decubitus ulcers or urinary tract infections caused by gram-negative bacteria. Acute heart failure, especially when secondary to myocardial infarction, may cause sudden hypotension. Since these patients generally have intravenous and urinary catheters, there may be initial confusion about whether the shock is cardiogenic or bacteremic. Likewise, electrocardiographic abnormalities associated with the metabolic myocardial depression seen in bacteremic shock may be confused with those of acute myocardial infarction. Some patients with suspected bacteremic shock may have adrenal insufficiency with associated fever and hypotension; adrenal insufficiency usually can be identified on the basis of the typical electrolyte abnormalities and eosinophilia. The tachypnea, tachycardia, agitation, and pulmonary infiltrates associated with acute pulmonary embolization may initially be confused with bacteremia with early shock. Whenever bacteremia cannot be excluded by careful clinical evaluation, empiric administration of antibiotics is indicated until this diagnosis is excluded by culture results and additional clinical data.

Complications

The primary infection may not respond to antibiotic therapy, and continued bacteremia and widespread infection may result. Prolonged hypoxia and hypotension may lead to acute tubular necrosis and renal failure or serious cardiac sequels—heart failure, arrhythmias, and infarction. Hemorrhages into the skin and subcutaneous tissue, the gastrointestinal tract, and various organs may occur in association with disseminated intravascular coagulation. One of the most serious complications is pulmonary failure associated with adult respiratory distress syndrome ("shock lung"). Any of these complications may lead to death.

Prevention

As with many other infectious diseases, the optimal treatment of gram-negative bacteremia is its prevention. A major effort should be made to prevent and control hospital-acquired gram-negative bacillary infections at primary sites. Control measures should be directed especially toward the 3 most frequent sources of infection: indwelling urinary catheters, intravenous catheters, and ventilatory equipment. These devices should be used only when absolutely necessary and withdrawn as soon as possible. Transurethral diagnostic and surgical procedures should not be performed, especially in male patients, unless the urine is sterile and preventive antimicrobial therapy is employed. Strict aseptic technique should be used during insertion of bladder catheters, and only closed drainage systems should be used. Intravenous catheters must be inspected regularly for early signs of infection and removed promptly or changed regularly every 48–72 hours. Special care of ventilatory equipment is required; disposable devices should be used whenever possible, and nondisposable materials must be kept clean and sterile. Care must be taken to minimize infection associated with wounds, tracheostomies, tube drainage, and catheters. Every effort must be made to prevent bed sores and to minimize inadvertent transmission of bacterial pathogens from patient to patient or from hospital devices and equipment to patients.

Treatment

Prompt diagnosis and treatment of bacteremia are essential, especially to prevent septic shock, severe morbidity, and an increased risk of death. The clinician must be alert to early signs of bacteremia in high-risk patients, especially those who have recently undergone urethral instrumentation. Since the diagnosis of bacteremia is confirmed only by blood cultures, treatment often must be initiated only on the basis of clinical findings. However, the need for prompt recognition and treatment of bacteremia does not negate the need for bacteriologic studies to confirm the identity of the infecting pathogen and its susceptibility to antimicrobial agents. Before antibiotics are administered, appropriate specimens must be collected for Gram staining and culture. Bacteremia typically develops from localized infections; therefore, before the initiation of empiric antimicrobial therapy, specimens for microscopic examination and culture must be obtained from blood, urine, sputum, intravenous catheters, wound drainage, and other sites or sources of local infection.

The general therapeutic aims in the management of septic shock are to combat infection, restore circulating blood volume, and improve perfusion of vital organs (heart, brain, and lungs).

A. Specific Measures:

1. Initial measures–

a. Establish the diagnosis of bacteremia (collect blood, urine, and other appropriate specimens for Gram staining and culture), and rule out other causes of shock.

b. Insert an indwelling urethral or punch suprapubic catheter to monitor hourly urinary output. A closed drainage system should be used.

c. Insert a central venous pressure catheter into the superior vena cava or right atrium, or insert a Swan-Ganz catheter into the pulmonary artery to monitor pulmonary capillary wedge pressure. Placement of both catheters permits optimal monitoring and control of volume expansion.

2. Antibiotics–If the organism from the primary site has been identified and its antimicrobial susceptibilities are known, the best drug or combination of drugs should be administered in maximal therapeutic dosage. If the pathogen has not yet been identified, infection with a gram-negative rod should be assumed. Empiric antibiotic therapy must be started immediately; treatment must not await the results of culture and sensitivity tests. An aminoglycoside (amikacin, gentamicin, or tobramycin) is the drug of choice. Give amikacin, 5 mg/kg intravenously every 8 hours; or gentamicin, 1.5 mg/kg intravenously every 8 hours; or tobramycin, 1.5 mg/kg intravenously every 8 hours. If P aeruginosa infection is suspected, give carbenicillin, 4–6 g intravenously every 4–6 hours, or ticarcillin, 3–6 g intravenously every 6 hours, in addition to the aminoglycoside, since these agents have synergistic activity with aminoglycosides against this organism. If sepsis arising from a primary urinary tract infection involving enterococci is suspected, therapy combining an aminoglycoside with ampicillin, 2 g intravenously every 4–6 hours, is indicated. For suspected polymicrobic infection involving gram-negative bacilli and anaerobes (especially Bacteroides species), optimal therapy consists of an aminoglycoside plus clindamycin, 450–600 mg intravenously every 6 hours. When the responsible pathogen or pathogens are identified, therapy is altered to continue the least toxic antibiotic that is most effective against the infecting organism and withdraw other antibiotic agents. The drug dosage must be adjusted appropriately if renal failure is present or develops during therapy (Table 13–4). Antibiotic therapy should continue for a minimum of 5 days after the patient becomes afebrile, or even longer if local infection persists. Diagnosis of local infections, removal of foreign bodies, and drainage of purulent accumulations is essential.

3. Measures to improve circulating blood volume and perfusion of vital organs–

a. Parenteral fluids–Once septic shock is suspected, give 1000 mL of crystalloid solution (eg, normal saline solution, lactated Ringer's injection) intravenously over a 20- to 30-minute period unless congestive heart failure is present. Colloid solutions (albumin or low-molecular-weight dextran) should be administered as soon as possible, because their oncotic pressure tends to draw plasma back into the capillaries; this lessens tissue and cellular edema and helps to wash sludged red and white cells and platelets into the general circulation. Low-molecular-weight dextran decreases blood viscosity and combats platelet adhesiveness. Absolute central venous pressure

(CVP) and pulmonary capillary wedge pressure (PCWP) values are not as important in fluid management as pressure changes in response to fluid infusions. As long as the CVP does not exceed 14 cm of water or the PCWP does not exceed 22 mm Hg, volume expansion with both crystalloid and colloid solutions is continued at a rate of 15–20 mL/min. A sudden or continuously progressive increase in CVP of over 5 cm of water or a CVP level greater than 14 cm of water, or an increase in PCWP of over 8 mm Hg or a PCWP level greater than 22 mm Hg, implies possible fluid overload and requires a cutback in infusion rates. The usual goal is to raise the blood pressure to a level about 20 mm Hg less than the normal systolic blood pressure observed before the onset of shock and to maintain it at this level. The urinary output should be maintained at 40–50 mL/h. CVP and PCWP monitoring should be accompanied by frequent auscultation of the chest and examination of the jugular pulse. Increased urinary output, clearing of mentation, and improved respiration are favorable signs. In most cases, antibiotic therapy plus correction of the circulating blood volume is all that is needed for complete recovery.

b. Corticosteroids–Despite extensive study during the past few decades, the use of corticosteroids in the therapy of septic shock remains highly controversial. Some studies suggest improved survival rates, while others demonstrate no benefit from the use of steroids in the management of bacteremia with shock. Patients with bacteremic shock randomly treated with 1–2 doses of methylprednisolone, 3 mg/kg, showed an increased survival rate compared with that of patients who received no steroids. Conversely, Kreger, Craven, and McCabe (1980) found that the mortality rate associated with the use of "pharmacologic" doses of corticosteroids in patients with septic shock was increased compared with that of controls. A more recent prospective study of the efficacy of high-dose corticosteroids was conducted by Sprung et al (1984), who concluded that corticosteroids do not improve the overall survival rate of patients with severe, late septic shock but may be helpful early in the course and in certain subgroups of patients.

c. Vasoactive agents–If volume expansion fails to produce prompt improvement, vasoactive agents are indicated to further enhance cardiac output. Although a variety of vasoactive drugs have been used in the past, few have been found ideal.

(1) Dopamine–The most widely used vasoactive agent in the treatment of bacteremic shock is dopamine. Its effects are clearly dose-related. At low doses (2–5 μg/kg/min), it activates β-adrenergic receptors and increases myocardial contractility more than heart rate; it also produces non-β-adrenergic dilatation of the renal and splanchnic vasculature. At high doses (> 10 μg/kg/min), it produces α-adrenergic effects of generalized vasoconstriction that intensify directly with increasing doses. Therefore, treatment with dopamine should begin at doses of 2–5 μg/kg/min, and the dosage should be titrated to pro-

duce the lowest possible infusion rate that will restore blood pressure and urinary output.

(2) Isoproterenol–Although isoproterenol increases cardiac output, its vasodilatory activity is undesirable in the treatment of early bacteremic shock; furthermore, it tends to cause tachycardia and cardiac arrhythmias. For these reasons, most clinicians avoid using isoproterenol in septic shock. The usual dose is 1–2 μg/min.

(3) Norepinephrine–The marked vasoconstriction caused by norepinephrine virtually eliminates its use in the treatment of septic shock. Its only usefulness may be in patients with septic shock who also have severe coronary insufficiency, because it enhances coronary arterial flow.

4. Support of vital organs–

a. Lungs–Since the pulmonary complications of shock interfere with normal oxygenation of the blood, they are the most serious. An initial step in management is to ensure an adequate airway and administer oxygen at a rate of 5–8 L/min. Intubation or tracheostomy may be required so that assisted or controlled mechanical ventilation can be employed, especially if the P_{O2} remains below 70 mm Hg. An attempt should be made to raise the P_{aO_2} to 70–90 mm Hg and hold the P_{aCO_2} between 32 and 40 mm Hg. The treatment of heart failure may reduce pulmonary edema and improve aeration.

b. Heart–Steps taken to raise the CVP and PCWP and increase myocardial contractility will improve cardiac output. If congestive heart failure is present, immediate digitalization is required. The deleterious effect of metabolic acidosis upon the myocardium may be counteracted by intravenous administration of sodium bicarbonate.

c. Kidneys–Volume expansion, with or without the additional use of vasoactive drugs, usually counteracts the oliguria associated with early bacteremic shock. Persistence of oliguria may imply acute renal tubular necrosis; it should be treated by intravenous infusion of mannitol, 12.5 g over 5 minutes and repeated after 2 hours if a urine flow of 30 to 40 mL/h is not achieved. Furosemide, 240 mg, is given intravenously at the time of the second infusion of mannitol. If the response to mannitol and furosemide is poor, furosemide, 480 mg, is given intravenously. If the response to this large second dose of furosemide is poor, no further attempts at diuresis are indicated, and standard therapy for acute renal failure is initiated. Dialysis may become necessary.

B. Other Measures:

1. Correction of fluid and electrolyte balance–Sodium bicarbonate can be used for total correction of moderate degrees of acidosis. One method is to give half the calculated base deficit intravenously, and then recheck the blood pH. Alternatively, 44 meq of sodium bicarbonate can be given for each 2 meq/L deficit from the normal bicarbonate level.

2. Treatment of disseminated intravascular coagulation (DIC)–Changes characteristic of disseminated intravascular coagulation probably occur to some degree in all cases of septic shock; however, successful treatment of the infection, its underlying cause, and the circulatory manifestations of shock generally corrects the consumption coagulopathy without the specific need for heparin. Low-molecular-weight dextran, in addition to expanding blood volume, decreases the blood viscosity. One or 2 units should be given during the initial 24 hours of treatment and 1 unit daily thereafter. When disseminated intravascular coagulation is unresponsive to therapy of other aspects of the infection-shock syndrome, treatment using heparin is indicated. The suggested dosage is 1000–2000 units intravenously every 4–6 hours. Appropriate blood products should be given concomitantly. Careful monitoring by means of blood clotting tests and alertness for evidence of increased hemorrhage is required.

3. Removal of foreign bodies and drainage of purulent collections–Local sites of infection responsible for the bacteremia must be identified and treated immediately. Any underlying obstructive uropathy must be detected and relieved by the simplest possible means. Abscesses or purulent collections must be drained. Foreign bodies, including urinary, intravenous, and intra-arterial catheters present before the onset of the bacteremia, must be removed. Such catheters should be removed, cultured, and replaced with sterile catheters. Although patients with septic shock are usually poor candidates for surgical procedures, operation may be necessary to control local sites of infection that perpetuate the bacteremia.

Prognosis

With prompt diagnosis and immediate institution of appropriate treatment, the prognosis is generally favorable, especially when bacteremia is controlled and septic shock is avoided. Recent studies indicate that the mortality rate tends to vary directly with the severity of the underlying disease. The prognosis is worst for patients who are least able to generate natural defenses (eg, those with severe granulocytopenia, advanced malignant neoplastic diseases, or severe cardiopulmonary diseases). In general, mortality rates for patients with septic shock are higher in large medical centers than in community hospitals; this undoubtedly reflects differences in the severity of the underlying diseases. In the USA, the overall mortality rate for patients with gram-negative rod bacteremia is about 25%, whereas that for patients with gram-negative rod bacteremia complicated by shock approximates 50%.

INTERSTITIAL NEPHRITIS & PAPILLARY NECROSIS

Etiology

Papillary necrosis is a result of ischemic necrosis of the papillary tip or the entire pyramid. It occurs in association with acute and chronic forms of interstitial nephritis of variable cause. Acute papillary necrosis is usually associated with urinary tract infection and

severe bacterial renal interstitial infection; it occurs mainly in diabetics. However, papillary necrosis is now most commonly seen in patients with chronic interstitial nephritis unrelated to infection but caused by chronic analgesic abuse (mainly of drugs containing phenacetin and its metabolites); this is called analgesic nephropathy. Other causes of chronic interstitial nephritis and papillary necrosis include renal vascular diseases, hypertension, obstructive nephropathy, nephrolithiasis, sickle cell disease, potassium depletion, disseminated intravascular coagulation, diabetes mellitus, hypercalcemia, radiation injury, lead nephropathy, and Balkan nephropathy. Papillary necrosis occurs mainly in adult women; it is rare in children and infants.

Pathogenesis & Pathology (Figs 13–5 and 13–6)

Interstitial nephritis with papillary necrosis generally occurs bilaterally, although acute symptoms related to the sloughing of a papilla may lateralize to one kidney. As the disease progresses, a few or all of the papillae and their corresponding calices may become more severely involved. Most patients have no acute or persistent renal bacterial infection; however, patients with chronic interstitial nephritis and papillary necrosis who have vesicoureteral reflux and recurrent urinary tract infections are at serious risk of rapidly progressive renal demage. The common denominator in the pathogenesis of all forms of papillary necrosis apparently is papillary vascular insufficiency.

Renal atrophy is characteristic; it may be rapid and symmetrically involve the entire kidney or irregular and associated with identifiable papillary injury. One or more papillae may be absent as a result of sloughing or total sclerosis. Retained or calcified papillae occasionally are found free in the renal pelvis. Typical gross and histologic changes of chronic interstitial nephritis are seen in the affected kidney. Severe ischemia of the pyramids may be observed. Infiltration of the site of the papillary slough by polymorphonuclear neutrophils, small round cells, and plasma cells may be observed microscopically.

Clinical Findings

A. Symptoms: The rare fulminant type of papillary necrosis generally associated with urinary tract infection is characterized by severe sepsis of rapid onset, with fever, hematuria, abdominal or loin pain, and, occasionally, signs and symptoms of bacteremic shock. Other patients present with classic symptoms of acute pyelonephritis, but the pyelonephritis responds poorly to antimicrobial therapy that normally is effective. In most cases, papillary necrosis occurs insidiously, without associated urinary tract infection; patients remain asymptomatic until symptoms of renal failure develop, or symptoms (pain and hematuria) develop acutely as a result of sloughing and migration of papillary material. Careful history taking, especially questions about the ingestion of analgesics, is needed to clarify the underlying cause. Unfortunately, most

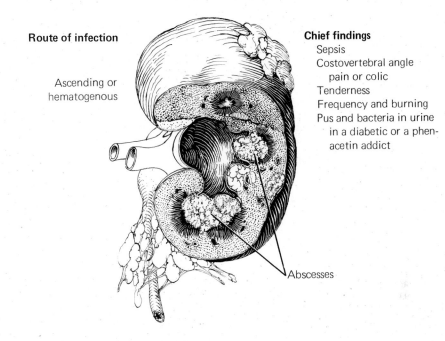

Route of infection

Ascending or
hematogenous

Chief findings
Sepsis
Costovertebral angle
    pain or colic
Tenderness
Frequency and burning
Pus and bacteria in urine
    in a diabetic or a phen-
    acetin addict

Abscesses

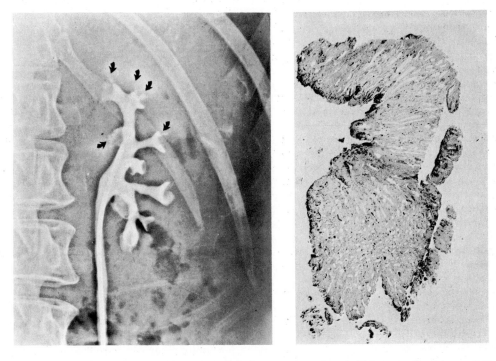

Figure 13–5. Papillary necrosis. *Top:* Pathogenesis. *Left:* Arrows point to "cracks" into parenchyma in a patient in the earliest stage of papillitis (medullary type). *Right:* Papilla passed spontaneously in urine, recovered by patient. (Reduced 30% from × 10.)

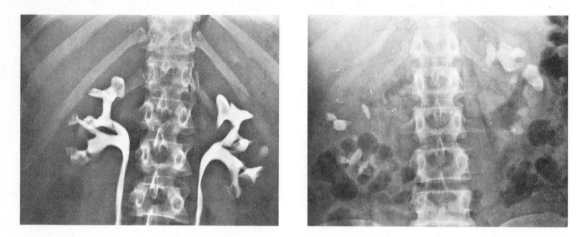

Figure 13–6. Papillary necrosis. *Left:* Retrograde urogram showing papillary necrosis. Calices seem enlarged because of sloughed papillae. "Negative" shadows in upper medial calices and in lowest calices on left represent sloughed papillae. *Right:* (Same patient 5 years later.) Multiple renal stones caused by calcification of retained sloughed papillae. The papillae are represented by the relatively translucent centers in peculiarly shaped stones.

patients will deny taking excessive amounts of analgesics. Most abusers of analgesic drugs are women who complain of chronic headaches and various other pain syndromes.

B. Signs: In acute papillary necrosis associated with renal bacterial infection, the patient usually experiences chills, fever, hematuria, abdominal or loin pain, and prostration. The picture may rapidly degenerate to one of bacteremic shock. There may be localized tenderness of the involved kidney. In acute papillary necrosis without accompanying bacterial infection, there are no signs of sepsis, but pain and hematuria may be present. Many patients have so few signs and symptoms that papillary necrosis goes undetected until azotemia is found.

C. Laboratory Findings: In acute papillary necrosis associated with renal bacterial infection, the usual findings are those of acute pyelonephritis. Leukocytosis with a marked shift to the left is typical. Urinalysis shows pyuria, hematuria, and bacteriuria. The infecting pathogen is often found in urine and blood cultures. Diabetics usually show glycosuria and hyperglycemia; metabolic acidosis may develop.

In patients with chronic interstitial nephritis and papillary necrosis secondary to abuse of analgesic drugs, laboratory evidence of urinary tract infection usually is absent. Sterile pyuria occurs in about 50% of these patients and often is a valuable clue in diagnosis. Most patients show signs of progressive renal failure, azotemia, and anemia.

D. X-Ray Findings: It is necessary to infuse large doses of radiographic contrast material to obtain satisfactory excretory urograms in azotemic patients. This may lead to nephrotoxicity, especially if dehydration is used in patient preparation. In the earliest stages of interstitial nephritis, before papillary slough, urograms often detect no caliceal abnormalities. Later, ulceration of the central portion of a papilla

(medullary necrosis; Fig 13–5) or cavities caused by papillary slough may be seen (Fig 13–6). At times "negative" shadows representing retained papillae are visible. During the late phases of papillary necrosis, irregular calcified bodies with radiolucent centers (the papillae) are diagnostic findings. In addition to the caliceal changes, segmental or total renal atrophy is characteristic. Medullary calcifications (nephrocalcinosis) of variable degree also are noted on occasion.

In patients with severe azotemia, excretory urography may be contraindicated. In such cases, retrograde urography performed under strict aseptic conditions may establish the diagnosis or reveal a treatable urologic disorder.

Differential Diagnosis

Because specific treatment varies according to the underlying disorder, the various causes of interstitial nephritis and papillary necrosis must be considered.

Diabetics with acute pyelonephritis unaccompanied by papillary necrosis generally respond rapidly to control of the infection and the associated metabolic derangement; those with papillary necrosis, especially when it is bilateral, generally respond poorly and often develop acute renal failure. Renal cortical abscesses, particularly in diabetics, at times are confused with papillary necrosis. Standard urograms made early in either condition may not be diagnostic; however, renal abscesses usually are detected readily by gallium scans, ultrasonography, and CT scan.

Negative filling defects within the collecting system and ureters, including blood clots, nonopaque stones, and uroepithelial tumors, are sometimes confused with sloughed papillae. Careful examination of urograms usually allows differentiation; however, differentiation may be difficult when these conditions occur in patients with preexisting caliceal abnormalities.

Complications

Sloughed papillae serve as a nidus for unresolved or persistent infection that causes bacteriuria. Acute papillary necrosis associated with fulminant renal infection (especially in diabetics) may lead to bacteremic shock, severe morbidity, and death. Patients with more insidious forms of papillary necrosis and interstitial nephritis (eg, abusers of analgesic drugs), develop progressive renal damage and renal insufficiency unless treatment is successful. Analgesic nephropathy has been a leading cause of renal failure resulting in a need for dialysis and kidney transplantation in Australia (Kincaid-Smith, 1978). Patients with analgesic nephropathy also have an increased incidence of transitional cell carcinoma (Bengtsson et al, 1978; Gonwa et al, 1980).

Prevention

Because interstitial nephritis and papillary necrosis typically lead to progressive renal damage and renal failure, prevention is important, particularly in diabetics and abusers of analgesic drugs, the 2 groups of patients most susceptible to this condition. Control of urinary infections and vascular disease is important in diabetics. Analgesic abusers must be identified and must stop taking analgesics. If analgesic abusers stop taking analgesics, their renal function usually improves and stabilizes; but if they continue, progressive renal damage and irreversible renal failure ensue.

Treatment

A. Specific Measures:

1. Medical measures–In cases of papillary necroses associated with urinary tract infections, intensive treatment with appropriate antimicrobial drugs and other appropriate measures is important.

2. Surgical measures–If the disease is unilateral and fulminating (as demonstrated by physical examination, urography, renal function tests, and other measures) and if drug therapy does not control the infection or produce prompt improvement, nephrectomy must be considered. Nephrectomy must be undertaken with caution, however, because the other kidney ultimately may become involved.

A sloughed papilla that migrates and obstructs a ureter usually can be removed by endoscopic manipulation.

B. General Measures: Diabetes must be carefully controlled, and prevention and prompt treatment of genitourinary tract infections is important in diabetic patients. Analgesic abusers must be identified and must stop taking analgesics; this often requires referral to an interested psychiatrist or a substance abuse center.

Prognosis

Unless successful therapy is instituted immediately, acute fulminating papillary necrosis associated with renal bacterial infection may be fatal. The morbidity and mortality rates associated with chronic forms of papillary necrosis vary directly with the cause, the rapidity with which it is diagnosed, and both the patient's and the clinician's interest and determination in control. Progressive renal failure leading to a need for dialysis and kidney transplantation is the rule in analgesic abusers who do not reform. The outlook for patients with analgesic nephropathy who develop transitional cell carcinoma generally is poor; diagnosis is difficult and often is delayed until cure is impossible.

RENAL ABSCESS
(Renal Carbuncle)

Etiology

Renal cortical abscesses develop primarily as a result of hematogenous spread of *Staphylococcus aureus* infections at distant sites (most often the skin). At times, foci of primary renal infections caused mainly by gram-negative bacteria (coliform organisms) coalesce in the renal medulla to form abscesses. In the past, most renal abscesses were caused by staphylococci; recently, coliform bacteria have become the predominant pathogens in renal abscesses. Renal abscesses caused by obligate anaerobic bacteria are rare.

Pathogenesis & Pathology
(Fig 13–7)

An abscess (carbuncle) caused by *S aureus* develops from hematogenous spread of the organism from a primary skin lesion. Intravenous drug abusers are especially prone to develop staphylococcal renal abscesses. Multiple focal abscesses evolve and eventually coalesce to form a multilocular abscess. Untreated cortical abscesses may rupture into the pyelocaliceal system or into the perinephric space (perinephric abscess). Urinary tract infection occurs only if the abscess communicates with pyelocaliceal system.

The more common type, renal medullary abscess, evolves from acute or chronic foci of pyelonephritis, often associated with ureteral obstruction or calculous disease (calculous pyonephrosis) (Malgieri, Kursh, and Persky, 1977). The infecting pathogens usually are gram-negative rods. Timmons and Perlmutter (1976) believe that gram-negative bacillary abscesses in children may be a complication of vesicoureteral reflux, with the pathogens invading the collecting tubules. In adults, the kidney usually is damaged by chronic suppurative pyelonephritis that may culminate in one or more abscesses. Medullary abscesses may also rupture into the perinephric space. One-third of affected patients are diabetics (Thorley, Jones, and Sanford, 1974).

Clinical Findings

A. Symptoms: Staphylococcal renal abscess is typified by an abrupt onset of chills, fever, and localized costovertebral pain. In the early stages, when the abscess does not communicate with the collecting system, symptoms of vesical irritability are absent and urinalysis is normal, although the patient may appear

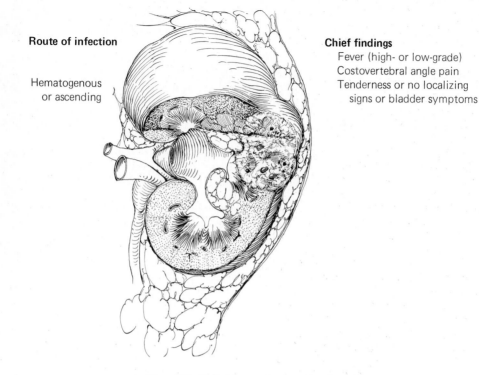

Route of infection

Hematogenous
or ascending

Chief findings
Fever (high- or low-grade)
Costovertebral angle pain
Tenderness or no localizing
signs or bladder symptoms

Figure 13–7. Pathogenesis of renal carbuncle.

quite septic. The clinical picture often mimics that of acute pyelonephritis.

In most patients with medullary abscesses due to gram-negative rods, there is a history of persistent or recurrent bouts of urinary tract infection, often associated with urolithiasis, obstructive uropathy, or renal surgery.

B. Signs: In acute cases, localizing signs are flank tenderness, possibly a palpable mass, and erythema and edema of the skin of the overlying loin. At times, however, abscesses associated with both acute and chronic infections present as febrile illnesses with few localizing signs.

C. Laboratory Findings: The hemogram usually shows marked leukocytosis with a shift to the left. With cortical abscesses that do not communicate with the collecting system, urinalysis shows no pyuria or bacteriuria, and urine culture is negative. Medullary abscesses generally are associated with heavy pyuria, bacteriuria, and positive urine cultures. The sudden appearance of heavy pyuria and bacteriuria may herald the rupture of a previously noncommunicating abscess into the collecting system. Blood cultures may be positive.

Depending upon the extent of renal involvement and associated renal abnormalities, the serum creatinine and urea nitrogen values may be normal or elevated. Since patients with renal abscesses often are diabetic, gylcosuria and hyperglycemia may be found.

D. X-Ray Findings: If the renal outline is visi-

ble, the plain film may show an enlarged kidney or a bulge of the external renal contour. With perinephric edema, however, often the renal outline is obliterated and the psoas shadow indistinct. Unless the abscess has ruptured into the perinephric space or is quite large, scoliosis generally is not observed. Renal stones may be noted.

When cortical abscesses are small, the excretory urogram may appear normal; most often, however, a space-occupying lesion (the abscess) is delineated (Fig 13–8). Pyelonephritic changes, hydronephrosis, and urolithiasis also may be observed. Delayed opacification or even a nonfunctioning kidney may be found.

Renal angiography may or may not be diagnostic. The abscess fails to opacify; its walls are irregular. Surrounding vessels are displaced, and hypervascularity is common. The most important sign is excessive capsular vessels overlying the abscess.

E. Ultrasonography: Renal echograms generally distinguish simple cysts (no internal echoes) from solid masses (many internal echoes) but often fail to distinguish renal abscesses from malignant lesions, particularly necrotic, cystic renal cell carcinomas. Percutaneous needle aspiration of the mass under ultrasonic guidance may confirm the diagnosis.

F. CT Scans: CT scanning is probably the most accurate diagnostic study. The attenuation coefficient value (CT number) varies considerably with the amount of liquid pus or solid debris within the abscess,

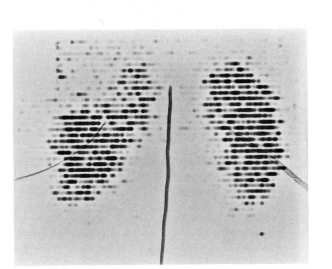

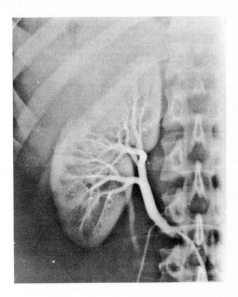

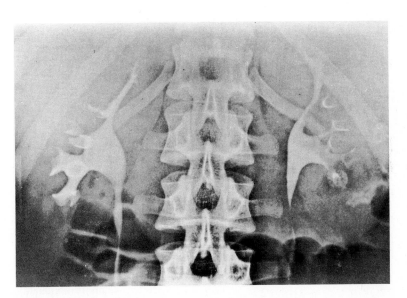

Figure 13–8. Renal carbuncle. *Upper left:* Renal scan revealing absence of functional renal tissue in superolateral portion, right kidney. *Upper right:* Selective renal angiogram, same patient, showing avascular mass in superolateral portion, right kidney. Surgical diagnosis: renal carbuncle. *Bottom:* Excretory urogram. Elongation of upper calix, right kidney. Carbuncle was a complication of measles.

and abscesses cannot be differentiated from hemorrhagic cysts or solid neoplasms with certainty. Percutaneous needle aspiration of the mass under CT control may confirm the diagnosis.

G. Isotope Scanning: The rectilinear scan will depict a space-occupying lesion (Fig 13–8). With the use of technetium and iodine compounds, the Anger camera will show an avascular mass lesion. These findings also are compatible with simple cyst. Gal-

lium-67 localizes in inflammatory tissue; an abscess will therefore "light up" on dynamic scanning. Gallium scanning may demonstrate an abscess even when excretory urograms are normal (Hopkins, Hall, and Mende, 1976).

Differential Diagnosis

In acute pyelonephritis, symptoms and signs may be similar to those of abscess; however, no space-occupying lesion is shown on the urogram, and a gallium scan will not show an abscess.

When symptoms of vesical irritability are absent and urinalysis is normal, renal abscess may be confused with acute cholecystitis. The presence of a palpable and tender gallbladder may make the diagnosis. Radiographic visualization of the gallbladder and kidneys should be definitive.

Acute appendicitis may be confused with renal abscess, because renal pain often radiates to the lower abdominal quadrant. The findings on physical examination, laboratory studies, and radiographic studies should allow differentiation.

At times, renal cell carcinoma may be confused with renal abscess, especially when there is fever related to tumor necrosis. Radiographic studies and scans usually will allow differentiation; however, percutaneous needle aspiration may be required in some cases.

Complications

Complications of renal abscess include both bacteremia with generalized sepsis and rupture of the abscess into the perinephrium.

Treatment

Staphylococcal abscesses should be treated with a penicillin resistant to β-lactamase. In the early stages, antibiotics alone may cure the abscess (Schiff et al, 1977). When the abscess is caused by gram-negative rod infection, therapy should consist of an aminoglycoside alone or in combination with a cephalosporin or other agent. Aminoglycosides are important in therapy because they are concentrated in renal parenchyma and thus may obviate the need for surgical drainage (Hoverman et al, 1980). Drainage by percutaneous means or surgical incision may be necessary. Relief of complicating urinary obstruction is mandatory. Nephrectomy and partial nephrectomy are required less often today than in the past.

Prognosis

The outlook is good provided the diagnosis is made promptly and effective therapy is instituted immediately.

PERINEPHRIC ABSCESS

Etiology

Perinephric abscesses lie between the renal capsule and the perirenal (Gerota's) fascia. Most result from rupture of an intrarenal abscess into the perinephric space; the causative organisms are usually coliform bacteria and *Pseudomonas,* less often staphylococci and obligate anaerobes.

Pathogenesis & Pathology
(Fig 13–9)

Staphylococcal perinephric abscesses probably originate from rupture of a small renal cortical abscess

or, less commonly, from a renal carbuncle. The primary renal lesion may heal, although the perinephric abscess progresses.

Usually, however, perinephric cellulitis and abscess complicate severe renal parenchymal infection caused by gram-negative bacteria in association with calculous pyonephrosis or infected hydronephrosis. It is presumed that spontaneous extravasation of infected material occurs. In this instance, pus and bacteria usually are found in the urine.

Perinephric abscesses may become quite large. When advanced, they tend to point over the iliac crest (Petit's triangle) posterolaterally.

Clinical Findings

A. Symptoms: The most common symptoms of perinephric abscess include chills, fever, unilateral flank pain, and abdominal pain. Malaise and prostration occur variably. Only about one-third of patients complain of dysuria.

B. Signs: Fever tends to be low-grade unless generalized sepsis evolves. There is usually marked tenderness over the affected kidney and costovertebral angle. A large mass may be felt or percussed in the flank. Abdominal tenderness accompanied by variable rebound tenderness may be elicited. The diaphragm on the affected side may be elevated and fixed. Ipsilateral pleural effusion is common. Scoliosis with the concavity to the affected side usually is seen; this results from spasm of the psoas muscle, which also causes the patient to lie with the ipsilateral leg flexed on the abdomen. Erythema and edema of the overlying skin may be evident. Minimal edema is best demonstrated by having the patient lie on a rough towel for a few minutes.

C. Laboratory Findings: Leukocytosis is usual but may be mild; a shift to left is commonly seen. The erythrocyte sedimentation rate usually is elevated; anemia may be present. Pyuria and bacteriuria are found commonly but not routinely. Blood cultures may be positive. Unless bilateral renal disease is present, the serum creatinine and blood urea nitrogen values generally are normal.

D. X-Ray Findings: A plain film of the abdomen typically shows evidence of a flank mass. Surrounding edema often results in obliteration of the renal and psoas shadows on the affected side. Scoliosis with the concavity to the affected side is common. The presence of a calcified body in this area suggests an abscess resulting from calculous pyonephrosis. Occasionally, a localized collection of gas caused by infection with gas-forming (coliform) organisms may be observed in the perirenal area.

Excretory urograms may show delayed visualization or nonfunction related to obstructive uropathy or parenchymal disease. Changes suggesting a space-occupying lesion (eg, carbuncle) may be noted; however, evidence of advanced hydronephrosis or calculous pyonephrosis is seen most commonly. Lack of mobility of the kidney with change in position of the patient or with respiration strongly suggests acute or

Route of infection

Direct extension
from kidney

Chief findings
Sepsis or low-grade fever
Costovertebral angle pain
Tenderness
Psoas spasm

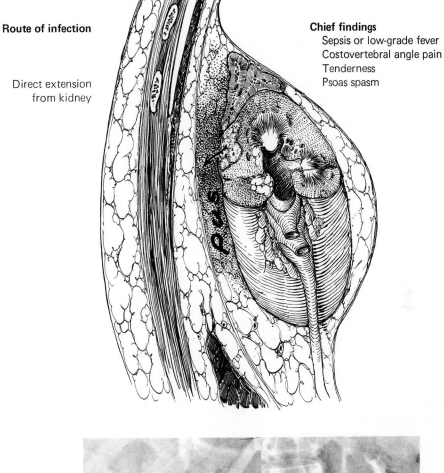

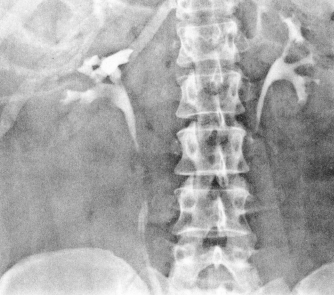

Figure 13–9. Perinephric abscess. *Top:* Pathogenesis. *Bottom:* Excretory urogram showing lateral displacement of lower pole of right kidney, scoliosis of spine, and absence of right psoas shadow. Note compression of upper right ureter by abscess.

chronic perinephritis. The entire kidney or only one pole may be displaced laterally by the abscess (Fig 13–9).

A barium enema may show displacement of the bowel anteriorly, laterally, or medially. Paralytic ileus may be observed on plain films of the abdomen or on upper gastrointestinal series.

Chest films may demonstrate an elevated diaphragm on the ipsilateral side; fluoroscopy often shows fixation on respiration. Some free pleural fluid and platelike atelectasis may be observed.

When the findings of excretory urography are equivocal, the performance of retrograde urograms may be helpful.

Gallium-67 localizes in inflammatory tissue; hence, the diagnosis often may be confirmed by use of the scintillation camera.

Echograms, CT scans, and renal angiograms may assist in diagnosis, especially when combined with percutaneous needle aspiration.

Differential Diagnosis

Acute renal infections cause many of the symptoms that accompany perinephric abscess: fever, localized pain, and tenderness. In acute pyelonephritis, the urine uniformly shows evidence of infection; in perinephric abscess, the urine may or may not show evidence of infection. X-ray studies and scans, however, should facilitate differentiation of these 2 conditions.

Infected hydronephrosis may cause fever and localized pain and tenderness and may account for the presence of a flank mass. Again, x-ray studies and scans should make the differentiation.

Paranephric abscess is a collection of pus external to the perirenal fascia and often is secondary to inflammatory disease of the spine (eg, tuberculosis). Many of the signs of perinephric abscess may be seen on a plain x-ray film, but the finding of a lesion in bone in the low thoracic area should suggest the correct diagnosis. Urograms are normal.

Complications

Unless the correct diagnosis is made promptly and effective therapy is initiated early, the mortality rate from generalized sepsis is quite high. Rarely, the perinephric abscess may point just above the iliac crest posterolaterally or extend downward into the iliac fossa and inguinal region. It is most unusual for the phlegmon to extend within the perirenal fascia across the midline to involve the opposite side of the body.

The abscess may produce considerable ureteral compression, giving rise to hydronephrosis. Even after drainage of the abscess, ureteral stenosis from periureteritis may evolve during the healing process.

Prevention

Early, effective treatment of urinary tract disease is the only means of preventing perinephric abscess. Appropriate therapy of urinary tract infection and removal of calculi and other obstructive conditions are of highest priority.

Treatment

Generally, treatment is similar to treatment for renal abscesses, except that surgical drainage usually is required for perinephric abscesses but may not be required for intrarenal abscesses. Intensive antimicrobial therapy, based upon culture and sensitivity testing of the pathogen isolated from urine, blood, or pus obtained by needle aspiration of the lesion, is mandatory. Unless adequate percutaneous drainage can be established, surgical drainage usually is needed. Because of underlying renal disease, nephrectomy may be required, either acutely or subsequent to initial control of the abscess. When nephrectomy is not required—indeed, even if the kidney itself is normal—excretory urography should be performed about 3 months after therapy is completed to make certain that late complications (eg, ureteral stenosis) are not missed.

Prognosis

Perinephric abscess often is fatal when diagnosis and appropriate therapy are delayed. A high index of suspicion and improved methods of diagnosis and treatment should offer a better prognosis than the 44% mortality rate observed by Thorley, Jones, and Sanford (1974).

NONSPECIFIC INFECTIONS OF THE URETER

Isolated infection of the lumen of the ureter does not occur. Ureteritis may accompany bacterial pyelonephritis or vesicoureteral reflux of infected bladder urine but causes few symptoms and generally is of little clinical importance. Ureteral infection caused by certain bacterial pathogens may interfere with normal peristaltic activity and result in ureteral dilatation of variable degree. On rare occasions, ureteral fibrosis may evolve. When the renal or bladder infection is cured, the ureteral inflammation usually subsides without sequels.

NONSPECIFIC INFECTIONS OF THE BLADDER

ACUTE CYSTITIS

Etiology & Pathogenesis

Acute bacterial cystitis is an infection of the urinary bladder caused mainly by coliform bacteria (usually strains of *E coli*) and less often by gram-positive aerobic bacteria (especially *Staphylococcus saprophyticus* and enterococci). The infection usually ascends to the bladder from the urethra. The pathogenesis and susceptibility factors involved in cystitis have been reviewed in detail earlier in this chapter. The incidence of acute cystitis is much greater in girls and women than in boys and men. Adenovirus infection may lead to hemorrhagic cystitis in children; however, viral cystitis rarely is found in adults.

Pathology

In the early stages of acute cystitis, the bladder mucosa typically shows hyperemia, edema, and infiltration by neutrophils. As the process advances, the mucosa is replaced by a friable, hemorrhagic, granular surface focally pitted with shallow ulcers containing exudate. The muscularis generally remains uninvolved.

Clinical Findings

A. Symptoms: Irritative voiding symptoms prevail: frequency, urgency, nocturia, burning on urination, and dysuria. Low back and suprapubic pain and discomfort are common complaints. Urge incontinence and hematuria occur commonly, but significant fever is unusual. The onset in women frequently follows sexual intercourse ("honeymoon cystitis").

B. Signs: Although suprapubic tenderness is sometimes elicited, no specific physical signs are characteristic. Possible associated contributing factors should be sought: vaginal, introital, or urethral abnormalities (eg, urethral diverticulum) or vaginal discharge in female patients; urethral discharge or a swollen, tender prostate or epididymis in male patients.

C. Laboratory Findings: The hemogram may be normal or show mild leukocytosis. Urinalysis typically shows pyuria and bacteriuria; gross or microscopic hematuria is seen on occasion. The infecting pathogen will be found on urine culture. Unless the patient has associated urologic disorders, the serum creatinine and blood urea nitrogen values are normal.

D. X-Ray Findings: Radiographic evaluation is warranted only if renal infection or genitourinary tract abnormalities are suspected. In patients with *Proteus* infections that do not respond promptly to therapy or that relapse, x-rays should be taken to investigate the possibility of infected struvite calculi.

E. Instrumental Examination: Cystoscopy usually is indicated when hematuria is prominent; however, the procedure should be delayed until the acute phase is over and the infection has been treated adequately.

Differential Diagnosis

In female patients, acute bacterial cystitis must be distinguished from several other infectious processes. Vulvovaginitis may mimic the symptoms of cystitis but can be diagnosed accurately by pelvic examination coupled with proper examination of vaginal discharge for pathogens. Acute urethral syndrome causes frequency and dysuria, but urine cultures show low counts or no growth of bacteria. Acute pyelonephritis

often causes symptoms of vesical irritability but typically produces loin pain and significant fever. In children, vulval and urethral irritation caused by detergents in bubble bath or by pinworms may mimic the symptoms of cystitis.

In male patients, acute bacterial cystitis must be distinguished mainly from infections of the urethra, prostate, and kidney. Appropriate physical examination and laboratory tests usually enable the physician to make a specific diagnosis.

Noninfectious types of cystitis produce symptoms that exactly mimic those of bacterial cystitis. Some of these conditions include cystitis resulting from anticancer therapy (eg, irradiation, cyclophosphamide), interstitial cystitis, eosinophilic cystitis ("allergic" cystitis), bladder carcinoma (especially carcinoma in situ), and psychosomatic disorders.

Complications

The main complication of acute cystitis is infection that ascends to the kidneys. Children with vesicoureteral reflux and pregnant women are especially prone to this complication.

Prevention

Patients prone to recurrent bouts of acute cystitis should be evaluated for factors that may contribute to enhanced susceptibility, and these should be corrected whenever possible. Failing this, antimicrobial prophylaxis may prove necessary (see Antimicrobial Treatment of Urinary Tract Infections, p 232).

Treatment

A. Specific Measures: Although its efficacy has not been proved in men, the use of short-term antimicrobial therapy (1–3 days or even a single dose) is effective in acute uncomplicated cystitis in women. Ideally, an antimicrobial agent should be selected on the basis of culture and sensitivity testing. Since most uncomplicated infections occurring outside the hospital environment are due to strains of *E coli* sensitive to many antibiotics, sulfonamides, trimethoprim-sulfamethoxazole, nitrofurantoin, or ampicillin usually is effective. Urologic evaluation is warranted when the response is unsatisfactory.

B. General Measures: Because acute uncomplicated cystitis responds rapidly to proper antimicrobial therapy, additional measures usually are unnecessary. Hot sitz baths, anticholinergics (eg, propantheline bromide), and urinary analgesics (eg, phenazopyridine hydrochloride) are occasionally warranted for relief of symptoms.

Prognosis

Acute uncomplicated bacterial cystitis usually resolves rapidly in response to appropriate antimicrobial therapy. Permanent bladder injury is unusual.

ACUTE URETHRAL SYNDROME IN WOMEN

Acute urethral syndrome consists of dysuria and frequency (plus variable other bladder or urethral symptoms) in women whose bladder urine shows "no growth" or low bacterial counts on culture. Gallagher, Montgomerie, and North (1965) found that, in a general practice setting, 41% of women with such irritative voiding symptoms had urine cultures deemed nondiagnostic of bacterial cystitis; however, documented bacteriuria of significance occurred in about a third of these women within the ensuing few months. Fihn and Stamm (1983) were able to categorize acutely dysuric women into groups with specific therapeutic implications, as follows:

(1) Vaginitis (32%).

(2) Typical cystitis, with growth of $\geq 10^5$ bacteria per milliliter of midstream urine (32%).

(3) Acute urethral syndrome (36%).

(a) Pyuria present (22%) (bladder bacteriuria in 15%, and chlamydial infection in 7%).

(b) Pyuria absent; sterile urine (12%).

(c) Other pathogens, including herpes simplex and *N gonorrhoeae* (2%).

In evaluating an acutely dysuric woman, the physician should check routinely for the presence of vaginitis, obtain vaginal specimens for diagnosis, and treat any recognized infection. Women in whom dense bacteriuria is found on culture clearly have bacterial cystitis that usually responds promptly to appropriate antimicrobial therapy. Acutely dysuric women without vaginitis or classic bacterial cystitis generally have acute urethral syndrome.

Acute urethral syndrome itself is not a homogeneous group. Many women with pyuria and "low-count" bacteriuria actually have bacterial urethrocystitis and should be treated appropriately with the usual antimicrobial agent of choice. In a second group, cultures are positive for organisms that may be sexually transmitted. These women and their sexual partners should be treated with an appropriate antibiotic: a tetracycline or erythromycin for *C trachomatis* infection; a penicillin or tetracycline (see p 265) for gonorrhea. In a third group, no causative pathogen is identifiable, but, curiously, the dysuria will respond to antimicrobial therapy. A small group of women with no pyuria or identifiable pathogen will respond poorly to antimicrobial therapy; some clinicians believe that these women may suffer from some type of functional voiding dysfunction.

CHRONIC CYSTITIS

Etiology & Pathogenesis

Like "chronic pyelonephritis," the term "chronic cystitis" is confusing because it means different things to different people: some physicians use this term exclusively to mean unresolved or persistent bladder infection, whereas others use it to mean 3 or more bouts of bladder infection occurring in the course of 1 year.

Chronic infectious cystitis is caused by the same pathogens that cause acute cystitis and acute and chronic pyelonephritis. The factors implicated in chronic bladder infections are reviewed on p 200.

Pathology

Persistence of bladder infection beyond the acute stage leads to chronic cystitis, which differs from the acute form mainly in the character of the inflammatory infiltrate. In the early stages of chronic cystitis, the bladder mucosa becomes progressively more edematous, erythematous, and friable; it may ulcerate. In the later stages of chronic infection, the submucosa is infiltrated by fibroblasts, plasma cells, and lymphocytes; the bladder wall eventually becomes thickened, fibrotic, and inelastic.

Clinical Findings

A. Symptoms: Patients with chronic cystitis are asymptomatic or have variable symptoms of vesical irritability. If the bladder infection is caused by a persistent source of infection in the kidneys or prostate, there may also be symptoms associated with the primary infection. Pneumaturia suggests an enterovesical fistula or infection caused by a gas-forming pathogen (usually a coliform organism). The latter is seen most often in diabetics.

B. Signs: Physical findings often are absent and usually are sparse and nonspecific.

C. Laboratory Findings: Unless chronic cystitis is associated with a serious primary genitourinary tract disorder, the hemogram and renal function studies usually are normal. Urinalysis typically shows significant bacteriuria but may show surprisingly little pyuria. Urine culture generally is positive.

D. X-Ray Findings: Unless chronic cystitis is associated with other genitourinary tract disease, radiographic studies usually are normal. Excretory and retrograde urograms and voiding cystograms may demonstrate associated conditions (eg, obstructive uropathy, vesicoureteral reflux, atrophic pyelonephritis, vesicoenteric or vesicovaginal fistulas).

E. Instrumental Examination: Urethral calibration, catheterization, and urethrocystoscopy may be indicated to evaluate whether contributing conditions (eg, urethral stricture, prostatic obstruction) exist.

Differential Diagnosis

Infectious types of chronic cystitis must be distinguished from other infectious diseases of the genitourinary tract in men and women. Sometimes these conditions mimic cystitis; sometimes they are associated with or contribute to chronic cystitis. Examples include infectious vaginitis, prostatitis, and urethritis and renal infections. Tuberculosis of the kidney or bladder must be considered in the differential diagnosis of chronic cystitis characterized by "sterile" pyuria.

Noninfectious conditions that must be considered

in the differential diagnosis include senile vaginitis and urethritis related to hormonal deficiency, noninfectious urethral disease, nonbacterial forms of prostatitis, interstitial cystitis, "allergic" cystitis, radiation cystitis, cystitis secondary to the use of chemotherapeutic (including anticancer) agents, and various psychosomatic syndromes.

Complications

Chronic bladder infections may lead to ascending infection of the kidneys, the development of infected calculi in the upper urinary tract and bladder, or secondary infection of the prostate or epididymis.

Prevention

The prevention of chronic cystitis depends upon the identification of causative and contributing factors and the relative success of correcting these factors.

Treatment

The causative organism should be identified by culture, and the infection should be treated with appropriate antimicrobial therapy based upon susceptibility testing. Long-term preventive therapy or suppressive therapy with agents such as nitrofurantoin, trimethoprim-sulfamethoxazole, or methenamine plus an acidifier may prove necessary.

The most important aspect of treatment is thorough evaluation for underlying causes and appropriate correction of contributing factors when possible.

Prognosis

Uncomplicated chronic cystitis may produce annoying illness but seldom leads to serious sequels unless infection ascends to the kidney. The outlook varies considerably with the nature and severity of underlying causes and contributing factors.

NONSPECIFIC INFECTIONS OF THE PROSTATE GLAND

ACUTE BACTERIAL PROSTATITIS

Etiology

Acute bacterial prostatitis is mainly caused by aerobic gram-negative rods. The coliforms (especially strains of *E coli*) and *Pseudomonas* predominate. Most authorities agree that enterococci (*S faecalis*) cause bacterial prostatitis; however, whether other gram-positive aerobic bacteria cause prostatitis is doubtful. Current evidence suggests that obligate anaerobic bacteria rarely cause prostate infections.

Pathogenesis & Pathology

The possible routes of prostatic infection include (1) ascent from the urethra, (2) reflux of infected urine into prostatic ducts that empty into the posterior urethra, (3) direct extension or lymphatogenous spread of bacteria from the rectum, and (4) hematogenous spread. Ascending infection and reflux of infected urine into prostatic ducts are probably the most common routes of prostatic infection.

Acute bacterial infection of the prostate usually is associated with acute cystitis and often results in acute urinary retention. The acute infection may resolve completely in response to appropriate therapy or may progress to abscess formation. Marked inflammation of part or all of the prostate gland is characteristic. Numerous polymorphonuclear leukocytes are noted within and around the acini, along with intraductal desquamation and cellular debris and varying degrees of tissue invasion by lymphocytes, plasma cells, and macrophages. Diffuse edema and hyperemia of the stroma are seen. Microabscesses may occur early; large abscesses are late complications.

Clinical Findings

A. Symptoms: Acute bacterial prostatitis is an acute febrile illness characterized by chills, low back and perineal pain, urinary urgency and frequency, nocturia, dysuria, and varying degrees of bladder outlet obstruction. Both myalgia and arthralgia are common.

B. Signs: Moderate or high-grade fever usually is present. Rectal palpation typically discloses an exquisitely tender, swollen prostate gland that is firm, indurated, and warm to the touch. The acute inflammatory process may affect all or only part of the gland. Since acute cystitis often accompanies acute bacterial prostatitis, the urine may be cloudy and malodorous. Initial, terminal, or even total gross hematuria may be observed occasionally.

C. Laboratory Findings: The hemogram typically shows leukocytosis with a shift to the left. The voided urine usually shows significant pyuria, microscopic hematuria, and bacilluria. The infecting pathogen can usually be identified by culture of the voided urine. The prostatic expressate is purulent and yields the infecting pathogen in heavy growth on culture plates. However, because massage of an acutely infected prostate is painful for the patient and can produce bacteremia, prostatic massage is generally contraindicated.

D. Instrumental Examination: Transurethral instrumentation should be avoided during the acute stage of bacterial prostatitis. Acute urinary retention requiring bladder drainage is best managed by placement of a punch suprapubic tube under local anesthesia. Transurethral catheterization should be avoided.

Differential Diagnosis

Acute pyelonephritis may be accompanied by severe bladder irritability; in prostatitis, however, the backache is usually sacral, while in pyelonephritis, it is lumbar. The characteristic findings on rectal examination in acute prostatitis easily allow differentiation from acute upper urinary tract infection.

Acute diverticulitis involving the rectosigmoid

may at times be confused with acute prostatitis, especially if an inflammatory mass or abscess is present. However, careful history taking and physical examination generally will differentiate these 2 conditions.

Acute nonspecific granulomatous prostatitis must be differentiated from simple acute bacterial prostatitis. The acute eosinophilic variety of granulomatous prostatitis occurs mainly in men with a history of severe allergy or bronchial asthma. It usually presents as one of several manifestations of a generalized vasculitis; it is also characterized by a high number of eosinophils in the bloodstream. The noneosinophilic variety of nonspecific granulomatous prostatitis at times is associated with coliform infection of the prostate. Diagnosis should usually be confirmed by histologic examination of biopsy specimens.

The intense tissue reaction to acute bacterial infection within the prostate may be confused with prostatic carcinoma. However, as the inflammatory reaction resolves following appropriate treatment of an infection, the palpable abnormalities of the prostate revert to normal findings; in prostatic carcinoma, abnormal findings on prostatic palpation persist.

Complications

The marked swelling of the prostate gland associated with acute prostatitis may lead to acute urinary retention. The urinary retention usually resolves without the need for surgical intervention as the prostatitis responds to therapy. One or more large abscesses may evolve and rupture spontaneously into the urethra, rectum, or perineum. Acute bacterial cystitis usually accompanies acute bacterial prostatitis; acute pyelonephritis eventually may evolve. Unilateral or bilateral acute bacterial epididymitis may develop. The most serious complication of acute bacterial prostatitis is bacteremia and possible septic shock.

Prevention

A better understanding of the biologic factors that increase the susceptibility of some men to ascending genitourinary tract infection is essential before acute bacterial prostatitis can be effectively prevented. Iatrogenic infection can be minimized by use of strict aseptic technique during urethral instrumentation. Furthermore, urethral instrumentation should never be undertaken unless the urine is known to be sterile.

Treatment

A. Specific Measures: Patients with acute bacterial prostatitis often respond dramatically to therapy with antimicrobial agents that normally diffuse poorly from plasma into prostatic fluid. The intense and diffuse inflammatory reaction of acute bacterial prostatitis undoubtedly enhances the passage of antimicrobial agents into prostatic tissues and secretions. An appropriate drug should be selected by in vitro susceptibility testing and administered in doses that produce bactericidal levels in the bloodstream. Since the causative organisms are usually gram-negative rods, preferred initial therapy is with trimethoprim-sulfamethoxazole (trimethoprim, 160 mg, and sulfamethoxazole, 800 mg, orally twice daily) until the results of culture and sensitivity testing are known. If the pathogen is sensitive to these drugs and the clinical response is favorable, this regimen should be continued for at least 30 days to prevent the development of chronic bacterial prostatitis. Alternatively, initial therapy with gentamicin or tobramycin, 3–5 mg/kg/d divided into 3 intravenous or intramuscular doses, plus ampicillin, 2 g intravenously every 6 hours, is recommended until the results of culture and sensitivity tests are known. A suitable oral antimicrobial agent can be substituted after about 1 week and continued for at least 30 days in full dosage. After completion of successful therapy, the patient should be followed for at least 4 months with periodic examinations and cultures of prostatic fluid to ensure that the infection was cured.

Transurethral instrumentation is contraindicated during acute infection. Acute urinary retention requiring bladder drainage is best managed by the insertion of a punch suprapubic tube until the inflammation subsides and the patient can void without assistance. If a large prostatic abscess develops, perineal needle drainage in addition to antimicrobial drugs may lead to resolution of the infection. Incisional perineal drainage or transurethral unroofing of the abscess may be necessary. Transrectal prostatic ultrasonography and pelvic CT scan may help confirm the diagnosis of a prostatic abscess and prove useful in drainage procedures.

B. General Measures: Hospitalization may be required, especially if acute urinary retention develops. General supportive measures such as bed rest, hydration, medication for fever and pain, and stool softeners are indicated.

Prognosis

Unless the patient develops septicemia and septic shock, the prognosis generally is good with prompt and appropriate therapy. When antibacterial management is effective, most patients with acute bacterial prostatitis do not develop chronic bacterial prostatitis.

PROSTATIC ABSCESS

In recent years, the incidence of prostatic abscess has decreased and the type of infecting organism has changed. Fifty years ago, 75% of prostatic abscesses were caused by gonococci; more recently, about 70% of prostatic abscesses have been caused by coliform bacteria, mostly *E coli* (Dajani and O'Flynn, 1968; Pai and Bhat, 1972).

Although the pathogenesis remains unclear, most cases of prostatic abscess are probably complications of acute bacterial prostatitis. Prostatic abscess has been reported in a 46-day-old infant; however, most cases occur in men in the fifth or sixth decade of life. Diabetics seem especially prone to prostatic abscess.

The signs and symptoms of prostatic abscess can exactly mimic those of acute bacterial prostatitis. The findings on rectal examination are variable; however, the gland usually is tender and enlarged, with the affected lobe predominating. Fluctuation is an important diagnostic clue; unfortunately, it often is not apparent until after several days of therapy for acute prostatitis. An initial favorable clinical response to the treatment of acute bacterial prostatitis followed by a worsening of the clinical picture is always suggestive of abscess formation. The abscess can rupture spontaneously into the urethra. Once the diagnosis of prostatic abscess is made, preferred treatment consists of surgical drainage combined with appropriate antimicrobial therapy. Drainage by transperineal insertion of a large-bore needle sometimes suffices; however, transurethral resection or perineal incision often is necessary for adequate drainage. With proper diagnosis and therapy, the overall prognosis is good; recurrent abscesses are rare.

CHRONIC BACTERIAL PROSTATITIS

Etiology

Chronic bacterial prostatitis is a nonacute infection of the prostate caused by one or more specific bacteria. As in acute bacterial prostatitis, the causative agents typically are gram-negative aerobes: the coliforms (mainly strains of *E coli*) and *Pseudomonas*. Some clinicians believe that gram-positive bacteria (eg, staphylococci, streptococci, diphtheroids) cause prostatitis; unlike prostatic infections due to gram-negative organisms, however, those due to gram-positive bacteria rarely persist and lead to relapsing recurrent urinary tract infection. A notable exception is *S faecalis* prostatitis. Most authorities agree that gram-positive organisms other than *S faecalis* play a doubtful role in chronic bacterial prostatitis. Current evidence also suggests that mycoplasmas, ureaplasmas, and chlamydiae are infrequent causes of prostatic infections (see Nonbacterial Prostatitis, p 227).

Pathogenesis & Pathology

The possible routes of infection are the same in acute and chronic bacterial prostatitis (see p 224). At times, chronic bacterial prostatitis clearly evolves from unresolved acute prostatitis; sometimes, however, there is no history of acute prostatitis.

The histologic findings in chronic bacterial prostatitis are nonspecific: the inflammatory reaction is less intense and more focal than in acute bacterial prostatitis. Variable infiltration within and around the acini and in the stroma by plasma cells, macrophages, and lymphocytes is typical. Kohnen and Drach (1979) observed similar histologic findings in 98% of the specimens from 162 men who underwent prostatectomy for hyperplastic prostates. Few of their patients had clinical or bacteriologic evidence of infected prostatic tissue; therefore, a definitive diagnosis of chronic bacterial prostatitis cannot be confirmed by histologic means.

Clinical Findings

A. Symptoms: The symptoms of chronic bacterial prostatitis are variable. Some patients are asymptomatic and are diagnosed eventually only because asymptomatic bacteriuria is found incidentally; most have varying degrees of irritative voiding dysfunction (eg, urgency, frequency, nocturia, dysuria) and low back or perineal pain or discomfort. Chills and fever are unusual and most often indicate an acute flare-up of a chronic prostatic infection. Occasionally, myalgia and arthralgia accompany the other symptoms.

B. Signs: On rectal examination, the prostate may feel normal, boggy, or focally indurated. Crepitation may be felt when large prostatic stones are present. Initial or terminal hematuria, hemospermia, and urethral discharge are unusual findings. Secondary epididymitis sometimes is associated with chronic bacterial prostatitis.

C. Laboratory Findings: Unless secondary epididymitis is present or the patient experiences an acute flare-up of the chronic infection, the hemogram usually is normal, without leukocytosis. The prostatic secretions obtained by prostatic massage typically show excessive numbers of inflammatory cells. Many researchers and clinicians believe that more than 10 white cells per high-power field in prostatic fluid is excessive; most agree that the presence of more than 15 white cells per high-power field represents leukocytosis. The presence of large numbers of lipid-laden macrophages in prostatic fluid correlates particularly well with the presence of prostatic inflammation. When secondary cystitis is present, the midstream urine may show pyuria and bacteriuria caused by the organism infecting the prostate.

When the urine itself is not infected, the location of the infecting organism can be determined by obtaining for culture essentially simultaneous segmented specimens from the urethra, midstream urine, and prostatic secretions obtained by prostatic massage (Meares and Stamey, 1968). With this technique, the physician carefully obtains from the patient the first voided 10 mL of urine (urethral specimen), a late midstream urine sample (bladder specimen), a specimen of uncontaminated pure prostatic secretions (by means of prostatic massage), and the first voided 10 mL of urine immediately following prostatic massage (prostatic specimen). The specimens are surface-streaked onto both blood agar and MacConkey agar and incubated for 24–48 hours. Standard microbiologic methods are used to identify specific bacterial growth. When the bladder specimen is sterile or nearly so, the bacterial colony counts of the other specimens are compared to localize the site of infection to the urethra or prostate: If the bacterial count of the urethral specimen significantly exceeds (by at least 10-fold) those of the prostatic specimens, the organisms are localized to the urethra; if the reverse is true, the infection is localized to the prostate.

D. X-Ray Findings: Plain films or excretory urograms are normal unless there are complications (eg, prostatic calculi, prostatic enlargement, urethral stricture, renal infection).

E. Instrumental Examination: Cystoscopy and

urethroscopy may reveal normal findings or erythema and edema of the prostatic urethra, with or without inflammatory polyps. These findings are not specifically diagnostic of chronic bacterial prostatitis and may be seen in other forms of prostatic inflammation. Endoscopy is indicated mainly to evaluate whether complicating factors (eg, prostatic enlargement, urethral stricture, renal infection) exist.

Differential Diagnosis

The symptoms of acute or chronic urethritis may suggest prostatitis; however, stained smears and cultures of segmented specimens from the urethra, bladder urine, and prostatic secretions generally identify the site of inflammation and infection.

Cystitis may be confused with chronic bacterial prostatitis and at times is a complication of prostatic infection. Again, segmented specimens for microscopic examination and culture as outlined above will identify the site of infection. If cystitis accompanies an underlying bacterial prostatitis, the presence of prostatic infection can be confirmed by repeating the localization cultures after the bladder urine has been sterilized by means of an appropriate antimicrobial agent that is bactericidal at urinary levels but diffuses poorly into prostatic secretions (eg, nitrofurantoin, penicillin G).

Diseases of the anus (eg, fissure, thrombosed hemorrhoid) may cause perineal pain and even urinary urgency; physical examination, however, should make the diagnosis obvious.

Complications

Relapsing recurrent urinary tract infection is the hallmark of chronic bacterial prostatitis. Although the signs and symptoms of urinary tract infection generally clear quickly as the urine is sterilized during appropriate antibacterial therapy, recurrent infection with the same pathogen at variable intervals following completion of therapy is the rule; the pathogen remains unaltered in the prostate despite sterilization of the urine because most standard antibacterial agents diffuse poorly into prostatic fluid, and after completion of therapy, the bacteria that persist within the prostatic secretions can eventually reinfect the urine.

Ascending bacterial infection of the upper urinary tract and bacterial epididymitis are both potential complications of chronic bacterial prostatitis. Infected prostatic calculi may develop and result in chronic infection that is incurable by medical therapy. Bladder outlet obstruction due to bladder neck contracture sometimes accompanies chronic bacterial prostatitis, but whether there is a causal relationship remains unclear.

Prevention

Prevention is difficult because susceptibility factors are not well defined. Prostatic fluid normally contains a zinc compound that is a potent antibacterial factor, but this is markedly reduced in men with chronic bacterial prostatitis (Fair, Couch, and Wehner, 1976).

Fair and associates believe that this prostatic antibacterial factor may serve as a natural defense mechanism against ascending genital and urinary tract infection in men, but they have been unable to stimulate this factor or raise the level of zinc in prostatic secretions by oral administration of zinc to male patients. Preventing chronic bacterial prostatitis by means of vigorous treatment of acute bacterial prostatitis is always indicated. Strict aseptic technique must be used during urethral instrumentation and in the management of inlying urethral catheters to prevent iatrogenic prostatic infection.

Treatment

A. Specific Measures:

1. Medical measures – Pharmacokinetic studies in dogs confirm the clinical experience in humans: few antimicrobial agents achieve therapeutic levels in prostatic secretions in instances of nonacute inflammation (Meares, 1982; Sharer and Fair, 1982). Trimethoprim does diffuse into prostatic fluid and has the best-documented success in curing chronic bacterial prostatitis due to susceptible pathogens. Long-term therapy (12 weeks) has proved more successful than short-term therapy (2 weeks) in achieving cures.

For nonazotemic men with chronic bacterial prostatitis, one of the following is recommended (the causative organism must be proved by culture to be susceptible to the drug chosen):

a. Trimethoprim-sulfamethoxazole, 1 double-strength tablet (trimethoprim, 160 mg, and sulfamethoxazole, 800 mg) orally twice daily for 12 weeks.

b. Trimethoprim, 2 tablets (each containing 100 mg) orally twice daily for 12 weeks.

c. Carbenicillin indanyl sodium, 2 tablets (each containing 383 mg) orally 4 times daily for at least 4 weeks.

d. Minocycline, 100 mg orally twice daily for at least 4 weeks.

e. Erythromycin, 500 mg orally 4 times daily for at least 4 weeks.

Specific therapy must always be individualized to meet the patient's needs and drug tolerance.

Most men whose chronic bacterial prostatitis is not cured by medical therapy may be kept relatively comfortable if the bladder urine is kept sterile by continuous use of low-dose daily suppressive therapy with an appropriate oral agent (eg, nitrofurantoin, 100 mg once a day; or trimethoprim-sulfamethoxazole, 1 single-strength tablet daily). If suppressive therapy is discontinued, the bladder urine will eventually be reinfected and symptoms will return.

2. Surgical measures – Patients whose chronic bacterial prostatitis is not cured or adequately controlled by medical therapy may be candidates for surgical treatment. Indeed, men with chronic bacterial infection of the prostate and prostatic stones often are candidates for operation, since infected prostatic calculi cannot be sterilized by means of antimicrobial therapy alone. Radical prostatovesiculectomy is curative; unfortunately, the sequels of this operation (sexual impotence and possible urinary incontinence) seldom make this a desirable choice. Transurethral prostatectomy can be curative provided that all infected stones and tissue are successfully removed; unfortunately, this may be difficult to achieve, especially since the peripheral zone of the prostate usually contains the most foci of infection.

B. General Measures: Symptoms can be relieved by the liberal use of hot sitz baths. Irritative voiding discomfort and pain often respond to the use of anti-inflammatory agents (eg, indomethacin, ibuprofen) and anticholinergic drugs (eg, oxybutynin chloride, propantheline bromide).

Prognosis

Chronic bacterial prostatitis is difficult to cure permanently, but its symptoms and tendency to cause recurrent urinary tract infections generally can be controlled by suppressive antimicrobial therapy.

NONBACTERIAL PROSTATITIS

Etiology

Nonbacterial prostatitis clearly is the most common of the prostatitis syndromes; its cause is unknown. Men with nonbacterial prostatitis have abnormal numbers of inflammatory cells in their prostatic expressates, but no causative infectious agent can be found by culture or other means. Efforts to prove that unusual pathogens (eg, obligate anaerobic bacteria, mycoplasmas, ureaplasmas, chlamydiae, trichomonads or other protozoons, and viruses) cause nonbacterial prostatitis generally have been unsuccessful. There has been much speculation but little proof that chlamydial infection is responsible for many cases of apparent nonbacterial prostatitis. Indeed, careful studies using cultures and serologic tests (eg, Mardh et al, 1978) have shown no causal relationship between chlamydial infection and prostatitis. Likewise, Weidner et al (1980) found little evidence that infection due to *U urealyticum* plays an important role in prostatitis. Some researchers believe that nonbacterial prostatitis is an autoimmune disease of the prostate. The diagnosis of nonbacterial prostatitis is confirmed only by exclusion of other specific forms of prostatitis.

Pathogenesis & Pathology

The cause and pathogenesis of nonbacterial prostatitis are unknown. The histopathologic findings are nonspecific and resemble those seen in chronic bacterial prostatitis.

Clinical Findings

The signs and symptoms of nonbacterial and bacterial prostatitis are similar except that documented urinary tract infection almost never occurs in the former. Although excessive numbers of inflammatory cells are characteristically present in the prostatic secretions of patients with nonbacterial prostatitis, no causative agent can be identified by localization cultures or other

methods. X-ray and endoscopic examination are not helpful in diagnosis except to rule out associated nonspecific conditions.

Differential Diagnosis

Nonbacterial prostatitis must be differentiated from other specific forms of prostatitis, especially chronic bacterial prostatitis. At times, urethritis and cystitis must be considered in the differential diagnosis. In middle-aged and older men with irritative voiding symptoms and negative results of cultures for prostatitis or cystitis, the possibility of a bladder tumor, especially carcinoma in situ, must be carefully evaluated. In such cases, although cytologic examination of the urine may be helpful, cystoscopy with bladder biopsy often is indicated.

Complications

Nonbacterial prostatitis causes no known organic complications, but the anxiety, depression, and other emotional stress that often accompany the recurrent symptoms of this poorly understood condition can result in significant morbidity.

Prevention

Since the cause of nonbacterial prostatitis is unknown, prevention is not possible.

Treatment

A. Specific Measures: When bacteriologic localization cultures fail to demonstrate a causative pathogen in a patient with symptoms of chronic prostatitis and prostatic secretions indicative of inflammation, the clinician is left with a diagnosis of nonbacterial prostatitis. Because it is not known with certainty whether mycoplasmas, chlamydiae, and ureaplasmas cause apparent nonbacterial prostatitis, a clinical trial of antimicrobial therapy directed against these agents is recommended. Either minocycline, 100 mg orally twice daily, or erythromycin, 500 mg orally 4 times daily, should be tried for at least 4 weeks. Trimethoprim and carbenicillin are not effective.

Because nonbacterial prostatitis does not usually respond to antibiotic therapy, the continued empiric use of antibiotics is not justified; instead, therapy must be directed toward control of symptoms. Symptomatic flare-ups often respond to anti-inflammatory agents (eg, ibuprofen, 400–600 mg orally 3 times daily).

Most authorities agree that prostatectomy is not indicated in the management of nonbacterial prostatitis. Patients must be made to understand that they have a noninfectious inflammatory disorder of the prostate (similar to noninfectious arthritis) that tends to be chronic and may cause annoying symptoms but has no serious sequels and is not life-threatening.

B. General Measures: The liberal use of hot sitz baths usually affords symptomatic relief. Dietary restrictions, especially of alcoholic beverages, coffee, and spicy foods, are not necessary unless the patient has noted exacerbation of symptoms in association with such foods. The patient should be encouraged to live as normal a life as possible. Normal sexual activity should be encouraged. Some clinicians advocate periodic "therapeutic" prostatic massage, but others question its efficacy.

Prognosis

Nonbacterial prostatitis causes annoying intermittent symptoms but no known serious sequels. Until the cause of this condition is known, prevention and cure are not possible.

PROSTATODYNIA

In some men with symptoms suggestive of prostatitis, especially "prostatic" or "pelvic" pain and discomfort, there is no documented history of urinary tract infection and no apparent prostatic inflammation, and microscopy and culture disclose no abnormality of the prostatic expressates. These men suffer from prostatodynia, a syndrome of variable cause (Drach et al, 1978).

In some patients with prostatodynia, urodynamic testing discloses voiding dysfunction associated with apparent functional obstruction of the bladder neck and prostatic urethra near the external urethral sphincter (Meares and Barbalias, 1983). This "spasm" during voiding results in a higher than normal pressure within the prostatic urethra that may produce intraprostatic reflux and chemical irritation of the prostate by urine. In such cases, there is a favorable response to α-blocking agents (eg, prazosin, 2–4 mg orally twice daily).

In other cases, there is apparent tension myalgia of the pelvic floor; this responds best to treatment using diathermy, muscle relaxants, and physiotherapy, with or without the use of diazepam, 5 mg orally 3 times daily (Segura et al, 1979).

In still others, emotional problems seem primary; psychiatric consultation is warranted for these patients.

NONSPECIFIC GRANULOMATOUS PROSTATITIS

Nonspecific granulomatous prostatitis is seen occasionally; it may be eosinophilic or noneosinophilic. The eosinophilic variety typically occurs in men who are asthmatic or prone to allergies. The apparent underlying cause is a type of vasculitis. The noneosinophilic variety probably results from a granulomatous reaction within the prostate that is caused by extravasation of prostatic secretions from the ducts and acini into the stroma. Both varieties present clinically as acute, febrile illnesses characterized by irritative and obstructive voiding dysfunction. The prostate often is markedly swollen and indurated, simulating advanced carcinoma. Prostatic biopsy is required to confirm the diagnosis. Both varieties usually respond dramatically to therapy with steroids.

NONSPECIFIC INFECTIONS OF THE SEMINAL VESICLES

Although infections of the seminal vesicles undoubtedly occur, clinical proof generally is not possible with currently available diagnostic methods. It is not known whether such infections occur without concomitant infection of the prostate. Random histopathologic studies at autopsy suggest that the incidence of seminal vesiculitis is low; however, its incidence in men with clinical signs and symptoms of prostatitis apparently has not been well documented by histopathologic study.

It is not now possible to obtain "pure" seminal vesicular fluid for culture and analysis. Semen analyses that show a low volume of ejaculate and subnormal fructose levels suggest secretory dysfunction of the seminal vesicles but do not confirm an infectious cause of this dysfunction. Moreover, a positive culture or abnormal results of cytologic examination of the semen cannot be used to confirm a diagnosis of seminal vesiculitis with certainty.

Suspected cases of seminal vesiculitis are probably best managed by the regimens used to treat chronic bacterial prostatitis.

NONSPECIFIC INFECTIONS OF THE MALE URETHRA

See Chapter 15.

NONSPECIFIC INFECTIONS OF THE EPIDIDYMIS

ACUTE EPIDIDYMITIS

Etiology

Although occasional cases of epididymal inflammation are caused by trauma or reflux of sterile urine from the urethra through the vas deferens, most cases can be divided into 2 groups: (1) a sexually transmitted form associated with urethritis and commonly caused by *C trachomatis* and *N gonorrhoeae* (singly or in combination), and (2) a primarily non-sexually transmitted form associated with urinary tract infections and prostatitis and caused mainly by Enterobacteriaceae or *Pseudomonas*. The hydrostatic pressure associated with voiding or physical strain may force urine containing pathogens from the urethra or prostate up the ejaculatory ducts and through the vas deferens to reach the epididymis, or infection may reach the epididymis through the perivasal lymphatics. Recurrent epididymitis in a young boy suggests the possibility of ureteral drainage into a seminal vesicle. Tuberculous epididymitis now occurs infrequently in the USA; however, it is common in areas where pulmonary tuberculosis is still a public health problem.

Pathogenesis & Pathology

In its early stages, epididymitis is a cellular inflammation (cellulitis). It generally begins in the vas deferens and descends to the lower pole of the epididymis.

In the acute stage, the epididymis is swollen and indurated. The infection spreads from the lower to the upper pole. On section, small abscesses may be seen. The tunica vaginalis often secretes serous fluid (inflammatory hydrocele), which may become purulent. The spermatic cord becomes thickened. The testis becomes swollen secondarily from passive congestion but rarely becomes involved in the infectious process.

Histologically, changes range from edema and infiltration with neutrophils, plasma cells, and lymphocytes to actual abscess formation. The tubular epithelium may show necrosis. The infection may resolve completely without residual injury, but peritubular fibrosis often develops and occludes the ducts. Bilateral epididymitis may result in sterility or low levels of fertility.

Clinical Findings

A. Symptoms: Epididymitis may follow severe physical strain (eg, lifting a heavy object) or considerable sexual excitement. The patient may have experienced signs or symptoms of urethritis or prostatitis. At times, pathogens from the urethra or prostate are transmitted to the epididymis as a consequence of urethral instrumentation or prostatic surgery. Postprostatectomy bacterial epididymitis may evolve unless the urine is kept sterile throughout prostatectomy and the convalescent period.

Pain that is usually quite severe develops suddenly in the scrotum and may radiate along the spermatic cord and even reach the flank. The epididymis is exquisitely sensitive. Swelling is rapid and may cause the organs to double their normal size in the course of 3–4 hours. The temperature may reach 40 °C (104 °F). Urethral discharge may be seen. Symptoms of cystitis or prostatitis, with cloudy urine, may accompany the painful scrotal swelling.

B. Signs: There may be tenderness over the groin (spermatic cord) or in the lower abdominal quadrant on the affected side. The scrotum usually is enlarged, and the overlying skin may be reddened. If an abscess is present, the overlying skin may appear dry, flaky, and thinned; the abscess may rupture spontaneously. Early in the course of acute epididymitis, the enlarged, indurated, tender epididymis may be distinguished from the testis; but after a few hours, the testis and epididymis typically become one mass.

The spermatic cord is thickened by edema; a reactive hydrocele secondary to the inflammation may develop within a few days. Urethral discharge may be seen.

Palpation of the prostate may reveal changes suggesting acute or chronic prostatitis. The prostate should not be massaged during acute epididymitis, because the epididymitis may worsen.

C. Laboratory Findings: The hemogram typically shows marked elevation of the white blood cell count, with a shift to the left. In preschool children, epididymitis is frequently associated with urinary tract infection due to coliform organisms or *Pseudomonas;* therefore, urinalysis and urine culture are important in the diagnosis of these children. The cause of epididymitis can be differentiated by examination of Gram-stained smears or cultures of a midstream urine specimen and a urethral specimen. If coliform bacteria, *Pseudomonas, N gonorrhoeae,* or *C trachomatis* is found, a presumptive diagnosis of epididymitis due to that organism is justified.

Differential Diagnosis

Tuberculous epididymitis seldom is associated with pain or significant fever. The epididymis usually is distinguishable from the testis on palpation. "Beading" of the vas deferens may be observed. Induration of the prostate and a thickened ipsilateral seminal vesicle usually are found in tuberculous epididymitis. The diagnosis can be established by finding tubercle bacilli in cultures of the urine or prostatic fluid.

Testicular tumors generally cause painless swelling of the affected testis; on occasion, however, acute hemorrhage within the tumor may cause sudden distention of the tunica albuginea and pain. Careful palpation generally detects a mass separate from a normal epididymis rising from the testicle. Prostatic examination and urinalysis are normal. Scrotal ultrasonography may be helpful in differential diagnosis. If the diagnosis is still in doubt, surgical exploration is mandatory.

Torsion of the spermatic cord occurs primarily in prepubertal boys but occasionally may be seen in young adults. In men 30 years of age or older, epididymitis is common but torsion of the spermatic cord occurs infrequently. In the early phase of torsion, the epididymis may be palpated anterior to the testis. The testis is apt to be retracted. Later, however, the testis and epididymis become one enlarged, tender mass. **Prehn's sign** (when the scrotum is gently lifted onto the symphysis, pain due to epididymitis is relieved but that due to torsion is worsened) may be helpful in the differential diagnosis but is not totally reliable. Use of the Doppler stethoscope or radionuclide scanning may confirm the diagnosis of epididymitis but should not be allowed to delay surgical exploration of possible torsion.

Torsion of the appendages of the testis or epididymis occurs occasionally in prepubertal boys.

These pedunculated bodies may become twisted, causing localized pain and swelling. In the early stages, palpation discloses a tender nodule of the upper pole of the testicle; the epididymis is normal. Later, the entire testis becomes swollen, making the differential diagnosis between epididymitis and torsion of the cord or its rudimentary appendages difficult. Early surgery is necessary in this case, since torsion of the cord must be treated promptly.

Testicular trauma may simulate acute epididymitis in every way, but the history of injury and the absence of pyuria or abnormal urethral discharge will help in differentiation.

Mumps orchitis usually is accompanied by parotitis. There are no urinary symptoms, and the urinary sediment is free of excessive numbers of white cells and bacteria. If diagnosis and appropriate therapy are delayed, an abscess may form and drain spontaneously through the scrotum; it may require surgical drainage.

Complications

Epididymal abscess may extend into and destroy the testis (epididymo-orchitis), but this is rare. Chronic epididymitis may evolve.

Prevention

In order to prevent recurrence of sexually transmitted forms of epididymitis, infected sexual partners must be identified and treated. Identification and treatment of underlying causes of urinary tract infections and prostatitis can prevent non-sexually transmitted forms of epididymitis. Recurrent acute attacks may indicate the need for ipsilateral vasoligation.

Treatment

A. Specific Measures: Sexually transmitted acute epididymitis occurs mainly in young adults in association with urethritis without underlying genitourinary disease or abnormalities. For treatment, tetracycline hydrochloride, 500 mg orally 4 times daily for 21 days, or doxycycline, 100 mg orally twice daily for 21 days, is recommended. Alternative treatment for gonococcal urethritis and epididymitis is ampicillin, 500 mg orally 4 times daily for 21 days, or a 10-day course of a parenteral second- or third-generation cephalosporin. For nongonococcal urethritis and epididymitis, alternative therapy may consist of erythromycin, 500 mg orally 4 times daily for 21 days.

Non-sexually transmitted acute epididymitis is most often a consequence of infection with Enterobacteriaceae or *Pseudomonas,* especially in middle-aged or older men. Prompt treatment with antimicrobial drugs selected on the basis of culture and sensitivity tests is indicated. Provided that the pathogens are susceptible to these drugs, trimethoprim-sulfamethoxazole (trimethoprim, 160 mg, and sulfamethoxazole, 800 mg) orally twice daily for 4 weeks, is recommended, especially if an underlying bacterial prostatitis is suspected. The patient should be evaluated for underlying genitourinary tract disease.

B. General Measures: Bed rest is necessary during the acute phase (3–4 days). Support for the enlarged, heavy testicle partially relieves the discomfort; the more roomy athletic supporter is preferred to standard scrotal supports. Local injection of 20 mL of 1% lidocaine or other local anesthetic agent into the spermatic cord at the pubic tubercle (just above the testicle) may produce marked relief of pain and discomfort. This may be repeated on a daily basis as needed. Oral analgesics and antipyretics are usually indicated. In the early phase, an ice bag helps prevent swelling. Afterward, local heat affords comfort and probably hastens resolution of the inflammatory process.

Sexual activity or physical strain may exacerbate the infection and worsen the symptoms and therefore should be avoided.

Prognosis

When diagnosed promptly and treated appropriately, acute epididymitis usually resolves slowly without complications. Complete resolution of pain and symptoms often takes up to 2 weeks, and 4 or more weeks may be required for the epididymis to return to normal size and consistency. Complications are unusual, although lowered fertility and even sterility may ensue, especially when the process is bilateral.

CHRONIC EPIDIDYMITIS

Chronic epididymitis usually represents the irreversible end stage of a severe acute epididymitis that has been followed by frequent mild attacks.

In chronic epididymitis, fibroplasia leads to induration of part or all of the organ. Histologically, the scarring is extensive and tubular occlusion is common. The tissues are infiltrated with lymphocytes and plasma cells.

Except during a mild exacerbation, at which time variable degrees of local discomfort are the rule, chronic epididymitis is not associated with specific symptoms. The patient may notice a lump in the scrotum.

The epididymis usually is thickened and somewhat enlarged; it may or may not be tender. It is easily distinguished from the testis on palpation. The spermatic cord is often thickened, and the diameter of the vas deferens may be increased. The prostate may be firm or may contain areas of fibrosis. When chronic epididymitis is associated with chronic prostatitis, the prostatic expressate shows excessive numbers of inflammatory cells. The voided urine may show pyuria, and cultures may be positive for an underlying prostatitis or urinary tract infection.

Tuberculous epididymitis mimics nonspecific chronic epididymitis in every way. Beading of the vas deferens, thickening of the ipsilateral seminal vesicle, and the finding of "sterile" pyuria and tubercle bacilli in the urine generally make the diagnosis of tuberculous epididymitis. Urograms may show typical changes associated with tuberculous involvement of the urinary tract. Cystoscopy may reveal ulcers involving the bladder lining.

Testicular tumors may present as a "lump in the testicle." Careful palpation, however, will show a thickened epididymis or a hard, insensitive testicular tumor.

Except in infants and elderly men, tumors of the epididymis are rare. Differentiation from chronic epididymitis ultimately may be made only by the surgical pathologist.

If chronic epididymitis is bilateral, sterility or relative infertility may result.

When it is suspected that an exacerbation of chronic epididymitis is associated with active bacterial infection, the use of appropriate antibacterial agents is indicated. However, the scarring associated with chronic epididymitis can impede diffusion of the antimicrobial agents into the tissues. Appropriate treatment of underlying urinary tract infection or prostatitis is always indicated. At times, vasoligation on the affected side may prevent recurrent bouts of ascending epididymitis. Surgical excision of the epididymis and attached vas deferens may prove necessary.

Except for recurring pain and the threat of infertility (when involvement is bilateral), chronic epididymitis is of little consequence. Once the stage of diffuse fibrosis is reached, little can be done other than epididymectomy to resolve the problem.

NONSPECIFIC INFECTIONS OF THE TESTIS & SCROTUM

ACUTE ORCHITIS

Etiology

Inflammation of the testis may occur as a result of hematogenous spread of various systemic infectious diseases. It is thought that orchitis without epididymitis originates in this way.

Epididymo-orchitis, a fearful complication of mumps, is generally seen only in adolescent boys and young men. The factors that predispose to this complication are unknown; however, mumps orchitis occurs in 20–35% of cases of mumps in males in this age range and is bilateral in 10%. The onset is usually 3–4 days after the development of parotitis.

Tuberculous orchitis may result from hematogenous spread of tubercle bacilli from a pulmonary focus of infection or, more commonly, by direct extension from tuberculous epididymitis.

The testis may be involved in syphilis; gummas with large areas of necrosis occasionally complicate advanced stages of syphilis.

Granulomatous orchitis, a nonspecific inflammatory process in the testis, occurs occasionally in middle-aged and older men. It apparently is of noninfectious origin. Evidence suggests that it is an autoimmune disease which represents a granulomatous response to spermatozoa.

Pathogenesis & Pathology

On gross inspection, the testis involved by nonspecific orchitis is variably enlarged, congested, and tense; on section, small abscesses may be seen. Histologically, edema of the connective tissue and diffuse infiltration by neutrophils are characteristic. The seminiferous tubules also may be involved, and frank necrosis may be present. The seminiferous tubules are replaced by caseous tubercles in tuberculous orchitis and by an infiltrate of mononuclear cells (plasma cells, lymphocytes, multinucleated giant cells, and epithelioid cells) in nonspecific granulomatous orchitis. The outline of the seminiferous tubules remains, but spermatogenic activity is absent. In the healed stage, the seminiferous tubules and the interstitial cells usually are preserved.

Mumps is the most common infectious cause of orchitis. Interestingly, mumps orchitis occurs only in postpubertal males. Grossly, the testis is greatly enlarged and bluish in color. On section, because of the interstitial reaction and edema, the tubules do not extrude. Histologically, edema and dilatation of blood vessels are observed; neutrophils, lymphocytes, and macrophages are abundant; and tubular cells show varying degrees of degeneration. In the healed stage, the testis is small and soft. Histologic study at this stage shows marked tubular atrophy but preservation of the interstitial cells of Leydig. The epididymis often is similarly involved.

Clinical Findings

A. Symptoms: The onset of mumps orchitis is sudden; it usually occurs about 3–4 days after the onset of parotitis. The scrotum becomes erythematous and edematous. Unlike the findings in epididymitis, urinary symptoms characteristically are absent. Fever may reach 40 °C (104 °F), and prostration may be marked.

B. Signs: The parotitis of mumps may be present, or evidence of other infectious disease may be found. One or both testicles are enlarged and very tender. Often the epididymis cannot be distinguished from the testis by palpation. The scrotal skin may be reddened. An acute hydrocele that transilluminates may develop.

C. Laboratory Findings: The hemogram usually shows leukocytosis. Mild proteinuria and microhematuria have been described, but the urinalysis usually is normal. During acute episodes of viral orchitis, the infective organism can be recovered from the urine.

Differential Diagnosis

When seen early, acute epididymitis easily is distinguished from acute orchitis because only the epididymis is involved in the inflammatory reaction. Later, as passive congestion of the testicle develops, the differentiation between epididymitis and orchitis becomes more difficult. The presence of urethral discharge and pyuria, positive results of urine and prostatic fluid cultures, and the absence of a generalized infectious disease suggest epididymitis, not orchitis.

Torsion of the spermatic cord at times presents difficulty in the differential diagnosis. During the early stages of torsion, the epididymis is felt anterior to the testis. Absence of laboratory and physical findings suggesting an infectious disease tends to rule out orchitis.

Nonspecific granulomatous orchitis easily is confused with testicular tumors on the basis of clinical findings. The differentiation usually is made by the surgical pathologist following radical orchiectomy.

Posttraumatic rupture of the testis and acute hemorrhage into the testis due to minor trauma are conditions that must be distinguished from orchitis. Spontaneous hemorrhage into the testicle may occur in men with polyarteritis nodosa. Orchiectomy is often required because these conditions cannot be distinguished from testicular tumors.

Complications

Spermatogenesis is irreversibly damaged in about 30% of testes involved in mumps orchitis. Marked atrophy of the affected testis is the rule. If both testes are involved, permanent sterility may result, but androgenic function usually is maintained.

Prevention

Live attenuated mumps virus vaccine is highly effective in preventing parotitis and complicating orchitis; it is recommended for all susceptible persons over age 1 year. The incidence of mumps orchitis may possibly be reduced by the administration of mumps hyperimmune globulin, 20 mL, during the incubation period or very early stages of the disease. Routine administration of estrogens or corticosteroids to all postpubertal males who develop mumps has been suggested as prophylaxis against orchitis; however, the efficacy of this practice is controversial.

Treatment

A. Specific Measures: Orchitis due to bacterial infections should be treated with appropriate antimicrobial drugs, but these drugs are useless against mumps orchitis. Rapid resolution of swelling and relief of pain often results after infiltration of the spermatic cord immediately superior to the involved testis with 20 mL of 1% lidocaine. This also may protect spermatogenic activity by improving the blood supply to the testicle. In proved cases of nonspecific granulomatous orchitis, the use of corticosteroids is indicated.

B. General Measures: Bed rest is necessary during the acute phase of orchitis. Local heat is helpful and may relieve the pain. Support to the organ affords comfort; a towel placed under the scrotum or the use of an athletic supporter may be helpful. Medication for relief of pain and fever is advised.

Prognosis

Bilateral orchitis may result in irreversible damage to spermatogenesis and permanent sterility. The acute phase of mumps orchitis lasts for about 1 week. Noticeable atrophy may occur in 1 or 2 months.

• • •

ANTIMICROBIAL TREATMENT OF URINARY TRACT INFECTIONS

Choice of Drug

A. Type of Infecting Organism and Confirmation of Diagnosis: The diagnosis of urinary tract infection is made by proper examination of the urine. The differential diagnosis often requires examination of urethral and vaginal specimens in female patients and urethral and prostatic specimens in male patients. Proper techniques of specimen collection (see p 46) and processing are essential to an accurate diagnosis. A clean-catch midstream specimen is usually examined; this generally is reliable in boys and men but is less reliable in girls and women because of possible vaginal contamination. A more reliable urine sample may be obtained from females by properly performed transurethral catheterization, but this procedure may introduce infection, especially in bedridden or hospitalized female patients. Suprapubic needle aspiration of the bladder is recommended in children, especially newborns; samples thus obtained are diagnostic of infection even when small numbers (10^2–10^4) of pathogenic bacteria are identified.

Microscopic examination of a fresh specimen should be performed immediately to avoid artifacts. The urine should be centrifuged at 2000 rpm for 5 minutes, the supernatant discarded, and the sediment examined under the high-power objective. The presence of bacteria and excessive numbers of leukocytes suggests urinary tract infection. The presence of any bacteria in a stained or unstained smear from a centrifuged sample indicates 10^4–10^5 bacteria per milliliter of urine; the presence of one organism per oil-immersion field of an uncentrifuged, unstained sample indicates 10^6 bacteria per milliliter of urine.

Although a variety of chemical tests have been devised to screen for "significant" bacteriuria, none are completely reliable. Quantitative urine culture is the standard method for diagnosis of urinary tract infection. The traditional diagnostic criterion for urinary tract infection has been the presence of 10^5 or more bacteria of a single kind per milliliter. It is now recognized that a culture showing a known urinary pathogen in counts less than 10^5/mL in an acutely symptomatic patient probably represents an infection that warrants treatment. Since most acute, uncomplicated, nonnosocomial urinary tract infections in healthy adolescent girls and women are caused by sensitive strains of *E coli,* urine culture for definitive identification of the causative organism is not always mandatory in initial treatment. However, careful follow-up, including culture and sensitivity testing, is required when the response to therapy is poor or when infection recurs rapidly.

B. Identification of the Site of Infection: The initial clinical picture (presence or absence of chills, fever, and toxic signs) suggests whether deep tissue infection (kidney or prostate) or superficial mucosal infection (urethra or bladder) is more likely. The most accurate of the various tests currently available to localize the site of infection to the upper or lower urinary tract are the most invasive (Table 13–3). Although such tests may have important applications in research, they are seldom necessary in routine clinical practice. However, performing segmented quantitative cultures to localize the site of infection to the urethra or prostate is valuable in the management of recurrent urinary tract infection in men.

Uncomplicated infections of the lower urinary tract (urethra and bladder) tend to respond more rapidly to antimicrobial therapy than infections of the kidneys and generally require less intense and less prolonged treatment. The former generally respond quickly to short-term therapy with antimicrobial agents that achieve high concentrations in the urine, without the need for high systemic drug levels. Effective drug levels in the urine are produced by urinary antiseptics and low doses of systemic drugs that are excreted into the urine in high concentration.

Acute symptomatic infections of the kidney or prostate that produce chills and fever may be associated with bacteremia; in such cases, initial therapy must achieve a high blood level of drugs effective against the pathogen.

C. Acute Versus Chronic and Initial Versus Recurrent Infection: Although some uncomplicated acute urinary tract infections subside and clear spontaneously, most require treatment with antimicrobial drugs. Because septicemia is found in nearly one-third of cases of urinary tract infection in newborns, intravenous therapy using gentamicin plus ampicillin is recommended for initial treatment of children 1 day to 3 months of age. In children over 3 months of age, an oral sulfonamide, ampicillin alone, or a cephalosporin usually is satisfactory. Acute, symptomatic, uncomplicated lower urinary tract infections in children and women require only short-course antimicrobial therapy—even single-dose treatment. Agents used successfully in single-dose regimens include ampicillin or amoxicillin, 2 double-strength trimethoprim-sulfamethoxazole (TMP-SMX) tablets, and 2 g of sulfisoxazole. A single intramuscular dose of kanamycin or gentamicin has also proved efficacious. Long-standing or complicated lower urinary tract infections generally require prolonged therapy with systemic agents and careful follow-up; the same is true for infections of the kidneys or prostate. When prolonged suppressive or preventive therapy is indicated, a drug

that exerts minimal pressure upon the fecal flora (eg, trimethoprim-sulfamethoxazole, nitrofurantoin, nalidixic acid, cinoxacin) should be selected.

D. Adverse Reaction to Drugs: If a patient has a history of hypersensitivity to a particular drug, a substitute drug is usually required. Patients with a history of a reaction to penicillin should receive no form of penicillin and probably no cephalosporin for urinary tract infections—although they might well tolerate either. Similarly, patients who have reacted adversely to nitrofurantoin or sulfonamides should not be given these drugs. However, a history of reactions probably caused by changes in microbial flora following the use of tetracyclines or ampicillin is not a definite contraindication to use of these drugs. Unlike hypersensitivity reactions, adverse side effects may be dose-related; if so, they may be minimized by proper alteration of dosing schedules.

E. Antimicrobial Drug Susceptibility Tests: In urologic office practice, proper microscopic examination of the urine is often an adequate guide to drug selection in many acute, uncomplicated infections. Screening cultures are inexpensive, provide an approximate quantification of bacterial numbers, and may provide a culture for subsequent testing if this is required. Culture for precise quantitation and identification of the organism often is reserved for recurrent or complicated urinary tract infections. In such cases, disk sensitivity tests usually are performed. However, results of disk tests commonly indicate susceptibility of the organism to *blood* concentration of drug, which is many times lower than the *urine* concentration of drug, and the latter is the most important therapeutic concern in urinary tract infections. Results of disk tests for nitrofurantoin, nalidixic acid, cinoxacin, and sometimes sulfonamides do indicate bacterial susceptibility to urine concentrations of these drugs, but the disk test results for many systemically employed antimicrobial drugs have limited relevance to the selection of drugs for urinary tract infection.

The recent commercial availability of microtiter plates with measured drug concentrations and simple inoculation methods has made possible a return to sensitivity testing of drug in broth dilution. Results are stated as **minimal inhibitory concentration (MIC)** of a given drug. This permits interpretations in terms of usual urine concentrations and is helpful in treatment of urinary tract infections that did not respond to or relapsed following initial treatment. Microtiter broth dilution assays can also reveal the **minimal bactericidal concentration (MBC)** of a drug for the infecting organism.

Drug Dosage
& Renal Function

Most antimicrobial drugs are excreted by the kidneys and appear in the urine in much higher concentration than in blood or tissues. So-called "urinary doses" are a fraction of the usual systemic dose and result in urinary drug levels inhibitory for many bacteria in the urine. The urine must not become too dilute to maintain adequate drug levels. Fluid intake should be between 1500 and 2000 mL/d for an adult.

The excretion of many drugs is greatly reduced with renal insufficiency. This results in drug retention and added nephrotoxicity. To avoid accumulation of the drug in the bloodstream and tissues, either the dose must be reduced or the interval between doses increased. In Table 13–4, the half-life of drugs in serum of normal subjects is compared with that in patients with creatinine clearance of 10 mL/min, and possible dosage adjustments are suggested. The kidneys of uremic individuals do not excrete some drugs in sufficient quantities to reach antibacterial concentrations in the urine. Nitrofurantoin, methenamine salts, polymyxin B, colistimethate, nalidixic acid, tetracyclines, and trimethoprim-sulfamethoxazole generally should *not* be given in renal failure.

Duration of Treatment & Follow-Up

A. Infants and Children: Newborns and young children with urinary tract infections are best treated with systemic antimicrobial drugs for the standard course of 10–14 days. Careful evaluation for possible complicating factors (eg, congenital genitourinary tract abnormalities) is important, and follow-up cultures at 1, 4, and 6 weeks are mandatory to be certain that the infection has been cured. Relapse with the same organism is managed best by a prolonged course of therapy (4–6 weeks) with an appropriate drug.

A different approach is possible in children 2–14 years of age. Fang et al (1982) have treated children with a single dose of amoxicillin, 1 g/20 kg body weight, and achieved cure in most cases. Radiologic abnormalities were found in 80% of the children not cured by a single dose of amoxicillin. Indeed, failure of cure following single-dose therapy in children suggests underlying abnormalities and tends to identify children who need careful urologic evaluation or reevaluation. Children with bacteriuria 2–3 days after single-dose therapy require treatment for 2 weeks with an agent selected on the basis of sensitivity testing. Children who have no correctable urologic abnormalities but experience relapsing recurrent infection after conventional 2-week therapy should receive a 4- to 6-

Table 13–4. Use of antibiotics in patients with renal failure.

	Principal Mode of Excretion or Detoxification	Approximate Half-Life in Serum		Proposed Dosage Regimen In Renal Failure		Significant Removal of Drug by Dialysis (H = Hemodialysis; P = Peritoneal Dialysis)
		Normal	Renal Failure*	Initial Dose†	Give Half of Initial Dose at Interval of	
Penicillin G	Tubular secretion	0.5 h	6 h	6 g IV	8–12 h	H, P no
Ampicillin	Tubular secretion	1 h	8 h	6 g IV	8–12 h	H yes, P no
Carbenicillin	Tubular secretion	1.5 h	16 h	4 g IV	12–18 h	H, P yes
Ticarcillin	Tubular secretion	1.5 h	16 h	3 g IV	12–18 h	H, P yes
Nafcillin	Kidney 20%, liver 80%	0.5 h	2 h	2 g IV	4–6 h	H, P no
Cephalothin	Tubular secretion	0.8 h	8 h	4 g IV	18 h	H, P yes
Cephalexin Cephradine	Tubular secretion and glomerular filtration	2 h	15 h	2 g orally	8–12 h	H yes, P no
Cefazolin	Tubular secretion and glomerular filtration	2 h	30 h	2 g IM	24 h	H yes, P no
Cefoxitin, cefamandole	Tubular secretion and liver	1 h	16–20 h	2 g IV	12–18 h	H, P yes
Amikacin	Glomerular filtration	2.5 h	3 d	15 mg/kg IM	3 d	H, P yes
Gentamicin	Glomerular filtration	2.5 h	2–4 d	3 mg/kg IM	2–3 d	H, P yes‡
Tobramycin	Glomerular filtration	2.5 h	3 d	3 mg/kg IM	2 d	H, P yes
Vancomycin	Glomerular filtratrion	6 h	6–9 d	1 g IV	5–8 d	H, P no
Polymyxin B	Glomerular filtration	6 h	2–3 d	2.5 mg/kg IV	3–4 d	P yes, H no
Tetracycline	Glomerular filtration	8 h	3 d	1 g orally or 0.5 g IV	3 d	H, P no
Chloramphenicol	Mainly liver	3 h	4 h	1 g orally or IV	8 h	H, P no
Erythromycin	Mainly liver	2.5 h	5 h	1 g orally or IV	8 h	H, P no
Clindamycin	Glomerular filtration and liver	2.5 h	4 h	600 mg IV or IM	8 h	H, P no

*Considered here to be marked by creatinine clearance of 10 mL/min or less.
†For a 60-kg adult with a serious systemic infection. The "initial dose" listed is administered as an intravenous infusion over a period of 1–8 hours, or as 2 intramuscular injections during an 8-hour period, or as 2–3 oral doses during the same period.
‡Aminoglycosides are removed irregularly in peritoneal dialysis. Gentamicin is removed 60% in hemodialysis.

week course of treatment. Since infants and children are at great risk for developing renal scars and permanent functional loss in association with urinary tract infections, careful management and follow-up are mandatory. Children prone to rapid reinfection or persistent infection unresponsive to treatment are best managed by use of long-term (months or years) preventive or suppressive therapy.

B. Adult Nonpregnant Women: Acute, uncomplicated, symptomatic urinary tract infection in adult women is cured just as often with single-dose therapy as with conventional therapy for 7–10 days, and single-dose therapy is less expensive and causes fewer adverse reactions (Fang et al, 1982). Agents proved effective in single-dose therapy include amoxicillin or ampicillin, trimethoprim-sulfamethoxazole, sulfisoxazole, and aminoglycosides. If single-dose therapy fails, a 2-week course of treatment with a drug chosen on the basis of culture and sensitivity testing is required. Relapsing recurrent infections suggest the need for thorough evaluation for possible sources of persistent infection (eg, infected calculi). Recurrent reinfections may be managed by long-term preventive therapy (eg, nitrofurantoin, 100 mg orally daily, or trimethoprim-sulfamethoxazole, 1 regular-strength tablet orally daily) after initial sterilization of the urine.

C. Pregnant Women: Because women who have significant bacteriuria during pregnancy, especially during early pregnancy, are at considerable risk of developing symptomatic pyelonephritis at some time during or immediately after that pregnancy, screening for bacteriuria is recommended throughout the course of pregnancy. Any detected infections must be treated appropriately.

Although the safety of many antimicrobial agents for the fetus remains uncertain, it is known that some drugs should not be used during pregnancy. For example, tetracyclines should not be given after the fourth month of pregnancy because they produce hypoplasia and staining of bones and teeth in the fetus. Parenteral tetracyclines can be severely toxic to the liver of a pregnant woman. Sulfonamides and trimethoprim-sulfamethoxazole should be avoided during the third trimester, because they may contribute to kernicterus in the newborn. Likewise, the use of agents that interfere with DNA synthesis (eg, nalidixic acid, oxolinic acid, and cinoxacin) is questioned because their effects upon the fetus are unknown. In general, the penicillins are thought to be safe for use in pregnant women.

D. Adult Men: Although single-dose therapy for acute, uncomplicated urinary tract infections in men has not been studied adequately, it is not currently recommended. Indeed, several investigators have found that a 6-week course of therapy often is required in the management of recurrent urinary tract infections in men (Gleckman et al, 1980; Smith et al, 1979). Relapsing recurrent infections in men often are associated with chronic bacterial prostatitis, and they may require a 12-week course of therapy for cure, suppres-

sive therapy for an indefinite period, or attempts at cure by surgical means (Meares, 1982).

E. Acute Infections of the Kidney: Initial therapy for acute pyelonephritis often requires hospitalization of the patient and parenteral administration of large doses of antimicrobial drugs. If the clinical response is favorable, a suitable oral agent may be substituted for the parenteral drug when the patient becomes afebrile; it must be continued for at least 2 weeks. Urine cultures should be repeated 1, 4, and 6 weeks after completion of therapy. Evidence of recurrent infection on follow-up cultures generally indicates the need for an additional 6-week course of therapy and careful evaluation for complicating factors. An unfavorable response to initial therapy (persistent symptoms and fever) warrants immediate evaluation for complicating factors and reevaluation of urine culture and sensitivity tests.

SYSTEMIC ANTIMICROBIAL DRUGS

Sulfonamides

This large group of drugs inhibits the growth of many bacteria by blocking the uptake of extracellular p-aminobenzoic acid required for synthesis of folate. The most soluble sulfonamides, sulfisoxazole and trisulfapyrimidines, rarely (if ever) precipitate in urine to cause crystalluria. However, they may cause other side effects of sulfonamides (rash, fever, hematologic disturbances, vasculitis, etc). Soluble sulfonamides are among the drugs of choice for the initial treatment of a first urinary tract infection, which is commonly caused by coliform bacteria, because many coliform bacteria are still susceptible to sulfonamides, although other bacteria (eg, streptococci) have become resistant. Sulfisoxazole or trisulfapyrimidines, 2–4 g/d (150 mg/kg/d for children), are given orally for 7–10 days. Long-acting sulfonamides should never be given for urinary tract infections. Whenever sulfonamides are administered, the urine should be kept alkaline and the urine volume kept above 1500 mL/d. Sulfonamides are not ideal for long-term use, because they exert pressure upon the fecal flora and select out resistant strains of pathogens.

Trimethoprim

This substituted pyrimidine inhibits bacterial dihydrofolate reductase thousands of times more efficiently than it inhibits the same enzyme of mammalian cells and thus blocks synthesis of purines in bacteria. It inhibits many gram-negative enteric bacteria that commonly cause urinary tract infection (eg, *E coli, Proteus, Klebsiella, Enterobacter*). About 2–8% of organisms carry plasmids that make them resistant to trimethoprim. The usual dose of trimethoprim, 100 mg orally every 12 hours, gives urine levels of 50–180 μg/mL. This is sufficient for the treatment of urinary tract infections due to susceptible bacteria. The dosage may be doubled to treat difficult or serious infections (eg, bacterial prostatitis). Trimethoprim also concentrates by nonionic diffusion in prostatic and vaginal fluids and thus may be effective in bacterial prostatitis or vaginitis. Side effects include fever, rashes, gastrointestinal symptoms, and hematologic abnormalities attributable to folate deficiency. Trimethoprim alone or in combination (see below) should not be given to patients with a creatinine clearance below 15 mL/min.

Trimethoprim-Sulfamethoxazole

Fixed-dose combinations of sulfamethoxazole, 400 mg, and trimethoprim, 80 mg, are available for the treatment of urinary tract and other infections. The 2 drugs interrupt sequential steps in the synthesis of purines and demonstrate synergistic activity in vitro.

The usual dose is 2 regular-strength tablets or 1 double-strength tablet orally twice daily. For single-dose therapy of acute symptomatic urinary tract infections in women, 2 double-strength tablets are usually given. In children, pregnant women, or patients with renal failure, the usual dosage must be reduced. A dose of 1 single-strength tablet daily or even 3 times a week has a prophylactic effect in sexually active women and others who tend to have recurrent urinary tract infections. An intravenous formulation of trimethoprim-sulfamethoxazole is available for use in serious illness due to bacteria not susceptible to other drugs (eg, *Serratia*). The side effects include those mentioned for each component of the mixture plus others.

Penicillins

All penicillins share the same chemical nucleus, which contains the β-lactam ring necessary for biologic activity, and act on bacteria by inhibiting the final step (transpeptidation) in the synthesis of cell wall mucopeptide. Part of the bactericidal action of penicillins is due to activation of lytic enzymes in the cell wall. The most common cause of resistance to some penicillins is bacterial production of enzymes (β-lactamases) that break the lactam ring and inactivate the drug. Penicillin resistance on this basis is common among staphylococci and gram-negative rods.

All penicillins taken by mouth must be given 1 hour before or after a meal. Penicillin G remains a drug of choice for streptococci, non-β-lactamase-producing staphylococci and gonococci, treponemes, clostridia and other anaerobes, and certain gram-negative aerobic organisms. Penicillin G or ampicillin, 500 mg orally 4 times daily, or amoxicillin, 250 mg orally 4 times daily, may be effective in acute cystitis caused by *E coli* or *P mirabilis*. Each drug, until and unless it is inactivated by β-lactamase, appears in the urine in sufficiently high concentration to suppress the causative bacteria. Carbenicillin indanyl sodium, 1–2 tablets orally every 6 hours, can be effective in urinary tract infections, especially those caused by *Proteus, Pseudomonas,* or enterococci.

For severe systemic infection, these lactamase-susceptible penicillins are injected intravenously in doses 5–50 times larger than those given above (Table 13–5). Carbenicillin or ticarcillin often is combined with gentamicin to treat major infections caused by *Pseudomonas*. Ampicillin plus either gentamicin, tobramycin, or amikacin is the drug of choice for systemic infections caused by enterococci.

The β-lactamase-resistant penicillins are used mainly against lactamase-producing staphylococci. For minor infections, nafcillin or dicloxacillin can be given orally; for major infections, nafcillin, 3–12 g, is injected intravenously (Table 13–5).

All penicillins cross-react in hypersensitive patients, and persons with a history of penicillin reactions are also about 4 times more likely to have hypersensitivity reactions to a cephalosporin than persons without such a history. However, a history of penicillin reaction is far from reliable in predicting a patient's response. Penicillin excretion is reduced in renal failure; thus, the usual dose should be adjusted downward (Table 13–4).

Cephalosporins

Cephalosporins are chemically similar to penicillins, cross-react to a certain extent with them, and have a similar mode of action. Cephalosporins, particularly the new agents, are relatively resistant to β-lactamases and can be effective against bacteria that produce these enzymes. Numerous changes in the basic cephalosporin nucleus have been made since the first clinically useful cephalosporins were introduced about 2 decades ago. These modifications have been designed to produce new agents possessing different pharmacokinetic properties, greater activity against susceptible pathogens, or wider spectrums of antibacterial activity. As new cephalosporins with different activities were produced (eg, cefoxitin, cefamandole, cefuroxime, cefonicid, ceforanide), they were arbitrarily called second-generation cephalosporins to distinguish them from first-generation cephalosporins (eg, cephalothin, cephaloridine, cefazolin, cephalexin). Subsequently, still newer compounds were designated third-generation cephalosporins (eg, cefotaxime, ceftizoxime, ceftriaxone, ceftazidime, cefoperazone, moxalactam).

In general, first-generation cephalosporins have significantly greater activity against gram-positive bacterial pathogens than do third-generation compounds. In contrast, third-generation cephalosporins generally have significantly greater activity against gram-negative uropathogens than do first-generation compounds. Indeed, most organisms resistant to cephalothin and cefamandole (first- and second-generation cephalosporins) and to aminoglycosides are inhibited by third-generation cephalosporins. Although the third-generation cephalosporins have some activity against *P aeruginosa*, the most active agent is ceftazidime, followed by cefoperazone. The cephalosporins with the greatest activity against anaerobes are cefoxitin and ceftizoxime.

Oral cephalosporins, including cefadroxil, cephalexin, cephradine, and cefaclor, are sufficiently

Table 13–5. Antimicrobials often used in urology.

Drug	Route	Daily Adult Dose	Daily Pediatric Dose	Untoward Effects
Soluble sulfonamide (sulfisoxazole, trisulfapyrimidines)	Oral	1 g 4 times	100–150 mg/kg	Rashes, fever, nausea, vomiting, diarrhea, arthritis, stomatitis, thrombocytopenia, hemolytic or aplastic anemia, granulocytopenia, hepatitis, vasculitis, Stevens-Johnson syndrome, psychosis, etc. Crystalluria and hematuria rare.
Trimethoprim	Oral	100 mg twice	15–30 mg/kg	
Trimethoprim-sulfamethoxazole	Oral	4 tablets	Trimethoprim, 15 mg/kg, and sulfamethoxazole, 150 mg/kg	
Ampicillin	Oral	2–4 g	50–100 mg/kg	Hypersensitivity: rashes, fever, anaphylaxis, dermatitis, serum sickness, nephritis, eosinophilia, vasculitis, hemolytic anemia, granulocytopenia. Nausea, vomiting, diarrhea especially with oral penicillins. CNS toxicity with very high doses and renal insufficiency.
	IV	2–10 g	100–300 mg/kg	
Amoxicillin	Oral	0.75–1.5 g	20–40 mg/kg	
Carbenicillin	Oral	1.5–3 g	50–70 mg/kg	
Mezlocillin	IV	200–300 mg/kg	300 mg/kg	
Piperacillin	IV	12–24 g	?	
Ticarcillin	IV	200–300 mg-kg	200–300 mg/kg	
Nafcillin	Oral	2–4 g	50–100 mg/kg	
	IV	3–12 g	100–200 mg/kg	
Dicloxacillin	Oral	1–2 g	25–50 mg/kg	
Penicillin G	Oral	1.6–3.2 million units	0.05–0.1 million units/kg	
	IV	1.2–20 million units	0.05–0.3 million units/kg	
Cefamandole	IV	4–12 g	50–150 mg/kg	Same as with penicillins.
Cefazolin	IV	3–6 g	25-100 mg/kg	
Cefoperazone	IV	2–12 g	?	
Ceforanide	IV	1-2 g	20-40-mg/kg	
Cefotaxime	IV	4–12 g	50–300 mg/kg	
Cefoxitin	IV	4–12 g	80–160 mg/kg	
Ceftriaxone	IV	1-4 g	50-75 mg/kg	
Ceftizoxime	IV	2-12 g	150-200 mg/kg	
Cefuroxime	IV	2-4 g	50-100 mg/kg	
Cephalothin	IV	4–12 g	80–160 mg/kg	
Cephapirin	IV	4–12 g	40–80 mg/kg	
Cephradine	IV	2–8 g	50–100 mg/kg	
Cefadroxil	Oral	1–2 g	30 mg/kg	
Cefaclor	Oral	1–4 g	20–40 mg/kg	
Cephalexin	Oral	1–4 g	25–50 mg/kg	
Cephradine	Oral	1–4 g	50–100 mg/kg	
Tetracycline	Oral	1–2 g	20–40 mg/kg	Fever, rashes, anorexia, nausea, diarrhea, yellow mottling of teeth and bones, liver damage, vestibular reactions, renal tubular damage.
Oxytetracycline	Oral	1–2 g	20–40 mg/kg	
Doxycycline	Oral	200 mg	2.5–4 mg/kg	
Minocycline	Oral	200 mg	2.5–4 mg/kg	
Erythromycin	Oral	1–2 g	30–50 mg/kg	Anorexia, nausea, diarrhea; cholestatic hepatitis as a hypersensitivity reaction.
Gentamicin	IM or IV	3–5 mg/kg	3–5 mg/kg	Nephrotoxicity and ototoxicity.
Tobramycin	IM or IV	3–5 mg/kg	3–5 mg/kg	
Amikacin	IM or IV	15 mg/kg	15 mg/kg	
Netilmicin	IV	3-6 mg/kg	5-8 mg/kg	
Kanamycin	IM or IV	15 mg/kg	15 mg/kg	
Polymyxin B	IV	2.5 mg/kg	1.5–2.5 mg/kg	Paresthesias, dizziness, nephrotoxicity.
Colistimethate	IM	2.5–5 mg/kg	2.5 mg/kg	
Nitrofurantoin	Oral	200–400 mg	5–7 mg/kg	Nausea, vomiting, rashes, pulmonary infiltrates, rare neurotoxicity.
Methenamine hippurate	Oral	2 g	75 mg/kg	Vesical irritation.
Methenamine mandelate	Oral	4 g	75 mg/kg	
Nalidixic acid	Oral	4 g	30–60 mg/kg	Rashes, gastrointestinal disturbances, visual and CNS disturbances, photosensitization (rare).
Cinoxacin	Oral	1 g	?	

well absorbed so that 0.25—1 g every 6 hours results in high urine levels, suitable for treatment of acute, uncomplicated urinary tract infection with coliform organisms. Parenteral cephalosporins, including second-generation agents (eg, cefoxitin, cefamandole, cefuroxime, cefonicid, ceforanide) or third-generation compounds (eg, cefotaxime, ceftizoxime, ceftriaxone, ceftazidime, cefoperazone) in appropriate dosage (Table 13–5), should be given intravenously for major systemic infections or severe pyelonephritis caused by gram-negative enteric bacteria. Cefoxitin, 3–12 g/d intravenously, and ceftizoxime, 2–12 g/d intravenously, are active against anaerobes as well. Cefazolin, 1 g every 6 hours pre- and postoperatively for 24 hours, has found favor in surgical prophylaxis. All cephalosporins can induce hypersensitivity reactions, but hematologic or renal disorders are rare. A notable exception is moxalactam, which has been implicated in severe hematologic dysfunction. The toxic potential of cephalosporins may be enhanced by diuretics or aminoglycosides. All cephalosporins are expensive; this tends to limit their usefulness in treating uncomplicated urinary tract infections.

Tetracyclines

This large group of drugs is active against many organisms. Tetracycline hydrochloride and oxytetracycline are most commonly used in oral doses of 0.5 g 4 times daily; doxycycline and minocycline are given orally in doses of 100 mg twice daily. Because of a high frequency of resistance among coliform bacteria and enterococci, these drugs are not preferred in urinary tract infections. However, many gonococcal infections are cured by treatment with tetracyclines for 5 days, and nongonococcal urethritis and other chlamydial infections are cured by treatment with tetracyclines for 10–14 days. The tetracyclines are especially useful in treating uncomplicated urinary tract infections caused by *P aeruginosa*.

The absorption of tetracyclines is impaired by divalent cations (milk, antacids, ferrous sulfate), and a large proportion of the oral drug is excreted in feces and modifies normal flora in the gut. Because they are deposited in bone and teeth, tetracyclines should not be given to pregnant women or children under age 7. Tetracyclines, except doxycycline, accumulate in renal insufficiency.

Table 13–6. Choices of drugs for microorganisms commonly encountered in infections of the urinary and genital tracts.

Microorganism	Oral Therapy Choices	Parenteral Therapy Choices
Gram-positive cocci		
Staphylococcus aureus	Nafcillin, nitrofurantoin	Nafcillin, vancomycin
Staphylococcus epidermidis	Ampicillin, nitrofurantoin	Ampicillin, penicillin G
Staphylococcus saprophyticus	Ampicillin, nitrofurantoin	Ampicillin, penicillin G
Streptococcus, group D Streptococcus faecalis (enterococci)	Ampicillin, nitrofurantoin	Ampicillin plus gentamicin or amikacin
Streptococcus bovis	Penicillin G, ampicillin	Ampicillin, vancomycin
Streptococcus, group B	Ampicillin, cephalosporin	Ampicillin, cephalosporin
Gram-negative cocci		
Neisseria gonorrhoeae	Ampicillin plus probenecid, tetracycline	Penicillin G plus probenecid or ceftriaxone
Neisseria gonorrhoeae (β-lactamase–producing)	Tetracycline (may not be effective)	Spectinomycin, ceftriaxone
Gram-negative rods		
Escherichia coli	TMP-SMX, sulfonamide, ampicillin, nitrofurantoin	Gentamicin, amikacin, tobramycin
Enterobacter sp	TMP-SMX, cinoxacin, carbenicillin	Gentamicin plus carbenicillin
Gardnerella vaginalis (Haemophilus vaginalis)	Metronidazole, ampicillin	Metronidazole
Klebsiella sp	TMP-SMX, cinoxacin, carbenicillin	Gentamicin ± cephalosporin
Proteus mirabilis	Ampicillin, TMP-SMX, cinoxacin	Ampicillin, gentamicin
Proteus sp (indole-positive)	TMP-SMX, cinoxacin, carbenicillin	Gentamicin ± carbenicillin
Pseudomonas aeruginosa	Carbenicillin, tetracycline	Gentamicin plus ticarcillin or carbenicillin
Serratia sp	TMP-SMX, carbenicillin, cinoxacin	TMP-SMX, amikacin
Chlamydiae (Chlamydia trachomatis)	Tetracycline, erythromycin	Tetracycline, erythromycin
Mycoplasmas, ureaplasmas	Erythromycin, tetracycline	Erythromycin, tetracycline
Fungi (Candida sp)	Flucytosine	Amphotericin B
Obligate anaerobes	Metronidazole, clindamycin	Metronidazole, clindamycin
Trichomonas vaginalis	Metronidazole	Metronidazole

Chloramphenicol

This bacteriostatic drug is effective against many bacteria, but because of its potential serious toxicity (aplastic anemia, gray syndrome in infants), it is only used for very specific indications. Oral doses of 0.5 g 4 times daily are sometimes used for serious anaerobic infections or gram-negative sepsis. However, chloramphenicol has little place in general urologic practice.

Aminoglycosides

Drugs in this group share antimicrobial, pharmacologic, and toxic features. They act as potent inhibitors of protein synthesis in bacteria and are often bactericidal. All aminoglycosides are ototoxic and nephrotoxic, and all are more effective at alkaline pH. All can accumulate in renal failure; to avoid serious toxicity, adjustments must be made in dosage or the time interval between injections when the serum creatinine level is elevated. No aminoglycosides are absorbed from the gut; they must be injected intramuscularly or intravenously to yield systemic or urinary levels. The usefulness of a given aminoglycoside varies with time and place, since susceptible bacterial populations are replaced by resistant ones owing to overuse of the drug. Susceptibility testing is essential.

A. Neomycin and Kanamycin: These 2 aminoglycosides are too ototoxic and nephrotoxic to be used systemically. When taken orally, they remain principally in the gut lumen and affect the gut flora. To sterilize the bowel in preparation for intestinal surgery, neomycin (or, less often, kanamycin) plus erythromycin base is given orally in addition to mechanical cleansing. Occasionally, solutions of these drugs are used for irrigation of contaminated or infected spaces, but the total daily dose must not exceed 10 mg/kg. Placement of 2–4 g of either drug into the peritoneal cavity may result in respiratory arrest.

B. Gentamicin, Netilmicin, and Tobramycin: These agents are active against many gram-negative bacteria in concentrations of 1–5 μg/mL, but streptococci and *Bacteroides* are unaffected. Cross-resistance between the drugs is significant, and strains of *Pseudomonas, Serratia, Proteus,* and *Enterobacter* must be tested for individual susceptibility. After injection of 3–5 mg/kg/d in divided doses, serum levels reach 3–8 μg/mL—sufficient to treat gram-negative systemic and bacteremic infections. With injected doses of 2–3 mg/kg/d, urine drug levels are ample to control most of the common infecting organisms in urinary tract infection.

Upon prolonged use, these agents may affect both the auditory and vestibular portions of the eighth nerve. The loss of high-frequency sound perception is often a premonitory sign on audiograms. These drugs are nephrotoxic, particularly in renal failure, and dose adjustment is required. This can be done best by laboratory monitoring of drug levels (which must be kept below peak levels of 10 μg/mL) or by adjustments suggested in Table 13–4. The initial dose of tobramycin for a patient with renal insufficiency can be estimated as follows: 1 mg/kg intramuscularly every (6 × serum creatinine level [in mg/dL]) hours. Tobramycin is believed to be less nephrotoxic than gentamicin, but this is not established. These agents often are given intravenously rather than intramuscularly.

These drugs sometimes act synergistically with carbenicillin or ticarcillin against gram-negative rods, especially *Pseudomonas,* but laboratory confirmation is required in individual cases.

C. Amikacin: Give this derivative of kanamycin in doses of 15 mg/kg/d intramuscularly (or intravenously) to achieve peak serum levels of 10–30 μg/mL. In systemic infections, some gram-negative bacteria that are resistant to gentamicin or tobramycin respond to amikacin. In urinary tract infection caused by such resistant bacteria, amikacin, 5–8 mg/kg/d intramuscularly (or intravenously), provides urine drug levels sufficient to suppress the bacteria. Like all aminoglycosides, amikacin is nephrotoxic and ototoxic. Its levels should be monitored in patients with renal insufficiency.

Spectinomycin

This drug, related to aminoglycosides, is used only for treatment of penicillinase-producing gonococci. A single intramuscular injection of 2 g cures up to 95% of such gonorrhea. Pain at the injection site is significant.

Polymyxins

Polymyxin B and polymyxin E (colistin) are bactericidal for many gram-negative bacteria. Polymyxin B sulfate, 2.5 mg/kg/d, can be given intravenously in serious infections with resistant gram-negative organisms. Colistimethate (polymyxin E) produces little pain on intramuscular injection, and 2.5–5 mg/kg/d can be given to achieve very high drug levels in urine. *Pseudomonas* and *Serratia* are often susceptible.

In closed catheter drainage, mixtures of polymyxin B, 20 mg/L, plus neomycin, 40 mg/L, can be used for continuous irrigation to delay establishment of bacterial infection in the bladder. Polymyxins are bound and inactivated by purulent exudates and have no effect in deep tissue or organ infections. Their side effects—dizziness, paresthesias, incoordination, and proteinuria—tend to disappear upon cessation of the drug. Instillation of 300 mg or more of these drugs into the peritoneal cavity can result in respiratory arrest.

Erythromycins & Lincomycins

These drugs are active mainly against gram-positive bacteria and serve as substitutes for penicillins in allergic patients. Clindamycin is effective against anaerobic infections, particularly *B fragilis*. It is given orally or intravenously in doses of 300 mg 2–4 times daily, but there is a substantial risk of developing antibiotic-associated colitis with prolonged use. These drugs diffuse well into the prostate but have limited activity against the usual gram-negative genitourinary tract pathogens. Erythromycin is used mainly in urology to treat infections caused by mycoplasmas, ureaplasmas, and chlamydiae.

URINARY ANTISEPTICS

Urinary antiseptics are drugs that exert antibacterial activity in the urine but have few or no systemic antibacterial effects. Their usefulness is limited to the treatment of urinary tract infections, and they rarely affect the microbial flora in other parts of the body.

Nitrofurantoin

Nitrofurans are inhibitory and can be bactericidal for both gram-positive and gram-negative bacteria in concentrations of $10-100$ μg/mL. This is well within the range of concentrations achieved in the urine with the usual doses (100 mg 4 times daily by mouth). Disk sensitivity tests determine bacterial susceptibility in the urine. Most *P aeruginosa, P mirabilis,* and many indole-positive *Proteus* organisms are resistant to nitrofurantoin; however, there is no cross-resistance between nitrofurantoin and other antimicrobial drugs. In susceptible microbial strains, resistant mutants are very rare, and clinical resistance emerges slowly if at all. The activity of nitrofurantoin is enhanced at pH 5.5 or lower.

Nitrofurantoin is absorbed rapidly and completely after oral administration and is completely bound to protein in the bloodstream. The carrier protein is split off in the kidney, so the free drug can act in the urine. Excretion is by both glomerular filtration and tubular secretion. In the presence of renal failure, excretion is markedly reduced, and antibacterial drug levels in the urine are not reached. Thus, the drug is ineffective and toxic in uremia.

Nitrofurantoin, 400 mg daily for $7-10$ days, can be effective in urinary tract infection. In chronic urinary tract infection, after initial suppression of the large bacterial population, 200 mg daily may be given for many weeks or months. In women subject to frequently recurring urinary tract infection, nitrofurantoin, 100 mg daily, is often effective prophylaxis.

The most frequent side effects are gastrointestinal intolerance and allergic reactions ranging from rashes to pulmonary infiltrates. In glucose-6-phosphate dehydrogenase deficiency, hemolytic anemia or hepatic insufficiency may occur. Other side effects (neuropathies, vasculitis) are rare.

Methenamine Salts of Organic Acids

Methenamine is absorbed readily after oral intake and is excreted into the urine. In acidic urine, methenamine liberates formaldehyde, which is antibacterial. Methenamine is usually administered as the salt of mandelic, sulfosalicylic, or hippuric acid. Each of these acids can be antibacterial by itself. The dosage of methenamine mandelate or sulfosalicylate is 1 g 4 times daily orally; that of mandelamine hippurate is 1 g twice daily orally.

The urinary pH must be 5.5 or lower to achieve antibacterial efficacy, and the urine volume should be limited by fluid restriction to 1200 mL daily in order to permit a formaldehyde concentration of 100 μg/mL. This concentration of formaldehyde, however, may result in irritation of mucous membranes and even hematuria. Urine should be tested daily to ascertain that its pH is suitably low. If necessary, methionine or ascorbic acid can be given to acidify the urine.

Methenamine drugs can be effective for suppression of bacteriuria in chronic infections, but they are less commonly effective in acute infections with very large bacterial populations. The efficacy of the 3 salts is similar, but the dosage of hippurate calls for fewer tablets to be swallowed daily. Gastrointestinal intolerance and dysuria or bladder pain are the commonest side effects. Allergic reactions can occur. Laboratory tests with methenamine salts are meaningless, because the liberated formaldehyde is antibacterial.

Nalidixic Acid

In concentrations of $1-30$ μg/mL, nalidixic acid and other synthetic organic acids inhibit many gram-negative bacteria both by making the urine acid and by inhibiting bacterial DNA synthesis. Because emergence of resistant variants (chromosomal mutants) is relatively common in susceptible populations, there is a substantial failure rate of this drug during prolonged use in urinary tract infection unless proper dosing is maintained. The drug is absorbed rapidly after oral intake but is metabolized in a complex fashion so that only a small portion of active drug appears in the urine. With oral doses of 1 g 4 times daily, urine levels of active drug reach $20-200$ μg/mL. For children, the dose is $30-60$ mg/kg/d in $2-4$ divided doses, but the drug is not recommended for young children. In several studies, the cure rate with this drug in acute urinary tract infection has been as high as with any other drug.

Prominent side effects are gastrointestinal intolerance, hemolytic anemia in glucose-6-phosphate dehydrogenase deficiency, rashes, photosensitization, visual disturbances, dizziness, and restlessnes. Nalidixic acid greatly increases the effect of oral anticoagulants.

Nalidixic acid in urine may give false-positive tests for glucose, but true hyperglycemia with glycosuria has also been observed.

Cinoxacin

Cinoxacin is a new chemotherapeutic agent that inhibits bacterial DNA synthesis during replication and is approved for treatment of initial and recurrent urinary tract infections. Cinoxacin is closely related to nalidixic acid but offers certain advantages: rapid attainment of therapeutic urinary levels and greater activity against strains of Enterobacteriaceae that cause urinary tract infection. It is not effective against grampositive bacteria or *P aeruginosa.* The usual dosage in patients with normal renal function is 500 mg orally twice daily. The dose must be reduced in patients with impaired renal function. During standard dosing in patients with normal renal function, about 50–60% of the drug is excreted intact in urine; thus, the urinary drug levels attained generally exceed significantly the MICs for most enteric gram-negative bacteria. However, cinoxacin is highly bound to plasma proteins and achieves low levels of activity in the blood, and it is poorly soluble in lipids; thus, its clinical usefulness is limited mainly to the treatment of uncomplicated urinary tract infections.

Resistance to cinoxacin, like that to nalidixic acid, is not transferred by means of plasmids carrying R factors or transposons—a clear advantage in the therapy of urinary tract infection caused by multiply-resistant bacteria. This drug also exerts minimal pressure upon fecal bacteria, a characteristic that makes it suitable for long-term preventive or suppressive therapy in the management of recurrent urinary tract infection. Its adverse reactions are similar to those of nalidixic acid.

REFERENCES

Pathogenesis

Beachey EH: Bacterial adherence: Adhesin-receptor interactions mediating the attachment of bacteria to mucosal surfaces. *J Infect Dis* 1981;**143**:325.

Cox CE, Hinman F Jr.: Experiments with induced bacteriuria, vesical emptying and bacterial growth on the mechanism of bladder defense to infection. *J Urol* 1961;**66**:739.

Domingue GJ et al: Pathogenic significance of P-fimbriated *Escherichia coli* in urinary tract infections. *J Urol* 1985;**133**:983.

Fair WR, Couch J, Wehner N: Prostatic antibacterial factor: Identity and significance. *Urology* 1976;**7**:169.

Fairley KF et al: Simple test to determine the site of urinary-tract infection. *Lancet* 1967;**2**:427.

Fowler JE Jr, Pulaski ET: Excretory urography, cystography, and cystoscopy in the evaluation of women with urinary-tract infection: A prospective study. *N Engl J Med* 1981;**304**:462.

Gander RM, Thomas VL, Forland M: Mannose-resistant hemagglutination and P receptor recognition of uropathogenic *Escherichia coli* isolated from adult patients. *J Infect Dis* 1985;**151**:508.

Hodson CJ, Heptinstall RH, Winberg J (editors): *Reflux Nephropathy Update—1983*. Karger, 1984.

Jacobson SH et al: P fimbriated *Escherichia coli* in adults with acute pyelonephritis. *J Infect Dis* 1985;**152**:426.

Kallenius G et al: Occurrence of P-fimbriated *Escherichia coli* in urinary tract infections. *Lancet* 1981;**2**:1369.

Kunin CM, McCormack RC: Bacteriuria and blood pressure among nuns and working women. *N Engl J Med* 1968;**278**:635.

Kuriyama SM, Silverblatt FJ: Effect of Tamm-Horsfall urinary glycoprotein on phagocytosis and killing of Type I-fimbriated *Escherichia coli*. *Infect Immun* 1986;**51**:193.

Lomberg H et al: Correlation of P blood group, vesicoureteral reflux, and bacterial attachment in patients with recurrent pyelonephritis. *N Engl J Med* 1983;**308**:1189.

Parsons CL et al: Role of surface mucin in primary antibacterial defense of bladder. *Urology* 1977;**9**:48.

Schaeffer AJ: Bladder defense mechanisms against urinary tract infections. *Semin Urol* 1983;**1**:106.

Schaeffer AJ, Jones JM, Dunn JK: Association of in vitro *Escherichia coli* adherence to vaginal and buccal epithelial cells with susceptibility of women to recurrent urinary-tract infections. *N Engl J Med* 1981;**304**:1062.

Shortliffe LMD, Stamey TA: Infections of the urinary tract: Introduction and general principles. Pages 738–796 in: *Campbell's Urology*, 5th ed. Vol 1. Walsh PC et al (editors). Saunders, 1986.

Shortliffe LMD, Stamey TA: Urinary infections in adult women. Pages 797–830 in: *Campbell's Urology*, 5th ed.

Vol 1. Walsh PC et al (editors). Saunders, 1986.

Smellie JM: Urinary tract infection, vesicoureteric reflux, and renal scarring. *Semin Urol* 1986;**4**:82.

Stamey TA: *Pathogenesis and Treatment of Urinary Tract Infections*. Williams & Wilkins, 1980.

Stamey TA et al: The immunologic basis of recurrent bacteriuria: Role of cervicovaginal antibody in enterobacterial colonization of the introital mucosa. *Medicine* 1978;**57**:47.

Stamm WE et al: Diagnosis of coliform infection in acutely dysuric women. *N Engl J Med* 1982;**307**:463.

Tullus K et al: Epidemic outbreaks of acute pyelonephritis caused by nosocomial spread of P fimbriated *Escherichia coli* in children. *J Infect Dis* 1984;**150**:728.

Uehling DT, Iversen P: Urinary tract infections—female. *Curr Trends Urol* 1982;**2**:114.

Uehling DT, Mizutani K, Balish E: Inhibitors of bacterial adherence to urothelium. *Invest Urol* 1980;**18**:40.

Urinary tract infection during pregnancy. (Editorial). *Lancet* 1985;**2**:190.

Winberg J: Urinary tract infections in infants and children. Pages 831–867 in: *Campbell's Urology*, 5th ed. Vol 1. Walsh PC et al (editors). Saunders, 1986.

Meares EM Jr: Prostatitis syndromes: New perspectives about old woes. *J Urol* 1980;**123**:141.

O'Hanley P et al: Gal-Gal binding and hemolysin phenotypes and genotypes associated with uropathogenic *Escherichia coli*. *N Engl J Med* 1985;**313**:414.

Nonspecific Infections of the Kidneys

Ahlering TE et al: Emphysematous pyelonephritis: A 5-year experience with 13 patients. *J Urol* 1985;**134**:1086.

Asscher AW: *The Challenge of Urinary Tract Infections*. Grune & Stratton, 1980.

Braun G, Moussali L, Balanzar JL: Xanthogranulomatous pyelonephritis in children. *J Urol* 1985;**133**:236.

Cardiff-Oxford Bacteriuria Study Group: The sequelae of urinary tract infections in schoolgirls: A four-year follow-up study. *Lancet* 1978;**1**:889.

Davidson AJ, Talner LB: Urographic and angiographic abnormalities in adult-onset acute bacterial nephritis. *Radiology* 1973;**106**:249.

Elder JS: Xanthogranulomatous pyelonephritis: The great imitator. *Infect Surg* 1984;**3**:145.

Goldman SM et al: CT of xanthogranulomatous pyelonephritis: Radiologic-pathologic correlation. *AJR* 1984;**142**:963.

Huland H, Busch R: Pyelonephritis scarring in 213 patients with upper and lower tract infections: Long-term follow-up. *J Urol* 1984;**132**:936.

Hurwitz SR et al: Gallium-67 imaging to localize urinary-tract infections. *Br J Radiol* 1976;**49**:156.

Losse H, Asscher AW, Lison AE (editors): *Pyelonephritis.* Thieme-Stratton, 1980.

Pazin GJ, Braude AI: Pyelonephritis. Pages 545–557 in: *Infectious Diseases,* 3rd ed. Hoeprich PD (editor). Harper & Row, 1983.

Rolleston GI, Mailing TMJ, Hodson CJ: Intrarenal reflux and the scarred kidney. *Arch Dis Child* 1974;**49**:531.

Silver TM et al: The radiological spectrum of acute pyelonephritis in adults and adolescents. *Radiology* 1976;**118**:65.

Steinhardt GF: Reflux nephropathy. *J Urol* 1985;**134**:855.

Thomas V, Shelokov A, Forland M: Antibody-coated bacteria in the urine and the site of urinary tract infection. *N Engl J Med* 1974;**290**:588.

Winberg J et al: Clinical pyelonephritis and focal renal scarring: A selected review of pathogenesis, prevention, and prognosis. *Pediatr Clin North Am* 1982;**29**:801.

Zinner SH: Bacteriuria and babies revisited. *N Engl J Med* 1979;**300**:853.

Bacteremia & Septic Shock

Gleckman R, Hibert D: Afebrile bacteremia: A phenomenon in geriatric patients. *JAMA* 1982;**248**:1478.

Kalter ES et al: Activation and inhibition of Hageman factor-dependent pathways and the complement system in uncomplicated bacteremia or bacterial shock. *J Infect Dis* 1985;**151**:1019.

Kaplan RHL, Sahn SA, Petty TL: Incidence and outcome of the respiratory distress syndrome in gram-negative sepsis. *Arch Intern Med* 1979;**139**:867.

Kreger BE, Craven DE, McCabe WR: Gram-negative bacteremia. 4. Reevaluation of clinical features and treatment in 612 patients. *Am J Med* 1980;**68**:344.

Krieger JN, Kaiser DL, Wenzel RP: Urinary tract etiology of bloodstream infections in hospitalized patients. *J Infect Dis* 1983;**148**:57.

McCabe WR, Olans RN: Shock in gram-negative bacteremia: Predisposing factors, pathophysiology, and treatment. Pages 121–150 in: *Current Clinical Topics in Infections Diseases.* Vol 2. Remington JS, Swartz MN (editors). McGraw-Hill, 1981.

McCue JD: Improved mortality in gram-negative bacillary bacteremia. *Arch Intern Med* 1985;**145**:1212.

McGowan JE Jr: Changing etiology of nosocomial bacteremia and fungemia and other hospital-acquired infections. *Rev Infect Dis* 1985;**7(Suppl)**:S357.

Mizock B: Septic shock: A metabolic perspective. *Arch Intern Med* 1984;**144**:579.

Robinson MRG et al: Bacteraemia and bacteriogenic shock in district hospital urological practice. *Br J Urol* 1980;**52**:10.

Siegel JD, McCracken GH Jr: Sepsis neonatorium. *N Engl J Med* 1981;**304**:642.

Sprung CL et al: The effects of high-dose corticosteroids in patients with septic shock: A prospective, controlled study. *N Engl J Med* 1984;**311**:1137.

Wolff SM: The treatment of gram-negative bacteremia and shock (Editorial.) *N Engl J Med* 1982;**307**:1267.

Young LS: Combination or single drug therapy for gram-negative sepsis. Pages 177–205 in: *Current Clinical Topics in Infectious Diseases.* Vol 3. Remington JS, Swartz MN (editors). McGraw-Hill, 1982.

Ziegler EJ et al: Treatment of gram-negative bacteremia and shock with human antiserum to a mutant *Escherichia coli.* *N Engl J Med* 1982;**307**:1225.

Interstitial Nephritis & Papillary Necrosis

Bengtsson U et al: Malignancies of the urinary tract and their relation to analgesic abuse. *Kidney Int* 1978;**13**:107.

Burry A: Pathology of analgesic nephropathy: Australian experience. *Kidney Int* 1978;**13**:34.

Eknoyan G et al: Renal papillary necrosis: An update. *Medicine* 1982;**61**:55.

Flaster S, Lome LG, Presman D: Urologic complications of renal papillary necrosis. *Urology* 1975;**5**:331.

Gonwa TA et al: Analgesic-associated nephropathy and transitional cell carcinoma of the urinary tract. *Ann Intern Med* 1980;**93**:249.

Heptinstall RH: Interstitial nephritis. *Am J Pathol* 1976;**83**:214.

Husband P, Howlett KA: Renal papillary necrosis in infancy. *Arch Dis Child* 1973;**48**:116.

Kincaid-Smith P: Analgesic nephropathy. *Kidney Int* 1978;**13**:1.

Lindvall N: Radiological changes of renal papillary necrosis. *Kidney Int* 1978;**13**:93.

Murray RM: Analgesic nephropathy: Removal of phenacetin from proprietary analgesics. *Br Med J* 1972;**4**:131.

Murray TG, Goldberg M: Analgesic-associated nephropathy in the USA: Epidemiologic, clinical and pathogenic features. *Kidney Int* 1978;**13**:64.

Murray TG, Goldberg M: Chronic interstitial nephritis: Etiologic factors. *Ann Intern Med* 1975;**82**:453.

Pandya KK et al: Renal papillary necrosis in sickle cell hemoglobinopathies. *J Urol* 1976;**115**:497.

Poynter JD, Hare WSC: Necrosis in situ: A form of renal papillary necrosis seen in analgesic nephropathy. *Radiology* 1974;**111**:69.

Renal & Perinephric Abscesses

Anderson KA, McAninch JW: Renal abscesses: Classification and review of 40 cases. *Urology* 1980;**16**:333.

Brugh R 3rd et al: Gallium-67 scanning and conservative treatment in acute inflammatory lesions of the renal cortex. *J Urol* 1979;**121**:232.

Cronan JJ, Amis ES Jr, Dorfman GS: Percutaneous drainage of renal abscesses. *AJR* 1984;**142**:351.

Fallon B, Gershon C: Renal carbuncle: Diagnosis and management. *Urology* 1981;**17**:303.

Goldman SM et al: Renal carbuncle: The use of ultrasound in its diagnosis and treatment. *J Urol* 1977;**118**:525.

Hampel N, Class RN, Persky L: Value of 67 Gallium scintigraphy in diagnosis of localized renal and perirenal inflammation. *J Urol* 1980;**124**:311.

Hoddick W et al: CT and sonography of severe renal and perirenal infections. *AJR* 1983;**140**:517.

Hopkins GB, Hall RL, Mende CW: Gallium-67 scintigraphy for the diagnosis and localization of perinephric abscesses. *J Urol* 1976;**115**:126.

Hoverman IV et al: Intrarenal abscess: Report of 14 cases. *Arch Intern Med* 1980;**140**:914.

Koehler PR, Nelson JA: Arteriographic findings in inflammatory mass lesions of the kidney. *Radiol Clin North Am* 1976;**14**:281.

Malgieri JJ, Kursh ED, Persky L: The changing clinico-pathological pattern of abscesses in or adjacent to the kidney. *J Urol* 1977;**118**:230.

Morgan WR, Nyberg LM Jr: Perinephric and intrarenal abscesses. *Urology* 1985;**26**:529.

Mulligan ME, Rose JG, Finegold SM: Intrarenal and perirenal abscess. Pages 559–565 in: *Infectious Diseases,* 3rd ed. Hoeprich PD (editor). Harper & Row, 1983.

Rives RK, Harty JI, Amin M: Renal abscesses: Emerging

concepts of diagnosis and treatment. *J Urol* 1980; **124:**446.

Saiki J, Vaziri ND, Barton C: Perinephric and intranephric abscesses: A review of the literature. *West J Med* 1982; **136:**95.

Schiff M Jr et al: Antibiotic treatment of renal carbuncle. *Ann Intern Med* 1977;**87:**305.

Thorley JD, Jones SR, Sanford JP: Perinephric abscess. *Medicine* 1974;**53:**441.

Timmons JW, Perlmutter AD: Renal abscess: A changing concept. *J Urol* 1976;**115:**299.

Nonspecific Infection of the Bladder

Anderson RU, Hsieh-Ma ST: Association of bacteriuria and pyuria during intermittent catheterization after spinal cord injury. *J Urol* 1983;**130:**299.

Fair WR, McClennan BL, Jost RG: Are excretory urograms necessary in evaluating women with urinary tract infections? *J Urol* 1979;**121:**313.

Fihn SD, Stamm WE: The urethral syndrome. *Semin Urol* 1983;**1:**121.

Gallagher DJA, Montgomerie JZ, North JDK: Acute infections of the urinary tract and the urethral syndrome in general practice. *Br Med J* 1965;**1:**622.

Hashida Y, Gaffney PC, Yunis EJ: Acute hemorrhagic cystitis of childhood and papovavirus-like particles. *J Pediatr* 1976;**89:**85.

Larsen S et al: Mast cells in interstitial cystitis. *Br J Urol* 1982;**54:**283.

Meares EM Jr: Urinary catheters and nosocomial infection. *Urology* 1985;**26(1 Suppl):**12.

Messing EM: Interstitial cystitis and related syndromes. Pages 1070–1092 in: *Campbell's Urology*, 5th ed. Vol 1. Walsh PC et al (editors). Saunders, 1986.

Mufson MA, Belshe RB: A review of adenovirsues in the etiology of acute hemorrhagic cystitis. *J Urol* 1976;**115:**191.

Neu HC: Urinary tract infections in the 1980s. *Semin Urol* 1983;**1:**130.

Powell NB et al: Allergy of the lower urinary tract. *J Urol* 1972;**107:**631.

Rein MF: Current therapy of vulvovaginitis. *Sex Transm Dis* 1981;**8(Suppl):**316.

Ronald AR: The management of urethrocystitis in women. *Semin Urol* 1983;**1:**114.

Ronald AR, Harding GKM: Urinary infection prophylaxis in women. *Ann Intern Med* 1981;**94:**268.

Shortliffe LMD, Stamey TA: Urinary infections in adult women. Pages 797–830 in: *Campbell's Urology*, 5th ed. Vol 1. Walsh PC et al (editors). Saunders, 1986.

Stamey TA: *Pathogenesis and Treatment of Urinary Tract Infections*. Williams & Wilkins, 1980.

Stamm WE et al: Diagnosis of coliform infection in acutely dysuric women. *N Engl J Med* 1982;**307:**463.

Stamm WE et al: Treatment of the acute urethral syndrome. *N Engl J Med* 1981;**304:**956.

Winberg J: Urinary tract infections in infants and children. Pages 831–867 in: *Campbell's Urology*, 5th ed. Vol 1. Walsh PC et al (editors). Saunders, 1986.

Nonspecific Infections of the Prostate Gland

Brunner H et al (editors): *Chronic Prostatitis: Clinical, Microbiological, Cytological and Immunological Aspects of Inflammation*. Schattauer Verlag, 1985.

Brunner H et al (editors): *Therapy of Prostatitis: Experimental and Clinical Data*. Zuckschwerdt Verlag, 1986.

Dajani MD, O'Flynn JD: Prostatic abscess. *Br J Urol*

1968;**40:**736.

Drach GW et al: Classification of benign diseases associated with prostatic pain: Prostatitis or prostatodynia? *J Urol* 1978;**120:**266.

Fair WR, Cordonnier JJ: The pH of prostatic fluid: A reappraisal and therapeutic implications. *J Urol* 1978;**120:**695.

Fair WR, Couch J, Wehner N: Prostatic antibacterial factor: Identity and significance. *Urology* 1976;**7:**169.

Kohnen PW, Drach GW: Patterns of inflammation in prostatic hyperplasia: Histologic and bacteriologic study. *J Urol* 1979;**121:**755.

Mardh P-A et al: Role of *Chlamydia trachomatis* in nonacute prostatitis. *Br J Vener Dis* 1978;**54:**330.

Meares EM Jr: Prostatitis: Review of pharmacokinetics and therapy. *Rev Infect Dis* 1982;**4:**475.

Meares EM Jr: Prostatitis and related disorders. Pages 868–887 in: *Campbell's Urology*, 5th ed. Vol 1. Walsh PC et al (editors). Saunders, 1986.

Meares EM Jr, Barbalias GA: Prostatitis: Bacterial, nonbacterial, and prostatodynia. *Semin Urol* 1983;**1:**146.

Meares EM, Stamey TA: Bacteriologic localization patterns in bacterial prostatitis and urethritis. *Invest Urol* 1968;**5:**492.

O'Dea MJ, Hunting DB, Greene LF: Non-specific granulomatous prostatitis. *J Urol* 1977;**118:**58.

Orland SM, Hanno PM, Wein AJ: Prostatitis, protatosis, and prostatodynia. *Urology* 1985;**25:**439.

Pai MG, Bhat HS: Prostatic abscess. *J Urol* 1972;**108:**599.

Schacter J: Is *Chlamydia trachomatis* a cause of prostatitis? (Editorial.) *J Urol* 1985;**134:**711.

Schaeffer AJ et al: Prevalence and significance of prostatic inflammation. *J Urol* 1981;**125:**215.

Segura JW et al: Prostatosis, prostatitis or pelvic floor tension myalgia? *J Urol* 1979;**122:**168.

Sharer WC, Fair WR: The pharmacokinetics of antibiotic diffusion in chronic bacterial prostatitis. *Prostate* 1982;**3:**139.

Shortliffe LMD, Wehner N, Stamey TA: The detection of a local prostatic immunologic response to bacterial prostatitis. *J Urol* 1981;**125:**509.

Taylor EW et al: Granulomatous prostatitis: Confusion clinically with carcinoma of the prostate. *J Urol* 1977;**117:**316.

Towfighi J et al: Granulomatous prostatitis with emphasis on the eosinophilic variety. *Am J Clin Pathol* 1972;**58:**630.

Weidner W et al: Quantitative culture of *Ureaplasma urealyticum* in patients with chronic prostatitis or prostatosis. *J Urol* 1980;**124:**622.

Nonspecific Infections of the Epididymis

Berger RE: Urethritis and epididymitis. *Semin Urol* 1983; **1:**138.

Berger RE et al: Clinical use of epididymal aspiration cultures in management of selected patients with acute epididymitis. *J Urol* 1980;**124:**60.

Berger RE et al: Etiology, manifestations and therapy of acute epididymitis: Prospective study of 50 cases. *J Urol* 1979;**121:**750.

Gierup J, von Hedenberg C, Osterman A: Acute nonspecific epididymitis in boys: A survey based on 48 consecutive cases. *Scand J Urol Nephrol* 1975;**9:**5.

Levy OM et al: Diagnosis of acute testicular torsion using radionuclide scanning. *J Urol* 1983;**129:**975.

Miller HC: Local anesthesia for acute epididymitis. *J Urol* 1970;**104:**735.

Resnick MI: Imaging techniques and testicular abnormalities. (Guest editorial.) *J Urol* 1983;**129**:984.

Sufrin G: Acute eqpididymitis. *Sex Transm Dis* 1981; **8(Suppl)**:132.

Wilson SK, Hagan KW, Rhamy RK: Epididymectomy for acute and chronic disease. *J Urol* 1974;**112**:357.

Nonspecific Infections of the Testis & Scrotum

Beard CM et al: The incidence and outcome of mumps orchitis in Rochester, Minnesota, 1935 to 1974. *Mayo Clin Proc* 1977;**52**:3.

Biswas M et al: Necrotizing infection of scrotum. *Urology* 1979;**14**:576.

Chilton CP, Smith PJB: Steroid therapy in the treatment of a granulomatous orchitis. *Br J Urol* 1979;**51**:404.

Fauer RB et al: Clinical aspects of granulomatous orchitis. *Urology* 1978;**12**:416.

Krieger JN: Epididymitis, orchitis, and related conditions. *Sex Transm Dis* 1984;**11**:173.

Nickel WR, Plumb RT: Cutaneous diseases of external genitalia. Pages 956–982 in: *Campbell's Urology*, 5th ed. Vol 1. Walsh PC et al (editors). Saunders, 1986.

Antimicrobial Treatment of Urinary Tract Infections

A clinical perspective of antibiotic therapy: Aminoglycosides vs broad-spectrum beta-lactams. (Symposium.) Gilbert DN, Sanford JP (editors). *Rev Infect Dis* 1983;**5(Suppl)**:1–398.

Acar JF, Neu HC (editors): Gram-negative aerobic bacterial infections: A focus on directed therapy, with special reference to aztreonam. (Symposium.) *Rev Infect Dis* 1985;**7(Suppl 4)**:S537.

Appel GB, Neu HC: The nephrotoxicity of antimicrobial agents. (3 parts.) *N Engl J Med* 1977;**296**:663, 722, 784.

Ball AP: Clinical uses of penicillins. *Lancet* 1982;**2**:197.

Bartlett JG: Anti-anaerobic antibacterial agents. *Lancet* 1982;**2**:478.

Bennett WM et al: Drug therapy in renal failure: Dosing guidelines for adults. 1. Antimicrobial agents, analgesics. *Ann Intern Med* 1980;**93**:62.

Bergan T: The role of broad-spectrum antibiotics and diagnostic problems in urinary tract infections. *Arch Intern Med* (Oct 25) 1982;**142**:1993. [Special issue.]

Buckwold FJ et al: Therapy for acute cystitis in adult women: Randomized comparison of single-dose sulfisoxazole vs trimethoprim-sulfamethoxazole. *JAMA* 1982;**247**:1839.

Calderwood SB, Moellering RC Jr: Common adverse effects of antibacterial agents on major organ systems. *Surg Clin North Am* 1980;**60**:65.

Chodak GW, Plaut ME: Systemic antibiotics for prophylaxis in urologic surgery: Critical review. *J Urol* 1979;**121**:695.

Chow AW, Jewesson PJ: Pharmacokinetics and safety of antimicrobial agents during pregnancy. *Rev Infect Dis* 1985;**7**:287.

Cohen J: Antifungal chemotherapy. *Lancet* 1982;**2**:532.

Fair WR et al: Three-day treatment of urinary tract infections. *J Urol* 1980;**123**:717.

Fang LST et al: Clinical management of urinary tract infection. *Pharmacotherapy* 1982;**2**:91.

Fihn SD, Stamm WE: Interpretation and comparison of treatment studies for uncomplicated urinary tract infections in women. *Rev Infect Dis* 1985;**7**:468.

Fihn SD, Stamm WE: The urethral syndrome. *Semin Urol* 1983;**1**:121.

Fowler JE Jr: Office bacteriology: Techniques and interpretations. *Semin Urol* 1983;**1**:97.

Gleckman R et al: Recurrent urinary tract infections in men: An assessment of contemporary treatment. *Am J Med Sci* 1980;**279**:31.

Greenberg RN et al: Randomized study of single-dose, three-day, and seven-day treatment of cystitis in women. *J Infect Dis* 1986;**153**:277.

Hausman MS: Treatment of urinary infections with cefadroxil: Controlled comparison of high-compliance oral dosage regimens. *Urology* 1980;**15**:40.

Holmberg L et al: Adverse reactions to nitrofurantoin: Analysis of 921 reports. *Am J Med* 1980;**69**:733.

Jabbar A et al: Use of oral carbenicillin in urinary tract infection. *Curr Ther Res* 1978;**23**:22.

Kucers A: Chloramphenicol, erythromycin, vancomycin, tetracyclines. *Lancet* 1982;**2**:425.

Kunin CM: Duration of treatment of urinary tract infections. *Am J Med* 1981;**71**:849.

Lesar TS et al: Gentamicin dosing errors with four commonly used nomograms. *JAMA* 1982;**248**:1190.

Light RB et al: Trimethoprim alone in the treatment and prophylaxis of urinary tract infection. *Arch Intern Med* 1981; **141**:1807.

Meares EM Jr: Prostatitis: Review of pharmacokinetics and therapy. *Rev Infect Dis* 1982;**4**:475.

Moellering RC Jr, Siegenthaler WD (editors): Aminoglycoside therapy—the new decade: A worldwide perspective. (Symposium.) *Am J Med* 1986;**80(Suppl 6B)**:1. [Entire issue.]

Neu HC (editor): Advances in cephalosporin therapy: Beyond the third generation. *Am J Med* 1985;**79(Suppl 2A)**:1. [Entire issue.]

Neu HC: Urinary tract infections in the 1980s. *Semin Urol* 1983;**1**:130.

New trends in antimicrobial susceptibility testing. (Symposium of the XIII international Congress of Microbiology, Boston, Massachusetts, August 9, 1982.) *Diagn Microbiol Infect Dis* 1983;**1**:v–47.

Rahal JJ: Antibiotic combinations: The clinical relevance of synergy and antagonism. *Medicine* 1978;**57**:179.

Reeves D: Sulphonamides and trimethoprim. *Lancet* 1982; **2**:370.

Remington JS (editor): Carbapenems: A new class of antibiotics. (Symposium.) *Am J Med* 1985;**78(Suppl 6A)**:1. [Entire issue.]

Ronald AR: The management of urethrocystitis in women. *Semin Urol* 1983;**1**:114.

Scavone JM, Gleckman RA, Fraser DG: Cinoxacin: Mechanism of action, spectrum of activity, pharmacokinetics, adverse reactions, and therapeutic indications. *Pharmacotherapy* 1982;**2**:266.

Shortliffe LMD, Stamey TA: Urinary infections in adult women. Pages 797–830 in: *Campbell's Urology*, 5th ed. Vol 1. Walsh PC et al (editors). Saunders, 1986.

Smith CR et al: Double-blind comparison of the nephrotoxicity and auditory toxicity of gentamicin and tobramycin. *N Engl J Med* 1980;**302**:1106.

Smith JW et al: Recurrent urinary tract infections in men: Characteristics and response to therapy. *Ann Intern Med* 1979;**91**:544.

Stamey TA: *Pathogenesis and Treatment of Urinary Tract Infections*. Williams & Wilkins, 1980.

Stamm WE et al: Is antimicrobial prophylaxis of urinary tract infections cost-effective? *Ann Intern Med* 1981;**94**:251.

Tolkoff-Rubin NE et al: Single-dose therapy with trimethoprim-sulfamethoxazole for urinary tract infection in
women. *Rev Infect Dis* 1982;**4**:444.

Trimethoprim-sulfamethoxazole revisited. (Symposium.)
Finland M, Kass EH, Platt R (editors). *Rev Infect Dis*
1982;**4**:1–618.

Winberg J: Urinary tract infections in infants and children.
Pages 831–867 in: *Campbell's Urology,* 5th ed. Vol 1.
Walsh PC et al (editors). Saunders, 1986.

14

Specific Infections of the Genitourinary Tract

Emil A. Tanagho, MD

"Specific" infections are those caused by "specific" organisms, each of which causes a clinically unique disease. See also Chapter 15.

TUBERCULOSIS

Tubercle bacilli may invade one or more (or even all) of the organs of the genitourinary tract and cause a chronic granulomatous infection that shows the same characteristics as tuberculosis in other organs. Urinary tuberculosis is a disease of young adults (60% of patients are between the ages of 20 and 40) and is a little more common in males than in females.

Etiology

The infecting organism is *Mycobacterium tuberculosis,* which reaches the genitourinary organs by the hematogenous route from the lungs. The primary site is often not symptomatic or apparent.

The kidney and possibly the prostate are the primary sites of tuberculous infection in the genitourinary tract. All other genitourinary organs become involved either by ascent (prostate to bladder) or descent (kidney to bladder; prostate to epididymis). The testis may become involved by direct extension from epididymal infection.

Pathogenesis
(Fig 14–1)

A. Kidney and Ureter: When a shower of tubercle bacilli hits the renal cortex, the organisms may be destroyed by normal tissue resistance. Evidence of this is commonly seen in autopsies of persons who have died of tuberculosis; only scars are found in the kidneys. However, if enough bacteria of sufficient virulence become lodged in the kidney and are not overcome, a clinical infection is established.

Tuberculosis of the kidney progresses slowly; it may take 15–20 years to destroy a kidney in a patient having good resistance to the infection. As a rule, therefore, there is no renal pain and little or no clinical disturbance of any type until the lesion has involved the calices or the pelvis, at which time pus and organisms may be discharged into the urine. It is only at this stage that symptoms (of cystitis) are manifested. The infection then proceeds to the pelvic mucosa and the ureter, particularly its upper and vesical ends. This

may lead to stricture and back pressure (hydronephrosis).

As the disease progresses, a caseous breakdown of tissue occurs until the entire kidney is replaced by cheesy material. Calcium may be laid down in the reparative process. The ureter undergoes fibrosis and tends to be shortened and therefore straightened. This change leads to a "golf-hole" (gaping) ureteral orifice, typical of an incompetent valve.

B. Bladder: Vesical irritability develops as an early clinical manifestation of the disease as the bladder is bathed by infected material. Tubercles form later, usually in the region of the involved ureteral orifice, and finally coalesce and ulcerate. These ulcers may bleed. With severe involvement, the bladder becomes fibrosed and contracted; this leads to marked frequency. Ureteral reflux or stenosis and, therefore, hydronephrosis may develop. If contralateral renal involvement occurs later, it is probably a separate hematogenous infection.

C. Prostate and Seminal Vesicles: The passage of infected urine through the prostatic urethra will ultimately lead to invasion of the prostate and one or both seminal vesicles. There is no local pain.

On occasion, the primary hematogenous lesion in the genitourinary tract is in the prostate. Prostatic infection can ascend to the bladder and descend to the epididymis.

D. Epididymis and Testis: Tuberculosis of the prostate can extend along the vas or through the perivasal lymphatics and affect the epididymis. Because this is a slow process, there is usually no pain. If the epididymal infection is extensive and an abscess forms, it may rupture through the scrotal skin, thus establishing a permanent sinus, or it may extend into the testicle.

Pathology

A. Kidney and Ureter: The gross appearance of the kidney with moderately advanced tuberculosis is often normal on its outer surface, although it is usually surrounded by marked perinephritis. Usually, however, there is a soft, yellowish localized bulge. On section, the involved area is seen to be filled with cheesy material (caseation). Widespread destruction of parenchyma is evident. In otherwise normal tissue, small abscesses may be seen. The walls of the pelvis, calices, and ureter may be thickened, and ulceration ap-

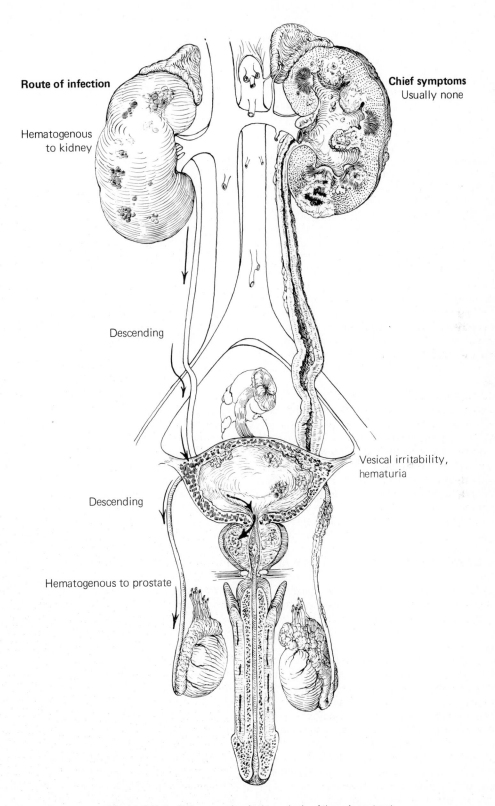

Route of infection

Hematogenous
to kidney

Descending

Descending

Hematogenous to prostate

Chief symptoms
Usually none

Vesical irritability,
hematuria

Figure 14–1. Pathogenesis of tuberculosis of the urinary tract.

pears frequently in the region of the calices at the point at which the abscess drains. Ureteral stenosis may be complete, causing "autonephrectomy." Such a kidney is fibrosed and functionless. Under these circumstances, the bladder urine may be normal and symptoms absent.

Tubercle foci appear close to the glomeruli. These are an aggregation of histiocytic cells possessing a vesicular nucleus and a clear cell body that can fuse with neighboring cells to form a small mass called an epithelioid reticulum. At the periphery of this reticulum are large cells with multiple nuclei (giant cells). This pathologic reaction, which can be seen macroscopically, is the basic lesion in tuberculosis. It can heal by fibrosis or coalesce and reach the surface and ulcerate, forming an ulcerocavernous lesion. Tubercles might undergo a central degeneration and caseate, creating a tuberculous abscess cavity that can reach the collecting system and break through. In the process, progressive parenchymal destruction occurs. Depending on the virulence of the organism and the resistance of the patient, tuberculosis is a combination of caseation and cavitation and healing by fibrosis and scarring.

Microscopically, the caseous material is seen as an amorphous mass. The surrounding parenchyma shows fibrosis with tissue destruction, small round cell and plasma cell infiltration, and epithelial and giant cells typical of tuberculosis. Acid-fast stains will usually demonstrate the organisms in the tissue. Similar changes can be demonstrated in the wall of the pelvis and ureter.

In both the kidney and ureter, calcification is common. It may be macroscopic or microscopic. Such a finding is strongly suggestive of tuberculosis but, of course, is also observed in bilharzial infection. Secondary renal stones occur in 10% of patients.

In the most advanced stage of renal tuberculosis, the parenchyma may be completely replaced by caseous substance or fibrous tissue. Perinephric abscess may develop, but this is rare.

B. Bladder: In the early stages, the mucosa may be inflamed, but this is not a specific change. The bladder is quite resistant to actual invasion. Later, tubercles form and can be seen easily, especially through the cystoscope, as white or yellow raised nodules surrounded by a halo of hyperemia. With severe vesical contracture, reflux may occur.

Microscopically, the nodules are typical tubercles. These break down to form deep, ragged ulcers. At this stage the bladder is quite irritable. With healing, fibrosis develops that involves the muscle wall.

C. Prostate and Seminal Vesicles: Grossly, the exterior surface of these organs may show nodules and areas of induration from fibrosis. Areas of necrosis are common. In rare cases, healing may end in calcification. Large calcifications in the prostate should suggest tuberculous involvement.

D. Spermatic Cord, Epididymis, and Testis: The vas deferens is often grossly involved; fusiform swellings represent tubercles that in chronic cases are

characteristically described as beaded. The epididymis is enlarged and quite firm. It is usually separate from the testis, although occasionally it may adhere to it. Microscopically, the changes typical of tuberculosis are seen. Tubular degeneration may be marked.

The testis is usually not involved except by direct extension of an abscess in the epididymis.

E. Female Genital Tract: Infections are usually carried by the bloodstream; rarely, they are the result of sexual contact with an infected male. The incidence of associated urinary and genital infection in females ranges from 1 to 10%. The uterine tubes may be affected. Other presentations include endarteritis, localized adnexal masses (usually bilateral), and tuberculous cervicitis, but granulomatous lesions of the vaginal canal and vulva are rare.

Clinical Findings

Tuberculosis of the genitourinary tract should be considered in the presence of any of the following situations: (1) chronic cystitis that refuses to respond to adequate therapy, (2) the finding of pus without bacteria in a methylene blue stain or culture of the urinary sediment, (3) gross or microscopic hematuria, (4) a nontender, enlarged epididymis with a beaded or thickened vas, (5) a chronic draining scrotal sinus, or (6) induration or nodulation of the prostate and thickening of one or both seminal vesicles (especially in a young man). A history of present or past tuberculosis elsewhere in the body should cause the physician to suspect tuberculosis in the genitourinary tract when signs or symptoms are present.

The diagnosis rests upon the demonstration of tubercle bacilli in the urine by culture. The extent of the infection is determined by (1) the palpable findings in the epididymides, vasa deferentia, prostate, and seminal vesicles; (2) the renal and ureteral lesions as revealed by excretory urograms; (3) involvement of the bladder as seen through the cystoscope; (4) the degree of renal damage as measured by loss of function; and (5) the presence of tubercle bacilli in one or both kidneys.

A. Symptoms: There is no classic clinical picture of renal tuberculosis. Most symptoms of this disease, even in the most advanced stage, are vesical in origin (cystitis). Vague generalized malaise, fatigability, low-grade but persistent fever, and night sweats are some of the nonspecific complaints. Even vesical irritability may be absent, in which case only proper collection and examination of the urine will afford the clue. Active tuberculosis elsewhere in the body is found in less than half of patients with genitourinary tuberculosis.

1. Kidney and ureter–Because of the slow progression of the disease, the affected kidney is usually completely asymptomatic. On occasion, however, there may be a dull ache in the flank. The passage of a blood clot, secondary calculi, or a mass of debris may cause renal and ureteral colic. Rarely, the presenting symptom may be a painless mass in the abdomen.

2. Bladder—The earliest symptoms of renal tuberculosis may arise from secondary vesical involvement. These include burning, frequency, and nocturia. Hematuria is occasionally found and is of either renal or vesical origin. At times, particularly in a late stage of the disease, the vesical irritability may become extreme. If ulceration occurs, suprapubic pain may be noted when the bladder becomes full.

3. Genital tract—Tuberculosis of the prostate and seminal vesicles usually causes no symptoms. The first clue to the presence of tuberculous infection of these organs is the onset of a tuberculous epididymitis.

Tuberculosis of the epididymis usually presents as a painless or only mildly painful swelling. An abscess may drain spontaneously through the scrotal wall. A chronic draining sinus should be regarded as tuberculous until proved otherwise. In rare cases, the onset is quite acute and may simulate an acute nonspecific epididymitis.

B. Signs: Evidence of extragenital tuberculosis may be found (lungs, bone, lymph nodes, tonsils, intestines).

1. Kidney—There is usually no enlargement or tenderness of the involved kidney.

2. External genitalia—A thickened, nontender, or only slightly tender epididymis may be discovered. The vas deferens often is thickened and beaded. A chronic draining sinus through the scrotal skin is almost pathognomonic of tuberculous epididymitis. In the more advanced stages, the epididymis cannot be differentiated from the testis upon palpation. This may mean that the testis has been directly invaded by the epididymal abscess.

Hydrocele occasionally accompanies tuberculous epididymitis. The "idiopathic" hydrocele should be tapped so that underlying pathologic changes, if present, can be evaluated (epididymitis, testicular tumor). Involvement of the penis and urethra is rare.

3. Prostate and seminal vesicles—These organs may be normal to palpation. Ordinarily, however, the tuberculous prostate shows areas of induration, even nodulation. The involved vesicle is usually indurated, enlarged, and fixed. If epididymitis is present, the ipsilateral vesicle usually shows changes as well.

C. Laboratory Findings: Proper urinalysis affords the most important clue to the diagnosis of genitourinary tuberculosis. .

1. Persistent pyuria without organisms on culture or on the smear stained with methylene blue means tuberculosis until proved otherwise. Acid-fast stains done on the concentrated sediment from a 24-hour specimen are positive in at least 60% of cases. However, this must be corroborated by a positive culture.

About 15–20% of patients with tuberculosis have secondary pyogenic infection; the clue ("sterile" pyuria) is thereby obscured. If clinical response to adequate treatment fails and pyuria persists, tuberculosis must be ruled out by bacteriologic and roentgenologic means.

2. Cultures for tubercle bacilli from the first morning urine are positive in a very high percentage of cases of tuberculous infection. If positive, sensitivity tests should be ordered. In the face of strong presumptive evidence of tuberculosis, negative cultures should be repeated.

The blood count may be normal or may show anemia in advanced disease. The sedimentation rate is usually accelerated.

Tubercle bacilli may often be demonstrated in the secretions from an infected prostate. Renal function will be normal unless there is bilateral damage: as one kidney is slowly injured, compensatory hypertrophy of the normal kidney develops. It can also be infected with tubercle bacilli, or it may become hydronephrotic from fibrosis of the bladder wall (ureterovesical stenosis) or vesicoureteral reflux.

If tuberculosis is suspected, perform the tuberculin test. A positive test, particularly in an adult, is hardly diagnostic; but a negative test in an otherwise healthy patient speaks against a diagnosis of tuberculosis.

D. X-Ray Findings: (Fig 14–2.) A chest film that shows evidence of tuberculosis should cause the physician to suspect tuberculosis of the urogenital tract in the presence of urinary signs and symptoms. A plain film of the abdomen may show enlargement of one kidney or obliteration of the renal and psoas shadows due to perinephric abscess. Punctate calcification in the renal parenchyma may be due to tuberculosis. Renal stones are found in 10% of cases. Calcification of the ureter may be noted, but this is rare (Fig 6–2). Small prostatic stones the size of grape seeds in the region of the pubic symphysis are ordinarily not due to tuberculosis, but large calcific bodies may be.

Excretory urograms can be diagnostic if the lesion is moderately advanced. The typical changes include (1) a "moth-eaten" appearance of the involved ulcerated calices, (2) obliteration of one or more calices, (3) dilatation of the calices due to ureteral stenosis from fibrosis, (4) abscess cavities that connect with calices, (5) single or multiple ureteral strictures, with secondary dilatation, with shortening and therefore straightening of the ureter, and (6) absence of function of the kidney due to complete ureteral occlusion and renal destruction (autonephrectomy).

If the excretory urograms demonstrate gross tuberculosis in one kidney, there is no need to do a retrograde urogram on that side. In fact, there is at least a theoretical danger of hematogenous or lymphogenous dissemination resulting from the increased intrapelvic pressure. Retrograde urography may, however, be carried out on the unsuspected side as a verification of its normality. This is further substantiated if the urine from that side is free of both pus cells and tubercle bacilli.

E. Instrumental Examination: Thorough cystoscopic study is indicated even when the offending organism has been found in the urine and excretory urograms show the typical renal lesion. This will clearly demonstrate the extent of the disease. Cystoscopy may reveal the typical tubercles or ulcers of tuberculosis. Biopsy can be done if necessary. Severe

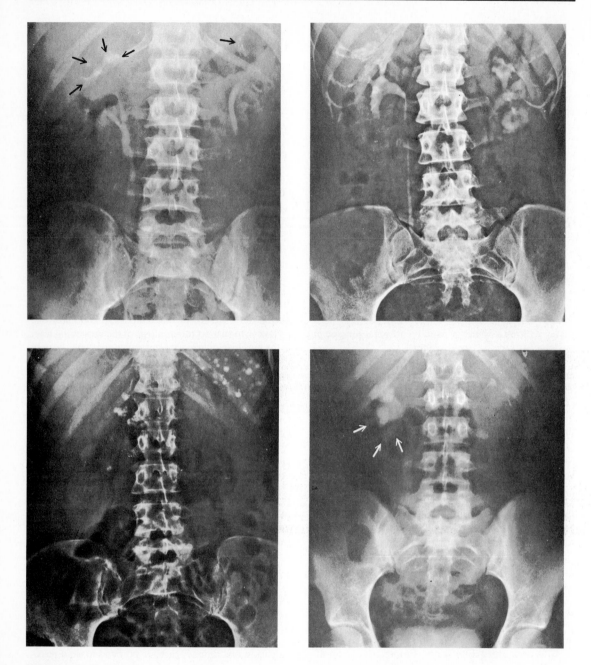

Figure 14–2. Radiologic evidence of tuberculosis. *Upper left:* Excretory urogram showing "moth-eaten" calices in upper renal poles. Calcifications in upper calices; right upper ureter is straight and dilated. *Upper right:* Excretory urogram showing ulcerated and dilated calices on the left. *Lower left:* Plain film showing calicifications in right kidney, adrenals, and spleen (tuberculosis of right kidney and Addison's disease). *Lower right:* Excretory urogram. Dilatation of calices; upper right ureter dilated and straight. Arrows point to poorly defined parenchymal abscesses.

contracture of the bladder may be noted. A cystogram may reveal ureteral reflux. A clean specimen of urine should also be obtained for further study.

Differential Diagnosis

Chronic nonspecific cystitis or pyelonephritis may mimic tuberculosis perfectly, especially since 15–20% of cases of tuberculosis are secondarily in-

vaded by pyogenic organisms. If nonspecific infections do not respond to adequate therapy, a search for tubercle bacilli should be made. Painless epididymitis points to tuberculosis. Cystoscopic demonstration of tubercles and ulceration of the bladder wall means tuberculosis. Urograms are usually definitive.

Acute or chronic nonspecific epididymitis may be confused with tuberculosis, since the onset of tuberculosis is occasionally quite painful. It is rare to have palpatory changes in the seminal vesicles with nonspecific epididymitis, but these are almost routine findings in tuberculosis of the epididymis. The presence of tubercle bacilli on a culture of the urine is diagnostic. On occasion, only the pathologist can make the diagnosis by microscopic study of the surgically removed epididymis.

Amicrobic cystitis usually has an acute onset and is often preceded by a urethral discharge. "Sterile" pyuria is found, but tubercle bacilli are absent. Cystoscopy may reveal ulcerations, but these are acute and superficial. Although urograms show mild hydroureter and even hydronephrosis, there is no ulceration of the calices as seen in renal tuberculosis.

Interstitial cystitis is typically characterized by frequency, nocturia, and suprapubic pain with vesical filling. The urine is usually free of pus. Tubercle bacilli are absent.

Multiple small renal stones or nephrocalcinosis seen by x-ray may suggest the type of calcification seen in the tuberculous kidney. In renal tuberculosis, the calcium is in the parenchyma, although secondary stones are occasionally seen.

Necrotizing papillitis, which may involve all of the calices of one or both kidneys or, rarely, a solitary calix, shows caliceal lesions (including calcifications) that simulate those of tuberculosis. Careful bacteriologic studies will fail to demonstrate tubercle bacilli.

Medullary sponge kidneys may show small calcifications just distal to the calices. The calices, however, are sharp, and no other stigmas of tuberculosis can be demonstrated.

In disseminated coccidioidomycosis, renal involvement may occur. The renal lesion resembles that of tuberculosis (Connor, Drach, and Bucher, 1975). Coccidioidal epididymitis may be confused with tuberculous involvement (Cheng, 1974).

Urinary bilharziasis is a great mimic of tuberculosis. Both present with symptoms of cystitis and often hematuria. Vesical contraction, seen in both diseases, may lead to extreme frequency. Schistosomiasis must be suspected in endemic areas; the typical ova are found in the urine; cystoscopic and urographic findings are definitive in differential diagnosis.

Complications

A. Renal Tuberculosis: Perinephric abscess may cause an enlarging mass in the flank. A plain film of the abdomen will show obliteration of the renal and psoas shadows. Sonograms and CT scans may be more helpful. Renal stones may develop if secondary nonspecific infection is present. Uremia is the end stage if both kidneys are involved.

B. Ureteral Tuberculosis: Scarring with stricture formation is one of the typical lesions of tuberculosis and most commonly affects the juxtavesical portion of the ureter. This may cause progressive hydronephrosis. Complete ureteral obstruction may cause complete nonfunction of the kidney (Feldstein, Sullivan, and Banowsky, 1975).

C. Vesical Tuberculosis: When severely damaged, the bladder wall becomes fibrosed and contracted. Stenosis of the ureters or reflux occurs, causing hydronephrotic atrophy.

D. Genital Tuberculosis: The ducts of the involved epididymis become occluded. If this is bilateral, sterility results. Abscess of the epididymis may rupture into the testis, through the scrotal wall, or both, in which case the spermatogenic tubules may slough out.

Treatment

Tuberculosis must be treated as a generalized disease. Even when it can be demonstrated only in the urogenital tract, one must assume activity elsewhere. (It is theoretically possible, however, for the primary focus to have healed spontaneously.) This means that basically the treatment is medical. Surgical excision of an infected organ, when indicated, is merely an adjunct to overall therapy.

A. Renal Tuberculosis: A strict medical regimen should be instituted. The following drugs are usually considered only in cases of resistance to first-line drugs and when expert medical personnel are available to treat toxic side effects, should they occur: aminosalicylic acid (PAS), capreomycin, cycloserine, ethionamide, pyrazinamide, viomycin. See note below on pyrazinamide.

The following combinations of drugs can be utilized. The choice can be governed by the results of sensitivity tests. (1) Cycloserine, aminosalicylic acid (PAS), and isoniazid (INH). (2) Cycloserine, ethambutol, and INH. (3) Rifampin, ethambutol, and INH. The latter group is probably the most efficacious. The oral dose of each is as follows: cycloserine, 250 mg twice daily; PAS, 15 g in divided doses; INH, 300 mg; ethambutol, 1.2 g; rifampin, 600 mg. Sensitivity testing may indicate the use of streptomycin intramuscularly. Administer 1 g/d the first month, 1 g 3 times a week for the next month, and then 1 g twice a week. Since INH may cause peripheral neuropathy, give pyridoxine, 100 mg/d orally. Wechsler and Lattimer (1975) prefer the combination of INH, ethambutol, and cycloserine.

While most authorities advise appropriate medication for 2 years (or longer if cultures remain positive), Gow (1979) finds that a 6-month course of drugs is adequate. He recommends 600 mg of rifampin, 300 mg of INH, 1 g of pyrazinamide, and 1 g of vitamin C daily for 2 months, followed by 900 mg of rifampin, 600 mg of INH, and 1 g of vitamin C 3 times a week for 4 months. *Pyrazinamide may cause serious liver damage.*

If, after 3 months, cultures are still positive and gross involvement of the affected kidney is radiologically evident, nephrectomy should be considered. Gow (1979) recommends that nonfunctioning kidneys be removed after 1–2 months of medical therapy.

If bacteriologic and radiographic studies demonstrate bilateral disease, only medical treatment can be considered. The only exceptions are (1) severe sepsis, pain, or bleeding from one kidney (may require nephrectomy as a palliative or lifesaving measure); and (2) marked advance of the disease on one side and minimal damage on the other (consider removal of the badly damaged organ).

B. Vesical Tuberculosis: Tuberculosis of the bladder is always secondary to renal or prostatic tuberculosis; it tends to heal promptly when definitive treatment for the "primary" genitourinary infection is given. Vesical ulcers that fail to respond to this regimen may require transurethral electrocoagulation. Vesical instillations of 0.2% monoxychlorosene (Clorpactin) may also stimulate healing.

Should extreme contracture of the bladder develop, it may be necessary to divert the urine from the bladder or perform subtotal cystectomy and anastomose a patch of ileum, ileocecal segment, or sigmoid to the remainder (ileocystoplasty, ileocecocystoplasty, sigmoidocystoplasty) in order to afford comfort (Abel and Gow, 1978).

C. Tuberculosis of the Epididymis: This is never an isolated lesion; the prostate is always involved and usually the kidney as well. Only rarely does the epididymal infection break through into the testis. Treatment is medical. If after months of treatment an abscess or a draining sinus exists, epididymectomy is indicated.

D. Tuberculosis of the Prostate and Seminal Vesicles: Although a few urologists advocate removal of the entire prostate and the vesicles when they become involved by tuberculosis, the majority opinion is that only medical therapy is indicated. Control can be checked by culture of the semen for tubercle bacilli.

E. General Measures for All Types: Optimal nutrition is no less important in treating tuberculosis of the genitourinary tract than in the treatment of tuberculosis elsewhere. Bladder sedatives may be given for the irritable bladder.

F. Treatment of Other Complications: Perinephric abscess usually occurs when the kidney is destroyed, but this is rare. The abscess must be drained, and nephrectomy should be done either then or later to prevent development of a chronic draining sinus. Prolonged antimicrobial therapy is indicated. If ureteral stricture develops on the involved side, ureteral dilatations offer a better than 50% chance of cure (Murphy et al, 1982; Cos and Cockett, 1982). The severely involved bladder may cause incompetence of the ureterovesical junction on the uninvolved side. Ureteroneocystostomy cannot be done in such a bladder; some form of urinary diversion may be required. For this reason, serial excretory urograms are necessary even under medical treatment.

Prognosis

The prognosis varies with the extent of the disease and the organs involved, but the overall control rate is 98% at 5 years. The urine must be studied bacteriologically every 6 months during treatment and then every year for 10 years (Wechsler and Lattimer, 1975). Relapse will indicate the need for reinstitution of treat-

ment. Nephrectomy is rarely necessary. In the healing process, ureteral stenosis or vesical contraction may develop. Appropriate surgical intervention may be necessary.

AMICROBIC (ABACTERIAL) CYSTITIS

Amicrobic cystitis is a rare disease of abrupt onset with a marked local vesical reaction. Although it acts like an infectious disease, bacterial search for the usual urinary pathogens is negative. It affects adult men and occasionally children, usually boys.

Etiology

The patient usually gives a history of recent sexual exposure. Mycoplasmas and chlamydiae have been isolated or suspected as etiologic agents. An adenovirus has been isolated from the urine in children suffering from acute hemorrhagic cystitis.

Pathogenesis & Pathology

Whatever the source and identity of the invader, the disease is primarily manifested as an acute inflammation of the bladder. Vesical irritability is severe and often associated with terminal hematuria. The mucosa is red and edematous, and superficial ulceration is occasionally seen. A thin membrane of fibrin often lies upon the wall. Similar changes may be noted in the posterior urethra. The renal parenchyma is not involved, although the pelvic and ureteral mucosa may show mild inflammatory changes. Some dilatation of the lower ureters is apt to develop. This may be due to an inflammatory reaction about the ureteral orifices, for these changes regress after successful treatment.

Microscopically, there is nothing specific about the reaction. The mucosa and submucosa are infiltrated with neutrophils, plasma cells, and eosinophils. Submucosal hemorrhages are common; superficial ulceration of the mucosa may be noted.

Clinical Findings

A. Symptoms: All symptoms are local. Urethral discharge, which is usually clear and mucoid but may be purulent, may be the initial symptom in men. Symptoms of acute cystitis come on abruptly. Urgency, frequency, and burning may be severe. Terminal hematuria is not uncommon. Suprapubic discomfort or even pain may be noted; it is most apt to be present as the bladder fills and is relieved somewhat by voiding. There is no fever or malaise.

B. Signs: Some suprapubic tenderness may be found. Urethral discharge may be profuse or scanty, and purulent or thin and mucoid. The prostate is usually normal to palpation. Massage is contraindicated during the acute stage of urinary tract infection. When massage is done later, infection is usually not present.

C. Laboratory Findings: Some leukocytosis may develop. The urine is grossly purulent and may contain blood as well. Stained smears reveal an absence of bacteria. Routine cultures are uniformly negative. In a few cases, mycoplasmas and TRIC agent (*Chlamydia trachomatis*) have been identified, but the significance of this is not yet clear. Search for tubercle bacilli is not successful.

Urethral discharge reveals no bacteria. Renal function is not impaired.

D. X-Ray Findings: Excretory urograms may demonstrate some dilatation of the lower ureters, but these changes regress completely when the disease is cured. The bladder shadow is small because of its markedly diminished capacity. Cystograms may reveal reflux.

E. Instrumental Examination: Cystoscopy is not indicated in acute inflammation of the bladder. It has been done, however, when the diagnosis was obscure and tuberculosis suspected. In such cases it reveals redness and edema of the mucosa. Superficial ulceration may be noted. Bladder capacity is markedly diminished. Biopsy of the wall shows nonspecific changes.

Differential Diagnosis

Tuberculosis causes symptoms of cystitis, which, however, usually come on gradually and become severe only in the stage of ulceration. A painless, nontender enlargement of an epididymis suggests tuberculosis. Although both tuberculosis and amicrobic cystitis produce pus without bacteria, thorough laboratory study will demonstrate tubercle bacilli only in the former. On cystoscopy, the tuberculous bladder may be studded with tubercles. The ulcers in this disease are deep and of a chronic type. The changes in amicrobic cystitis are more acute; ulceration, if present, is superficial. Excretory urograms in tuberculosis may show "moth-eaten" calices typical of infection with acid-fast organisms.

Nonspecific (pyogenic) cystitis may mimic amicrobic cystitis perfectly, but pathogenic organisms are easily found on a smear stained with methylene blue or on culture.

Cystitis secondary to chronic nonspecific prostatitis occasionally produces pus without bacteria. The findings on rectal examination, the pus in the prostatic secretion, and the response to antibiotics point to the proper diagnosis.

Vesical neoplasm may ulcerate, become infected, and bleed; hence it may mimic amicrobic cystitis. Bacteriuria, however, will be found. In case of doubt, cystoscopy is indicated.

Interstitial cystitis may be accompanied by severe symptoms of vesical irritability. However, it usually affects women past the menopause, and urinalysis is entirely negative except for a few red cells. Cystoscopy should be diagnostic.

Complications

Amicrobic cystitis is usually self-limited. Rarely, secondary contracture of the bladder develops. Under these circumstances, vesicoureteral reflux may be noted.

Treatment

A. Specific Measures: One of the tetracyclines or chloramphenicol, 1 g/d orally in divided doses for 3–4 days, is said to be curative in 75% of cases. Streptomycin, 1–2 g/d intramuscularly for 3–4 days, may be tried. Neoarsphenamine is also effective and appears to be the drug of choice, but arsenicals are hard to find. The first dose is 0.3 g intravenously; subsequent dosage is 0.45 g intravenously every 3–5 days for a total of 3–4 injections.

Penicillin and the sulfonamides are without effect.

In the cases reported in children, cure occurred spontaneously.

B. General Measures: Bladder sedatives are usually of little help if symptoms are severe. Analgesics or narcotics may prove necessary to combat pain. Hot sitz baths may relieve spasm.

Wettlaufer (1976) recommends the instillation of a 0.1% solution of sodium oxychlorosene (Clorpactin WCS-90).

Prognosis

The prognosis is excellent.

CANDIDIASIS

Candida albicans is a yeastlike fungus that is a normal inhabitant of the respiratory and gastrointestinal tracts and the vagina. The intensive use of potent modern antibiotics is apt to disturb the normal balance between normal and abnormal organisms, thus allowing fungi such as *Candida* to overwhelm an otherwise healthy organ. The bladder and, to a lesser extent, the kidneys have proved vulnerable; candidemia has been observed. Anogenital candidiasis is discussed on p 600.

The patient may present with vesical irritability or symptoms and signs of pyelonephritis. Fungus balls may be passed spontaneously. The diagnosis is made by observing mycelial or yeast forms of the fungus microscopically in a properly collected urine specimen. The diagnosis may be confirmed by culture. Excretory urograms may show caliceal defects and ureteral obstruction (fungus masses).

Vesical candidiasis usually responds to alkalinization of the urine with sodium bicarbonate. A urinary pH of 7.5 is desired; the dose is regulated by the patient, who checks the urine with indicator paper. Should this fail, amphotericin B should be instilled via catheter 3 times a day. Dissolve 100 mg of the drug in 500 mL of 5% dextrose solution.

If there is renal involvement, irrigations of the renal pelvis with a similar concentration of amphotericin B are efficacious. In the presence of systemic manifestations or candidemia, flucytosine (Ancobon) is the drug of choice. The dose is 100 mg/kg/d orally in divided doses given for 1 week. In the face of serious involvement, give 600 mg intravenously on the first day and then shift to the oral form of the drug. Grüneberg and Leaky (1976) recommend nifuratel, a nitrofuran antibiotic, which they claim is superior to flucytosine. The recommended dose is 400 mg 3 times daily for 1 week. The dose must be modified in the face of renal impairment. The drug is more active in acid urine. Graybill et al (1983) reported good results with ketoconazole. The dose is 200–400 mg/d for 2–3 weeks or more depending upon the effect as reflected by serial cultures. Its toxicity is relatively low. Amphotericin B (Fungizone) has the disadvantages of requiring parenteral administration and being highly nephrotoxic. It is given intravenously in a dosage of 1–5 mg/d in divided doses dissolved in 5% dextrose. The concentration of the solution should be 0.1 mg/mL.

ACTINOMYCOSIS

Actinomycosis is a chronic granulomatous disease in which fibrosis tends to become marked and spontaneous fistulas are the rule. On rare occasions, the disease involves the kidney, bladder, or testis by hematogenous invasion from a primary site of infection. The skin of the penis or scrotum may become involved through a local abrasion. The bladder may also become diseased by direct extension from the appendix, bowel, or oviduct.

Etiology
Actinomyces israelii (A bovis) is the causative organism.

Clinical Findings
There is nothing specifically pathognomonic about the symptoms or signs in actinomycosis. The microscopic demonstration of the organisms, which are visible as yellow bodies called "sulfur granules," makes the diagnosis. If persistently sought for, these may be found in the discharge from sinuses or in the urine. Pollock et al (1978) recommend aspiration biopsy performed by a thin needle. They found that in addition to the discovery of sulfur granules, both Gram's stain and a modified Ziehl-Neelsen stain were useful in diagnosis. Definitive diagnosis is established by culture.

Urographically, the lesion in the kidney may resemble tuberculosis (eroded calices) or tumor (space-occupying lesion).

Treatment
Penicillin G is the drug of choice. Give 10–20 million units/d parenterally for 4–6 weeks. Follow this with penicillin V orally for a prolonged period. If secondary infection is suspected, add a sulfonamide; streptomycin is also efficacious. Broad-spectrum antibiotics are indicated only if the organism is resistant to penicillin. Surgical drainage of the abscess or, better, removal of the involved organ is usually indicated (Patel, Moskowitz, and Hashmat, 1983).

Prognosis
Removal of the involved organ (eg, kidney or

testis) may be promptly curative. Drainage of a granulomatous abscess may cause the development of a chronic draining sinus. Chemotherapy is helpful.

SCHISTOSOMIASIS
(Bilharziasis)*

Schistosomiasis, caused by a blood fluke, is a disease of warm climates. In its 3 forms, it affects about 350 million people. *Schistosoma mansoni* is widely distributed in Africa, South and Central America, Pakistan, and India; *Schistosoma japonicum* is found in the Far East; and *Schistosoma haematobium (Bilharzia haematobia)* is limited to Africa (especially along its northern coast), Saudi Arabia, Israel, Jordan, Lebanon, and Syria.

Schistosomiasis is on the increase in endemic areas because of the construction of modern irrigation systems that provide favorable conditions for the intermediate host, a certain freshwater snail. This disease principally affects the urogenital system, especially the bladder, ureters, seminal vesicles, and, to a lesser extent, the male urethra and prostate gland. Because of emigration of people from endemic areas, the disease is being seen with increasing frequency in both Europe and the USA. Infection with *S mansoni* and *S japonicum* mainly involves the colon.

Etiology
Humans are infected when they come in contact with larva-infested water in canals, ditches, or irrigation fields during swimming, bathing, or farming procedures. Fork-tailed larvae, the cercariae, lose their tails as they penetrate deep under the skin. They are then termed schistosomules. They cause allergic skin reactions that are more intense in people infected for the first time. These schistosomules enter the general circulation through the lymphatics and the peripheral veins and reach the lungs. If the infection is massive, they may cause pneumonitis. They pass through the pulmonary circulation, to the left side of the heart, and to the general circulation. Those worms that reach the vesicoprostatic plexus of veins survive and mature, whereas those that go to other areas die.

Pathogenesis
The adult *S haematobium* worm, a digenetic trematode, lives in the prostatovesical plexus of veins. The male is about 10 × 1 mm in size, is folded upon itself, and carries the long, slim 20 × 0.25 mm female in its "schist," or gynecophoric canal. In the smallest peripheral venules, the female leaves the male and partially penetrates the venule to lay her eggs in the subepithelial layer of the affected viscus, usually in the form of clusters that form tubercles. The ova

---

* This section was contributed by Mohamed M. Al Ghorab, MB, ChB, DS, MCh, FICS.

are only rarely seen within the venules; they are almost always in the subepithelial or interstitial tissues. The female returns to the male, which carries her to other areas to repeat the same process.

The living ova, by a process of histolysis and helped by contraction of the detrusor muscle, penetrate the overlying urothelium, pass into the cavity of the bladder, and are extruded with the urine. If these ova reach fresh water, they hatch, and the contained larvae, ciliated miricidia, find a specific freshwater snail that they penetrate. There they form sporocysts that ultimately form the cercariae which leave the snail hosts and pass into fresh water to repeat their life cycle in the human host.

Pathology

The fresh ova excite little tissue reaction when they leave the human host promptly through the urothelium. The contents of the ova trapped in the tissues and death of the organisms cause a severe local reaction, with infiltration of round cells, monocytes, eosinophils, and giant cells that form tubercles, nodules, and polyps. These are later replaced by fibrous tissue that causes contraction of different parts of the bladder and strictures of the ureter. Fibrosis and massive deposits of eggs in subepithelial tissues interfere with the blood supply of the area and cause chronic bilharzial ulcerations. Epithelial metaplasia is common, and squamous cell carcinoma is a frequent sequela. Secondary infection of the urinary tract is a common complication and is difficult to overcome. The trapped dead ova become impregnated with calcium salts and form sheets of subepithelial calcified layers in the ureter, bladder, and seminal vesicles.

Clinical Findings

A. Symptoms: Penetration of the skin by the cercariae causes certain allergic reactions, with cutaneous hyperemia and itching that are more intense in people infected for the first time. During the stage of generalization or invasion, the patient complains of malaise, fatigue and lassitude, low-grade fever, excessive sweating, headache, backache, etc. When the ova are laid in the bladder wall and begin to be extruded, the patient complains of terminal, slightly painful hematuria that is occasionally profuse. This may remain the only complaint for a long time until complications set in, when vesical symptoms become exaggerated and progressive. Increasing frequency, suprapubic and back pain, urethralgia, profuse hematuria, pyuria, and necroturia are likely to occur, with secondary infection, ulceration, or malignancy. Renal pain may be due to ureteral stricture, vesicoureteral reflux, or secondary stones obstructing the ureter. Fever, rigor, toxemia, and uremia are manifestations of renal involvement.

B. Signs: In early uncomplicated cases, there are essentially no clinical findings. Later, a fibrosed, pitted, bilharzial glans penis, urethral stricture or fistula, or a perineal fibrous mass may be found. A suprapubic bladder mass or a renal swelling may be felt abdominally. Rectal examination may reveal a fibrosed prostate, an enlarged seminal vesicle, or a thickened bladder base.

C. Laboratory Findings: Urinalysis usually reveals the terminal-spined dead or living ova, blood and pus cells, and bacteria. Malignant squamous cells may be seen. The hemogram usually shows leukocytosis with eosinophilia and hypochromic normocytic anemia. Serum creatinine and blood urea nitrogen measurements may demonstrate some degree of renal impairment.

A variety of immunologic methods have been used to confirm the diagnosis of schistosomiasis. Positive immunologic tests indicate previous exposure but not whether schistosomiasis is currently present. The cercariae, schistosomules, adult worms, and eggs are all potentially antigenic. Adult worms, however, acquire host antigen on their integument that circumvents the immunologic forces of the host. Antibody production may be manifested as hypergammaglobulinema.

D. X-Ray Findings: A plain film of the abdomen may show areas of grayness in the flank (enlarged hydronephrotic kidney) or in the bladder area (large tumor). Opacifications (stones) may be noted in the kidney, ureter, or bladder. Linear calcification may be seen in the ureteral and bladder walls (Fig 14–3). Punctate calcification of the ureter (ureteritis calcinosa) and a honeycombed calcification of the seminal vessels may be obvious (Fig 14–3).

Excretory urograms may show either normal or diminished renal function and varying degrees of dilatation of the upper urinary tracts (Fig 14–4). These changes include hydronephrosis, dilated and tortuous ureters, ureteral strictures, or a small contracted bladder having a capacity of only a few milliliters. Gross irregular defects of the bladder wall represent cancer (Fig 14–4).

Retrograde urethrography may reveal a bilharzial urethral stricture. Cystograms often reveal vesicoureteral reflux, particularly if the bladder is contracted.

E. Instrumental Examination: Urethral calibration with a sound may reveal stricture formation.

Cystoscopy may show fresh conglomerate, grayish tubercles surrounded by a halo of hyperemia, old calcified yellowish tubercles, sandy patches of mucous membrane, and a lusterless ground-glass mucosa that lacks the normal vascular pattern. Other obvious lesions include bilharzial polyps, chronic ulcers on the dome that bleed when the bladder is deflated (weeping ulcers), vesical stones, malignant lesions, stenosed or patulous ureteric orifices, and a distorted, asymmetric trigone. All are signs of schistosomal infestation.

Differential Diagnosis

Bilharzial cystitis is unmistakable in endemic areas. The presence of schistosomal ova in the urine, together with radiographic and cystoscopic findings, usually confirms the diagnosis. Nonspecific cystitis usually responds to medical treatment unless there is a complicating factor. Tuberculous cystitis may mimic

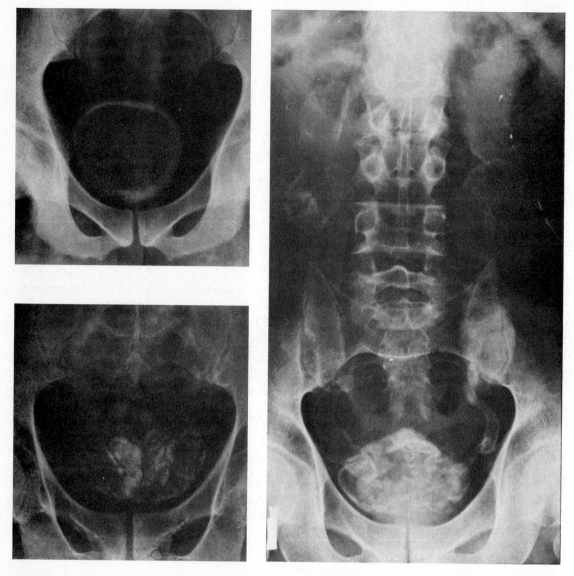

Figure 14–3. Schistosomiasis. Plain films. *Upper left:* Extensive calcification in the wall of a contracted bladder. *Right:* Extensive calcification of the bladder and both ureters up to the renal pelves. The ureters are dilated and tortuous. *Lower left:* Extensive calcification of seminal vesicles and ampullae of vasa.

bilharzial cystitis; the detection of tubercle bacilli, together with the radiographic picture, is confirmatory, but tuberculosis may occur in a bilharzial bladder. Vesical calculi and malignancy should be diagnosed by thorough urologic examination, although both conditions are common in association with bilharzial bladder. Complications of schistosomiasis are the result of fibrosis, which may be extreme and causes contraction of the bladder neck as well as the bladder itself. It also causes strictures of the urethra and ureter that are usually bilateral. Vesicoureteral reflux is a frequent sequela. Secondary persistent infection and stone formation usually complicate the picture still further. Squamous cell tumors of the bladder are common.

They are seen as early as the second or third decade of life and are much more common in men than in women.

Treatment

A. Medical Measures: Praziquantel, metrifonate, and oxamniquine are the drugs of choice in treating schistosomiasis. These drugs do not have the serious side effects associated with the older drugs (eg, antimonials).

1. Praziquantel is unique in that it is effective against all human schistosome species. It is given orally and is effective in adults and children. Patients

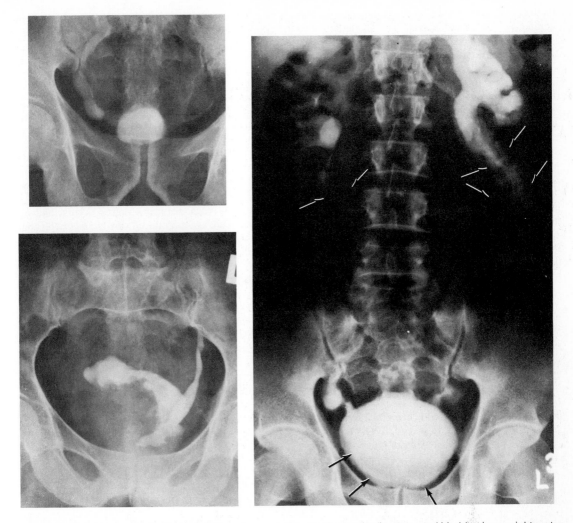

Figure 14–4. Schistosomiasis. *Upper left:* Excretory urogram showing markedly contracted bladder. Lower right ureter dilated probably secondary to vesicoureteral reflux. *Right:* Excretory urogram at 2 hours showing a fairly normal right kidney. The upper ureter is distorted. Arrows point to calcified wall. The lower ureter is quite abnormal. The calices and pelvis of the left kidney are dilated, but the kidney shows atrophy secondary to nonspecific infection. The upper ureter is dilated and displaced by elongation due to obstruction. Arrows show calcification. Linear calcification can be seen in the periphery of the lower half of the bladder wall (*arrows*). *Lower left:* Nodular squamous cell carcinoma of the bladder. Dilated left lower ureter probably secondary to obstruction by tumor. Nonvisualization of the right ureter caused by complete occlusion.

in the hepatosplenic stage of advanced schistosomiasis tolerate the drug well. The recommended dosage for all forms of schistosomiasis is 20 mg/kg 3 times daily for one day.

2. Metrifonate is also a highly effective oral drug. It is the drug of choice for treatment of *S haematobium* infections but is not effective against *S mansoni* or *S japonicum*. For treatment of *S haematobium* infections, the dosage is 7.5–10 mg/kg (maximum 600 mg) once and then repeated twice at 2-week intervals.

3. Oxamniquine is a highly effective oral drug and is the drug of choice for treatment of *S mansoni* infections. It is safe and effective in advanced disease. It is not effective in *S haematobium* or *S japonicum* infec-

tions. The dosage is 12–15 mg/kg given once; for children under 30 kg, 20 mg/kg is given in 2 divided doses in one day, with an interval of 2–8 hours between doses. Cure rates are 70–95%.

4. Niridazole, a nitrothiazole derivative, is effective in treating *S mansoni* and *S haematobium* infections. It may be tried against *S japonicum* infections. It is given orally and should be administered only under close medical supervision. The dosage is 25 mg/kg (maximum, 1.5 g) daily in 2 divided doses for 7 days. Side effects may occur, including nausea, vomiting, anorexia, headache, T wave depression, and temporary suppression of spermatogenesis.

5. Antimonial drugs are no longer used in the

treatment of schistosomiasis if praziquantel, oxamniquine, or metrifonate is available. The antimonials (eg, sodium antimony dimercaptosuccinate [stibocaptate], stibophen, tartar emetic) are much more toxic, and a longer course of therapy is needed. Tartar emetic is nonetheless occasionally needed as a third alternative drug in the treatment of *S japonicum* infection.

B. General Measures: Antibiotics or urinary antiseptics are needed to overcome or control secondary infection. Supportive treatment in the form of iron, vitamins, and a high-calorie diet is indicated in selected cases.

C. Complications: Treatment of the complications of schistosomiasis of the genitourinary tract makes demands on the skill of the physician. Juxtavesical ureteral strictures require resection of the stenotic segment with ureteroneocystostomy. If the ureter is not long enough to reimplant, a tube of bladder may be fashioned, turned cephalad, and anastomosed to the ureter. Should the ureter be widely dilated, it must be tailored to approach normal size. Vesicoureteral reflux requires a suitable surgical repair. A contracted bladder neck may need transurethral anterior commissurotomy or a suprapubic Y-V plasty.

A chronic "weeping" bilharzial bladder ulcer necessitates partial cystectomy. The contracted bladder is treated by enteroplasty (placing a segment of bowel as a patch on the bladder), preferably with an isolated portion of sigmoid colon. This procedure, which significantly increases vesical capacity, is remarkably effective in lessening the severity of symptoms associated with contracted bladder. Preoperative vesicoureteral reflux may disappear.

The most dreaded complication, squamous cell carcinoma, requires total cystectomy with supravesical urinary diversion if the lesion is deemed operable. Unfortunately, late diagnosis is the rule.

Prognosis

With energetic treatment, mild and early cases of schistosomiasis are not likely to result in severe damage to the urinary tract. On the other hand, massive repeated infections undermine the function of the urinary tract to such an extent that patients are disabled and become chronic invalids whose life spans are shortened by 1 or 2 decades.

In many endemic areas, attempts have been made to control the disease by mass treatment of patients, proper education, mechanization of agriculture, and various methods of eradication or control of the snail population. All these efforts have failed to be fully effective.

FILARIASIS

Filariasis is endemic in the countries bordering the Mediterranean, in South China and Japan, the West Indies, and the South Pacific islands, particularly Samoa. Limited infection, as seen in American soldiers during World War II, gives an entirely different clinical picture from that seen in the frequent reinfections usually encountered among the native population.

Etiology

Wuchereria bancrofti is a threadlike nematode about 0.5 cm or more in length that lives in the human lymphatics. In the lymphatics, the female gives off microfilariae, which are found, particularly at night, in the peripheral blood. The intermediate host (usually a mosquito), biting an infected person, becomes infested with microfilariae, which develop into larvae. These are in turn transferred to another human, in whom they reach maturity. Mating occurs, and microfilariae are again produced. *Brugia malayi,* a nematode that causes filariasis in Southeast Asia and adjacent Pacific islands, acts in a similar fashion.

Pathogenesis & Pathology

The adult nematode in the human host invades and obstructs the lymphatics; this leads to lymphangitis and lymphadenitis. In long-standing cases, the lymphatic vessels become thickened and fibrous; there is a marked reticuloendothelial reaction.

Clinical Findings

A. Symptoms: In mild cases (few exposures), the patient suffers recurrent lymphadenitis and lymphangitis with fever and malaise. Not infrequently, inflammation of the epididymis, testis, scrotum, and spermatic cord occurs. These structures then become edematous, boggy, and at times tender. Hydrocele is common. In advanced cases (many exposures), obstruction of major lymph channels may cause chyluria and elephantiasis.

B. Signs: Varying degrees of painless elephantiasis of the scrotum and extremities develop as obstruction to lymphatics progresses. Lymphadenopathy is common.

C. Laboratory Findings: Chylous urine may look normal if minimal amounts of fat are present, but in an advanced case or following a fatty meal, it is milky. On standing, the urine layers: the top layer is fatty, the middle layer is pinkish, and the lower layer is clear. In the presence of chyluria, large amounts of protein are to be expected. Hypoproteinemia is found, and the albumin:globulin ratio is reversed. Both white and red blood cells are found. The fat will be dissolved by chloroform; the urine will therefore become clear.

Marked eosinophilia is the rule in the early stages. Microfilariae may be demonstrated in the blood, which should preferably be drawn at night. The adult worm may be found by biopsy. When filariae cannot be found, an indirect hemagglutination titer of 1:128 and a bentonite flocculation titer of 1:5 in combination are considered diagnostic.

D. Cystoscopy: Following a fatty meal, endoscopy to observe the efflux of milky urine from the ureteral orifices may differentiate between unilateral and bilateral cases.

E. X-Ray Findings: Retrograde urography and lymphangiography may reveal the renolymphatic connections in patients with chyluria.

Prevention

In endemic areas, mosquito abatement programs must be intensively pursued.

Treatment

A. Specific Measures: Diethylcarbamazine (Hetrazan) is the drug of choice, but it is toxic (Nelson, 1979). The dose is 2 mg/kg orally 3 times daily for 12 days. This drug kills the microfilariae but not the adult worms. Several courses of the drug may be necessary. Antibiotics may be necessary to control secondary infection.

B. General Measures: Prompt removal of recently infected patients from the endemic area almost always results in regression of the symptoms and signs in early cases.

C. Surgical Measures: Elephantiasis of the external genitalia may require surgical excision.

D. Treatment of Chyluria: Mild cases require no therapy. Spontaneous cure results in 50% of cases (Ohyama, Saita, and Miyasato, 1979). If nutrition is impaired, the lymphatic channels may be sealed off by irrigating the renal pelvis with 2% silver nitrate solution. Should this fail, renal decapsulation and resection of the renal lymphatics should be performed (Okamoto and Ohi, 1983).

Prognosis

If exposure has been limited, resolution of the disease is spontaneous, and the prognosis is excellent. Frequent reinfection may lead to elephantiasis of the scrotum or chyluria.

ECHINOCOCCOSIS
(Hydatid Disease)

Involvement of the urogenital organs by hydatid disease is relatively rare in the USA. It is common in Australia, New Zealand, South America, Africa, Asia, the Middle East, and Europe. Livestock are the intermediate hosts. Canines, especially dogs, are the final hosts.

Etiology

The adult tapeworm (*Echinococcus*) inhabits the intestinal tracts of carnivorous animals. Its eggs pass out with the feces and may be ingested by such animals as sheep, cattle, pigs, and occasionally humans. Larvae from these eggs pass through the intestinal wall of the various intermediate hosts and are disseminated throughout the body. In humans, the liver is principally involved, but about 3% of infected humans develop echinococcosis of the kidney.

If a cyst of the liver should rupture into the peritoneal cavity, the scoleces (tapeworm heads) may directly invade the retrovesical tissues, thus leading to the development of cysts in this area.

Clinical Findings

If renal hydatid disease is closed (not communicating with the pelvis), there may be no symptoms until a mass is found. With communicating disease, there may be symptoms of cystitis, and renal colic may occur as cysts are passed from the kidney. X-ray films may show calcification in the wall of the cyst (Fig 14–5), and urograms often reveal changes typical of a space-occupying lesion. The cystic nature of the lesion will be demonstrated on sonograms and CT scans. Calcification in the cyst wall may be noted. Scintillation scanning or angiography can also suggest the presence of a cyst. Serologic tests that should be done include immunoelectrophoresis and indirect hemagglutination. The Casoni intracutaneous procedure is unreliable.

Retroperitoneal (perivesical) cysts may cause symptoms of cystitis, or acute urinary retention may develop secondary to pressure. The presence of a suprapubic mass may be the only finding. It may rupture into the bladder and cause hydatiduria, which establishes the diagnosis.

Treatment

Nephrectomy is generally the treatment of choice for renal hydatid disease. Aspiration of the cyst is unwise; leakage or rupture may occur. Retroperitoneal cysts are best treated by marsupialization and curettage.

Prognosis

Echinococcosis of the kidney usually has a good prognosis. The problem presented by perivesical cysts is more troublesome. After surgical intervention, drainage may be prolonged. It must be remembered, too, that involvement of other organs, especially the liver, is usually present.

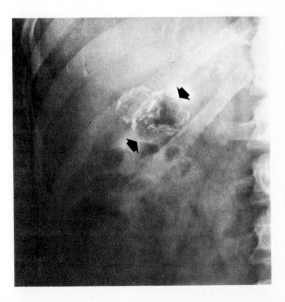

Figure 14–5. Hydatid disease, right kidney. Plain film showing 2 calcified hydatid cysts.

REFERENCES

Tuberculosis

Abel BJ, Gow JG: Results of caecocystoplasty for tuberculous bladder contracture. *Br J Urol* 1978;**50:**511.

Agarwalla B et al: Tuberculosis of the penis: Report of 2 cases. *J Urol* 1980;**124:**927.

Bjorn-Hansen R, Aakhus T: Angiography in renal tuberculosis. *Acta Radiol [Diagn] (Stockh)* 1971;**11:**167.

Bowersox DW et al: Isoniazid dosage in patients with renal failure. *N Engl J Med* 1973;**289:**84.

Cheng SF: Bilateral coccidioidal epididymitis. *Urology* 1974;**3:**362.

Cinman AC: Genitourinary tuberculosis. *Urology* 1982;**20:**353.

Conner WT, Drach GW, Bucher WC Jr: Genitourinary aspects of disseminated coccidioidomycosis. *J Urol* 1975;**113:**82.

Cos CR, Cockett ATK: Genitourinary tuberculosis revisited. *Urology* 1982;**20:**111.

Ehrlich RM, Lattimer JK: Urogenital tuberculosis in children. *J Urol* 1971;**105:**461.

Feldstein MS, Sullivan MJ, Banowsky LH: Ureteral involvement in genitourinary tuberculosis: Review of 20 cases encountered over three years. *Urology* 1975;**6:**175.

Gow JG: Genitourinary tuberculosis: A 7-year review. *Br J Urol* 1979;**51:**239.

Gow JG: The management of genitourinary tuberculosis. Chap 7, pp 91–105, in: *Recent Advances in Urology/Andrology,* 3rd ed. Hendry WF (editor). Churchill Livingstone, 1981.

Griffith DP, Saccomani MN, Johnson CF: Sensitivity studies in bacteriologic diagnosis of urinary tuberculosis. *Urology* 1975;**6:**182.

Kollins SA et al: Roentgenographic findings in urinary tract tuberculosis: A 10-year review. *Am J Roentgenol* 1974;**121:**487.

Murphy DM et al: Tuberculous stricture of ureter. *Urology* 1982;**20:**382.

Narayana AS: Overview of renal tuberculosis. *Urology* 1982;**19:**231.

Pagani JJ, Barbaric ZL, Cochran ST: Augmentation enterocystoplasty. *Radiology* 1979;**131:**321.

Simon HB et al: Genitourinary tuberculosis: Clinical features in a general hospital population. *Am J Med* 1977;**63:**410.

Symes JM, Blandy JP: Tuberculosis of the male urethra. *Br J Urol* 1973;**45:**432.

Wechsler H: Update on chemotherapy of renal tuberculosis. *J Urol* 1980;**124:**319.

Wechsler M, Lattimer JK: An evaluation of the current therapeutic regimen for renal tuberculosis. *J Urol* 1975;**113:**760.

Wong SH, Lau WY: The surgical management of non-functioning tuberculous kidneys. *J Urol* 1980;**124:**187.

Amicrobic (Abacterial) Cystitis

Hewitt CB, Stewart BH, Kiser WS: Abacterial pyuria. *J Urol* 1973;**109:**86.

Moore T, Parker C, Edwards EC: Sterile non-tuberculous pyuria. *Br J Urol* 1971;**43:**47.

Numazaki Y et al: Acute hemorrhagic cystitis in children: Isolation of adenovirus type II. *N Engl J Med* 1968;**278:**700.

Parsons CL, Schmidt JD, Pollen JJ: Successful treatment of interstitial cystitis with sodium pentosanpolysulfate. *J Urol* 1983;**130:**51.

Wettlaufer JN: Abacterial cystitis: Treatment with sodium oxychlorosene. *J Urol* 1976;**116:**434.

Candidiasis

Graybill JR et al: Ketoconazole therapy for fungal urinary tract infections. *J Urol* 1983;**129:**68.

Grüneberg RN, Leaky A: Treatment of candidal urinary tract infection with nifuratel. *Br Med J* 1976;**2:**908.

Hamory BH, Wenzel RP: Hospital-associated candiduria: Predisposing factors and review of the literature. *J Urol* 1978;**120:**444.

Kozinn PJ et al: Advances in the diagnosis of renal candidiasis. *J Urol* 1978;**119:**184.

Michigan S: Genitourinary fungal infections. *J Urol* 1976;**116:**390.

Schönebeck J: Studies on *Candida* infection of the urinary tract and on the antimycotic drug 5-fluorocytosine. *Scand J Urol Nephrol* 1972;**Suppl 11.**

Schönebeck J, Segerbrand E: *Candida albicans* septicaemia during first half of pregnancy successfully treated with 5-fluorocytosine. *Br Med J* 1973;**4:**337.

Wise GJ, Goldberg P, Kozinn PJ: Genitourinary candidiasis: Diagnosis and treatment. *J Urol* 1976;**116:**778.

Actinomycosis

Crosse JEW, Soderdahl DW, Schamber DT: Renal actinomycosis. *Urology* 1976;**7:**309.

Fass RJ et al: Clindamycin in the treatment of serious anaerobic infections. *Ann Intern Med* 1973;**78:**853.

Patel BJ, Moskowitz H, Hashmat A: Unilateral renal actinomycosis. *Urology* 1983;**21:**172.

Pollock PG et al: Rapid diagnosis of actinomycosis by thin-needle aspiration biopsy. *Am J Clin Pathol* 1978;**70:**27.

Sarosdy MF, Brock WA, Parsons CL: Scrotal actinomycosis. *J Urol* 1979;**121:**256.

Schistosomiasis (Bilharziasis)

Abdel-Halim RE: Ileal loop replacement and restoration of kidney function in extensive bilharziasis of the ureter. *Br J Urol* 1980;**52:**280.

Al Ghorab MM: Radiological manifestations of genitourinary bilharziasis. *Clin Radiol* 1968;**19:**100.

Al Ghorab MM: Ureteritis calcinosa: A complication of bilharzial ureteritis and its relation to primary ureteric stone formation. *Br J Urol* 1962;**34:**33.

Al Ghorab MM, El-Badawi AA, Effat H: Vesico-ureteric reflux in urinary bilharziasis: A clinico-radiological study. *Clin Radiol* 1966;**17:**41.

Bazeed MA et al: Ileal replacement of the bilharzial bladder: Is it worthwhile? *J Urol* 1983;**130:**245.

Bazeed MA et al: Partial flap ureteroneocystostomy for bilharzial strictures of the lower ureter. *Urology* 1982;**20:**237.

El-Bolkainy MN et al: Carcinoma of the bilharzial bladder: Diagnostic value with urine cytology. *Urology* 1974;**3:**319.

El-Mahrouky A et al: The predictive value of 2, 4-dinitrochlorobenzene skin testing in patients with bilharzial bladder cancer. *J Urol* 1983;**129:**497.

Farid Z et al: Symptomatic, radiological, and functional improvement following treatment of urinary schistosomiasis. *Lancet* 1967;**2:**1110.

Ghoneim MA, Ashamallah A, Khalik MA: Bilharzial strictures of the ureter presenting with anuria. *Br J Urol* 1971;**43:**439.

Ghoneim MA et al: Staging of the carcinoma of bilharzial bladder. *Urology* 1974;**3:**40.

Hanafy MH, Youssef TK, Saad MS: Radiographic aspects of (bilharzial) schistosomal ureter. *Urology* 1975;**6:**118.

Khafagy MM, El-Bolkainy MN, Mansour MA: Carcinoma of the bilharzial urinary bladder. *Cancer* 1972;**30**:150.

Lamki LM, Lamki N: Radionuclide studies of chronic schistosomal uropathy. *Radiology* 1981;**140**:471.

Wagenknecht LV: Carcinoma of bilharzial bladder and urogenital bilharziasis (author's translation). *Urologe (A)* 1974;**13**:59.

Webbe G: Schistosomiasis: Some advances. *Br Med J* 1981; **283**:1104.

Young SW et al: Urinary tract lesion of *Schistosoma haematobium* with detailed radiographic consideration of the ureter. *Radiology* 1974;**111**:81.

Zahran MM et al: Bilharziasis of urinary bladder and ureter: Comparative histopathologic study. *Urology* 1976;**8**:73.

Filariasis

Crane DB, Wheeler WE, Smith MJV: Chyluria. *Urology* 1977;**9**:429.

Iturregui-Pagán JR, Fortuño RF, Noy MA: Genital manifestation of filariasis. *Urology* 1976;**8**:207.

Lang EK, Redetzki JE, Brown RL: Lymphangiographic demonstration of lymphaticocalyceal fistulas causing chyluria (filariasis). *J Urol* 1972;**108**:321.

Nelson GS: Current concepts in parasitology: Filariasis. *N Engl J Med* 1979;**300**:1136.

Ohyama C, Saita H, Miyasato N: Spontaneous remission of chyluria. *J Urol* 1979;**121**:316.

Okamoto K, Ohi Y: Recent distribution and treatment of filarial chyluria in Japan. *J Urol* 1983;**129**:64.

Onchocerciasis

Awadzi K: The chemotherapy of onchocerciasis. 2. Quantitation of the clinical reaction to microfilaricides. *Ann Trop Med Parasitol* 1980;**74**:189.

Gibson DW, Heggie C, Connor DH: Clinical and pathologic aspects of onchocerciasis. *Pathol Annu* 1980;**15**:195.

Echinococcosis (Hydatid Disease)

Amir-Jahed AK et al: Clinical echinococcosis. *Ann Surg* 1975;**182**:541.

Baltaxe HA, Fleming RJ: The angiographic appearance of hydatid disease. *Radiology* 1970;**97**:599.

Birkhoff JD, McClennan BL: Echinococcal disease of the pelvis: Urologic complication, diagnosis and treatment. *J Urol* 1973;**109**:473.

Diamond HM et al: Echinococcal disease of the kidney. *J Urol* 1976;**115**:742.

Haines JG et al: Echinococcal cyst of the kidney. *J Urol* 1977;**117**:788.

Martorana G, Giberi C, Pescatore D: Giant echinococcal cyst of the kidney associated with hypertension evaluated by computerized tomography. *J Urol* 1981;**126**:99.

15

Sexually Transmitted Diseases in Males

Bruce M. Mayer, MD, & Richard E. Berger, MD

GONOCOCCAL URETHRITIS

Gonococcal urethritis, the most extensively studied sexually transmitted disease over the last 20 years, reached a peak incidence in 1975 and is now declining in frequency, while the incidence of nongonococcal urethritis is rising.

On a gram-stained smear of urethral scrapings, *Neisseria gonorrhoeae* are gram-negative diplococci located within the neutrophils. The intracellular diplococcus causes neutrophil, lymphocyte, and plasma cell infiltration of the tissues.

Concurrent infections with *Chlamydia* and other organisms are common. The urethra is the most common site of infection in all men. In heterosexual men, the pharynx is infected in 7%, and in homosexual men, the pharynx is infected in 40% and the rectum in 25% (Handsfield et al, 1980). A single episode of intercourse with an infected female partner carries a transmission risk of 17–20% for the male; however, the female partner of an infected male will contract the disease about 80% of the time (Harrison, 1984; Thin, Williams, and Nicol, 1971).

Clinical Findings

A. Symptoms: In males, the usual symptoms of gonorrhea are urethral discharge and dysuria. There may be only urethral itching. The usual incubation period is 3–10 days but may be any time from 12 hours to 3 months. Without treatment, urethritis will persist for 3–7 weeks, with 95% of men becoming asymptomatic after 3 months. Gonococcal urethritis may be asymptomatic in 40–60% of contacts of partners with known gonorrhea (Harrison, 1984). Complications such as involvement of the prostate may lead to urinary frequency, urgency, and nocturia. Spread down the vas deferens to the epididymis may lead to acute epididymitis.

B. Signs: The discharge with gonococcal urethritis is usually yellow or brown. There may be meatal edema and erythema. The pendulous urethra may exhibit tenderness. Inspect the pharynx and rectum if, by history, there was contact in those regions. Anoscopy will show easy bleeding from rectal mucosa and pus with proctitis. Pharyngeal infections are often asymptomatic.

C. Laboratory Findings: The patient is best examined 1 hour, preferably 4 hours, after last voiding, so that the discharge will not be washed away (Fig

15–1). A calcium alginate swab is then inserted 2–3 cm into the urethra and rotated gently. Do not use cotton-tipped swabs, as they are bactericidal. The swab is then rolled onto a slide for gram staining, and the swab is plated immediately onto a culture medium or placed in a transport medium. The gram-stained smear should show evidence of urethritis, with 4 or more leukocytes per high-power field (magnification $\times$ 400). Cultures of pharyngeal and rectal scrapings are required if there is a history of oral or rectal intercourse.

Do not swab the anal epithelium but instead obtain a swab from the rectal mucosa by anoscopy. A gram-stained smear is positive if gram-negative diplococci are seen within polymorphonuclear leukocytes. The smear is negative if no gram-negative diplococci are seen. The examination is equivocal if diplococci are only extracellular or if they are intracellular but atypical. The specificity of a gram-stained smear in gonococcal urethritis is 95%. The sensitivity is nearly 100% in urethritis and 60% in rectal gonorrhea. Although cultures are not always necessary for diagnosis, they should be obtained to determine antibiotic sensitivities, especially in populations with a high percentage of resistant organisms. Alternative diagnostic methods based on detection of the gonococcal enzymes, antigens, DNA, and liposaccharides are available (Hook and Holmes, 1985).

Differential Diagnosis

The discharge in nongonococcal urethritis is often more scant and clearer than in gonococcal urethritis; however, the discharge may appear identical in both diseases. Gram-stained smear of the urethral swab will show only leukocytes in a male with nongonococcal urethritis.

Complications

Periurethritis is one of the more common complications and may lead to abscess formation, urethral fibrosis, and, finally, urethral stricture. Prostatitis may develop and may cause perineal pain and low backache; if this is left untreated, an abscess may occur. Epididymitis may occur and could lead to infertility or testicular atrophy.

Proctitis presents as anal discharge, bleeding, pain, tenesmus, or constipation. Anoscopy will reveal pus and easy bleeding from the mucosal surface. One polymorphonuclear leukocyte or more per high-power field (magnification $\times$ 400) on gram-stained smear is

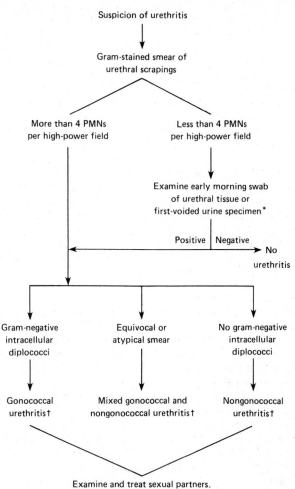

Suspicion of urethritis

↓

Gram-stained smear of
urethral scrapings

More than 4 PMNs
per high-power field

Less than 4 PMNs
per high-power field

↓

Examine early morning swab
of urethral tissue or
first-voided urine specimen*

| Positive | Negative |

→ No
urethritis

Gram-negative
intracellular
diplococci

Equivocal or
atypical smear

No gram-negative
intracellular
diplococci

↓

Gonococcal
urethritis†

Mixed gonococcal and
nongonococcal urethritis†

Nongonococcal
urethritis†

Examine and treat sexual partners.
Repeat positive cultures at follow-up.

Figure 15–1. Diagnosis and treatment for suspected urethritis. *First-voided urine specimen is the first 10 mL of urine passed. The presence of more than 15 white blood cells per high-power field is evidence of urethritis. †Diagnosis is made by culture. (Modified and reproduced, with permission, from Berger RE: Page 907 in: *Campbell's Urology,* 5th ed. Vol 1. Saunders, 1986.)

consistent with proctitis. Gram-stained smear of the rectal mucosa is 60% sensitive but 100% specific if intracellular diplococci are seen (Klein et al, 1977). The differential diagnosis includes infection due to *Chlamydia,* herpes simplex virus, and other agents.

Infection may become disseminated. Fever and leukocytosis are uncommon. Small, tender papules or petechiae may appear on the arms and legs and may quickly develop into pustules, becoming hemorrhagic or necrotic. Tenosynovitis and arthritis may occur. The knees are more commonly involved than other joints. Synovial effusion is present in approximately 33% of patients with joint involvement. A culture for gonococci will be positive if the synovial fluid reveals leukocytes, more than 80,000/μL (Handsfield, Wiesner, and Holmes, 1976). Florid monarticular arthritis may require open drainage and irrigation.

Also rarely seen are hepatitis, myocarditis, endocarditis, and meningitis.

Prevention

Condoms, if properly used, will prevent the spread of *N gonorrhoeae.* Nonoxynol-9, a vaginal spermicide, has been shown to kill gonococcus (Jick et al, 1982). It is even more effective if used with a contraceptive diaphragm (Barlow, 1977). Antibiotic prophylaxis may be effective but may lead to selection of resistant strains (Singh, Cutler, and Utidjian, 1972). Currently, control of gonorrhea depends on case finding. Contacts, whether symptomatic or not, should be examined, cultured, and treated.

Treatment

The growth of plasmid-mediated beta-lactamase-

Table 15–1. Current approaches to therapy for uncomplicated gonorrhea and selected complications of gonorrhea.*

Type of Gonorrhea	Group A Regimens†	Group B Regimens‡
Uncomplicated gonorrhea	Amoxicillin, 3 g, plus probenecid, 1 g, both orally; or ampicillin, 3.5 g, plus probenecid, 1 g, both orally; or aqueous procaine penicillin G, 4.8 million units intramuscularly, plus probenecid, 1 g orally (drug of choice only for pharyngeal infection or infection in homosexual men); or spectinomycin, 2 g intramuscularly (recommended for patients allergic to penicillin or for whom penicillin has failed).§	Ceftriaxone, 250 mg intramuscularly; or cefotaxime, 1 g intramuscularly, plus probenecid, 1 g orally; or cefoxitin, 2 g intramuscularly, plus probenecid, 1 g orally; or spectinomycin, 2 g intramuscularly.§
Gonococcal pelvic inflammatory disease	Cefoxitin and probenecid plus doxycycline (ambulatory or hospitalized patients); or gentamicin or tobramycin plus clindamycin (hospitalized patients only).	Cefoxitin and probenecid plus doxycycline (ambulatory or hospitalized patients); or gentamicin or tobramycin plus clindamycin (hospitalized patients only).
Gonococcal epididymitis	Single-dose therapy for gonorrhea as above plus either tetracycline, 500 mg 4 times a day orally for 10 days, or doxycycline, 100 mg twice a day orally for 10 days.	Cefoxitin, 2 g intramuscularly, plus probenecid, 1 g orally, plus doxycycline, 100 mg orally twice a day for 10 days.
Disseminated gonococcal infection	Crystalline penicillin G until improved, then ampicillin to complete a 7-day course.	Cefoxitin, 1 g 4 times a day intravenously for 7 days; or cefotaxime, 500 mg 4 times a day intravenously for 7 days, or spectinomycin, 2 g twice a day intramuscularly for 7 days.

*Reproduced, with permission, from Hook EW III, Holmes KK: Gonococcal infections. *Ann Intern Med* 1985;**102**:229.
†For use in areas where gonococci have maintained chromosomal sensitivity to antimicrobial agents and penicillinase-producing strains of *N gonorrhoeae* comprise less than 1% of isolates.
‡For use in areas where chromosomal resistance to antimicrobial agents results in cure rates of less than 95% with group A regimens or where penicillinase-producing strains of *N gonorrhoeae* are prevalent (5% or more than 1% and increasing).
§Add doxycycline, 100 mg twice a day orally for 7 days, to therapy for uncomplicated gonorrhea when treating possible *C trachomatis* coinfection. Tetracycline hydrochloride, 500 mg 4 times a day orally, is cheaper and can be substituted when treating compliant patients. Because of increasing chromosomal resistance and decreasing cure rates for tetracycline regimens, tetracycline or doxycycline is no longer recommended as the sole treatment for gonorrhea.

producing *N gonorrhoeae* and chromosome-mediated penicillin- and tetracycline-resistant *N gonorrhoeae* has stimulated the development of more effective antimicrobials and faster diagnostic methods. As infection does not confer immunity, the search for a vaccine continues.

Because of regional differences in antibiotic susceptibility, no single therapeutic regimen can any longer be prescribed. The latest WHO (World Health Organization) report gives 2 lists of recommendations applicable to industrialized countries (Centers for Disease Control, 1982). The Group A regimen is for areas where resistant strains are not known to have developed. The Group B regimen is for areas where resistant strains are more prevalent.

A. Specific Measures: Specific recommendations for antibiotic treatment are listed in Table 15–1.

B. General Measures: Sexual intercourse should be avoided until cure has been established.

C. Treatment of Complications: The WHO treatment for gonococcal epididymitis is a single dose of amoxicillin, 3 g given intramuscularly; ampicillin, 3.5 g given intramuscularly; or aqueous procaine penicillin, 4.8×10^6 units given intramuscularly; **plus** either tetracycline, 500 mg orally 4 times a day for 10 days; or doxycycline, 100 mg orally twice a day for 10 days.

The treatment for disseminated gonococcal infection is crystalline penicillin G, 10 million units given intravenously daily for 3 days or until symptoms improve. Then, amoxicillin, 3 g orally daily, or ampicillin, 3.5 g orally daily, is given to complete the 5- to 7-day course.

Urethral strictures require urethral dilations or surgical intervention.

Treatment regimens for rectal and pharyngeal gonorrhea are the same as for uncomplicated gonococcal infection described above, except that amoxicillin and doxycycline are ineffective (Klein et al, 1977).

Prognosis

Once the infection has been treated properly, the discharge should disappear within 12 hours. In the 10–35% of patients with concurrent infection due to *Chlamydia* who do not receive a 7-day regimen of tetracycline or doxycycline, there may remain a thin, clear urethral discharge (**postgonococcal urethritis**), which should be treated as a chlamydial infection.

Cure of gonococcal urethritis should be established by gram-stained smear of urethral tissue in 10 days. If the infection has not been cured, spectinomycin is commonly selected; it is not affected by penicillinase-producing microorganisms. The recommended dose is 2 g given intramuscularly once only. The cure rate is about 95% (Centers for Disease Control, 1982).

NONGONOCOCCAL URETHRITIS

Etiology

In most sexually transmitted disease clinics and student health services, urethritis is nongonococcal more than 50% of the time. Nongonococcal urethritis is usually not reported to health authorities, and sexual contacts are not often examined or treated. This condition more commonly affects men of higher socioeconomic status and heterosexual men more often than homosexual men. The morbidity of nongonococcal urethritis is probably equal to or greater than that associated with gonococcal urethritis (Table 15–2).

Nongonococcal urethritis is a syndrome with several microbial causes. The most important and potentially dangerous is *Chlamydia trachomatis* (Stamm et al, 1984). Within the last decade, *C trachomatis* has been recognized as being responsible for an increasing number of genital syndromes. Since many practitioners did not have access to means of isolating this organism, infections were often diagnosed and treated without confirmation. Now there is usually access to immunofluorescent staining, so that chlamydial infections can be confirmed (Table 15–2).

C trachomatis is a small bacterium and an obligate intracellular parasite of columnar or pseudocolumnar epithelium. Two species of *Chlamydia* exist: *Chlamydia psittaci*, which causes psittacosis, and *C trachomatis*, which has 15 serotypes. Serotypes A–C cause hyperendemic blinding trachoma; serotypes D–K cause genital tract infection; and serotypes L1–L3 cause lymphogranuloma venereum.

C trachomatis can be recovered from the urethra in 25–60% of heterosexual men with nongonococcal urethritis, in 4–35% of men with gonorrhea, and in 0–7% of men in sexually transmitted disease clinics without symptoms of urethritis (Stamm et al). Asymptomatic infection occurs in 28% of the contacts of women with chlamydial cervical infections (Lycke et al, 1980).

Postgonococcal urethritis occurs in patients who probably acquire gonorrhea and chlamydial infection simultaneously but develop biphasic illness due to the longer incubation period of the latter. This occurs in 15–35% of heterosexuals with gonorrhea (Stamm et al, 1984).

Table 15–2. Diseases associated with *N gonorrhoeae* and *C trachomatis.**

N gonorrhoeae	*C trachomatis*
Urethritis	Urethritis
Cervicitis	Cervicitis
Salpingitis	Salpingitis
Bartholinitis	Bartholinitis
Perihepatitis	Perihepatitis
Arthritis	Reiter's syndrome
Urethral syndrome	Urethral syndrome
Proctitis	Proctitis
Conjunctivitis	Conjunctivitis
Endocarditis	Endocarditis
Asymptomatic disease	Asymptomatic disease
	Pneumonia
	Otitis media

*Reproduced, with permission, from Berger RE: Nongonococcal urethritis and related syndromes. *Monogr Urol* 1982;**3**:99.

Ureaplasma urealyticum may be the cause of nongonococcal urethritis in 20–50% of cases. The pathogenic role of *U urealyticum* in nongonococcal urethritis is difficult to interpret because genital colonization increases with an increasing number of sexual partners. In men with few sexual partners and no history of urethritis, the rate of *U urealyticum* colonization is low (Stamm et al, 1984). Urethral cultures from 40% of men with a history of 3–5 sexual partners will yield *U urealyticum* whether or not they have urethritis.

Evidence for *U urealyticum* as a urethral pathogen comes from several sources. The rate of isolation is higher in men with nongonococcal urethritis with negative *C trachomatis* cultures compared to those with positive cultures (Stamm et al, 1984). In men with *C trachomatis*-negative cultures and *U urealyticum*-positive cultures, the urethritis responds poorly to sulfonamides but well to aminocyclitols (eg, spectinomycin) (to which *U urealyticum* but not *C trachomatis* is sensitive) (Stamm et al, 1984). Nongonococcal urethritis persists in a group of *C trachomatis*-negative patients who have persistence of *Ureaplasma* during treatment with tetracycline. Endourethral inoculation of *U urealyticum* into humans and nonhuman primates has produced colonization and urethritis. Some of the 14 different serotypes of *U urealyticum* may be more pathogenic than others (Stamm et al, 1984).

Twenty to 30% of men with acute urethritis are negative for *N gonorrhoeae, C trachomatis,* and *U urealyticum.* Some of these men respond to antibiotic treatment, but persistence and recurrence of infection are common. Herpes simplex virus, cytomegalovirus, *Trichomonas vaginalis,* and other organisms have not been convincingly associated with most of these cases (Stamm et al, 1984).

Clinical Findings

A. Symptoms and Signs: Clinically, *Chlamydia*-positive and *Chlamydia*-negative nongonococcal urethritis cannot be differentiated on the basis of signs and symptoms alone. Both usually present after a 7- to 21-day incubation period, with dysuria and mild to moderate whitish or clear urethral discharge. Urethral discharge is often scant; however, it may be thick and purulent. Discharge may be absent, and the patient may only complain of urethral itching. Asymptomatic infection is common, especially among contacts of women with known cervical chlamydial infection. Examination reveals no abnormalities other than discharge in most cases; associated adenopathy, focal urethral tenderness, and meatal or penile lesions should suggest herpetic urethritis. Tenderness on palpation of the prostate has not been convincingly linked to chlamydial urethritis.

B. Laboratory Findings: Diagnosis of nongonococcal urethritis requires demonstration of urethritis and exclusion of infection with *N gonorrhoeae* (Fig 15–1). The man suspected of having urethritis ideally should be examined after 4 hours of urinary continence so that the discharge may be reliably demonstrated. On gram-stained smear of a urethral swab, the presence of more than 4 PMNs per oil-immersion field confirms urethritis. Alternatively, the presence of 15 or more PMNs in 5 random high-power fields (magnification × 400) of spun urine sediment correlates with urethritis. Many men with asymptomatic chlamydial urethral infection have urethral leukocytosis (4 PMNs per high-power field) on gram-stained smear of urethral secretions. When urethritis is suspected but urethral inflammation cannot be detected, the urethral swab should be obtained in the early morning before voiding.

Because *C trachomatis* is an intracellular parasite of columnar epithelium, the best specimen for culture is an endourethral swab rather than urethral exudate or urine. This specimen must be taken carefully from an area 2–4 cm inside the urethra. Preliminary culture results are available 2–3 days after inoculation. A fluorescein conjugated monoclonal antibody has been used in the diagnosis of chlamydial nongonococcal urethritis. It requires less than 30 minutes to perform and is based on the detection of extracellular chlamydial bodies. It has a sensitivity of 93% and a specificity of 96% (Tam et al, 1984). Although many physicians believe that cultures are unnecessary, *C trachomatis* is a dangerous pathogen, and culture results will serve both as a guide to therapy and as documentation of the disease.

Treatment

Since nongonococcal urethritis is a syndrome that can be caused by different organisms that respond differently to treatment, results of therapy are inconsistent. The current recommendations from the Centers for Disease Control are based on chlamydial infection (Table 15–3).

Depending on the organism causing urethritis, there are different responses to therapy. Patients with *C trachomatis* have the best response, and those with neither *C trachomatis* nor *U urealyticum* have the poorest response to therapy.

Nongonococcal urethritis not confirmed by culture should be assumed to be caused by *C trachomatis.* Ev-

Table 15–3. Management of nongonococcal urethritis.*

Initial management of diagnosed urethritis
  Give tetracycline, 500 mg orally 4 times a day for 7 days; or monocycline or doxycycline, 100 mg twice daily for 7 days; or erythromycin, 500 mg 4 times a day for 7 days.
  Examine and treat sexual partners with the same regimen.
Management of persistent or recurrent urethritis
  Question the patient about compliance with treatment and reexposure to infection.
  Examine the patient carefully for less common causes of urethritis.
  Confirm urethritis.
  Treat any specific cause that can be elucidated.
  If a specific cause is not found or if *U urealyticum* is present, treat with erythromycin base, 500 mg 4 times a day for 14 days.

*Modified and reproduced, with permission, from Bowie WR: Nongonococcal urethritis. *Urol Clin North Am* 1984;**11**:55.

ery attempt should be made to treat the patient's sexual partner promptly. In general, the same regimen is used to treat the male and the female.

In most cases, infection due to *Chlamydia* is easily treated. No tetracycline resistance has been documented. However, complications such as epididymitis, prostatitis, proctitis, or Reiter's syndrome do occur.

Complications

C trachomatis has been shown to cause most cases of epididymitis in heterosexual men less than 35 years of age. Men with epididymitis who are older than 35 years generally have coliform infections accompanied by a history of urologic disease or instrumentation (Berger, 1983).

The possibility of *C trachomatis* causing nonbacterial prostatitis is still controversial. In Mårdh's study in 1978, only 13% of patients with nonbacterial prostatitis had antibodies to *C trachomatis* and none had positive cultures from expressed prostatic secretions.

A recent prospective evaluation indicated that *C trachomatis* may be found in 15% of cases of proctitis in homosexual men (Stamm et al, 1982; Quinn et al, 1981). Lymphogranuloma venereum immunotypes can produce a primary ulcerative proctitis and a histopathologic picture of giant cell formation in granulomas identical to those seen in acute Crohn's disease. Symptoms and signs may include rectal pain, bleeding, mucus discharge, and diarrhea. Most *C trachomatis*-infected patients have abnormally high numbers of PMNs in their stool and on sigmoidoscopy have friable rectal mucosa.

Reiter's syndrome (urethritis, conjunctivitis, arthritis, and characteristic mucocutaneous lesions), reactive tenosynovitis, and arthritis without the other components of Reiter's syndrome have been associated with genital infection with *C trachomatis*. Preceding or concurrent infection with *C trachomatis* may be present in more than 80% of patients with Reiter's syndrome, which occurs with increased frequency in patients with the HLA-B27 haplotype (Brewerton et al, 1973).

Prognosis

Most nongonococcal urethritis responds promptly to tetracycline. Vigorous treatment of the man's sexual partner or partners is imperative.

TRICHOMONIASIS

Etiology

Trichomonas vaginalis was described by Donne in 1836 and was long regarded as a harmless inhabitant of the vagina. Of the 3 species of trichomonads that infect humans, only *T vaginalis* causes clinical disease. The prevalence of colonization in control male populations ranges from nil in asymptomatic men to 18% in men with gonococcal urethritis (Krieger, 1981). The median prevalence in control male populations is 2%.

The highest prevalence in both men and women is at ages 15–40 years.

There is a consensus that *T vaginalis* is sexually transmitted in almost all instances. *T vaginalis* has been isolated from 14–60% of male partners of infected women and in 67–100% of female partners of infected men. The difference is most likely attributable to the difficulty of demonstrating trichomonads in the male genital tract, as well as the spontaneous clearance in many men (Krieger, 1981).

Many European investigators feel that trichomoniasis may be a major cause of morbidity in men (Krieger, 1981). The cause is unknown in 30–50% of cases of nongonococcal urethritis. The evidence for trichomoniasis as a sole cause of urethritis is poor. *T vaginalis* has been claimed to cause some cases of balanoposthitis, epididymitis, urethral stricture, prostatitis, pyelonephritis, and, rarely, infertility (Lewis and Carrol, 1928). Most infections due to *T vaginalis* in men are asymptomatic, and some feel that men serve primarily as vectors for transmission of symptomatic disease to women.

Clinical Findings

Urethral discharge should be mixed immediately with 1–2 mL of saline and studied microscopically. This examination has less accuracy in men than the 60–70% accuracy that it has in women (Rothenberg et al, 1976; Fleury, 1979).

Liquid and semisolid media cultures have proved to be most accurate for diagnosis of trichomoniasis (Nielsen, 1973; Rothenberg et al, 1976; Cox and Nicol, 1973).

Treatment

Most cases of trichomoniasis in men are discovered and treated on the basis of contact with women with trichomoniasis vaginitis. Once the diagnosis has been made, a condom should be used during intercourse until treatment has been successful.

Metronidazole, 2 g orally as a single dose, should be given to patient and partner whether they are symptomatic or not.

Prognosis

Most trichomonad infections respond promptly to metronidazole. Vigorous treatment of the man's sexual partner or partners is imperative.

PRIMARY SYPHILIS

Clinical Findings

A. Symptoms and Signs: Syphilis is caused by *Treponema pallidum,* a spirochete, which gains access through the intact or abraded skin or mucous membranes. The patient usually presents with a painless penile sore (**chancre**) 2–4 weeks after sexual exposure. The chancre begins as a hyperemic or erythematous spot. This painless papule, or pustule, develops on the glans, corona, foreskin, shaft, suprapubic area, or scrotum. It may break down to form an indurated, punched-out lesion. The syphilitic (hard) chancre is relatively deep, has indurated edges and a clean base, and is not tender on pressure. The lesion may be so small and transient that it may be missed. Without treatment, the lesion will heal spontaneously and slowly. Discrete enlarged inguinal nodes may be palpable. These may be in a unilateral or bilateral satellite formation. They are not tender unless secondarily infected (Table 15–4).

B. Laboratory Findings: The diagnosis is made by finding the spirochetes on darkfield examination of scrapings of the base of the chancre or by fluorescent antibody techniques. Where the darkfield examination is not available, a reagin (RPR) card test may be used (Kraus, 1984). This is equivalent to and is replacing the VDRL test. Repeated examinations daily for 3 days without local or systemic treatment and aspiration of the enlarged nodes may be necessary to demonstrate the organism. The serologic tests may remain negative for 1–3 weeks after the appearance of the chancre. The quickest and least expensive examination, the fluorescent treponema antibody-absorption test (FTS-ABS), is also the most specific and sensitive. The more expensive and more difficult *Treponema pallidum* immobilization test has been replaced by the microhemagglutination test, which can be automated and quantitated (Garner et al, 1972).

Differential Diagnosis

Chancroid, lymphogranuloma venereum, granuloma inguinale, balanitides of varying cause, carcinoma, scabies, psoriasis, lichen planus, leukoplakia, erythroplasia, and infection due to herpes simplex virus may resemble syphilis. *Borrelia refringens* is difficult to distinguish from *T pallidum*. Erythroplasia of Queyrat may resemble a hard chancre. All penile lesions should be considered syphilis until proved otherwise.

Complications

Urologic complications are rare and occur in the tertiary form of the disease. They include gummas of the testis and neurogenic bladder secondary to neurosyphilis.

Prevention

If exposure has occurred, give benzathine penicillin G, 2.4 million units intramuscularly in a single dose.

Treatment

Patients with early syphilis (primary, secondary, or latent of less than 1 year's duration) should receive benzathine penicillin G, 2.4 million units intramuscularly in a single dose. Patients allergic to penicillin should receive tetracycline hydrochloride, 500 mg orally 4 times daily for 15 days, or erythromycin, 500 mg orally 4 times daily for 15 days.

Prognosis

The prognosis is excellent; relapse is rare. If it occurs, more intensive penicillin therapy is required.

CHANCROID

Chancroid is a sexually transmitted disease caused by *Haemophilus ducreyi*.

Clinical Findings

A. Symptoms: A papule is the first lesion of chancroid, usually seen a few days after sexual exposure. One or more painful, dirty-appearing chancroid ulcers then appear. These are deep with flat, rugged, erythematous borders that extend into the dermis and subcutaneous tissue of the surrounding skin. Chancroid ulcers often have purulent secretions. About 50% of patients will have fever, malaise, and headache.

B. Signs: Ulcers caused by chancroid may be indurated but are usually soft and malleable. The base is friable and bleeds easily. Lesions may be painful. Untreated ulcers slowly enlarge, rupture, and coalesce with other ulcers. Confluent ulcers enlarge by peripheral extension. Painful chronic inguinal inflammation seen with chancroid may cause lymphatic obstruction. Genital lymphedema may ensue, with the end stage being elephantiasis.

C. Laboratory Findings: A gram-stained smear reveals *H ducreyi* in 50% of cases. Selective culture for *H ducreyi* has greater sensitivity and specificity than clot cultures and gram-stained smears. Biopsy is always diagnostic.

Differential Diagnosis

Chancroid must be differentiated from other ulcerative lesions of the external genitalia (eg, genital herpes, syphilis, granuloma inguinale, lymphogranuloma venereum, traumatic ulcer, and lesions associated with drug reactions).

Complications

Uncommonly, secondary infection with aerobic and anaerobic bacteria may cause marked destruction of tissue.

Treatment

A. Specific Measures: Response with tetracycline is excellent. The dose is 500 mg orally 4 times daily for 10 days. Erythromycin, 500 mg orally 4 times daily, is also effective, as is trimethoprim-sulfamethoxazole, one double-strength tablet orally twice daily. Therapy should be continued for a minimum of 10 days and until ulcers or nodes have disappeared. Sexual partners should be examined and treated identically.

B. General Measures: Cleanliness is important; washing the genitalia carefully with green soap and water immediately after intercourse has been shown to be effective (Moore, 1920).

Table 15–4. Genital ulcers.*

Disease	Cause	Preferred Test	Type of Ulcer	Ancillary Tests	Type of Adenopathy	Drug of Choice	Alternative Drug
Genital herpes	Herpes simplex virus type 1 or 2	Viral culture.	Grouped vesicles; small, painful when scraped; soft.	Tzanck smear.	Firm, tender when palpated.	Acyclovir ointment 5% 6 times a day for 7 days (initial episode). Acyclovir, 200 mg orally 4 times a day for 10 days. Acyclovir, 5 mg/kg intravenously every 8 hours for 5 days.	
Chancroid	*Haemophilus ducreyi*	Selective medium culture.	Deep, undermined border; painful, soft or indurated, purulent.		Fluctuant, tender overlying erythema.	Erythromycin, 500 mg orally 4 times a day for 10 days.	Trimethoprim-sulfamethoxazole, 1 double-strength tablet twice a day for 10 days.
Granuloma inguinale	*Calymmatobacterium granulomatis*	Crush preparation.	Firm, painless; rolled elevated border; chronic, spreading.	Histology.	No adenopathy.	Tetracycline, 500 mg orally 4 times a day for 2 weeks or until healed.	Erythromycin, 500 mg orally 4 times a day for 2 weeks; or trimethoprim-sulfamethoxazole, 1 double-strength tablet twice a day for 2 weeks or until healed.
Lymphogranuloma	*Chlamydia trachomatis* (L1, L2, L3 subtypes)	Complement fixation or immunofluorescence.	Usually absent.	*C trachomatis* culture.	Fluctuant, tender.	Tetracycline, 500 mg 4 times a day for 2 weeks.	Erythromycin, 500 mg orally 4 times a day for 2 weeks.
Traumatic ulcer		None.	Onset during sexual activity.				
Fixed drug reaction		None.	Recurrences associated with the same systemic medicine.				
Syphilis (primary)	*Treponema pallidum*	Darkfield microscopy	Painless, firm, "hard," indurated.	RPR, VDRL, FTS-ABS, MHA-TP.	Firm, nontender or tender, "rubbery."	Benzathine penicillin G, 2.4 million units intramuscularly.	Tetracycline, 500 mg orally 4 times a day for 15 days.

*Modified and reproduced, with permission, from Kraus SJ: Evaluation and management of acute genital ulcers in sexually active patients. *Urol Clin North Am* 1984;11:155.

C. Treatment of Complications: If a superinfection complicates the picture, use penicillin or clindamycin in addition to the antibiotics described above.

Prognosis

With proper antibiotic therapy, the prognosis is excellent.

LYMPHOGRANULOMA VENEREUM

Chlamydia trachomatis immunotypes L1, L2, and L3 cause lymphogranuloma venereum. The disease is characterized by a transient genital lesion followed by lymphadenitis and, possibly, rectal strictures. The inguinal and subinguinal lymph nodes may become matted, undergo suppuration, and form multiple sinuses.

Clinical Findings

A. Symptoms and Signs: A papule or pustule appears 5–21 days after sexual exposure. The genital lesion of lymphogranuloma venereum is so small and transient that it often goes unnoticed. It may simply be a vesicle or a superficial erosion. An initial lesion that erodes to form an ulcer is usually superficial.

Painful nodes may become fluctuant. Unilateral lymphadenopathy is most common and may be the initial symptom. At the stage of bubo formation, constitutional symptoms are commonly present (eg, chills, fever, headache, generalized joint pains, nausea, and vomiting). Skin rashes are frequent.

B. Laboratory Findings: The white blood count may reach 20,000/μL if the lymph nodes are invaded. Anemia may be present. Proteins (globulin) are elevated. Skin lesions show acute and subacute inflammation; there is nothing specific or diagnostic in their appearance. The nodes show abscesses with heavy infiltration by neutrophils. Hyperplasia of lymphoid elements takes place, and plasma cells appear.

The most specific test in the diagnosis of lymphogranuloma venereum is culture of *C trachomatis* from an inguinal node aspirate. Serologic tests, including the lymphogranuloma venereum complement fixation and microimmunofluorescent antibody tests, are commonly used and have replaced the Frei skin test. The complement fixation test is not specific for lymphogranuloma venereum because it also detects other chlamydial infections, including urethritis and psittacosis.

Differential Diagnosis

All other causes of penile ulcers should be differentiated, especially syphilis, infection due to herpes simplex virus, and chancroid. Always suspect lymphogranuloma venereum in patients with a rectal stricture. The inguinal syndrome of lymphogranuloma venereum is indistinguishable from that of chancroid in that both are unilateral in two-thirds of cases, and in both, an inguinal bubo (a firm, slightly painful mass) may appear in 1–2 weeks (Kraus, 1982).

Complication

Rupture of inguinal nodes in lymphogranuloma venereum can lead to draining sinuses. Chronic inguinal inflammation may cause lymphatic obstruction and elephantiasis. Rectal stricture is a late complication.

Treatment

A. Specific Measures: Lymphogranuloma venereum is treated with antibiotics that are effective in other chlamydial infections. Tetracycline is the drug of choice, 500 mg orally 4 times daily for 2 weeks. Alternatives include erythromycin, 500 mg orally 4 times daily, and sulfamethoxazole, 1 g orally twice daily. Treatment with any of these medications should continue for at least 2 weeks.

B. Treatment of Complications: Aspiration of fluctuant nodes is indicated. Draining sinuses can be excised. Rectal stenosis may require surgery.

Prognosis

The prognosis is excellent if the disease is treated promptly. The late complications are genital elephantiasis and rectal stricture.

GRANULOMA INGUINALE

This sexually transmitted chronic infection of the skin and subcutaneous tissue of the genitalia, perineum, and inguinal area has an incubation period of 2–3 months. The infective agent, *Calymmatobacterium granulomatis,* is related to *Klebsiella pneumoniae* and grows with difficulty on an egg yolk medium.

Clinical Findings

A. Symptoms and Signs: A papule is the first sign of granuloma inguinale. This may form an ulcer protruding above the level of the surrounding skin. The ulcer base is erythematous and may have hemorrhagic secretions. It is firm, indurated, and nontender. The inguinal swelling or pseudobubo is a subcutaneous granulomatous process rather than a true lymphadenopathy. Untreated, it enlarges by direct extension or erodes through the skin. Chronic inguinal inflammation may cause lymphatic obstruction and elephantiasis. The microscopic picture includes nonspecific infiltrates of plasma cells, giant cells, neutrophils, and large monocytes. The monocyte cytoplasm contains Donovan bodies, the intracellular stage of *C granulomatis.*

B. Laboratory Findings: Identification of **Donovan bodies** in monocytes on a stained smear makes the diagnosis. These organisms appear as bipolar staining rods within the monocytes. A crush preparation for cytologic study is prepared by obtaining a small fragment of tissue from the ulcer base and crushing it between 2 slides. Giemsa's stain, Wright's stain, or Leishman's stain can be used. Serial sections are done, as histologic visualization of Donovan bodies may not be seen on only one study. Crush preparation test results are available in minutes, whereas results of histologic studies cannot be obtained for days. In case of doubt, biopsy may be performed. A reliable culture for *C granulomatis* is not available.

Complications

Secondary infection may cause deep ulceration and tissue destruction. Sinuses may result. Phimosis may occur. A change in bowel habits suggests a rectal stricture.

Prevention

The use of a condom does not prevent perigenital spread.

Treatment

Neither controlled granuloma inguinale therapy trials nor in vitro susceptibilities of *C granulomatis* are available. Treatment has been successful with tetracycline, 500 mg orally 4 times daily, or trimethoprim-sulfamethoxazole, one double-strength tablet orally twice daily. These doses are continued until the lesion has healed. Gentamicin and chloramphenicol, although more toxic, are also effective.

Prognosis

The antibiotics are effective, the complications few, and the prognosis good.

GENITAL HERPES INFECTIONS

Etiology

Genital herpes is a disease of great concern to physicians and patients. The increasing prevalence of infection in men and women, the risk of transmission to sexual partners, the high rates of morbidity and even death associated with infections in infants, the possible association with cervical cancer, and the absence of curative therapy have made it imperative that all physicians be able to diagnose, counsel, and treat patients with genital herpes.

Herpes simplex virus is a double-stranded DNA virus that may cause persistent or latent infections. Most genital herpes infections are due to type 2 virus, although infection due to type 1 herpes virus, which is commonly associated with oral infections, has been reported in 10–25% of cases of genital herpes. Herpes simplex is seen in 5% of patients seeking help at clinics for sexually transmitted disease (Corey and Holmes, 1983). In college students, herpes simplex virus infections are 10 times more common than gonorrhea or syphilis (Corey et al, 1983). Although it is not inevitable that the sexual partner of an infected patient will also become infected, partners are at risk even when the infection is asymptomatic.

Clinical Findings

A. Symptoms and Signs: Retrospective studies suggest that 50–70% of herpes type 2 infections are asymptomatic, but prospective studies to deter-

mine the percentage of asymptomatic infections have not been undertaken. Herpes simplex virus types 1 and 2 produce primary genital lesions of equal severity. The first episode of disease is much more severe in persons without prior oral herpes. The incubation period is 2–10 days. Approximately 2% of patients with primary genital herpes develop severe sacral or autonomic nervous system dysfunction resulting in urinary retention (Corey et al, 1983). Vesicles grouped on an erythematous base, not following a neural distribution, and associated with a previous history of such eruptions are pathognomonic for genital herpes. The lesions are tender to touch. Adenopathy is usually bilateral, and the lymph nodes are mildly tender, nonfixed, and slightly firm. Dysuria is present in 44% of men. Herpes simplex virus can be isolated from the urethra in most of these patients (Corey and Holmes, 1983). Extragenital skin lesions, usually from autoinoculation, are found in approximately 10% of men with primary genital herpes.

B. Laboratory Findings: Virus isolation by culture is the most sensitive of techniques for diagnosing herpes infections. In recurrent disease, urethral isolation can be obtained in fewer than 2% of men. Results can be available in 5 days. Tzanck or Papanicolaou smears of lesions will demonstrate intranuclear inclusions in 50–60% of culture-positive cases. Immunofluorescent techniques will reveal 57% of culture-positive cases (Moseley et al, 1981). Serum antibody to herpes simplex virus infections can be measured by a number of methods. No test presently available is completely reliable in differentiating type 1 from type 2 infections. Serologic tests are now used only to document a history of past infection.

Treatment

Acyclovir is the only drug that has shown efficacy in the treatment of genital herpes. Topical, intravenous, and oral forms are effective for first-episode genital herpes.

Acyclovir acts on viral thymidine kinase as a guanine analog. It is selectively phosphorylated in the virus, acts as an inhibitor of viral DNA polymerase, and acts as a chain terminator (Colby et al, 1980). Oral acyclovir, 200 mg 5 times daily for 5–10 days, and intravenous acyclovir appear more effective than topical therapy in the treatment of primary genital herpes. Acyclovir decreases the duration of viral shedding, the time to crusting of lesions, and the time to healing of lesions, during which there is pain or itching, or both. Only the oral and intravenous forms decrease dysuria, vaginal discharge, systemic symptoms, and the development of new lesions (Corey and Holmes, 1983). Prophylactic treatment with acyclovir, 200 mg orally 2–5 times daily, may sufficiently decrease recurrence, but more information on the long-term side effects is needed before this form of therapy can be recommended (Bryson et al, 1983).

Table 15–5. Sexually transmitted diseases that cause infections of the the liver, intestines, and rectum.*

Organ	Agents
Liver	Hepatitis B virus Hepatitis A virus Hepatitis non-A, non-B agents
Intestines	*Giardia lamblia* *Entamoeba histolytica* *Cryptosporidium* species *Shigella* species *Campylobacter jejuni* *Strongyloides* species
Rectum	*Neisseria gonorrhoeae* *Chlamydia trachomatis* *Treponema pallidum* Herpes simplex virus Human papillomavirus

*Reproduced, with permission, from Judson FN: Sexually transmitted viral hepatitis and enteric pathogens. *Urol Clin North Am* 1984;**11**:178.

HEPATITIS & ENTERIC INFECTIONS

In the past, viral hepatitis and enteric infections were not viewed as sexually transmitted diseases. Now, however, many of these infections are known to be sexually transmitted in some cases (Table 15–5). Hepatitis A and B may be transmitted by sexual contact and through other close physical contact. Enteric infections such as amebiasis, giardiasis, shigellosis, and campylobacteriosis may be transmitted sexually. Most of these sexually transmitted enteric infections occur in homosexual men. Contact is made through anal intercourse or anilingus. Enteric disease contracted by homosexual contact may also be transmitted to female partners.

Approximately one-third of hepatitis B cases may be attributable to homosexual contacts. Thirty to 80% of homosexual men test seropositive for hepatitis B (Schreeder et al, 1982). Hepatitis A is also spread by sexual contact and is more prevalent in homosexual men than in heterosexual men. At this time, there is little evidence that non-A, non-B hepatitis has a sexual mode of transmission (Hentzer et al, 1980).

ACQUIRED IMMUNODEFICIENCY SYNDROME

Acquired immunodeficiency syndrome **(AIDS),** first reported in 1981, has as its basis acquired im-

munoincompetence. The retrovirus (human T cell leukemia virus, lymphotropic virus type 3, or human immunodeficiency virus [HIV] appears to be transmitted by sexual contact, contaminated syringes, or blood transfusion. Most patients are homosexuals with multiple partners, abusers of intravenous drugs, hemophiliacs receiving factor VIII concentrate, or recipients of multiple transfusions. Vertical transmission from mother to fetus has been reported, as well as female-to-male and male-to-female penile-vaginal transmission (Harris et al, 1983). The disease is transmitted only by sexual contact; normal physical contact, even within a household, will not spread disease (Curran, Gold, and Jaffe, 1984).

The prodromal syndrome includes fatigue, weight loss, fever, and diarrhea. Four AIDS syndromes have been reported: lymphadenopathy syndrome, Kaposi's sarcoma, increased susceptibility to opportunistic infections, and cancer (lymphoma, squamous cell carcinoma, or Burkitt's lymphoma) (Ziegler et al, 1984).

The physician may find generalized lymphadenopathy, multiple purple "bruises" on the legs **(Kaposi's sarcoma),** or recurring infections (bacterial, viral, or fungal). Be on the alert for the chronic cough of *Pneumocystis carinii* pneumonia.

Laboratory data reveal the depressed immune system. There is an abnormal ratio or even a reversal in the ratio of helper T cells to suppressor T cells. One should search for antibodies to hepatitis B virus and cytomegalovirus, as these organisms infect compromised hosts. An enzyme-linked immunosorbent assay (ELISA) has been developed to detect antibodies to HIV. Serum antibody to HIV was found in 95% of patients with AIDS, 87% of those with lymphadenopathy syndrome, and less than 1% of controls (Sarngadharan et al, 1984).

The spermicide nonoxynol-9 is inhibitory to HIV and, if used in combination with condoms, may decrease transmission of the virus. There is no therapeutic intervention to date that has permanently reversed the immunodeficiency. The patients often succumb to aggressive Kaposi's sarcoma or other runaway infections, such as *P carinii* pneumonia.

The overall mortality rate in the first 1500 cases is close to 40%; this rate will probably increase on follow-up studies (Curran, Gold, and Jaffe, 1984).

REFERENCES

General

Bardin E, Berger RE: Sexually transmitted disease in men. *Primary Care* 1985;**12**:761.

Centers for Disease Control: Sexually transmitted diseases treatment guidelines 1982. *MMWR* 1982;**31(Suppl)**:35f.

Mandell GL, Sande MA: Antimicrobial agents. Chap 50, pp 1115–1149, and Chap 52, pp 1170–1198, in: *The Pharmacological Basis of Therapeutics,* 7th ed. Gilman AG et al (editors). Macmillan, 1985.

Rothenberg RB et al: Efficacy of selected diagnostic tests for sexually transmitted diseases. *JAMA* 1976;**235:**49.

Smith DR: Sexually transmitted diseases in males. Chap 14, pp 244–252, in: *General Urology*, 11th ed. Smith DR (editor). Lange, 1984.

World Health Organization: *Report of WHO Expert Committee on Sexually Transmitted Diseases—Geneva, Switzerland*. World Health Organization, 1985.

Gonococcal Urethritis

Barlow D: The condom and gonorrhoea. *Lancet* 1977;**2:**811.

Brewerton DA et al: Reiter's disease and HL-A 27. *Lancet* 1973;**2:**996.

Centers for Disease Control: Chromosomally mediated resistant *Neisseria gonorrhoeae*—United States. *MMWR* 1984;**33:**408.

Centers for Disease Control: Penicillin-resistant gonorrhea—North Carolina. *MMWR* 1983;**32:**273.

Handsfield HH, Wiesner PJ, Holmes KK: Treatment of the gonococcal arthritis-dermatitis syndrome. *Ann Intern Med* 1976;**84:**661.

Handsfield HH et al: Asymptomatic gonorrhea in men: Diagnosis, natural course, prevalence and significance. *N Engl J Med* 1974;**290:**117.

Handsfield HH et al: Correlation of auxotype and penicillin susceptibility of *Neisseria gonorrhoeae* with sexual preference and clinical manifestations of gonorrhea. *Sex Transm Dis* 1980;**7:**1.

Harrison WO: Gonococcal urethritis. *Urol Clin North Am* 1984;**11:**45.

Hook EW 3rd, Holmes KK: Gonococcal infections. *Ann Intern Med* 1985;**102:**229.

Jick H et al: Vaginal spermicides and gonorrhea. *JAMA* 1982;**248:**1619.

Klein EJ et al: Anorectal gonococcal infection. *Ann Intern Med* 1977;**86:**340.

Singh B, Cutler JC, Utidjian HM: Studies on the development of a vaginal preparation providing both prophylaxis against venereal disease and other genital infections and contraception: 2. Effect in vitro of vaginal contraceptive and noncontraceptive preparations on *Treponema pallidum* and *Neisseria gonorrhoeae*. *Br J Vener Dis* 1972; **48:**57.

Thin RNT, Williams IA, Nicol CS: Direct and delayed methods of immunofluorescent diagnosis of gonorrhoeae in women. *Br J Vener Dis* 1971;**47:**27.

Wiesner PJ et al: Clinical spectrum of pharyngeal gonococcal infection. *N Engl J Med* 1973;**288:**181.

William DC, Felman YM, Riccardi NB: The utility of anoscopy in the rapid diagnosis of symptomatic anorectal gonorrhea in men. *Sex Transm Dis* 1981;**8:**16.

Nongonococcal Urethritis

Berger RE: Epididymitis. Chap 57, pp 650–662, in: *Sexually Transmitted Diseases and Etiologic Agents*. Holmes KK et al (editors). McGraw-Hill, 1984.

Berger RE: Urethritis and epididymitis. *Semin Urol* 1983; **1:**138.

Bowie WR: Nongonococcal urethritis. *Urol Clin North Am* 1984;**11:**55.

Bowie WR et al: Etiology of nongonococcal urethritis: Evidence for *Chlamydia trachomatis* and *Ureaplasma urealyticum*. *J Clin Invest* 1977;**59:**735.

Brewerton DA et al: Reiter's disease and HL-A 27. *Lancet* 1973;**2:**996.

Kraus SJ: Semiquantitation of urethral polymorphonuclear leukocytes as objective evidence of nongonococcal urethritis. *Sex Transm Dis* 1982;**9:**52.

Lycke E et al: The risk of transmission of genital *Chlamydia trachomatis* infection is less than that of genital *Neisseria gonorrhoeae* infection. *Sex Transm Dis* 1980;**7:**6.

Mårdh PA et al: Role of *Chlamydia trachomatis* in nonacute prostatitis. *Br J Vener Dis* 1978;**54:**330.

Quinn TC et al: *Chlamydia trachomatis* proctitis. *N Engl J Med* 1981;**305:**195.

Stamm WE, Holmes KK: *Chlamydia trachomatis* infections of the adult. Chap 24, pp 258–270, in: *Sexually Transmitted Diseases and Etiologic Agents*. Holmes KK et al (editors). McGraw-Hill, 1984.

Stamm WE et al: *Chlamydia trachomatis* proctitis in chlamydial infections. Pages 111–114 in: *Sexually Transmitted Diseases*. Mårdh PA et al (editors). Elsevier, 1982.

Stamm WE et al: Effect of treatment regimens for *Neisseria gonorrhoeae* on simultaneous infection with *Chlamydia trachomatis*. *N Engl J Med* 1984;**310:**545.

Tam MR et al: Culture-independent diagnosis of *Chlamydia trachomatis* using monoclonal antibodies. *N Engl J Med* 1984;**310:**1146.

Trichomoniasis

Cox PJ, Nicol CS: Growth studies of various strains of *T vaginalis* and possible improvements in the laboratory diagnosis of trichomoniasis. *Br J Vener Dis* 1973;**49:**536.

Fleury FJ: Diagnosis of *Trichomonas vaginalis* infection. (Letter.) *JAMA* 1979;**242:**2556.

Krieger JN: Urologic aspects of trichomoniasis. *Invest Urol* 1981;**18:**411.

Lewis B, Carrol G: A case of *Trichomonas vaginalis* infection of the kidney pelvis. *J Urol* 1928;**19:**337.

Nielsen R: *Trichomonas vaginalis*. 2. Laboratory investigations in trichomoniasis. *Br J Vener Dis* 1973;**49:**531.

Perl G, Nagazzoni DV: Further studies in treatment of female and male trichomoniasis with metronidazole. *Obstet Gynecol* 1963;**22:**376.

Underhill RA, Peck JE: Causes of therapeutic failure after treatment of trichomonal vaginitis with metronidazole: Comparisons of single-dose treatment with a standard regimen. *Br J Clin Pract* 1974;**28:**134.

Primary Syphilis

Garner MF et al: *Treponema pallidum* haemagglutination test for syphilis: Comparison with TPI and FTA-ABS tests. *Br J Vener Dis* 1972;**48:**470.

Kraus SJ: Evaluation and management of acute genital ulcers in sexually active patients. *Urol Clin North Am* 1984;**11:**155.

Chancroid

Moore JE: The diagnosis of chancroid and the effect of prophylaxis upon its incidence in the American expeditionary forces. *J Urol* 1920;**4:**169.

Lymphogranuloma Venereum

Kraus SJ: Semiquantitation of urethral polymorphonuclear leukocytes as objective evidence of nongonococcal urethritis. *Sex Transm Dis* 1982;**9:**52.

Granuloma Inguinale

Kraus SJ: Evaluation and management of acute genital ulcers on sexually active patients. *Urol Clin North Am* 1984;**11:**55.

Kraus SJ et al: Pseudogranuloma inguinale caused by *Haemophilus ducreyi*. *Arch Dermatol* 1982;494.

Genital Herpes Infections

Bryson YJ et al: Treatment of first episodes of genital herpes simplex virus infections with oral acyclovir: A randomized double-blind controlled trial in normal subjects. *N Engl J Med* 1983;**308:**916.

Colby BM et al: Effect of acyclovir [9-(2-hydroxyethoxymethyl)guanine] on Epstein-Barr virus DNA replication. *J Virol* 1980;**34:**560.

Corey L, Holmes KK: Genital herpes simplex virus infections: Current concepts in diagnosis, therapy, and prevention. *Ann Intern Med* 1983;**98:**973.

Corey L et al: Genital herpes simplex infection: Clinical manifestations, course and complications. *Ann Intern Med* 1983;**98:**958.

Kraus SJ: Evaluation and management of acute genital ulcers in sexually active patients. *Urol Clin North Am* 1984;**11:**155.

Moseley RC et al: Comparison of viral isolation, direct immunofluorescence, and indirect immunoperoxidase techniques for detection of genital herpes simplex virus infection. *J Clin Microbiol* 1981;**13:**913.

Oriel JD: Genital warts. Chap 46, pp 496–507, in: *Sexually Transmitted Diseases and Etiologic Agents*. Holmes KK et al (editors). McGraw-Hill, 1984.

Hepatitis & Enteric Infections

Hentzer B et al: Viral hepatitis in a venereal clinic population: Relation to certain risk factors. *Scand J Infect Dis* 1980;**12:**245.

Judson FN: Sexually transmitted viral hepatitis and enteric pathogens. *Urol Clin North Am* 1984;**11:**177.

Quinn TC et al: The polymicrobial origin of intestinal infections in homosexual men. *N Engl J Med* 1983;**309:**576.

Schreeder MT et al: Hepatitis B in homosexual men: Prevalence of infection and factors related to transmission. *J Infect Dis* 1982;**146:**7.

Acquired Immunodeficiency Syndrome

Curran JW, Gold J, Jaffe HW: The acquired immunodeficiency syndrome (AIDS). In: *Sexually Transmitted Diseases and Etiologic Agents*. Holmes KK et al (editors). McGraw-Hill, 1984.

Fauci AS: Immunologic abnormalities in the acquired immunodeficiency syndrome (AIDS). *Clin Res* 1984;**32:**491.

Harris C et al: Immunodeficiency in female sexual partners of men with the acquired immunodeficiency syndrome. *N Engl J Med* 1983;**308:**1181.

Landesman SH, Ginzburg HM, Weiss SH: The AIDS epidemic. *N Engl J Med* 1985;**312:**521.

Redfield RR et al: Frequent transmission of HTLV-III among spouses of patients with AIDS-related complex and AIDS. *JAMA* 1985;**253:**1571.

Sarngadharan MG et al: Antibodies reactive with human T-lymphotropic retroviruses (HTLV-III) in the serum of patients with AIDS. *Science* 1984;**224:**506.

Sonnabend J, Witkin SS, Purtilo DT: Acquired immunodeficiency syndrome, opportunistic infections, and malignancies in male homosexuals: A hypothesis of etiologic factors in pathogenesis. *JAMA* 1983;**249:**2370.

Ziegler JL et al: Non-Hodgkin's lymphoma in 90 homosexual men: Relation to generalized lymphadenopathy and the acquired immunodeficiency syndrome. *N Engl J Med* 1984;**311:**565.

Urinary Stones

16

J. Patrick Spirnak, MD, & Martin I. Resnick, MD

Archeologic studies show that urinary tract stone disease was an affliction of humans earlier than 4800 BC (Shattock, 1905). Ancient Greek and Roman physicians recorded the symptoms and treatment of urologic stone disease, but little attention was directed to localization of the stone or to the cause of its formation. For a complete review of the historical aspects of urinary stone disease, see Resnick and Boyce (1979).

In the 20th century, advances in technology and microscopic techniques have led to a better understanding of the structural characteristics of calculi, their chemical composition, and the various components of urine. Many theories have been proposed to explain the cause and development of urologic calculi, but none have been able to answer fully the questions concerning stone formation. In all probability, stone disease will be found to result from the interaction of multiple factors, many of which are as yet unknown.

Theories of Stone Formation

A. Nucleation Theory: Stone formation is initiated by the presence of a crystal or foreign body in urine supersaturated with a crystallizing salt that favors growth of a crystal lattice.

B. Stone Matrix Theory: An organic matrix of serum and urinary proteins (albumin; α_1- and α_2- globulins and occasionally γ- globulins; mucoproteins; and matrix substance A) provides a framework for deposition of crystals.

C. Inhibitor of Crystallization Theory: Some urinary substances, eg, magnesium, pyrophosphate, citrate, phosphocitrate, diphosphonate, mucoproteins, and various peptides, inhibit crystal formation. Absence or low concentration of inhibitors permits crystallization.

Most investigators acknowledge that these 3 theories describe the 3 basic factors influencing urinary stone formation. It is likely that more than one factor operates in causing stone disease. A generalized model of stone formation combining these 3 basic theories has been proposed. A period of abnormal crystalluria is required during which large crystals or aggregates of crystals are produced in the urine. In order for these crystals to continue to grow and propagate, a certain number of chemical factors must be present, ie, the urine must be supersaturated with the salt of the stone-forming crystal, certain inhibitors of crystallization must be reduced or absent from the urine, and a certain concentration of nucleating matrix material must be present.

Additional risk factors can influence the degree and severity of clinical stone disease. These include the metabolic state of the patient, which is influenced by genetic background as well as the presence of certain hormonal imbalances; environmental factors, which could lead to supersaturation of already saturated urine; dietary excesses; and anatomic abnormalities, which could lead to chronic infection or actually enhance the deposition of crystals in the upper urinary tract.

Anatomic Site of Stone Formation

There are several different theories as to where stone formation occurs in the kidney: (1) deposition of calcium on the basement membrane of collecting tubules and on the surface of papillae; (2) deposition of linear precipitates of calcium within the renal lymphatics to produce obstruction and breakdown of the membrane separating the lymphatics from the collecting tubules; and (3) intratubular deposits of amorphous necrotic calcific cellular debris or organized microcalculi (or both).

DIAGNOSTIC EVALUATION

Medical History

A personal as well as a family history should be obtained for all patients. A history of inflammatory bowel disease, recurrent urinary tract infection, prolonged periods of immobilization, gout, or familial occurrence of certain inherited renal diseases, eg, renal tubular acidosis or cystinuria, should be sought. Calcium oxalate stone disease is inherited in a multifactorial manner, and hypercalciuria has been shown to be inherited as an autosomal dominant trait. The presence of other endocrine or metabolic disorders should also be considered.

A complete list of all medications taken should be obtained. Acetazolamide, useful in the treatment of glaucoma, has been implicated as a cause of calcium stones. Absorbable silicates, usually found as part of an antacid preparation, may rarely be implicated in the formation of silicon calculi. Ascorbic acid in amounts greater than 2 g/d may increase urinary excretion of oxalate and contribute to formation of calcium oxalate stones. Any drug that decreases the urinary pH may contribute to the formation of uric acid stones. Orthophosphates prescribed to decrease calcium stone formation have been associated with an increase in the size of struvite stones. The diuretic hydrochlorothiazide may cause uricosuria and formation of uric acid stones, and allopurinol, a potent xanthine oxidase inhibitor useful in the treatment of gout, may also cause precipitation and formation of xanthine stones in certain individuals. In patients with a history of stone disease, all methods of previous treatment, including surgery, should be documented and details of stone composition sought.

Symptoms & Signs at Presentation

It is generally accepted that renal stones are initially formed in the proximal urinary tract and pass progressively into the calices, renal pelvis, and ureter. Their presentation may therefore vary from an incidental opaque shadow found on x-ray to fulminant pyelonephrosis if obstruction and infection have occurred.

A. Symptoms Related to Stones at Specific Sites:

1. Caliceal stones–Small, asymptomatic, nonobstructing caliceal stones are usually discovered as incidental findings on radiograms obtained for the evaluation of other organ systems. Patients with nonobstructing caliceal stones are often asymptomatic but may consult the physician after an episode of gross hematuria. If the stone becomes large enough to obstruct an infundibulum, flank pain, recurrent infection, or persistent hematuria may result.

2. Renal pelvic stones–A small stone in the renal pelvis may remain there asymptomatically, pass into the ureter, or become impacted at the ureteropelvic junction. If obstruction occurs at the level of the ureteropelvic junction, the pain may be intermittent, corresponding to the obstruction of urine flow, and may be localized to the flank or the costovertebral angle. When urinary infection accompanies obstruction, the patient may present with florid pyelonephritis or gram-negative septicemia.

3. Proximal ureteral stones–A calculus small enough to pass into the ureter can produce ureteral colic and hematuria. Beyond the ureteropelvic junction, the ureter assumes a diameter of about 10 mm (30F), and small calculi can easily pass to the level at which the ureter crosses over the iliac vessels. At this point, the diameter of the ureter narrows to about 4 mm (12F), and stones at this level commonly obstruct urine flow (Fig 16–1). The patient who presents with a stone in the upper ureter will frequently experience a sharp, spasmodic pain of acute onset, localized to the flank. As the stone passes down the ureter to the level of the pelvic brim, the pain remains sharp and intermittent, corresponding to peristalsis of the ureter. The pain frequently will radiate to the lateral flank and abdominal area and may be accompanied by nausea and vomiting. The pain is typically intermittent, with intense episodic intervals followed by periods of relief ("renal colic").

4. Distal ureteral stones–As the stone passes into the distal ureter, the pain remains intermittent and

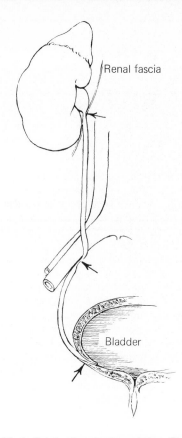

Figure 16–1. Points of ureteral narrowing. The ureter is narrow at 3 points: (1) at the ureteropelvic junction, (2) at the point where the ureter crosses over the iliac vessels, and (3) in the ureterovesical zone. A stone that passes the ureteropelvic junction has an excellent chance, therefore, of continuing the whole distance. If it becomes arrested, it is usually in the lower 5 cm of the ureter.

sharp, corresponding to the intermittence of ureteral peristalsis. In males, the pain frequently radiates along the inguinal canal into the groin and corresponding testicle. In females, the pain may radiate to the labia (Fig 16–2).

A third area of ureteral narrowing exists at the level of the ureterovesical junction. At this point, the ureter narrows to a diameter of 1–5 mm and it is here that most stones become lodged. Once a calculus reaches the distal ureter and approaches the bladder, symptoms of vesical irritation frequently are noted.

B. Associated Nonrenal Symptoms: Owing to the arrangement of the autonomic nervous system, which transmits visceral pain, and the similar neurologic innervation of the kidneys and stomach by the celiac ganglia (see pp 29–34), it is not unusual for ureteral colic to be accompanied by nausea and vomiting. Abdominal distention resulting from reflex ileus or intestinal stasis may also be present and confuse the diagnosis. It is therefore necessary to consider other pathologic entities that may mimic the presentation of a ureteral stone. Among these are gastroenteritis,

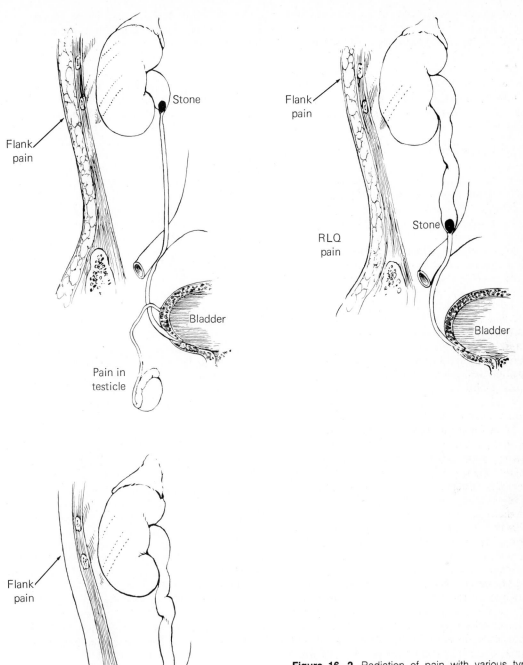

Figure 16-2. Radiation of pain with various types of ureteral stone. *Upper left:* Ureteropelvic stone. Severe costovertebral angle pain from capsular and pelvic distention; acute renal and ureteral pain from hyperperistalsis of smooth muscle of calices, pelvis, and ureter, with pain radiating along the course of the ureter (and into the testicle, since the nerve supply to the kidney and testis is the same). The testis is hypersensitive. *Upper right:* Midureteral stone. Same as above but with more pain in the lower abdominal quadrant. *Left:* Low ureteral stone. Same as above, with pain radiating into bladder, vulva, or scrotum. The scrotal wall is hyperesthetic. Testicular sensitivity is absent. When the stone approaches the bladder, urgency and frequency with burning on urination develop as a result of inflammation of the bladder wall around the ureteral orifice.

acute appendicitis, colitis, diverticulitis, salpingitis, and cholecystitis.

C. Variability of Symptoms: Less frequently, the passage of a stone may not be as dramatic as noted above. Such patients may describe a "dull" ache in the flank area that may have been present for several weeks without interfering with their daily routine. This pain is not as localized as acute colic and may be confused with other visceral pain.

Other less dramatic forms of presentation include persistent hematuria, either gross or microscopic, and persistent urinary tract infection. These patients will frequently have a struvite stone (see below).

Patients with asymptomatic stone disease may present initially for the evaluation of hypertension, azotemia, or symptoms referable to the gastrointestinal tract.

D. Findings on Physical Examination: A thorough physical examination is an essential part of the initial evaluation of the patient who may have a urinary calculus. Upon presentation to the emergency room, most patients will be experiencing severe colic and will be in obvious distress. In contradistinction to patients with acute peritonitis or abdominal pain, patients with ureteral colic will toss about and be unable to find comfort in any position. Diaphoresis, tachycardia, and tachypnea are frequent signs. Hypertension secondary to the discomfort may also be present. Fever is usually not present unless infection is associated with obstruction.

The abdomen should be examined carefully, with particular attention directed to palpation of the flank, where ureteral obstruction may produce an acutely hydronephrotic kidney. The kidney or the costovertebral angle is frequently tender to palpation. The abdomen should be carefully palpated to rule out surgical causes of abdominal pain. It is not unusual for the bowel sounds to be hypoactive and for an ileus to be present on radiographic examination. The bladder should also be palpated, since urinary retention can occur secondary to acute ureteral colic.

E. Laboratory Findings: Urinalysis and urine culture are required for all patients in whom stone disease is suspected. Microscopic or gross hematuria is frequently present in patients with acute ureteral colic. However, the absence of hematuria does not rule out renal stone disease. Pyuria may be present even without urinary tract infection, and bacteriuria is frequently seen in female patients with acute stone disease. Findings suggestive of infection may alter the therapeutic approach. The presence of crystals should also be noted, since they often occur in the acute phase of stone disease and may accurately reveal the type of stone present. The urinary pH should be noted, because patients with uric acid or cystine stones usually have acidic urine and those with struvite stones have alkaline urine.

F. Radiographic Findings: At least 90% of all renal stones are radiopaque and therefore readily visible on a plain film of the abdomen. Stones composed of calcium phosphate (apatite) are the most radiopaque

and have a density similar to that of bone. Calcium oxalate is slightly less dense, followed by magnesium ammonium phosphate (struvite) and cystine (Table 16–1). Stones composed solely of uric acid or matrix are considered to be radiolucent and would not appear on a plain film of the abdomen. Other calcifications that may appear on the plain film and be confused with a urinary calculus include calcified mesenteric lymph nodes, calcium in rib cartilage, gallstones, foreign bodies (pills), and pelvic phleboliths. Oblique films may show whether the calcification is in line with the normal anatomic position of the kidney or ureter.

1. Intravenous urography – Patients whose history and physical examination are compatible with urinary stone disease should undergo an intravenous urogram unless they are allergic to the contrast medium. In a patient with acute colic, the most common finding on intravenous urography is a delay in visualization of the collecting system on the affected side. In the absence of complete ureteral obstruction or a nonfunctional kidney, a dense nephrogram will appear, followed by visualization of the collecting system (Fig 16–3). Delayed films should be obtained until the complete collecting system is opacified down to the area of ureteral obstruction. Frequently, stones located in the intramural portion of the ureter may be obscured by dye collected in the bladder. An oblique film obtained after voiding will often show the calculus.

2. Tomography – In patients who present with acute ureteral colic, the plain film of the abdomen often shows a paralytic ileus that may obscure existing calculi. Plain-film tomograms may help to identify a stone otherwise obscured by overlying gas or feces.

It is not uncommon to see perirenal or periureteral extravasation of contrast medium in patients with obstructing ureteral calculi. The extravasation is believed to originate from a forniceal tear and is associated with the increased pressure caused by the obstructing stones. In the absence of infection, the condition is self-limiting and does not require further therapy. If infection is suspected, antibiotic therapy should be instituted.

3. Retrograde urography – Retrograde urograms are rarely needed to diagnose a stone; however, they are indicated when the diagnosis is suspect or the patient is allergic to contrast medium (Fig 16–4).

Table 16–1. Stone density as related to degree of radiopacity.

	Density	Degree of Radiopacity
Calcium phosphate	22.0	Very opaque
Calcium oxalate	10.8	Opaque
Magnesium ammonium phosphate	4.1	Moderately opaque
Cystine	3.7	Slightly opaque
Uric acid	1.4	Nonopaque
Xanthine	1.4	Nonopaque

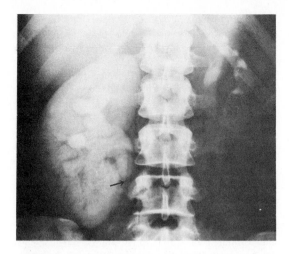

Figure 16–3. Ureteral stone. "Nephrogram" caused by acute ureteral obstruction. Marked density of renal parenchyma with moderate hydronephrosis. Arrow points to nonopaque (uric acid) stone.

4. Ultrasonography–In patients in whom it is not possible to obtain an intravenous urogram, ultrasonic evaluation of the kidneys may aid in the diagnosis of renal stones. In pregnant women with flank pain in whom it is desirable to limit radiation exposure or in anuric patients or patients with chronic renal failure, the presence of hydronephrosis and acoustic shadowing may be diagnostic.

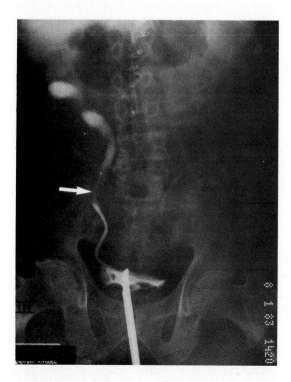

Figure 16–4. Retrograde urogram obtained in patient with kidney that did not visualize on intravenous urogram. Arrow points to a poorly calcified stone in the mid ureter.

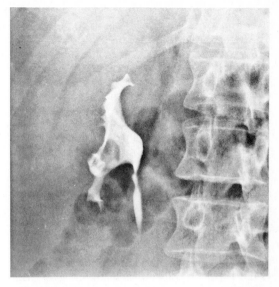

Figure 16–5. Excretory urogram showing uric acid stone as "negative" shadow because radiopaque medium is more dense than the stone.

5. CT scanning–CT scanning is seldom indicated as the first diagnostic study for the evaluation of a patient with a suspected urinary calculus. However, in cases where the presence of a nonopaque stone or a urinary tract tumor is being considered, CT scans have proved diagnostic.

Although a radiolucent stone cannot be detected on the plain film alone, the diagnosis should be suspected when hydronephrosis and a radiolucent filling defect are found on sonograms or urograms (Fig 16–5). A CT scan may help to differentiate a stone from a blood clot or tumor.

CALCIUM STONES

Calcium-containing stones can occur as calcium phosphate or calcium oxalate or, more commonly, as a mixture of the 2. Calcium oxalate is the sole or major component of about 80% of all stones and may be present as the monohydrate, the dihydrate, or both. Calcium phosphate can be present as either the more common apatite ($Ca_{10}[PO_4]_6[OH]_2$) or relatively unusual brushite ($CaHPO_4 \cdot 2H_2O$). Under the normal ionic conditions of urine, calcium oxalate and calcium phosphate both are highly insoluble salts, which probably accounts for their being the most frequent components of calcium stones.

Epidemiology

Calcium-containing stones are the most common stones found in North America. Epidemiologic studies have shown that the incidence of stone disease is highest at 30–50 years of age, with the initial manifestation of clinical stone disease occurring in the third decade in most patients. When all forms of renal stones are considered, the incidence in men and women is approximately equal, but calcium-containing stones occur in men 3 times more often than in women. Blacks in the USA experience less stone disease than whites.

Geographically, the highest incidence of stone disease in the USA occurs in the mountainous northwest, the tropical southeast, and the arid southwest. A study in the southeastern USA showed that the highest incidence of stone disease occurs during the months of July, August, and September, when presumably dehydration due to perspiration is common and the urine contains high concentrations of lithogenic substances.

Other epidemiologic observations have been made: Individuals with a sedentary life-style are known to be more susceptible to calcium stone disease, as are those with professional or managerial occupations; calcium stones occur much less frequently in unskilled or manual workers.

The type of food and the amount of water consumed are important considerations in the evaluation of stone-forming patients. The incidence of stone disease is increased in patients with persistently low urinary volumes. Diets rich in calcium-, phosphate-, and oxalate-containing foods may lead to increased renal excretion of those substances and an increased incidence of stone formation in susceptible individuals.

It has been estimated that after the initial stone has formed, a patient has approximately a 60% chance of forming a second stone within the next 7 years. With selective medical treatment based on the type of stone and the metabolic abnormality, it is possible to decrease the recurrence rate.

Diagnostic Evaluation

A. Screening Studies: All patients who form a single calcium stone should undergo screening laboratory studies, including a complete blood count, urinalysis and urine culture (see Chapter 5), a serum chemistry survey, an intravenous urogram, and measurement of calcium, phosphorus, uric acid, and creatinine levels in a 24-hour urine specimen. In major centers treating urinary stones, urinary oxalate levels are also obtained. However, because of difficulties in measuring oxalate, routine clinical measurement is not recommended. Urinary citrate is a known inhibitor of calcium crystallization. A subset of chronic stone-forming patients has been identified, with low urinary citrate (< 300 mg/d) being their only metabolic abnormality. In many centers, urinary citrate levels are routinely obtained. A more thorough metabolic evaluation is performed only if abnormalities are detected.

B. Complete Metabolic Evaluation: Only patients with evidence of metabolically active stone dis-

ease, ie, radiologic evidence of new stone formation or stone growth or documented passage of gravel within 1 year, require full metabolic evaluation. A complete metabolic evaluation can be performed on either an outpatient or a hospitalized patient. The diagnosis of hypercalciuria can be made correctly in either case, but there is some difficulty in differentiating between absorptive hypercalciuria and renal hypercalciuria when the outpatient protocol is used. The outpatient protocol appears to detect hyperuricosuria better than does the inpatient protocol, and the former is also less costly.

1. Outpatient protocol (Pak et al, 1980)–

a. Urine examination–The patient is initially instructed to collect two 24-hour urine specimens while maintaining a regular diet at home. Analysis of these initial specimens is important for 2 reasons: (1) to provide baseline data against which results of further tests can be compared, and (2) to detect hypercalciuria or hyperuricosuria—or both—which may be evident only while the patient is on a regular diet. Urinary oxalate and citrate levels are also determined from these specimens.

The patient is then placed on a calcium- and sodium-restricted diet (400 mg of calcium and 100 meq of sodium daily) for 1 week, after which an additional 24-hour urine specimen is collected for determination of calcium, phosphorus, uric acid, and creatinine levels. The sodium nitroprusside test, a qualitative test for cystine, is performed on two 24-hour urine specimens, and a quantitative amino acid analysis is performed on all positive specimens. The pH of all voided urine is measured using Nitrazine paper.

b. Blood examination–Serum calcium, phosphorus, uric acid, and creatinine levels are determined in blood samples obtained while the patient is on the regular diet and on the restricted diet. Because the serum calcium level may be elevated postprandially or owing to prolonged occlusion of blood vessels by a tourniquet, it is best to obtain blood samples in the morning following an overnight fast and, if possible, without using a tourniquet. If the serum calcium level is high, a blood sample should be sent to the laboratory for determination of the immunoreactive parathyroid hormone level. The serum parathyroid hormone level should also be determined if hyperparathyroidism is suspected.

c. Fasting and calcium loading tests–These tests are always a routine part of the metabolic evaluation. The patient is instructed to fast from 9:00 PM to 7:00 AM, drinking only distilled water during this period, and to report to the physician's office at 7:00 AM. At the physician's office, the patient voids and the urine is discarded. A fasting 2-hour urine specimen is then collected from 7:00 AM to 9:00 AM. At 9:00 AM, the patient is given calcium gluconate, 1 g orally. Urine representing the calcium loading sample is then collected from 9:00 AM to 1:00 PM. The volume of each sample (fasting and calcium loading) is recorded, and the calcium and creatinine levels in each are determined. A normal fasting specimen will have a calcium to creatinine ratio less than 0.11; a higher ratio is indicative of renal hypercalciuria. Absorptive hypercalciuria is considered to be present if the calcium to creatinine ratio in the calcium loading sample is greater than 0.2. The pH of all fasting specimens is also determined; if it is above 5.3, the presence of renal tubular acidosis must be ruled out by performing an ammonium chloride acid loading test. Using this simple outpatient protocol, Pak and coworkers (1978) have been able to differentiate between resorptive, renal, and absorptive hypercalciuria and also to detect hyperuricosuria and enteric hyperoxaluria. This method is useful in differentiating 90% of cases of recurrent stone disease.

2. Other protocols–Other protocols, both outpatient and inpatient, have been used for metabolic evaluation of patients with calcium stone disease (Pitts and Resnick, 1980; Boyce and Resnick, 1979; Pak et al, 1975). It is important that the chosen protocol be used uniformly in order to allow comparison of patients and systematic following of patients and monitoring of their responses to specific forms of therapy.

C. Criteria for Hypercalciuria: Although the etiology of calcium stone disease is diverse, most patients with calcium stones demonstrate hypercalciuria of the absorptive, renal, or resorptive type (see below). What constitutes hypercalciuria varies according to the amount of calcium in the diet. For practical clinical purposes a urinary excretion of calcium in amounts greater than 300 mg/d is considered abnormal for patients on unrestricted diets. Breslau and Pak (1981) define hypercalciuria as urinary excretion of calcium in amounts greater than 4 mg/kg/d in a patient on an unrestricted diet.

Treatment

Medical methods for prevention and management of specific types of stone disease are discussed in the following sections. For manipulative and surgical treatment of stones, see pp 288 and 291–297.

HYPERCALCIURIA

The average dietary intake of calcium is 500–1000 mg/d. Calcium is absorbed from the gastrointestinal tract mostly in the duodenum and upper jejunum. Active absorption by a vitamin D-dependent calcium-binding protein is responsible for most calcium uptake, although some occurs by passive diffusion. Vitamin D acting independently from the effect of parathyroid hormone appears to be essential for calcium absorption.

Absorptive Hypercalciuria

A. General Considerations: Absorptive hypercalciuria, the most common metabolic abnormality detected in patients with calcium oxalate stones, is present in 50–60% of such patients. These patients are believed to have an altered intestinal response to vita-

min D that causes increased absorption of calcium, elevated serum calcium levels, and depression of parathyroid function, with the result that increased amounts of calcium are delivered to the kidney and excreted in the urine.

Urinary excretion of calcium level is frequently elevated in these patients when the diet is unrestricted but may fall to 225 mg/d when dietary calcium is restricted to 150 mg/d. With fasting, the urinary calcium level returns to normal; after calcium loading, the urinary calcium level again becomes abnormally high, often rebounding to 2–3 times the resting level. A rebound in the urinary calcium level may also occur in normocalcemic patients who are given a calcium load after being maintained on a calcium-restricted diet; such patients are likely to have absorptive hypercalciuria and may demonstrate excessive calcium excretion when on their normal diet.

B. Medical Treatment:

1. Diet–Patients with absorptive hypercalciuria should be placed on a calcium-restricted diet. Because it is known that a low-sodium diet also helps to reduce intestinal absorption of calcium, sodium should be restricted to 100 meq/d and calcium to 400 mg/d. An attempt should also be made to limit the intake of refined carbohydrates and animal proteins, both of which are known to cause hypercalciuria. In addition, patients should be encouraged to eat foods rich in natural fiber content and bran, which provide phytic acid (inositol hexaphosphate) to bind dietary calcium in an insoluble and unabsorbable complex.

2. Hydration–Patients with calcium stone disease should be encouraged to drink enough fluid to maintain a urine output of 3–4 L/d. It is helpful to measure the urine volume before treatment and repeat this measurement periodically to ensure that the urine volume is adequate. Follow-up urinalyses should include measurement of the urine specific gravity to ascertain that significant hydration is occurring. Patients should be encouraged to increase fluid intake when they are at the greatest risk of having the urine supersaturated with calcium, ie, 2–4 hours after meals, during periods of heavy physical activity and dehydration, and at night. Water is probably the best fluid if stones are to be avoided. Colas, fruit juices, and tea are high in oxalate and should be avoided or taken in moderation.

3. Cellulose phosphate–Sodium cellulose phosphate, a nonabsorbable ion exchange resin, has recently been approved for use in the USA. When used in conjunction with a calcium-restricted diet, it effectively reduces the incidence of stone recurrence in patients with absorptive hypercalciuria. As an ion exchange resin, it acts in the gastrointestinal tract by exchanging sodium for calcium and thus inhibiting calcium absorption. In addition to effectively lowering the urine concentration of calcium, cellulose phosphate is known to cause an increase in the urinary phosphate level, a decrease in the serum magnesium level, and an increase in urinary excretion of oxalate. In order for cellulose phosphate to be effective, it must be taken with meals; the usual dose is 5 g 2–3 times per day. Oral magnesium supplementation should be given and dietary oxalate restricted. Although expensive, the drug may prove valuable in treating patients with recurrent calcium stones who have hypercalciuria due to abnormal absorption of calcium and continue to form stones in spite of dietary restrictions and maintenance of dilute urine.

4. Orthophosphates–Orthophosphates have been shown to decrease the incidence of recurrent stone formation in patients with hypercalciuria. Orthophosphates act by decreasing urinary excretion of calcium and increasing urinary excretion of pyrophosphate and citrate, 2 potent inhibitors of calcium stone formation in urine. Orthophosphates are available in a number of different preparations as potassium acid phosphate, a neutral mixture consisting of potassium and sodium phosphates; as potassium phosphate alone; or as an alkaline mixture of disodium and dipotassium phosphates. Acid phosphates should be avoided, and one study has shown that they may predispose to rather than protect from recurrent stone disease. Patients with absorptive hypercalciuria should first be placed on an adequate diet (see above). The diet may then be supplemented with an orthophosphate preparation in amounts sufficient to increase urinary excretion of phosphate to 1200–1400 mg/d or to produce a urinary calcium to phosphorus ratio in the range of 0.1–0.125. A dosage of 3–6 g/d is usually required. Diarrhea is the most frequently noted side effect. Often mild diarrhea is noted with the onset of phosphate therapy and subsequently subsides. Persistent diarrhea may sometimes be reduced if the medication is taken after rather than before meals. Phosphates should not be used in patients with urinary tract infection, because the added phosphate load may lead to increased stone formation. Antacids containing phosphate-binding aluminum gels should be avoided while phosphates are being taken.

Renal Hypercalciuria

A. General Considerations: Renal hypercalciuria, due to inability of the kidney to conserve calcium, occurs in about 10% of all stone-forming patients. The cause of the "renal leak" of calcium is unknown, but evidence indicates that an abnormality in tubular function may be responsible. The loss of calcium via the urine results in a low serum calcium level, which causes stimulation of parathyroid hormone secretion, increased synthesis of vitamin D_3, and increased absorption of calcium from the gastrointestinal tract and resorption from bone.

The urinary calcium level does not decrease in these patients following fasting, and it may increase in response to calcium loading.

B. Medical Treatment:

1. Thiazides–Thiazides effectively decrease renal excretion of calcium and are the drugs of choice in this condition. The hypocalciuric effect usually begins 2–3 days after starting the medication, becomes maximal within 6 days, and is nearly always sustained. It is believed that thiazides function by increasing calcium reabsorption in the distal tubule and by causing extracellular volume depletion, which further stimulates reabsorption of calcium in the proximal tubule. Thiazides are also known to reduce urinary excretion of oxalate and to increase the urinary concentration of zinc and magnesium; this may enhance their effectiveness.

Hydrochlorothiazide in doses of 50 mg twice a day is the agent most frequently used. Side effects, reported to occur in about 30% of patients, may frequently be related to hypokalemia and include weakness, fatigue, loss of energy, and lassitude. Gout, diabetes mellitus, loss of libido, and a decrease in the serum magnesium level may also occur.

Some investigators now believe that it is not necessary to differentiate between absorptive and renal hypercalciuria. Instead, hydrochlorothiazide is used to treat both groups of patients.

2. Orthophosphates–In difficult situations involving secondary hyperparathyroidism, orthophosphates (see above) may be used in conjunction with thiazides and a calcium-restricted diet, without adverse side effects.

Resorptive Hypercalciuria

A. General Considerations: Resorptive hypercalciuria, which is relatively uncommon, is found primarily in patients with hyperparathyroidism. These patients may be identified easily by finding hypercalcemia on routine blood chemistry studies. Hyperparathyroidism accounts for 4–6% of all patients with calculi and is seen more often in females than in males. Excessive secretion of parathyroid hormone stimulates bone destruction and increases intenstinal absorption of calcium, both of which contribute to hypercalciuria.

Other causes of resorptive hypercalciuria include Cushing's disease, hyperthyroidism, and disorders such as multiple myeloma, metastatic cancer, and prolonged periods of immobilization.

B. Treatment: Treatment of resorptive hypercalciuria due to hyperparathyroidism requires surgical removal of the abnormal parathyroid tissue. Urinary and serum calcium levels should return to normal after parathyroidectomy.

Treatment of resorptive hypercalciuria due to other causes consists of treatment of the underlying problem.

NORMOCALCIURIA

Normocalciuric patients who continue to form stones should be encouraged to maintain their optimal weight, drink 10 glasses of water a day, and maintain a moderate intake of calcium. If the urinary phosphorus level is low, treatment with neutral phosphates is often beneficial. Urinary excretion of phosphorus in amounts above 800 mg/d is desirable. Treatment with thiazide diuretics has also resulted in a decrease in the incidence of stone formation in these patients.

OTHER METABOLIC DISORDERS ASSOCIATED WITH CALCIUM STONES

Other metabolic disorders can contribute to the formation of calcium stones. Proper diagnosis is essential, because each patient may require a different combination of therapy to achieve satisfactory control.

Sarcoidosis

A. General Considerations: Patients with sarcoidosis usually form mixed calcium stones composed of calcium oxalate and calcium phosphate. These patients frequently have hypercalciuria owing to increased sensitivity of the intestinal epithelium to vitamin D_3. Increased serum levels of vitamin D_3 have been reported in these patients.

B. Medical Treatment: Corticosteroids usually correct the hypercalciuria; however, patients who form stones usually continue to do so.

Renal Tubular Acidosis

A. General Considerations: Renal tubular acidosis is a clinical syndrome characterized by persistent metabolic acidosis. Three types of renal tubular acidosis have been described, 2 of which are not associated with stone formation.

Type I, distal renal tubular acidosis, may occur as an autosomal dominant trait or may arise spontaneously. About 70% of patients are female, and about 70% of patients form calcium stones. The complete form of distal renal tubular acidosis is associated with diminished serum levels of bicarbonate and potassium and a decreased urinary citrate level. Patients with distal renal tubular acidosis also have an elevated serum alkaline phosphatase level and mild to moderate hypercalciuria, are acidotic, and have a low arterial pH, with resultant bone demineralization. These patients are unable to acidify their urine below a pH of 6.0. Stone formation is related to the hypercalciuria and low urinary citrate level, and the stones frequently are composed of pure calcium phosphate. Patients with this type of renal tubular acidosis are prone to the development of nephrocalcinosis. Incomplete distal renal tubular acidosis is not associated with systemic acidosis but is associated with stone formation. These patients are able to acidify their urine to a pH of 5.4 but not below.

Type II, proximal renal tubular acidosis, results from impaired reabsorption of bicarbonate from the proximal renal tubule. These patients do not form renal calculi and do not develop nephrocalcinosis.

The third type of renal tubular acidosis, designated **type IV,** may be the most common form. The renal defect is believed to be in the renal collecting tubules and ducts and is characterized by reduced secretion of both hydrogen and potassium ions. Patients with this disorder do not develop nephrolithiasis or nephrocalcinosis.

B. Medical Treatment: Treatment of type I renal tubular acidosis includes increasing the fluid intake and giving either sodium bicarbonate or sodium potassium citrate to alkalinize the urine. The therapeutic effect can be monitored by measuring urinary excretion of citrate and the plasma bicarbonate level.

HYPEROXALURIA

Because calcium oxalate stones are the most common type of renal calculi identified in the USA, accounting for 70–80% of all renal stones, a brief review of oxalate metabolism is warranted.

Oxalic acid is a nonessential end product of metabolism. Its major significance in humans is due to the extreme insolubility of the calcium salt of oxalate. At a neutral pH, only 0.67 mg of the calcium salt will dissolve per 100 mL of water; the solubility is minimally affected by changes in the pH of urine. It is therefore not surprising that urine is often supersaturated with calcium oxalate and stone formation occurs.

Oxalic acid is found in a variety of foods and beverages, including a number of green leafy vegetables, citrus fruits, rhubarb, Concord grapes, cranberries, plums, tea, cocoa, almonds, cashews, carbonated beverages, and decaffeinated and instant coffee. In a typical Western diet, the daily intake of oxalate ranges from 70 to 920 mg/d. When the diet is predominantly vegetarian, the daily intake of oxalate can range from 80 to 2000 mg/d.

Oxalate is poorly absorbed from the gastrointestinal tract. Approximately half of ingested oxalate is destroyed by enteric bacteria, and about 25% is excreted unchanged in the feces. Studies have shown that although absorption can occur anywhere along the gastrointestinal tract, including the colon, only 2.3–12% of ingested oxalate is absorbed (Archer et al, 1957; Earnest et al, 1974).

Daily oxalate excretion in urine is normally 10–50 mg. All of the absorbed and the endogenously produced oxalate is filtered by the kidney and secreted unchanged in the urine. Since the amount of exogenous oxalate absorbed from the gastrointestinal tract is quite small, most oxalate that appears in the urine is derived from endogenous sources. Endogenous oxalate is produced from 2 major sources: ascorbic acid and glyoxalic acid. Approximately 40% of the excreted oxalate comes from the metabolism of ascorbic acid, and about 40–50% comes from metabolic reactions involving glyoxalic acid. The conversion of ascorbic acid to oxalate is poorly understood, but that of glyoxalic acid is well defined (Fig 16–6).

Primary Hyperoxaluria

A. General Considerations: Primary hyperoxaluria is a rare autosomal recessive disorder that can cause recurrent calcium oxalate stones in children (Fig 16–7) and result in nephrocalcinosis and eventually death from renal failure, usually before age 40. In type I hyperoxaluria, a deficiency of the enzyme glyoxalate carboligase leads to increased conversion of glyoxalic

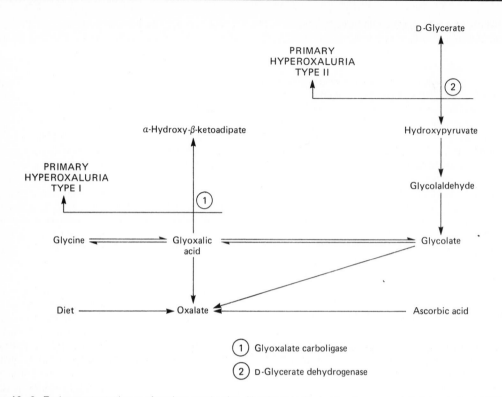

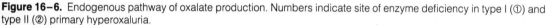

Figure 16–6. Endogenous pathway of oxalate production. Numbers indicate site of enzyme deficiency in type I (①) and type II (②) primary hyperoxaluria.

acid to glycolate and oxalate. In type II, there is a deficiency of the enzyme D-glycerate dehydrogenase. Diagnosis is based on the persistent finding of increased urinary excretion of oxalate, usually greater than 100 mg/d.

Patients with the genetic form of hyperoxaluria usually progress to chronic renal failure. Unfortunately, if renal transplantation is performed, calcium oxalate usually reaccumulates rapidly in the new kidney, with eventual loss of the transplant. Chronic hemodialysis has not proved to be of significant value. Although uremia can be readily controlled by dialysis, the deposition of oxalate in soft tissues and blood vessels persists, with the development of infarcts in subcutaneous tissues.

B. Medical Treatment: Studies have shown that in some patients with primary hyperoxaluria, the urinary oxalate level can be reduced when large doses of pyridoxine (100–400 mg/d) are ingested in divided doses. Maintenance of large urine volumes should be encouraged, and restriction of foods rich in oxalate may be helpful. The use of magnesium and phosphate, urinary inhibitors of stone formation, has also been reported to be of some therapeutic benefit.

Ingestion & Inhalation Hyperoxaluria

Hyperoxaluria may occur secondary to ingestion or inhalation of substances that, when metabolized, yield oxalate.

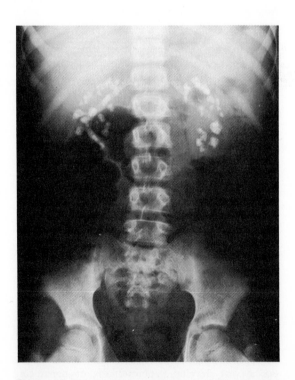

Figure 16–7. Intravenous urogram in child who had passed multiple stones. Metabolic evaluation revealed primary hyperoxaluria.

A. Ethylene Glycol: The acute ingestion of ethylene glycol, a common ingredient of antifreeze solutions, can result in massive hyperoxaluria and intrarenal obstructive uropathy, presumably owing to its rapid conversion to glyoxalate and oxalate.

Treatment is by hemodialysis

B. Ascorbic Acid: Chronic ingestion of ascorbic acid in doses greater than 5 g/d may cause hyperoxaluria and lead to stone formation.

C. Methoxyflurane: Methoxyflurane, a fluorinated 2-carbon inhalational anesthetic agent, can be converted to oxalate in the liver. This can cause intrarenal deposition of oxalate and the development of acute renal failure. Renal failure is discussed in Chapter 25.

Enteric Hyperoxaluria

A. General Considerations: Hyperoxaluria may occur secondary to inflammatory diseases of the gastrointestinal tract or to small-bowel bypass surgery for the treatment of morbid obesity. Hyperabsorption of dietary oxalate has been consistently demonstrated in these 2 groups of patients.

Hyperoxaluria may also occur secondary to intestinal malabsorption syndromes. Patients with intestinal malabsorption syndromes characteristically have low urinary calcium levels. In the normal intestinal tract, most of the oxalate binds to calcium and exists as the insoluble and nonabsorbable calcium salt. However, in patients with malabsorption syndromes, excessive amounts of unabsorbed fatty acids are present in the intestine; they bind intraluminal calcium and are excreted as calcium salts. Therefore, such patients have less calcium available to bind enteric oxalate; thus, oxalate absorption is increased. In addition, the increase in bile salts and fatty acids that frequently occurs in these syndromes may alter the mucosal permeability of the colon and lead to increased absorption of oxalate in the colon.

B. Medical Treatment: The treatment of enteric hyperoxaluria is based on decreasing the amount of oxalate available for absorption by the gastrointestinal tract. Measures may include institution of a low-oxalate diet, an increase in the fluid intake to maintain a urine output of 3–4 L/d, and maintenance of a low-fat diet, with the use of medium-chain triglycerides to decrease steatorrhea and calcium binding. Calcium supplements may be given to increase the amount of calcium available to bind oxalate and form a nonabsorbable salt so that the urinary oxalate level will decrease. However, the benefit achieved by reducing the urinary oxalate level may be offset by the increase in calcium excretion. Aluminum-containing antacids bind oxalate and provide the same benefit as calcium supplements but avoid the potential risk of hypercalciuria. Cholestyramine binds oxalate and may be helpful in reversing hyperoxaluria in patients with inflammatory bowel disease. When all else fails, patients who have had an ileal bypass procedure may require reversal of the bypass.

HYPERURICOSURIA

Uric acid stones are discussed on p 289.

General Considerations

Hyperuricosuria has been reported in approximately 20% of patients who form calcium oxalate stones. Two possible mechanisms have been proposed to explain the association between increased urinary excretion of uric acid and stone formation: (1) Heterogeneous nucleation may occur when uric acid crystals act as a nucleus or seed core for the precipitation of calcium oxalate crystals (Coe, 1978). (2) Uric acid may counteract the inhibitory effects of acid mucopolysaccharides, which are normally present in urine and interfere with the formation of calcium oxalate crystals (Robertson, Knowles, and Peacock, 1976).

Medical Treatment

Allopurinol, a xanthine oxidase inhibitor, should be given to reduce urinary uric acid levels. Patients should maintain a high level of fluid intake. Urinary levels of uric acid are often increased after consumption of excessive amounts of food containing purines; therefore, treatment should include limiting purine-containing foods in the diet. Hypercalciuria that exists in addition to hyperuricosuria should also be treated.

MILD HYPERCYSTINURIA (Heterozygous Cystinuria)

General Considerations

An unexpectedly high incidence of heterozygous cystinuria has been found in patients who form calcium oxalate stones. The incidence of this associated metabolic abnormality is greater in females (17.1%) than in males (11.8%). It has been proposed, though not proved, that cystine has a role analogous to that of uric acid in inducing the formation of calcium oxalate stones.

Medical Treatment

Alkalinizing agents and a high level of fluid intake may effectively decrease stone formation in patients with this metabolic abnormality.

HYPOCITRATURIA

General Considerations

Hypocitraturia has been implicated as a possible contributing factor in 19–63% of all patients with nephrolithiasis (Pak et al, 1985). Citrate is known to inhibit the crystallization of calcium oxalate and calcium phosphate presumably by complexing urinary calcium and thereby reducing the saturation of calcium oxalate and phosphate. It may also act by inhibiting crystal nucleation.

Medical Treatment

Potassium citrate (20 meq 3 times daily) administered as a slow-release preparation (Urocit-K) has been shown to significantly increase urinary citrate levels and to decrease the risk of new stone formation without untoward side effects (Pak et al, 1985). When hypercalciuria or hyperuricosuria is also present, hydrochlorothiazide, allopurinol, or both may also be given.

CYSTINE STONES
(Severe Hypercystinuria, Homozygous Cystinuria)

Cystinuria is a relatively rare autosomal recessive inborn error of metabolism characterized by impaired reabsorption of dibasic amino acids (cystine, lysine, ornithine, and arginine) from the renal tubule and gastrointestinal tract. About one in 20,000 individuals in the general population is affected, and about 1–4% of urinary stones are cystine calculi.

If it were not for the low solubility of cystine in urine, cystinuria would be of no clinical significance. It has been estimated that when the urinary pH is 4.5–7.0, the solubility of cystine is about 300–400 mg/L; it is higher in more alkaline urine. Individuals with homozygous cystinuria excrete 500–1000 mg of cystine in the urine daily, those with heterozygous cystinuria usually excrete 100–300 mg/d, and normal individuals typically excrete less than 100 mg/d. Therefore, only those with homozygous cystinuria excrete sufficient amounts of cystine to form stones.

Diagnostic Evaluation

Cystine stones may become clinically manifest at any age; however, the first episode usually occurs soon after puberty. It is not unusual for patients with cystine stone disease to undergo multiple surgical procedures for removal of symptomatic renal calculi before the correct diagnosis is made. In one series, the average interval between the initial stone episode and establishment of the correct diagnosis was about 6 years (Evans, Resnick, and Boyce, 1982).

A. Medical History: The diagnosis of cystinuria should be considered in individuals with an early onset of clinical stone disease, a family history of recurrent stone disease, and recurrent stone formation unresponsive to the usual forms of therapy.

B. Symptoms and Signs: See p 276.

C. Laboratory Findings: The urine is often acidic and contains classic hexagonal cystine crystals. The nitroprusside test may be used as a rapid screening procedure to detect cystine in urine (Grant and Kachmar, 1976). If the nitroprusside test is positive, a 24-hour urine specimen should be analyzed for total cystine content. Analysis of a stone, if one is available, will also provide the correct diagnosis.

D. X-Ray Findings: The diagnosis of cystine stones should be considered in patients with renal colic and radiographic evidence of a slightly dense, laminated, obstructing calculus of ground-glass appearance (Fig 16–8).

Medical Treatment

The medical management of patients with clinical cystine stone disease is based on 3 principles: decreasing the total cystine concentration in urine, increasing the solubility of cystine in urine, and decreasing urinary excretion of cystine.

A. Hydration: Fluid diuresis is the cornerstone of management. Patients with mild to moderate cystinuria (excretion of less than 1000 mg of cystine daily) have been successfully managed by maintaining a urine output of approximately 2 mL/min. A regimen of 2 glasses of water every 2 hours while awake plus 2 glasses before bedtime and 2 glasses during the night is usually sufficient to maintain a urine output of 3–4 L/d. Unfortunately, compliance with this regimen is sometimes difficult, and stone formation recurs in patients who do not maintain an adequate urine volume.

B. Alkalinization of Urine: The solubility of cystine in urine can be doubled to more than 800 mg/L simply by increasing the pH of the urine to 7.5. Sodium bicarbonate in a daily dose of 15–20 g; sodium-potassium citrate solution, 10–15 mL 4 times daily; or potassium citrate, 60–80 meq/d, may be used to accomplish this. However, it is often difficult to sustain a urinary pH of 7.5–8.0 throughout the day.

Direct irrigation of the stone with an alkaline solution via retrograde or percutaneous catheters has also been helpful in dissolution of stones.

C. Cystine-Binding Drugs:

1. Penicillamine– D-Penicillamine, a derivative

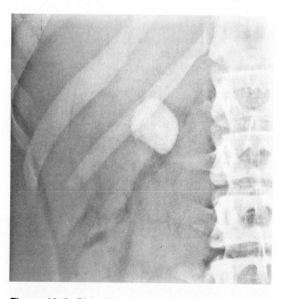

Figure 16–8. Plain film showing homogeneous, mildly opaque cystine stone.

of penicillin, may be used to decrease urinary excretion of cystine. Penicillamine acts by binding with cystine to form a cystine–S–penicillamine complex 50 times more soluble than cystine. Daily doses of 1–2 g of penicillamine have proved successful in dissolving existing stones. Side effects associated with the use of D-penicillamine include rash, fever, agranulocytosis, iron depletion, proteinuria, and, on occasion, the nephrotic syndrome. The occurrence of side effects may be minimized by beginning with a low dose of penicillamine (150 mg 3 times a day) and by stopping treatment when side effects first appear. The more toxic L- or DL- forms of the drug should not be used.

2. α-Mercaptopropionylglycine– This newer agent has an action similar to penicillamine but produces fewer side effects. It may be added to the therapeutic regimen in patients with severe recurrent or nondissolving stones. Further clinical experience with this drug is needed.

D. Methionine Restriction: Methionine is the dietary precursor of cystine; therefore, restriction of methionine-containing foods is in theory a sound way to decrease the cystine level in urine. Although methionine restriction results in a bland, unpalatable, poorly tolerated diet, it may be useful for the patient who is difficult to treat otherwise.

STONES ASSOCIATED WITH INFECTION
(Struvite Stones)

Stones associated with chronic urinary tract infection occur about twice as often in women as in men and account for approximately 15–20% of all urinary calculi. They are referred to as struvite or triple phosphate stones.

Struvite is a geologic term for a crystalline substance composed of magnesium ammonium phosphate ($MgNH_4PO_4 \cdot 6H_2O$). The term "triple phosphate" is used interchangeably with struvite. Modern crystallographic analysis has shown that these stones are actually a mixture of magnesium ammonium phosphate and carbonate apatite ($Ca_{19}[PO_4]_6 \cdot CO_3$).

The association of urinary tract infection and struvite stone formation has long been recognized; however, it is not known whether the infection or the stone is the initiating factor. If analysis of a stone proves it to be struvite, this is evidence of a current or past urinary tract infection with urea-splitting bacteria. In order for struvite stones to form, the urine must be supersaturated with magnesium, ammonium, phosphate, and carbonate apatite. Uninfected urine remains unsaturated, and struvite crystals will not form. If a urinary tract infection is present but the urinary pH remains at 5.85, the normal physiologic mean, struvite stones will not form. However, struvite stones tend to form in urinary tract infections with urea-splitting bacteria, because these organisms both alkalinize the urine to a pH above 7.0 and produce increased concentrations of bicarbonate and ammonium ions; thus, the urine becomes supersaturated with the components of struvite, and struvite stones form.

Common urea-splitting bacteria include *Proteus, Pseudomonas, Klebsiella,* and *Staphylococcus. Escherichia coli* does not produce urease and, when associated with this type of stone, most likely represents a superinfection. The incidence of struvite stones is increased in patients who have undergone urinary diversion and those with infections associated with chronic catheter drainage. Patients with spinal cord injuries or neurogenic vesical dysfunction are also more prone to develop struvite stones. When the stone forms in the kidney, it frequently assumes a staghorn configuration and may fill the entire collecting system (Fig 16–9). Only 60–90% of staghorn stones result solely from urinary tract infection with urea-splitting organisms, and it is not uncommon to find staghorn stones of mixed composition resulting from metabolic stone disease associated with a secondary infection with urea-splitting bacteria. The secondary infection may result in the deposition of magnesium ammonium phosphate over a core of cystine or calcium oxalate.

Diagnostic Evaluation
A. History, Symptoms and Signs, and Physical Examination: See p 275.

B. Laboratory Studies: Urinalysis, urine cultures, and antimicrobial drug sensitivity studies should be performed to document the presence of infection, identify the causative organism, and determine which antimicrobial drugs will be effective in treatment.

C. Radiographic Studies: A plain film of the abdomen should be taken to determine the number, size, and location of stones. Struvite stones involving the upper collecting system are often poorly mineralized owing to a large protein matrix; because such

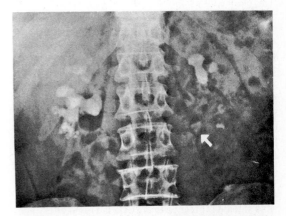

Figure 16–9. Plain film showing bilateral staghorn calculi and left upper ureteral stone. Arrow points to ureteral stone.

stones are relatively nonopaque, they may be difficult to visualize on routine x-ray studies. Nephrotomograms obtained before injection of contrast medium may be invaluable in locating small fragments and inapparent caliceal extensions of stones. An excretory urogram including oblique films is essential to evaluate the uninvolved kidney and determine whether there are surgically correctable anatomic abnormalities in the involved kidney that may be responsible for the persistence of infections. Retrograde urograms are sometimes helpful in delineating caliceal and infundibular abnormalities not evident on routine contrast studies. Cystograms are useful in evaluating the lower urinary tract and determining whether reflux is present. Voiding cystourethrograms and urodynamic studies should be performed.

Radionuclide renal scans should be performed to evaluate the function of a chronically obstructed kidney.

D. Instrumental Examination: Cystoscopy may be performed to evaluate the integrity of the lower urinary tract and determine whether reflux is present.

Treatment

The indications for stone removal include recurrent urinary tract infection, progressive renal damage, urinary obstruction, and persistent pain. Surgical removal of struvite stones is the procedure of choice, but stone dissolution and lithotripsy (see below and Chapter 7) are useful alternatives. Medical therapy has only an adjunctive role in the management of these patients and is directed primarily at controlling the urinary tract infection before, during, and after surgical removal of the stones.

Staghorn struvite calculi must be removed, or the patients can be expected to experience significant morbidity as a result of persistent urinary tract infection and the development of perinephric abscess and sepsis. Patient survival is also reduced if staghorn calculi are left in place; the 10-year survival rate ranges from 50 to 72%. In approximately half of patients who do not have staghorn calculi removed, renal function will deteriorate and eventually cease even when the character and size of the stone appear unchanged on x-rays.

A. Surgical Measures: The objectives of surgery to remove struvite calculi include (1) removal of all calculi; (2) repair of anatomic abnormalities; (3) eradication of urinary tract infection; (4) preservation of functioning renal tissue; and (5) prevention of recurrent infection and stone formation.

1. Preoperative antibiotics–Appropriate preoperative antibiotics, selected on the basis of culture and sensitivity tests, should be started 24–48 hours before surgery. Nephrotoxic agents such as aminoglycosides must be used with care in patients with compromised renal function and should be avoided if possible when it is planned to occlude the renal artery and cool the kidney during stone removal.

2. Types of surgery–(See also p 291.)

a. Nephrectomy–This procedure should be reserved for patients with staghorn calculi in a nonfunctioning kidney or for patients who are considered too poor a risk for a more lengthy surgical procedure.

b. Partial nephrectomy–Partial nephrectomy should be performed only in patients with severe obstruction and parenchymal loss, in whom the recovery of renal function in the damaged segment is expected to be minimal.

c. Pyelolithotomy–Pyelolithotomy and extended pyelolithotomy may be performed when the stone is confined to the renal pelvis or extends minimally into the calices.

d. Anatrophic nephrolithotomy–When the stone is large and completely fills the renal pelvis and caliceal system, intersegmental anatrophic nephrolithotomy (Boyce procedure; Smith and Boyce, 1967) affords excellent exposure to the internal collecting system, allows for maximal reconstructive procedures, and minimizes parenchymal loss.

3. Follow-up and prognosis–Long-term follow-up should include repeat urine cultures obtained at 1- to 2-month intervals for the first year and periodically thereafter. All recurrent urinary tract infections require intensive antimicrobial therapy and long-term antimicrobial prophylaxis in some cases.

It is often impossible to completely remove all stone fragments. In spite of recent improvements in intraoperative x-ray techniques that allow for identification of calculi as small as 1–2 mm in diameter, intraoperative use of nephroscopy and ultrasonography, and the use of hypothermia to minimize the effects of renal ischemia, there is a residual stone rate of about 5–30%. Moreover, urinary tract infections are completely eradicated in only 60–80% of patients, in spite of complete stone removal and intensive antimicrobial therapy. Therefore, it is not surprising that a stone recurrence rate of 30% within 6 years has been reported. It is likely that the development of new, less nephrotoxic antimicrobial drugs will result in decreases in the incidence of persistent urinary tract infection and stone recurrence.

B. Stone Dissolution: (See also Chapter 7.) The dissolution of struvite calculi confined to the upper collecting system has been attempted for a number of years. Many physicians have now successfully used hemiacidrin, a solution containing citric acid, anhydrous D-gluconic acid, magnesium hydroxycarbonate, magnesium acid citrate, and calcium carbonate, as the irrigant for dissolving struvite stones. Hemiacidrin acts by an ion exchange mechanism in which the calcium of the stone is replaced by magnesium to form a magnesium salt that is soluble in the gluconocitrate present in the solution. Ureteral catherters, nephrostomy tubes, and recently, percutaneous nephrostomy tubes have been used successfully to deliver and completely bathe the stone with the irrigant.

The urine must be sterilized with appropriate systemic antimicrobial drugs before stone dissolution is attempted. Urine cultures must be performed daily to ascertain that the urine remains sterile. In order to be certain that the irrigation system is patent and operates properly, sterile saline solution should be used to irrigate the stone for at least 24 hours before hemiacidrin irrigation is begun. If leakage or pain occurs, irrigation should be discontinued until healing is complete. A 10% solution of hemiacidrin should be started at a slow infusion rate, which may be increased to a maximum of 120 mL/h. Plain films of the abdomen and nephrotomograms should be obtained during stone dissolution. The patient should be closely monitored for evidence of obstruction, hypermagnesemia, and renal failure. If pain or fever develops, the irrigation should be discontinued.

Routine use of hemiacidrin following surgical removal of renal calculi via a nephrostomy tube has been reported to reduce the incidence of stone recurrence.

C. Urease Inhibitors: Attention has recently focused on the use of urease inhibitors—acetohydroxamic acid and hydroxyurea—as agents that might be effective in the prevention of struvite stones. Acetohydroxamic acid, a compound of low toxicity, and hydroxyurea inhibit the bacterial enzyme urease and thereby inhibit alkalinization of urine by urea-splitting organisms and subsequent precipitation of struvite. These drugs may prove useful in inhibiting the growth of residual stones when complete surgical removal is unsuccessful and in preventing new stone formation in patients with intractable urinary tract infections. Although further clinical evaluation is required, it appears that long-term treatment with antimicrobial drugs and urease inhibitors can be expected to reduce stone growth and the incidence of stone recurrence in patients with residual stone disease.

URIC ACID STONES
(See also p 285.)

Uric acid stones account for 5–10% of urinary stones found in the USA. Humans and dalmatian dogs are the only mammals prone to the development of uric acid stones. Uric acid, which is very insoluble in water, is the major end product of purine metabolism in humans. Other mammals possess the hepatic enzyme uricase, which converts uric acid to allantoin, a highly water-soluble substance. (Dalmatian dogs possess uricase, but their proximal renal tubules do not reabsorb all filtered uric acid; thus, uric acid is excreted in their urine.)

All uric acid in the serum is filtered by the glomeruli and, except in dalmatian dogs, readily reabsorbed by the proximal renal tubule. In humans, the reabsorbed uric acid is secreted by the distal renal tubule; in other mammals, it is recirculated to the liver and there transformed into allantoin, which is excreted by the kidneys. The average man excretes about 400 mg of uric acid daily, approximately 10 times more that most other mammals.

Uric acid is insoluble in water, which accounts for the formation of uric acid calculi. Once uric acid is secreted into the urine, it exists in 2 forms: insoluble uric acid and urate salt, which is 20 times more soluble than the free acid form. Uric acid is a weak acid, with a pK_a of 5.75; ie, in a solution with a pH of 5.75, half of the uric acid will exist in the insoluble un-ionized form and half in the ionized form. As the urine becomes more acidic, more of the uric acid exists in the un-ionized form. Humans secrete predominantly acidic urine, and therefore most of the uric acid secreted is in the insoluble un-ionized state. At a pH of 5.0 and at 37 °C, urinary saturation occurs with only 60 mg of uric acid per liter of urine, but if the pH is increased to 6.0, the urine does not become saturated until it contains 220 mg of uric acid per liter. Individuals who are prone to uric acid calculi tend to maintain a constant urinary pH in the acidic range.

A decrease in urine volume can also lead to oversaturation with uric acid and an increased incidence of stone formation. Patients with an inflammatory disease of the bowel, eg, ulcerative colitis, ordinarily excrete highly concentrated urine and have an increased incidence of uric acid stone formation.

Classification

There are 4 categories of uric acid calculous disease.

A. Idiopathic Uric Acid Lithiasis: Patients with idiopathic calculi do not have elevated serum levels of uric acid or increased urinary excretion of uric acid. They tend to excrete a persistently acidic urine without the normal variations in urinary pH.

B. Calculi Associated With Hyperuricemia: Patients with a metabolic abnormality such as primary gout or Lesch-Nyhan syndrome may form uric acid calculi. The upper limit of normal for serum uric acid concentration is generally accepted to be 7 mg/dL in men and 5.5 mg/dL in women. About 25% of patients with symptomatic gout form uric acid stones, and about 25% of patients who have formed uric acid stones will prove to have gout. Individuals with myeloproliferative disorders such as lymphoma may also exhibit hyperuricemia and hyperuricosuria, presumably as a result of increased cell turnover. Patients receiving chemotherapy for other neoplastic disease may also have increased serum levels and urinary excretion of uric acid.

C. Calculi Associated With Chronic Dehydration: Patients with chronic diarrhea or those with ileostomies are known to be more prone to formation of uric acid stones. Excessive perspiration may also lead to decreased urinary volume if fluids are not adequately replaced.

D. Calculi Associated With Hyperuricosuria Without Hyperuricemia: In men, hyperuricosuria is defined as the presence of more than 800 mg of uric acid in a 24-hour urine specimen, and in women, as the presence of more than 750 mg of uric acid in such a specimen. Drugs such as thiazide diuretics and salicylates can cause hyperuricosuria and lead to uric acid stone formation.

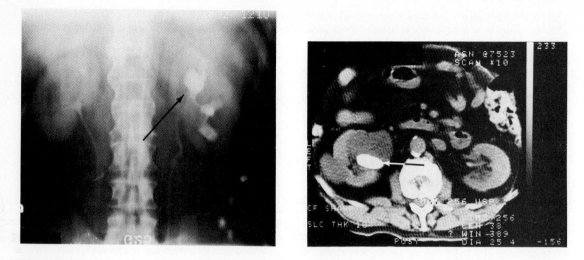

Figure 16–10. *Left:* Intravenous urogram showing large filling defect, initially thought to represent a tumor, in left renal pelvis. *Right:* CT scan obtained without contrast medium showing uric acid stone (*arrow*) and large left renal cyst.

Diagnostic Evaluation

Pure uric acid stones are radiolucent and will not be seen on plain films. Excretory urograms frequently demonstrate a filling defect in the renal pelvis or collecting system. Retrograde urograms, sonograms, and occasionally CT scans may be helpful in differentiating a radiolucent uric acid stone from a urothelial tumor (Fig 16–10).

Medical Treatment

While surgical intervention may occasionally be indicated for the relief of pain or urinary obstruction, many uric acid stones can be treated medically.

A. Hydration: As in the treatment of cystine stones, a dilute urine is essential if the dissolution of uric acid calculi is to be successful. It is desirable to maintain a urine output of at least 2 L/d.

B. Alkalinization of Urine:

1. Oral measures–Sodium bicarbonate in doses of 650–1000 mg every 6–8 hours, potassium bicarbonate, potassium citrate, or Polycitra (a commercially available mixture of sodium citrate and potassium citrate), given orally, have all been used successfully. The urinary pH should be checked regularly with Nitrazine paper and drug dosages adjusted to maintain a urinary pH of 6.5–7.0. Uric acid stones can be completely dissolved using this regimen, but dissolution may require 3–4 months of intensive medical therapy.

2. Ureteral irrigation–In patients in whom a rapid response to alkalinization is desired, irrigation of the renal pelvis with sodium bicarbonate solution via transureteral or percutaneous catheter has been successful.

3. Intravenous alkalinization–Lewis et al (1981) described a regimen of rapid alkalinization using lactate, 1 mol/L, intravenously. Kursh and Resnick (1984) have employed a modification of this

regimen, using 0.167 molar lactate, 40–50 mL/h by continuous intravenous infusion until stones dissolve completely (usually several days to 1 week), to dissolve large, obstructing, intrapelvic uric acid stones and bilateral uric acid stones without complication.

C. Diet: Patients with hyperuricosuria should be instructed to consume a diet low in purine-rich foods and to limit protein intake to about 90 g/d.

D. Allopurinol: Hyperuricemic patients or those unresponsive to the above forms of treatment will often respond to the xanthine oxidase inhibitor allopurinol given in doses of 200–600 mg/d. By inhibiting the formation of uric acid, allopurinol diminishes its concentration in serum as well as in urine. Side effects include skin rash, drug fever, diarrhea, and abdominal cramps. Formation of xanthine stones has been reported as a rare complication.

E. Prophylactic Measures: In patients with gout, prophylactic measures may prevent stone formation. Patients should be encouraged to maintain a urine volume greater than 2 L/d and to restrict protein intake. If uricosuric agents are to be used, it is prudent to alkalinize the urine for the first 10 days of treatment.

Patients with neoplastic disorders who have hyperuricemia should be instructed to maintain a large urine volume. Alkalinization of the urine and allopurinol therapy should be instituted if the patient is to receive cytotoxic therapy.

URINARY STONES IN PREGNANCY

Urinary stone disease complicating pregnancy occurs infrequently. The reported incidence varies from

1:188 to 1:3800 obstetric hospital admissions (average, 1:1500 deliveries). An acute attack of ureteral colic with flank or lower quadrant pain is the usual presentation. Of those with renal colic, only 12% are in the first trimester of pregnancy and the remaining 88% equally distributed between the second and third trimesters (Lattanzi and Cook, 1980).

A number of physiologic changes affect the urinary tract during pregnancy and might contribute to stone formation. Hydronephrosis and dilatation of the proximal and mid ureter occur early in the second trimester and progress to become most marked immediately before delivery. The right ureter tends to become more dilated than the left. These changes are believed to be results both of hormonal changes and mechanical obstruction caused by the enlarging uterus. With the resultant increase in urinary stasis, one might expect an increase in urinary tract infection and stone production.

Diagnostic Evaluation

The diagnosis of renal stone disease should be entertained in women who present with severe pyelonephritis, recurrent urinary tract infections, urinary tract infections unresponsive to usual antimicrobial drug therapy, or symptoms not classic for renal stone disease but a history of calculi.

Diagnostic procedures are similar to those used in nonpregnant patients. Since hydronephrosis of a pregnancy does not occur before the tenth week of gestation, an ultrasound examination may be diagnostic in

the first trimester but difficult to interpret if obtained in the second or third trimester. During pregnancy it is desirable to avoid the use of radiologic studies if possible. However, if other means of diagnosis and evaluation are unavailable or inconclusive, a limited intravenous urogram consisting of a preliminary abdominal scout film and a delayed film obtained 30–60 minutes after the injection of contrast medium should be obtained (Fig 16–11).

Treatment

The management of stone in a pregnant patient should be conservative. With hydration and analgesia, about 50% of stones will pass spontaneously. In the presence of severe obstruction or sepsis, urinary drainage—either by the placement of a double "J" ureteral catheter or by percutaneous nephrostomy—must be provided. If urinary diversion is unsuccessful or unavailable and surgical intervention is absolutely necessary, the stone should be removed operatively, with the obstetrician present.

TREATMENT OF URINARY STONES

SURGICAL TREATMENT OF RENAL STONES

Renal stones that must be surgically removed may be located in the pelvis, infundibula, calices, or combinations thereof. In the past, specific surgical techniques have been required to manage each of these situations. With the widespread availability of extracorporeal shock-wave lithotripsy (ESWL), many of these procedures are no longer being performed and are mentioned only out of historical interest.

Indications

Indications for surgical removal of urinary stones confined to the upper collecting system include intractable urinary tract infection, progressive renal damage, urinary obstruction, and persistent pain. In most cases, surgery can be delayed until a metabolic evaluation is completed. However, if severe obstruction or sepsis occurs, urinary drainage should be provided by placement of a ureteral catheter or by percutaneous nephrostomy.

Hypothermia in Urologic Surgery

Hypothermia reduces renal metabolism and prevents cellular damage during periods of ischemia associated with intraoperative occlusion of the renal artery. Renal cooling reduces cellular metabolic activity, so that the parenchymal cells, especially those of the proximal convoluted tubule, are better able to tolerate ischemia. The temperature needed to prevent ischemic changes is controversial, but experimental

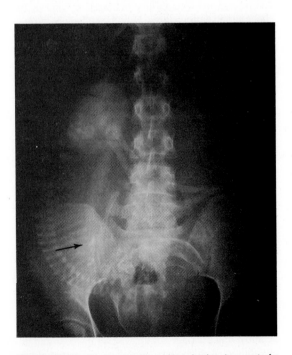

Figure 16–11. Six-hour delayed film obtained as part of a limited intravenous urogram in a pregnant patient with right flank pain. Arrow points to midureteral stone.

studies and clinical experience indicate that the kidney is optimally protected when it is maintained at approximately 15–20 °C. Packing the kidney in an ice slush prepared from physiologic salt solutions, applying external cooling coils, and other methods are acceptable ways of cooling the kidney.

Intraoperative X-Rays

Intraoperative x-rays as well as sonograms obtained using portable ultrasonographic equipment greatly aid the urologist in locating and removing small stone fragments. Intraoperative nephroscopy and pulsatile irrigation are also helpful in the removal of small stone fragments.

Open Surgical Procedures

A. Nephrectomy and Partial Nephrectomy: Nephrectomy meets many objectives of surgery for removal of stones but cannot be endorsed for treatment of stone disease, because renal tissue is needlessly sacrificed. Indiscriminate partial nephrectomy often sacrifices salvageable renal tissue and should be performed only in patients with severe obstruction and parenchymal damage in whom the recovery of renal function of that segment is expected to be minimal.

B. Pyelolithotomy: Simple pyelolithotomy is used for removal of calculi confined to the renal pelvis. Minimal dissection of the renal sinus is usually needed, and exposure of the entire kidney is not required. This procedure is not indicated for the removal of entrapped caliceal stones or large, branched renal calculi.

C. Extended Pyelolithotomy: Trapped caliceal and branched stones usually cannot be adequately removed through a simple pyelotomy. Dissection of the renal sinus and exposure of the infundibula permit access to larger stones. Advocates of extended pyelolithotomy consider it superior to anatrophic nephrolithotomy because it is less traumatic to the renal parenchyma. Operative blood loss is usually minimal, so that occlusion of the renal vessels is rarely required.

D. Pyelonephrolithotomy: The removal of branched calculi located within the lower pole infundibulum may be facilitated by extending a routine pyelotomy incision through the renal parenchyma overlying the lower pole infundibulum posteriorly. This procedure is also indicated for the removal of stones in the lower pole of a kidney with a small intrarenal renal pelvis. The procedure is relatively bloodless, and clamping of the renal artery is usually not necessary.

E. Coagulum Pyelolithotomy: Coagulum pyelolithotomy consists of use of a mixture of pooled human fibrinogen and thrombin to form a clot within the renal collecting system that effectively traps stones and facilitates their removal. The mixture is injected into the renal pelvis before the latter is opened. The renal pelvis is opened after 10 minutes, when the clot has formed. The main application of this technique is in the removal of multiple small calculi in a large ex-

trarenal renal pelvis. It may also be useful in the removal of soft calculi that are likely to crumble during removal.

F. Anatrophic Nephrolithotomy: Intersegmental anatrophic nephrolithotomy (Boyce procedure; Smith and Boyce, 1967) is indicated for the removal of multiple or branched calculi associated with infundibular stenosis. It is also indicated in situations where pyelolithotomy is technically impossible, eg, in a kidney with a small intrarenal renal pelvis and in cases where prior surgery has obliterated access to the renal sinus. An incision is made within the avascular plane or division between the anterior and posterior vascular segments, the renal artery is clamped, and the kidney is cooled to prevent ischemic changes. When the procedure is properly performed, large renal calculi can be easily removed with minimal trauma to the kidney. Reconstruction of the collecting system should also be done to facilitate drainage and reduce the incidence of recurrent stone formation.

G. Radial Nephrotomy: Radial nephrotomy may be used as a primary procedure or in conjunction with any of the other surgical procedures discussed above. It is indicated for the removal of a solitary caliceal stone or a caliceal stone associated with a larger intrapelvic stone. In order to decrease intraoperative blood loss, it is helpful to clamp the main renal artery and cool the kidney. The radial parenchymal incisions should be made on the convex border of the posterior surface whenever possible, thereby minimizing damage to the intralobar vessels.

H. Ex Vivo, or "Bench," Surgery and Autotransplantation: Nearly all patients with renal stone disease can be successfully managed by one of the above surgical procedures. However, "bench" surgery with autotransplantation of the kidney may have a role in treatment of patients with recurrent stone disease and a history of multiple surgical procedures, stenosis of the pelvis or proximal ureter, or calculi associated with congenital renal anomalies or of patients with intractable ureteral colic.

PERCUTANEOUS STONE REMOVAL

Cooperative efforts between urologists and radiologists have led to the development of endourology (see Chapter 7). A nephroscope may be inserted through a nephrostomy tract to remove a stone from the renal pelvis. An ultrasound probe may be used to fragment a large (> 1.5 cm) or branched calculus.

The advantages of percutaneous methods are obvious. No incision is required, and many of the procedures can be performed under local anesthesia. Recovery time is shortened, and the patient can usually return to full activity in a short period of time.

Disadvantages include the occasional need for nephrostomy drainage for up to several weeks and the possibility of bleeding secondary to percutaneous stone manipulation. These are new techniques, and long-term effects are still uncertain, as is the success rate compared with that of more conventional surgical methods.

The criteria for percutaneous stone removal are identical to those for open procedures for stone removal. Patients should have complete laboratory studies, and all stones should be identified and located preoperatively. Antimicrobial drugs should be used to treat urinary tract infections before stone manipulation.

The cornerstone of percutaneous manipulative procedures is the accurate intrarenal placement of a percutaneous nephrostomy tube and the establishment of a nephrostomy tube tract of adequate caliber to accommodate the nephroscope. Intrarenal access may be achieved by either the antegrade or retrograde technique. Immediate dilation of the nephrostomy tract and delayed dilation of the tract over a 1- to 2-week period have both been successfully employed.

The methods of stone removal are varied, and the choice is based on the experience of the surgeon and the needs of the patient. Stones can be grasped or flushed out under fluoroscopic control or under direct vision using a nephroscope. Stone baskets or specially designed forceps may be employed. Large stones may be fragmented using either an ultrasonic or electrohydraulic lithotrite under direct vision.

Before ESWL was widely available, percutaneous stone removal was the treatment of choice for nearly all surgical stones. Complications and long-term morbidity have been minimal with this technique.

EXTRACORPOREAL SHOCK-WAVE LITHOTRIPSY (ESWL)

Extracorporeal shock-wave lithotripsy permits removal of renal stones without direct surgical intervention (Chaussy, 1981; Chaussy, Brendel, and Schmidt, 1980). The patient is given an epidural local or general anesthetic and lowered into a tank of distilled water at the bottom of which is placed the shock-wave electrode used to produce the shock waves that fragment the renal stone. The shock waves produced by the electrode are focused and directed at the stone by a 2-dimensional radiographic scanning system and are keyed to follow the R wave of the patient's ECG. The average patient receives 1000–1500 shock-wave pulses. After about 200 pulses, the stone begins to fragment. Small particles are passed in the urine over the next several days.

In studies performed on dogs, the shock waves caused no tissue damage except to the lungs, but the dosage was 50 times greater than that used on humans. The shock waves did not damage bone tissue, because of the large protein matrix of bone.

This technique is being successfully used to treat nearly all renal calculi. Side effects are minimal. Contraindications to the procedure include urinary tract obstruction and active urinary tract infection. Patients with heart disease requiring cardiac pacemakers are not candidates for ESWL. Staghorn calculi may be managed using a combination of percutaneous and ESWL techniques. However, multiple procedures may be required. Patients with associated infundibular stenosis require surgical reconstruction in addition to stone removal and are not good candidates for ESWL therapy.

TREATMENT OF URETERAL STONES

Ureteral stones originate in the renal collecting system and pass into the ureter, where they frequently become lodged and cause symptoms of ureteral colic (Fig 16–12). The right and left ureters are involved with equal frequency. Management depends on the size and location of the stone, age of the patient, presence or absence of urinary tract infection, anatomy of the urinary tract, and degree of symptoms. Treatment may be expectant, manipulative, or surgical.

Studies have shown that 31–93% of ureteral stones pass spontaneously. Size and location of the stone need to be considered when planning a course of therapy. Ninety percent of stones located in the distal ureter and measuring less than 4 mm in diameter were found to pass spontaneously, whereas only 50% of stones 4–5.9 mm in diameter passed spontaneously. Only 20% of stones greater than 6 mm in diameter passed without surgical intervention. Stones located in the proximal ureter are much less likely to pass spontaneously.

Expectant Therapy

Most ureteral stones are less than 5 mm in diameter and pass spontaneously. Expectant management consists of hydration and the liberal use of analgesics. Patients are instructed to strain all urine and to save the stone for analysis. Plain films of the abdomen and pelvis are obtained at 1- to 2-week intervals to monitor progress of the stone down the ureter. If the patient develops fever associated with a urinary tract infection, severe ureteral colic unresponsive to oral medications, severe nausea and vomiting, complete obstruction of a solitary kidney, or impaction of the stone, hospital admission and surgical or manipulative treatment are indicated.

Manipulative Treatment

In the past, it was generally accepted that stone manipulation should not be attempted when the stone was above the rim of the bony pelvis (Anderson, 1974). With the use of fluoroscopy to guide stone extraction, small stones lodged in the upper and mid ureter may be safely approached endoscopically with double-balloon stone catheters and a ureteroscope. Large stones in the renal pelvis or proximal ureter have been removed using the ureteroscope and ultrasonic lithotriptor to disintegrate impacted stones. Stones 5–8 mm in diameter usually pass into the distal ureter to lodge at the ureterovesical junction; this location is ideal for transurethral manipulation.

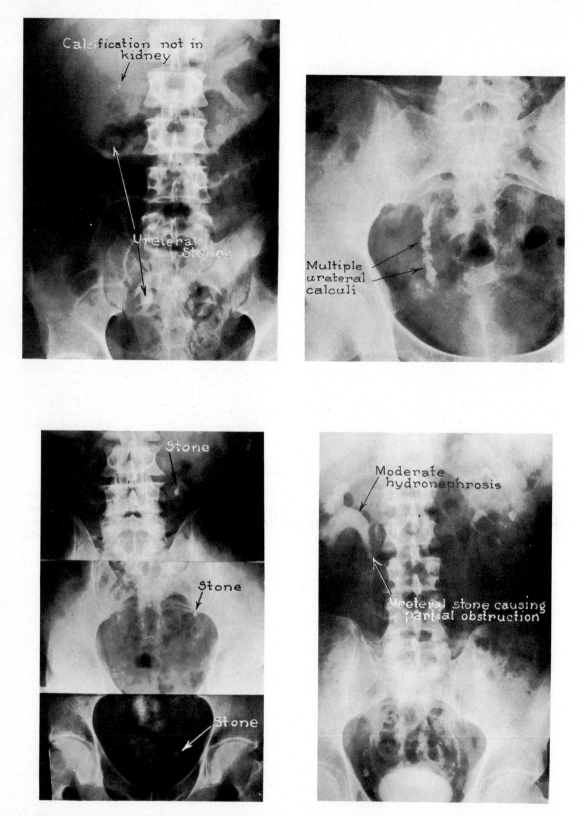

Figure 16–12. Multiple radiograms showing ureteral stones. *Upper left:* Two stones in right ureter, mildly radiopaque: cystine. *Upper right:* Multiple stones, right ureter. *Lower left:* Plain films showing progress of stone down ureter. *Lower right:* Stone in upper right ureter causing moderate obstruction.

Instruments used with varying success for the removal of ureteral stones include Councill and Johnson baskets, expandable Robinson baskets, retractable Dormia and Pfister-Schwartz baskets, end-loop and side-loop Davis catheters, balloon catheters including double-balloon catheters, and multiple ureteral catheters. Success rates vary according to the skill of the surgeon and the instrument used. There is a reported 93% success rate when the loop catheter is used and allowed to pass spontaneously. Wire stone baskets have been successful in about 60–70% of cases.

Complications resulting from stone manipulation are relatively rare and range from 0.3% with loop catheters to 2% with wire stone baskets. Complications include urinary tract infection, hematuria, ureteral perforation, breakage and entrapment of the stone basket, and complete avulsion of the ureter.

Ureteral stones have been successfully removed using percutaneous techniques (see p 292). ESWL may also be used to treat proximal and mid ureteral stones with a moderate degree of success. Distal ureteral stones are still best managed by stone basketing or ureteroscopic stone manipulation.

Surgical Measures

Patients that do not respond to expectant, manipulative, or ESWL therapy require open surgical stone removal. A number of different approaches to the ureter have been described, including the modified dorsal lumbar approach or the anterior kidney incision for stones located in the proximal ureter. Midureteral stones may be approached by a McBurney or Gibson incision, while stones in the distal ureter may be removed through a Pfannenstiel or lower midline incision. In carefully selected patients, the transvesical or transvaginal approach may be useful in removing distal ureteral calculi.

● ● ●

BLADDER STONES

Primary stones of the bladder are relatively rare in the USA but occur commonly in children in parts of India, Indonesia, the Middle East, and China. These stones usually occur in sterile urine. They are uncommon in girls. It is believed that the incidence is related to diets low in protein and phosphate. Dehydration due to hot weather and diarrhea further compounds the problem. In areas where bladder stones are endemic, they are usually composed of ammonium acid urate.

Secondary vesical stones form as a result of other urologic conditions. They nearly always occur in men and are frequently associated with urinary stasis and chronic urinary tract infection. Urinary obstruction may be due to prostatic hyperplasia or urethral stricture. Neurogenic vesical dysfunction may be a cause of chronic infection and urinary retention with eventual stone formation. Patients with chronic indwelling catheters frequently develop encrustations on the catheter and bladder calculi. Ureteral stones may pass into the bladder but fail to pass through the urethra. Foreign bodies in the urinary tract may act as a nidus for calcium deposition and stone formation.

The composition of bladder stones varies according to urinary pH and the concentration of stone-forming elements in the urine. In the USA, calcium oxalate is the most common constituent, whereas in European countries, uric acid and urate stones predominate.

Diagnostic Evaluation

Patients with bladder stones frequently give a history of hesitancy, frequency, dysuria, hematuria, dribbling, or chronic urinary tract infection unresponsive to antimicrobial drug therapy. Sudden interruption of the urinary stream associated with the acute onset of pain radiating down and along the penis may occur when the stone intermittently obstructs the bladder neck (Fig 16–13).

Most vesical stones are radiopaque and apparent on a plain film of the pelvis (Fig 16–14). Oblique films may be helpful in differentiating bladder stones from calcifications in ovaries, lymph nodes, or uterine fibroids.

Cystoscopy is the most accurate means of diagnosis.

Treatment

Small bladder stones may be removed by transurethral irrigation. Larger stones may be crushed by one of a variety of different manual lithotrites and removed from the bladder by irrigation. Ultrasonic and electrohydraulic lithotriptors are available to fragment large bladder calculi.

Stones that are too large to manage transurethrally and stones associated with prostatic hypertrophy should be removed by a suprapubic surgical procedure which allows for contemporaneous prostatectomy. Other urologic conditions that contribute to formation of stones must be corrected if recurrence is to be prevented. Chemolysis using hemiacidrin or Suby's solution G administered via a catheter may be an effective form of treatment in patients who cannot tolerate general anesthetics.

URETHRAL STONES

Primary urethral calculi are formed in the urethra and are rare. They are usually found in association with an abnormality of the lower urinary tract that typically causes stasis of urine or chronic urinary tract in-

Obstruction with infection
by urea-splitting organisms

Other less common causes:
    Renal stone
    Foreign body
    Parasites

Symptoms and signs:
    Sudden interruption of urinary stream
      with radiation of pain down urethra
    Urinary symptoms of underlying disease
      (eg, prostatism, secondary cystitis)

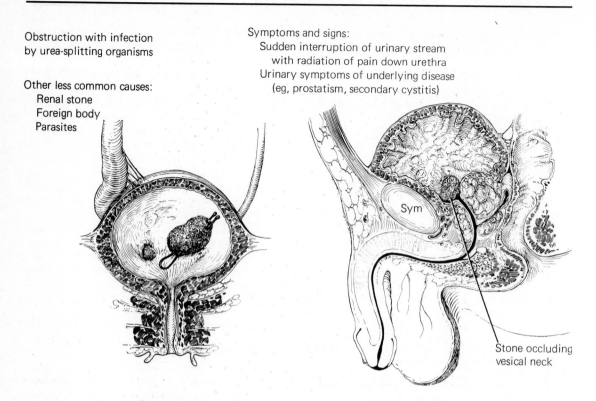

Sym

Stone occluding
vesical neck

Figure 16–13. Genesis and symptoms and signs of vesical calculus.

fection and leads to stone formation. Patients with ure-thral diverticula, strictures, foreign bodies in the urethra, chronic urethral fistulas, benign prostatic hyperplasia, and meatal stenosis are more prone to the development of urethral stones.

Secondary urethral calculi are more common; they are formed in the kidney or bladder and become lodged in the urethra as they progress down the urinary tract (Fig 16–15).

Most urethral calculi (59–63%) are located in the anterior urethra and up to 11% at the fossa navicularis.

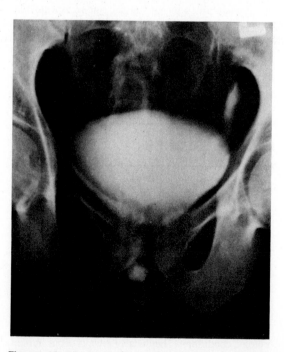

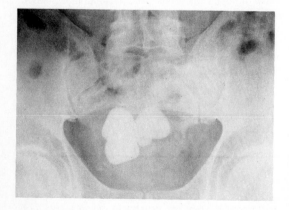

Figure 16–14. Plain film showing multiple radiopaque vesical calculi.

Figure 16–15. Excretory urogram showing multiple stones lodged in urethra. (Courtesy of MM Al Ghorab.)

However, up to 42% may become impacted at the membranous urethra or external urinary sphincter.

Diagnostic Evaluation

A urethral calculus should be considered when there is a history of acute urinary retention preceded by sharp perineal pain. Careful palpation of the urethra may disclose the presence of a pendulous or distal urethral stone. In females, the stone should be evident from transvaginal palpation of the urethra. Retrograde urethrography in males will identify the presence and location of the stone.

Treatment

Management of impacted urethral stones is surgical. Therapeutic goals should include not only removal of the stone but also repair of any urethral abnormality leading to stone formation.

REFERENCES

Historical Perspective

Butt AJ: Historical survey. Pages 3–47 in: *Etiologic Factors in Renal Lithiasis*. Butt AJ (editor). Thomas, 1956.

Joly JS: *Stones and Calculous Disease of the Urinary Organs*. Mosby, 1929.

Keyser LD: The etiology of urinary lithiasis: An experimental study. *Arch Surg* 1923;**6**:525.

Murphy LJ: *The History of Urology*. Thomas, 1972.

Resnick MI, Boyce WH: Aetiological theories of renal lithiasis: A historical review. Chap 1, pp 1–20, in: *Urinary Calculous Disease*. Wickham JEA (editor). Churchill Livingstone, 1979.

Shattock SG: A prehistoric or predynastic Egyptian calculus. *Trans Path Soc London* 1905;**61**:275.

Theories of Stone Formation

Baumann JM et al: The role of inhibitors and other factors in the pathogenesis of recurrent calcium-containing renal stones. *Clin Sci* 1977;**53**:141.

Boyce WH: Organic matrix of human urinary concretion. *Am J Med* 1968;**45**:673.

Boyce WH: Ultrastructure of human renal calculi. Pages 247–255 in: *International Symposium on Renal Stone Research*. Fuentes-Delate LC, Rapada A, Hodgkinson A (editors). Karger, 1973.

Boyce WH, Garvey FK: The amount and nature of the organic matrix in urinary calculi: A review. *J Urol* 1956;**76**:213.

Brockis JG, Levitt AF, Cruthers SM: The effects of vegetable and animal protein diets on calcium, urate and oxalate excretion. *Br J Urol* 1982;**54**:590.

Carr RJ: A new theory on the formation of renal calculi. *Br J Urol* 1954;**26**:105.

Coe FL et al: Urinary macromolecular crystal growth inhibitors in calcium nephrolithiasis. *Miner Electrolyte Metab* 1980;**3**:268.

Drach GW, Boyce WH: Nephrocalculosis as a source for renal stone nuclei: Observations on human and squirrel monkeys and on hyperparathyroidism in the squirrel monkey. *J Urol* 1972;**107**:897.

Finlayson B: Where and how does urinary stone disease start? An essay on the expectation of free and fixed particle urinary stone disease. Pages 7–32 in: *Idiopathic Urinary Bladder Stone Disease*. Van Reen R (editor). DHEW Publication No. (NIH) 77–1063. US Department of Health, Education, and Welfare, 1977.

Menon M, Mahle CJ: Urinary citrate excretion in patients with renal calculi. *J Urol* 1983;**129**:1158.

Oliver J et al: The renal lesions of electrolyte imbalance. 4. The intranephronic calculosis of experimental magnesium depletion. *J Exp Med* 1966;**124**:263.

Peacock M, Robertson WG: The biochemical aetiology of renal lithiasis. Chap 4, pp 69–95, in: *Urinary Calculous Disease*. Wickham JEA (editor). Churchill Livingstone, 1979.

Posey LC: Urinary concretions. 2. A study of the primary calculous lesions. *J Urol* 1942;**48**:300.

Prien EL: The riddle of Randall's plaques. *J Urol* 1975;**11**:500.

Randall A: Origin and growth of renal calculi. *Ann Surg* 1937;**105**:1009.

Randall A: Papillary pathology as a precursor of primary renal calculus. *J Urol* 1940;**44**:580.

Resnick MI: Urinary stone matrix. Pages 73–82 in: *Idiopathic Urinary Bladder Stone Disease*. Van Reen R (editor). DHEW Publication No. (NIH) 77–1063. US Department of Health, Education, and Welfare, 1977.

Resnick MI, Boyce WH: Aetiological theories of renal lithiasis: A historical review. Chap 1, pp 1–20, in: *Urinary Calculous Disease*. Wickham JEA (editor). Churchill Livingstone, 1979.

Resnick MI, Oliver J, Drach GW: Intranephronic calculosis in the squirrel monkey. *Invest Urol* 1978;**15**:295.

Robertson WG, Peacock M: Calcium oxalate crystalluria and inhibitors of crystallization in recurrent renal stone-formers. *Clin Sci* 1972;**43**:499.

Robertson WG, Peacock M, Nordin BEC: Crystalluria. Pages 243–254 in: *Urolithiasis: Physical Aspects*. Finlayson B, Hench LL, Smith LH (editors). National Academy of Sciences, 1972.

Rosenow EC Jr: Renal calculi: A study of papillary calcification. *J Urol* 1940;**44**:119.

Spector AR, Gray A, Prien EL: Kidney stone matrix: Differences in acidic protein composition. *Invest Urol* 1976;**13**:387.

Vermeulen CW, Ellis JE, Hsu TC: Experimental observations on the pathogenesis of urinary calculi. *J Urol* 1966;**95**:681.

Radiographic Examination

Dourmaskin RL: Cytoscopic treatment of stones in the ureter with special references to large calculi based on a study of 1550 cases. *J Urol* 1945;**54**:245.

Resnick MI, Kursh ED, Cohen AM: Use of computerized tomography in the delineation of uric acid calculi. *J Urol* 1984;**131**:9.

Roth R, Finlayson B: Observations on the radiopacity of stone substances with special reference to cystine. *Invest Urol* 1973;**11**:186.

Calcium Stones

Archer HE et al: Studies on the urinary excretion of oxalate by normal subjects. *Clin Sci* 1957;**16**:405.

Bernstein DS, Newton R: The effect of oral sodium phosphate on the formation of renal calculi and on idiopathic hypercalciuria. *Lancet* 1966;**2**:1105.

Blacklock NF: The epidemiology of renal lithiasis. Chap 2, pp 21–39, in: *Urinary Calculous Disease.* Wickham JEA (editor). Churchill Livingstone, 1979.

Boyce WH, Garvey FK, Strawcutter HE: Incidence of urinary calculi among patients in general hospitals: 1948–1952. *JAMA* 1956;**161**:1437.

Boyce WH, Resnick MI: Biochemical profiles of stone forming patients: A guide to treatment. *J Urol* 1979;**121**:706.

Brenner RJ et al: Incidence of radiographically evident bone disease, nephrocalcinosis, and nephrolithiasis in various types of renal tubular acidosis. *N Engl J Med* 1982;**307**:217.

Breslau NA, Pak CYC: Practical outpatient evaluation for recurrent nephrolithiasis. *Urol Clin North Am* 1981;**8**:253.

Briggs MH, Garcia-Webb P, Davies P: Urinary oxalate and vitamin-C supplements. *Lancet* 1973;**2**:201.

Burdette DC, Thomas WC, Finlayson B: Urinary supersaturation with calcium oxalate before and during orthophosphate therapy. *J Urol* 1976;**115**:418.

Burkland CE, Rosenberg M: Survey of urolithiasis in the United States. *J Urol* 1955;**73**:198.

Chadwick VS, Modha K, Dowling RH: Pathogenesis of secondary hyperoxaluria in ileal resection. *Gut* 1972;**13**:840.

Clark PB, Nordin BEC: The problem of calcium stones. Pages 1–5 in: *Renal Stone Research Symposium.* Hodgkinson A, Nordin BC (editors). Churchill, 1969.

Coe FL: Hyperuricosuric calcium oxalate nephrolithiasis. *Kidney Int* 1978;**13**:418.

Coe FL, Raisen L: Allopurinol treatment of uric acid disorders in calcium stone formers. *Lancet* 1973;**1**:129.

Coe FL et al: Evidence for secondary hyperparathyroidism in idiopathic hypercalciuria. *J Clin Invest* 1973;**52**:134.

Dent CE, Stamp TCB: Treatment of primary hyperoxaluria. *Arch Dis Child* 1970;**45**:735.

Dobbins JW, Binder HJ: Effect of bile salts and fatty acids on the colonic absorption of oxalate. *Gastroenterology* 1976;**70**:1096.

Drach GW: Urinary lithiasis. Chap 22, pp 779–878, in: *Campbell's Urology.* Harrison JH et al (editors). Saunders, 1978.

Earnest DL et al: Hyperoxaluria in patients with ileal resection: An abnormality in dietary oxalate absorption. *Gastroenterology* 1974;**66**:1114.

Edwards NA, Russell RGG, Hodgkinson A: The effect of oral phosphate in patients with renal calculus. *Br J Urol* 1965;**37**:390.

Finlayson B: Renal lithiasis in review. *Urol Clin North Am* 1974;**1**:181.

Frank M, DeVries A: Prevention of urolithiasis. *Arch Environ Health* 1966;**13**:625.

Gibbs D, Watts RWE: The action of pyridoxine in primary hyperoxaluria. *Clin Sci* 1970;**38**:277.

Gregory JG: Hyperoxaluria and stone disease in the gastrointestinal bypass patient. *Urol Clin North Am* 1981;**8**:331.

Griffith DP: Patient evaluation: The initial stone former. Page 132 in: *Urolithiasis Update, 1983.* Office of Education, American Urological Association, Houston, Texas, 1983.

Hallson PC, Kasidas GP, Rose GA: Urinary oxalate in summer and winter in normal subjects and in stone forming patients with idiopathic hypercalciuria both untreated and treated with thiazides and/or cellulose phosphate. *Urol Res* 1976;**4**:169.

Herring LC: Observations of 10,000 urinary calculi. *J Urol* 1962;**88**:545.

Hockaday TDR et al: Studies on primary hyperoxaluria. 2. Urinary oxalate, glycolate, and glyoxalate measurement by isotope dilution method. *J Lab Clin Med* 1965;**65**:677.

Hodgkinson A, Heaton FW: The effect of food ingestion on the urinary excretion of calcium and magnesium. *Clin Chim Acta* 1965;**2**:354.

Hodgkinson A, Peacock M, Nicholson M: Quantitative analysis of calcium-containing urinary calculi. *Invest Urol* 1969;**6**:549.

King JS, Jackson R, Ashe B: Relation of sodium intake to urinary calcium excretion. *Invest Urol* 1964;**1**:555.

Lindeman RD et al: Influence of various nutrients in urinary divalent cation excretion. *J Lab Clin Med* 1967;**70**:236.

Lyles KW, Drezner MK: An overview of calcium homeostasis in humans. *Urol Clin North Am* 1981;**8**:209.

Menon M: Calcium oxalate stones: Management. Page 6 in: *Urolithiasis Update, 1983.* Office of Education, American Urological Association, Houston, Texas, 1983.

Menon M: Renal tubular acidosis and medullary sponge kidney. Page 116 in: *Urolithiasis Update, 1983.* Office of Education, American Urological Association, Houston, Texas, 1983.

Menon M, Mahle CJ: Oxalate metabolism and renal calculi. *J Urol* 1982;**127**:148.

Menon M, Mahle CJ: Urinary citrate excretion in patients with renal calculi. *J. Urol* 1983;**129**:1158.

Nicar MJ et al: Low urinary citrate excretion in nephrolithiasis. *Urology* 1983;**21**:8.

Pak CYC: Medical management of nephrolithiasis. *J Urol* 1982;**128**:1157.

Pak CYC: The spectrum and pathogenesis of hypercalciuria. *Urol Clin North Am* 1981;**8**:245.

Pak CYC, Delea CS, Barter FC: Successful treatment of recurrent nephrolithiasis (calcium stones) with cellulose phosphate. *N Engl J Med* 1979;**290**:175.

Pak CYC, Fuller C: Idiopathic hypocitraturic calcium-oxalate nephrolithiasis successfully treated with potassium citrate. *Ann Intern Med* 1986;**104**:32.

Pak CYC, Peterson R: Successful treatment of hyperuricosuric calcium oxalate nephrolithiasis with potassium citrate. *Arch Intern Med* 1986;**146**:863.

Pak CYC et al: Ambulatory evaluation of nephrolithiasis: Classification, clinical presentation, and diagnostic criteria. *Am J Med* 1980;**69**:19.

Pak CYC et al: Dietary management of idiopathic calcium urolithiasis. *J Urol* 1984;**131**:850.

Pak CYC et al: Estimation of the state of saturation of brushite and calcium oxalate in urine: A comparison of three methods. *J Lab Clin Med* 1977;**89**:891.

Pak CYC et al: Evaluation of calcium urolithiasis in ambulatory patients. *Am J Med* 1978;**64**:979.

Pak CYC et al: Is selective therapy of recurrent nephrolithiasis possible? *Am J Med* 1981;**71**:615.

Pak CYC et al: Long-term treatment of calcium nephrolithiasis with potassium citrate. *J Urol* 1985;**134**:11.

Pak CYC et al: A simple test for the diagnosis of absorptive, resorptive, and renal hypercalciurias. *N Engl J Med* 1975;**292**:497.

Papapoulos SE et al: Dihydroxycholecalciferol in the pathogenesis of the hypercalcemia of sarcoidosis. *Lancet* 1979;**1**:627.

Pitts GW, Resnick MI: Urinary stone formation: Patient evaluation and management. *Urol Clin North Am* 1980;**7**:45.

Preminger GM, Harvey JA, Pak CYC: Comparative efficacy of "specific" potassium citrate therapy versus conservative management in nephrolithiasis of mild to moderate severity. *J Urol* 1985;**134**:658.

Preminger GM et al: Prevention of recurrent calcium stone

formation with potassium citrate therapy in patients with distal renal tubular acidosis. *J. Urol* 1985;**134:**20.

Prince CL, Scardino PL: A statistical analysis of ureteral calculi. *J Urol* 1960;**83:**561.

Prince CL, Scardino PL, Wolan TC: The effect of temperature, humidity, and dehydration on the formation of renal calculi. *J Urol* 1956;**75:**209.

Resnick MI, Goodman HO, Boyce WH: Heterozygous cystinuria and calcium oxalate urolithiasis. *J Urol* 1979;**122:**52.

Resnick MI, Rush WH, Boyce WH: Metabolic evaluation of the renal stone patient. *J Cont Educ Urol* 1978;**17:**11.

Robertson WG, Knowles F, Peacock M: Urinary acid mucopolysaccharide inhibitors of calcium oxalate crystallization. Page 331 in: *Urolithiasis Research.* Fleisch H et al (editors). Plenum Press, 1976.

Singh PP et al: Nutritional value of foods in relation to their oxalic acid contents. *Am J Clin Nutr* 1972;**25:**1147.

Smith LH: Calcium-containing renal stones. *Kidney Int* 1978;**13:**383.

Smith LH, Williams HE: Treatment of primary hyperoxaluria. *Mod Treat* 1967;**4:**522.

Stauffer JQ, Humphreys MH, Weir GJ: Acquired hyperoxaluria with regional enteritis after ileal resection: Role of dietary oxalate. *Ann Intern Med* 1973;**79:**383.

Sutor DJ, Wooley SE, Illingworth JJ: Some aspects of the adult urinary stone problem in Great Britain and Northern Ireland. *Br J Urol* 1974;**46:**275.

Thomas WC: Use of phosphates in patients with calcareous renal calculi. *Kidney Int* 1978;**13:**390.

Williams HE: Oxalic acid and the hyperoxaluric syndromes. *Kidney Int* 1978;**13:**410.

Williams HE, Smith LH Jr: Primary hyperoxaluria. Page 204 in: *The Metabolic Basis of Inherited Disease,* 5th ed. Stanbury JB et al (editors). McGraw-Hill, 1983.

Yendt ER, Cohanim M: Prevention of calcium stones with thiazides. *Kidney Int* 1978;**13:**397.

Yendt ER, Guay FG, Garcia DA: The use of thiazides in the prevention of renal calculi. *Can Med Assoc J* 1970;**102:**614.

Cystine Stones

Adams DA et al: Nephrotic syndrome associated with penicillamine therapy of Wilson's disease. *Am J Med* 1964;**36:**330.

Burns JR, Hamrick LC Jr: In vitro dissolution of cystine urinary calculi. *J Urol* 1986;**136:**850.

Crawhall JC, Watts RWE: Cystinuria. *Am J Med* 1968;**45:**736.

Dahlberg PJ et al: Clinical features and management of cystinuria. *Mayo Clin Proc* 1977;**52:**533.

Day AT, Golding JR: Hazards of penicillamine in the treatment of rheumatoid arthritis. *Postgrad Med J* 1974;**50:**71.

Dent CE, Senior B: Studies on the treatment of cystinuria. *Br J Urol* 1955;**27:**317.

Dent CE et al: Treatment of cystinuria. *Br Med J* 1965;**1:**403.

Dretler SP et al: Percutaneous catheter dissolution of cystine calculi. *J Urol* 1984;**131:**216.

Evans WP, Resnick MI, Boyce WH: Homozygous cystinuria: Evaluation of thirty-five patients. *J Urol* 1982;**127:**707.

Grant G, Kachmar JF: Nitroprusside test. Page 389 in: *Fundamentals of Clinical Chemistry,* 2nd ed. Teitz NW (editor). Saunders, 1976.

Lotz M et al: D-Penicillamine therapy in cystinuria. *J Urol* 1966;**95:**257.

MacDonald WB, Fellers FX: Penicillamine in the treatment

of patients with cystinuria. *JAMA* 1966;**197:**396.

Saltzamn N, Gittes RF: Chemolysis of cystine calculi. *J Urol* 1986;**136:**846.

Stones Associated With Infection

Blandy JP, Singh M: The case for a more aggressive approach to staghorn stones. *J Urol* 1976;**115:**505.

Boyce WH, Elkins IB: Reconstructive renal surgery following anatrophic nephrolithotomy: Follow-up for 100 consecutive cases. *J Urol* 1974;**111:**307.

Comarr AE, Kawaichi GK, Bors E: Renal calculosis of patients with traumatic cord lesions. *J Urol* 1962;**87:**647.

Comarr AE et al: Dissolution of renal stone by renacidin in patients with spinal cord injury. *Proc Annu Clin Spinal Cord Inj Conf* 1971;**18:**174.

Dana ES: *Descriptive Minerology.* Wiley, 1920.

Dretler SP, Pfister RC: Primary dissolution therapy of struvite calculi. *J Urol* 1984;**131:**861.

Dretler SP, Pfister RC, Newhouse JH: Renal stone dissolution via percutaneous nephrostomy. *N Engl J Med* 1979;**300:**341.

Elliot JS, Sharp RF, Lewis L: The solubility of struvite in urine. *J Urol* 1959;**81:**366.

Griffith DP: Infection-induced stones. Pages 203–228 in: *Nephrolithiasis: Pathogenesis & Treatment.* Coe FL (editor). Year Book, 1978.

Griffith DP: Struvite stones. *Kidney Int* 1978;**13:**372.

Griffith DP, Musher DM, Campbell JW: Inhibitor of bacterial urease. *Invest Urol* 1973;**11:**234.

Griffith DP, Musher DM, Itin C: Urease: The primary cause of infection-induced urinary stones. *Invest Urol* 1976;**13:**346.

Krieger JN, Rudd TG, Mayo ME: Current treatment of infection stones in high risk patients. *J Urol* 1984;**132:**874.

Nemoy NJ, Stamey TA: Surgical, bacteriological and biochemical management of infection stones. *JAMA* 1971;**215:**1470.

Resnick MI: Evaluation and management of infection stones. *Urol Clin North Am* 1981;**8:**265.

Russell M: Dissolution of bilateral renal staghorn calculi with renacidin. *J Urol* 1962;**88:**141.

Sant GR, Blaivas JG, Meares EM Jr: Hemiacidrin irrigation in the management of struvite calculi: Long-term results. *J Urol* 1983;**130:**1048.

Shattock SG: A prehistoric or predynastic Egyptian calculus. *Trans Path Soc London* 1905;**61:**275.

Singh M et al: The fate of the unoperated staghorn calculus. *Br J Urol* 1973;**45:**581.

Smith MJV, Boyce WH: Anatrophic nephrotomy and plastic calyorrhaphy. *Trans Am Assoc Genitourin Surg* 1967;**59:**18.

Suby HI, Albright F: Dissolution of phosphatic urinary calculi by the retrograde introduction of a citrate solution containing magnesium. *N Engl J Med* 1943;**228:**81.

Sutherland JW: Residual postoperative upper urinary tract stone. *J Urol* 1981;**126:**573.

Wickham JP, Coe N, Ward JP: One hundred cases of nephrolithotomy under hypothermia. *J Urol* 1974;**112:**702.

Uric Acid Stones

Bogash M, Dowben RM: Low protein diet in the management of uric acid stones. *J Urol* 1954;**72:**1057.

Burns JR, Gauthier JF, Finlayson B: Dissolution kinetics of uric acid calculi. *J Urol* 1984;**131:**708.

Drach GW: Urinary lithiasis. Chap 22, pp 779–878, in: *Campbell's Urology.* Harrison JH et al (editors). Saunders, 1978.

Elliot JS, Sharp RF, Lewis L: Urinary pH. *J Urol* 1959;**81**:339.

Freiha FS, Hemady K: Dissolution of uric acid stones: Alternative to surgery. *Urology* 1976;**8**:334.

Gutman AB, Yu TF: Benemid [*p*-(di-N-propylsulfamyl)-benzoic acid] as uricosuric agent in chronic gouty arthritis. *Trans Assoc Am Physicians* 1951;**64**:279.

Gutman AB, Yu TF: Uric acid nephrolithiasis. *Am J Med* 1968;**45**:756.

Hardy B, Klein LA: In situ dissolution of ureteral calculus. *Urology* 1976;**8**:444.

Herring LC: Observation in the analysis of ten thousand urinary calculi. *J Urol* 1962;**88**:545.

Kursh ED, Resnick MI: Dissolution of uric acid calculi with systemic alkalinization. *J Urol* 1984;**132**:286.

Lewis RW et al: Molar lactate in the management of uric acid renal obstruction. *J Urol* 1981;**125**:87.

Peters JP, Van Slyke DD: *Quantitative Clinical Chemistry.* 2nd ed. Vol 1. Williams & Wilkins, 1946.

Rodman JS, Williams JJ, Peterson CM: Dissolution of uric acid calculi. *J Urol* 1984;**131**:1039.

Sadi MV et al: Experimental observations on dissolution of uric acid calculi. *J Urol* 1985;**134**:575.

Seegmiller JE: Xanthine stone formation. *Am J Med* 1968;**45**:780.

Smith LH: Medical evaluation of urolithiasis: Etiologic aspects and diagnostic evaluation. *Urol Clin North Am* 1974;**1**:242.

Thomas WC: Medical aspects of renal calculous disease: Treatment and prophylaxis. *Urol Clin North Am* 1974;**1**:261.

Uhlir K: The peroral dissolution of renal calculi. *J Urol* 1970;**104**:239.

Vermeulen CW, Fried FA: Observations on dissolution of uric acid calculi. *J Urol* 1965;**94**:293.

Stones in Pregnancy

Cumming D, Taylor PJ: Urologic and obstetric significance of urinary calculi in pregnancy. *Obstet Gynecol* 1979;**53**:505.

DiSaia PJ, Nolan JF, Arneson AN: Radiation therapy in gynecology. Chap 60, pp 1214–1230, in: *Obstetrics and Gynecology,* 4th ed. Danforth DN (editor). Harper & Row, 1982.

Drago JR, Rohner TJ, Chez RA: Management of urinary calculi in pregnancy. *Urology* 1982;**20**:578.

Fainstat T: Ureteral dilatation in pregnancy: A review. *Obstet Gynecol Surv* 1963;**18**:845.

Houston CS: Diagnostic irradiation of women during the reproductive period. *Can Med Assoc J* 1977;**117**:648.

Lattanzi DR, Cook WA: Urinary calculi in pregnancy. *Obstet Gynecol* 1980;**56**:462.

McVann RM: Urinary calculi associated with pregnancy. *Am J Obstet Gynecol* 1964;**89**:314.

Simon L: Exposure to radiation or chemotherapy. Pages 20–21 in: *Obstetrical Decision Making.* Friedman EA (editor). BC Decker/Stratton, 1982.

Strong DW, Murchison RJ, Lynch DF: The management of ureteral calculi during pregnancy. *Surg Gynecol Obstet* 1978;**146**:604.

Treatment of Renal Stones

Burns JR, Finlayson B: Coagulum pyelolithotomy. *Curr Trends Urol* 1982;**2**:31.

Chaussy C: Shattering renal calculi without surgery. *Wellcome Trends Urol* 1981;**3**:7.

Chaussy C, Brendel W, Schmidt E: Extracorporeally induced destruction of kidney stones by shock waves. *Lancet* 1980;**2**:1265.

Chaussy C et al: Extracorporeal shock-wave lithotripsy (ESWL) for treatment of urolithiasis. *Urology* 1984;**23**:59.

Dees JE: The use of an intrapelvic coagulum in pyelolithotomy. *South Med J* 1943;**36**:167.

Ekelund L et al: Studies on renal damage from percutaneous nephrolitholapaxy. *J Urol* 1986;**135**:682.

Elder JS, Gibbons RP, Bush WH: Ultrasonic lithotripsy of a large staghorn calculus. *J Urol* 1984;**131**:1152.

Gillenwater JY: Notes on visiting the shock-wave machine for kidney stones. *Year Book of Urology Newsletter* (May) 1983;**1**(10).

Kahnoski RJ et al: Combined percutaneous and extracorporeal shock wave lithotripsy for staghorn calculi: Alternative to anatrophic nephrolithotomy. *J Urol* 1984;**135**:679.

Kurth KH, Hohenfellner R, Altwein JE: Ultrasound litholapaxy of a staghorn calculus. *J Urol* 1977;**117**:242.

Lawson RK et al: Retrograde method for percutaneous access to kidney. *Urology* 1983;**22**:580.

Novick AC: Role of bench surgery and autotransplantation in renal calculous disease. *Urol Clin North Am* 1981;**8**:299.

Resnick MI: Pyelonephrolithotomy for removal of calculi from the inferior renal pole. *Urol Clin North Am* 1981;**8**:585.

Resnick MI, Grayhack JT: Simple and extended pyelolithotomy. *Urol Clin North Am* 1974;**1**:319.

Rupel E, Brown NR: Nephroscopy with removal of stone following nephrostomy for obstructive calculous anuria. *J Urol* 1941;**46**:177.

Segura JW et al: Percutaneous removal of kidney stones: Review of 1000 cases. *J. Urol* 1985;**134**:1077.

Smith MJV, Boyce WH: Anatrophic nephrotomy and plastic calyorrhaphy. *Trans Am Assoc Genitourin Surg* 1967;**59**:18.

Snyder JA, Smith AD: Staghorn calculi: Percutaneous extraction versus anatrophic nephrolithotomy. *J Urol* 1986;**136**:351.

Treatment of Ureteral Stones

Abdelsayed M, Onal E, Wax SH: Avulsion of the ureter caused by stone basket manipulation. *J Urol* 1977;**118**:868.

Anderson EE: The management of ureteral calculi. *Urol Clin North Am* 1974;**1**:357.

Bowers L: Loop catheter delivery of ureteral calculi. *J Urol* 1973;**110**:178.

Carstensen HE, Hansen TS: Stones in the ureter. *Acta Chir Scand [Suppl]* 1973;**433**:66.

Drach GW: Stone manipulation. *Urology* 1978;**12**:286.

Dretler SP, Keating MA, Riley J: Algorithm for management of ureteral calculi. *J Urol* 1986;**136**:1190.

Fox M, Pyran LN, Raper FP: Management of ureteric stone: A review of 292 cases. *Br J Urol* 1965;**37**:660.

Huffman JL et al: Transurethral removal of large ureteral and renal pelvis calculi using ureteroscopic ultrasonic lithotripsy. *J Urol* 1983;**130**:31.

Kahn RI: Endourological treatment of ureteral calculi. *J Urol* 1986;**135**:239.

Mueller SC et al: Extracorporeal shock wave lithotripsy of ureteral stones: Clinical experience and experimental findings. *J Urol* 1986;**135**:831.

O'Boyle PJ, Gibbon NOK: Vaginal ureterolithotomy. *J Urol* 1976;**48**:231.

Sandegard E: Prognosis of stone in the ureter. *Acta Chir*

Scand [Suppl] 1956;**219**:1.

Shihata AA, Greene JE: Ureteric stone extraction by a new double-balloon catheter: An experimental study. *J Urol* 1983;**129**:616.

Young HH: Treatment of calculus of the lower end of the ureter in the male. *Am Med* 1902;**4**:209.

Bladder Stones

Thalut K et al: The endemic bladder stones of Indonesia: Epidemiology and clinical features. *Br J Urol* 1976;**48**:617.

Urethral Stones

Amin HA: Urethral calculi. *Br J Urol* 1973;**45**:192.

Bridges CH et al: Urethral calculi. *J Urol* 1982;**128**:1036.

Debenham RK: Urethral calculi. *Br J Urol* 1930;**2**:113.

Englisch J: Ueber einngelagerte und einngesackte Steine der Harnröhre. *Arch Klin Chir* 1904;**72**:487.

Maatman TJ, Spirnak JP, Resnick MI: Impacted membranous urethral calculus. *J Urol (Paris)* 1984;**90**:405.

17 Injuries to the Genitourinary Tract

Jack W. McAninch, MD

EMERGENCY DIAGNOSIS & MANAGEMENT

About 10% of all injuries seen in the emergency room involve the genitourinary system to some extent. Many of them are subtle and difficult to define and require great diagnostic expertise. Early diagnosis is essential to prevent serious complications.

Initial assessment should include control of hemorrhage and shock along with resuscitation as required. Resuscitation may require intravenous lines and a urethral catheter in the seriously injured patient. In men, before the catheter is inserted, the urethral meatus should be examined carefully for the presence of blood. Once the intravenous lines are established, if any suspicion of renal or ureteral injury is entertained, contrast material should be injected intravenously for later x-ray study.

The history should include a detailed description of the accident. In cases involving gunshot wounds, the type and caliber of the weapon should be determined, since high-velocity projectiles cause much more extensive damage.

The abdomen and genitalia should be examined for evidence of contusions or subcutaneous hematomas, which might indicate deeper injuries to the retroperitoneum and pelvic structures. Fractures of the lower ribs are often associated with renal injuries and pelvic fractures with bladder and urethral injuries. Diffuse abdominal tenderness is consistent with perforated bowel, free intraperitoneal blood or urine, or retroperitoneal hematoma. As an aid to diagnosis of intraperitoneal injuries, a small catheter inserted percutaneously into the abdomen followed by irrigation will help detect free intraperitoneal blood.

Initial radiographic studies should be done in the trauma unit, if possible, before moving the patient. Plain films of the abdomen will disclose early excretion of contrast material injected at the time intravenous lines were inserted. Lower rib fractures, vertebral body and transverse process fractures, and pelvic fractures may be associated with severe urinary tract injuries. Early extravasation of contrast material may be noted with renal, ureteral, or bladder injuries.

Patients who do not have life-threatening injuries and whose blood pressure is stable can undergo more deliberate radiographic studies. This provides more definitive staging of the injury.

Special Examinations (Fig 17–1)

When genitourinary tract injury is suspected on the basis of the history and physical examination, additional studies are required to establish its extent.

A. Catheterization and Assessment of Injury: Assessment of the injury should be done in an orderly fashion, so that accurate and complete information is obtained. This process of defining the extent of injury is termed "staging." The algorithm (Fig 17–1) outlines the staging process for urogenital trauma.

1. Catheterization– Blood at the urethral meatus in men indicates urethral injury; catheterization should not be attempted if blood is present, but retrograde urethrography should be done immediately. If no blood is present at the meatus, a urethral catheter can be carefully passed to the bladder to recover urine; microscopic or gross hematuria indicates urinary system injury. If catheterization is traumatic despite the greatest care, the significance of hematuria cannot be determined, and other studies must be done to investigate the possibility of urinary system injury.

2. Excretory urography– Immediately after intravenous lines have been established and the resuscitation process has begun, 150 mL (2 mL/kg) of contrast material can be injected intravenously by push technique. As hypotension is overcome and renal perfusion improves, plain abdominal films will permit adequate visualization of the kidneys. This technique allows evaluation of renal injuries without undue delay before emergency operations, if indicated. If renal injury seems likely from the urogram, nephrotomography should be done immediately. In most cases, it is not necessary to inject more contrast medium, since adequate contrast medium remains, and tomography will give additional information regarding parenchymal injuries.

3. Retrograde cystography– Filling of the bladder with contrast material is essential to establish whether bladder perforations exist. At least 300 mL of contrast medium should be instilled for full vesical distention. A film should be obtained with the bladder filled and a second one after the bladder has emptied itself by gravity drainage. These 2 films will establish the degree of bladder injury as well as the size of the surrounding pelvic hematomas.

4. Urethrography– A small (12F) catheter can

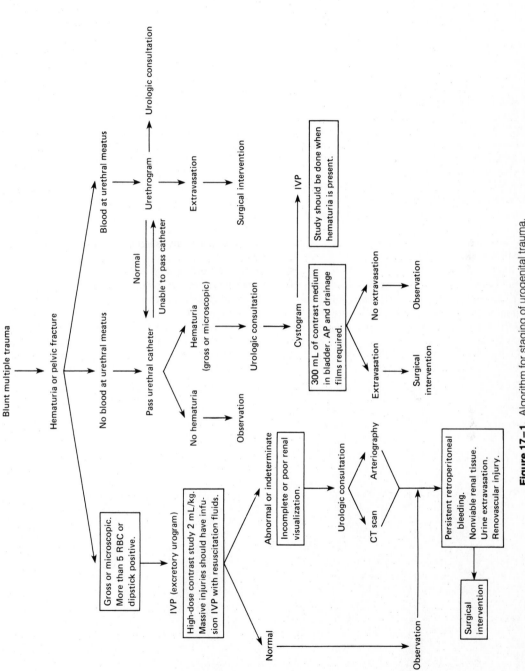

Figure 17–1. Algorithm for staging of urogenital trauma.

be inserted into the urethral meatus and 3 mL of water placed in the balloon to hold the catheter in position. After retrograde injection of 20 mL of water-soluble contrast material, the urethra will be clearly outlined on film, and extravasation in the deep bulbar area in case of straddle injury—or free extravasation into the retropubic space in case of prostatomembranous disruption—will be visualized.

5. Arteriography–Arteriography may help define renal parenchymal and renal vascular injuries. It is also useful in the detection of persistent bleeding from pelvic fractures for purposes of embolization with Gelfoam or autologous clot.

6. Computed tomography–CT scans can help in assessing the size and extent of retroperitoneal hematomas and renal parenchymal trauma. It is a noninvasive test that gives accurate and fast information when excretory urography does not adequately establish the degree and extent of renal injury.

B. Cystoscopy and Retrograde Urography: These studies are seldom necessary, since information can be obtained by less invasive techniques.

INJURIES TO THE KIDNEY

Renal injuries are the most common injuries of the urinary system. The kidney is well protected by heavy lumbar muscles, vertebral bodies, ribs, and the viscera anteriorly. Fractured ribs and transverse vertebral processes may penetrate the renal parenchyma or vascula-

ture. Most injuries occur from automobile accidents or sporting mishaps, chiefly in men and boys. Kidneys with existing pathologic conditions such as hydronephrosis or malignant tumors are more readily ruptured from mild trauma.

Etiology
(Fig 17–2)

Blunt trauma directly to the abdomen, flank, or back is the most common mechanism, accounting for 80–85% of all renal injuries. Trauma may result from motor vehicle accidents, fights, falls, and contact sports. Vehicle collisions at high speed may result in major renal trauma from rapid deceleration and cause major vascular injury. Gunshot and knife wounds cause most penetrating injuries to the kidney; any such wound in the flank area should be regarded as a cause of renal injury until proved otherwise. Associated abdominal visceral injuries are present in 80% of renal penetrating wounds.

Pathology & Classification
(Fig 17–3)

A. Early Pathologic Findings: Lacerations from blunt trauma usually occur in the transverse plane of the kidney. The mechanism of injury is thought to be force transmitted from the center of the impact to the renal parenchyma. In injuries from rapid deceleration, the kidney moves upward or downward, causing sudden stretch on the renal pedicle and sometimes complete or partial avulsion. Acute thrombosis

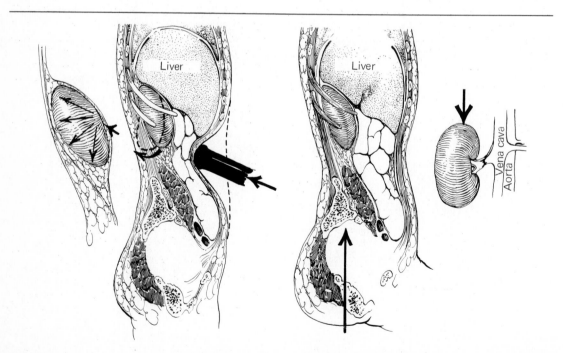

Figure 17–2. Mechanisms of renal injury. *Left:* Direct blow to abdomen. Smaller drawing shows force of blow radiating from the renal hilum. *Right:* Falling on buttocks from a height (contrecoup of kidney). Smaller drawing shows direction of force exerted upon the kidney from above. Tear of renal pedicle.

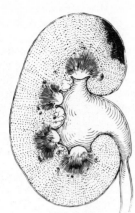

Ecchymosis

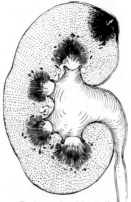

Ecchymosis with small
subcapsular hematoma

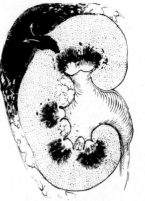

Superficial cortical laceration
of parenchyma and capsule
with perirenal hematoma;
no extravasation

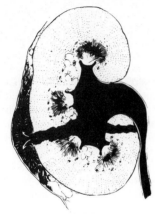

Deep corticomedullary laceration
of parenchyma and pelvis;
gross hematuria often present

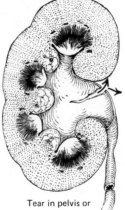

Tear in pelvis or
ureter; urinary
extravasation

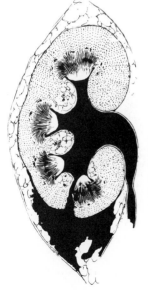

Deep corticomedullary
laceration of parenchyma
and pelvis; extravasation
of blood and urine;
gross hematuria usual

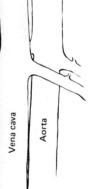

Laceration of renal
vascular pedicle with
severe perirenal
hemorrhage

Figure 17–3. Types and degrees of renal injury.

of the renal artery may be caused by an intimal tear from rapid deceleration injuries owing to the sudden stretch.

Pathologic classification of renal injuries is as follows:

1. Minor renal trauma–(85% of cases.) Renal contusion or bruising of the parenchyma is the most common lesion. Subcapsular hematoma in association with contusion is also noted. Superficial cortical lacerations are also considered minor trauma. These injuries rarely require surgical exploration.

2. Major renal trauma–(15% of cases.) Deep corticomedullary lacerations may extend into the collecting system, resulting in extravasation of urine into the perirenal space. Large retroperitoneal and perinephric hematomas often accompany these deep lacerations. Multiple lacerations may cause complete destruction of the kidney. Laceration of the renal pelvis without parenchymal laceration from blunt trauma is rare.

3. Vascular injury–(About 1% of all blunt trauma cases.) Vascular injury of the renal pedicle is rare but may occur, usually from blunt trauma. There may be total avulsion of the artery and vein or partial avulsion of the segmental branches of these vessels. Stretch on the main renal artery without avulsion may result in renal artery thrombosis. Vascular injuries are difficult to diagnose and result in total destruction of the kidney unless the diagnosis is made promptly.

B. Late Pathologic Findings: (Fig 17–4.)

1. Urinoma–Deep lacerations that are not repaired may result in persistent urinary extravasation and late complications of a large perinephric renal mass and, eventually, hydronephrosis and abscess formation.

2. Hydronephrosis–Large hematomas in the retroperitoneum and associated urinary extravasation may result in perinephric fibrosis engulfing the ureteropelvic junction, causing hydronephrosis. Follow-up excretory urography is indicated in all cases of major renal trauma.

3. Arteriovenous fistula–Arteriovenous fistulas may occur after penetrating injuries but are not common.

4. Renal vascular hypertension–The blood flow in tissue rendered nonviable by injury is compromised; this results in renal vascular hypertension in about 1% of cases. Fibrosis from surrounding trauma has also been reported to constrict the renal artery and cause renal hypertension.

Clinical Findings

Microscopic or gross hematuria following trauma to the abdomen indicates injury to the urinary tract. It bears repeating that stab or gunshot wounds to the flank area should alert the physician to possible renal injury whether or not hematuria is present. Some cases of renal vascular injury are not associated with hematuria. These cases are almost always due to rapid deceleration accidents and are an indication for intravenous urography.

The degree of renal injury does not correspond to the degree of hematuria, since gross hematuria may occur in minor renal trauma and only mild hematuria

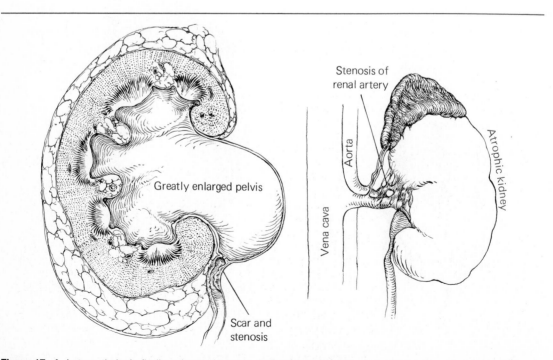

Figure 17–4. Late pathologic findings in renal trauma. *Left:* Ureteropelvic stenosis with hydronephrosis secondary to fibrosis from extravasation of blood and urine. *Right:* Atrophy of kidney caused by injury (stenosis) of arterial blood supply.

in major trauma. The presence of hematuria demands evaluation.

A. Symptoms: There is usually visible evidence of abdominal trauma. Pain may be localized to one flank area or over the abdomen. Associated injuries such as ruptured abdominal viscera or multiple pelvic fractures also cause acute abdominal pain and may obscure the presence of renal injury. Catheterization will usually reveal hematuria. Retroperitoneal bleeding may cause abdominal distention, ileus, and nausea and vomiting.

B. Signs: Initially, shock or signs of a large loss of blood from heavy retroperitoneal bleeding may be noted. Ecchymosis in the flank or upper quadrants of the abdomen is often noted. Lower rib fractures are frequently found. Diffuse abdominal tenderness may be found on palpation; and "acute abdomen" indicates free blood in the peritoneal cavity. A palpable mass may represent a large retroperitoneal hematoma or perhaps urinary extravasation. If the retroperitoneum has been torn, free blood may be noted in the peritoneal cavity but no palpable mass will be evident. The abdomen may be distended and bowel sounds absent.

C. Laboratory Findings: Microscopic or gross hematuria is usually present. The hematocrit may be normal initially, but a drop may be found when serial studies are done. This finding represents persistent retroperitoneal bleeding and development of a large retroperitoneal hematoma. Persistent bleeding may require operation.

D. Staging and X-Ray Findings: Staging of renal injuries allows a systematic approach to these problems (Fig 17–1). Adequate studies help define the extent of injury and dictate appropriate management. For example, blunt trauma to the abdomen associated with gross hematuria and a normal urogram requires no additional renal studies; however, nonvisualization of the kidney will require immediate arteriography or CT scan to determine whether renal vascular injury exists. Ultrasonography and retrograde urography are of little use initially in the evaluation of renal injuries.

Staging begins with excretory urography as soon as the intravenous lines are established and resuscitation has begun. This procedure avoids the delay involved in requesting a plain film of the abdomen but does not deprive the examiner of information that would be obtained on the plain film, ie, whether bone fracture, free air, or displaced bowel is present. The urogram should establish the presence or absence of both kidneys, clearly define the renal outlines and cortical borders, and outline the collecting systems and ureters (Fig 17–5).

Nephrotomography is indicated if the urogram does not fully define the extent of injury. Tomograms outline the cortical borders and establish the presence of cortical lacerations, intrarenal hematomas, and areas of poor vascular perfusion. Excretory urography combined with tomography will adequately stage 85% of renal injuries.

Arteriography defines major arterial and parenchy-

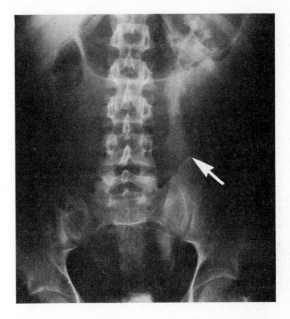

Figure 17–5. Blunt renal trauma to left kidney demonstrating extravasation (*at arrow*) on intravenous urogram.

mal injuries when previous studies have not fully done so. Arterial thrombosis and avulsion of the renal pedicle are best diagnosed by arteriography and are likely when the kidney is not visualized on the excretory urogram (Fig 17–6). The major causes of nonvisualization on an excretory urogram are total pedicle avulsion, arterial thrombosis, severe contusion causing vascular spasm, and absence of the kidney (either congenital or from operation).

Computed tomography (CT scan) has proved to be an effective means of staging renal trauma. This noninvasive technique provides excellent definition of parenchymal lacerations, clearly defines extravasa-

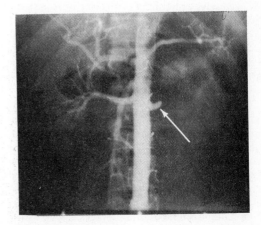

Figure 17–6. Arteriogram following blunt abdominal trauma shows typical findings of acute renal artery thrombosis (*arrow*) of left kidney.

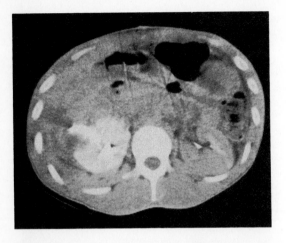

Figure 17–7. CT scan of right kidney following knife stab wound. Laceration with urine extravasation is seen. Large right retroperitoneal hematoma is present.

tion, shows extension of perirenal hematoma, defines nonviable renal tissue, and outlines surrounding organs such as the pancreas, liver, and major vessels (Fig 17–7).

Radionuclide renal scans have been used in staging renal trauma. However, in emergency management, this technique is less sensitive than arteriography or CT scan.

Differential Diagnosis

Trauma to the abdomen and flank areas is not always associated with renal injury. In such cases, there is no hematuria, and the results of excretory urography are normal.

Complications

A. Early Complications: Hemorrhage is perhaps the most important immediate complication of renal injury. Heavy retroperitoneal bleeding may result in rapid exsanguination. Patients must be observed closely, with careful monitoring of blood pressure and hematocrit. Complete staging must be done early (Fig 17–1). The size and expansion of palpable masses must be carefully monitored. Bleeding will cease spontaneously in 80–85% of cases. Persistent retroperitoneal bleeding or heavy gross hematuria may require early operation.

Urinary extravasation from renal fracture may show as an expanding mass (urinoma) in the retroperitoneum. These collections are prone to abscess formation and sepsis. A resolving retroperitoneal hematoma may cause slight fever (38.3 °C [101 °F]), but higher temperatures suggest infection. A perinephric abscess may form, resulting in abdominal tenderness and flank pain. Prompt operation is indicated.

B. Late Complications: Hypertension, hydronephrosis, arteriovenous fistula, calculus formation, and pyelonephritis are important late complications. Careful monitoring of blood pressure for several months is necessary to watch for hypertension. At 3–6 months, a follow-up excretory urogram should be obtained to be certain that perinephric scarring has not caused hydronephrosis or vascular compromise; renal atrophy may occur from vascular compromise and will be detected by follow-up urography.

Heavy late bleeding may occur 1–4 weeks after injury.

Treatment

A. Emergency Measures: The objectives of early management are prompt treatment of shock and hemorrhage, complete resuscitation, and evaluation of associated injuries.

B. Surgical Measures:

1. Blunt injuries–Minor renal injuries from blunt trauma account for 85% of cases and do not usually require operation. Bleeding stops spontaneously with bed rest and hydration. Cases in which operation is indicated include those associated with persistent retroperitoneal bleeding, urinary extravasation, evidence of nonviable renal parenchyma, and renal pedicle injuries (15% of all renal injuries). Aggressive preoperative staging allows complete definition of injury before operation.

2. Penetrating injuries–Penetrating injuries should be surgically explored. A rare exception to this rule is when staging has been complete and only minor parenchymal injury, with no urinary extravasation, is noted. In 80% of cases of penetrating injury, associated organ injury requires operation; thus, renal exploration is only an extension of this procedure.

C. Treatment of Complications: Retroperitoneal urinoma or perinephric abscess demands prompt surgical drainage. Malignant hypertension requires vascular repair or nephrectomy. Hydronephrosis may require surgical correction or nephrectomy.

Prognosis

With careful follow-up, most renal injuries have an excellent prognosis, with spontaneous healing and return of renal function. Follow-up excretory urography and monitoring of blood pressure will ensure detection and appropriate management of late hydronephrosis and hypertension.

INJURIES TO THE URETER

Ureteral injury is rare but may occur, usually during the course of a difficult pelvic surgical procedure or as a result of gunshot wounds. Rapid deceleration accidents may avulse the ureter from the renal pelvis. Endoscopic basket manipulation of ureteral calculi may also result in injury. Injury to the intramural ureter during transurethral resections also occurs.

Etiology

Large pelvic masses (benign or malignant) may displace the ureter laterally and engulf it in reactive fibrosis. This may lead to ureteral injury during dissection, since the organ is anatomically malpositioned. Inflammatory pelvic disorders may involve the ureter in a similar way. Extensive carcinoma of the colon may invade areas outside the colon wall and directly involve the ureter; thus, resection of the ureter may be required along with resection of the tumor mass. Devascularization may occur with extensive pelvic lymph node dissections or after radiation therapy to the pelvis for pelvic cancer. In these situations, ureteral fibrosis and subsequent stricture formation may develop along with ureteral fistulas.

Endoscopic manipulation of a ureteral calculus with a stone basket or ureteroscope may result in ureteral perforation or avulsion. Passage of a ureteral catheter beyond an area of obstruction may perforate the ureter. This is usually secondary to the acute inflammatory process in the ureteral wall and surrounding the calculus.

Pathogenesis & Pathology

The ureter may be inadvertently ligated and cut during difficult pelvic surgery. In such cases, sepsis and severe renal damage usually occur postoperatively. If a partially divided ureter is unrecognized at operation, urinary extravasation and subsequent buildup of a large urinoma will ensue, which will usually lead to ureterovaginal or ureterocutaneous fistula formation. Intraperitoneal extravasation of urine can also occur, causing ileus and peritonitis. After partial transection of the ureter, some degree of stenosis and reactive fibrosis develops, with concomitant mild to moderate hydronephrosis.

Clinical Findings

A. Symptoms: If the ureter has been completely or partially ligated during operation, the postoperative course is usually marked by fever of 38.3–38.8 °C (101–102 °F) as well as flank and lower quadrant pain. Such patients often experience paralytic ileus with nausea and vomiting. If ureterovaginal or cutaneous fistula develops, it usually does so within the first 10 postoperative days. Bilateral ureteral injury will be manifested by postoperative anuria.

Ureteral injuries from external violence should be suspected in patients who have sustained stab or gunshot wounds to the retroperitoneum. The mid portion of the ureter seems to be the most common site of penetrating injury. There are usually associated vascular and other abdominal visceral injuries.

B. Signs: The acute hydronephrosis of a totally ligated ureter will result in severe flank pain and abdominal pain with nausea and vomiting early in the postoperative course and with associated ileus. Signs and symptoms of acute peritonitis may be present if there is urinary extravasation into the peritoneal cavity. Watery discharge from the wound or vagina may be identified as urine by determining the creatinine concentration of a small sample—urine has many times the creatinine concentration found in serum— and by intravenous injection of 10 mL of indigo carmine, which will appear in the urine as dark blue.

C. Laboratory Findings: Ureteral injury from external violence is manifested by microscopic hematuria in 90% of cases. Urinalysis and other laboratory studies are of little use in diagnosis when injury has occurred from other causes. The serum creatinine level usually remains normal except in bilateral ureteral obstruction.

D. X-Ray Findings: Diagnosis is by excretory urography. A plain film of the abdomen may demonstrate a large area of increased density in the pelvis or in an area of retroperitoneum where injury is suspected. After injection of contrast material, delayed excretion is noted with hydronephrosis. Partial transection of the ureter will result in more rapid excretion, but persistent hydronephrosis is usually present and contrast extravasation at the site of injury will be noted on delayed films (Fig 17–8).

In acute injury from external violence, the excretory urogram usually appears normal, with very mild fullness down to the point of extravasation at the ureteral transection.

Retrograde ureterography will demonstrate the exact site of obstruction or extravasation.

E. Ultrasonography: Ultrasonography will outline hydroureter or urinary extravasation as it develops into a urinoma and is perhaps the best means of ruling out ureteral injury in the early postoperative period. It has the advantages of being noninvasive and rapid.

F. Radionuclide Scanning: Radionuclide scanning will demonstrate delayed excretion on the injured side, with evidence of increasing counts owing to accumulation of urine in the renal pelvis. Its great benefit, however, is to assess renal function after surgical correction.

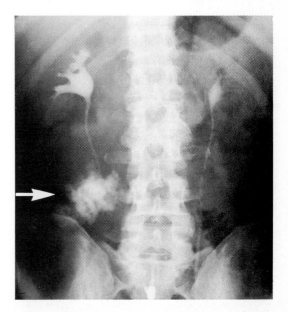

Figure 17–8. Stab wound of right ureter shows extravasation (*at arrow*) on intravenous urogram.

Differential Diagnosis

Postoperative bowel obstruction and peritonitis may cause symptoms similar to those of acute ureteral obstruction from injury. Fever, "acute abdomen," and associated nausea and vomiting following difficult pelvic surgery are definite indications for screening sonography or excretory urography to establish whether ureteral injury has occurred.

Deep wound infection must be considered postoperatively in patients with fever, ileus, and localized tenderness. The same findings are consistent with urinary extravasation and urinoma formation.

Acute pyelonephritis in the early postoperative period may also result in findings similar to those of ureteral injury. Sonography is normal, and urography shows no evidence of obstruction.

Drainage of peritoneal fluid through the wound from impending evisceration may be confused with ureteral injury and urinary extravasation. The creatinine concentration of the transudate will be similar to that of serum, whereas urine will contain very high creatinine levels.

Complications

Ureteral injury may be complicated by stricture formation with resulting hydronephrosis in the area of injury. Chronic urinary extravasation from unrecognized injury may lead to formation of a large retroperitoneal urinoma. Pyelonephritis from hydronephrosis and urinary infection may require prompt proximal drainage.

Treatment

Prompt treatment of ureteral injuries is required. The best opportunity for successful repair is in the operating room when the injury occurs. If the injury is not recognized until 10–14 days after the event and no infection, abscess, or other complications exist, immediate reexploration and repair are indicated. Proximal urinary drainage by percutaneous nephrostomy or formal nephrostomy should be considered if the injury is recognized late or if the patient has significant complications that make immediate reconstruction unsatisfactory. The goals of ureteral repair are to achieve complete debridement, a tension-free spatulated anastomosis, watertight closure, ureteral stenting (in selected cases), and retroperitoneal drainage.

A. Lower Ureteral Injuries: Injuries to the lower third of the ureter allow several options in management. The procedure of choice is reimplantation into the bladder combined with a psoas-hitch procedure to minimize tension on the ureteral anastomosis. An antireflux type procedure should be done when possible. Primary ureteroureterostomy can be utilized in lower third injuries when the ureter has been ligated without transection. The ureter is usually long enough for this type of anastomosis. Bladder tube flap can be utilized when the ureter is shorter.

Transureteroureterostomy may be utilized in lower third injuries if extensive urinoma and pelvic infection have developed. This procedure allows anastomosis and reconstruction in an area away from the pathologic processes.

B. Mid Ureteral Injuries: Mid ureteral injuries usually result from external violence and are best repaired by primary ureteroureterostomy or transureteroureterostomy.

C. Upper Ureteral Injuries: Injuries to the upper third of the ureter are best managed by primary ureteroureterostomy. If there is extensive loss of the ureter, autotransplantation of the kidney can be done as well as bowel replacement of the ureter.

D. Stenting: Most anastomoses after repair of ureteral injury should be stented. The preferred technique is to insert a silicone internal stent through the anastomosis before closure. These stents are "double-J'd" to prevent their migration in the postoperative period. After 3–4 weeks' healing, stents can be endoscopically removed from the bladder. The advantages of internal stenting are maintenance of a straight ureter with a constant caliber during early healing, the presence of a conduit for urine during healing, prevention of urinary extravasation, maintenance of urinary diversion, and easy removal.

Prognosis

The prognosis for ureteral injury is excellent if the diagnosis is made early and prompt corrective surgery is done. Delay in diagnosis worsens the prognosis because of infection, hydronephrosis, abscess, and fistula formation.

INJURIES TO THE BLADDER

Bladder injuries occur most often from external force and are often associated with pelvic fractures. (About 15% of all pelvic fractures are associated with concomitant bladder or urethral injuries.) Iatrogenic injury may result from gynecologic and other extensive pelvic procedures as well as from hernia repairs and transurethral operations.

Pathogenesis & Pathology
(Fig 17–9)

The bony pelvis protects the urinary bladder very well. When the pelvis is fractured by blunt trauma, fragments from the fracture site may perforate the bladder. These perforations usually result in extraperitoneal rupture. If the urine is infected, extraperitoneal bladder perforations may result in deep pelvic abscess and severe pelvic inflammation.

When the bladder is filled to near capacity, a direct blow to the lower abdomen may result in bladder disruption. This type of disruption ordinarily is intraperitoneal. Since the reflection of the pelvic peritoneum covers the dome of the bladder, a linear laceration will allow urine to flow into the abdominal cavity. If the diagnosis is not established immediately and if the urine is sterile, no symptoms may be noted for several days. If the urine is infected, immediate peritonitis and acute abdomen will develop.

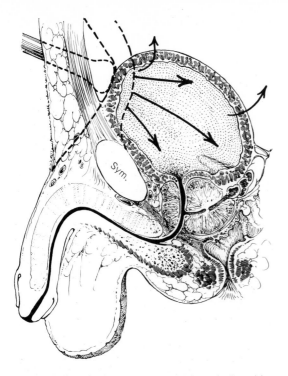

Figure 17–9. Mechanism of vesical injury. A direct blow over the full bladder causes increased intravesical pressure. If the bladder ruptures, it will usually rupture into the peritoneal cavity.

Clinical Findings

Pelvic fracture accompanies bladder rupture in 90% of cases. The diagnosis of pelvic fracture can be made initially in the emergency room by lateral compression on the bony pelvis, since the fracture site will show crepitus and be painful to the touch. Lower abdominal and suprapubic tenderness is usually present. Pelvic fracture and suprapubic tenderness with acute abdomen suggest intraperitoneal bladder disruption.

A. Symptoms: There is usually a history of lower abdominal trauma. Blunt injury is the usual cause. Patients ordinarily are unable to urinate, but when spontaneous voiding occurs, gross hematuria is usually present. Most patients complain of pelvic or lower abdominal pain.

B. Signs: Heavy bleeding associated with pelvic fracture may result in hemorrhagic shock, usually from venous disruption of pelvic vessels. Evidence of external injury from a gunshot or stab wound in the lower abdomen should make one suspect bladder injury, manifested by marked tenderness of the suprapubic area and lower abdomen. Acute abdomen indicates intraperitoneal bladder rupture. A palpable mass in the lower abdomen usually represents a large pelvic hematoma. On rectal examination, landmarks may be indistinct because of a large pelvic hematoma.

C. Laboratory Findings: Catheterization usually is required in patients with pelvic trauma but not if bloody urethral discharge is noted. Bloody urethral

discharge indicates urethral injury, and a urethrogram is necessary before catheterization (Fig 17–1). When catheterization is done, gross or, less commonly, microscopic hematuria is usually present. Urine taken from the bladder at the initial catheterization should be cultured to determine whether infection is present.

D. X-Ray Findings: A plain abdominal film will generally demonstrate pelvic fractures. There may be haziness over the lower abdomen from blood and urine extravasation. An intravenous urogram should be obtained to establish whether kidney and ureteral injuries are present.

Bladder disruption will be shown on cystography (Fig 17–1). The bladder should be filled with 300 mL of contrast material and a plain film of the lower abdomen obtained. Contrast medium should then be allowed to drain out completely, and a second film of the abdomen should be obtained. The drainage film is extremely important, because it will demonstrate areas of extraperitoneal extravasation of blood and urine that may not appear on the filling film (Fig 17–10). With intraperitoneal extravasation, free contrast medium will be visualized in the abdomen, highlighting bowel loops (Fig 17–11).

E. Instrumental Examination: If urethral injury is suspected (bloody discharge), a urethrogram should be obtained before any attempt is made to catheterize the patient. If there is no evidence of urethral injury, catheterization can be safely accomplished.

Cystoscopy is not indicated, since bleeding and clots obscure visualization and prevent accurate diagnosis.

Differential Diagnosis

Abdominal trauma with hematuria may cause in-

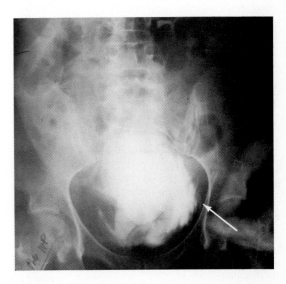

Figure 17–10. Extraperitoneal bladder rupture. Extravasation (*at arrow*) seen outside the bladder in the pelvis on cystogram.

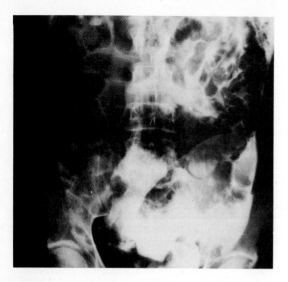

Figure 17–11. Intraperitoneal bladder rupture. Cystogram shows contrast surrounding loops of bowel.

jury to the kidney and ureter as well as the bladder. A urogram is indicated for all patients with trauma-related hematuria. Associated injuries to the pelvic vessels and bowel should also be considered.

The urethra may be injured as well as the bladder; this possibility should be considered in any patient with blunt trauma and pelvic fractures. Urethrography will demonstrate disruption of the urethra.

Complications

A pelvic abscess may develop from extraperitoneal bladder rupture; if the urine becomes infected, the pelvic hematoma becomes infected too.

Intraperitoneal bladder rupture with extravasation of urine into the abdominal cavity will cause delayed peritonitis.

Partial incontinence may result from bladder injury when the laceration extends into the bladder neck. Meticulous repair may ensure normal urinary control.

Treatment

A. Emergency Measures: Shock and hemorrhage should be treated.

B. Surgical Measures: A lower midline abdominal incision should be made. As the bladder is approached in the midline, a pelvic hematoma, which is usually lateral, should be avoided. Entering the pelvic hematoma can result in increased bleeding from release of tamponade and in infection of the hematoma, with subsequent pelvic abscess. The bladder should be opened in the midline and carefully inspected. After repair, a suprapubic cystostomy tube is usually left in place to ensure complete urinary drainage and control of bleeding.

1. Extraperitoneal rupture–Extraperitoneal rupture should be repaired intravesically. As the bladder is opened in the midline, it should be carefully in-

spected and lacerations closed from within. Polyglycolic acid or chromic absorbable sutures should be used.

Extraperitoneal bladder lacerations occasionally extend into the bladder neck and should be repaired meticulously. Fine absorbable sutures should be used to ensure complete reconstruction, so that the patient will have urinary control after injury. Such injuries are best managed with indwelling urethral catheterization and suprapubic diversion.

Peritoneotomy should be done and the intra-abdominal fluid inspected before completing the procedure. If abdominal fluid is bloody, complete abdominal exploration should be done to rule out associated injuries.

2. Intraperitoneal rupture–Intraperitoneal bladder ruptures should be repaired via a transperitoneal approach after careful transvesical inspection and closure of any other perforations. The peritoneum must be closed carefully over the area of injury. The bladder is then closed in separate layers by absorbable suture. All extravasated fluid from the peritoneal cavity should be removed before closure. At the time of closure, care should be taken that the suprapubic cystostomy is in the extraperitoneal position.

3. Pelvic fracture–Stable fracture of the pubic rami is usually present. In such cases, the patient can be ambulatory within 4–5 days without damage or difficulty. Unstable pelvic fractures requiring external fixation have a more protracted course.

4. Pelvic hematoma–There may be heavy uncontrolled bleeding from rupture of pelvic vessels even if the hematoma has not been entered at operation. At exploration and bladder repair, packing the pelvis with laparotomy tapes often controls the problem. If bleeding persists, it may be necessary to leave the tapes in place for 24 hours and operate again to remove them. Embolization of pelvic vessels with Gelform or skeletal muscle under angiographic control is useful in controlling persistent pelvic bleeding.

C. Medical Measures: The patient whose cystogram shows only a small degree of extravasation can be managed by placing a urethral catheter into the bladder, without operation or suprapubic cystostomy. The urine must be free of infection. Hayes, Sandler, and Corriere (1983) have reported success with such management. Careful observation is necessary because of the potential for pelvic hematoma infection, continued bleeding from the bladder, and clot retention (Cass et al, 1983).

Prognosis

With appropriate treatment, the prognosis is excellent. The suprapubic cystostomy tube can be removed within 10 days, and the patient can usually void normally. Patients with lacerations extending into the bladder neck area may be temporarily incontinent, but full control is usually regained. At the time of discharge, urine culture should be performed to determine whether catheter-associated infection requires further treatment.

INJURIES TO THE URETHRA

Urethral injuries are uncommon and occur most often in men, usually associated with pelvic fractures or straddle type falls. They are rare in women.

Various parts of the urethra may be lacerated, transected, or contused. Management varies according to the level of injury. The urethra can be separated into 2 broad anatomic divisions: the posterior urethra, consisting of the prostatic and membranous portions; and the anterior urethra, consisting of the bulbous and pendulous portions.

1. INJURIES TO THE POSTERIOR URETHRA

Etiology
(Fig 17–12)

The membranous urethra passes through the urogenital diaphragm and is the portion of the posterior urethra most likely to be injured. The urogenital diaphragm contains most of the voluntary urinary sphincter. It is attached to the pubic rami inferiorly, and when pelvic fractures occur from blunt trauma, the membranous urethra is sheared from the prostatic apex at the prostatomembranous junction. The urethra can also be transected by the same mechanism at the interior surface of the membranous urethra.

Pathogenesis & Pathology

Injuries to the posterior urethra commonly occur from blunt trauma and pelvic fractures. The urethra usually is sheared off just proximal to the urogenital diaphragm, and the prostate is displaced superiorly by the developing hematoma in the periprostatic and perivesical spaces.

Clinical Findings

A. Symptoms: Patients usually complain of lower abdominal pain and inability to urinate. A history of crushing injury to the pelvis is usually obtained.

B. Signs: Blood at the urethral meatus is the single most important sign of urethral injury. The importance of this finding cannot be overemphasized, because an attempt to pass a urethral catheter may result in infection of the periprostatic and perivesical hematoma and conversion of an incomplete laceration to a complete one. The presence of blood at the external urethral meatus indicates that immediate urethrography is necessary to establish the diagnosis.

Suprapubic tenderness and the presence of pelvic fracture will be noted on physical examination. A large developing pelvic hematoma may be palpated. Perineal or suprapubic contusions are often noted. Rectal examination may reveal a large pelvic hematoma with the prostate displaced superiorly. Rectal examination can be misleading, however, because a tense pelvic hematoma may resemble the prostate on palpation. Superior displacement of the prostate does

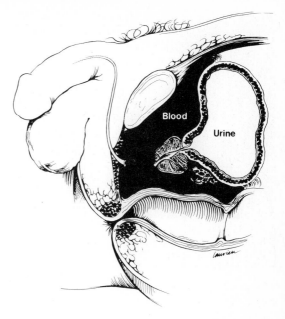

Figure 17–12. Injury to the posterior (membranous) urethra. The prostate has been avulsed from the membranous urethra secondary to fracture of the pelvis. Extravasation occurs above the triangular ligament and is periprostatic and perivesical.

not occur if the puboprostatic ligaments remain intact. Partial disruption of the membranous urethra (currently 10% of cases) is not accompanied by prostatic displacement.

C. Laboratory Findings: Anemia due to hemorrhage may be noted. Urine cannot usually be obtained initially, since the patient should not void and catheterization should not be attempted.

D. X-Ray Findings: Fractures of the bony pelvis are usually present. A urethrogram (using 20–30 mL of water-soluble contrast material) will show the site of extravasation at the prostatomembranous junction. Ordinarily, there is free extravasation of contrast material into the perivesical space (Fig 17–13). Incomplete prostatomembranous disruption will be seen as minor extravasation, with a portion of contrast material passing into the prostatic urethra and bladder.

E. Instrumental Examination: The only instrumentation involved should be for urethrography. Catheterization or urethroscopy should not be done, because these procedures pose an increased risk of hematoma and infection and further damage to partial urethral disruptions.

Differential Diagnosis

Bladder rupture may be associated with posterior urethral injuries. An intravenous urogram should be considered part of the assessment. Delayed films should be obtained to demonstrate the bladder and note extravasation. Cystography cannot be done preoperatively, since a urethral catheter should not be

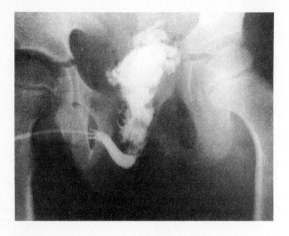

Figure 17-13. Ruptured prostatomembranous urethra shows free extravasation on urethrogram. No contrast medium is seen entering the prostatic urethra.

passed. Careful evaluation of the bladder at operation is necessary.

The anterior portion of the urethra may be injured as well as the prostatomembranous urethra.

Complications

Stricture, impotence, and incontinence as complications of prostatomembranous disruption are among the most severe and debilitating mishaps that result from trauma to the urinary system.

Stricture following primary repair and anastomosis occurs in about half of cases. If the preferred transpubic approach with delayed repair is used, the incidence of stricture can be reduced to about 5%.

The incidence of impotence after primary repair is 30-80% (mean, about 50%). This can be reduced to 10-15% by suprapubic drainage with delayed urethral reconstruction.

Incontinence in primary reanastomosis is noted in one-third of patients. Delayed reconstruction reduces the incidence to less than 5%.

Treatment

A. Emergency Measures: Shock and hemorrhage should be treated.

B. Surgical Measures: Urethral catheterization should be avoided.

1. Immediate management-Initial management should consist of suprapubic cystostomy to provide urinary drainage. A midline lower abdominal incision should be made, care being taken to avoid the large pelvic hematoma. The bladder and prostate are usually elevated superiorly by large periprostatic and perivesical hematomas. The bladder will often be distended by a large volume of urine accumulated during the period of resuscitation and operative preparation. The urine is often clear and free of blood, but gross hematuria may be present. The bladder should be opened in the midline and carefully inspected for lacerations.

If a laceration is present, the bladder should be closed with absorbable suture material and a cystostomy tube inserted for urinary drainage. This approach involves no urethral instrumentation or manipulation. The suprapubic cystostomy is maintained in place for about 3 months. This allows resolution of the pelvic hematoma, and the prostate and bladder will slowly return to their anatomic positions.

Incomplete laceration of the posterior urethra will heal spontaneously, and the suprapubic cystostomy can be removed within 2-3 weeks. The cystostomy tube should not be removed before voiding cystourethrography shows that no extravasation persists.

2. Urethral reconstruction-Reconstruction of the urethra after prostatic disruption can be undertaken within 3 months, assuming there is no pelvic abscess or other evidence of persistent pelvic infection. Before reconstruction, a combined cystogram and urethrogram should be done to determine the exact length of the resulting urethral stricture. This stricture usually is 1-2 cm long and situated immediately posterior to the pubic bone. The preferred approach is transpubic urethroplasty with direct excision of the strictured area and anastomosis of the bulbous urethra directly to the apex of the prostate. A 16F silicone urethral catheter should be left in place along with a suprapubic cystostomy. Catheters are removed within a month, and the patient is then able to void (Fig 17-14).

3. Immediate urethral realignment-Some surgeons prefer to realign the urethra immediately. Direct suture reconstruction of the prostatomembranous disruption in the acute injury is extremely difficult. Persistent bleeding and surrounding hematoma create technical problems. The incidence of stricture, impotence, and incontinence appears to be higher than with immediate cystostomy and delayed reconstruction.

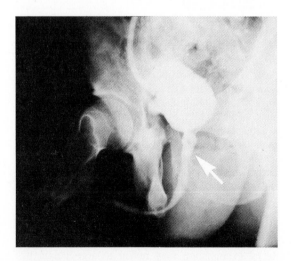

Figure 17-14. Delayed repair of urethral injury. Normal voiding urethrogram after transpubic repair of stricture following prostatomembranous urethral disruption. Arrow indicates area of repair.

However, Patterson et al (1983) have reported success with immediate urethral realignment.

C. General Measures: After delayed reconstruction by a transpubic approach, patients are allowed ambulation by the fifth postoperative day. No abnormality in gait or persistent pain due to removal of the pubic bone will be noted.

D. Treatment of Complications: Approximately 1 month after the delayed transpubic reconstruction, the urethral catheter can be removed and a voiding cystostogram obtained through the suprapubic cystostomy tube. If the cystogram shows a patent area of reconstruction free of extravasation, the suprapubic catheter can be removed; if there is extravasation or stricture, suprapubic cystostomy should be maintained. A follow-up urethrogram should be obtained within 2 months to watch for stricture development.

Stricture, if present, is usually very short, and urethrotomy under direct vision offers easy and rapid cure.

The patient may be impotent for several months after delayed repair. Impotence is permanent in about 10% of cases. Implantation of a penile prosthesis is indicated if impotence is still present 2 years after reconstruction (see Chapter 36).

Incontinence seldom follows transpubic reconstruction. If present, it will usually resolve slowly.

Prognosis

If complications can be avoided, the prognosis is excellent. Urinary infections ultimately resolve with appropriate management.

2. INJURIES TO THE ANTERIOR URETHRA

Etiology
(Fig 17–15)

The anterior urethra is that portion distal to the urogenital diaphragm. Straddle injury may cause laceration or contusion of the urethra. Self-instrumentation or iatrogenic instrumentation may cause partial disruption.

Pathogenesis & Pathology

A. Contusion: Contusion of the urethra is a sign of crush injury without urethral disruption. Perineal hematoma usually resolves without complications.

B. Laceration: A severe straddle injury may result in laceration of part of the urethral wall, allowing extravasation of urine. If the extravasation is unrecognized, it may extend into the scrotum, along the penile shaft, and up to the abdominal wall. It is limited only by Colles' fascia and often results in sepsis, infection, and serious morbidity.

Clinical Findings

A. Symptoms: There is usually a history of a fall, and in some cases a history of instrumentation. Bleeding from the urethra is usually present. There is local pain into the perineum and sometimes massive perineal hematoma. If voiding has occurred and extravasation is noted, sudden swelling in the area will be present. If diagnosis has been delayed, sepsis and severe infection may be present.

B. Signs: The perineum is very tender, and a mass may be found. Rectal examination reveals a normal prostate. The patient usually has a desire to void, but voiding should not be allowed until assessment of the urethra is complete. No attempt should be made to pass a urethral catheter, but if the patient's bladder is overdistended, percutaneous suprapubic cystostomy can be done as a temporary procedure.

When presentation of such injuries is delayed, there is massive urinary extravasation and infection in the perineum and the scrotum. The lower abdominal wall may also be involved. The skin is usually swollen and discolored.

C. Laboratory Findings: Blood loss is not usually excessive, particularly if secondary injury has occurred. The white count may be elevated with infection.

D. X-Ray Findings: A urethrogram, with instillation of 15–20 mL of water-soluble contrast material, will demonstrate extravasation and the location of injury (Fig 17–16). The contused urethra will show no evidence of extravasation.

E. Instrumental Examination: If there is no evidence of extravasation on the urethrogram, a urethral catheter may be passed into the bladder. Extravasation is a contraindication to further instrumentation at this time.

Differential Diagnosis

Partial or complete disruption of the prostatomembranous urethra may occur if pelvic fracture is present. Urethrography will usually demonstrate the location and extent of extravasation and its relationship to the urogenital diaphragm.

Complications

Heavy bleeding from the corpus spongiosum injury may occur in the perineum as well as through the urethral meatus. Pressure applied to the perineum over the site of the injury usually controls bleeding. If hemorrhage cannot be controlled, immediate operation is required.

The complications of urinary extravasation are chiefly sepsis and infection. Aggressive debridement and drainage are required if there is infection.

Stricture at the site of injury is a common complication, but surgical reconstruction may not be required unless the stricture significantly reduces urinary flow rates.

Treatment

A. General Measures: Major blood loss usually does not occur from straddle injury. If heavy bleeding does occur, local pressure for control, followed by resuscitation, is required.

B. Specific Measures:

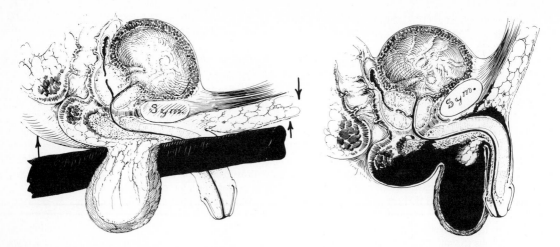

Figure 17–15. Injury to the bulbous urethra. *Left:* Mechanism: Usually a perineal blow or fall astride an object; crushing of urethra against inferior edge of pubic symphysis. *Right:* Extravasation of blood and urine enclosed within Colles' fascia (see Fig 1–9).

1. Urethral contusion–The patient with urethral contusion shows no evidence of extravasation, and the urethra remains intact. After urethrography, the patient is allowed to void; and if the voiding occurs normally, without pain or bleeding, no additional treatment is necessary. If bleeding persists, urethral catheter drainage can be done.

2. Urethral lacerations–Instrumentation of the urethra following urethrography should be avoided. A small midline incision in the suprapubic area readily exposes the dome of the bladder so that a suprapubic cystostomy tube can be inserted, allowing complete urinary diversion while the urethral laceration heals. If only minor extravasation is noted on the urethrogram, a voiding study can be performed within 7 days after suprapubic catheter drainage to search for extravasa-

tion. In more extensive injuries, one should wait 2–3 weeks before doing a voiding study through the suprapubic catheter. Healing at the site of injury may result in stricture formation. Most of these strictures are not severe and do not require surgical reconstruction. The suprapubic cystostomy catheter may be removed if no extravasation is documented. Follow-up with documentation of urinary flow rates will show whether there is urethral obstruction from stricture.

3. Urethral laceration with extensive urinary extravasation–After major laceration, urinary extravasation may involve the perineum, scrotum, and lower abdomen. Drainage of these areas is indicated. Suprapubic cystostomy for urinary diversion is required. Infection and abscess formation are common and require antibiotic therapy.

4. Immediate repair–Immediate repair of urethral lacerations can be performed, but the procedure is difficult and the incidence of associated stricture is high.

C. Treatment of Complications: Strictures at the site of injury may be extensive and require delayed reconstruction.

Prognosis

Urethral stricture is a major complication but in most cases does not require surgical reconstruction. If, when stricture resolves, urinary flow rates are poor and urinary infection and urethral fistula are present, reconstruction is required.

INJURIES TO THE PENIS

Disruption of the tunica albuginea of the penis (penile fracture) can occur during sexual intercourse. At presentation, the patient has penile pain and hematoma. This injury should be surgically corrected.

Gangrene and urethral injury may be caused by ob-

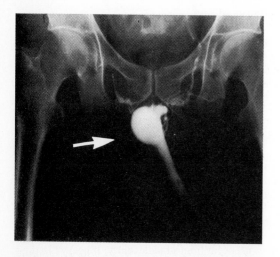

Figure 17–16. Ruptured bulbar (anterior) urethra following straddle injury. Extravasation (*at arrow*) on urethrogram.

structing rings placed around the base of the penis. These objects must be removed without causing further damage. Penile amputation is seen occasionally, and in a few patients the penis can be surgically replaced successfully by microsurgical techniques.

Total avulsion of the penile skin occurs from machinery injuries. Immediate debridement and skin grafting are usually successful in salvage.

Injuries to the penis should suggest possible urethral damage, which should be investigated by urethrography.

INJURIES TO THE SCROTUM

Superficial lacerations of the scrotum may be debrided and closed primarily. Blunt trauma may cause local hematoma and ecchymosis, but these injuries resolve without difficulty. One must be certain that testicular rupture has not occurred.

Total avulsion of the scrotal skin may be caused by machinery accidents or other major trauma. The testes and spermatic cords are usually intact. It is important to provide coverage for these structures: this is best done by immediate surgical debridement and by placing the testes and spermatic cords in the subcutaneous tissues of the upper thighs. Later reconstruction of the scrotum can be done with a skin graft or thigh flap.

INJURIES TO THE TESTIS

Blunt trauma to the testis causes severe pain and, often, nausea and vomiting. Lower abdominal tenderness may be present. A hematoma may surround the testis and make delineation of its margin difficult. Ultrasonography can be used as an aid to better define the organ. If rupture has occurred, the sonogram will delineate the injury, which should be surgically repaired.

REFERENCES

Emergency Diagnosis & Management

Ahmed S, Morris LL: Renal parenchymal injuries secondary to blunt abdominal trauma in childhood: A 10-year review. *Br J Urol* 1982;**54:**470.

Baker WNW, Mackie DB, Newcombe JF: Diagnostic paracentesis in the acute abdomen. *Br Med J* 1967;**3:**146.

Barlow B, Gandhi R: Renal artery thrombosis following blunt trauma. *J Trauma* 1980;**20:**614.

Cass AS: Blunt renal trauma in children. *J Trauma* 1983;**23:**123.

Cass AS: Renal trauma in multiple-injured child. *Urology* 1983;**21:**487.

Danto LA: Paracentesis and diagnostic peritoneal lavage. Pages 45–58 in: *Trauma Management.* Vol 1. Thieme-Stratton, 1982.

Shaftan GW: The initial evaluation of the multiple-injured patient. *World J Surg* 1983;**7:**19.

Injuries to the Kidney

Bernath AS et al: Stab wounds of the kidney: Conservative management in flank penetration. *J Urol* 1983;**129:**468.

Carini M et al: Surgical treatment of renovascular hypertension secondary to renal trauma. *J Urol* 1981;**126:**101.

Carroll PR, McAninch JW: Operative indications in penetrating renal trauma. *J Trauma* 1985;**25:**587.

Cass A et al: Renal pedicle injury in patients with multiple injuries. *J Trauma* 1985;**25:**892.

Cass AS, Luxenberg M: Conservative or immediate surgical management of blunt renal injuries. *J Urol* 1983;**130:**11.

Cosgrove MD, Mendez R, Morrow JW: Traumatic renal arteriovenous fistula: Report of 12 cases. *J Urol* 1973;**110:**627.

Erturk E et al: Renal trauma: Evaluation by computerized tomography. *J Urol* 1985;**133:**946.

Guice K et al: Hematuria after blunt trauma: When is pyelography useful? *J Trauma* 1983;**23:**305.

Kuzmarov IW, Morehouse DD, Gibson S: Blunt renal trauma in the pediatric population: A retrospective study. *J Urol* 1981;**126:**648.

McAninch JW, Carroll PR: Renal trauma: Kidney preservation through improved vascular control: A refined approach. *J Trauma* 1982;**22:**285.

McAninch JW, Federle MP: Evaluation of renal injuries with computerized tomography. *J Urol* 1982;**128:**456.

Nicolaisen GS et al: Renal trauma: Re-evaluation of the indications for radiographic assessment. *J Urol* 1985;**133:**183.

Peterson NE: Fate of functionless posttraumatic renal segment. *Urology* 1986;**27:**237.

Sagalowsky AI, McConnell JD, Peters PC: Renal trauma requiring surgery: An analysis of 185 cases. *J Trauma* 1983;**23:**128.

Skinner DG: Traumatic renal artery thrombosis: A successful thrombectomy and revascularization. *Ann Surg* 1973;**177:**264.

von Knorring J, Fyhrquist F, Ahonen J: Varying course of hypertension following renal trauma. *J Trauma* 1981;**126:**798.

Injuries to the Ureter

Cass AS: Ureteral contusion with gunshot wounds. *J Trauma* 1984;**24:**59.

Drago JR et al: Bilateral ureteropelvic junction avulsion after blunt abdominal trauma. *Urology* 1981;**27:**169.

Fackler ML et al: Bullet fragmentation: A major cause of tissue disruption. *J Trauma* 1984;**24:**35.

Liroff SA, Pontes JE, Pierce JM Jr: Gunshot wounds of the ureter: 5 year experience. *J Urol* 1977;**118:**551.

Peterson NE, Pitts JC III: Penetrating injuries to the ureter. *J Urol* 1981;**126:**587.

Stutzman RE: Ballistics and the management of ureteral injuries from high velocity missiles. *J Urol* 1977;**118:**947.

Injuries to the Bladder

Carroll PR, McAninch JW: Major bladder trauma: The accuracy of cystography. *J Urol* 1983;**130:**887.

Carroll PR, McAninch JW: Major bladder trauma: Mechanisms of injury and a unified method of diagnosis and repair. *J Urol* 1984;**132**:254.

Cass AS et al: Nonoperative management of bladder rupture from external trauma. *Urology* 1983;**22**:27.

Hayes EE, Sandler CM, Corriere JN Jr: Management of the ruptured bladder secondary to blunt abdominal trauma. *J Urol* 1983;**129**:946.

Montie J: Bladder injuries. *Urol Clin North Am* 1977;**4**:59.

Injuries to the Urethra

Devine PC, Devine CJ Jr: Posterior urethral injuries associated with pelvic fractures. *Urology* 1982;**20**:467.

Gibson GR: Impotence following fractured pelvis and ruptured urethra. *Br J Urol* 1970;**42**:86.

Johanson B: Reconstruction of male urethral strictures. *Acta Chir Scand [Suppl]* 1953;**176**:1. [Entire issue.]

Malloy TR, Wein AJ, Carpiniello L: Transpubic urethroplasty for prostatomembranous urethral disruption. *J Urol* 1980;**124**:359.

McAninch JW: Traumatic injuries to the urethra. *J Trauma* 1981;**21**:291.

Morehouse DD, MacKinnon KJ: Management of prostatomembranous urethral disruption: 13 year experience. *J Urol* 1980;**123**:173.

Patterson DE et al: Primary realignment of posterior urethral injuries. *J Urol* 1983;**129**:513.

Waterhouse K, Laugani G, Patil U: The surgical repair of membranous urethral strictures: Experience with 105 consecutive cases. *J Urol* 1980;**123**:500.

Webster GD, Mathes GL, Selli C: Prostatomembranous urethral injuries: A review of the literature and a rational approach to their management. *J Urol* 1983;**130**:898.

Injuries to the Penis

Bergner DM, Wilcox ME, Frentz GD: Fractures of penis. *Urology* 1982;**20**:278.

Flowerdew R, Fishman IJ, Churchill BM: Management of penile zipper injury. *J Urol* 1977;**117**:671.

Mendez R, Kiely WF, Morrow JW: Self-emasculation. *J Urol* 1972;**107**:981.

Nicolaisen GS et al: Rupture of the corpus cavernosum: Surgical management. *J Urol* 1983;**130**:917.

Tuerk M, Weir WH Jr: Successful replantation of a traumatically amputated glans penis. *Plast Reconstr Surg* 1971;**48**:499.

Injuries to the Scrotum

McAninch JW et al: Major traumatic and septic genital injuries. *J Trauma* 1984;**24**:291.

McDougal WS: Scrotal reconstruction using thigh pedicle flaps. *J Urol* 1983;**129**:757.

Injuries to the Testis

Anderson KA et al: Ultrasonography for the diagnosis and staging of blunt scrotal trauma. *J Urol* 1983;**130**:933.

Cass AS: Testicular trauma. *J Urol* 1983;**129**:299.

Fournier GR Jr et al: High resolution scrotal ultrasonography: A highly sensitive but nonspecific diagnostic technique. *J Urol* 1985;**134**:490.

McConnell JD, Peters PC, Lewis SE: Testicular rupture in blunt scrotal trauma: Review of 15 cases with recent application of testicular scanning. *J Urol* 1982;**128**:309.

Pollen JJ, Funckes C: Traumatic dislocation of the testes. *J Trauma* 1982;**22**:247.

Schulman CC: Traumatic rupture of the testicle: An underestimated pathology. *Urol Int* 1974;**29**:31.

Immunology of Genitourinary Tumors

18

Perinchery Narayan, MD

The term immune derives from the Latin *immunis,* meaning "exempt from charges (taxes)." For nearly a century, the term immunity has meant resistance to illness, usually infection. Current understanding of the immune system, however, reveals that it is much more complex than previously believed. The immune system not only provides defenses against infectious disease but is also intricately involved in defense against neoplastic disease and, more importantly, in the maintenance of normal homeostasis and health.

The immune system exerts control over the entire body by an extensive network of cellular and humoral components. The response of the system to antigenic challenge by an infection or neoplasm is complex and integrated and affects the whole organism. Several aspects of the immune response are still incompletely understood; however, certain broad concepts have been tested and several mechanisms clarified.

This chapter will describe briefly the major components of the immune system, the immunologic concepts of oncogenesis, the experimental and established techniques of immunologic diagnosis, and various types of immunotherapy as they apply to genitourinary cancer.

COMPONENTS OF THE IMMUNE SYSTEM

The communication network of the immune system may be considered as having 2 components: a humoral component, mediated by biochemical molecules, and a cellular component, composed of a few distinct cell types.

Cellular Immunity

The major cellular elements are macrophages and lymphocytes.

A. Macrophages: Macrophages are derived from monocytes and are found ubiquitously throughout the body. They may be found in the circulatory and lymphatic systems or may be specialized and relatively immobile in tissues. Examples of tissue macrophages are Kupffer cells of the reticuloendothelial system of the liver, alveolar macrophages of the lung, microglia of the brain, and histiocytes of connective tissue. Macrophages have the following functions:

1. Macrophages secrete biologically active mediators, which govern the type and magnitude of the T (thymus-derived) and B (bone marrow-derived) cell response to antigenic challenge. The mediators include several proteins of the complement system, lysosomal proteases, and other enzymes and lymphokines such as interferon and interleukin.

2. Macrophages are the principal phagocytic cells that phagocytize and destroy foreign cells. Phagocytosis is stimulated by specialized proteins called opsonins that adsorb to surfaces of foreign cells and render them susceptible.

3. Macrophages possess the ability to be antigen-presenting cells. This is a specialized function requiring processing of antigen and presentation of the antigenic determinant on the cell surface for reaction with lymphocytes.

4. The macrophage surface has several markers, including receptors for antigens, antibodies, complement, and specialized proteins (Ia antigens) involved in T cell interactions. Based on the presentation of antigens, the lymphocytic reaction may be stimulatory or suppressive.

B. Lymphocytes: Lymphocytes are antigen-specific and act via receptors on their surfaces. Each receptor is highly specific, and clones of cells express similar specificity. The origin of lymphocyte clones and their receptor specificity is a matter of debate. There is evidence for both genetic regulation as well as somatic mutation, and there is controversy as to which factor is predominant.

T lymphocytes may be classified as regulatory T cells (helper or suppressor T cells) and effector T cells (cells mediating delayed hypersensitivity; mixed lymphocyte reactivity or cytotoxic killer T cells). Killer T cells may be natural killer cells (NK) or antibody-dependent (K) killer cells.

B lymphocytes are precursors of antibody-forming cells and may be designated on the basis of the immunoglobulin classes as B γ, α, μ, δ, or ϵ. Mature antibody-producing B cells are also called plasma cells. There are also a group of B cells important in the rapid secondary response to antigen challenge (anamnestic reaction) called memory B cells.

C. Lymphokines: While antibody molecules are principally products of B cells, several other low-molecular-weight proteins are secreted by lymphocytes and macrophages in response to antigenic stimulation. These products are termed lymphokines. Lymphokines are active in low concentrations and interact with a variety of cells, including somatic cells, other lymphocytes, and macrophages to bring about biologic effects. Although initially discovered to be products of lymphocytes, lymphokines such as interferon (IFN) are now known to be produced by many other cells in the body.

D. Other Cellular Elements: Apart from lymphocytes and macrophages, several other circulating cells participate in immune activity. These cells are not as specialized, and their actions are nonspecific. These include neutrophils, basophils, eosinophils, platelets, and mast cells, among others.

Humoral Immunity

The basic component of humoral immunity is the immunoglobulin (Ig) molecule. Structurally, Ig molecules are composed completely of glycoproteins. Almost all functional activity resides in the polypeptide portion. Each Ig molecule is composed of 4 polypeptide chains: 2 identical light (L) chains and 2 identical heavy (H) chains. Each chain has a constant (C) region and a variable (V) region. The C region determines the biologic function. The V region determines the antigenic receptor site and the idiotype specificity, which in part helps to control the magnitude and duration of antibody response. The H chain determines the Ig class of the molecule (IgG, IgA, IgM, IgD, IgE). Even though there are only 5 major classes of Ig molecules, the total number of potentially available antibodies is increased tremendously by variability in the number and sequence of amino acids in the V regions.

Ig molecules have the following functions:

(1) Ig molecules form the antibodies released by mature B cells in response to antigenic challenge.

(2) Ig molecules function as antigen-specific receptors on the surface of B lymphocytes (there are also antigen-specific receptors on the surface of T cells, but it is unclear whether they are similar to Ig molecules).

(3) When Ig molecules bind to antigens, they initiate a variety of secondary immune phenomena such as complement fixation and release of biologic mediators by interaction with lymphocytes and macrophages. These biologic mediators have several functions in maintaining immune surveillance and in mounting the immune response to antigenic and neoplastic challenge. Some of them have pharmacologic actions (see Biologic Response Modifiers, below).

Genetic Control of the Immune System & Immune Regulation

Several mechanisms of genetic control of the immune system have been elucidated at a molecular level. One is the mechanism of generation of antibody diversity, which allows a few distinct immunocompetent cell types to generate 10^6–10^8 different antibody molecules. This is achieved in part by 2 separate structural genes collaborating to form a single Ig molecule. Another mechanism is regulation of the im-

mune system by the genes of the major histocompatibility complex (MHC). Genes within the MHC modulate the production of 3 classes of molecules: those involved in antigen "typing," lymphocyte interaction, and complement activation. These molecules regulate the response to antigens, graft-versus-host reactions, susceptibility to autoimmune diseases, allergic reactions, resistance to viruses, and many other functions. The capacity to reject tumors (transplant antigens) appears to be located in the D region at one end of the MHC complex.

The various components of the immune system function in an integrated manner. Several mechanisms have been postulated to explain the cell-cell communication and recognition that is the basis of the controlled immune response. One mechanism is idiotype-anti-idiotype recognition postulated by Jerne in 1974. This theory proposes that following the first wave of antibody production (idiotypes), several successive sets of anti-antibodies (anti-idiotypes) are produced that enhance or suppress further antibody production. A second proposed mechanism important in immune regulation is the presence of T cell suppressor circuits. Suppressor T cells, by their presence or absence, can suppress or enhance the B cell antibody response. Other postulated mechanisms of immune regulation include antigen processing by macrophages, regulation by suppressor determinants on some proteins, and production of blocking antibodies by neoplastic cells and products of the MHC. The complexity of reactivity is governed by the type of antigen, prior exposure to it, and the presence or absence of normal immunity in the host.

IMMUNOLOGIC CONCEPTS OF ONCOGENESIS

Immune Surveillance

The concept of immune surveillance was first proposed by Thomas and popularized by Burnet (1970) as the normal mechanism for prevention of tumor development. The rationale is that tumor cells arise frequently in all individuals by mutation but are usually recognized as "foreign" and destroyed by the immune system. There is experimental evidence that tumor cells dislodged into the circulating system in normal individuals are rapidly destroyed by the immune system. In the absence of a normal immune system, therefore, the incidence of tumors and metastases should be higher. Several clinical observations confirm a high incidence of tumors in immunodeficient states. For example, patients with congenital immunodeficiency diseases (eg, agammaglobulinemia, ataxia-telangiectasia, Wiskott-Aldrich syndrome, Chédiak-Higashi syndrome) have a 100-fold increase in the incidence of cancer, even at an early age. Similarly, patients with induced long-term immunosuppression, such as renal transplant patients, have a 100- to 200-fold increase in the incidence of cancer. Acquired immunodeficiency syndrome (AIDS) has also clearly been associated with an increased incidence of Kaposi's sarcoma and other cancers not normally found in this age group of patients. Most of these cancers involve lymphoreticular tissue, although some epithelial neoplasms have also been noted. Cancer patients with poor immunity (as determined by skin test reactivity or in vitro laboratory tests) have more rapid progression of disease and a poorer prognosis than patients with normal immune systems.

Tumor-Associated Antigens

There are extensive data showing that tumor-associated antigens exist in human tumors. A variety of biochemical and immunologic techniques have identified the presence of tumor-associated antigens on tumor cells and in serum, urine, and other body fluids. Tumor-associated antigens should be distinguished from tumor-specific antigens, which have not been conclusively demonstrated to have a role in human tumors. Tumor-associated antigens, while preferentially expressed by tumor cells, are not necessarily unique to them. The tumor-associated antigens that have been most useful clinically have the oncodevelopmental antigens (so called because they are also expressed normally by fetal cells). Notable examples of oncodevelopmental antigens are alpha-fetoprotein (AFP), the β subunit of human chorionic gonadotropin (β-hCG) and carcinoembryonic antigen. Recently, the discovery of monoclonal antibodies has added considerable data attesting to the existence of restricted cell surface antigens on tumors. Some of the most convincing evidence has been presented by Vessella and associates, who have isolated a monoclonal antibody restricted to high-grade renal cell carcinomas. Whether these and others will prove to be truly tumor-specific remains to be seen.

Host Immunity

If tumor-associated antigens exist, then the logical response of the host to a tumor would be production of antitumor antibodies and development of antitumor cell-mediated immune responses. There are both clinical and laboratory data to support the theory of host immunity in human cancers.

A. Renal Cancer: Patients with renal cancer have exhibited several features of natural host immunity. A dramatic example is the rare but definite occurrence of spontaneous regression in 0.3–0.8% of patients with metastatic renal cancer. Also, renal cancers exhibit varying growth patterns, with "quiescent" metastases for several years. While the median survival rate for patients with metastatic renal cancer is 11 months, 20% of patients live for 3 years or longer. Similarly, 11% of recurrences are seen 10 years or longer after removal of the primary tumor. Other indications of immune modulation in patients with renal cancer are the relatively good prognosis of patients following removal of tumors extending into large veins, including the vena cava, and the long-term survival of patients with bilateral renal cancer following parenchymal-sparing resections. The 5-year survival

rate following bilateral partial nephrectomy is 70%, with a recurrence rate of 10% (the same rates as for unilateral total nephrectomy for unilateral renal carcinoma). Finally, renal cancer is one of the few cancers in which resection of a solitary metastasis results in long-term cures.

There is laboratory evidence for both cellular and humoral immunity in patients with renal cancer. Hakala et al found complement-dependent, tumor-specific cytotoxic antibodies in patients with metastatic renal cancer. These antibodies were specific for renal cancer-associated antigens, since the cytotoxicity could be eliminated by absorption with autologous tumor cells but not autologous normal kidney cells. Also, high titers of complement-fixing antibodies have been demonstrated in patients with metastatic renal cancer. Antibody titers in these patients decrease after surgical excision of renal cancer and reappear when renal cancer recurs.

Evidence for cell-mediated immunity in renal cancer is available both from clinical studies and in vitro studies. Several investigators have noted a relation between cutaneous sensitivity to recall antigen dinitrochlorobenzene (DNCB) and tumor burden in patients with renal cancer. Several investigators have used cytotoxicity assays to measure cell-mediated immune responses in patients with renal cancer. Hellström, Cummings, and Bubenik have reported the cytotoxicity of lymphocytes from renal cancer patients using in vitro cultured renal cancer cell lines. Cole and Elhilali have extended these studies and shown a relationship between the presence of cytotoxic lymphocytes and the clinical stage of renal cancer. Other studies have noted changes in effector cell populations with disease progression in patients with renal cancer. Also, cell-mediated immunity in renal cancer has been demonstrated by use of leukocyte migration inhibition assays.

B. Bladder Cancer (Transitional Cell Carcinoma): Evidence of host immunity in transitional cell carcinoma has been studied in several ways. In the past, skin test reactivity was used to measure clinical response. In Catalona's study of 38 patients with potentially curable bladder cancer, 13 of 19 patients with poor DNCB reactivity developed recurrences and 11 died; in contrast, only 5 of 19 who had good DNCB reactivity developed recurrences and none died during the same period. However, other studies have not been able to demonstrate similar correlations. Other clinical evidence for immune reactivity of transitional cell carcinoma has come from the excellent response of superficial transitional cell carcinoma to treatment with intravesical live attenuated tubercle bacilli (bacillus Calmette-Guérin [BCG]). Intravesical BCG causes both systemic and local effects. The systemic effect is noted by the conversion of skin reactivity to purified protein derivative (PPD). Patients who are PPD-negative prior to BCG therapy become PPD-positive after several weeks of therapy. Also, the conversion of a negative PPD to a positive one during therapy denotes a favorable prognosis to therapy. Local effects of intravesical BCG are observed in the form of a localized inflammatory reaction in the bladder mucosa and the formation of "granulomas." The therapy is still experimental, however, and the therapeutic contributions of local versus systemic effects of BCG on superficial transitional cell carcinoma are still unclear.

Laboratory evidence of cellular immunity in transitional cell carcinoma has been obtained by cytotoxicity assays; which have demonstrated altered immune responses in patients with transitional cell carcinoma when compared to normal controls. Evidence of humoral immunity to transitional cell carcinoma has been noted by the presence of complement-dependent antibodies in the sera of transitional cell carcinoma patients.

C. Carcinoma of the Prostate: The immune status of patients with carcinoma of the prostate has been difficult to interpret because of the older age of patients and the slow growth of tumors. In one study, skin test reactivity to DNCB antigen was depressed in all patients tested, regardless of the stage of the disease. In vitro cytotoxicity assays have also produced conflicting results. A major problem has been the inability to artificially culture long-term cell lines of carcinoma of the prostate to conduct extensive cytotoxicity assays. Humoral immunity in carcinoma of the prostate has been identified in patients with carcinoma of the prostate and reportedly has caused regression of metastases in patients after cryosurgery. However, these reports have not been confirmed by other studies.

D. Carcinoma of the Testis: Human carcinoma of the testis has not been extensively investigated for immune reactivity for several reasons: (1) Carcinoma of the testis is rare, accounting for less than 5% of all genitourinary cancers; (2) seminoma, the most common histologic variant, cannot be cultured in vitro; and (3) carcinoma of the testis is sensitive to chemotherapy and irradiation and therefore has not been considered for immunotherapy. On the other hand, murine teratocarcinoma has been extensively studied morphologically and immunologically as a model to understand embryonic development as well as malignant transformation. Shared oncodevelopmental and embryonic antigens have been identified on murine and human teratocarcinoma cells. Also, work on the murine teratocarcinoma model has shown that regions within the MHC may influence neoplastic transformation. In humans, a relationship between the MHC and carcinoma of the testis has been shown by DeWolf and associates, who noted an increased prevalence of HLA-D locus Dw7 in patients with nonseminomatous carcinomas of the testis.

Tumor Heterogeneity & Adaptation to Host Responses

If antitumor antibody and cell-mediated immunity exist in human tumors, why is the body unable to destroy tumors more effectively? One speculation is that tumor-associated antigens may exist in close proximity to stronger antigens such as histocompatibility antigens and therefore may be masked and not adequately exposed to the body's defense systems. However, there is evidence that tumor cells are recognized and rapidly destroyed in the circulatory system, with its abundant immune factors, but because clones of metastatic cells are inherently chromosomally unstable, they mutate rapidly and by a process of selection establish themselves and grow in receptive tissue environments. The ultimate landing site is governed by a complex interrelated set of factors, currently the object of intense research. Factors that have been implicated include the composition of the tumor cell surface, the presence of basement membrane receptors, type IV collagenase, and circulating levels of prostaglandins, lymphokines, and other biologic modulators.

Other explanations are also available to account for the ability of tumor cells to escape immune surveillance. At early stages of tumor development, small foci of tumor cells may elaborate too small a quantity of tumor antigens to stimulate a strong antitumor immune response. By the time the host is fully sensitized, the tumor may be too large and growing too rapidly to be rejected.

It has also been suggested that tumor-bearing hosts possess factors that depress their immunocompetence in a nonspecific manner. Perhaps tumors themselves elaborate immunosuppressive factors. This suppression seems to be reversible, since normal immunity is often restored if the tumor is removed or otherwise treated. This concomitant immunity is, at least in some tumors, a problem of logistics; the quantity of tumor cells and tumor doubling time exceeds the cytolytic and cytostatic capacity of a finite immune response.

True immunoselection may also occur, whereby host immune responses may be altered or genetic variants of reduced or altered antigenicity may emerge. Immunoselection may also be important in determining whether or not metastases occur.

IMMUNOLOGIC METHODS IN TUMOR DIAGNOSIS

Immunologic methods in tumor diagnosis may be classified as (1) measurements of cellular or humoral host immunity and (2) serologic or histochemical measurements of tumor-associated antigens on tumor cells. Most assays of cellular and humoral immunity are experimental and not useful clinically. Measurements of tumor-associated antigens, however, are useful clinically in the diagnosis and management of patients with genitourinary cancers.

Tests of Cellular Immunity

Cellular immunity in cancer patients has been measured in the following ways: (1) Standard recall antigen panels such as DNCB, PPD, mumps antigen, *Candida* antigen, and streptokinase-streptodornase

(SKSD) antigens have been used to measure delayed cutaneous hypersensitivity reactions. (2) In vitro transformations of peripheral blood lymphocytes, as in mixed lymphocyte cultures, autologous tumor stimulation assays, and lymphocyte proliferation assays, have been used to measure T cell response to neoplastic cells. (3) Measurements of T cell subsets and their ratio in patients with cancer as opposed to normal controls have been performed using the sheep red blood cell "E" receptor rosette assay, as well as the OKT group of monoclonal antibodies. (4) Cytotoxicity assays have been used, in which antitumor cell cytotoxicity of antibody-dependent killer (K) T cells and antibody-independent natural killer (NK) T cells is measured in vitro. (5) Migration-inhibition assays have been used to measure the degree of lymphocyte activation by their ability to inhibit in vitro migration of macrophages and leukocytes. (6) Leukocyte-adherence inhibition assays have been performed to measure the ability of tumor cell extracts to prevent adherence of activated leukocytes in vitro.

Most of these techniques and their variants require sophisticated equipment or trained personnel and therefore are not available outside a research setting. Further, their diagnostic accuracy and specificity are variable in clinical settings. Thus, they have not enjoyed wide clinical application.

Tests of Humoral Immunity

Humoral immunity in cancer patients has been difficult to measure because of the polyclonality of antibodies and the logistics of developing assays to separate these antibodies. Tests have been adapted from conventional serologic assays and have included complement fixation, immunodiffusion, immunofluorescence, radioimmunoassays, and enzyme-linked immunoassays. These assays are usually insensitive and nonspecific. Old and colleagues have recently reaffirmed the existence of serologic reactivity to various cancers and have suggested a useful way of classifying antitumor antibodies based on 3 classes of antigens: (1) class I antigens, unique to the patient's tumor and not present on other tumors of the same histologic variety; (2) class II antigens, found on all tumors with similar histology and a few other tumors but not found in normal cells; and (3) class III antigens, found on a variety of tumor cells and in some normal cells. The availability of monoclonal antibodies should further clarify the existence and role of humoral immunity in cancer.

Measurement of Tumor-Associated Antigens

Measurement of tumor-associated antigens in serum and their detection in histologic specimens has been of practical value in the diagnosis and management of genitourinary cancers. The most commonly employed tests measure AFP and β-hCG. Both are oncodevelopmental antigens expressed by 60–80% of testicular cancers.

A. Alpha-Fetoprotein (AFP): AFP is a glycoprotein (MW 70,000) produced by the liver, yolk sac, and gastrointestinal tract of the fetus. It was first noted to be elevated in tumors by Abelev in 1963. In normal adults, levels of this marker are below 11 ng/mL. AFP has a half-life of 5 days. AFP levels are raised in most patients with hepatomas, in 75% of patients with nonseminomatous cancer of the testis, and occasionally in patients with gastrointestinal cancers of gastric, pancreatic, or biliary origin. Levels may also be elevated occasionally in patients undergoing hepatocellular regeneration (eg, patients with hepatitis). Serum AFP levels are of practical value in the management of patients with cancer of the testis.

Histochemical stains of AFP are important in distinguishing pure seminomas from those containing nonseminomatous elements and in the differential diagnosis of extragonadal germ cell carcinomas.

B. β Subunit of Human Chorionic Gonadotropin (β-hCG): Human chorionic gonadotropin (hCG) is a glycoprotein (MW 38,000) normally elevated in the first trimester of pregnancy. It is composed of 2 subunits, α and β. The α subunit is identical to the α subunit of luteinizing hormone, follicle-stimulating hormone, and thyroid-stimulating hormone. The β subunit is immunologically distinct from those of the other hormones and is therefore measurable. In normal adult males, the level of β-hCG is below 3 ng/mL. Its half-life is 2 days. The discovery that β-hCG was elevated in choriocarcinomas was made in 1930 by Zondek. In cancers of the testis, β-hCG is produced by syncytiotrophoblast cells. It is elevated in 50–60% of nonseminomatous cancers of the testis and in 10% of seminomatous tumors that contain these elements. It is useful in both serologic and histochemical assays.

Prostate-Specific Antigen

Prostate-specific antigen (PSA) is a recently identified biologic marker for prostate cancer. It is a protein of MW 34,000 and has no subunits. PSA is chemically and immunologically distinct from prostatic acid phosphatase (PAP). Several recent studies have suggested that PSA is not only of value in prostate cancer but that it may be prognostically more significant that PAP. Killian et al analyzed 602 serum specimens from 70 patients with prostate cancer and found that in those with PSA levels of 88 ng/mL, an average time of less than 2 months elapsed before clinical recurrence was evident. In a series of 64 patients, Ercole et al found that the presence of normal PSA levels preoperatively indicated localized prostatic cancer and that PSA levels were 50% more accurate in predicting recurrence than were PAP levels.

Other Tumor Markers

Several other serologic and immunohistochemical markers have been described for diagnosis and staging of genitourinary cancers (eg, placental alkaline phosphatase, ABO blood group antigens, serum pregnancy-associated antigens). Their usefulness is limited by the technical complexity and relative insensitivity of assay systems.

IMMUNOTHERAPY & BIOTHERAPY

Two recent advances in molecular biology have caused a resurgence of interest in the immune modulation of tumors. First, the discovery of monoclonal antibody technology has provided new insights into cell surface molecules of both tumor cells and cells of the immune system. Second, rapid growth in recombinant DNA technology has led to the commercial production of several biologic mediators, which have antitumor activity in pharmacologic doses. Many of these biologic mediators have actions that extend beyond the immune system, and they have therefore been termed biologic response modifiers. Therapy with biologic response modifiers is termed biologic therapy, or biotherapy. The term initially referred to naturally occurring biologic mediators and their synthetic counterparts. However, it is now replacing the term immunotherapy, as we begin to understand that the actions of the classic immunotherapeutic agents may extend beyond the immune system.

1. IMMUNOTHERAPY

For descriptive purposes, the classic forms of immunotherapy may be categorized as active immunotherapy (specific or nonspecific), passive immunotherapy, adoptive immunotherapy, and restorative immunotherapy.

Active Immunotherapy

Active immunotherapy, like active immunization, implies the use of vaccines to achieve immunity. Inactivated tumor cells or cell products are injected, with or without a nonspecific immunoadjuvant, to stimulate the immune response. The concept was first introduced by Prehn and Main in 1957 when they noted that chemically induced sarcomas in mice could specifically be made resistant to rechallenge by briefly growing these tumors and then excising them. The first human trial of active specific immunotherapy used intradermal injections of autologous homogenized tumor cells polymerized with ethylchlorformiate, along with PPD or *Candida* antigen. The most favorable responses to therapy were noted in patients with metastatic renal cell carcinoma. Since then, other trials have been conducted. The main criticism of these studies has been the uncontrolled nature of the trials, the cachexic patient population, and the large tumor burden expected to respond. Recently, Hoover et al conducted a controlled trial of active specific immunotherapy in colon cancer patients. This trial addressed drawbacks of earlier trials and was preceded by several years of careful, intensive animal studies. Preliminary results from this trial at 4 years of follow-up revealed statistically significant survival rates

among treated patients when compared with untreated controls. A similar trial of active specific immunotherapy in renal cancer is currently under way.

Active nonspecific immunotherapy utilizes powerful immunoadjuvants such as BCG to nonspecifically enhance the immune response to tumors. The advantages of this type of therapy are that it is simple and uncomplicated and does not require tumor tissue for vaccine. The obvious disadvantage is that it is nonspecific and can induce a powerful nonspecific immune response that may, in fact, deplete the immune system's capacity to respond to specific antigens. Several trials of active nonspecific immunotherapy have failed to show any significant survival advantage. Immunotherapy using BCG is further discussed under Biologic Response Modifiers, below.

Passive Immunotherapy

Passive immunotherapy, like passive immunization, is short-lived and has been the least successful type of immunotherapy for cancer. Passive immunotherapy involves the transfer of preformed antibodies into the host. Since tumor-specific antigens have not been conclusively identified, it has not been possible to obtain specific antibodies from serum for use in passive immunotherapy. Also, the polyclonal nature of the immune response has precluded the generation of pure high-affinity antibodies to any antigen.

Monoclonal Antibodies

A major advance in immunology was the development of monoclonal antibody techniques by Kohler and Milstein in 1975. Using the hybridoma technology of fusing specifically activated antibody-producing B lymphocytes to myeloma cells, scientists are now able to obtain large quantities of pure high-titer antibody of defined specificity consistently from single clones of cells. This has revolutionized the study of antibody structure and function and the antigenic composition of cells. The enormous potential of this technique has been realized in several ways. Monoclonal antibodies have already been useful in defining several new functions of lymphocytes and macrophages. They have identified new tumor-associated antigens and oncofetal antigens and have aided in histopathologic diagnosis, classification, and in vivo tumor detection. In vitro studies suggest that monoclonal antibodies are highly effective anticancer agents, especially when used in combination with chemotherapeutic and radioactive agents. Therapeutically, monoclonal antibodies have been used to remove T cells from bone marrow to improve bone marrow transplantation. While several problems still remain, especially with the currently available mouse monoclonal antibodies, the future is likely to see monoclonal antibodies as active immunotherapeutic agents.

Adoptive Immunotherapy

Adoptive immunotherapy implies transfer of immunocompetent cells and cell products that are able to functionally direct the host immune system. This type of therapy has been very effective in rodent leukemias and lymphomas. In humans, use of bone marrow transplants in patients with leukemias may be considered a form of adoptive immunotherapy. Use of "immune" RNA (a cell extract of RNA) is another form of adoptive immunotherapy. Immune RNA therapy has been attempted in renal cancer, although with minimal success. Adoptive immunotherapy using lymphokine-activated T cells is another technique that has shown promise in therapy of melanomas and renal cancer. This is further discussed under Biologic Response modifiers, below.

Restorative Immunotherapy

Restorative immunotherapy refers to functional repletion of immunocompetent cells by use of stimulants such as thymic hormones and agents such as levamisole. The rationale for its use is to stimulate precursor cells of the immune system to differentiate into activated cells. Use of agents such as cyclophosphamide in low doses to block the effects of suppressor T cells and prostaglandin synthetase inhibitors to block suppressor macrophages is also restorative immunotherapy. Restorative immunotherapy may become more widely used as we understand the intricacies of the immune system and learn to manipulate the various subpopulations of cells and their products.

2. BIOTHERAPY
(Biologic Response Modifiers)

Biologic response modifiers are a group of agents with widely varying actions that involve many cell types in the body. The term is broad enough to include all classic immunotherapeutic agents, as well as products of the immunocompetent cells (lymphokines, cytokines), thymic factors, antibodies, growth inhibitors, pharmacologic agents, and chemotherapeutic agents (Table 18–1). The primary therapeutic potential of biologic response modifiers is modulation of the

Table 18–1. Biologic response modifiers.

Complex biologics
  Bacillus Calmette-Guérin, *Corynebacterium parvum*
Pharmaceuticals
  Acridines, aziridines, tilorone, cimetidine, pyrimidinones, prostaglandin inhibitors, imidazoles, levamisole; polyribonucleotides (poly I · **C**, poly **L** · **C**)
Anticancer agents
  Cyclophosphamide, doxorubicin, vincristine, vinblastine, thiotepa, mitomycin
Naturally occurring biologic mediators and their synthetic counterparts
  Cytokines and lymphokines (interferons, interleukins, lymphotoxins, tumor necrosis factor); thymic factors (thymosin factor 5, α_1-thymosin)
Tumor-differentiating agents and growth inhibitors
  Cytarabine, dimethyl sulfoxide, hexamethylene bis-acetamide, retinoic acid, phorbol esters, neutrophil colony-stimulating factor, pluriprotein
Monoclonal antibodies

host immune response. Although biologic response modifiers have been known to exist for several years, the advent of recombinant DNA technology has made their pharmacologic use more feasible and valuable.

Complex Biologics

Microorganisms and microbial products have been studied extensively as biologic response modifiers. The first biologic response modifier used in large-scale studies was BCG. BCG is a live attenuated form of the tubercle bacillus and has been an integral part of several trials of nonspecific active immunotherapy. While systemic BCG has not been found useful for disseminated tumors, BCG seems to have some antitumor activity when injected directly into the tumor or in close proximity to it. Intradermal BCG for melanoma of the skin has been successful both in experimental animals and in humans. Recently, the usefulness of intravesical BCG for superficial bladder cancer has been confirmed by several trials. That the local effect of BCG is important is seen from the fact that transitional cell carcinomas of the prostatic urethra are not eradicated by intravesical BCG unless a prior transurethral resection allows BCG to come into contact with the prostatic urethra. That there is a systemic component to intravesical BCG is demonstrated by the fact that patients who are PPD-negative prior to therapy become PPD-positive after several weeks of therapy. Also, this conversion is related to a favorable prognosis of therapy. Five separate mechanisms have been advanced to explain the immunopotentiation of tumor immunity by BCG vaccine. These include enhancement of macrophage cytotoxicity, stimulation of lymphocyte trapping, activation of T lymphocytes, direct action on B lymphocytes, and immunostimulation because of shared antigens between BCG and tumor cell. There is evidence to support each of these mechanisms of action of BCG, and more than one mechanism may be involved in a specific tumor type.

Pharmaceuticals

Chemically defined immunomodulators have several advantages over complex biologics. They may be produced by chemical methods, purified to homogeneity, and studied by conventional pharmacologic approaches. The synthetic analogs of naturally occurring molecules also fall into this category. These include muramyl dipeptide, the smallest active component of mycobacterial cell walls; microbial polysaccharides; and polyribonucleotides. Two agents that have been studied clinically in this group include levamisole and poly I·C. Levamisole is an orally active synthetic phenylimidazole that affects T cell and macrophage function. In trials with colorectal cancer patients, levamisole was found to prolong survival when used as an adjunct to surgery and chemotherapy with 5-fluorouracil. Similar results have been noted with levamisole as an adjunct to chemotherapy in leukemia and multiple myeloma.

Poly I·C is a synthetic double-stranded complex of polyribonucleotides. It stimulates both antibody-mediated and cellular immune responses. In patients with breast cancer, poly I·C was found to prolong survival when used as an adjuvant to surgery and irradiation.

Anticancer Agents

Traditionally, it has been known that anticancer agents suppress immune reactivity by general inhibition of cell proliferation. However, certain anticancer drugs cause selective immunopotentiation. In humans, cyclophosphamide has been an immunopotentiator when used in combination with autologous tumor vaccines in patients with melanoma. The mechanism seems to be selective toxicity for suppressor T cells and their precursors. Other drugs such as thiotepa, mitomycin, doxorubicin, vincristine, and methotrexate have been shown to have immunopotentiative effects in animal experiments. The most important variable in determining immunopotentiation seems to be the timing of therapy. Administration of chemotherapy 3–4 days before antigen exposure is associated with the greatest immunopotentiation. This may have implications in the future for the design of clinical trials using chemotherapy and tumor vaccines.

Lymphokines & Cytokines

Lymphokines and cytokines are products of immunocompetent cells, which, in physiologic concentrations, function in cell-cell interaction and regulation of the immune response. However, in pharmacologic doses, they have several antitumor effects, including augmentation of T cell response and antiproliferative activity against neoplastic cells. Lymphokines that have been used clinically include interferons, interleukins, and lymphotoxins.

Interferons

Interferons (IFNs) are a family of naturally occurring small proteins (MW 15,000–21,000) secreted by virtually all cells in response to viral infections, tumors, and synthetic inducers. IFN was first identified by Isaacs and Lindemann (1957) as an excretory product of T cells produced in response to viral antigens. Although viruses are potent IFN inducers, a variety of other agents, including bacteria, rickettsiae, parasites, bacterial endotoxins, complex polysaccharides, chemicals, and antineoplastic agents such as dactinomycin, will induce IFN secretion. The molecular stimulant for IFN production is thought to be double-stranded RNA, either from natural inducers or from cell products of chemolysis. Synthetic RNA pairs such as polymers of polyinosinic acid and polycytidylic acid have been found to be potent stimulants of IFN secretion and have provided further evidence of the role of double-stranded RNA in IFN secretion.

Three major classes of IFN that have been identified on the basis of antigenic properties are IFN α, IFN β, and IFN γ. There are several subspecies within these 3 classes. Gene-splicing techniques have revealed 8 different genes coding for IFN α and 5 for IFN β. IFN α is normally produced by leukocytes, IFN β by fibroblasts, and IFN γ by T lymphocytes.

IFNs function as true biologic response modifiers in that they can modulate cell proliferation and differentiation, affect antibody formation, influence macrophage function, and augment cytotoxicity of T cells. IFNs have biologic activity against several cancers, including multiple myeloma, lymphomas, leukemias, and melanomas. In genitourinary cancers, preliminary studies have revealed IFN α to be active against renal cancer and superficial transitional cell carcinoma, including carcinoma in situ. Combining IFN α and IFN γ seems to potentiate antitumor activity, and clinical trials are under way to test the combination of these agents.

Interleukins

Interleukin-1 (IL-1), originally known as lymphocyte-activating factor, is a macrophage-derived cytokine. It was originally identified as a nonspecific enhancer of lymphocyte proliferation and is now known to be essential in the activation of T cell growth factor. Interleukin-2 (IL-2) is another lymphokine produced by human T cells. In murine tumor models, IL-2 has substantial antineoplastic activity alone or in combination with the adoptive transfer of lymphokine-activated killer T (LAK) cells. The mechanisms of action of this combination are not completely understood. Changes in immune system activity have included a redistribution of lymphoid cells in the peripheral vascular system, a 1- to 16-fold expansion of lymphoid cells in the peripheral blood, and the presence of IFN γ in the serum. The induction of secretion of other lymphokines may also play a role. In human trials, IL-2 derived from natural (human T cell tumors) and recombinant DNA sources has been active against a variety of tumors, including renal cancer, melanomas, colon cancer, Kaposi's sarcoma, and breast carcinoma. A multi-institutional trial of IL-2 along with LAK cells for these cancers is currently in progress.

Lymphotoxins are products of mitogen-stimulated leukocytes. A variety of inducers, both specific and nonspecific, can stimulate lymphocytes to release lymphotoxins. Several forms of lymphotoxins are released by different subpopulations of lymphocytes, depending on the inducer. Certain lymphotoxin forms have cytolytic and growth-inhibitory effects on transformed cells in vitro and in vivo. Synergy between lymphotoxin forms and IFN has also been noted and will be important for the design of future trials. These agents are involved in several aspects of the immune response, including T cell-mediated cytotoxicity.

Recently, a group of molecules termed tumor necrosis factors, similar in activity to lymphotoxins, have been isolated. Lymphotoxin activity may be potentiated when used in combination with other lymphokines and chemotherapeutic agents.

Thymic Factors

Several thymic extracts have biologic activity in the immune system. Thymosin factor 5 and α_1-thymosin have been studied in some detail. Thymosins correct immunodeficiency states and augment T cell responses in patients with cancer. α_1-Thymosin has been made synthetically and is currently undergoing clinical trials.

Chalones, Endogenous Growth Inhibitors, & Differentiation Agents

A. Chalones: Just as there are growth factors responsible for and involved in cell growth, there are growth inhibitors, or chalones, involved in preventing cell proliferation. The word chalone is derived from the Greek word for "to lower." The function of chalones was first postulated to be maintenance of balance between cell growth and attrition among hemopoietic and epithelial cells by tissue-specific growth inhibition (acting in concert with growth promotion in a feedback system). More recent research reveals that growth inhibitors are tissue-nonspecific, that they may be involved in the control mechanisms of several organ systems, and that their primary action may be in promoting cell maturation rather than inhibition of cell division. Response of tumors to chalones has been described in skin cancer, myelocytic leukemias, and lymphomas in animal models and in a small series of patients with lymphocytic leukemias.

B. Differentiation Agents: Other growth inhibitors of tumor cells have been termed differentiation agents. The differentiation agents that have been studied clinically include chemotherapeutic agents, polar compounds, phorbol diesters, vitamin analogs, and cytokines. Among chemotherapeutic agents, cytarabine has been shown to promote differentiation of leukemic cells. Among polar-planer compounds, dimethyl sulfoxide (DMSO) and hexamethylene bisacetamide are active agents that promote cell differentiation. Retinoic acid, a metabolite of vitamin A, is of critical importance in the maturation of epithelial cells and promotes in vitro differentiation of embryonal cancer cells. Similarly, vitamin D promotes mat-

uration of hemopoietic cells. Phorbol esters that bind to protein kinase C can induce a spectrum of cell differentiations, and this is being exploited clinically. Among cytokines, a specific type of neutrophil colony-stimulating factor (G-CSF) in murine systems and a human counterpart termed pluriprotein have been described. Differentiation agents are an important group of potential biologic response modifiers.

The era of biologic therapy is just beginning. More than 100 types of biologic response modifiers have been described. With recombinant DNA technology, more of these agents are likely to be developed and used in clinical trials.

SUMMARY

In summary, the accumulated knowledge of immunology of tumors suggests that the immune system can and does combat cancer to varying degrees and that it is possible to modify the system to increase its effectiveness. However, application of these concepts to clinical therapy of human cancers has so far met with only limited success. Among the factors that may be responsible are the wide variation in the immune response of each individual to similar cancers; varying age, general health, and nutritional status of individuals with similar cancers; incomplete understanding of the complexity of the immune response; and availability of alternate modes of therapy.

The future of immunotherapy and biologic response modification is bright. As trials of immunotherapy are refined, therapeutic activity will be enhanced and toxicity diminished. It is clear that successful cancer therapy requires a multimodal approach and that immunotherapy will take its proper place in the armamentarium of the oncologist. Eventually, modulation of the immune response will not only combat existing cancers but may prevent new occurrences, the ultimate goal of all therapy.

REFERENCES

Components of the Immune System

Bellanti JA (editor): *Immunology*, 2nd ed. Saunders, 1978.

Bloom W, Fawcett DW (editors): *A Textbook of Histology*, 10th ed. Saunders, 1975.

Burnett FM: *The Clonal Selection Theory of Acquired Immunity*. Columbia Univ Press, 1959.

Dreyer WJ, Bennett JC: The molecular basis of antibody formation: A paradox. *Proc Natl Acad Sci USA* 1965;**54:**864.

Golub ES: *The Cellular Basis of the Immune Response*. Sinauer, 1977.

Holborow JE, Reeves GW (editors): *Immunology in Medicine* 2nd ed. Grune & Stratton, 1983.

Hood LE et al (editors): *Immunology*. Benjamin/Cummings, 1984.

Jerne NK: Toward a network theory of the immune system. *Ann Immunol* 1974;**125C:**373.

Paul WE (editor): *Fundamental Immunology*. Raven Press, 1983.

Stites DP, Stobo JD, Wells JV (editors): *Basic & Clinical Immunology*, 6th ed. Appleton & Lange, 1987.

Immunologic Concepts of Oncogenesis

Alexander P, Eccles SA: Host mediated mechanisms in the elimination of circulating cancer cells. Chap 20, pp 293–308, in: *Cancer Invasion and Metastases: Biologic and Therapeutic Aspects*. Nicholson GL, Milas L (editors). Raven Press, 1983.

Artzt K et al: Surface antigens common to mouse cleavage embryos and primitive teratocarcinoma cells in culture. *Proc Natl Acad Sci USA* 1973;**70:**2988.

Bean MA et al: Cytotoxicity of lymphocytes from patients with cancer of the urinary bladder: Detection by a 3-H-proline microcytotoxicity test. *Int J Cancer* 1974;**14:**186.

Bloom HJG: Hormone-induced and spontaneous regression of metastatic renal cancer. *Cancer* 1973;**32:**1066.

Brosman S, Hausman M, Shacks S: Immunologic alterations in patients with prostatic carcinoma. *J Urol* 1975; **113:**841.

Bubenik JJ et al: Demonstration of cell mediated immunity in renal carcinoma in man. *Int J Cancer* 1971;**8:**503.

Burnet FM: The concept of immunological surveillance. *Progr Exp Tumor Res* 1970;**13:**1.

Catalona WJ, Chretien PB, Trahan EE: Abnormalities of cell-mediated immunocompetence in genitourinary cancer. *J. Urol* 1974;**111:**229.

Catalona WJ, Smolev JK, Harty JI: Prognostic value of host immunocompetence in urologic cancer patients. *J Urol* 1975;**114:**922.

Cole AT et al: Cell-mediated immunity in renal cell carcinoma: Preliminary report. *J Urol* 1975;**115:**234.

Cummings KB, Peter JB, Kaufman JJ: Cell-mediated immunity to tumor antigens in patients with renal cell carcinoma. *J Urol* 1973;**110:**31.

Daly JJ et al: Specificity of cellular immunity to renal cell carcinoma. *J Urol* 1974;**111:**448.

Decenzo JM, Leadbetter GW Jr: The interaction of host immunocompetence and tumor aggressiveness in superficial bladder carcinoma. *J Urol* 1976;**115:**262.

DeKernion JB, Ramming KP, Smith RB: The natural history of metastatic renal cell carcinoma: Computer analysis. *J Urol* 1980;**124:**148.

DeWolf WC et al: HLA and testicular cancer. *Nature* 1979;**5693:**216.

Eccles SA: Host immune mechanisms in the control of tumor metastases. Chap 3, p 37, in: *Tumor Immunity in Prognosis.* Haskill S (editor). Marcel Dekker, 1982.

Elhilali MM, Nayak SK: Immunologic evaluation of human bladder cancer: In vitro studies. *Cancer* 1975;**35:**419.

Elhilali MM, Nayak SK: In vitro cytotoxicity studies in bladder and renal cancer. *Urology* 1976;**7:**488.

Evans MJ: Are teratocarcinomas formed from normal cells? Chap 3, p 24, in: *Germ Cell Tumors.* Anderson TK et al (editors). AR Liss, 1981.

Hakala TR et al: Humoral cytotoxicity in human renal cell carcinoma. *Invest Urol* 1974;**11:**405.

Hellström I, Hellström KE, Sjögren HO: Serum factors in tumor-free patients cancelling the blocking of cell-mediated tumor immunity. *Int J Cancer* 1971;**8:**185.

Jacobs SC, Berg SI, Lawson RK: Synchronous bilateral renal cell carcinoma: Total surgical excision. *Cancer* 1980; **46:**2341.

Kajaer M, Bendixen G: Tumor-directed cellular hypersensitivity detected by leukocyte migration in patients with renal carcinoma. *Ann NY Acad Sci* 1976;**276:**260.

Levine AS: The epidemic of acquired immune dysfunction in homosexual men and its sequelae: Opportunistic infections, Kaposi's sarcoma, and other malignancies: An update and interpretation. *Cancer Treat Rep* 1982;**66:**1391.

McNichols DW, Segura JW, DeWeerd JH: Renal cell carcinoma: Long-term survival and late recurrence. *J Urol* 1981;**126:**17.

Morales A, Eidinger D: Immune reactivity in renal cancer: A sequential study. *J Urol* 1976;**115:**510.

Schellhammer PF et al: Immune evaluation with skin testing: A study of testicular, prostatic, and bladder neoplasms. *Cancer* 1976;**38:**149.

Stemsward J et al: Tumor distinctive cellular immunity to renal cancer. *Clin Exp Immunol* 1970;**6:**963.

Stewart T, Mintz B: Successive generations of mice produced from an established culture line of euploid teratocarcinoma cells. *Proc Natl Acad Sci USA* 1981;**78:**6314.

Sugarbaker EV, Cohen AM: Altered antigenicity in spontaneous pulmonary metastases from an antigenic murine sarcoma. *Surgery* 1972;**72:**155.

Vessella RL et al: Monoclonal antibodies to human renal cell carcinoma: Recognition of shared and restricted tissue antigens. *Cancer Res* 1985;**45:**6131.

Immunologic Methods

Abelev GI et al: Production of embryonal globulin by transplantable mouse hepatoma. *Transplantation* 1963;**1:**174.

Ercole C et al: The superiority of serum determinations of prostatic specific antigen (PSA) over prostatic acid phosphatase (A) as a serum marker in carcinoma of the prostate (CAP): AUA Abstract 975. *J Urol* 1986;**135(4-Part 2):**103A.

Javadpour N: The role of biologic tumor markers in testicular cancer. *Cancer* 1980;**45(7 Suppl):**1755.

Killian CS et al: Prognostic importance of prostate-specific antigen for monitoring patients with stages B_2 and D_1 prostate cancer. *Cancer Res* 1985;**45:**886.

Kurman RJ, Scardino PT: Immunoperoxidase localization of alpha-fetoprotein and human chorionic gonadotropin in malignant germ cell tumors of the ovary and testis. In: *Diagnostic Immunocytochemistry.* DeLellis RA, Sternberg SS (editors). Masson, 1981.

Lange PH et al: Serum alpha-fetoprotein and human chorionic gonadotropin in patients with seminoma. *J Urol* 1980;**124:**472.

Old LJ: Cancer immunology: The search for specificity. GHA Clowes Memorial Lecture. *Cancer Res* 1981; **41:**361.

Waldmann TA, McIntire KR: The use of a radioimmunoassay for alpha-fetoprotein in the diagnosis of malignancy. *Cancer* 1974;**34(Suppl):**1510.

Wang MC et al: Purification of a human prostate specific antigen. *Invest Urol* 1979;**17:**159.

Immunotherapy & Biotherapy

Berd D, Maguire HC Jr, Mastrangelo MJ: Immunopotentiation by cyclophosphamide and other cytotoxic agents. Pages 39–61 in: *Immune Modulating Agents and Their Mechanisms.* Fenichel R, Chirigos M (editors). Marcel Dekker, 1984.

Berd D et al: Augmentation of the human immune response by cyclophosphamide. *Cancer Res* 1982;**42:**4862.

Bloch A: Induced cell differentiation in cancer therapy. *Cancer Treat Rep* 1984;**68:**199.

Borden EC, Hawkins MJ: Biologic response modifiers as adjuncts to other therapeutic modalities. *Semin Oncol* 1986;**13:**144.

Borden EC, Verma AK, Wolberg WH: Potential role of polyribonucleotides in human neoplastic disease. *J Biol Response Mod* 1985;**4:**676.

Borden EC et al: Interim analysis of a trial of levamisole and 5-fluorouracil in metastatic colorectal carcinoma. Pages 231–235 in: *Immunotherapy of Human Cancer.* Terry WD, Rosenberg SA (editors). Elsevier, 1982.

Braun DP, Harris JE: Modulation of the immune response by chemotherapy. *Pharmacol Ther* 1981;**14:**89.

Brosman SA: Experience with bacillus Calmette-Guérin in patients with superficial bladder carcinoma. *J Urol* 1982;**128:**27.

Gabrilove JL: Differentiation factors. *Semin Oncol* 1986; **13:**228.

Gutterman JU et al: Pharmacokinetic study of partially pure gamma-interferon in cancer patients. *Cancer Res* 1984; **44:**4164.

Hanna MG Jr, Brandhorst J, Peters LC: Active-specific immunotherapy of residual micrometastasis: An evaluation of sources, doses and ratios of BCG with tumor cells. *Cancer Immunol Immunother* 1979;**7**:165.

Hanna MG Jr, Peters LC: Specific immunotherapy of established visceral micrometastases by BCG-tumor cell vaccine alone or as an adjunct to surgery. *Cancer* 1978;**42**:2613.

Harris JE, Vera R, Sandler S: Randomized trial of two doses of leukocyte interferon in metastatic renal cell carcinoma. *Proc Am Assoc Cancer Res* 1983;**24**:146.

Herscowitz HH: Immunophysiology, cellular function and cellular interaction in antibody formation. In: *Immunology III*. Bellanti JA (editor). Saunders, 1985.

Hoover HC Jr et al: Prospectively randomized trial of adjuvant active-specific immunotherapy for human colorectal cancer. *Cancer* 1985;**55**:1236.

Isaacs A, Lindemann J: Virus interference. 1. The interferon. *Proc R Soc Lond (Biol)* 1957;**147**:258.

Krown SE: Interferon and interferon inducers in cancer treatment. *Semin Oncol* 1986;**13**:207.

Lacour J et al: Adjuvant treatment with polyadenylic-polyuridylic acid in operable breast cancer: Updated results of a randomised trial. *Br Med J* 1984;**288**:589.

McCune CS, Schapira DV, Henshaw EC: Specific immunotherapy of advanced renal carcinoma: Evidence for the polyclonality of metastases. *Cancer* 1981;**47**:1984.

Mitchell M, Oettgen HF (editors): *Hybridomas in Cancer Diagnosis and Treatment*. Raven Press, 1982.

Morales A: Long-term results and complications of intracavitary baccillus Calmette-Guérin therapy for bladder cancer. *J Urol* 1984;**132**:457.

Morales A, Eidinger D, Bruce AW: Intracavitary bacillus Calmette-Guérin in the treatment of superficial bladder tumors. *J Urol* 1976;**116**:180.

Morton DL: Active immunotherapy against cancer: Present status. *Semin Oncol* 1986;**13**:180.

Morton DL et al: Adjuvant immunotherapy of malignant melanoma: Results of a randomized trial in patients with lymph node metastases. Pages 245–249 in: *Immunotherapy of Human Cancer*. Terry WD, Rosenberg SA (editors). Elsevier, 1982.

Neidhart JA et al: Active specific immunotherapy of stage IV renal carcinoma with aggregated tumor antigen adjuvant. *Cancer* 1980;**46**:1128.

Prehn RT, Main JM: Immunity to methylocholanthrene-induced sarcomas. *J Natl Cancer Inst* 1957;**18**:769.

Quesada JR et al: Renal cell carcinoma: Antitumor effects of leukocyte interferon. *Cancer Res* 1983;**43**:940.

Rosenberg SA et al: Biological activity of recombinant human interleukin-2 produced in *Escherichia coli*. *Science* 1984;**223**:1412.

Rosenberg SA et al: Observations on the systemic administration of autologous lymphokine-activated killer cells and recombinant interleukin-2 to patients with metastatic cancer. *N Engl J Med* 1985;**313**:1485.

Salmon SE et al: Alternating combination chemotherapy and levamisole improves survival in multiple myeloma: A Southwest Oncology Group study. *J Clin Oncol* 1983;**1**:217.

Schmidt JA et al: Interleukin-1, a potential regulator of fibroblast proliferation. *J Immunol* 1982;**128**:2177.

Sells S, Reisfeld R (editors): Monoclonal antibodies in cancer. Pages 1–485 in: *Contemporary Biomedicine*. Humana, 1985.

19

Tumors of the Genitourinary Tract

Douglas E. Johnson, MD, David A. Swanson, MD, & Andrew C. von Eschenbach, MD

Neoplasms of the prostate gland, bladder, and kidney are among the most common abnormal growths that afflict the human body. They are often silent, so that diagnosis may not be possible until quite late. Tumors of the testis are highly malignant and afflict young men. Neoplasms of the ureter, urethra, penis, scrotum, epididymis, and seminal vesicle are rare.

Adrenal tumors are discussed in Chapter 22.

MANIFESTATIONS OF UROGENITAL TRACT NEOPLASMS

Hematuria

Gross or microscopic hematuria is common when ulceration of a vesical, ureteral, or renal pelvic neoplasm occurs or when a renal parenchymal tumor breaks through the pelvic lining. It is seen often with benign prostatic hyperplasia, in which case bleeding is usually from dilated veins in the region of the bladder neck. Symptoms of prostatism plus hematuria do not, therefore, necessarily mean prostatic cancer; in fact, bleeding from the malignant prostate does not occur until the tumor grows through the mucosa of the bladder or urethra.

Pain

A. Renal Pain: Renal carcinoma can incite pain in the costovertebral angle (from renal capsular distention) if the tumor bleeds into its own substance. Renal and ureteral colic may occur if a blood clot or a mass of cells passes down the ureter. This type of pain is caused by hyperperistalsis of the pelvis or ureter.

B. Ureteral Pain: Ureteral tumors (rare) usually cause ureteral obstruction and occasionally colic.

C. Vesical Pain: Ulceration of a vesical tumor predisposes to midtract (bladder) infection, which causes symptoms of cystitis. With extravesical extension, constant suprapubic pain that increases with urination may be experienced.

D. Low Back Pain: Pain low in the back with radiation down one or both legs in an elderly man strongly suggests metastases to the pelvis and lumbar spine from cancer of the prostate. Local (perineal) pain is seldom a symptom of cancer of the prostate.

E. Testicular Pain: Testicular neoplasm typically causes little or no pain, but if spontaneous bleeding occurs into the tumor, it can mimic painful lesions (eg, torsion of the spermatic cord, acute epididymitis).

Dysuria

Hesitancy, impaired caliber and force of the urinary stream, and terminal dribbling are most commonly caused by benign prostatic hyperplasia, but cancer of the prostate produces the same difficulties. A tumor of the bladder on or near the internal vesical orifice may cause similar symptoms. Cystoscopy is therefore necessary in all cases of bladder neck obstruction.

Tumor of the urethra causes progressive diminution of the urinary stream. A palpable urethral mass suggests tumor or stricture. Biopsy may be needed for positive differentiation.

Skin Lesions

Tumors or ulcers of the penile and scrotal skin may be benign or malignant but can be caused by infection. If there is the slightest doubt, a specimen should be obtained for pathologic study.

Palpable Mass

A. Renal Mass: Renal tumors frequently present no symptoms other than the discovery of a tumor mass by the patient or the physician. Neoplasms can be confused with simple renal cysts, polycystic kidney, hydronephrosis, cyst of the pancreas, or an enlarged spleen.

B. Abdominal Mass: An intra-abdominal mass near the umbilical region should suggest metastases to the preaortic lymph nodes from tumor of the testis. A suprapubic midline mass may represent a dilated (obstructed) bladder or may be caused by gastrointestinal or gynecologic tumor. It is not common for a vesical neoplasm to be palpable suprapubically except on bimanual (abdominorectal or abdominovaginal) examination with the patient under anesthesia.

C. Prostatic Mass: When the prostate is diffusely stony-hard and fixed, it is almost certainly cancerous, but a hard area in the gland may pose a problem in differential diagnosis. The possibilities include early cancer, fibrosis from chronic infection, prostatic calculi, granulomatous prostatitis, and tuberculosis. At times the differentiation can only be made by biopsy.

D. Testicular Mass: A painless, firm testis should be regarded as neoplastic until proved otherwise. Gummas may cause induration, but they are rare; serologic tests will be helpful in differentiation.

Fever

Tumors of the kidney may excite no symptoms other than fever. Tumors of the urinary organs may also cause obstruction and be complicated by sepsis.

Hypertension

Hypertension is noted in about half of patients with Wilms' tumor, in some with renal adenocarcinoma, and in patients with juxtaglomerular adenomas.

Anemia

With advanced cancer in any urologic organ, anemia is to be expected even in the absence of blood loss. This is particularly true with prostatic cancer, when bone marrow may be extensively involved.

Erythrocytosis

Erythrocytosis occurs in association with 4% of renal cancers, including Wilms' tumor. It may also be noted with certain benign renal lesions.

Transitional Cells in Urine

In most individuals with vesical neoplasms and transitional cell tumors of the ureter or renal pelvis, examination of the urinary sediment stained with methylene blue will reveal round (transitional) epithelial cells; therefore, the presence of these cells should always arouse suspicion of tumor. Cytologic examination of urinary sediment is discussed in Chapter 5.

SYMPTOMS & SIGNS OF METASTASES

Tumors of the genitourinary tract often cause no local symptoms or definite signs. Clinical manifestations may arise only from metastases.

Central nervous system. Tumors of the kidney or prostate may metastasize to the central nervous system. The first symptoms may therefore be neurologic.

Lungs. Tumors of the kidney, prostate, and testis often spread to the lungs. Pleuritic pain may suggest secondary pleural involvement.

Liver. Renal tumors frequently metastasize to the liver, which then becomes enlarged and nodular. If compression of the common duct occurs, jaundice will be noted.

Lymph nodes. Enlargement of the left supraclavicular lymph nodes may be the only finding in cancer of the kidney or testis. Palpable para-aortic abdominal masses in a young man may mean tumor of the testis. Edema of one or both legs may develop from compression of the iliac vessels by masses of lymph nodes containing tumor cells from cancer of the prostate or bladder (Figs 19–1 and 19–2).

Bones. Metastasis to the skeletal system is most common from cancer of the prostate and kidney. This may cause pain in the bone, spontaneous fracture, or neurologic manifestations due to metastasis to the spine.

TUMORS OF THE RENAL PARENCHYMA

BENIGN TUMORS

Most benign tumors of the kidney are mesenchymal in origin. They are usually found incidentally or at autopsy, and few are important clinically (Bennington and Beckwith, 1975). They include the leiomyoma, lipoma, myolipoma, angiomyolipoma, hemangioma, juxtaglomerular tumor, lymphangioma, cortical fibroma, medullary fibroma, and renomedullary interstitial cell tumor. Rarely can these tumors be diagnosed without nephrectomy, even if they are large enough to cause symptoms. The exceptions are juxtaglomerular tumor and angiomyolipoma.

Juxtaglomerular Tumor

Juxtaglomerular tumors secrete renin, thus causing hypertension (Dennis et al, 1985). Plasma renin levels are elevated, particularly in the ipsilateral renal vein, and urinary aldosterone levels are high. Hypokalemia is present. The tumors, which are small and slightly gray, have well-circumscribed or encapsulated cortical neoplasms. On x-ray, they are solid and hypovascular (Dunnick et al, 1983). Histologically, they are composed of many cytoplasmic granules containing renin, as determined by immunofluorescence studies. Nephrectomy cures the hypertension in younger patients with juxtaglomerular tumor (Squires et al, 1984).

Angiomyolipoma (Renal Hamartoma)

Although angiomyolipoma is relatively uncommon, it has received much attention because of its interesting clinical spectrum and the controversy over its management. At the Mayo Clinic during a 50-year period, only 23 angiomyolipomas were found among over 400 renal tumors discovered at surgical exploration; 9 more were found at autopsy (Farrow et al, 1968). Angiomyolipoma commonly occurs in association with tuberous sclerosis (Bourneville's disease), adenoma sebaceum, and other lesions such as retinal phakomas and hamartomas of the kidney, brain, and other viscera (Bissada et al, 1975). At least 50% of patients with angiomyolipoma have tuberous sclerosis. In this combination, the tumors are often bilateral and multiple; however, when tuberous sclerosis is absent, lesions are usually solitary and unilateral and occur predominantly in females.

Angiomyolipomas are typically round to oval, and their growth tends to be expansile, although local invasion can occur (Bennington and Beckwith, 1975). Hemorrhage, necrosis, cystic changes, and calcification may be present. The cut surface is yellow to gray, depending on the mixture of mature fat, thick-walled blood vessels, and smooth muscle, which can

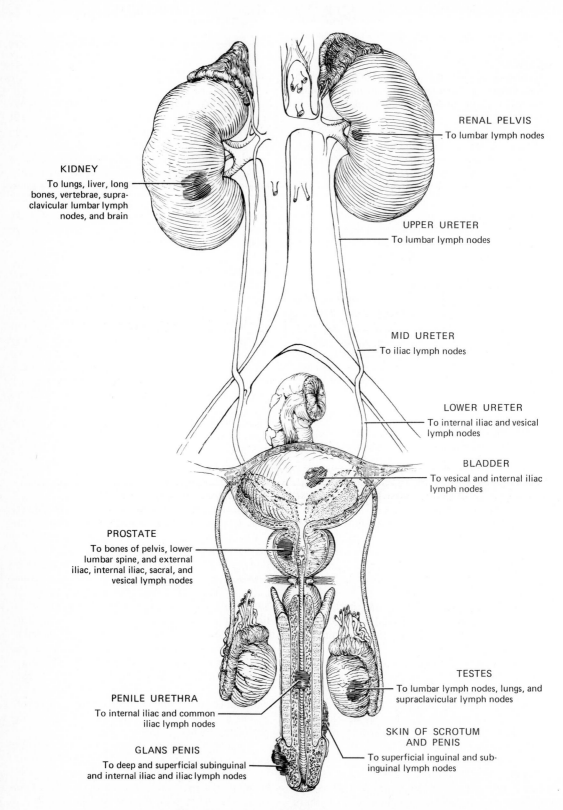

KIDNEY
To lungs, liver, long bones, vertebrae, supra-clavicular lumbar lymph nodes, and brain

RENAL PELVIS
To lumbar lymph nodes

UPPER URETER
To lumbar lymph nodes

MID URETER
To iliac lymph nodes

LOWER URETER
To internal iliac and vesical lymph nodes

BLADDER
To vesical and internal iliac lymph nodes

PROSTATE
To bones of pelvis, lower lumbar spine, and external iliac, internal iliac, sacral, and vesical lymph nodes

TESTES
To lumbar lymph nodes, lungs, and supraclavicular lymph nodes

PENILE URETHRA
To internal iliac and common iliac lymph nodes

SKIN OF SCROTUM AND PENIS
To superficial inguinal and sub-inguinal lymph nodes

GLANS PENIS
To deep and superficial subinguinal and internal iliac and iliac lymph nodes

Figure 19–1. Sites of tumor origin and metastases in the male.

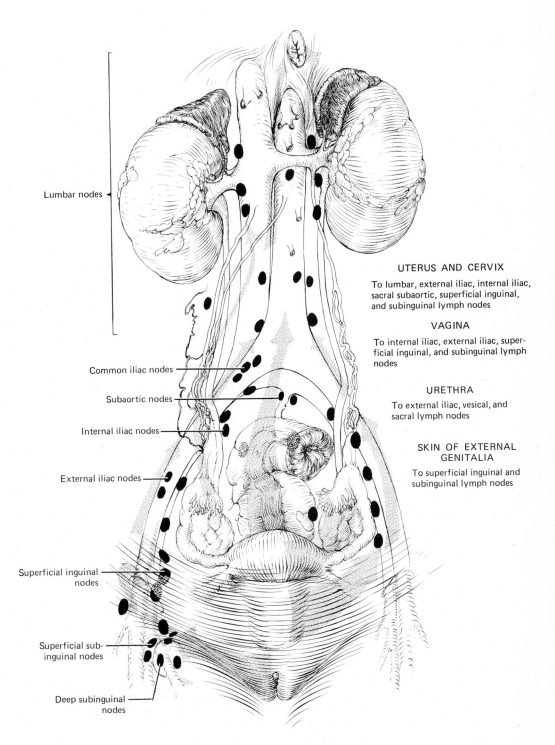

Lumbar nodes

UTERUS AND CERVIX

To lumbar, external iliac, internal iliac, sacral subaortic, superficial inguinal, and subinguinal lymph nodes

VAGINA

To internal iliac, external iliac, superficial inguinal, and subinguinal lymph nodes

URETHRA

To external iliac, vesical, and sacral lymph nodes

SKIN OF EXTERNAL GENITALIA

To superficial inguinal and subinguinal lymph nodes

Common iliac nodes

Subaortic nodes

Internal iliac nodes

External iliac nodes

Superficial inguinal nodes

Superficial sub-inguinal nodes

Deep subinguinal nodes

Figure 19–2. Sites and routes of tumor metastases in the female.

be found in varying proportions on microscopic examination.

The clinical presentation varies. The fact that symptoms may be absent, particularly if the lesions are small, obscures the true incidence of the disease. When present, symptoms are usually produced by intrarenal or perirenal hemorrhage. Pain is reported frequently and is usually severe, although a chronic dull flank pain may occur. Massive bleeding may cause shock. Hypertension and hematuria may be present.

Preoperative diagnosis may be difficult. Unless the tuberous sclerosis complex is present, angiomyolipoma is hard to differentiate from renal cell carcinoma. Even among patients with tuberous sclerosis, renal cell carcinoma—occasionally bilateral—has been reported. Excretory urography reveals only the presence of a renal mass. Ultrasonography may reveal high-intensity internal echoes, suggestive of fat; CT scanning demonstrates the fat if it is present in sufficient quantity. Arteriographic findings in angiomyolipoma are similar to those in renal cell carcinoma.

Various therapeutic approaches have been recommended, including observation, arterial embolization, conservative surgery (enucleation or partial nephrectomy), and nephrectomy. Since many of these tumors grow slowly (if at all) and remain asymptomatic, observation is usually preferable to surgery. Oesterling et al (1986) recommend observation or conservative treatment, depending on the size of the lesion and the associated symptoms. If bleeding occurs, conservative management with blood transfusions and, possibly, selective arterial embolization may obviate surgery (Jardin et al, 1980; Zerhouni et al, 1984). Nephrectomy is rarely recommended, except in cases of life-threatening hemorrhage that cannot be otherwise controlled. In selected patients, enucleation or partial nephrectomy may be considered for treatment of polar or peripheral lesions, especially when there is persistent hematuria, calcification, or an enlarging mass. Shapiro et al (1984) recommend aggressive surgery in these cases, with preservation of the parenchyma.

ADENOCARCINOMA OF THE KIDNEY (Renal Cell Carcinoma)

In the USA, adenocarcinoma accounts for 86% of all malignant tumors of the renal parenchyma and constitutes approximately 2% of all new cancers found each year. Described in 1883 by Grawitz, the tumor has since been known by such names as Grawitz's tumor, hypernephroma, and clear cell carcinoma. Because it originates from the epithelial cells of the proximal convoluted tubule, the most accurate name for this tumor is renal cell carcinoma or adenocarcinoma of the kidney.

The incidence of these tumors correlates strongly with both age and sex. The greatest number of cases occur when patients are in their 60s, and tumors develop 2–3 times more frequently in men than in women. The incidence rate has increased steadily through the years. Renal cell carcinoma occasionally occurs in children and adolescents; 155 cases were reported by 1979. Wilms' tumor is more common than renal cell carcinoma in children, but a renal tumor in an adolescent is likely to be an adenocarcinoma.

Although no data permit reliable comparison of the frequency of renal cell carcinoma among different racial populations, it appears to be the same among Caucasians, Mexicans, and blacks. However, frequency varies considerably from country to country, with the highest rates reported for Scandinavian countries, more moderate rates for Europe and North America, lower rates for Spain and South America, and the lowest rates for India, Japan, and parts of Africa. The incidence is higher among urban dwellers, but this does not seem to be related to socioeconomic status.

Renal cell carcinoma has occurred in more than one family member in 18 cases, including 2 in which 3 generations were affected. This suggestion of a possible genetic factor is supported by the findings of Cohen et al (1979), who reported a balanced reciprocal translocation between chromosomes 3 and 8 in patients with renal cell carcinoma. Ten family members in 3 consecutive generations had the tumor. The translocation was present in all 8 patients with cancer whose karyotype was known, while no family member with a normal karyotype (22 people tested) had renal cancer.

Renal tumors, both benign and malignant, are strongly associated with von Hippel-Lindau disease, an autosomal dominant disease. In this association, the tumors are usually bilateral, may be benign or cystic, and are clinically diagnosed in 25% of patients (Horton, Wong, and Eldridge, 1976). The incidence of malignant tumors at autopsy may be as high as 40–60%.

Etiology

The cause of renal cell carcinoma is not known, although similar tumors have been produced experimentally in numerous animal models by a large assortment of agents, including chemicals, natural agents such as cycasin and aflatoxins, and antibiotics. Exposures to lead, cadmium, radiation, and viruses have all produced renal tumors.

The relationship between renal tumors and hormones has been particularly interesting because of the observed difference in incidence rates in men and women and because of the possible role of hormones in the clinical management of renal cell carcinoma. Investigators discovered that use of exogenous estrogens in Syrian golden hamsters could produce renal carcinomas in the female during periods of low progestational activity and in the castrated male (Kirkman, 1959). The most frequently used method of tumor induction is subcutaneous implantation or injections of diethylstilbestrol, which must be continued to maintain the tumors.

Although human renal cell tumors have not been causally linked to any of the agents mentioned above, a definite correlation has been established with smoking and a probable one with diet (Bennington and Beckwith, 1975). The risk of developing renal cell carcinoma was found to be over 5 times higher in men who used any form of tobacco at all than in men who did not use tobacco (Bennington and Laubscher, 1968). Coffee drinking has also been mentioned as a possible causative agent, but Wynder, Mabuchi, and Whitmore (1974) noted no significant influence when the study was controlled for smoking.

A worldwide positive correlation exists between death from renal cell carcinoma and per capita consumption of fats (particularly animal fats), oils, milk, and sugar. The fact that Japanese immigrants to the USA have a higher incidence of renal cell carcinoma than native Japanese may possibly be explained on the basis of dietary influences. Perhaps cigarette smoking and diet are cofactors, which would explain why there is a positive correlation between cigarette smoking and death from renal cell carcinoma in the USA but not worldwide.

Recently, it has become apparent that the kidneys of patients on long-term hemodialysis frequently demonstrate multiple cysts and, occasionally, renal cell carcinoma (Cho, Friedland, and Swensen, 1984; Levine et al, 1984; Hughson, Buchwald, and Fox, 1986). The incidence of acquired cystic disease correlates with the duration of hemodialysis. Patients with transplanted kidneys seem to be spared both acquired cystic disease and malignant tumors. The natural history of acquired cystic disease and neoplasms in patients with chronic renal failure remains largely unknown.

Pathogenesis & Pathology

Despite Grawitz's 1883 assertion that renal cell carcinoma arose from adrenal rests, Sudek proposed in 1893 that its source was renal tubular cells (Bennington and Beckwith, 1975). This was confirmed in 1960 when electron microscopy demonstrated the similarity between cells of the proximal convoluted tubules and renal adenocarcinoma cells (Oberling, Riviere, and Haguenau, 1960), and the finding was supported later by immunofluorescence studies (Wallace and Nairn, 1972).

The renal cell carcinoma usually bulges from the surface and distorts the normal contour of the kidney. It is roughly spherical and generally contained by a pseudocapsule of condensed connective tissue at its periphery. The cut surface typically appears variegated, and fibrous septa often create rough lobulations. Cells rich in lipids give it a yellow-to-orange color, while necrotic areas may be gray and areas containing granular cells tan to rich brown. Hemorrhage and necrosis are common. Calcification may be present, and tumor degeneration may lead to a gelatinous, cystic, or fibrous appearance.

Histologic examination reveals clear, granular, or sarcomatoid cells arranged in solid, papillary, tubular, and cystic patterns (Bennington and Beckwith, 1975). Individual cells are generally uniform, have a distinct cytoplasmic membrane, and are tightly adherent to adjacent cells. Clear cells are rounded or polygonal and contain abundant cytoplasm. Although they stain poorly on routine processing, they stain well with periodic acid-Schiff because of their intracellular glycogen and also stain well with stains for neutral lipids or phospholipids. Granular cells contain less glycogen and lipids but more mitochondria and other organelles.

Oncocytoma, a special presentation of the granular cell tumor, has received a lot of attention since Klein and Valensi (1976) suggested that it might be a benign clinicopathologic entity. Although it is not entirely clear why patients with this tumor have all done well clinically, it may be due to the fact that oncocytomas, strictly defined, are all well-differentiated (grade I) renal cell carcinomas. It is apparent, however, that as the criteria of Klein and Valensi are more loosely applied, permitting some tumors of higher grade to be included, more variable clinical behavior can be expected (Lieber, Tomera, and Farrow, 1981; Barnes and Beckman, 1983). The oncocytomas are often quite large, are uniformly tan to mahogany brown, are invariably well circumscribed, and are devoid of hemorrhage or necrosis. They are composed solely of eosinophilic epithelial cells without mitotic figures and containing no more than focal nuclear pleomorphism. Ultrastructurally, the oncocytic cells have very few organelles except for the striking number of mitochondria, which accounts for their color and appearance on gross and microscopic examination.

The pathogenesis of renal cell carcinoma is unclear. Very small primary tumors sometimes metastasize, and very large tumors may still be encapsulated. Most tumors develop as a solitary expanding mass that compresses the renal tissue at its periphery, distorts the renal contour and collecting system, and then "breaks through" the renal capsule to invade perinephric fat, Gerota's fascia, and, eventually, contiguous organs. As it grows, the tumor may invade and destroy the peripheral collecting system (although gross invasion of the renal pelvis is not common), invade intrarenal veins, and enter the intrarenal lymphatic network. Some authors speculate that macroscopic growth into the main renal vein and inferior vena cava may represent only a "prolapse" of the tumor and does not have the same significance as it does in other tumors. Certainly, however, the characteristic hypervascularity of this tumor suggests little barrier to the bloodstream.

The kidney has 2 lymphatic networks—an intrarenal network, in which lymphatics run parallel to and are intimately related to the venous system, and a capsular network—and these networks are known to communicate (Rouvière, 1938; Cockett, 1977). Since lymphovenous communications exist, cancer cells can metastasize widely via lymphatic and hematogenous routes. Lymphatic dissemination does not proceed in a stepwise manner in renal cell carcinoma; because of the extensive neovascularity and parasitization of blood supply, "skip" metastases (isolated positive lymph nodes in the supraclavicular, iliac, and contralateral lumbar region) have been identified (Hulten et al, 1969). The overall incidence of lymph node metastases reported in an autopsy series was 34% (Bennington and Beckwith, 1975), and that reported in various clinical series was about the same.

The lateral aortic and interaortocaval lymph nodes lie in close proximity to the cisterna chyli, and thus malignant cells within the lymphatic system can easily pass into the thoracic duct and into the superior vena cava. After passing through the heart, the tumor cells may lodge in the lungs, or if they are not filtered out by the pulmonary capillaries, they may enter the left heart and be pumped into the arterial circulation. Likewise, malignant cells entering the venous drainage of the kidney may pass in a similar fashion to the lungs and subsequently the left heart, or they may pass along the axial skeleton by way of the paravertebral venous plexus of Batson. The percentages of cases with metastases at autopsy are as follows: in the lungs (55%), liver (33%), bone (32%, predominantly in the axial skeleton), adrenal (19%), contralateral kidney (11%), brain (5.7%), heart (5%), and other organs (less frequently).

Tumor cells may also pass retrograde down the gonadal vein to the pelvic structures or even antegrade down the ureter to implant in the ureter or bladder (Swanson and Liles, 1982). Bennington and Beckwith (1975) reported that renal cell carcinoma accounted for 11% of penile, 9% of vaginal, 4% of uterine, and 15% of ureteral metastatic lesions.

Tumor Staging & Grading

A. Tumor Staging: Our traditional staging systems for renal cell carcinoma are all surgical, ie, based on information that can only be obtained from complete histopathologic examination of the specimen. Petkovic (1956) published the first staging classification, but most of the classification systems in the USA originated with the system reported by Flocks and Kadesky (1958). Robson, Churchill, and Anderson (1969) first published the staging system which, with minor modifications, is the one most widely used in the USA:

Stage I: Tumor is confined to the kidney parenchyma; if present, the pseudocapsule may have ruptured, although the true renal capsule is intact.

Stage II: Renal capsule has been broken through and perirenal fat is involved, but the tumor is still confined within the envelope of Gerota's fascia.

Stage IIIA: Renal vein or inferior vena cava is grossly involved.

Stage IIIB: Lymphatic involvement.

Stage IIIC: Combination of both A and B above.

Stage IVA: Tumor involves adjacent organs other than the adrenal.

Stage IVB: Distant metastases.

Holland's (1973) popular modification simplifies the scheme of Robson et al by dropping the letter subclassifications.

These staging systems provide valuable prognostic information, but the relative importance of the various risk factors (eg, perinephric fat, venous or lymphatic involvement) is still controversial. Data are conflicting, owing partly to the relatively small numbers of patients, the tendency to "lump" risk factors into a single classification (eg, stage III is characterized by either venous or lymphatic involvement or by both), and the failure to control for one variable when higher-stage variables are being tested (eg, stage III venous involvement may be with or without tumor in perinephric fat).

The TNM system (tumor growth [T], spread to primary lymph nodes [N], and metastasis [M] used by the American Joint Committee on Cancer (AJCC) and the International Union Against Cancer (Union Internationale Contre le Cancer [UICC]) addresses some of these objections (Beahrs and Myers, 1983; Spiessl, Scheibe, and Wagner, 1982). The TNM system indicates when and how the staging was performed and thus guards against confusing clinical and pathologic stages. It also specifies whether lymph nodes are involved and whether distant metastases are present by use of separate N and M notations, as well as a supplemental notation for grade (G) and venous involvement (V). The TNM system, with or without its supplemental notations, is very precise, permitting accurate comparison of data (results) and providing the framework for reliable estimation of prognosis. It is very unwieldy, however; perhaps that is why it is rarely used in the USA.

B. Tumor Grading: Classification of renal cell carcinoma on the basis of cell type or patterns of organization (papillary, tubular, cystic) seems to have no prognostic significance. Although many authors have observed a correlation between prognosis and the histologic appearance of the tumor, they do not agree on which cytologic or histologic features are the most important. Grading is difficult and reproducibility often low. For this reason, and because careful staging confers much of the same prognostic information, grading has not been widely practiced in renal cell carcinoma.

Clinical Findings

A. Symptoms: Very few symptoms, none pathognomonic, are secondary to renal cell carcinoma. In fact, in at least one-third of patients, the symptoms and signs are unrelated to the primary tumor, and because of their nonurologic nature, the patient is often referred to his or her primary care physician or to a specialist other than a urologist—hence, the tumor is often called the "internist's tumor." When symptoms and signs are not secondary to the primary tumor in the kidney, they may reflect the systemic toxic or endocrine effects, some of which constitute the so-called paraneoplastic syndromes commonly associated with this disease, or the presence of metastatic lesions. About one-third of patients have metastases at the time of initial diagnosis.

Pain is the most common symptom, although it is caused by the primary tumor only 40–50% of the time. Tumor-related pain is usually described as a dull ache or a vague discomfort in the flank. If there is hemorrhage into the tumor or if clots pass down the ureter, the pain may become more severe and even colicky. Invasion into adjacent structures such as the posterior abdominal wall usually produces severe and unrelenting pain. Metastatic lesions quite commonly cause pain, particularly if they are osseous in nature.

Far more commonly, however, the symptoms are more subtle. Weakness, weight loss, and anemia were recognized by Berg as early as 1913 to be among the earliest symptoms and signs (Bennington and Kradjian, 1967). In one series, 61% of patients experienced nonspecific abdominal or gastrointestinal complaints such as anorexia, nausea and vomiting, flatulence, and a change in bowel habits (Gibbons et al, 1976). When metastases are absent, many of these symptoms may be reflex in origin, secondary to retroperitoneal irritation by the tumor. Malaise, fatigue, and lassitude are relatively common complaints; polyneuritis and myositis have been reported but are rare.

B. Signs: This disease is accompanied by far more signs than symptoms, but again they can be nonspecific. Hematuria, its cardinal sign, may be microscopic but is usually gross, intermittent, and painless unless ureteral colic results from clots passing. A late sign, it is present at some time in up to 60% of patients.

A palpable flank mass, another characteristically late finding, is present in about one-third of patients. The triad of hematuria, flank pain, and a palpable mass was at one time considered to be the classic mode of presentation. It is now realized that no more than 50% of patients present with this combination and that 35% have none of the triad findings. This complex of signs and symptoms appears late, and up to 47% of patients already have metastatic disease.

Weight loss as a single sign occurs in 30–45% of patients. Fever occurs in about 20% of patients and is the only sign in about 2–4%. An endogenous pyrogen appears to be responsible.

Hypertension has been reported in 43% of patients (Morlock and Horton, 1936), but perhaps 25% is a better estimate. Elevated blood pressure may be secondary to elevated renin levels (Sufrin et al, 1977), although renal artery stenosis and arteriovenous fistulas have also been reported to be responsible for hypertension.

Other signs include a bruit or even high-output cardiac failure secondary to arteriovenous fistulas within the tumor or within a large metastatic lesion. Complete obstruction of the vena cava by tumor thrombus may produce edema in the legs and genitalia, dilated surface veins on the abdominal wall, and ascites. If the thrombus obstructs the hepatic veins, a Budd-Chiari-like syndrome (edema, portal hypertension, and abnormal liver function) may develop. Obstruction of the spermatic vein can produce a varicocele that does not collapse when the patient reclines. Finally, a peripheral neuromyopathy may be present.

Signs secondary to metastatic lesions cannot be ignored. The obvious ones include pathologic fractures, focal neurologic deficit secondary to a central nervous system space-occupying lesion, hemoptysis, and vaginal bleeding. Endocrine dysfunction may manifest as gynecomastia, decreased libido, hirsutism, amenorrhea, and cushingoid features.

C. Laboratory Findings: The importance of urinalysis in diagnosing renal cell carcinoma is somewhat blunted by the fact that hematuria is so often gross and not microscopic. Nonetheless, some patients with only microscopic hematuria may be diagnosed this way. It is important to remember that normal findings on urinalysis do not exclude renal cell carcinoma. Proteinuria may indicate either renal vein thrombosis or be part of the nephrotic syndrome, which may be due to amyloidosis.

The most common hematologic abnormality is anemia, which occurs in about 30% of patients. It is generally normocytic and normochromic and is probably the result of bone marrow depression caused by a tumor-toxic effect. Removing the primary tumor may correct the anemia. Polycythemia (or, more accurately, erythrocytosis) occurs in up to 5% of patients. Erythropoietin has been produced by some renal cell carcinomas, but its production does not necessarily correlate clinically with the degree of erythrocytosis (Sufrin et al, 1977). An elevated erythrocyte sedimentation rate is common, and a leukemoid reaction has also been reported.

A syndrome of abnormal findings on liver function tests may be present in 10–15% of patients, even in the absence of metastatic disease within the liver. First described by Stauffer (1961), the syndrome bearing his name may include hepatosplenomegaly, altered serum protein values (increased α_2-globulin and decreased albumin), increased serum alkaline phosphatase levels, increased thymol turbidity, prolonged prothrombin time, and retention of sulfobromophthalein. Histologically, a nonspecific reactive hepatitis of varying severity is seen. The return to normal of abnormal liver function test findings after removal of the primary tumor appears to correlate with better survival rates (Warren, Kelalis, and Utz, 1970).

Hypercalcemia is seen in up to 15% of patients with renal cell carcinoma. Although it may be due to osseous metastases, it can also occur in their absence. Radioimmunoassays have detected within the tumor a substance indistinguishable from parathyroid hormone (Goldberg et al, 1964; Lytton, Rosof, and Evans, 1965). High concentrations of prostaglandin-like materials in a metastatic lesion have also been found (Brereton et al, 1974).

In fact, this tumor produces many biologically active hormonelike materials measurable in the laboratory. Renin has already been mentioned, but other substances produce specific clinical syndromes, including adrenocorticotropic hormone (Cushing's syndrome), enteroglucagon (protein enteropathy), prolactin (galactorrhea), insulin (hypoglycemia), and gonadotropins (gynecomastia and decreased libido; or hirsutism, amenorrhea, and receding hairline) (Altaffer and Chenault, 1979).

D. X-Ray Findings: The easiest radiographic study to obtain is the plain film of the abdomen (kidney, ureter, and bladder film). Exposed without contrast material, it shows the contour of the kidney by demonstration of the perinephric fat. Unilateral enlargement or distortion of the renal contour or a shift in its axis suggests a possible mass lesion. Calcification overlying the renal shadow, although not pathognomonic for malignant growth, is present in 7–10% of renal carcinomas (Daniel et al, 1972).

Distortion of the collecting system seen on the excretory urogram is the hallmark of a mass lesion within the kidney (Fig 19–3). If portions of the collecting system are compressed by the mass, these portions may not be visualized at all, or they may be dilated behind a partial obstruction. Excretory urography with tomography may help define subtle mass lesions of the kidney (Fig 19–4).

Arteriography is the mainstay of diagnosis of renal cell carcinoma. It characteristically shows neovascularity with irregular vessels of varied calibers (Fig 19–5), venous lakes within the tumor, aneurysms, arteriovenous shunting and premature venous filling, a mottled staining quality due to puddling of contrast material in necrotic portions of the tumor on late-phase films, and poor demarcation of the boundary between tumor and adjacent normal tissue. When the neovascularity is subtle and the diagnosis difficult, epinephrine injected prior to instillation of the contrast material causes constriction of normal vessels but not of neoplastic vessels. Although a positive arteriogram is virtually diagnostic, it is not as accurate in necrotic renal malignant tumors or the 10% that are hypovascular. Furthermore, although Lang (1973) noted excellent correlation of arteriographic stage with pathologic stage, multiple reports since then conclude that correlation is poor with arteriography.

Arteriography is invaluable in diagnosing distant metastatic lesions, since metastases characteristically are hypervascular if the primary tumor is hypervascular. It can identify lesions as small as 5 mm in the contralateral kidney or the liver and can even identify suspected soft tissue lesions or osseous lesions. In one series, extended angiography demonstrated metastases in 20 of 115 patients (17%), 10 of whom had no other known metastases (Hellekant and Nyman, 1979). For this reason, at our institution a complete workup routinely includes flush aortography, bilateral selective renal arteriography, celiac and selective hepatic arteriography, and (usually) inferior venacavography.

The risk of serious complications from arteriography is very low, but the procedure is expensive be-

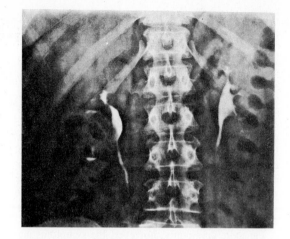

Figure 19–3. Space-occupying lesion (adenocarcinoma) of the kidney. Excretory urogram showing distortion of pelvis and middle and lower calices of right kidney. Left kidney is normal.

cause the patient must be hospitalized. Digital subtraction angiography, which requires only venous injection of contrast material and can be performed on an outpatient basis, may eventually replace the angiographic studies. It may be particularly suitable as a complement to ultrasonography or CT scanning (Engelmann et al, 1984; Zabbo et al, 1985).

Finally, the pattern of metastases necessitates a routine chest x-ray (Fig 19–6) and bone survey (or bone scan; see below). Whole lung tomography can clarify the nature of suspicious or indistinct findings;

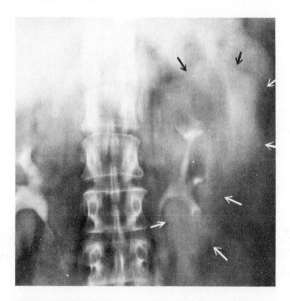

Figure 19–4. Adenocarcinoma of the kidney. Excretory urogram with tomography showing marked expansion of upper pole and elongated upper calix, left kidney.

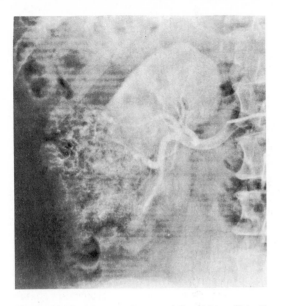

Figure 19–5. Adenocarcinoma of the kidney. Selective renal angiogram showing marked neovascularity of mass in lower portion of right kidney, typical of malignant tumor.

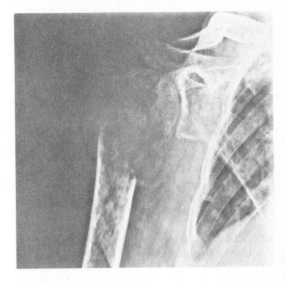

Figure 19–7. Adenocarcinoma of the kidney. Bone survey showing osteolytic metastases to humerus.

routine tomography can detect lesions as small as 6 mm in diameter and CT scanning as small as 3 mm (Schaner et al, 1978). A bone survey may reveal osteolytic metastases (Fig 19–7), which occur primarily in the pelvis and axial skeleton (Swanson et al, 1981).

E. Ultrasonography: The cheapest and safest method to distinguish between a renal cyst and tumor is ultrasonography. Abdominal pansonography of a solid renal mass may demonstrate inferior vena cava thrombus, retroperitoneal nodal masses, or hepatic metastases. Realtime ultrasonography increases the flexibility and usefulness of this modality. A major

disadvantage of ultrasonography is its ineffectiveness when excessive abdominal gas is present.

F. CT Scanning: In addition to accurately differentiating between a cystic and solid mass, the CT scan measures the density of the mass (in Hounsfield units) (Fig 19–8). Unlike cysts, which do not change appearance following the injection of contrast material, renal tumors are generally "enhanced" by contrast. The CT scan is superior to arteriography in preoperatively staging renal cell carcinoma, with accuracy as high as 91% (Cronan, Zeman, and Rosenfield, 1982; Richie et al, 1983; Lang, 1984). It can also be used to follow patients postoperatively for residual disease or recurrent tumor (Parienty et al, 1984) and to demonstrate otherwise "silent" osseous metastases not seen on plain x-rays or bone scans

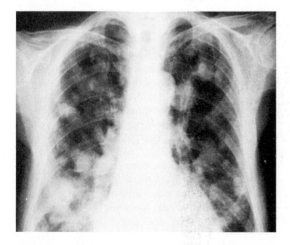

Figure 19–6. Adenocarcinoma of the kidney. Chest film showing metastases to lung. Note typical "cannonball" lesions.

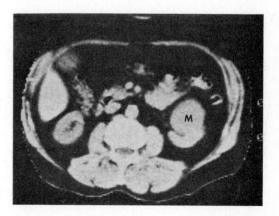

Figure 19–8. Carcinoma of the kidney. CT scan showing mass (M) arising from anterior aspect of left kidney. The mass has a density similar to that of adjacent normal renal parenchyma, indicating it is not a simple cyst.

(Swanson and Bernardino, 1982). The CT scan, unlike an ultrasonogram, will reveal a mass even though excessive gas is present in the bowel, but a very thin patient may yield suboptimal study results because of insufficient retroperitoneal fat to define adjacent structures. Some authors suggest that the CT scan may obviate the need for arteriography before nephrectomy in selected patients. Because larger tumors are more likely to be associated with occult metastases that might be demonstrated by arteriography, this recommendation is less controversial for small tumors.

G. Radionuclide Imaging: Dynamic plus static radionuclide imaging may offer information about the vascularity and function of a renal mass. It may effectively replace excretory urography in cases in which the patient is allergic to iodine or has compromised renal function. A radionuclide scan may demonstrate that a suspected mass is only a pseudotumor or hypertrophied column of Bertin.

More often, however, isotope scanning is used in the staging workup. Although liver, brain, and bone scans may show focal abnormalities suggesting metastatic lesions, they have a low yield.

H. Magnetic Resonance Imaging (MRI): Although clinical experience with this relatively new modality is still limited, several advantages over conventional radiologic imaging are immediately apparent: (1) MRI does not require ionizing radiation: (2) iodinated contrast medium is not required; and (3) no bone artifact or image distortion secondary to metal objects (such as surgical clips) is seen. Already, spatial resolution comparable to the latest generation of CT scanners has been demonstrated, and no short- or medium-term harmful biologic effects have been identified (Williams and Hricak, 1984). MRI distinguishes between solid and cystic renal masses and has an accuracy rate of 96% in tumor staging (Hricak et al, 1985). It seems to be particularly good for evaluating vascular structures, since blood flow produces a characteristic signal that helps differentiate between vessels and hilar or perivascular adenopathy. Recent technical advances (eg, extending MRI to other atoms) and the use of contrast agents to enhance the anatomic information make researchers in this field optimistic about the future role of MRI in clinical medicine.

I. Percutaneous Needle Aspiration and Biopsy: If the ultrasonogram or CT scan shows an apparent cystic mass, fluid from the cyst may be aspirated and examined to confirm the benign nature of the lesion. Fluoroscopy, ultrasonography, or CT scanning guides the needle into the lesion. Fluid is withdrawn and examined grossly for clarity, biochemically for fat, and cytologically for malignant cells. To exclude tumor, the aspirated fluid must be clear and straw-colored, contain no malignant cells, and have a low lipid and cholesterol level (Petersson et al, 1982). After the fluid is aspirated, contrast medium is usually injected and x-rays are taken to demonstrate the cyst wall, which should be smooth.

Needle aspiration can also be performed in the indeterminate or apparently solid lesion to provide material for cytologic evaluation; in selected patients, cores of tissue suitable for histologic examination can be removed by appropriate biopsy needles. Seeding of the needle tract with malignant cells has been reported twice (Bush, Burnett, and Gibbons, 1977; Wehle and Grabstald, 1986).

J. Instrumental Examination: Cystoscopy is the only appropriate instrumental procedure, and it should be performed if the patient presents with hematuria. Bloody efflux from the ureteral orifice identifies the origin of bleeding from the upper tract and rules out any concomitant lower tract lesion. Retrograde pyelography is not routinely performed, and washings of the upper tract are not necessary (see below).

K. Cytologic Examination: Cytologic examination of samples aspirated from within the tumor may be diagnostic, but because invasion of the collecting system is a late sign, cytologic examination of voided urine or even washings of the renal pelvis have rarely helped to diagnose this disease.

L. Tumor Markers: Renal cell carcinoma has no pathognomonic markers, although some of the biologically active substances it produces have already been mentioned. Serum erythropoietin levels were found to be elevated in 63% of 57 patients in one series, but elevation did not correlate with tumor histologic type, grade, stage, or prognosis (Sufrin et al, 1977).

Levels of plasma or urinary carcinoembryonic antigen and urinary polyamines (eg, spermine, spermidine, and putrescine) may be elevated, but these are nonspecific tumor markers. The level of serum haptoglobin, an α_2-globulin produced in the liver, has been shown to be elevated in patients with renal cell carcinoma and to correlate with the stage of disease, particularly the presence or absence of metastases (Vickers, 1974; Babaian and Swanson, 1982). At best, however, it is only a nonspecific tumor marker.

Recently, mouse monoclonal antibodies to cell surface antigens on human renal cancer both in vivo and in vitro have defined several different phenotypes (Bander, 1984; Finstad et al, 1985). The clinical importance of these findings has not yet been determined.

Two ways in which a marker may be helpful are in monitoring therapy and maintaining surveillance after therapy. In this sense, there are many "markers" in renal cell carcinoma, because many of the hematologic and biochemical abnormalities and the clinical signs and symptoms revert to normal after therapy. Thus, if a particular patient with fever at presentation has no fever postnephrectomy, that patient's tumor may have produced a useful "marker," and return of fever may indicate recurrent disease even though disease is not otherwise clinically apparent. Some of the more common examples of this are anemia or erythrocytosis, elevated sedimentation rate, abnormal liver function test findings, hypertension, and hypercalcemia.

Differential Diagnosis

The differential diagnosis of renal cell carcinoma is

that of the renal mass. As discussed earlier, the diagnosis can usually be determined radiographically, but it should remain axiomatic that unless the possibility of cancer can be reasonably excluded by standard radiographic workup, including needle aspiration or biopsy, surgery needs to be performed (Balfe et al, 1982). The apparent renal mass may be a lobulation that occurred during embryonic development, a distortion secondary to a scarred, pyelonephritic kidney (Fig 19–9), or a hypertrophied column of Bertin—diagnoses that might become evident with nephrotomography or a radionuclide scan.

Routine CT scans indicate that many normal kidneys have one or more simple cysts; this precludes surgical exploration or even cyst puncture for all patients with cysts. When symptoms are absent and an ultrasonogram or CT scan demonstrates the classic criteria for a cyst, routine cyst puncture is not recommended. Further evaluation is necessary in cases of symptomatic lesions, calcified lesions, and lesions that deviate from the rigidly defined criteria for a simple cyst.

A variety of space-occupying lesions are solid yet hypovascular. A carbuncle or abscess may be associated with a history of infection, fever, and leukocytosis, and needle aspiration may yield pus. Granulomas may occur in the kidney. Xanthogranulomatous pyelonephritis may mimic renal cell carcinoma and even have some neovascularity as a result of chronic infection; history and radiographic findings suggesting a diffuse process may be helpful. Angiomyolipomas may be virtually impossible to distinguish from renal cell carcinoma on arteriography, but CT scanning may identify the intralesional fat that should suggest the diagnosis. Any patient who presents with a renal mass or

bilateral masses and signs of tuberous sclerosis should obviously be suspected of having an angiomyolipoma because of the strong association.

A renal carcinoma may be a metastatic lesion, most frequently from the lung or breast or from malignant melanoma (Bracken et al, 1979). These metastatic tumors tend to be bilateral, multiple, and less than 3 cm in diameter. Arteriography may help make the diagnosis, and needle biopsy is often necessary. A more diffuse, infiltrative pattern of involvement sometimes suggests leukemia or lymphoma.

Renal pelvic tumors may cause confusion in diagnosis, especially if the excretory urogram shows a nonfunctional tumor. Ultrasonography or CT scanning may show the lesion within the renal pelvis and collecting system; otherwise, arteriography may be helpful. Needle aspiration may yield cells compatible with transitional cell carcinoma.

Extrarenal masses such as pancreatic pseudocysts, enlarged spleen, enlarged retroperitoneal lymph node, and adrenal tumors can be differentiated from a renal mass by radiographic studies, although large adrenal tumors make this difficult. Biochemical abnormalities and the clinical signs due to overproduction of adrenal hormones may identify these lesions.

Treatment
A. Specific Measures:
1. Localized disease–Although there is little hard data to support the clear superiority of radical (extrafascial) over simple (intrafascial) nephrectomy, clinicians almost universally agree that radical nephrectomy is the treatment of choice for non-metastatic renal cell carcinoma. A radical nephrectomy implies early control of the renal vascular pedicle and en bloc removal of the kidney, tumor, and intact Gerota's capsule. It can be performed via either a thoracoabdominal or transabdominal route. Although traditionally the homolateral adrenal gland has also been removed, its routine removal has recently been questioned (Robey and Schellhammer, 1986).

Whether or not lymphadenectomy is integral to the operation remains controversial. Although the overall incidence of lymph node metastases can be higher than 30%, Hulten et al (1969) showed that patients can have isolated lymphatic metastases on the other side of the great vessels, in the iliac nodes, or even in the supraclavicular nodes. DeKernion (1980) points out that the diffuse neovascularity characteristic of this tumor means that lymphatics along these vessels may bear tumor cells to any point in the retroperitoneum from the diaphragm to the pelvis; this makes an attempt to surgically remove all lymph nodes at risk an exercise in futility. Furthermore, a patient who has significant lymphatic regional metastases almost always has distant lymphatic or nonlymphatic metastases as well. Consequently, lymphadenectomy is a staging procedure that is most useful when it identifies unrecognized disease in a patient without demonstrable metastases. It is rarely therapeutic. Only Golimbu et al (1986) have shown higher survival rates following

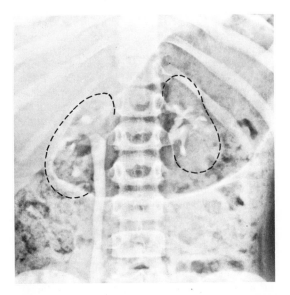

Figure 19–9. Pseudotumor of the kidney. Bilateral healed pyelonephritis secondary to vesicoureteral reflux. Radiogram shows that localized compensatory hypertrophy in lower pole of left kidney displaces calices, suggesting presence of space-occupying lesion.

lymphadenectomy; among patients with stage II and III tumors, the 5-year survival rate was about 15% higher if lymphadenectomy was performed and all lymph nodes were normal than if all lymph nodes were grossly normal and no lymphadenectomy was performed.

Survival rates for patients with lymph node involvement are poor whether or not lymphadenectomy is performed. Multiple studies report 5-year survival rates of less than 10% when regional lymph nodes are involved. Petkovic (1980) demonstrated that patients with early nodal involvement (N_1 and N_2) did better than those with advanced nodal disease (N_3 and N_4), but these nodes, the first-echelon drainage, are usually removed by a standard radical nephrectomy without formal lymphadenectomy.

In the rare instance when tumor is in a solitary kidney, partial nephrectomy (either in situ or ex vivo) should be considered. When all gross tumor is successfully removed, the survival rates have been surprisingly good—at least 65% for this highly selected group of patients (Topley, Novick, and Montie, 1984; Zincke et al, 1985). For in situ surgery, the local recurrence rate is reported to be only 4–16% and even lower for ex vivo operations sparing the parenchyma. For carefully selected patients, enucleation appears to be safe and can yield excellent tumor control (Novick et al, 1986). When bilateral tumors present synchronously, the same surgical principles apply. Bilateral partial nephrectomies or nephrectomy of one kidney plus partial nephrectomy of the other may yield reasonable survival rates in patients who do not have clinically apparent metastases. Some patients have undergone bilateral nephrectomies and chronic hemodialysis or transplantation (Jacobs, Berg, and Lawson, 1980), but total renal ablation in these circumstances is not recommended by everyone (Johnson, von Eschenbach, and Sternberg, 1978).

Radical nephrectomy should also be offered to patients with tumor thrombi extending into the inferior vena cava (estimated incidence is about 3–6%). These thrombi, some of which may extend all the way into the atrium, generally do not "invade" the vessel wall and can be coaxed out surgically. However, because of the mortality rate of 4–14%, the risks of complications (primarily renal failure and sepsis), and the low long-term survival rates, it is now generally accepted that thrombectomy should be attempted only in the absence of clinically apparent metastatic disease; (Kearney et al, 1981; Cherrie et al, 1982; Pritchett, Lieskovsky, and Skinner, 1986).

For tumors extending into the atrium or for very large retroperitoneal tumors, profound hypothermia with cardiac arrest and temporary exsanguination in conjunction with cardiopulmonary bypass permits surgery to proceed in a bloodless field (Marshall, Reitz, and Diamond, 1984; Krane et al, 1984). More experience with this technique will be necessary before it can be determined whether this more efficient surgical technique will yield better long-term results.

Two adjuncts to radical nephrectomy have been recommended for the patient with no evidence of metastasis: radiation therapy and preoperative embolization. The benefits of radiation therapy have been controversial since 1951, when Riches, Griffiths, and Thackray demonstrated tumor reduction after preoperative irradiation. Numerous researchers in the USA and Europe have tried various amounts and schedules for preoperative irradiation, but no results have shown conclusive benefit. Postoperative irradiation has also produced conflicting results, including death from radiation hepatitis. Postoperative irradiation may reduce the incidence of local tumor recurrence in patients with gross residual disease, but it can do nothing to prevent distant metastases.

Preoperative arterial embolization, or infarction, of the primary tumor can be accomplished with pieces of sterile cellulose or with polyvinyl alcohol, ethyl alcohol, or the Gianturco stainless steel coil (Chuang, Wallace, and Swanson, 1981). Preoperative embolization reduces blood loss and decreases operating time by collapsing collateral (tumor) vasculature, creating a zone of edema around the tumor, and preligating the renal artery—a particular advantage when performing transabdominal transperitoneal nephrectomy through an anterior incision (Swanson, 1982). It is invariably followed by pain and fever and sometimes by nausea and vomiting. Because more severe complications are possible, embolization should be restricted to large hypervascular tumors or tumors with thrombus in the renal vein or inferior vena cava. Its benefits, as mentioned above, are only technical; it has not improved survival rates. Embolization can also be used to palliate intractable pain or hematuria in a patient who is not a candidate for nephrectomy.

2. Disseminated disease—The large number of patients who either present with metastatic disease already clinically apparent or develop it subsequent to initial therapy (the poor long-term survival rates for all but patients with stage I tumors largely reflect this progression) makes treatment of disseminated disease particularly compelling. Both the metastatic lesions and the resulting paraneoplastic syndromes (such as hypercalcemia), which threaten not only the patients' lives but also their short-term comfort and sense of well-being, must be treated.

Therapy for the patient who presents with an untreated primary tumor and disseminated disease includes a number of options. Until recently, nephrectomy was recommended almost routinely and was believed to (1) prolong survival, (2) promote regression of metastatic lesions, (3) enhance the effectiveness of other forms of therapy, (4) control local symptoms, and (5) reduce the psychologic impact of the cancer. However, clinical experience does not support these arguments (Maldazys and deKernion, 1986), except when a patient has a solitary metastasis. Although this occurs rarely (in 1.6–3.6% of patients), 5-year survival rates up to 35% have been reported following nephrectomy plus resection of the metastasis (O'Dea et al, 1978). However, before excising the metastasis, the surgeon must prove that the lesion is solitary and be aware that cure is unlikely, since virtually all patients described so far have later developed additional metastases.

Approximately 50 cases of spontaneous regression after nephrectomy have been reported, but few have been histologically confirmed, and many have occurred following treatment other than nephrectomy (Freed, Halperin, and Gordon, 1977). In 1980, de-Kernion and Berry reported spontaneous regression in 0.8% of 571 patients. Nephrectomy does not appear to enhance the effectiveness of standard chemotherapeutic or hormonal agents available today. Furthermore, local symptoms such as pain and hematuria and systemic problems such as hypercalcemia or hypertension can usually be controlled medically or, if necessary, by transcatheter percutaneous arterial embolization of the primary or metastatic tumor (or both). Nephrectomy should generally be reserved for cases in which the patient cannot be controlled by nonoperative methods and is expected to survive for more than 6 months, since the reported operative mortality rate in patients with metastatic renal cell carcinoma is relatively high.

Almgard et al (1973) first reported the use of angioinfarction in patients with renal cell carcinoma, and data from several studies suggest that nephrectomy in the patient with metastatic disease may be more effective if preceded by angioinfarction (Almgard et al, 1973; Bracken et al, 1975). A recent analysis of 100 patients so treated, however, revealed that if there is any therapeutic benefit from such combination therapy, it is restricted to patients with only parenchymal pulmonary metastases, a highly selected group who did show statistically significant improvement in survival rates (Swanson et al, 1983). For no other patients did infarction plus nephrectomy prolong survival over nephrectomy alone. Angioinfarction without subsequent nephrectomy did not lengthen survival time either.

Nevertheless, embolization may have a role in total management. Combined with chemotherapy, it makes possible the delivery directly to the target tumor of substantially higher drug doses than could be delivered systemically (Kato et al, 1981). Another approach is to embolize nonresectable primary tumors and recurrent or metastatic lesions with radioactive iodine (^{125}I) seeds; according to Lang, Sullivan, and deKernion (1983), this procedure shrank all tumors and controlled pain and hemorrhage. Embolization of the metastatic site with inert materials can provide significant palliation for patients with large osseous metastases that become painful again following maximum radiation therapy (Chuang et al, 1979), and because the metastatic lesion is characteristically as hypervascular as the primary lesion, embolization of an osseous metastasis prior to orthopedic surgery has proved a valuable adjunct (Bowers et al, 1982).

Radiation therapy is used clinically to confer symptomatic relief from painful bone metastases. A linear accelerator is not needed; therapy with cobalt 60 (^{60}CO) is as effective. External-beam irradiation is also used for brain metastases, unless the lesion is soli-

tary and can be excised. The neurologic deficit can frequently be reversed (at least partially), even if treatment rarely prolongs survival time significantly. Whole brain irradiation should be supplemented by high-dose steroids. Low-energy irradiation delivered as electron-beam therapy may occasionally palliate painful and bleeding cutaneous metastases.

Ever since Kirkman (1959) demonstrated that testosterone or progestins block estrogen-induced renal cortical tumors in Syrian golden hamsters, hormonal therapy for renal cell carcinoma has excited interest. Bloom (1973) and other writers have championed the efficacy of progestins and androgens in several large series, reporting objective response rates of around 16%. However, in an extensive review, Hrushesky and Murphy (1977) reported that the objective response rate in over 400 patients treated with progestins, androgens, or both between 1971 and 1976 was less than 2%, and they theorized that response rates have diminished as stricter response criteria have been applied. Nonetheless, definite and well-documented objective responses have been reported (predominantly in the lungs in men), and a substantial number of patients with renal cell carcinoma obtain a subjective response and feel better. Since hormones have very few significant side effects and since no consistently effective cytotoxic agent is available for treatment of this disease, hormonal therapy (eg, with medroxyprogesterone acetate, 400 mg twice weekly) still deserves consideration in managing metastatic renal cell carcinoma as long as there are no false expectations.

Multiple reviews of cytotoxic chemotherapy through 1983 have failed to identify a single drug or combination of drugs that is consistently active in renal cell carcinoma (McDonald, 1982; Harris, 1983). Many agents or combinations produce response rates of 5–10%, but virtually all are partial or mixed responses, and they are generally of short duration. In many instances, the apparent success rate of a drug reflects simply the inadequate number of patients tested, and the initial promise exhibited by some drugs has evaporated as the clinical experience expanded.

The promising early experience with interferon must be viewed in this light. Partially purified human leukocyte interferon (IFN α) has been reported to produce at least a 50% reduction of tumors (and total reduction in rare cases) in 15–26% of patients (de-Kernion et al, 1983; Quesada, Swanson, and Gutterman, 1985), human lymphoblastoid interferon in 15% (Neidhart et al, 1984), and recombinant interferon (IFNα-2a) in 29%, but the development of neutralizing antibodies to IFNα-2a in 7 of 12 responders shortened the duration of remission (Quesada et al, 1985). Combinations of interferons are also being tested. Most responses have been in the skin and lung, but lesions in the retroperitoneal lymph nodes and liver have also responded. Various interferons appear to be active against renal cell carcinoma and deserve further testing, either alone or in conjunction with chemotherapeutic agents (Figlin et al, 1985; Neidhart, 1986; Fossá et al, 1986).

A definite therapeutic role is established for mithramycin. Hypercalcemia is common in renal cell carcinoma (estimated 10–12% of cases) and can occur whether or not bone metastases are present. Renal cell carcinomas themselves can produce a parathyroid hormone-like substance and prostaglandin E, both of which can raise the serum calcium level. Mithramycin, usually in an infusion of 25 μg/m^2 body surface area, effectively lowers the serum calcium level, although its peak effect is usually not manifest until 36–48 hours after infusion. The serum calcium level can be lowered immediately, however, by promoting a brisk diuresis with intravenous saline and furosemide (Lasix) (Swanson, 1983). Indomethacin, an antiprostaglandin, has also been reported to lower the serum calcium level (Brereton et al, 1974).

Since the report of the apparently successful transfer of serum from one cured patient to a family member with renal cell carcinoma (Horn and Horn, 1971), immunotherapy has been advocated experimentally for patients with advanced renal cell carcinoma. Homogenized, polymerized, and sometimes irradiated autologous tumor injected intradermally with an adjuvant has improved survival rates (Neidhart et al, 1980; McCune, Schapira, and Henshaw, 1981; Tallberg et al, 1985). Others have used immune RNA or bacille Calmette-Guérin (BCG) (deKernion and Ramming, 1980; Richie et al, 1984; Morales et al, 1982). More recent trials of biologic response modifiers are being performed using amplogen, tumor necrosis factor, interleukin-2, lymphokine-activated killer (LAK) cells, or various combinations of these (Rosenberg et al, 1985). However, no one has convincingly demonstrated that immunotherapy produces effective clinical regression of disease or prolongs survival time.

B. Follow-Up Care: Patients should be followed at regular intervals to monitor for disease recurrence or progression. Follow-up should include a physical examination to search for an abdominal mass or enlarged liver or lymph nodes, complete blood count to screen for anemia or erythrocytosis, and serum multiple analysis (SMA-12) to test for liver function and levels of serum creatinine and calcium. Nonspecific tumor markers such as serum haptoglobin, as well as biologically active substances that may be produced by renal cell carcinomas (see above), may be identified. Chest x-ray is mandatory. A plain film of the abdomen or a bone scan is rarely helpful unless complaints suggest a bony metastasis. A CT scan permits evaluation of the contralateral kidney and can rule out local recurrence in the renal fossa and metastases in the liver, although the yield is low unless the patient is symptomatic or at high risk for local recurrence (Parienty et al, 1984).

Prognosis

A number of factors correlate with survival expectations: clinical presentation, stage, histologic grade and size of tumor, erythrocyte sedimentation rate, and the sex of the patient. Recently, DNA content has been shown to correlate well with prognosis (Otto et al, 1984; Ljungberg et al, 1986). The best estimation of prognosis can be made from the surgical or histopathologic tumor stage.

The effect of the tumor on life expectancy was sharply defined at the Mayo Clinic by an analysis of 89 patients 20–40 years old for whom an age- and sex-matched cohort had a 97% likelihood of 10-year survival (Lieber et al, 1981). The 5- and 10-year survival rates, respectively, were 79% and 73% for patients with stage I disease (tumor confined to kidney); 40% and 24% for those with stage II or III disease (regional spread to perinephric fat or lymph nodes, or gross involvement of renal vein or inferior vena cava); and 8% (at 5 years) for those with stage IV disease (metastatic disease). Patients with stage I tumors had an excellent prognosis if they survived longer than 3 years; fewer than 50% of patients with stage IV tumors survived 1 year, and only 20% survived 3 years.

Despite earlier reports that venous involvement does not significantly affect survival rates, Hoehn and Hermanek, Sigel, and Chlepas (1983) found progressively poorer survival rates for patients with microscopic venous involvement or macroscopic involvement of intrarenal veins, the main renal vein, and the inferior vena cava. In their renal cell carcinoma study, the group from Rotterdam found that renal vein involvement significantly reduced the chance of cure (van der Werf-Messing, van der Heul, and Ledeboer, 1978). Perhaps the key lies in studies reporting that tumor in the inferior vena cava did not appear to influence the prognosis adversely unless the primary tumor also extended into the perinephric fat (Heney and Nocks, 1982; Cherrie et al, 1982; Golimbu et al, 1986).

Regional lymph node involvement conveys a poor prognosis. Only rare patients who present with stage IV disease survive 5 years, regardless of therapy.

NEPHROBLASTOMA
(Wilms' Tumor)

Nephroblastoma, or Wilms' tumor, is a malignant mixed renal tumor that occurs predominantly in children but can appear in adolescents and adults. The median age of incidence is 2 years 11 months (Lemerle et al, 1976). The tumor occurs with equal frequency in males and females, and racial or geographic factors do not significantly influence its incidence (Bennington and Beckwith, 1975). Tumors occur almost equally in right and left kidneys; about 5% are bilateral at diagnosis. Wilms' tumor is associated with congenital anomalies in 15% of patients (Pendergrass, 1976). Among 547 patients in the National Wilms' Tumor Study, the most common anomalies noted were aniridia (1% of children with Wilms' tumor), hemihypertrophy (2.9%), and genitourinary anomalies (4.4%).

Etiology

Wilms' tumor is believed to be at least in part congenital, as it is the only common tumor of mixed embryonic origin. Knudson and Strong (1972) have proposed that the tumor results from 2 separate mutational events, the first either prezygotic or postzygotic and the second always postzygotic. If the first mutation is prezygotic, the tumors are hereditary, but if it is postzygotic, they are nonhereditary. From this model, it is predicted that 38% of Wilms' tumors are hereditary and 62% are sporadic. A specific aberration of chromosome 11 has been reported to be present in patients with both aniridia and Wilms' tumor (Yunis and Ramsay, 1980).

Pathogenesis & Pathology

The 2-mutation hypothesis of Knudson and Strong (1972) may explain the induction of malignant transformation, but the origin of nephroblastoma is not known. Because of the higher incidence of persistent blastema in kidneys with nephroblastoma, Bove and McAdams (1976) and Rous et al (1976) have postulated that it arises from nodular renal blastema. There is some evidence that nodular blastema can progress to nephphroblastoma. Bennington and Beckwith (1975) speculate that blastema may persist as the result of a prezygotic mutation and can progress to nephroblastoma after the second (postzygotic) mutation.

The tumors are generally large and solitary, although multifocal disease is present in 7% of patients (Breslow and Beckwith, 1982). On cut section, nephroblastomas are typically soft and multilobulated, appear gray or tan, and bulge above the cut surface. Foral hemorrhage or necrosis may be present, and rare cystic changes may lead to the mistaken impression that the kidney is polycystic.

Histologically, the tumor is composed of a mixture of epithelial, stromal, and blastematous (immature mesenchyma) elements in varying proportions. Nephroblastomas have been divided into 2 broad categories based on histopathologic characteristics (Beckwith and Palmer, 1978). About 11% of tumors in patients entered in the National Wilms' Tumor Study had focal or diffuse anaplasia or sarcomatous features, and these findings were termed "unfavorable histology" (UH). The rest were designated "favorable histology" (FH), and prognosis correlated closely with whether the tumors were FH or UH. UH tumors are further subdivided into anaplastic tumors, rhabdoid tumors, and clear cell tumor variants. Each behaves clinically in a distinct fashion; they may, in fact, be separate entities (D'Angio et al, 1982).

Local spread occurs by direct invasion through the renal capsule and usually involves the retroperitoneal tissues, although penetration through the peritoneum and peritoneal seeding may occur. The tumor may propagate as a tumor thrombus in the renal vein and spread up the inferior vena cava even to the atrium; it usually does not invade the vessel. The collecting system may be infiltrated, filling the renal pelvis and ureter with polypoid tumor nodules. Lymph node involvement occurs in the hilar and periaortic regions. Distant metastases are present at diagnosis in about 11% of patients (D'Angio et al, 1981). The lungs are most frequently involved, with or without other organ involvement, and are the first site of metastasis after primary surgery in over 80% of patients. Metastases also occur in the liver, mediastinal lymph nodes, adrenal glands, diaphragm, retroperitoneum, and occasionally in other sites (Bennington and Beckwith, 1975). D'Angio et al (1982) reported that bone metastases are rare unless the tumor is the clear cell variant (sarcoma) and that brain metastases and independent small-cell brain tumors of the posterior fossa are found in association with rhabdoid tumors.

Tumor Staging

In the most widely used staging system, that proposed in 1976 by the National Wilms' Tumor Study Group (D'Angio et al, 1976), the patient's clinical "group" is decided by the surgeon in the operating room and is confirmed by pathologists. The proposed clinical "groups" have now been validated by retrospective analysis and can thus be considered "stages" (Farewell et al, 1981) as follows:

Stage I: Tumor limited to the kidney and completely excised. The surface of the renal capsule is intact; the tumor was not ruptured before or during removal. No residual tumor is apparent beyond the margins of excision.

Stage II: Tumor extends beyond the kidney but is completely excised. Tumor extends locally, ie, penetrates beyond the pseudocapsule into the perirenal soft tissues, or involves the periaortic lymph nodes. Renal vessels outside the kidney substance are infiltrated or contain tumor thrombus. No residual tumor is apparent beyond the margins of excision.

Stage III: Residual nonhematogenous tumor confined to the abdomen. One or more of the following occurs: (1) Tumor has been biopsied or ruptured before or during surgery; (2) implants are present on peritoneal surfaces; (3) lymph nodes beyond the abdominal periaortic chains are involved; (4) tumor is not completely removable, because of local infiltration into vital structures.

Stage IV: Hematogenous metastases. Deposits beyond stage III, eg, lung, liver, bone, brain.

Stage V: Bilateral renal involvement either initially or subsequently.

Clinical Findings

The following discussion of clinical manifestations is based on the observations of Bennington and Beckwith (1975) and D'Angio et al (1982).

A. Symptoms: Since most children with Wilms' tumor appear healthy and have no symptoms, the tumor is most commonly found by the physician during a well-baby examination or by a family member. However, pain has been reported in 20–30% of patients; anorexia, nausea, and vomiting in 15%; and fever in 10–20%. Constipation is occasionally seen.

B. Signs: An abdominal mass is by far the most common sign and is present in over 90% of cases. The mass may be extremely large and is usually firm and immobile. Hypertension occurs in up to 60% of cases and gross hematuria in about 10%. Signs secondary to the large mass, such as leg edema or varicocele, may also occur. Because of the high incidence of associated congenital anomalies, the presence of aniridia, hemihypertrophy, or some of the less common anomalies should alert the clinician to the possibility of Wilms' tumor.

C. Laboratory Findings: Urinalysis may show hematuria. Anemia may be present, particularly if hemorrhage into the tumor or rupture has occurred.

D. X-Ray Findings: Plain abdominal x-rays (kidney, ureter, and bladder film) may show a greatly enlarged renal shadow or displacement of abdominal organs by the mass. Calcifications, present in about 10% of Wilms' tumors, are usually spotlike or ringlike.

Excretory urography is the single most valuable and cost-effective diagnostic method, since only a small percentage of patients have a totally nonfunctioning kidney. The involved kidney is typically distorted and its collecting system displaced secondary to the intrarenal mass (Fig 19–10). Excretory urography also permits assessment of the contralateral kidney with regard to function, tumor involvement, and possible malformations.

Although inferior venacavography is used routinely by some clinicians, it should probably be reserved for cases in which the kidney does not visualize on excretory urography or prominent veins on the abdominal wall suggest the possibility of caval obstruction. Arteriography does not reliably contribute to diagnosis and is not indicated routinely.

Because of the high incidence of lung metastases, every patient with Wilms' tumor should have chest x-rays performed. Although whole lung tomography is indisputably more sensitive, it should not be performed routinely, because of the time, x-ray exposure, and cost involved and the lack of substantial effect on the ultimate outcome. Skeletal surveys are reserved for patients with clear cell sarcoma.

E. Ultrasonography and CT Scanning: These studies are being used with increased frequency, and their role is undergoing redefinition. Both demonstrate whether a renal mass is solid, whether the contralateral kidney is involved, whether tumor thrombus appears in the renal vein or inferior vena cava, whether retroperitoneal lymph nodes are enlarged, and whether the liver has tumor. Ultrasonography may assess the renal vein and inferior vena cava more easily, particularly with real-time imaging. CT scanning may be more sensitive in diagnosing and following tumor masses. CT scanning may ultimately replace arteriography in managing Wilms' tumor.

F. Radionuclide Imaging: All information provided by isotope scans is better obtained by other means.

G. Biopsy: Biopsy is virtually never indicated.

Differential Diagnosis

A flank mass in a child may be either benign or malignant. Hydronephrosis, the most common benign condition, is usually softer than a Wilms' tumor, may transilluminate, and can usually be differentiated by excretory urography. Ultrasonography or CT scanning demonstrates its cystic nature, and retrograde urography locates the obstruction.

Cystic kidneys accounted for 25% of the errors in diagnosis in the First National Wilms' Tumor Study (D'Angio et al, 1976). Ultrasonography can identify the cystic nature of these lesions; however, since some Wilms' tumors occur in association with cystic kidneys, surgery may be necessary to establish the correct diagnosis (D'Angio et al, 1982). A multicystic kidney is usually nonfunctioning, and a retrograde urogram demonstrates the complete obstruction of the ureter. Kidneys may be bilaterally polycystic. Congenital mesoblastic nephroma (hamartoma), as originally described by Bolande, Brough, and Izant (1967), is a benign tumor that is indistinguishable from Wilms' tumor by all present radiographic methods (Hartman et al, 1981), but surgery is appropriate and establishes the diagnosis.

The malignant tumor most commonly confused with Wilms' tumor is neuroblastoma. Neuroblastomas tend to displace the kidney downward and therefore are far less likely to distort the calices than Wilms' tumor, which is an intrinsic renal lesion. Neuroblas-

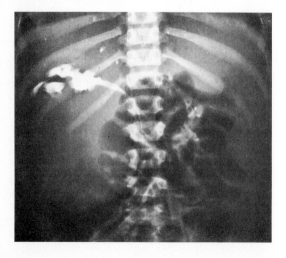

Figure 19–10. Wilms' tumor. Excretory urogram showing large globular mass in right upper quadrant, with displacement and distortion of calices. Upper right ureter is displaced over spine.

tomas are more likely to be calcified (about 30% of cases), and the calcification frequently exhibits a diffuse, fine stippling. If it is paravertebral, both kidneys may be displaced laterally. The child with neuroblastoma is more likely to appear chronically ill, pale, and irritable than one with nephroblastoma (Leape, 1978). At diagnosis, 70% of patients with neuroblastoma already have metastatic disease; bone metastases are common, and the liver may be massively enlarged owing to metastatic disease. The urinary level of vanilmandelic acid (VMA) is elevated in patients with neuroblastoma but is normal in patients with Wilms' tumor. It may be possible to diagnose an intrarenal neuroblastoma only after nephrectomy; 40% of the wrong diagnoses in the First National Wilms' Tumor Study were neuroblastomas (D'Angio et al, 1976).

Treatment

The survival rate for a patient with Wilms' tumor treated by surgery alone rose from under 10% early this century to a maximum of 40% by 1940 (D'Angio et al, 1980). It is a tribute to the concept of multimodal therapy—and to the National Wilms' Tumor Study Group, which championed its use and demonstrated its effectiveness—that the survival rate has improved so dramatically. Results of the first and second studies are now available (D'Angio et al, 1976, 1981), and final reports of the third, which has been completed, are awaited. The thrust of these studies has been first to lengthen survival time and then to seek refinements of therapy that would reduce toxicity and long-term sequels without decreasing survival rates in low-risk patients and that would be more effective in high-risk patients. The following is a summary of treatment recommendations of the study group.

A. Surgical Measures: Total nephrectomy for unilateral Wilms' tumor remains the cornerstone of management. The selected site of incision should permit careful exploration of the abdominal contents, exposure and formal exploration of the contralateral kidney, and safe, complete removal of the tumor with Gerota's fascia intact. Regional lymph nodes should be removed with the specimen and any suspicious-appearing nodes biopsied. Heroic efforts to remove all tumor by resecting major organs are to be avoided (Leape, Breslow, and Bishop, 1978). Likewise, tumor thrombus in the inferior vena cava should be removed only if removal is not unduly hazardous. Great care should be taken to avoid rupturing the tumor. If it is massive or is attached to other major organs, preoperative chemotherapy may shrink it and facilitate its removal (Bracken et al, 1982). When Wilms' tumors are bilateral, an attempt to surgically excise all gross tumor bilaterally is generally worthwhile, although such surgery is often deferred until after preliminary chemotherapy, radiation therapy, or both (Leape, Breslow, and Bishop, 1978; Lemerle, 1982).

B. Radiation Therapy: Few clinicians dispute that Wilms' tumor is very radiosensitive and that the early improvements in survival rate resulted from adding radiation therapy to surgery. The present trend,

however, is to omit postoperative irradiation in patients with low-stage disease and to decrease the dose of radiation therapy in those with high-stage disease by combining it with chemotherapy (D'Angio et al, 1982; Clouse et al, 1985); this is done in an attempt to spare the child the long-term functional and structural impairment of the skeleton seen in patients who received radiation therapy at a young age (Leape, Breslow, and Bishop, 1978). Radiation therapy is still used as part of the treatment of lung, liver, brain, and bone metastases.

C. Chemotherapy: The First National Wilms' Tumor Study Group established that use of the combination of vincristine and dactinomycin is better than use of either drug alone and that these 2 agents are the minimum needed postoperatively (D'Angio et al, 1982). The second study group found that doxorubicin (Adriamycin) is a valuable addition to the 2-drug regimen. The third study group is now investigating whether more intensive therapy with dactinomycin plus vincristine will give equally good results as the 3-drug regimen, since the long-term cardiac effects of doxorubicin are not known. The third study group is also evaluating whether shorter courses of postoperative chemotherapy are equally effective. Reports have indicated that preoperative use of either vincristine alone (Bracken et al, 1982) or vincristine plus dactinomycin (deKraker et al, 1982; Lemerle et al, 1983) markedly reduces tumor size, helps prevent intraoperative tumor rupture, and facilitates complete resection.

Prognosis

Several factors that strongly influence survival rates have been identified, but the most important are histologic type of tumor, lymph node involvement, and stage of disease (Lemerle et al, 1976; Beckwith and Palmer, 1978; D'Angio et al, 1982). The Second National Wilms' Tumor Study (D'Angio et al, 1981) reported that the 2-year relapse-free survival rates were 90% for patients with FH tumors versus 54% for those with UH tumors. Likewise, rates were significantly lower for patients with tumor involving lymph nodes, even if the nodes were excised: 82% without node involvement versus 54% with node involvement (all children in the study). Intraoperative spillage was closely related to abdominal recurrence and death even after accounting for the influence of histology and lymph nodes (Breslow et al, 1985). Patients in the second study had the following 2-year relapse-free survival rates and 2-year survival rates, respectively: stage I, 88% and 95%; stage II, 78% and 90%; stage III, 70% and 84%; and stage IV, 49% and 54%. Of 30 patients with stage V disease, 26 (87%) survived 2 years or more, indicating that even disease at this stage is treatable and has potentially good results (Bishop et al, 1977; Kay and Tank, 1986).

Although survival rates have improved dramatically, a substantial risk remains that patients cured of cancer will develop long-term sequels, including growth defects of the spine, radiation enteritis, radiation nephritis and hepatopathy, secondary malignant tumors, and sterility (Jaffe et al, 1980).

SARCOMA OF THE KIDNEY

Sarcomas of the kidney are rare, comprising only 2–3% of all malignant renal tumors. Leiomyosarcoma, liposarcoma, and hemangiopericytoma are discussed below; rhabdomyosarcoma, angiosarcoma, fibrosarcoma, fibroxanthosarcoma, and osteogenic sarcoma of the kidney have been reported but are even rarer than these 3 types. For an excellent review, see Bennington and Beckwith (1975).

Leiomyosarcoma

The most common sarcoma of the kidney is leiomyosarcoma, which accounts for over half of the renal sarcomas seen at the Mayo Clinic (Farrow et al, 1968) and 44% of those seen at the Memorial Sloan-Kettering Cancer Center (Srivnas et al, 1984). The incidence increases with age after 20 years. Leiomyosarcoma occurs more frequently in females than in males. The symptoms and signs result from the large and usually invasive tumor typically present at diagnosis. Leiomyosarcomas frequently extend into the pelvis to cause hematuria, and filling defects in the renal pelvis can be seen on excretory urography.

Nephrectomy is the treatment of choice if metastases are not clinically apparent, but local recurrence and metastatic disease usually develop. These tumors are relatively radioresistant, and combination cytotoxic chemotherapy has yielded rather poor results to date.

Liposarcoma

Liposarcomas are rare. Some retroperitoneal liposarcomas (the most common retroperitoneal sarcoma) have been confused with primary renal tumors, and angiomyolipomas have been mistakenly reported as liposarcomas. These tumors are typically large and bulky, and although they may appear well circumscribed, the extent of invasion is difficult to determine by gross examination. Histologically, these tumors may be confused with xanthogranulomatous pyelonephritis or poorly differentiated renal carcinoma.

Treatment is radical nephrectomy, but the chance for cure appears low. As with liposarcomas in other sites, local recurrence is more common than distant metastatic spread.

Hemangiopericytoma

Hemangiopericytoma is an uncommon, richly vascular tumor that apparently arises from the renal capsule or the retroperitoneum. It is believed that juxtaglomerular tumors are a specialized form of hemangiopericytoma that is able to secrete renin.

Five patients have been reported by the Mayo Clinic, and 4 died of their tumor despite nephrectomy (Farrow et al, 1968).

TUMORS OF THE RENAL PELVIS

Malignant tumors arising from the renal calices or pelves comprise approximately 7% of all renal neoplasms but represent fewer than 1% of all genitourinary tumors. They are seen approximately 3 times more frequently in men than in women. These tumors show no predilection for side, but they occur bilaterally in only 2–4% of patients.

Etiology

The causes of renal pelvic tumors are unknown but are believed to parallel those of bladder cancer (see p 355). The term urothelium was introduced by Melicow (1945) to emphasize the "oneness" of the membrane that lines the entire urinary tract and to reinforce the belief in a multicentric origin of urothelial tumors. Over 20% of patients with either renal pelvic, ureteral, or bladder tumors have multiple, rather than single, lesions at diagnosis. Over one-third of patients with renal pelvic tumors either have had, have, or will develop other urothelial tumors.

Chronic infection, urolithiasis, viruses, and environmental factors including cigarettes, coffee, and organic solvents used in the dye and leather industry have been implicated in the development of renal pelvic carcinoma. The interactions between irritants, promoters and initiators of tumor growth, carcinogens, and cocarcinogens are just now beginning to be understood.

Currently, 3 patient populations appear to be at high risk for developing renal pelvic tumors: (1) abusers of phenacetin, (2) patients with Balkan nephropathy, and (3) those in whom thorium dioxide (Thorotrast) was used for retrograde urography. Strong circumstantial evidence indicates a cause-and-effect relationship between heavy intake of phenacetin- and aspirin-containing analgesics and both papillary necrosis and transitional cell carcinoma of the renal pelvis. Renal pelvic carcinoma has developed in patients consuming from 1 to 25 kg of phenacetin over a period of 3–35 years (mean, 15 years). The period from analgesic ingestion to clinical recognition of the tumor (induction time) has ranged from 6 to 35 years (mean, 19 years). Tumors associated with analgesic nephropathy are usually of higher histologic grade and in a later stage of disease at diagnosis than those not associated with analgesic nephropathy.

It has been well documented that inhabitants of several well-defined areas of the Balkan countries, including Yugoslavia, Romania, Bulgaria, and Greece, who become afflicted with Balkan nephropathy are at high risk for developing renal pelvic tumors. These tumors have a different biologic behavior, however, from those usually seen in other parts of the world. They are usually small, comparatively benign, and frequently (10% of cases) bilateral.

Thorotrast, a 25% colloidal solution of thorium dioxide, was introduced in 1930 as an x-ray contrast medium for retrograde urography and was still used in some parts of the world in 1955. Reflux deposited the material in the renal parenchyma. The interval between its deposition and the development of renal pelvic tumors has ranged from 14 to 41 years. Most of the tumors have been squamous cell carcinomas of the renal pelvis; 4 of 5 patients in one series died of disease within 5 months of the diagnosis (Almgard et al, 1977). Consequently, prophylactic nephroureterectomy has been suggested for patients who have unilateral "Thorotrast kidney" without symptoms.

Pathogenesis & Pathology

Transitional cell carcinoma accounts for approximately 85% of renal pelvic tumors, and about two-thirds of these are papillary in type. Most of these papillary tumors are malignant; only 7 benign ones have been reported in the English literature (Toppercer, 1980). Patients with papillary tumors tend to have a better prognosis than those with nonpapillary tumors, but prognosis usually correlates more closely with amount of invasion and grade of the tumor.

Squamous cell carcinomas, which occur with equal frequency in men and women, account for 14% of the total number of renal pelvic tumors. They are usually associated with calculous disease and chronic irritation. They are invasive and highly malignant; only one 5-year survival had been reported up to 1960.

Adenocarcinoma accounts for fewer than 1% of renal pelvic carcinomas. The tumor occurs predominantly in women and is frequently associated with renal calculi (60% of cases), hydronephrosis (40%), and pyelonephritis (25%). Two-thirds of the cases involve the right side. The prognosis is poor.

Renal pelvic carcinoma spreads by (1) contiguous growth into the renal parenchyma, renal hilum, and peripelvic tissue; (2) lymphatic embolization to para-aortic, mediastinal, and supraclavicular lymph nodes; and (3) hematogenous metastasis to the lung, liver, and bones and, less frequently, the adrenals, opposite kidney, pancreas, and spleen. The presence of lymph node metastasis is usually indicative of systemic disease, and if visceral metastases are not already evident, they usually become clinically apparent within 6–9 months.

Tumor Staging

In the absence of accurate clinical staging procedures, classification of renal pelvic tumors has been based on pathologic findings. Grabstald, Whitmore, and Melamed (1971) and Batata et al (1975) evolved the following staging system for transitional cell tumors of the renal pelvis and ureter:

Stage 0: Neoplasms confined to the mucosa.
Stage A: Submucosal infiltration only.
Stage B: Muscular invasion without extension through the muscle wall of the calix, pelvis, or ureter.
Stage C: Invasion of the renal parenchyma or the peripelvic or periureteral fat.
Stage D: Extension outside the kidney or ureter into adjacent organs, regional lymph nodes, or distant metastases.

Clinical Findings

A. Symptoms: Gross painless hematuria, the most common complaint, is noted in 70–95% of patients with renal pelvic tumors. Flank pain has been reported in 8–40% of patients and may result from tumor obstructing the ureteropelvic junction, ureteral colic from passage of blood clots or tumor fragments, or local extension of the tumor to involve retroperitoneal structures. Symptoms of bladder irritation are present in 5–10% of patients. Constitutional symptoms (anorexia, weight loss, and lethargy) cause about 5% of patients to seek medical attention.

B. Signs: There may be tenderness over the kidney, particularly if ureteral obstruction has occurred or if infection has supervened. A flank mass secondary to the tumor or an associated hydronephrosis is present in 10–20% of patients.

C. Laboratory Findings: Anemia can be marked if bleeding is profuse. Gross or microscopic hematuria is to be expected, but at intervals the urine may be free of red cells. Renal infection can result from obstruction or can be associated with the primary tumor; in either case, pus and bacteria are present in the urine.

D. X-Ray Findings: The diagnosis is usually suspected on the basis of an excretory urogram, which almost always reveals abnormal findings in patients with renal pelvic carcinoma. The most common pyelographic finding is a filling defect in the renal pelvis, demonstrable in 50–75% of the urograms (Fig 19–11). Other radiographic findings include ureteropelvic or infundibular stenosis, hydronephrosis, or splaying of the calices, which may suggest a renal mass. Nonvisualization of the affected renal unit occurs in over 10% of patients.

Although several investigators (Boijsen and Falin, 1961; Mitty, Baron, and Fuler, 1969) have described a distinctive appearance of renal pelvic carcinoma on angiograms, false-positive interpretations have exceeded 40%. The most common error is mistaking inflammatory disease for the cancer. Selective angiograms may demonstrate one or more of the following features: (1) arterial encasement or amputation; (2) fine neovascularity and tumor staining; (3) enlarged prominent pelvic ureteral arteries; and (4) irregular diminished nephrograms, suggesting tumor invading the renal parenchyma. Angiography is most useful in demonstrating other pathologic conditions (renal artery aneurysms, vascular impressions, etc) that can cause a negative defect on urograms and mimic a renal pelvic tumor.

E. Ultrasonography: Ultrasonography may

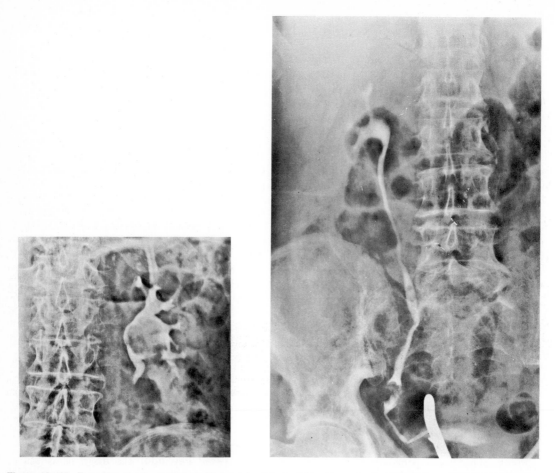

Figure 19–11. Transitional cell carcinoma of the renal pelvis. *Left:* Excretory urogram showing space-occupying lesion of left renal pelvis. *Right:* Retrograde urogram showing "negative" shadow caused by transitional cell carcinoma of lower right ureter without evidence of obstruction.

help define the nature of the lesion and distinguish a tumor from nonopaque calculi and blood clots.

F. Instrumental Examination: Cystoscopy should be done immediately when gross bleeding is present. Blood may be seen spurting from one ureteral orifice, which localizes the source of bleeding. During cystoscopy, the physician should search for other urothelial tumors on the bladder or urethral walls.

Transurethral ureteropyeloscopy is seldom required to establish a correct diagnosis and should only be considered in selected cases, since the procedure carries the risk of serious complications (eg, perforation, extravasation).

G. Cytologic Examination: Routine cytologic analysis of urine from a voided or catheterized bladder specimen is usually of limited value, since at least 30% of specimens are negative for malignant cells. Collecting a urine specimen after barbotage through a ureteral catheter greatly increases the chance for a positive diagnosis. A retrograde brush biopsy (Fig 19–12) provides specimens for both histologic and cy-

tologic studies leading to an accurate preoperative diagnosis.

Differential Diagnosis

Adenocarcinoma of the kidney also causes hematuria. Such a tumor, however, is apt to be palpable or may be visible on a plain film of the abdomen as an expansion of a portion of the kidney. Urograms show the intrarenal nature of the growth. However, blood clots in the renal pelvis can mimic pelvic tumor. If a transitional cell tumor invades the parenchyma, it simulates adenocarcinoma. Cytologic tests and angiography may make the differentiation.

A nonopaque renal stone may cause hematuria and renal pain. A mass may be palpable if hydronephrosis develops. Urograms show a space-occupying lesion of the pelvis, but the outline of the negative (black) shadow (representing the stone) tends to be smoothly round or oval for stone and irregular (papillary) for tumor (see Chapter 16 and Figs 16–4 and 16–8). When

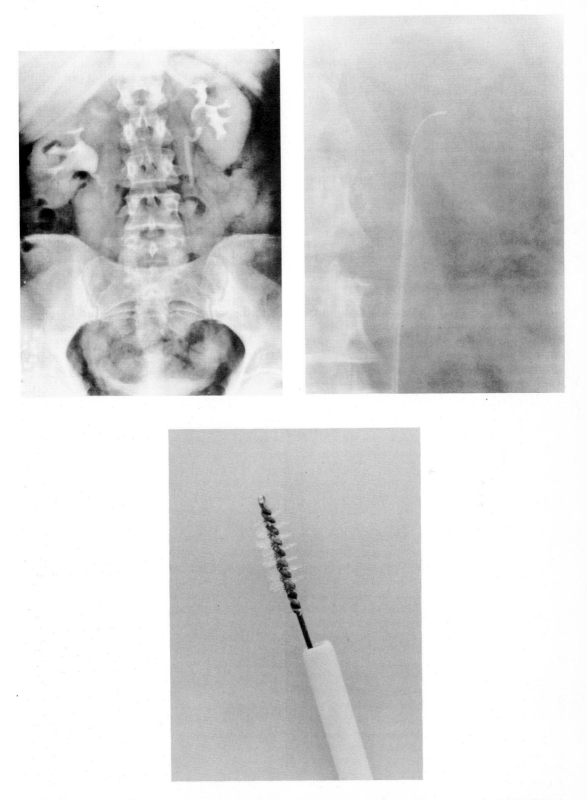

Figure 19–12. Carcinoma of the renal pelvis. *Upper left:* Excretory urogram showing filling defect typical of this disease. *Upper right:* Brush inserted and directed to site of lesion for biopsy. *Bottom:* Close-up of brush with bristles protruding from open-end catheter.

the mass is a tumor, cytologic studies usually yield positive results. Ultrasonography or CT scanning can help in differentiation.

An opaque renal stone may be associated with an epidermoid carcinoma of the renal pelvis. Under these circumstances, diagnosis may be difficult or may be possible only at the time of surgical exploration. Urinary cytology or ultrasonography may help in differentiation.

Renal tuberculosis may also mimic a pelvic neoplasm. The urogram may show irregularity of the pelvic outline caused by ulceration, which might suggest tumor. The patient with urinary tract tuberculosis usually complains of vesical irritability and has "sterile" pyuria. Acid-fast organisms can be demonstrated in the urine.

Cholesteatoma of the renal pelvis comprises a mass of keratinized squamous cells. Urography shows an intrapelvic mass. The urine is loaded with squamous cells. Angiography reveals no evidence of tumor.

An ectopic or aberrant renal papilla projecting into the renal pelvis appears on the urogram as a space-occupying lesion. Selective angiography is definitive.

Hemangioma, an occasional cause of hematuria involving the renal pelvis or submucosal parenchyma, is usually too small to be seen on a urogram. A large hemangioma appears on the urogram as a space-occupying lesion of the pelvis. Renal angiography establishes the diagnosis (Fig 19–13).

Treatment

A. Specific Measures: In the absence of demonstrable metastases, the optimal treatment is radi-

cal nephrectomy, which includes removal of the kidney and all perinephric tissue, keeping Gerota's capsule intact; removal of the ipsilateral adrenal gland; and complete excision of the ureter and adjacent vesical mucosa. When the distal ureter has not been completely excised, subsequent recurrent disease has been documented in one-third of the patients. Johansson and Wahlqvist (1979) found the 5-year survival rate to be significantly better for patients who underwent the radical procedure (84% rate) than for those treated by an intrafascial nephrectomy (51% rate).

The value of lymphadenectomy in treating this disease remains undetermined. Today, no improved rate of survival has been reported for patients with renal pelvic tumors who have been subjected to systematic en bloc lymphadenectomy. The age of many of these patients and the presence of atherosclerosis do not appear to justify the increased risk of additional surgery.

The role of radiotherapy in this disease has been inadequately studied. The unsuccessful attempts to improve survival rates of patients with renal cell carcinoma by either pre- or postoperative irradiation, the risks of radiation injuries to the liver and bowel, and the belief that lymph node involvement represents systemic disease have contributed to a lack of enthusiasm for using radiotherapy as an adjunct to surgery for treatment of renal pelvic tumors. However, a recent report by Brookland and Richter (1985) suggests that postoperative irradiation may improve local control in some high-risk patients.

B. Palliative Measures: Even though metastases are demonstrable, it may be advisable to remove the affected kidney if pain or infection from obstruc-

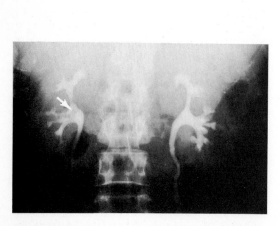
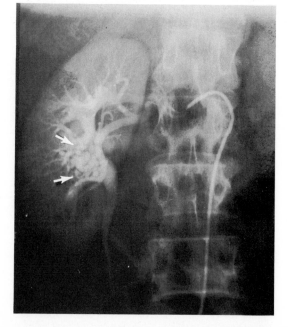

Figure 19–13. Hemangioma of the renal pelvis. *Left:* Excretory urogram showing filling defect in right renal pelvis. *Right:* Selective renal angiogram. Note multiple dilated arteries.

tion is severe or if bleeding is profuse. Occasionally, renal artery occlusion may be used to control these local symptoms. Chemotherapy is restricted to treating known metastatic lesions (lungs, liver, bones, etc); the drug programs parallel those currently used for patients with metastases from bladder cancer.

C. Follow-Up Care: The patient should be seen periodically to exclude the development of local recurrence (para-aortic lymph nodes), visceral metastases (lungs, liver, bones), and contralateral upper tract or vesical tumors. Careful physical examination, chest x-ray, cytologic studies of urine specimens, and cystoscopy should be performed at 3-month intervals for 3 years, then at 6-month intervals for 2 years, and then annually thereafter, provided no disease is demonstrated during that period of time.

Prognosis

The prognosis for patients with benign tumors is excellent. For patients with low-grade transitional cell carcinoma, the outlook is excellent (approaches 100%), but when the disease is poorly differentiated, fewer than 20% of patients are alive at 5 years. Similarly, the outlook for patients with low-stage malignant tumors is good but becomes fair to poor as the stage increases; few survivors are alive at 5 years if distant metastases occur. The prognosis is poor for patients with either adenocarcinoma or squamous cell carcinoma.

TUMORS OF THE URETER

Tumors of the ureter are uncommon, accounting for fewer than 1% of all genitourinary malignant lesions. They are seen twice as often in men as in women, and most patients are in the sixth or seventh decade of life at the time of diagnosis. Although there is no predilection to side, the lesion most commonly occurs in the lower ureter (70% of cases).

Etiology

The origin of these tumors is believed to be similar to that of other urothelial tumors. Schmauz and Cole (1974) have shown that the relative risks for developing ureteral carcinoma are increased in cigarette smokers, coffee drinkers, and leather workers. Only at high-level exposure are the carcinogens apt to be active, since their transit time through the ureter is so rapid.

Pathogenesis & Pathology

Most tumors arising primarily within the intact ureter are transitional cell carcinomas (93%); only 5% are squamous cell carcinomas. However, squamous cell carcinomas are seen more frequently when malig-

nant disease develops in the stump of the ureter following nephrectomy for nonmalignant disease. Primary adenocarcinoma of the ureter is rare. When adenocarcinoma is found in the ureter, it is probably metastatic from the gastrointestinal tract, uterine cervix, breast, lung, or prostate.

From 56 to 80% of ureteral tumors are papillary as opposed to solid. About 50% of the tumors are of intermediate grade (II), and only 10% are of low grade. The degree of anaplasia closely parallels the extent of invasion and is important in determining the prognosis.

Ureteral carcinomas spread by contiguous growth to invade neighboring structures and organs (intestines, psoas muscle, iliac vessels); through the lymphatics to invade the pelvic, para-aortic, inguinal, and supraclavicular lymph nodes; and through the vascular system to the lungs, bones, and liver. Distant metastases are usually observed within 2 years in all patients with regional lymph node metastases.

Tumor Staging

The staging system is based on surgical findings and is a modification of that suggested by Batata et al (1975). (See p 349.)

Clinical Findings

A. Symptoms: The most common symptom is hematuria, which occurs in 59–99% of patients and is usually intermittent and sometimes quite profuse. Flank pain is observed in 20–50% of patients. Chronic obstruction from the enlarged ureteral tumor causes dull flank pain, while passage of clots down the ureter causes acute and severe pain. Symptoms of bladder irritation (frequency, urgency, dysuria) are reported in 10–52% of patients. Less frequently, as a result of metastatic disease, patients may complain of leg edema, pain from nerve root involvement, or constitutional symptoms. The tumor is silent in 12–26% of patients and is discovered on excretory urograms or endoscopic examination in patients with a history of bladder cancer.

B. Signs: Physical findings are usually absent. A palpable mass, caused by ureteral obstruction and the resulting hydronephrosis, is present in 7–50% of patients. If renal infection has supervened, the renal mass may be tender. Supraclavicular adenopathy or hepatomegaly may be felt if metastasis has occurred.

C. Laboratory Findings: Anemia may be found if bleeding is prolonged or severe. Gross or microscopic hematuria is usually present. Evidence of infection may be seen on urinalysis. If metastasis has occurred, the results of liver profile studies or the serum alkaline phosphatase level may be abnormal.

D. X-Ray Findings: The excretory urogram usually shows abnormal findings in all patients with carcinoma of the ureter. The 2 most common urographic findings are an intraluminal filling defect and hydronephrosis, with or without hydroureter. In over one-third of patients, the kidney on the affected side is nonfunctioning and fails to visualize. Angiography is of little value because of the avascular nature of most urothelial tumors.

E. Ultrasonography and CT Scanning: Not enough patients have been evaluated with either ultrasonography or CT scanning to allow adequate assessment of these procedures in helping to establish a diagnosis.

F. Instrumental Examination: If the patient is actively bleeding, cystoscopy should be performed immediately in order to locate the source of the blood. At cystoscopy, the ureteral tumor is seen protruding from the ureteral orifice in 6–18% of patients. In these patients, biopsy confirms the diagnosis.

Ureteral catheterization, performed to collect urine for cytologic examination and to better delineate the ureteral lesion through retrograde ureterograms, is usually helpful in diagnosis. In retrograde studies, several signs have been considered diagnostic for ureteral tumors: (1) the Chevassu-Mock sign, ie, increased ureteral bleeding following manipulation at the site of the tumor; (2) Marion's sign, ie, drainage of clear urine after the ureteral catheter passes above the tumor; and (3) Bergman's sign, ie, coiling of the ureteral catheter in the distal area below the tumor. Usually, however, the occluding-tip ureteropyelogram remains the best method for demonstrating the nature and extent of the lesion.

The recent development of rigid, as well as flexible, ureteroscopes has permitted endoscopic access into the ureter, enabling tissue diagnosis and better preoperative cancer staging (Huffman et al, 1985). However, the procedure is not without risk, and the physician must weigh the benefits to be attained by the additional information against the risks that could ensue from complications (eg, perforation with intraperitoneal or retroperitoneal seeding).

G. Cytologic Examination: Urine should be collected either as a freshly voided specimen or through the retrograde catheter from the affected side prior to injecting the contrast medium. Unfortunately, cytologic studies, including those using retrograde urine collections, have significant (30%) false-negative results in patients with ureteral carcinoma. However, when the retrograde brushing technique developed by Gill, Lu, and Bibbo (1978) is used, the material obtained and examined histologically and cytologically usually confirms the diagnosis of ureteral carcinoma. Occasionally, tumor tissue may be procured by means of a Dormia stone basket (Kiriyama, Hironaka, and Fukuda, 1976).

Differential Diagnosis

Ureteral calculus may cause the same symptoms and signs as ureteral tumor if the calculus is radiolucent. The urogram in each instance shows a negative (black) shadow in the ureter and a dilated tract above it. Stone is suggested if a grating feeling is noted as a catheter is passed by it. Ultrasonography (Arger et al, 1979) or CT scanning should differentiate nonopaque stone from tumor. The correct diagnosis may be possible only at surgery.

Ureteral stenosis, often secondary to compression by masses of lymph nodes involved by cancer (eg, cervical), can mimic ureteral tumor. CT scanning may reveal the involved nodes.

A blood clot from a renal stone, a sloughed papilla, a renal adenocarcinoma, or a pelvic tumor also shows as a negative shadow within the ureter. The urograms should provide the differentiation. Air bubbles introduced through a ureteral catheter may be a source of confusion.

Treatment

A. Specific Measures: In the absence of demonstrable metastases, nephroureterectomy with resection of the periureteral bladder wall and adjacent vesical mucosa remains standard therapy. However, in patients with noninvasive low-grade tumors of the lower ureter, distal ureterectomy with reimplantation may be considered (Johnson and Babaian, 1979). Partial ureterectomy for lesions located elsewhere in the ureter (middle- or upper-third) carries with it a high risk of tumor developing later below the line of resection; therefore, local resection should be avoided. Resection of a tumor through a ureterotomy should be performed only for fibrous ureteral polyps (these are usually diagnosed by x-ray findings of a long, narrow, and generally smooth-filling ureteral defect without evidence of obstruction or renal damage).

Postoperative irradiation of the ureteral bed (4500 rads in 5 weeks) has been used successfully to reduce local recurrence in a small number of patients with high-grade invasive tumors of the distal ureter (Babaian, Johnson, and Chan, 1980). Radiotherapy has been well tolerated and has caused no long-term complications. Results of combination therapy for invasive tumors of the distal ureter, consisting of preoperative irradiation (5000 rads given in 25 fractions over 5 weeks) followed within 4–6 weeks by nephroureterectomy and excision of a bladder cuff, have likewise been encouraging, but further experience is still required.

B. Palliative Measures: If metastases are present, surgery is seldom justified unless it is required to relieve pain caused by obstruction or to control intractable bleeding. Radiotherapy, 6000 rads given in 30 fractions over 6 weeks, usually controls the local tumor. Chemotherapy is restricted to treating known metastatic lesions (lungs, liver, bones, etc); the drug programs parallel those in current use for patients with metastases from bladder cancer.

C. Follow-Up Care: The patient should be followed closely during the first several years to exclude local recurrences, visceral metastases, or late bladder tumors. Subsequent metastatic disease may be expected in approximately 40% of patients. In addition, the development of vesical malignant disease in more than 40% of patients requires that endoscopy be an integral part of the follow-up examinations. (See also the section on follow-up care for tumors of the renal pelvis, above.)

Prognosis

The prognosis for patients with ureteral carcinoma tends to be better than for patients with carcinoma of the renal pelvis (5-year survival rates of 67% and 53%, respectively), but the prognosis varies widely according to the grade of tumor and stage of disease. Patients presenting with metastatic disease usually die in less than 3 years.

TUMORS OF THE BLADDER

Tumors of the bladder are the second most common genitourinary neoplasm. (Only prostatic tumors occur more frequently.) Cancer of the bladder accounts for approximately 2% of all malignant disease, and its highest incidence is in industrialized countries. Bladder tumors are seen twice as often in men as in women. The average age of patients is 65 years, and fewer than 1% of cases have been reported in patients younger than 40 years.

Malignant disease is usually localized at the time of diagnosis; only 9% of new cases show regional metastasis, and 6% demonstrate distant metastasis (Silverberg, 1981). However, as many as 80% of patients develop recurrent tumors. When tumors recur, their biologic behavior is altered (increased cellular anaplasia and a greater degree of invasiveness) in about 30% of patients.

Etiology

Current clinical and laboratory investigations indicate that bladder carcinoma, like most malignant diseases, has a monoclonal origin; a single cell undergoes an inheritable change that permits future cellular duplication and an autonomous growth pattern (malignant transformation). The development of multiple tumors at different sites in the urothelium represents similar tumorigenic changes occurring either simultaneously or successively within single cells at multiple sites.

In the process of **initiation** of cell transformation, a normal cell is changed into a latent or dormant malignant cell. This is usually the result of multiple, complex interactions of a number of carcinogens acting over a period of time (Fig 19–14) rather than the result of exposure to a single specific carcinogen. The action of these carcinogens on the urothelial cell may be additive, synergistic, or antagonistic; ie, the total effect may be equal to, greater than, or less than the sum of the effects of each carcinogen alone. The effect of the carcinogens may also be modified by cofactors, which can enhance malignant transformation.

Once malignant transformation has occurred, the affected cell may lie quiescent for a variable period until **promotion** occurs, at which time the dormant initiated cell is stimulated to divide and grow into a recognizable tumor. While specific agents (**promoters**) may be required to cause latent or dormant tumor cells to grow, other agents (**propagators**) have been demonstrated than encourage rapid growth once promotion has gotten under way. For example, rapid tumor development has been seen in some patients with bladder cancer following urothelial trauma, during calculus development, or in the presence of a urinary tract infection. The reader is encouraged to consult the excellent review by Hicks (1980) for additional details.

Although much remains to be learned regarding the multistage development of bladder cancer, epidemiologic surveys have identified high-risk factors and potential causes for this malignant disease. Cigarette smoking appears to be the most important single factor, and as many as 50% of cases of bladder cancer in men and 33% in women may be attributed to this habit. It is estimated that 3 mg of 2-naphthylamine, one of the first proved bladder carcinogens, is absorbed from the smoke of 20 unfiltered cigarettes per day over 2 years (Wynder and Goldsmith, 1977).

Persons with occupational exposures to dyes, rubber, leather and leather products, paint, and organic chemicals are at risk for bladder cancer. Recent studies suggest that cooks, kitchen workers, clerical workers, and employees in aluminum and gas industries may also be at increased risk (Cole, Hoover, and Fridell, 1972; Wigle, 1977). The number of cases of bladder cancer identified as resulting from occupational exposure is 17% (early studies had suggested up to 25%). Current investigations have implicated an inherited predisposition in some instances of bladder

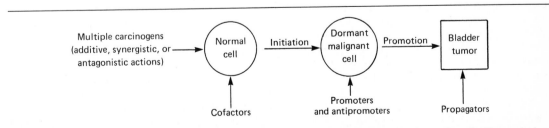

Figure 19–14. Diagram of multistage carcinogenesis of the urinary bladder. (Modified and reproduced, with permission, from Johnson DE, Boileau MA: Bladder cancer: Overview. Page 406 in: *Genitourinary Tumors: Fundamental Principles and Surgical Techniques.* Johnson DE, Boileau MA [editors]. Grune & Stratton, 1982.)

carcinoma, resulting in familial clusters (Purtilo et al, 1979). Other factors that may increase the risk of bladder cancer include treatment with isoniazid (INH), abuse of phenacetin, addiction to opium, and ingestion of bracken fern.

Although early studies suggested a causative role for the artificial sweeteners (saccharin, cyclamates, etc) in the development of bladder cancer, numerous subsequent reports have found no relationship between bladder cancer in humans and the consumption of artificial sweeteners (Newell, Hoover, and Kolbye, 1978; Connolly et al, 1978; Morrison and Buring, 1980). However, since these substances have been found to act as promoting agents, they should probably be avoided by patients with recurrent tumors (Hicks, Chowaniec, and Wakefield, 1978).

Pathogenesis & Pathology

The vast majority of bladder tumors (98%) are epithelial in origin; 92% of these are transitional cell carcinoma, 7% are squamous cell carcinoma, and 1–2% are adenocarcinoma. Sarcomas, pheochromocytomas, malignant lymphomas, mixed mesodermal tumors, and primary carcinoid tumors account for most of the nonepithelial tumors.

The World Health Organization (WHO) recommends classifying bladder carcinoma according to 4 primary histologic types: transitional cell, squamous cell, adenocarcinoma, and undifferentiated. When mixtures of the primary types occur, the different components should be listed in decreasing order of magnitude. The biologic behavior of mixed tumors as a group does not appear to be modified by the types involved (Koss, 1975). For treatment purposes, therefore, all 4 histologic types may be grouped together and treated similarly according to the stage of the disease (Johnson, 1974).

Most growths are papillary (80%) and malignant. WHO recognizes a papilloma as a papillary tumor with a delicate fibrovascular core covered by an epithelial layer that is indistinguishable from normal vesical mucosa and is less than 6 layers thick (Mostofi, 1979). Approximately 16% of patients with papilloma followed at least 5 years develop bladder carcinoma (Lerman, Hutter, and Whitmore, 1970). Management of papilloma is conservative, but semiannual surveillance is required for patients who have it.

Bladder carcinoma spreads by local extension, through lymphatics, or by hematogenous dissemination. The primary lymphatic drainage pattern from the bladder is to the external iliac (including the obturator chain), hypogastric, and presacral lymph nodes. The clinical sites in which metastases are most frequently diagnosed are (in decreasing order of occurrence) the pelvic lymph nodes, lungs, bones, and liver (Babaian et al, 1980). Although metastatic disease may develop at any time after diagnosis of the primary tumor, the median interval between this diagnosis and the clinical recognition of metastasis has generally been 11 months. Death usually ensues within 3 months of the diagnosis of metastasis.

Tumor Staging & Grading

A. Tumor Staging: The staging nomenclature generally used in the USA had its beginning in the autopsy findings reported by Jewett and Strong (1946), which related the depth of penetration of the bladder wall to the incidence of local extension and metastasis. Marshall modified this grouping in 1952, and his suggested staging classification for bladder cancer (Stages 0 through D_2; see below) remains essentially unchanged to the present. However, several weaknesses were inherent in Marshall's classification, such as failure to separate papillary noninvasive from nonpapillary noninvasive (carcinoma in situ) tumors and excessive emphasis on extent of invasion within the vesical wall. The Union Internationale Contre le Cancer (UICC) has tried to overcome these deficiencies by classifying bladder cancers on the basis of the 3 significant events in their life history: tumor growth (T), spread to primary lymph nodes (N), and metastasis (M). Although the TNM grouping according to tumor growth is somewhat similar to Marshall's staging, the reader is urged to consult the TNM classification of malignant tumors (International Union Against Cancer, 1978) for greater details. The following staging system is Marshall's system but with the UICC "T" numbers shown in parentheses:

Stage 0: Tumor is limited to the mucosa, including both papillary (Ta) and in situ (TIS) carcinoma.

Stage A: Lesions have invaded into the lamina propria but not into the muscle of the bladder wall (T1).

Stage B_1: Neoplasms have penetrated less than halfway through the muscle wall (T2).

Stage B_2: Tumors have invaded the muscle wall to a depth greater than halfway but are still confined to the muscularis (T3a).

Stage C: Neoplasms have invaded the perivesical fat (T3b).

Stage D_1: Malignant disease extends beyond the limits of the bladder and perivesical fat but is still confined to the pelvis either at or below the level of the sacral promontory; included are tumors invading contiguous organs (T4a), tumors involving the pelvic wall or rectus muscles below the level of the umbilicus (T4b), or lymph node metastases below the bifurcation of the common iliac artery.

Stage D_2: Tumors have metastasized to distant organs or to lymph nodes above the sacral promontory (bifurcation of the common iliac artery) or are external to the inguinal ligament.

B. Tumor Grading: Although many pathologists continue to employ Broder's 4 grades in evaluating the degree of anaplasia, Dart (1936) showed that the behavior of tumors of grades III and IV was so similar that deletion of grade IV was justified. Consequently, the following 3-grade system proposed by Mostofi has been in use by the American Bladder Tumor Registry and was adopted by WHO (Mostofi, Sobin, and Torlini, 1973):

Grade I: Tumors have the least degree of cellular anaplasia compatible with the diagnosis of malignancy.

Grade II: Tumors are intermediate between those of grades I and III.

Grade III: Tumors have the most severe degree of cellular anaplasia.

This system markedly reduces the variation in grade assignment from one observer to another, and it increases the interinstitutional comparability of cancer statistics. Its usefulness in predicting survival rates was recently demonstrated by Collan, Makinen, and Heikkinen (1979), who observed that 5-year survival rates were 70%, 37%, and 20%, respectively, for patients with tumors of grades I, II, and III.

Clinical Findings

A. Symptoms: The predominant symptom is hematuria, which is both painless and macroscopic in 75–80% of patients. Blood is usually noted throughout urination, although occasionally it may be present only at the beginning (initial hematuria) or at the end (terminal hematuria) of urination. In 17% of patients, bleeding may be so severe that clot retention develops. Symptoms of vesical irritability, usually the result of a secondary bacterial infection, are present in onefourth of patients presenting with bladder cancer. These symptoms include increased urinary frequency, dysuria, urgency, and nocturia. Pain in the flank may be noted if the growth obstructs a ureteral orifice and produces hydronephrosis. Twenty percent of patients have no specific symptoms, and malignant disease is discovered during an evaluation for occult hematuria, pyuria, etc.

B. Signs: Most patients have normal findings on physical examination. Only when the malignant disease has become deeply invasive or has penetrated the vesical wall does rectal or vaginal examination reveal an area of increased thickening or a definitive mass. Once the diagnosis has been established, bimanual abdominorectal palpation of the bladder and pelvis, performed when the patient is under anesthesia and the pelvis thoroughly relaxed, is mandatory. To ensure that all areas of the pelvis, pelvic viscera, and rectum are adequately examined, the clinician should first place the index finger of one hand in the rectum and the opposite hand on the abdomen, forcing the bladder and pelvic structures downward, and then reverse the hands and repeat the procedure.

When histologic examination demonstrates muscle invasion and bimanual examination reveals induration of the bladder wall, the disease is classified as stage B_2. Stage C is assigned to a definite mass that is palpable and can be moved in both anteroposterior and lateral directions. A mass that cannot be moved in both directions is considered to be fixed, and the tumor is classified as stage D_1. Also classified as stage D_1 are tumors extending directly into pelvic organs (prostate, vagina, rectum) and tumors fixed to the pelvic sidewall.

There may be signs of metastasis, such as palpable abdominal masses (liver metastases, involvement of iliac or para-aortic lymph nodes) or supraclavicular lymphadenopathy. Occasionally, edema may be present in one or both legs from occlusion of the iliac vessels.

C. Laboratory Findings: Results of laboratory studies are usually normal except for the findings of red blood cells, pus, and bacteria in the urine. Anemia is occasionally present and may be due to blood loss or chronic infection; if renal function has been compromised by ureteral obstruction, anemia may be due to azotemia.

D. X-Ray Findings: Although debate has been increasing in recent years regarding the cost-effectiveness of excretory urography in screening patients with various urologic disorders, the first step in diagnosing a bladder tumor is still an excretory urogram. The procedure aids in eliminating the upper urinary tract (renal parenchyma, ureters, pelves, and calices) as the source of the patient's symptoms. Ureteral obstruction at the time of initial diagnosis usually indicates muscle invasion (92%) or metastasis (55%) (Hatch and Barry, 1986). The excretory cystogram, which is an integral part of the urographic studies, frequently raises the suspicion of a bladder tumor by demonstrating an irregular radiolucent filling defect (Fig 19–15).

E. Ultrasonography, CT Scanning, and Magnetic Resonance Imaging: Radiologic procedures other than excretory urography are generally performed to aid in assessing the extent of the malignant growth rather than to help make a diagnosis. Transurethral ultrasonography is useful in determining the degree of tumor invasion of the bladder wall and aiding in selecting appropriate therapy (Resnick and Kursh, 1986). In addition, increasing experience with ultrasonographic assessment of bladder tumors suggests that ultrasonography may be helpful in diagnosing cases in which cystoscopy cannot be performed or is inconclusive, as in patients with tumors located in a diverticulum (Itzchak, Singer, and Fischelavitch, 1981).

Preliminary experience with magnetic resonance imaging suggests that it will increase senstivity for tumor detection and thereby improve staging of bladder neoplasms (Fisher, Hricak, and Tanagho, 1985).

As greater experience is gained with these new imaging techniques, staging of bladder neoplasms will most likely be much more accurate.

F. Instrumental Examination and Biopsy: Cystourethroscopy almost always reveals the tumor. Methodical inspection of the entire vesical and urethral urothelium should be performed before biopsy. Although McAninch, Kiesling, and Beck (1978) have suggested that adequate biopsies can be obtained without anesthesia, few nonanesthetized patients can tolerate both careful endoscopy and adequate removal of

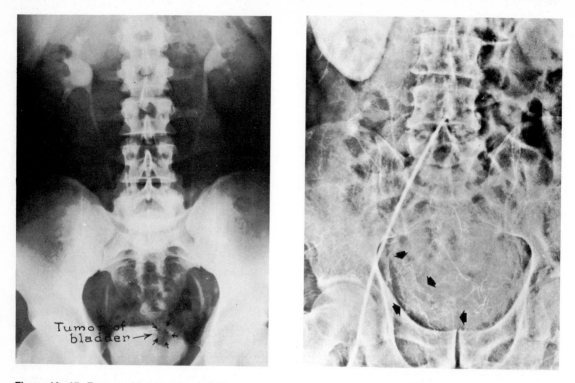

Figure 19–15. Tumors of the bladder. *Left:* Excretory urogram showing space-occupying lesion (transitional cell carcinoma) on left side of bladder; upper tracts are normal. *Right:* Vesical angiogram, delayed film, showing increased vascularity of a deeply invasive transitional cell carcinoma (grade IV, stage C), right vesical wall. Some of these vessels are presumed to be typical of tumor.

tissue. Ideally, tissue from the base of the tumor, including muscle, should be included with the specimen. In addition, biopsies of the primary tumor should include adjacent normal-appearing epithelium. Inadequate biopsies can severely restrict the pathologist's ability to assess the extent of the disease and can thereby adversely affect the patient's prognosis, since improper therapy is likely to result.

G. Cytologic Examination: The lack of cytologic abnormalities in cells collected either by a voided urine specimen or bladder washings limits the usefulness of urinary cytologic studies in patients with low-grade lesions (papilloma or papillary carcinoma, grade I or II). Urinary cytology does help in identifying carcinoma in situ and, in some patients, tumor in a bladder diverticulum. Its greatest usefulness, however, is in following patients after treatment or in screening industrial workers who are at high risk of developing bladder carcinomas.

H. Tumor Markers:

1. Cell surface antigen studies—Surface antigens identical to those that designate the ABO(H) blood groups are present on the surface of normal urothelial cells but are usually absent from high-grade or high-stage tumor cells (Javadpour, 1982). Specific red cell adherence testing (Stein et al, 1981) and the more reliable and recently available immunoperoxidase stains for detecting these antigens have proved useful in predicting which low-grade, low-stage tu-

mors will later progress to a higher grade and stage. The presence of these antigens has been associated with a low incidence (0–19%) of the ultimate development of invasive, high-grade lesions; the absence of the antigens correlates with a high incidence (60–76%) of subsequent multiple recurrences and invasive disease (Stein et al, 1981). The current state of knowledge, however, precludes recommending aggressive therapy when cell surface antigens are absent in low-stage disease, but their presence should provide added support for continued conservative management.

2. Flow cytometry—Flow cytometry of bladder washings has been established as a potentially useful technique for evaluating patients suspected of having bladder cancer and for monitoring response to therapy (Klein et al, 1982). Flow cytometry requires sophisticated and expensive instruments but nominal technical training to perform the test. Its value lies in its accuracy in detecting low-stage lesions. Using as a marker the presence of either a distinct aneuploid stem cell line or a tetraploid stem cell line containing greater than 15% hyperdiploid cells, the technician can recognize 92% of low-stage bladder tumors with only a 2% rate of false-positive results (Klein et al, 1982).

3. Chromosomal analysis—It appears that the presence of marker chromosomes in noninvasive bladder tumors indicates that recurrence is more than 90% likely; in contrast, when marker chromosomes are absent, the likelihood of recurrence is less than 5% (Sandberg, 1981). The triad of tetraploid cells, marker chromosomes, and submucosal invasiveness in moderately undifferentiated tumors carries such a poor prognosis that Falor and Ward (1977, 1978) have suggested that early radical cystectomy may be indicated. Difficulties in performing chromosomal analysis from bladder cancer tissue, however, limit the procedure's usefulness at present.

Treatment

A. Specific Measures:

1. Carcinoma in situ–Transurethral resection of the malignant areas, followed by a course of intravesical instillations of thiotepa, should be considered when (1) the lesion is confined to a relatively small (< 5 cm), reasonably well delineated area of the bladder; (2) the tumor does not involve the prostatic urethra, vesical neck, or either ureteral orifice; (3) the results of cytologic studies of urine specimens from the upper tracts are negative; and (4) the symptoms are not excessive (Utz and Farrow, 1980). If the lesions are too diffuse at initial presentation for local resection or if, after 3–6 months, they have not responded to thiotepa, other therapeutic methods such as intravesical instillation of mitomycin (Soloway, 1985), doxorubicin (Glashan, 1983; Jaske, Hofstadter and Marberger, 1984), or BCG (Brosman, 1985; de Kernion et al, 1985; Herr et al, 1986) should be considered. Preliminary experience with whole-bladder, hematoporphyrin-derivative photodynamic therapy appears to be effective in the treatment of diffuse, resistant carcinoma in situ (Benson, 1985). If the disease fails to respond to conservative therapy, is diffuse in the bladder mucosa, involves the prostatic urethra or distal ureters, or is marked by severe symptoms, radical cystectomy is required.

2. Superficial disease (stages 0 and A)– Superficial bladder carcinoma is usually managed by transurethral resection and fulguration. Unfortunately, tumors recur in 48–70% of patients. This rate can be significantly reduced if either thiotepa, mitomycin, or doxorubicin is instilled into the bladder during the first 24–48 hours postoperatively (Zincke et al 1985). In patients who have experienced several recurrences, multiple-dose thiotepa (Veenema et al, 1969; Byar and Blackard, 1977) significantly decreases the frequency of recurrences. Intravesical administration of bacille Calmette-Guérin (BCG) has recently been shown to reduce significantly the incidence of recurrent tumors and to prolong disease-free intervals (Lamm, 1985; Pinsky et al, 1985; Schellhammer, Ladaga, and Fillion, 1986).

In patients who present with multiple superficial lesions that involve much of the bladder mucosa and are not amenable to transurethral resection, an attempt to eradicate the lesions by intracavitary chemotherapy is usually warranted. While thiotepa has been used since 1962 (Veenema et al), mitomycin appears to be slightly more active (Henery, 1985). However, current experience with BCG suggests that it may be the preferred agent (Martinez-Pineiro, 1984; Lamm, 1985). Intravesical BCG is generally well tolerated, although severe, irritating side effects and systemic complications have occurred (Lamm et al, 1986).

Other methods of conservative treatment that have been tried but have met with limited success or applicability include interstitial radiotherapy employing either radium implants (van der Werf-Messing, 1978) or iridium wiring (Botto et al, 1980); hydrostatic pressure (England et al, 1973); hyperthermia (Hall, 1980); and intracavitary irradiation (Hewett, Babiszewski, and Antunez, 1981). Preliminary experience with whole-bladder, hematoporphyrin-derivative photodynamic therapy suggests that it is effective in the treatment of diffuse transitional cell carcinoma (Benson, 1985; Nseyo, 1985). When the number and extent of superficial tumors preclude definitive transurethral resection and other conservative measures have failed, cystourethrectomy with ileal conduit diversion remains the treatment of choice (Bracken, McDonald, and Johnson, 1981). External radiotherapy has not proved beneficial in this stage of disease.

3. Invasive disease (stages B₁, B₂, and C)–Endoscopic resection is indicated only in highly selected patients in whom the malignant disease is usually of intermittent grade and has penetrated only the most superficial portion of the muscularis. When the invasive tumor is solitary, has well-defined margins, occurs away from the fixed portion of the bladder (base, trigone, or neck), and allows for wide surgical excision, a partial or segmental resection may be employed. Fewer than 8% of patients presenting with bladder cancer have a tumor that meets these criteria (Utz et al, 1973; Masina, 1965). Although survival rates have been poor and local recurrence rates high when partial cystectomy has been used for high-stage or high-grade disease (Periss, Waterhouse, and Cole, 1977; Cummings et al, 1978; Resnick and O'Conor, 1973), a recent report by Ojeda and Johnson (1983) suggests that perhaps these results can be improved by combining preoperative irradiation (5000 rads over 5 weeks) with partial cystectomy.

Radical cystectomy with urinary diversion is usually the treatment of choice for invasive bladder carcinoma. Five-year survival rates following external radiotherapy alone have been in the range of 20–39% (Miller and Johnson, 1973; Rider and Evans, 1976; Hope-Stone et al, 1984; Shipley and Rose, 1985). When preoperative irradiation (ranging from 2000 rads given in 5 fractions over 5 days to 5000 rads given in 25 fractions over 5 weeks) was followed by cystectomy performed days to weeks later, the 5-year survival rates increased to 42–50% (Whitmore, 1980; Boileau et al, 1980; van der Werf-Messing, 1975; Wallace and Bloom, 1976). However, recent studies have suggested that similar survival rates can be achieved today with radical cystectomy alone (Mathur, Krahn, and Ramsey, 1981; Montie, Straffon, and Stewart, 1984). In a prospective randomized study comparing preoperative irradiation plus cystectomy to cystectomy alone as treatment for invasive bladder carcinoma, Anderstrom et al (1983) found no statistically significant differences in 5-year survival rates between the 2 approaches. Chemotherapy, given either preoperatively (neoadjuvant) or following cystectomy (adjuvant), is under investigation at several centers.

4. Metastatic disease limited to the pelvis (stage D₁) – Surgical treatment alone has proved highly unsatisfactory. In an evaluation of 97 consecutively treated patients who had pathologically demonstrable stage D bladder cancer, LaPlante and Brice (1973) reported that only 5 were clinically free of disease 5 years after radical cystectomy. (Of 22 patients who had demonstrable stage D_2 disease, none survived 5 years.) Likewise, there were no 5-year survivors among 23 patients whose disease invaded the prostate or among 13 patients whose vagina, cervix, uterus, or rectum was invaded. Dretler, Ragsdale, and Leadbetter (1973) reported that 6 (17%) of 35 patients who had stage D_1 disease and underwent radical cystectomy survived 5 years without recurrent disease. However, only 2 of their 23 patients who had more than 2 lymph nodes involved by tumor survived 5 years without evidence of recurrence. More recently, Zincke et al (1985) reported on 57 patients with stage D disease and demonstrated that radical surgery alone was associated with a 5-year survival rate of only 10%.

Treatment for stage D_1 disease traditionally has been irradiation alone, 6000 rads conventionally given in 30 fractions over 6 weeks (5 fractions of 200 rads per week). The 5-year survival rate for patients treated in this manner is 17% (Miller and Johnson, 1973). Attempts to use accelerated or split-course treatment programs have failed to improve survival rates and have resulted in increased numbers of gastrointestinal complications. Consequently, the preferred treatment today is combination chemotherapy consisting of cisplatin, cyclophosphamide, and doxorubicin (CISCA) or methotrexate, vinblastine, doxorubicin, and cisplatin (M-VAC); these and similar drug programs have resulted in long-term survivals with complete eradication of tumor (Logothetis et al, 1985; Sternberg et al, 1985; Meyers et al, 1985).

5. Disseminated disease (stage D₂) – See Chemotherapy of Urologic Malignant Disease, p 400.

B. Palliative Measures: If surgery is contraindicated because of the medical condition or disease status of a patient who presents either with severe intractable bladder hemorrhage related to tumor or with ureteral obstruction and progressive azotemia, the patient may benefit from a single dose of whole pelvic irradiation consisting of 1000 rads through the anterior and posterior portals (Chan, Bracken, and Johnson, 1979). In cases in which this proves ineffective or in which other conservative measures have failed and bleeding is life-threatening, an intravesical instillation of 10% formalin solution usually controls the hemorrhage. Percutaneous vascular occlusion techniques (see Chapter 7) may likewise be tried to control bleeding.

C. Follow-Up Care: Patients treated conservatively without radical cystectomy should be followed closely with periodic cystoscopy for at least 3 years. If no tumors have developed, the interval between examinations can be lengthened; after 5 years, only annual checkups may be needed. Urinary cytologic examinations are most beneficial when patients are suspected of having high-grade tumors or carcinoma in situ. There is little indication for frequent intravenous urograms, but the upper urinary tract should be checked whenever signs or symptoms suggest possible malignant disease.

Prognosis

The prognosis varies with the stage of disease. Patients who have superficial disease (stages 0 and A) and are treated appropriately should have excellent 5-year survival expectations, since disease becomes invasive in only about one-third of these patients. The 5-year survival rates for patients with documented muscle invasion range from 40 to 50%. When the disease has spread locally within the pelvis, 10–17% of patients may survive 5 years. There are few long-term survivors once visceral metastases have occurred.

TUMORS OF THE PROSTATE GLAND

As the prostate undergoes involution and atrophy in older men, hyperplastic and neoplastic alterations occur so often that the prostate has become the organ most frequently involved in tumor formation. It is estimated that 80% of men 50–60 years of age or older have benign prostatic hyperplasia, and approximately 10% of men over age 65 will eventually develop clinically apparent prostatic cancer.

This complex organ of acinar glands, excretory ducts, and supporting fibromuscular stroma begins in utero as a cluster of solid outgrowths from the prostatic urethra around the wolffian duct. Lowsley (1912), basing his comments on embryologic studies, described the prostate as composed of 5 lobes: anterior, middle, 2 lateral, and posterior. Although no histologic distinction can be recognized between these lobes in the adult, all areas of the prostate are not equally susceptible to hyperplastic and malignant changes. Franks (1954) described benign prostatic hyperplasia as occurring in the small inner glands immediately surrounding the prostatic urethra, while carcinoma appeared to occur in the outer protion of the gland in the posterior lobe (Fig 19–16). McNeil (1981) described the prostate as having 4 regions. The peripheral zone, the largest region of the glandular prostate, is the site of prostatic carcinoma and is immune to benign prostatic hyperplasia. Hyperplasia occurs exclusively in tissue located in the periurethral region extending from the verumontanum to the bladder

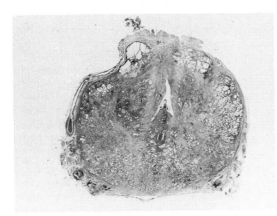

Figure 19–16. Cross section of prostate demonstrating the inner periurethral region in which benign hyperplasia occurs and the peripheral region that is the site of carcinoma. (Reproduced, with permission, from von Eschenbach AC: Cancer of the prostate. *Curr Probl Cancer* [June] 1981;5:1.)

neck. The discrete compartmentalization of benign prostatic hyperplasia and prostatic cancer makes attractive the hypothesis that the central and peripheral regions of the prostate differ in their embryologic derivation and have separate endocrine dependencies.

Benign prostatic hyperplasia and prostatic cancer are not sequential manifestations of the same pathologic process but, rather, are entirely different entities, each having its own specific mechanism of transformation. Nevertheless, both processes can exist simultaneously in the same gland. In a series of 450 patients with prostatic carcinoma, Geraghty (1922) reported a 75% incidence of hyperplastic changes, and carcinoma has been detected incidentally in 5–15% of patients undergoing surgery for benign prostatic hyperplasia.

Armenian et al (1974) have presented data to suggest that benign prostatic hyperplasia plays an important role in the pathogenesis of many prostatic cancers. In their study, 345 patients treated for benign prostatic hyperplasia had a death rate for prostatic cancer 3.7 times higher than that of a similar number of age-matched controls. However, these observations were refuted by Greenwald et al (1974), who followed 838 patients with benign prostatic hyperplasia and 802 age-matched controls for a mean of 11 years and found that prostatic cancer developed in only 2.9% of the patients and in 3.2% of the controls. At present, although the relationship between benign prostatic hyperplasia and prostatic cancer remains unsettled, physicians generally agree that these are 2 distinct disease entities that happen to occur during the same period of life in male adults (Hodges and Wan, 1983).

BENIGN PROSTATIC HYPERPLASIA (HYPERTROPHY)

A benign enlargement of the prostate associated with voiding dysfunction has been recognized for centuries. Although frequently described as benign prostatic hypertrophy, this process does not principally involve hypertrophy of cells but, rather, a hyperplastic development of any or all of the cellular components of the prostate. While the glands of the peripheral prostate undergo atrophy with aging, the inner glands grouped around the urethra undergo both stromal and epithelial hyperplasia. These hyperplastic regions take on a characteristic appearance: nodules containing tall columnar epithelial cells lining large convoluted alveolar glands. Hyperplastic mesenchymal elements of stroma or smooth muscle may surround these hyperplastic glands or may independently demonstrate stromal hyperplastic nodules. As these nodules increase in size and number, they compress the prostatic urethra and produce symptoms of bladder outlet obstruction, while the gland itself also increases in size.

Etiology

Although the exact cause of benign prostatic hyperplasia is unknown, the occurrence and progression of this disease with aging suggest a relationship to changes in the internal endocrine milieu associated with aging. The observation that benign prostatic hyperplasia does not occur in true eunuchs suggests that androgen is a necessary prerequisite for its development. However, administering testosterone to men over age 45 does not increase the incidence of the disease. Although testosterone is the principal circulating androgen, it is converted at the cellular level to dihydrotestosterone (DHT), which is twice as potent. Serum DHT levels had been reported to be increased in patients with benign prostatic hyperplasia. However, evidence by Walsh et al (1983) suggests that DHT levels are not elevated in benign prostatic hyperplasia and that the earlier measurements were subject to methodologic error. Estrogen may also have a causative role, because hyperplasia develops in an area of the gland considered to be especially sensitive to estrogen in utero, because at the time older men develop hyperplasia their estrogen:testosterone ratio has increased, and because estrogen can induce stromal hyperplasia. Experiments in dogs suggest that although testosterone is essential for hyperplasia to occur, the induction of hyperplastic changes is potentiated by estrogen. The exact mechanism of the postulated estrogen-androgen interaction is uncertain.

It further appears that a key element in the hyperplastic process is the interaction between stromal and epithelial elements. The stromal elements function as inductors of epithelial growth during embryonic life, and the reawakening of this process in the adult may be the mechanism of development of benign prostatic hyperplasia. Estrogen may exert its major effect on the stromal elements, and DHT may have a direct effect on the epithelial components.

Estrogen also has extraprostatic effects. By increasing the level of sex hormone-binding globulin (SHBG), which is preferentially concentrated in the cytosol of prostatic epithelial cells, a higher intracellular concentration of testosterone (as DHT) may be provided. In addition, estrogens increase the level of prolactin produced by the pituitary. Prolactin has the effect of potentiating the activity of testosterone at the cellular level. Thus, there is ample indirect evidence supporting the hypothesis that benign prostatic hyperplasia is a result of the influence of estrogen and androgen and the change that occurs in their relationship with aging, although the exact mechanism is unknown (Neubauer, 1983). The process may involve a complex interaction between stromal and epithelial elements in which there are paracrine effects from local prostatic growth factors.

Pathogenesis & Pathology

Enlargement of the prostate gland occurs as a silent (asymptomatic) process, only recognized by symptoms of bladder outlet obstruction resulting from associated compression of the prostatic urethral lumen. The onset of symptoms associated with voiding varies: Some patients have large prostate glands and few (if any) symptoms on voiding. In others, the gland may restrict the lumen without achieving large overall dimensions. The pathogenesis of the urinary obstruction caused by benign prostatic hyperplasia is described in Chapter 11.

Clinical Findings

A. Symptoms: As the hyperplastic nodule in the periurethral region increases in size, resistance to the flow of urine increases owing to compression of the prostatic urethra. Symptoms may be minimal at first, but eventually complete obstruction and urinary retention can occur. The mean age of onset of symptoms of benign prostatic hyperplasia is 65 years for whites and 60 years for blacks.

1. Symptoms on voiding–A decrease in the force and caliber of the urinary stream is the first and most frequent symptom encountered. As the urethral lumen decreases in size and intraurethral resistance increases, a greater voiding pressure must be generated by the bladder in order to achieve urine flow. Hesitancy or difficulty in initiating the stream may reflect the increasing latency period before the bladder is able to generate sufficiently high intravesical pressure. When flow is thus reduced, the time required to empty a fixed volume of urine from the bladder increases. If the bladder is not able to sustain such high pressure throughout this prolonged period of micturition, the urinary stream may be interrupted, and dribbling or squirting of urine may occur. In an effort to enhance micturition, the patient may use a Valsalva maneuver during flow.

The bladder musculature may eventually weaken, and the bladder may fail to empty completely. The retention of significant amounts of urine often results in urinary frequency and nocturia. Infection associated with the residual urine may further exacerbate the irritable symptoms and can increase obstruction by producing secondary inflammation and edema. Hematuria frequently occurs as the prostate continues to enlarge and as vessels in the prostatic urethra become friable. As the symptoms progress, the patient usually begins to sit rather than stand while voiding, either to wait out the inordinate delay or to relax the perineal muscles.

Acute urinary retention may occur after a prolonged period of putting off urination, allowing the bladder to become overdistended and atonic. Prostatic infarction or infection, which can cause edema within the gland, may also produce acute urinary retention. The patient then develops severe suprapubic pain and constant urgency, relieved only by catheterization and bladder drainage.

2. Generalized symptoms–Sustained bladder outlet obstruction plus hypertrophy or overdistention of the bladder may cause vesicoureteral reflux or obstruction of the upper tracts, resulting in hydroureteronephrosis. Flank pain may occur during the act of micturition. When obstruction is severe enough to produce renal failure, symptoms of uremia or azotemia occur: nausea and vomiting, somnolence or disorientation, fatigue, and weight loss. When the prostate becomes very large, the patient may become aware of a change in the caliber or shape of bowel movements.

B. Signs: When urinary retention occurs, the bladder, which is normally a pelvic organ, can rise above the level of the superior border of the symphysis pubis and become palpable up to the level of the umbilicus. Sometimes, especially in obese patients, palpation is difficult, but the full bladder can be detected by the presence of dullness to percussion in the suprapubic area.

The most conclusive sign of benign prostatic hyperplasia is an enlarged, smooth, symmetric prostate detected on digital rectal examination. The median sulcus, normally palpable in the midline of the prostate, is obliterated; as the gland continues to enlarge, it may assume a globular shape and encroach upon the lumen of the rectum. Longitudinal enlargement may occur, lifting the base of the bladder so that the examining finger in the rectum is not able to reach to the base of the prostate and the seminal vesicles. The gland may be soft or firm, and nodularity may be present; however, the nodules lack the stony-hard consistency associated with carcinoma (Fig 19–17).

C. Laboratory Findings: Urinalysis demonstrates white blood cells, bacteria, or microscopic hematuria when inflammation and infection are present. If obstruction has resulted in impairment of renal function, the creatinine and blood urea nitrogen levels may be elevated, and metabolic acidosis may occur.

D. X-Ray Findings: A plain film of the abdomen may demonstrate the presence of prostatic calculi outlining an enlarged prostate. Intravenous urography identifies hydroureteronephrosis, thickening and trabeculation of the bladder, and elevation of the bladder

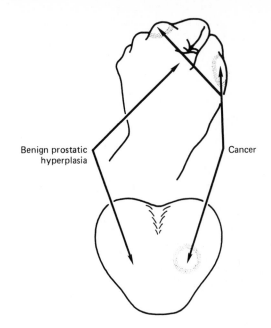

Figure 19–17. The normal or hyperplastic prostate has the consistency of the thenar eminence of the clenched fist. In contrast, the cancerous nodule has a stony-hard consistency similar to that of the bony prominence of the metacarpal phalangeal joints. (Reproduced, with permission, from von Eschenbach AC, Liles AE: The abnormal prostate. *Am Fam Physician* [Dec] 1981;**25**:61.)

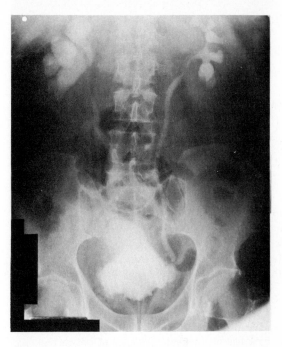

Figure 19–18. Benign prostatic hyperplasia. Preoperative 1-hour excretory urogram showing bilateral hydronephrosis and a heavily trabeculated bladder.

base and trigone by the enlarged prostate (Fig 19–18). The presence of residual urine on the postevacuation film further confirms the severity of obstruction. Abnormally dilated ureters may be apparent. When obstruction is severe, bladder diverticula and bladder calculi may develop. The intravenous urogram has been questioned, on the basis of cost-effectiveness, as an evaluative tool for patients with bladder outlet obstruction and benign prostatic hyperplasia, but most urologists continue to prefer this traditional method of evaluation.

E. Instrumental Examination: A postvoiding urethral catheterization can determine the amount of residual urine. The physician can roughly estimate the degree of obstruction by observing the patient void, but measuring the urinary flow rate provides a more accurate assessment. This can be done satisfactorily by noting the rising volume of urine in a graduated flask while measuring elapsed time by the sweep-second hand of a watch. More sophisticated methods, using urethral pressure profiles and uroflowmetry, have been developed to accurately and objectively assess the degree of voiding dysfunction.

Differential Diagnosis

Symptoms similar to those of benign prostatic hyperplasia can be caused by neurogenic dysfunction of the bladder and by anatomic abnormalities of the bladder outlet and urethra. Neurogenic bladder dysfunc-

tion may produce atony of the bladder musculature, resulting in diminished intravesical voiding pressures and low flow rates. Diabetic neuropathy or direct injury to the spinal cord or pelvic plexus can result in an atonic neurogenic bladder. Medications such as tranquilizers, ganglionic blocking agents, and parasympatholytic drugs can weaken detrusor contraction. The use of such drugs in the presence of a moderate degree of prostatism frequently results in acute urinary retention.

An atonic neurogenic bladder can be detected on physical examination by the presence of suprapubic dullness and a palpable suprapubic mass indicative of an overdistended bladder. Patients are frequently asymptomatic and unaware of their bladder distention. Neurologic examination may reveal perineal anesthesia or atonic relaxation of the anal sphincter. Cystoscopy does not provide any evidence of anatomic obstruction, although some degree of prostatic hypertrophy may be apparent. A cystometrogram confirms the presence of a large-capacity overdistended bladder with impaired sensitivity and inability to generate normal intravesical voiding pressure.

Spinal cord injury, causing hypertonicity of the musculature of the pelvis and lower extremity, can produce sphincter dyssynergia. During normal voiding, an increase in intravesical pressure is accompanied by relaxation of the external sphincter, which decreases resistance to flow; however, in syndromes of sphincter dyssynergia, the bladder neck or external sphincter contracts hypertonically, which results in increased intraurethral pressure on voiding. Urethral pressure profiles are able to detect such regions of hypertonicity.

Either contracture of the vesical neck secondary to surgery or the presence of urethral strictures secondary to trauma or infection can mimic the symptoms of prostatism by decreasing the size and caliber of the stream and reducing the urinary flow rate. These anatomic abnormalities can be identified by panendoscopy. Inflammatory conditions such as prostatitis may cause obstructive symptoms, but these conditions are usually acute, are accompanied by fever, and are identifiable on physical examination. When carcinomas and sarcomas of the prostate become large enough, they produce obstruction, distortion, and angulation of the urethra, resulting in bladder outlet obstruction. A ball-valve intravesical calculus or tumor may produce a sudden cessation of the urinary stream associated with pain radiating along the urethra and penis. Radiography and cystoscopy reveal such conditions.

In a group of 107 patients referred for evaluation of prostatism, Andersen and Nordling (1979) found that 25% had no anatomic evidence of obstruction. Another 3% had urethral strictures, and 5% had detrusor bladder neck dyssynergia. Before selecting patients for prostate surgery, the physician must be careful to determine that voiding symptoms are a direct consequence of the enlarged prostate and that no other pathologic condition exists.

Treatment

Benign prostatic hyperplasia is not necessarily a progressive process, and not all patients require immediate surgery. Lytton (1968) has estimated that the probability of a 40-year-old man requiring surgery for benign prostatic hyperplasia by the age of 80 is 10.9%. For those patients who present with severe obstruction and evidence of bladder or upper urinary tract dilatation, surgical relief of obstruction is mandatory. For the remaining large group of patients, the timing of surgery or intervention is highly variable.

A. Conservative Measures: Control of secondary infections by judicious use of antimicrobial agents may reduce local inflammatory response and relieve obstructive voiding symptoms. Patients should be cautioned to avoid dietary indiscretion, such as excessive intake of alcohol and highly seasoned or irritative foods. They should also avoid prolonged periods of urinary retention accompanied by excessive fluid intake, since overdistention of the bladder may result in atony and acute retention. Acute episodes of urinary retention frequently occur in men with minimal prostatism following pelvic or perineal surgery such as hemorrhoidectomy or herniorrhaphy. Once pain has subsided and the patient is ambulatory and no longer requires narcotic analgesics, a more normal urine flow is possible. Acute urinary retention is best managed by an indwelling Foley catheter left in place for 2–3 days. When the catheter is removed, the patient usually resumes a fairly normal voiding pattern, since

vesical tone has been reestablished and prostatic congestion relieved. Conservative therapy is often a stopgap measure, however, and many patients require further treatment to relieve outlet obstruction.

B. Medical Measures: The identification of adrenergic and cholinergic receptors present in the bladder and prostate and responsible for mediating micturition has offered hope of developing methods for medical management of urinary obstruction due to benign prostatic hyperplasia. Although medical management would probably not change the static anatomic obstruction resulting from prostatic enlargement, it might influence the dynamic process of micturition and relieve symptoms.

1. Blockade of α-adrenergic receptors – Because sympathomimetic drugs such as ephedrine, phenylpropanolamine, and phenylephrine, found in cold and cough remedies, have worsened the symptoms of prostatism, the logical assumption is that pharmacologic blockade of α-adrenergic receptors might reduce the dynamic obstructive component of benign prostatic hyperplasia and improve bladder emptying. The drug most commonly used for α-adrenergic blockade is phenoxybenzamine. It is administered orally and has a cumulative effect. Laboratory studies have demonstrated improvement in maximal urinary flow rate, reduction in the prostatic component of urethral pressure profile measurements, decrease in residual urine, and improvement in diurnal and nocturnal patterns of urination.

Caine, Perlberg, and Meretyk (1978) have reported that 80% of 200 consecutive patients who used phenoxybenzamine experienced symptomatic relief. Uroflowmetry in 102 patients showed the flow to be more than doubled in nearly one-half of patients and increased by more than 50% in another one-fourth. Improvement was noticed within the first 2 days of therapy and reached its maximum after 7 days of treatment. No effect was anticipated in the static component of obstruction, and indeed there was no effect; the drug did not reduce the size of the prostate and did not interrupt future growth.

Side effects are common with phenoxybenzamine and include hypostatic hypotension resulting in dizziness and tachycardia, retrograde ejaculation, fatigue, and nasal congestion. Less common side effects include dry mouth, difficulty with visual accommodation, and a feeling of tension. Side effects were reported by 30% of patients, but in only 10% were they considered sufficiently troublesome to stop treatment. However, when induced hypotension in older men could conceivably result in cerebral thrombosis or coronary insufficiency, the risk may be prohibitive.

Use of α-adrenergic receptor antagonists does not relieve the underlying anatomic obstruction and is considered only a temporary measure for symptomatic control. Drugs that can both improve voiding function and induce a regression in hyperplastic growth are under research.

2. Hormonal manipulation – Castration was observed to relieve urinary obstruction due to benign prostatic hyperplasia in the late 1800s, when White (1895) reported an 87% decrease in prostate size in 111 patients so treated. In a series of 61 patients, Cabot (1896) reported that urinary retention disappeared in 27 and that 50 showed overall marked improvement following castration. Experiments by Huggins and Stevens (1940) indicated that androgen deprivation significantly affects the prostate, but the process may require 3 months or more to complete. However, these early encouraging reports have not been confirmed, and a mere reduction in the serum testosterone level does not appear to be sufficient to produce significant prostatic involution or to relieve the obstructive symptoms of benign prostatic hyperplasia. For this reason, plus the implications of castration, orchiectomy is unacceptable today.

Androgen deprivation can also be achieved by the administration of estrogens, which inhibits pituitary gonadotropin release. However, estrogens may play a direct role in the development of benign prostatic hyperplasia and may also affect the smooth muscle of the bladder and urethra. No current studies suggest any appropriate role for estrogens in the management of established benign prostatic hyperplasia.

Cyproterone acetate, an antiandrogen that has marked progestational activity (inhibits androgen action by competitive binding with the androgen receptor), has caused subjective improvement in patients with benign prostatic hyperplasia. Scott and Wade (1969) reported that 11 of 13 patients treated with cyproterone acetate experienced subjective improvement, including an increased urinary flow rate and decreased volume of residual urine. An objective decrease in the epithelial cell size was apparent in 8 of 11 patients whose prostatic biopsies were available.

Flutamide, a nonsteroidal veterinary antiandrogen, has been found to be a potent inhibitor of testosterone-induced prostatic growth in experimental animals. Flutamide appears to act by directly competing for the intracellular androgen-receptor protein complex. In a double-blind placebo-controlled clinical trial, Caine, Perlberg, and Gordon (1975) reported early subjective improvement among 30 patients; however, the improvement was not maintained, and no significant change occurred in the size of the prostate or the volume of residual urine.

Megestrol acetate effectively blocks the action of androgen by reducing the activity of intracellular 5α-reductase and competing for androgen receptor protein in the cytosol. Geller et al (1979) demonstrated a decrease in prostate size and improved urinary flow rates in 8 of 13 patients; however, no statistically significant difference in subjective improvement could be demonstrated. Donkervoort et al (1975) reported similarly that subjective improvement was minimal, and changes in urinary flow rate were insignificant.

Other potential agents of endocrine manipulation, such as medrogestone, spironolactone, bromocriptine, candicidin, and amphotericin B, have not demonstrated any significant advantage. Because of the uncertainty about their mechanism of action and the difficulty in assessing subjective and objective improvement, the role of hormones in managing benign prostatic hyperplasia is difficult to assess. Future research must consider the interactions of the hormones and their effect on stromal and epithelial elements.

C. Surgical Measures: The most effective method of relieving obstruction due to benign prostatic hyperplasia is surgical extirpation. The objective of surgery is to remove the portion of the enlarged prostate that is causing the obstruction by a technique that is considered effective and safe. Removal of the adenoma can be achieved by transurethral resection of the prostate or by open prostatectomy.

Walsh et al (1983) have defined mandatory and optional indications for prostatectomy. Mandatory indications include cases in which there is total outflow obstruction due directly to enlargement of the prostate and cases in which there is chronic outflow obstruction impairing renal function or producing symptoms distressing to the patient. Chronic urinary tract infection accompanied by bouts of recurrent cystitis and prostatitis may require that the outlet obstruction be relieved before the infection can be managed properly. Bladder stones requiring litholapaxy may indicate the need for prostatectomy to obliterate obstruction and residual urine. Bladder tumors may necessitate transurethral resection of the prostate to provide easy access to the bladder for endoscopic inspection, resection of the tumors, and obliteration of residual urine. Recurrent gross hematuria or chronic congestive cardiac failure exacerbated by prostatic obstruction may likewise require surgical intervention. When chronic urinary retention produces severe symptoms such as overflow urinary incontinence, urgency, intense frequency, or severe nocturia, surgery is mandatory.

Optional indications for prostatectomy are relative to the circumstances of the individual patient. Although urinary frequency and nocturia may be inconsequential to one patient, another patient may find them so disruptive of life-style as to warrant surgery. The size of the prostate does not in itself determine the need for surgery, but larger prostates are more likely to develop prostatic infarctions and to produce episodes of acute urinary retention. If patients will require psychotropic, anticholinergic, or α-adrenergic drugs to control medical disorders and already have significant voiding symptoms, prostatectomy may be indicated.

1. Transurethral resection of the prostate— Transurethral resection is employed in over 90–95% of patients. The obstructing adenoma can be readily removed by endoscopic resection under general or spinal anesthesia. For the past 40 years, this method has been popular with both urologists and patients because of its safety. The mortality rate ranges from 0 to 1.3%, with 0.4% considered the average for experienced urologists; this rate is lower than that for open prostatectomy (Mebust and Valk, 1983).

Among those not recommended for transurethral resection are (1) patients with a life expectancy of less than 6 months who might best be treated by catheter drainage instead and (2) patients with a physical deformity such as ankylosis of the hips that would prevent proper positioning for endoscopic surgery.

Patients with chronic renal insufficiency can undergo transurethral resection, but they must be monitored carefully before, during, and after surgery. During resection, a patient absorbs (on the average) about 900 mL of irrigating fluid through the prostatic fossa and open veins. Preoperative assessment of renal function is therefore important. Patients with a serum creatinine level of 1.5 mg/kg have a 6-fold increase in postresection morbidity and mortality rates (Melchior et al, *J Urol* 1974;**112:**643), but they can be treated safely by transurethral resection as long as their fluid and electrolyte status is continually monitored. When azotemia is due to outlet obstruction, patients should be placed on indwelling catheter drainage for 10–14 days preoperatively in order to improve renal function. Fluid absorption during surgery can result in hypervolemia and dilutional hyponatremia; in the immediate postoperative period, patients may develop hypertension, tachycardia, weakness, confusion, and (in severe cases) seizures. Treatment of acute cases includes diuresis with furosemide and infusions of hypertonic saline solution. Other intraoperative complications include perforation of the prostatic capsule, accompanied by extravasation and hemorrhage.

Patients with active urinary tract infections should receive appropriate antimicrobial drugs in an effort to eradicate the infection before they undergo instrumentation and operation and to prevent subsequent sepsis and epididymitis.

The size of the prostate should be considered in determining whether transurethral resection is the most appropriate surgical technique. Preoperative estimations of size are highly subjective and prone to error: the examiner estimates the dimensions of the gland, calculates its volume in cubic centimeters, and estimates its weight by the formula $1 \text{ g} = 1 \text{ cm}^3$. (Although transurethral sonography is more exact, it is not readily available; in general, an estimation that is a few grams over or under the precise determination is not clinically relevant.) Many urologists limit their use of transurethral resection to prostates that weigh no more than 45 g, while other urologists are comfortable resecting 100 g of tissue or more. Melchior et al (*J Urol* 1974;**112:**634) have reported a greater morbidity and mortality rate among patients with glands 60 g or larger who undergo transurethral resection. Operative morbidity and mortality rates are also increased by prolonging the time of operation, since there is an increased risk of absorbing the nonelectrolyte irrigating fluid.

More than 90% of patients can anticipate a satisfactory result from surgery, with excellent urinary control and a satisfactory urinary stream. Total permanent urinary incontinence is a distressing postoperative complication that occurs in fewer than 1% of patients. Intermittent hematuria may occur in the first 4–6 weeks, during which time prostatic fossa is still undergoing reepithelialization. If bleeding is persistent or severe and associated with clots, reinsertion of a 24F Foley catheter may be necessary. Uretheral stricture has been reported in 6% of patients and epididymitis in 2%. Erectile impotence as a direct result of the surgery is considered rare. Retrograde ejaculation has been reported in 40–50% of patients and is an important issue for preoperative discussion.

2. Open prostatectomy–Enucleation of adenomatous hyperplastic tissue can be performed by one of the following approaches: (1) an anterior transcapsular incision (retropubic); (2) a posterior transcapsular incision (perineal); or (3) an incision above the pubis and through the bladder neck (suprapubic). In none of these procedures is the entire prostate removed; therefore, a more proper term would be "adenomectomy" rather than prostatectomy. Indications for open enucleation of the prostate are related to the size of the gland. For prostates in excess of 60 g, which may be beyond the endoscopic expertise of the urologist, an open surgical procedure is associated with less risk of morbidity and mortality. Other indications for an open prostatectomy include the presence of large bladder diverticula or calculi that can be corrected at the time of open surgery, the presence of a severe impassable urethral stricture, and orthopedic conditions that do not allow proper patient positioning for endoscopic surgery. Prolonged postoperative catheter drainage by a urethral catheter, a suprapubic tube, or both is generally necessary for 7–10 days or until healing is complete. Intraoperative bleeding is greater in open prostatectomy than in endoscopic surgery, and 15% of patients require blood replacement. Postoperative complications of delayed bleeding, urinary incontinence, erectile impotence, and urethral stricture are uncommon. Retrograde ejaculation occurs frequently.

Prognosis

Because the growth rate of benign prostatic hyperplasia is quite variable, the rate of progression of symptoms or deterioration of function is difficult to predict. About 50% of cases may remain clinically stable for years, and a few may even improve spontaneously. In most patients, progression of symptoms eventually requires removal of the obstructing adenoma. The prognosis following surgical correction is discussed above.

CARCINOMA OF THE PROSTATE

Although malignant transformation can involve any of the cellular components of the prostate gland, over 95% of prostatic cancers are adenocarcinomas of tubuloalveolar or acinar origin. Prostatic carcinoma was considered rare when first identified as a specific entity in the early 19th century, but it is now recognized as probably the most prevalent malignant transformation occurring in men. Not all prostatic cancers are clinically apparent, and even when recognized they do not all express the same biologic or malignant potential. This heterogeneity in expression of prostatic cancer has been the source of much confusion and controversy, affecting the selection of appropriate therapy and the evaluation of results.

Cancer of the prostate is a disease of aging. It is rarely diagnosed in a man younger than 50 years, and its incidence increases progressively thereafter until a peak occurs in the eighth decade. In the USA, about 75,000 cases are diagnosed annually, and about 24,000 deaths occur each year as a direct result of the disease. Because the male population over age 50 is steadily increasing in numbers and because there is some evidence to suggest an increase in the incidence of prostate cancer, the number of cases diagnosed yearly is expected to exceed 125,000 by the year 2000. Moreover, 3–8 times more cases go unrecognized clinically and are apparent only upon incidental autopsy examination of the prostate or at the time of prostatectomy for benign disease. These "latent," or clinically unrecognized, cases represent a much larger population of men in whom the disease is of a very low malignant potential or in whom death from other causes intervenes before sufficient time has elapsed to allow for full expression of the prostatic cancer. In the future, with more sophisticated methods of detection, many of these "subclinical" cases will be clinically diagnosed, adding even further to the magnitude of the problem of prostate cancer.

The exact size of the pool of men with prostatic cancer is difficult to determine. Rich (1935) reported that the disease was recognized clinically prior to death in only one-third of patients found to have prostatic cancer at the time of autopsy. By carefully examining step sections of the prostate gland, Franks (1954) observed that 30% of men older than 50 years who died of other causes had histologic evidence of prostatic carcinoma. The incidence was 40% in men 70–79 years of age and 67% in men 80–89 years. Similar results have been found in analyses of material obtained at the time of transurethral resection of the prostate for benign disease. Sheldon et al (1980) reviewed the literature and reported the following average incidence rates of prostatic cancer discovered incidentally in men undergoing transurethral resection of the prostate: 10.4% in those 50–59 years of age, 18.5% in those 60-69 years, and 28.7% in those 70–79 years.

The statistics on incidence, clinical occurrence, and death from prostatic cancer lead to the conclusion that this tumor has a spectrum of biologic behavior. On one end of the spectrum is the tumor whose growth is slow, with a long time interval from initiation to diagnosis. Progression of the tumor thereafter is likewise exceedingly slow. The lesion remains confined, and if it arises late in life, the host dies of other causes with the tumor only incidental. On the other extreme is the rapidly progressive tumor that has a high rate of cell division and mutation leading to clones with invasive and metastatic potential. As a result of this aggressive biologic behavior, the interval from inception of the tumor to widespread dissemination is short. Patients with this form of tumor usually have metastases at diagnosis and live a relatively short time between diagnosis and death. In between these 2 extremes is the tumor with intermediate malignant expression. A long period of local growth may precede the moment when a sufficient number of mutations have occurred to result in clones of cells with metastatic potential.

Awareness of this heterogeneity of clinical expression of prostatic cancer calls for a new perspective on its etiology, pathogenesis, clinical assessment, selection of therapy, and assessment of results (Johnson and von Eschenbach, 1980).

Etiology

The precise cause of prostatic cancer is unknown, but epidemiologic studies suggest that a variety of factors may play a role in its development (incidence) and that other factors are associated with its malignant expression (mortality). It seems apparent that these causative factors have a time-dose relationship with the cancer and are operative beginning as early as adolescence and continuing throughout life.

A. Genetic Factors: Cancer of the prostate occurs more frequently within some families, indicating a shared genetic predisposition. Racial propensity has been reported; in the USA, blacks are more susceptible than, and have nearly twice the mortality rate of, whites. The impact of commonly shared environmental factors on these genetic influences is difficult to determine.

B. Hormonal Factors: Hormones influence the induction and promotion of this cancer, but their exact mechanism of action and the precise endocrine factors responsible remain uncertain. Rotkin (1977) has suggested that hormonal factors may be operative as early as puberty and has noted that puberty begins later in patients who develop prostatic cancer than in controls. Throughout life the hormonal influence is reflected by differences between patients and controls in sexual drive and frequency of sexual experiences, with prostatic cancer patients appearing to be more sexually active, more promiscuous, and more fertile.

The appearance of prostatic cancer after age 50 suggests that its clinical expression is linked to changes in the endocrine milieu that occur with aging, as the level of serum testosterone declines and the estrogen:testosterone ratio increases. The response of prostatic carcinoma to androgen deprivation further suggests a direct relationship between this tumor and hormones. Men with prostatic cancer secrete smaller amounts of androsterone and have higher serum levels of estrogen and estradiol. Increased estrogen levels may also inhibit tumor development; this has been suggested as an explanation for the low incidence of prostatic cancer in patients with cirrhosis whose livers are defective and who, therefore, have higher circulating levels of estrogen (Winkelstein and Ernster, 1979).

C. Diet: The difference in mortality rates observed geographically between Occidentals and Orientals appears to be a direct result of differences in dietary habits. The low mortality rate in Japan is not due purely to racial differences, since the rate increases among Japanese who migrate to the USA. Hirayama's (1979) prospective study of 122,261 Japanese men 40 years of age or older suggests that a Westernized diet high in animal fat is associated with the higher mortality rate, while the traditional Japanese diet rich in green and yellow vegetables appears to have a protective effect. The high content of fat in the diet could conceivably alter cholesterol and steroid metabolism and also may be associated with such carcinogenic substances as nitrosamines, derived from the preparation and cooking of the meat. Green and yellow vegetables are known to have a high content of vitamins A and C, which may have a protective effect.

D. Chemical Carcinogens: Environmental factors may act as direct carcinogens or as cocarcinogens for tumor promotion (Bonar, 1982). Men who work with batteries and are chronically exposed to cadmium, a known antagonist of zinc, have been shown to have a higher incidence of prostatic carcinoma. Particulate air pollution may explain the higher incidence in urban than in rural areas. Occupations in the rubber, fertilizer, and textile industries have likewise been linked to higher rates of prostatic cancer.

E. Viruses: A direct causal relationship between viruses and prostatic carcinoma has not been established but is suggested. Virus particles have been observed by electron microscopy in carcinomatous prostatic tissue. A temporal relationship has been established between the incidence of gonorrhea and a subsequent increase in the incidence of prostatic cancer; the assumption is that these patients were exposed to virus infection as well. As the role of oncogenes in prostatic cancer is more fully explored, the role of viruses may become clearer.

The heterogeneity of prostate cancer suggests that no single specific causative factor is responsible for this malignant transformation. A complex interaction of a variety of substances with individual time-dose relationships is the most logical mechanism.

Pathogenesis & Pathology

Malignant transformation occurs in the stem cells of the acinar prostatic epithelium. The degree of aberration can impart a variety of appearances to prostatic cancer: Some tumors are difficult to distinguish from normal prostate, except that the glands are small and crowded. Others manifest bizarre alterations in cellular structure and form a solid pattern with no glandular differentiation. Variations in glandular structure can occur within different portions of the same tumor, which has been a source of difficulty and confusion in grading prostatic cancers.

Although abnormal cytologic features may be absent in well-differentiated tumors, most malignant prostatic epithelial cells have a large hyperchromatic nucleus with large prominent nucleoli. The nucleus in malignant cells is eccentric, in contrast to that of the normal epithelial cells located at the base in proximity to the basement membrane. Malignant glands may be small and arranged in clusters, frequently with a back-to-back configuration. Cells are in a single layer, and the dark-staining basal layer is absent.

Tumor Staging & Grading

A. Tumor Staging: In the staging system proposed by Whitmore (1956), tumors are categorized as follows:

Stage A: Tumors microscopic and intracapsular.
Stage B: Tumors macroscopic and intracapsular.
Stage C: Tumors macroscopic and extracapsular.
Stage D: Metastatic disease.

Within each of these categories, however, experience has demonstrated that tumors show a diversity of biologic behaviors, which makes selection of therapy for patients and comparison of treatment results imprecise. As a result, numerous investigators have introduced a variety of subdivisions for each stage, with these further divisions also based on size or extent of tumor (Fig 19–19). Some investigators, eg, those in the Veterans Administration Cooperative Urologic Research Group (1964), have used the biochemical determination of elevated serum levels of prostatic acid phosphatase as a criterion for assigning patients to a metastatic category.

The American Joint Committee on Cancer has proposed a classification that considers the primary tumor, nodal extension, and presence of distant metastases (TNM) (Table 19–1).

B. Tumor Grading: Since Broder (1926) observed that the behavior of malignant cells can be predicted by their histologic appearance, various attempts have been made to develop a uniform grading system for prostatic cancer. Mostofi (1975) proposed a 3-grade system that takes into account both the cytologic characteristics of nuclear size and shape and the glandular morphology. The grading system of Gleason, Mellinger, and the Veterans Administration Cooperative Urologic Research Group (1974), which was based on an analysis of a large number of cases, establishes 5 patterns of glandular morphology. In order to deal with the varied patterns present within these tumors, a primary and secondary pattern score is assigned to the 2 most frequent patterns, and the scores are added to arrive at a grade. The grades thus range from 2 to 10.

The grading system of Gleason and his colleagues is the one most widely employed at present because it has the most extensive clinical correlation. Certain problems exist, however, in its reproducibility and its ability to determine prognosis on the basis of grades. Other systems of grading have attempted to simplify application while preserving discrimination of malignant potential. The system employed at the University of Texas M.D. Anderson Hospital (MDAH system) is based simply on assessment of percentage of gland formation in the tumor. Using the MDAH system in evaluating 182 patients, all of whom had stage C prostatic carcinoma and underwent definitive external-beam megavoltage irradiation, the 5-year survival rate for patients whose tumors were grade I (contain-

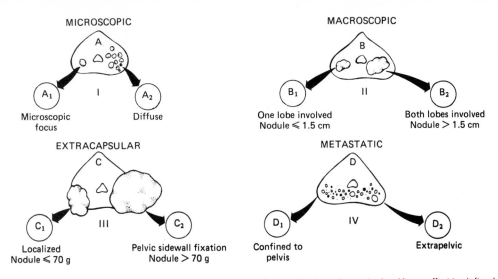

Figure 19–19. Various staging classifications of prostatic carcinoma that have been devised in an effort to define homogeneous groups for selection of therapy and analysis of results. (Reproduced, with permission, from von Eschenbach AC: Cancer of the prostate. *Curr Probl Cancer* [June] 1981;5:1.)

ing ≥ 75% glands) was 91%, while the 5-year survival rate for those with grade IV tumors (containing < 25% glands) was only 15% (Brawn et al, 1982).

Other systems of grading include Mostofi's system, which classifies tumors into 3 grades according to glandular morphology and degree of cellular anaplasia. The criteria of the Gaeta system and the Mayo Clinic system are similar.

Clinical Findings

A. Symptoms: In spite of the prevalence of prostatic cancer, the tumor usually escapes attention until disease is advanced, or it is discovered only incidentally at the time of surgery for benign disease. The failure to detect the tumor early is in part due to the lack of pathognomonic early warning signs or symptoms. Prostatic cancer does not necessarily progress in an orderly fashion from the stage of microscopic disease to local and regional growth and then to distant metastases; therefore, symptoms related to metastasis may precede any awareness of malignant growth in the prostate itself.

1. Local growth—Since benign prostatic hyperplasia occurs in the periurethral portion of the gland, it is usually responsible for the obstructive symptoms on voiding that occur with aging. Prostatic cancer begins in the periphery of the gland and usually produces compression of the urethra and impaired micturition only after the tumor reaches a considerable size. Obstruction due to cancer may present abruptly and progress rapidly in severity. When a patient can precisely date the onset of obstructive symptoms and the deterioration is rapid, cancer should be suspected. Local growth of the tumor may cause rectal obstruction re-

Table 19–1. TNM classification of prostatic carcinoma.

Primary tumor (T)

TX	Minimum requirements to assess the primary tumor cannot be met.
T_0	No tumor present.
T1a	No palpable tumor; in histologic sections, no more than 3 high-power fields of carcinoma found.
T1b	No palpable tumor; histologic sections reveal more than 3 high-power fields of prostatic carcinoma.
T2a	Palpable nodule less than 1.5 cm in diameter, with compressible, normal-feeling tissue on at least 3 sides.
T2b	Palpable nodule more than 1.5 cm in diameter, or nodule or induration in both lobes.
T3	Palpable tumor extending into or beyond the prostatic capsule.
T3a	Palpable tumor extending into the periprostatic tissues or involving 1 seminal vesicle.
T3b	Palpable tumor extending into the periprostatic tissues, involving one or both seminal vesicles; tumor diameter more than 6 cm.
T4	Tumor fixed or involving neighboring structures.

Nodal involvement (N)
The regional nodes are those within the true pelvis; all others are distant nodes. Histologic examination is required for stages N0 through N3.

Prostate

NX	Minimum requirements to assess the regional nodes cannot be met.
N_0	No involvement of regional lymph nodes.
N1	Involvement of a single homolateral regional lymph node.
N2	Involvement of contralateral, bilateral, or multiple regional lymph nodes.
N3	A fixed mass present on the pelvic wall with a free space between this and the tumor.

Distant Metastasis (M)

MX	Minimum requirements to assess the presence of distant metastasis cannot be met.
M_0	No (known) distant metastasis.
M1	Distant metastasis present. Specify _____.

sulting in a decreased caliber of stools and pain at defecation. Local extension of the tumor, especially with perineural invasion, may cause rectal or perineal pain. Difficulty with sexual function due directly to prostatic cancer does not usually occur, but pain on ejaculation may be described. Hematospermia and hematuria may accompany benign prostatic hyperplasia, but their presence in patients over age 50 should always warrant a careful assessment to rule out malignant disease.

2. Metastatic disease–Approximately 15–40% of patients present with symptoms caused by metastasis. In an elderly man, complaints of persistent bone pain (either localized or multifocal and especially in the spine or pelvis) should always prompt a search for prostatic cancer. Fatigue, weight loss, and malaise are nonspecific indications of extensive disease.

B. Signs: Changes in the size, shape, or consistency of the prostate in a man older than 50 years should alert the examining physician to the presence of malignant disease. Because epithelial cancers of the prostate evoke an intense stromal reaction, the area of malignant transformation assumes a stony-hard consistency; a normal prostate or a prostate with benign hyperplasia is much softer. A hard, discrete nodule in the prostate of a man over age 50 has about a 50% chance of being a malignant tumor. Loss of symmetry or the anatomic margins of the gland and extended induration place the chances of malignant disease in excess of 70%.

Other causes of induration in the gland include prostatic calculi or granulomatous inflammation, and nodularity does occur with benign prostatic hyperplasia. Unfortunately, early detection of prostatic cancer is hampered because 10–20% of the tumors are too small to be detected by digital rectal examination.

Metastases to bones may be recognized by localized areas of tenderness on palpation. On occasion, lymphadenopathy in the inguinal region, pelvic sidewall, or supraclavicular fossa may be detected by palpation.

C. Laboratory Findings: Routine laboratory studies to evaluate the patient with prostatic carcinoma include a complete blood count and serum multiple analysis (SMA-12). When metastatic disease is extensive, bone marrow involvement may be severe enough to produce anemia. Elevations in the levels of blood urea nitrogen and creatinine may reflect renal insufficiency caused by either bladder outlet obstruction or bilateral ureteral obstruction, either one the result of tumor extension. Results of liver function studies are abnormal in the presence of liver metastases. In approximately 85% of patients with advanced disease, the serum level of alkaline phosphatase is elevated. Isoenzyme fractionation of serum alkaline phosphatase is useful in determining whether the enzyme is of bone, liver, or tumor origin. Alterations in serum calcium levels can occur; hypocalcemia is reportedly the most common alteration and is a result of avid uptake of calcium by osteoblastic metastases (Jacobs,

1983). (See also Tumor Markers, below.)

D. X-Ray Findings: The initial evaluation of a patient with prostatic cancer usually includes posteroanterior and lateral chest x-rays, an excretory urogram, and a radionuclide bone scan. Complete skeletal surveys are not employed routinely, but specific bone films are obtained to confirm any abnormalities detected on the bone scan. Bilateral pedal lymphangiography and CT scanning are used to detect the presence of nodal metastases. Liver scans are obtained only when something else, such as abnormal liver enzyme levels, suggests that liver metastases are present.

1. Chest radiography–The Veterans Administration Cooperative Urologic Research Group found that, at autopsy, 24% of their patients had metastasis to the lung, most frequently as a result of lymphatic spread. Clinically, however, chest films are positive for metastatic disease in only 6–10% of patients. The principal pattern of clinically detected metastasis is nodular. The chest film may also demonstrate evidence of hilar nodal metastasis or the presence of osteoblastic metastasis in the ribs.

2. Excretory urography–Excretory urography is useful in searching for a number of abnormalities that may occur with prostatic carcinoma. The disease characteristically produces osteoblastic metastases in the bony skeleton; the sites most frequently involved are the ilium (83%), pubis and ischium (78%), and lumbosacral spine (71%). The scout radiograph of the urographic studies assesses the bones of the lumbar spine, sacrum, pelvis, and proximal femur—those most commonly involved by metastatic disease. This plain film plus a chest x-ray obviate the need for a routine bone survey. Following the injection of contrast medium, a delay in renal excretion may reflect the presence of obstructive uropathy due to local tumor extension into the trigone, or it may reflect deviation of the proximal ureters laterally or distal ureters medially due to enlarged lymph nodes. Bladder outlet obstruction and deformity of the base of the bladder, results of local tumor growth, may also be present.

3. Lymphangiography–Lymphatic capillaries arise in the glandular acini and form an intraprostatic network, which communicates with the periprostatic lymphatic network that drains into collecting trunks recognized as pedicles to the external iliac, hypogastric, and presacral lymph nodes. The frequency of lymph node metastasis from prostatic cancer is related to the clinical stage of the primary tumor and its histologic differentiation. Lymph node metastasis has been recognized in 24% of patients with stage A_2 prostatic tumors, 14% with stage B_1 tumors, 40% with stage B_2 tumors, and 50% with stage C tumors. High-grade prostatic cancers are associated with twice as much lymph node metastasis as low-grade cancers. McLaughlin et al (1976) reported that the incidence of lymph node metastasis in patients with stage B or C adenocarcinoma was 10% when tumors were well differentiated but 56% when tumors were undifferentiated.

Bilateral pedal lymphangiography is capable of assessing intranodal architecture and therefore can be a useful tool for detecting lymph node metastasis. By applying strict criteria for interpretation, ie, the presence of an intranodal filling defect not traversed by lymphatics on the flow phase, positive findings on the lymphangiogram can be 90–95% accurate. Nonetheless, lymphangiograms detect metastases in only 50–60% of patients with nodal disease. This is due partly to the fact that the bipedal lymphangiogram does not visualize all the lymph nodes that primarily drain the prostate. Presacral lymph nodes are not visualized, and the internal iliac or hypogastric lymph nodes are demonstrated in only about 50% of the patients studied. Understaging also results when micrometastases are too small to be resolved by lymphangiography or when lymph nodes have been completely replaced by metastatic disease and thus do not accept the contrast material. Although its sensitivity is limited, the lymphangiogram is still useful in demonstrating metastases in patients with large, poorly differentiated tumors who are likely to have nodal metastases; this may avoid the need for a staging pelvic lymphadenectomy. Bipedal lymphangiograms are no longer a routine method of staging, because of their poor sensitivity.

4. Staging pelvic lymphadenectomy–Surgical staging by pelvic lymphadenectomy has demonstrated that the incidence of understaging by lymphangiography is 15–24%. A staging pelvic lymphadenectomy is the most accurate method of assessing lymph node metastasis; however, the procedure has no therapeutic benefit and carries an operative morbidity rate of 20–34%. Complications include wound infection (5–15%), atelectasis, ileus, sepsis, pulmonary embolus (5–10%), thromobophlebitis, lymphoceles, and edema of the penis and lower extremities (5–10%). If external-beam megavoltage radiation is delivered to the prostate and pelvis postoperatively, it increases the incidence of morbidity (Johnson and von Eschenbach, 1981). In an effort to reduce the risk of postoperative lymphedema, some authors have proposed a modified node dissection. They preserve the lymphatics surrounding the external iliac artery and carry dissection from the circumflex iliac vessels distally to the common iliac artery proximally. Removing the lymph nodes around the hypogastric artery, obturator nerve, and external iliac vein provides a thorough sampling of the primary echelon of drainage from the prostate. Removing the hypogastric-obturator groups of nodes should identify almost all patients with nodal metastases; however, the extent of nodal disease may be underestimated in 55–80% of patients who undergo this limited operation.

Lymph nodes have been evaluated intraoperatively by frozen-section slides, but this technique has a false-negative rate of 20–40% when the nodes appear grossly normal (Catalona and Stein, 1982). Thus, great care must be taken by the pathologist when handling the specimen and multiple sections of each node, in order to reduce false-negative interpretations.

Lymph node metastasis occurs early in the dissemination of prostatic cancer and is indicative of systemic disease. Accurate assessment of the nodes is essential before therapy is selected, but such an assessment does not always demand surgical lymphadenectomy. It is now possible to select patients suitable for lymph node assessment by determining whether they are in a low-, high-, or intermediate-risk group. On one end of the spectrum of risk are those patients with small intracapsular well-differentiated tumors; they are at such low risk for nodal disease that the possible complications of surgical staging are unjustified. On the other hand, when the disease is extracapsular and poorly differentiated and the serum prostatic acid phosphatase (PAP) level is elevated, nodal metastases can often be easily identified by radiographic studies. Freiha, Pistenma, and Bagshaw (1979) reported that only 7% of patients with intracapsular tumors who had normal levels of serum PAP had evidence of nodal metastases, but when primary lesions were extracapsular, high-grade, and associated with elevated serum levels of PAP, 93% had nodal metastases. In their series of 100 consecutive patients, 42% fell clearly into one of these 2 groups and could be clinically staged, without a surgical procedure, with an accuracy rate of 93%. For the 58% of patients who fell into the intermediate group, the overall evidence of lymph node metastasis was 36%. Paulson (1979) reported that no patient with clinically localized disease who had a histologic Gleason score of 2, 3, or 4 had evidence of nodal metastasis, but when the Gleason score was 8, 9, or 10, 93% of patients had nodal metastasis. For patients in the intermediate-risk group, surgical lymphadenectomy is necessary before initiation of local or regional therapy.

Percutaneous aspiration and cytologic examination of the nodal site can spare approximately 50% of the patients an open surgical procedure. Thus, rather than routinely staging by pelvic lymphadenectomy, the physician can identify patients at high and low risk for lymph node metastasis and, when necessary, can evaluate them further by bilateral pedal lymphangiography, CT scanning, and percutaneous needle biopsy.

E. Ultrasonography and CT Scanning: The local extent of a prostatic tumor can be assessed by CT scanning or transrectal ultrasonography. The CT scan is unable to differentiate carcinoma from benign prostatic hyperplasia and is useful only for objective assessment of large tumors. Using transrectal ultrasonography in 100 consecutive patients, however, Braeckman and Denis (1983) reported no false-negative diagnoses among 27 patients with prostatic carcinoma and only 4 false-positive diagnoses of carcinoma among patients who had a pathologic diagnosis of adenoma. Thus, in addition to objectively assessing the size and shape of the prostate, transrectal ultrasonography may be useful in recognizing and localizing intracapsular prostatic tumors and monitoring the response of tumors to therapy.

The new probes with a frequency of 7 MHz provide greater resolution of the internal architecture of the prostate. This, along with the recognition by Lee et al (1985) that malignant tumors may be hypoechoic areas, should result in greater frequency of detection of small intraprostatic tumors, which can then be confirmed by ultrasonographically guided biopsy.

F. Radionuclide Imaging: Bone metastasis occurs in approximately 75–85% of patients with advanced prostatic carcinoma. Of these, osteoblastic lesions occur in approximately 80%, mixed osteoblastic and osteolytic lesions in 16%, and pure osteolytic lesions in 4%. Osteoblastic metastases are a result of calcification of osteoid formed by osteoblasts; this increased activity in the bone is detected by radionuclide bone scanning. Technetium-99m (^{99m}Tc) is an excellent scanning agent and is used to label phosphate, which is rapidly taken up by bone (Fig 19–20).

Bone scans are more sensitive than radiography and may detect lesions 6 months or more before abnormalities appear on the bone radiograph. For a lesion to be apparent on a conventional radiograph, 30–50% of the bone mass must be replaced, and the lesion must have a diameter of at least 10–15 mm. The more sensitive bone scans may detect 15–30% more metastatic lesions than the bone radiograph. Scans are less specific, however, and increased radionuclide uptake occurs with any process of increased bone metabolism, including trauma, arthritis, and metabolic diseases such as Paget's disease or hyperparathyroidism. Therefore, even though the pattern of diffuse focal lesions seen on a bone scan may be characteristic of metastatic disease, confirmation depends on a bone radiograph. When necessary, percutaneous needle aspiration and biopsy of a suspicious-appearing lesion can be performed, but when lesions are osteoblastic, the increased density of the bone makes needle biopsy difficult.

Since the radionuclide is excreted principally by the kidneys, the bone scan can also be a useful method of assessing renal function and may demonstrate the presence of hydronephrosis caused by obstruction.

G. Tumor Markers: The most important biochemical determination to be made in evaluating a patient with prostatic cancer is the serum level of acid phosphatase. Acid phosphatase is produced by a variety of tissues in the body and is not a tumor-specific marker; however, the prostate contains approximately 1000 times more acid phosphatase than any other organ, and there is a direct association between elevated

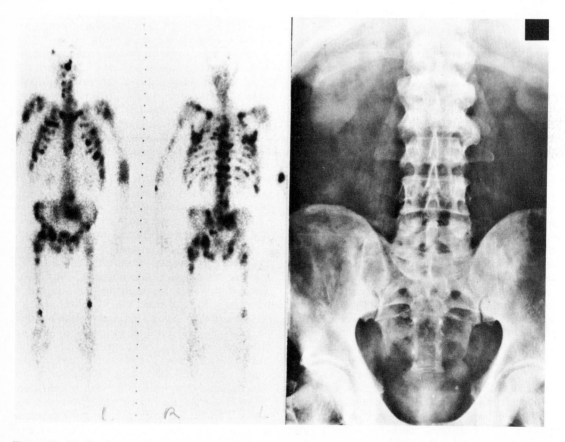

Figure 19–20. Carcinoma of the prostate. *Left:* Radionuclide scan demonstrates multiple focal areas of increased isotope uptake indicative of multiple metastases. *Right:* Plain radiograph of the lumbar spine and pelves demonstrates multiple osteoblastic lesions. (Reproduced, with permission, from von Eschenbach AC: Cancer of the prostate. *Curr Probl Cancer* [June] 1981;5:1.)

serum levels of PAP and the extent of prostatic cancer. By means of tartrate inhibition and the use of specific biochemical substrates such as *p*-nitrophenyl phosphate, β-glycerol phosphate, or thymolphthalein monophosphate, it is possible to isolate a fraction of serum acid phosphatase produced predominantly by prostatic epithelial cells. Elevated levels of PAP occur in 70–85% of patients with metastatic disease, but in only 10–30% are levels elevated when the tumor is locally confined. The usefulness of the PAP assay is to alert the examiner to the presence of metastatic disease. The assay is extremely limited as a screening tool to detect tumor, however, since a high number of false-negative results occur in patients who have small, locally confined tumors.

In an effort to provide a more sensitive test for localized disease, immunologic assays have been developed. Radioimmunoassay and counterimmunoelectrophoresis have proved to be more sensitive than biochemical assays, but unfortunately their specificity for the presence of malignant disease is lower. Foti et al (1977) reported that radioimmunoassays detected elevated levels of PAP in 33% of patients with stage A tumors, while biochemical assays detected elevated levels in only 12%. For those with stage D disease, elevated PAP levels were detected by radioimmunoassays in 92% of patients and by the enzymatic method in 60%. However, radioimmunoassays also identified elevated levels in 6% of patients with benign prostatic hyperplasia, 4% of those who had undergone total prostatectomy, and 5% of those with nonprostatic cancer, while biochemical assays detected no abnormal levels in these patients.

Although immunoassays are more sensitive than biochemical assays, their lower specificity has hampered their general acceptance. Serial determinations of PAP levels by either enzymatic or sensitive immunologic methods, however, can be an important technique for monitoring the course of disease and assessing the effectiveness of therapy.

Immunologic methods for identifying PAP within the cell are useful in making a histologic diagnosis of prostatic carcinoma. Immunoperoxidase identification of PAP in malignant epithelial cells obtained by biopsy of a metastatic site confirms the prostatic origin of the tumor.

Kuriyama et al (1982) detected another marker, prostate-specific antigen (PSA), which can also be used to confirm immunologically the presence of prostatic carcinoma. Preliminary experience with PSA suggests that its serum level is volume-dependent, and, therefore, it can be used as a parameter of tumor burden. This can make PSA an excellent marker to measure response to therapy. In a comparison of PSA and PAP, the sensitivity for detection of prostate cancer was 95% for PSA and 60% for PAP. For 35 patients with relapse of disease, the sensitivity of detection was 97% for PSA and 66% for PAP. Specificity was 96.8% for PSA and 98.9% for PAP (Seamonds et al, 1986).

Immunologic methods for identifying PAP or PSA within the cell are useful in making a histologic diagnosis of prostate carcinoma. Immunoperoxidase identification of PAP or PSA in malignant epithelial cells obtained by biopsy of a metastatic site can confirm the prostate origin of the tumor.

H. Percutaneous Needle Aspiration and Biopsy: When a malignant process is suspected, the diagnosis must be confirmed by biopsy. Access to the prostate can be accomplished by directly exposing the gland through the perineum; however, open perineal biopsy is seldom employed because of the possible adverse sequels. Instead, cores of prostate tissue adequate for histologic examination can be obtained easily by needle biopsy. A variety of biopsy needles based on the design of the Vim-Silverman needle are available to obtain tissue either by the direct transrectal route or transperineally. The transrectal approach affords the examiner a high degree of sampling accuracy, since the needle tip can be directly guided into the suspicious-appearing area by means of the finger in the rectum. However, transperineal biopsy is preferred by some because it avoids the risk of fecal contamination of the prostate, which is possible with the transrectal approach. Following transrectal needle biopsy, infection has been reported in approximately 15–40% of patients, although this has been reduced to less than 10% by using prophylactic antibiotics and mechanically cleansing the rectum prior to biopsy. Although many urologists perform needle biopsy of the prostate as an outpatient procedure, the diagnostic accuracy and usefulness of the procedure can be enhanced by anesthetizing the patient, taking multiple cores of tissues with a large-bore needle, and examining frozen sections to establish the diagnosis. The accuracy of needle biopsy is expected to be increased by the use of ultrasound for guidance, thereby avoiding the need for multiple samples and the necessity for anesthesia.

Following needle biopsy, hematuria or rectal bleeding may occur in approximately 5% of patients and urinary obstruction in 3%.

Transurethral resection of the prostate is not routinely considered as a method of biopsy, since tumors are usually located in the periphery of the gland. When transurethral resection is performed to remove obstructing tissue and the resection is extended to the peripheral capsule, prostatic cancer can be detected readily.

Fine-needle aspiration of the prostate is considered a safe and comfortable procedure, easily performed in the nonanesthetized patient. Aspirated material suitable for cytologic examination is prepared with a Papanicolaou, May-Grünwald, or Giemsa stain. Unfortunately, although cytologic evidence of malignant disease, such as atypical nuclei, may be found when tumors are poorly differentiated, it may be absent in well-differentiated carcinomas. Furthermore, with the increasing importance of histologic grading on the selection of therapy, biopsy is preferred to aspiration because it provides sufficient tissue for assessment of morphology.

Percutaneous fine-needle aspiration is also a useful tool for assessing possible metastatic sites. Percutaneous aspiration of lymph nodes that appear abnormal on CT scanning or lymphangiography can confirm the presence of metastasis and preclude an open surgical biopsy. Needle biopsy of bone lesions is hampered by the fact that most metastatic lesions are osteoblastic, and the calcified osteoid makes penetration by the needle and aspiration of tumor cells difficult. Bone marrow aspiration may confirm the presence of metastatic tumor, but findings are usually positive only when disease is widespread.

Differential Diagnosis

In benign prostatic hyperplasia, palpation of the prostate gland shows it to be enlarged but soft, firm, symmetric, and smooth. Nodules may be present, but these also are usually softer than those of prostatic carcinoma.

Firm nodules present difficulties in differential diagnosis. They can be caused by tuberculosis, granulomatous prostatitis, and calculi. Tuberculous nodules are multiple and are associated with induration and thickening of the seminal vesicles. Tuberculosis may also concomitantly involve the epididymis. Sterile pyuria is present. The diagnosis is confirmed by the finding of tubercle bacilli. Chronic prostatitis produces fibrous nodules and irregular, indurated glands. Inflammatory cells may be found in prostatic secretions, but biopsy is usually necessary to confirm the diagnosis. Granulomatous prostatitis causes a hard nodular prostate and is usually associated with chronic symptoms of prostatitis. Again, biopsy is necessary to establish the diagnosis. Prostatic calculi are frequently palpable as discrete, elevated, small, hard nodules just beneath the prostatic capsule. They are usually revealed on a plain film of the pelvis.

The differential diagnosis of osteoblastic lesions in bone must include mastocytosis and osteosclerosis. It is most important to rule out Paget's disease, which can be associated with elevated serum levels of alkaline and acid phosphatase, abnormal findings on the bone scan, and osteoblastic lesions visible on the bone x-ray. X-rays usually show the subperiosteal cortical thickening and enlargement characteristics of Paget's disease.

Treatment

Therapy for prostatic carcinoma includes transurethral resection of the prostate; radical prostatectomy; interstitial irradiation, external-beam megavoltage irradiation, or a combination of both; endocrine therapy; and chemotherapy. The recognition that the biologic behavior of prostatic carcinoma varies widely and that current staging methods fail to accurately predict its malignant potential has left both patients and practitioners confused about the selection of appropriate therapy. The status of the patient, the extent of disease at the time of diagnosis, the histologic characteristics of the tumor, and the limitations of each type of therapy determine whether the appropriate goals of therapy are eradication ("cure") of the disease or temporary control of local and distant disease ("palliation").

Approximately one-third of patients have metastatic disease at the time of diagnosis. In these patients, total eradication of disease has not been possible, and, thus, therapeutic efforts are more appropriately directed toward long-term palliation. In another one-third of patients, the tumor at diagnosis extends beyond the prostatic capsule, and half of these patients already have clinically unrecognizable metastases; therefore, total eradication of the disease by local therapy is possible only in the other half. In the remaining one-third of patients, tumors can be expected to be intracapsular and theoretically amenable to total eradication or "cure." Unfortunately, however, some of these small localized tumors are very virulent and disseminate rapidly. Whitmore (1973) has astutely pointed out that "appropriate treatment implies that therapy be applied neither to those patients for whom it is unnecessary nor to those for whom it will prove ineffective. Furthermore, the therapy should be that which will most assuredly permit the individual a qualitatively and quantitatively normal life. It need not necessarily involve an effort at cancer cure!"

The challenge for the physician is to provide the patient with a therapeutic option that is appropriate to the biologic threat posed by the cancer and to the desired goals (see decision-making matrix in Fig 19–21). More than one option may exist when more than one form of treatment has been demonstrated to be effective in achieving a goal or when the outcome is uncertain and the probabilities for success appear comparable.

A. Medical and Surgical Measures: (Fig 19–21.)

1. Transurethral resection of the prostate– In about 15% of patients undergoing surgery for the relief of bladder outlet obstruction due to benign prostatic hyperplasia, adenocarcinoma is detected histologically. When these tumors are focal, involving only a few of the prostatic chips, and histologically well differentiated, the biologic threat to the patient is exceedingly low: the 5- and 10-year survival rates of the untreated patient are comparable to those of normal age-matched controls. In evaluating 148 patients who had focal adenocarcinoma of the prostate and were treated with either placebo or endocrine manipulation, Byar (1972) and the Veterans Administration Cooperative Urologic Research Group reported that there were no deaths due to cancer and that disease progressed in only 6.8% of patients. This group's analysis of 4 other series plus their own revealed that in a total of 262 patients with stage A disease, only 5 (1.9%) died as a result of cancer.

However, transurethral resection of the prostate is not adequate therapy when the tumor is diffuse (stage A_2) or of high grade. Diffuse tumors have a greater malignant potential: 25–33% have already metastasized to the regional lymph nodes at diagnosis. As for histologic grade, Hanash et al (1972) followed 50 pa-

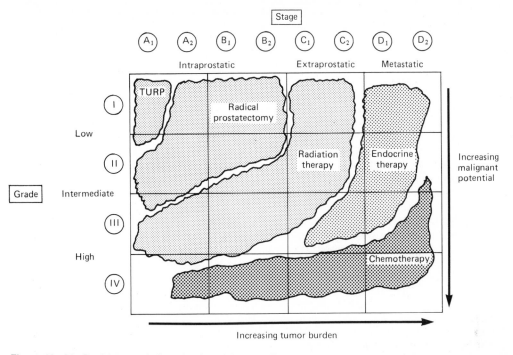

Figure 19–21. Decision matrix for selection of therapy. Tumor grade is correlated with increasing malignant potential, and tumor stage is correlated with increasing tumor burden. TURP = transurethral resection of the prostate.

tients with stage A disease and found no survivals at 15 years when the tumor was poorly differentiated.

The distinction between stage A_1 and stage A_2 disease is determined arbitrarily by the number of tissue fragments, or chips, that are involved by tumor on histologic examination. When only a few chips (eg, 3 or fewer) are involved or when 5% or less of the specimen is tumor, disease is designated as stage A_1. To be certain that no more tumor is present, some clinicians recommend a repeat transurethral resection of the prostate within 3 months of the initial diagnosis, based on a report of McMillen and Wettlaufer (1976). These investigators found that 26% of their patients originally classified as having stage A_1 disease had sufficient residual tumor in the tissue removed at the second transurethral resection to warrant reclassification as stage A_2. An additional 11% were found to have residual tumor that could still be considered focal. In a later report, Bridges et al (1983) assessed 40 patients with stage A_1 disease (defined as 5% or less of prostatic fragments positive for prostatic carcinoma) who underwent repeat transurethral resection of the prostate. No residual cancer was found in 28 patients (70%). In only 2 patients (5%) was reclassification as stage A_2 warranted.

These findings raise the question of whether repeat transurethral resection should be performed routinely. When transurethral resection of the prostate is thorough (resection down to the prostatic capsule) and only a few foci of well-differentiated carcinoma are found in careful examination of all the chips, it seems unlikely that a repeat resection will yield sufficient tu-

mor to justify further therapy. When the resection is less extensive, however, and a moderate amount of prostate remains, then a repeat transurethral resection is warranted.

2. Radical prostatectomy–The feasibility of achieving total eradication of prostatic cancer by complete excision of the prostate, seminal vesicles, and ampullae of the vasa deferentia was first demonstrated in the early 1900s. The procedure is performed by either the perineal or retropubic approach, and its efficacy appears to be related to the stage of the tumor and its histologic differentiation. The operative mortality rate is less than 1%. The most frequent postoperative complication, erectile impotence, occurs in 85–90% of patients, although Walsh and Donker (1982) have reported preservation of potency by sparing periprostatic autonomic nerves during dissection. Sparing the neurovascular bundle may result in a greater frequency of positive surgical margins, especially in patients with extensive tumors. Although this modification is successful in preservation of potency, its effectiveness for complete eradication of tumor will require careful assessment of the incidence of local failures, especially at 5–10 years after surgery. Urinary incontinence occurs postoperatively in almost all patients when the indwelling urethral catheter is removed, but leakage subsides, usually within 6 months, in 85–90% of patients. Since Byar, Mostofi, and the Veterans Administration Cooperative Urologic Research Group (1972) demonstrated that the tumor was present within 1 cm of the apex of the prostate in 75% of 208 radical prostatectomy specimens, any attempts to lessen this risk of urinary incontinence by leaving a portion of the apex of the gland seriously jeopardizes the effectiveness of this operation.

The criteria for selecting patients are extensive; as a result, the number suitable for radical prostatectomy is limited. Candidates should be those in whom long-term cancer-free survival is an appropriate expectation; ie, they should be free of serious medical problems (eg, cardiovascular disease) that would make them poor surgical risks and should have an expected survival of at least 10–15 years. The ideal patients are those in whom the disease is a discrete nodule that involves less than an entire lobe of the prostate (stage B_1). In an analysis of his experience with 103 patients who had a discrete nodule, Jewett (1975) reported that 27% lived 15–32 years without evidence of recurrent tumor. When an entire lobe or more was palpably involved (stage B_2), the 15-year survival rate dropped to 18%.

Total eradication of disease is limited, however, by clinical underestimation of tumor. Histologic examination demonstrated that in 17% of Jewett's patients with clinical stage B_1 disease, tumor had extended beyond the prostate (pathologic stage C). Of those with clinical stage B_2 disease, 50% had pathologic evidence of stage C disease, including invasion into the seminal vesicles, and approximately 40% had evidence of pelvic lymph node metastases (stage D). When disease was both clinically and pathologically confined to a single lobe, the 15-year disease-free survival rate was 33%. A more recent review by Walsh and Jewett (1980) indicates a 15-year disease-free survival rate of 51% for patients with a stage B_1 nodule. When a clinical stage B_2 tumor is found on pathologic examination to be confined within the gland, the survival rate is the same as for patients with stage B_1 disease (ie, 50% are disease-free at 15 years). Middleton and Smith (1982) have determined that the status of regional nodes is a reliable parameter for determining whether patients with stage B_2 tumors are suitable for radical prostatectomy. In 72% of their patients, the regional lymph nodes were free of tumor, and of these 50 patients, 86% had disease confined within the capsule of the prostate. As mentioned above, the number of patients who are suitable candidates for radical prostatectomy is small; of over 3700 patients with prostatic carcinoma seen at the Johns Hopkins Hospital up to January 1967, only 292 (8%) had clinical stage B_1 disease (Walsh and Jewett, 1980).

Histologic grade, as well as size, of the tumor must be considered in selecting appropriate patients. Among the 103 patients in Jewett's series, no long-term cancer-free survivals were achieved when tumors were poorly differentiated. For 33 patients with diffuse intracapsular microscopic tumors (stage A_2) treated by radical prostatectomy, Nichols, Barry, and Hodges (1977) have reported a 10-year survival rate of 60%, equal to that of age-matched normal controls. However, tumors were well differentiated in 86% of these patients. Patients who have moderately or poorly differentiated A_2 tumors are best treated at present

with external-beam megavoltage irradiation.

Some patients with stage A_2 disease have previously had a transurethral resection of the prostate. Some authors, including Jewett, consider total prostatectomy to be more difficult under these circumstances. However, Bass and Barrett (1980) have reported no increased morbidity rate, and various authors suggest waiting 6 weeks to 3 months before radical surgery.

Radical prostatectomy has been employed for local control of clinical stage C disease, but since the majority of patients involved are also treated with additional endocrine therapy or radiation therapy, the effect of surgery on survival is difficult to assess. Schroeder and Belt (1975) reported a 15-year survival rate of 20% for patients with stage C disease treated with radical prostatectomy plus estrogens. More recently, Zincke et al (1981) reported a 65% disease-free survival rate in 50 patients with stage C disease treated by radical prostatectomy, but adjunctive therapy was employed in some of these patients, presumably those with more advanced tumors. The high risk of metastasis in patients with clinical evidence of extracapsular disease makes cure by radical prostatectomy alone unlikely.

3. Radiation therapy–Radiation therapy has been employed in cases of prostatic cancer since the early 1900s, but its use was temporarily suspended because of poor results and excessive complications. Initially, prostatic cancer was considered to be radioresistant. However, after impressive tumor regression was reported following implantation of radioactive colloidal gold and after megavoltage sources of teletherapy were developed, irradiation became widely employed for patients with locally extensive tumors. Comparison of the efficacy of the 3 popular methods discussed below is difficult owing to wide differences in criteria for the selection of suitable patients, methods of staging employed, and the methods of follow-up.

a. Interstitial irradiation–Whitmore, Hilaris, and Grabstald (1972) of Memorial Sloan-Kettering Cancer Center have popularized implantation of ^{125}I for the control of locally advanced prostatic carcinoma. A pelvic lymphadenectomy is performed, and the prostate is implanted with ^{125}I seeds. A tumoricidal dose is considered to be approximately 15,000 rads delivered over 1 year. Because this isotope is of low energy and has a long half-life (60 days), the radiation extends only 5 mm from the source into surrounding tissue; thus, surrounding normal tissues receive little radiation, reducing the risk of radiation complications. However, this technique requires a very uniform distribution of radioactivity throughout the entire tumor volume to avoid "cold spots," since ^{125}I is the only source of radiation employed. Accordingly, patients must be selected carefully. The tumor must be discrete, and if extracapsular extension has occurred, the tumor must be small with well-defined borders. Patients are unsuitable for volume implantation if tumor has invaded the rectum or trigone or has extended to the pelvic sidewalls.

These guidelines for selecting patients suitable for radiation therapy produce a bias when results of interstitial implantation of ^{125}I are compared with results of other methods of irradiation. In follow-up studies of 91 patients with either stage B disease (57%) or stage C disease (43%), Whitmore (1980) reported that 71% were alive at 5 years, but only 33% were free of disease. Pelvic lymphadenectomy demonstrated lymph node involvement in 36%, and among these, 71% had developed distant metastases by 5 years. In contrast, only 38% of patients without lymph node involvement had developed metastatic disease by 5 years.

b. Combined interstitial and external-beam irradiation—

In this combined therapy, radioactive gold is implanted in the prostate to achieve a dose of approximately 3000–3500 rads and is then followed by external-beam irradiation, employing a linear accelerator to achieve a minimum tumor dose of 6500–7000 rads. Since ^{198}Au is of higher energy and has a half-life of 2.7 days, it delivers an effective dose within several weeks. Because delivering a tumoricidal dose by implanting ^{198}Au alone would severely damage surrounding normal tissue, combination therapy is used. Guerriero, Carlton, and Hudgins (1980) reported a 61% tumor-free survival rate at 7 years for 23 patients with stage B disease treated with this combination. Lymph node metastasis was detected in 24% of patients with stage A_2 disease, 19% with stage B, 31% with stage C_1 (tumor < 6 cm), and 86% with stage C_2 (tumor > 6 cm).

Complications of interstitial irradiation can be caused by radiation or related to the surgery. For ^{125}I therapy alone, Herr (1979) reported a 16% rate of early complications, including thrombophlebitis and lymphocele formation, and an 8% rate of late complications, including edema and irritative and obstructive symptoms on voiding. Guerriero, Carlton, and Hudgins (1980) reported similar complications following interstitial ^{198}Au combined with external-beam irradiation: postoperative penile and lower extremity edema (10%), proctitis (16%), cystitis or urethritis (17%), and rectal stenosis (4%). One major advantage of interstitial therapy is that over 90% of patients report no damage to erectile potency following therapy.

c. External-beam megavoltage irradiation—

When tumors are confined to the prostate and periprostatic tissue, tumoricidal doses of 6500–7000 rads are generally delivered at a rate of 175–200 rads daily. Teletherapy using ^{60}Co linear accelerators or betatron can produce photon beams with energies of 6–25 million electron volts. The higher the energy, the greater the depth of penetration of the maximum dose, making it possible to deliver a tumoricidal dose to the prostate deep in the pelvis while sparing surrounding tissue. Early follow-up studies of teletherapy reported actuarial survival rates at 5 years of 75% for 193 patients with stage B disease and 52% for 177 patients with stage C disease. The 10-year survival rates were 47% and 28%, respectively. A more recent analysis of the Stanford experience with radiation therapy for prostatic cancer over a period of 22 years (Bagshaw, 1984) reports actuarial survivals for intracapsular tumors (stages A and B) of 79.4% plus or minus 4 at 5 years, 57.5% plus or minus 5.8 at 10 years, and 37% plus or minus 8.2 at 15 years. For patients with extracapsular disease (stage C), the 5-, 10-, and 15-year survival rates are, respectively, 59.9% plus or minus 5.4, 36.1% plus or minus 6 and 22% plus or minus 7. Of the initial 775 patients reported in this analysis, only 36 patients have actually been followed for 15 years or more.

Local tumor control is dependent upon the size and grade of the tumor but overall has been reported as approximately 80–90% when determined clinically.

Assessment of local control by clinical parameters is controversial. Biopsy of the prostate has shown continued evidence of tumor in a high proportion of patients. Cox and Stoffel (1977) performed serial biopsies in 139 patients and found that 60% of biopsies taken at 6 months were positive for tumor, but only 19% of biopsies taken at 30 months were positive. In another study, positive biopsies were reported in 33% of 43 patients 12–18 months after ^{125}I treatment and in 13% of 23 patients 19–36 months after ^{125}I treatment. In 87 patients followed for 5 years, failure to locally control the disease occurred in 8% of those whose biopsy was negative and in 44% of those whose biopsy was positive, suggesting that histologic persistence of tumor 2½ years or more after ^{125}I implantation indicates treatment failure. However, because prostatic tumor may regress slowly after irradiation, histologic persistence of tumor in the absence of signs of progression within 1–2 years following therapy may not be clinically significant. Reporting on the Stanford experience, Freiha and Bagshaw (1984) observed that 61% of 72 patients had a positive biopsy 18 months after external-beam irradiation. Within 5–10 years, 16% of these remained free of local or distant progression, compared to 75% of those whose biopsies were negative. Although a positive biopsy must be considered an ominous sign, it does not universally indicate the presence of active progressive tumor.

Extended-field irradiation has been employed in an effort to improve survival results in patients with proved or suspected pelvic lymph node metastasis. Experience from a number of treatment centers has thus far failed to demonstrate any survival advantage for extended-field irradiation. Positive pelvic lymph nodes indicate systemic disease, and, regardless of local therapy, 75% or more of patients with positive nodes demonstrate distant metastases within 5 years.

4. Endocrine therapy (surgical, medical, or both)—

Recognizing that prostatic epithelial cells undergo atrophy when they are deprived of androgens, Huggins in the early 1940s elected to use castration and estrogen administration to treat patients with advanced prostatic carcinoma. The success that he and his colleagues achieved established endocrine manipulation as the principal form of therapy for advanced prostatic carcinoma.

The mechanisms of endocrine regulation have been the subject of numerous studies (Fig 19–22). About 95% of circulating serum androgen is in the form of testosterone, which originates in the Leydig cells of the testis. Once taken up by the prostatic cell, testosterone is converted by the enzyme 5α-reductase to dihydrotestosterone (DHT), which binds with the receptor complex in the cytosol and is translocated to the nucleus; there, its metabolites are responsible for promoting increased protein synthesis and cellular proliferation. Testosterone production by the testis is regulated by the pituitary gonadotropin luteinizing hormone (LH), which in turn is regulated by luteinizing hormone-releasing hormone (LHRH) produced by the hypothalamus. Serum testosterone is bound with high affinity (95%) to a serum β-globulin called sex hormone-binding globulin (SHBG), also known as testosterone-estrogen-binding globulin (TEBG), and with a much lower affinity to serum albumin.

Small amounts of the weak androgens androstenedione (3 mg/d) and dehydroepiandrosterone (24 mg/d) are produced by the adrenal gland under the control of adrenocorticotropic hormone (ACTH).

Applying knowledge of these pathways of endocrine regulation, clinicians have devised a variety of strategies for hormonal therapy (1) ablating the source of androgen production, (2) suppressing pituitary gonadotropin, (3) inhibiting androgen synthesis, and (4) inhibiting androgen action on the target tissue.

Bilateral scrotal orchiectomy is the most rapid and effective way to accomplish the first of these strategies. This procedure significantly reduces the serum testosterone concentration from normal adult male levels of 500–700 ng/dL to approximately 50 ng/dL. Through an incision in the midline scrotal raphe or through separate transverse incisions over each scrotal compartment, the testis is delivered and is then amputated at the level of the spermatic cord. An alternative to this guillotine amputation is the subcapsular technique in which the tunica albuginea of the testis is incised and the substance of the testis removed by blunt dissection, leaving behind the shell of the tunica albuginea and the structures of the distal spermatic cord. Clark and Houghton (1977) have confirmed that in spite of exogenous gonadotropin stimulation, circulating testosterone remains at a castrate level following this subcapsular procedure. Following orchiectomy, most patients are ambulatory and able to leave the hospital within a few days. Physical activity is limited for only a few weeks.

Estrogen, administered in the form of diethylstilbestrol, reduces the level of circulating serum testosterone by the second strategy, ie, by suppressing release of pituitary gonadotropins. However, its effectiveness is dose-dependent. Daily doses of less than 1 mg of diethylstilbestrol have no effect on the

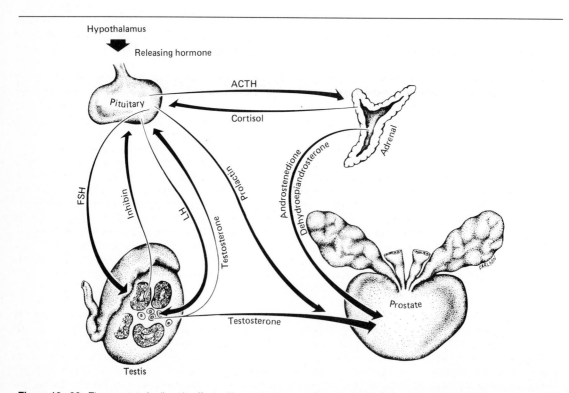

Figure 19–22. The prostate is directly affected by androgens produced principally by the testis. These various regulatory mechanisms provide numerous options for strategies of endocrine control. ACTH = adrenocorticotropic hormone; FSH = follicle-stimulating hormone; LH = luteinizing hormone.

serum testosterone level, and although 1 mg of diethylstilbestrol daily can reduce serum testosterone levels by about 50%, individual patterns vary widely. A dosage of 3 mg or more daily appears to be necessary to consistently achieve castrate serum levels of testosterone. However, even though they do not achieve maximal reduction of testosterone levels, daily doses of 1 mg have been able to effect clinical regression of metastatic disease.

Other estrogenic substances that can effectively reduce the serum testosterone level include conjugated estrogens such as Premarin, 2.5 mg orally 3 times daily, and ethinyl estradiol, 0.5 mg 3 times daily. Chlorotrianisene (Tace), a synthetic estrogen, has only a weakly suppressive effect on testosterone.

The direct role of estrogens on the prostate has been widely debated, but recent evidence indicates that estrogens can inhibit DNA polymerase and 5α-reductase activity in the prostatic cell in vitro, suggesting the possibility of direct action in vivo.

The third strategy of hormonal therapy, inhibiting androgen synthesis, can be accomplished by interfering with one or more of the 5 enzymes involved in synthesizing testosterone from cholesterol. Aminoglutethimide inhibits the conversion of cholesterol to pregnenolone, while cyproterone acetate, medrogestone, and spironolactone can inhibit androgen synthesis farther along the pathway. The antifungal agent ketoconazole has been found to be a potent inhibitor of androgen synthesis by both the testis and the adrenal gland.

Androgen action can be inhibited at the end organ. The progestational agent cyproterone acetate interferes with the DHT receptor complex in the prostatic nuclei. Flutamide, a nonprogestational, nonsteroidal antiandrogen (currently available only for veterinary use), does not suppress plasma testosterone itself but inhibits the direct action of androgen on the target cell. A recent strategy to reduce testosterone is to administer LHRH analogs such as buserelin or leuprolide in order to inhibit gonadotropin release at the hypothalamic-pituitary axis.

Nesbitt and Baum (1950) compared patients treated by endocrine manipulation with untreated controls from 1925 to 1940. Their studies in patients with metastatic disease demonstrated that 5-year survival rates ranged from 10% for those receiving diethylstilbestrol to 20% for those treated with diethylstilbestrol plus orchiectomy. In spite of the fact that ultimate survival rates of treated patients and controls appeared similar and the form of endocrine therapy employed did not influence the ultimate length of survival, the median duration of survival was longer among the patients treated with the combination of orchiectomy plus estrogen (36 months) than among those treated by orchiectomy alone (24 months) or estrogens alone (12 months).

The studies of the Veterans Administration Cooperative Urologic Research Group 20 years later confirmed the effectiveness of endocrine therapy in achieving objective and subjective improvement and demonstrated a reduction in the number of deaths due to cancer in patients treated with hormones. These studies, however, demonstrated no significant difference in survival rates between patients treated by orchiectomy alone, by estrogen alone, or by the combination of both. Furthermore, the Veterans Administration Cooperative Urologic Research Group study identified no difference in survival rate whether endocrine therapy was first administered at the time metastasis was diagnosed or was first administered at the time symptoms were noted.

The type of endocrine therapy varies widely among physicians. Use of estrogens has been curtailed because of potentially serious side effects of thromboembolic complications and fluid retention.

Estrogen use can be expected to induce gynecomastia in most patients. This is rarely severe enough to require mastectomy, and evidence suggests it can be prevented or minimized by giving radiation therapy before estrogen is administered. Gagnon, Moss, and Stevens (1979) reported a 70% incidence of gynecomastia, which could be prevented or minimized in 89% of the patients by delivering 300–500 rads to each breast on 3 consecutive days. These authors used orthovoltage equipment (140–300 kv) and treated a field no more than 5 cm in diameter that encompassed the nipple and areola area. Irradiation must be completed 2 days or more before estrogen therapy begins. When patients cannot tolerate oral diethylstilbestrol, polyestradiol phosphate (Estradurin) may be administered intramuscularly at a dosage of 40–80 mg every 3–4 weeks. A rapid estrogenic effect can be achieved by administering 500–1000 mg of diethylstilbestrol diphosphate (Stilphostrol) intravenously every 12 hours.

Synthetic compounds have been produced that are identical to the naturally occurring gonadotropin-releasing hormone (GnRH) found in the hypothalamus. These compounds, by modifying the sixth and tenth positions in the polypeptide chain, act as potent agonists of the naturally occurring hormone. When given daily in pharmacologic doses, these agonists saturate receptors in the pituitary and block the cyclic release of LH. After a transient rise in serum testosterone during the first few days of therapy, which results in initial stimulation of the tumor and a "flare" of symptoms in 25% of patients, testosterone levels progressively decrease over the next 1–2 weeks to castrate levels. In a report of the leuprolide study group (1984), 199 patients with advanced prostatic carcinoma (stage D_2) were randomized to receive either 1 mg/d subcutaneously of leuprolide or 3 mg/d of oral DES. Overall, 85% of the leuprolide group and 85% of the DES group had an objective response. Leuprolide produced a complete response in 1% and partial responses in 37% of patients, and DES produced complete response in 2% and partial responses in 44% of patients. Following the initial response to therapy, the median time to first progression of disease was 60 weeks for those taking leuprolide and 61 weeks for those taking DES. When comparing the leuprolide group to those treated with DES, researchers noted a significant decrease in the leuprolide group in the side effects of gynecomastia (3 patients versus 49 patients in the DES group), nausea and vomiting (5 patients versus 16 patients), edema (2 patients versus 16 patients), and thromboembolic phenomena (1 patient versus 7 patients).

Another LHRH agonist, buserelin, has been extensively evaluated in Europe and is currently undergoing study by a number of groups in the USA, including the National Prostate Cancer Project Study Group. Preliminary results indicate objective and subjective responses comparable to those achieved with orchiectomy, estrogens or both, with minimal side effects. Buserelin's effectiveness in achieving regression of the primary tumor has been demonstrated in one study of cytophotometry DNA histograms of prostate aspirates. Following therapy with buserelin, 17 of 21 patients (81%) demonstrated a significant regression of tumor according to a cytologic grading system (Borgman, 1983).

In an attempt to improve results of endocrine therapy, Labrie (1983) has proposed the concept of "total androgen blockage" by combining LHRH agonist with an antiandrogen. His initial reports suggested improved survival rates compared to historical perspectives; however, prospective randomized trials show no differences between the results of this strategy and those of orchiectomy or estrogen.

The role of adrenal androgens in the stimulation of prostate cancer appears to be insignificant. However, in a small subset of patients who demonstrate relapse following standard hormone therapy, subjective improvements in relief of pain and occasional objective regressions (especially fall in acid phosphatase levels) can be achieved by agents such as ketoconazole, which blocks the production of adrenal androgens.

After beginning any type of endocrine therapy, the disease status of 80–90% of patients can be expected to improve, but only in approximately 40% can the response be considered an objective regression according to the criteria established for chemotherapy programs. In spite of initial and often dramatic responses, most patients eventually relapse. In the Veterans Administration study (Jordan, 1977) of patients who had metastatic disease, only 10% lived longer than 10 years and 50% were dead within 36 months, regardless of therapy.

The relapse that eventually occurs after hormonal therapy was believed to be due to tumor reactivation, a result of stimulation by androgens of adrenal origin. Therefore, secondary forms of endocrine therapy such as hypophysectomy or adrenalectomy have been employed but have produced only short-lived responses, usually subjective. More recently, ketoconazole, 20 mg orally every 8 hours, has been employed as an alternative to surgical ablation of adrenal androgens and has produced excellent relief of pain in approximately 50% of patients.

5. Chemotherapy–(See above for chemotherapy with hormones.) In an effort to develop effective chemotherapy for patients with endocrine-resistant prostatic carcinoma, the National Prostatic Cancer Project began collaborative prospective randomized chemotherapy trials in the early 1970s (Murphy, 1977). These studies demonstrated that single agents such as cyclophosphamide, 5-fluorouracil, streptozocin, estramustine phosphate (Estracyt), and imidazole-carboxamide (DTIC) were able to produce subjective improvement and, in some instances, tumor regression or stabilization of disease. Responses to single-agent chemotherapy programs have been limited, however. Objective tumor regressions have occurred in 0–40% of patients, and in most patients, the response has been limited to approximately 6 months and has not lengthened the survival time beyond 1 year.

Because initial efforts demonstrated tumoricidal activity of single agents, a number of other studies have attempted to define combination chemotherapy programs that might be more effective.

Logothetis et al (1983) treated 62 hormone-refractory patients with a combination of doxorubicin, mitomycin C, and 5-fluorouracil and achieved an objective response rate of 48% with a median survival of 47.5 weeks for responding patients compared to 23.8 weeks for nonresponders. Other combination programs have had similar results. Thus far, in spite of occasional dramatic responses, the role of chemotherapy is limited to palliation.

B. Follow-Up Care: Following therapy for adenocarcinoma of the prostate, the patient should be examined every 3–4 months for the first 3 years to monitor the outcome of therapy. Digital rectal examination should be performed to detect local recurrence. In addition, serum levels of acid and alkaline phosphatase should be measured and a chest x-ray and plain abdominal x-ray (kidney, ureter, and bladder film) performed to monitor for metastasis. Periodic bone scans and CT scans of the abdomen and pelvis at 6-month intervals are necessary to monitor progression of metastasis in bones or regional lymph nodes.

Prognosis

Survival rates are discussed under the various forms of treatment (see above).

SARCOMA OF THE PROSTATE

Sarcomas of the prostate are uncommon tumors that constitute approximately 0.1% of all primary neoplasms of the prostate gland. In one-third of the cases, tumors appear early in childhood and are usually of the rhabdomyosarcoma type; later in life, leiomyosarcomas predominate. Other sarcomas that can involve the prostate include malignant fibrous histiocytoma, fibrosarcoma, angiosarcoma, and lymphoma.

Local growth of prostatic sarcoma causes urethral compression and produces symptoms of bladder outlet obstruction. As the tumor encroaches on the rectal lumen, it can cause constipation, obstipation, and a change in the caliber of stools. Extensive disease may produce edema of the genitalia and lower extremities. On rectal examination, the most impressive finding is the presence of a large, soft to firm mass involving the prostate and occupying a large portion of the pelvis. The mass frequently extends out of the pelvis and may be palpable on abdominal examination.

Intravenous pyelography may opacify a urinary bladder that is elevated out of the pelvis and has an elongated funnel-shaped base. Retrograde urography demonstrates an elongated compressed posterior urethra. The dimensions of the mass may be defined by ultrasonography or CT scanning. Lymph node metastasis occurs in 40% of patients with embryonal rhabdomyosarcoma and may be radiographically apparent. Cystoscopy or panendoscopy may not be feasible owing to angulation and compression of the urethra. Inspection of the prostatic urethra and bladder neck may reveal characteristic grapelike masses in children who have embryonal rhabdomyosarcoma.

Therapy of prostatic sarcomas depends upon the extent of disease and the histologic cell type. Results of treating localized disease with single-modality therapy such as radical surgery or irradiation have been disappointing and rates of local recurrence high. Similarly, chemotherapy has been disappointingly unable to achieve long-term survivals when disease is advanced or metastatic. In an effort to improve results, particularly in patients with localized disease, combination treatment programs have been employed. This strategy has thus far proved to be most effective in children with rhabdomyosarcomas. Chemotherapy combining vincristine, dactinomycin, and cyclophosphamide has been able to achieve tumor regression in over 50% of patients with extensive disease. This treatment is used either as an adjuvant following complete eradication of disease by surgery or preoperatively to diminish the size of the primary tumor, thus facilitating surgical excision or radiation therapy. Sarcomas of the prostate treated surgically require radical cystoprostatectomy and urinary diversion.

TUMORS OF THE PROSTATIC DUCTS

DUCTAL CARCINOMA

Adenocarcinomas of ductal origin without associated acinar carcinoma are rare, comprising only 1.3% of 4286 cases of prostatic adenocarcinoma seen at the Mayo Clinic from 1950 to 1970 (Dube, Farrow, and Greene, 1973).

Carcinomas of the primary ducts are papillary in configuration and appear as polypoid or villous intraurethral lesions. Obstructive urinary symptoms, gross hematuria, and pain are presenting complaints. The prostate may feel normal on rectal examination, especially if stromal invasion has not occurred.

Carcinomas of the secondary ducts are multicentric and have a comedo or cribriform appearance. Invasion of the stroma is usual, and the prostate may be enlarged and hard on palpation. In reviewing the Mayo Clinic experience, Greene (1979) concluded that survival of patients treated conservatively was poor and that carcinomas of the secondary ducts were less responsive to endocrine manipulation than were those of the primary ducts.

TRANSITIONAL CELL CARCINOMA

Transitional cell carcinoma of the prostatic ducts may occur in association with malignant transformation of the bladder urothelium or as a distinct and separate entity. The lesion may be discovered incidentally or may present with symptoms of obstruction and hematuria. Invasion into the stroma of the prostate may produce enlargement and induration of the gland.

Although successful conservative therapy by surgical excision has been reported, the lack of adequate means to evaluate the amount of ductal involvement and the degree of invasiveness usually demands radical cystoprostatectomy combined with urethrectomy. Radiation therapy has not proved effective.

TUMORS OF THE SEMINAL VESICLES

Primary carcinoma of the seminal vesicle is exceedingly rare but has been reported in elderly men. When it is suspected, it is frequently difficult to differentiate from a tumor metastasized from a primary prostatic carcinoma. The most common clinical finding is a palpable mass in the seminal vesicle. Hematuria, hematospermia, local pain, or obstructive uropathy may also occur. Metastases are frequently present.

Surgical extirpation should be performed either through a transcoccygeal approach to remove a limited lesion or through a perineal approach to perform radical prostatectomy and seminal vesiculectomy. For more advanced lesions, definitive radiotherapy may be employed. Endocrine therapy has likewise been suggested, since the seminal vesicle, like the prostate, is androgen-dependent (Lathem, 1975).

TUMORS OF THE URETHRA

Malignant urethral tumors developing in patients who have neither a concomitant nor an antecedent history of bladder cancer are rare. The causes of the disease are poorly understood, but the frequent presence of infection and chronic inflammation suggests that they may be predisposing or promoting factors. It is noteworthy that this is the only urothelial malignant disease that occurs more commonly in women than in men. Since the clinical presentation, method of diagnosis, and preferred treatment for urethral carcinoma differ markedly according to the patient's sex, the disease in women and in men is discussed separately below.

TUMORS OF THE FEMALE URETHRA

Malignant disease arising in the female urethra accounts for fewer than 1% of cases of cancer in the female genital tract and 0.02% of all neoplasms occurring in women. Malignant tumors may occur at any age but are seen most commonly during the seventh decade of life. They arise most frequently in the distal urethra and vulvourethral junction and less often in the proximal urethra.

Pathogenesis & Pathology

Most primary urethral carcinomas are squamous cell carcinoma (68%); adenocarcinoma (18%), transitional cell carcinoma (8%), melanoma (4%), and undifferentiated tumor (2%) account for the remainder (Zeigerman and Gordon, 1970). Rare tumors occurring in the female urethra have included mucoid carcinoma, transitional cloacogenic carcinoma, mesonephroma, and granular cell myoblastoma.

It has been suggested that adenocarcinoma responds more favorably to treatment, but analysis of histologic cell types and survival rates suggests that these differences probably represent differences in the extent of the disease at presentation. Prognosis depends largely on the clinical stage at presentation and is influenced little by cell type. Consequently, the various cell types can be considered as a single group for treatment purposes.

Primary urethral carcinoma spreads initially by contiguous growth and local invasion. The tumor metastasizes chiefly through the lymphatics to the inguinal and external iliac nodes. Visceral metastases are infrequent (14%), but when they occur, the most common sites are the lungs, liver, bones, and brain.

Tumor Staging

The staging system used predominantly in the USA was proposed originally by Grabstald et al (1966):

Stage 0: In situ (tumor limited to mucosa).

Stage A: Tumor does not extend beyond the submucosa.

Stage B: Tumor infiltrates periurethral muscle.

Stage C_1: Tumor infiltrates the muscular wall of the vagina.

Stage C_2: Tumor infiltrates the muscular wall of the vagina and invades the vaginal mucosa.

Stage C_3: Tumor infiltrates other adjacent structures such as the bladder, labia, or clitoris.

Stage D_1: Metastasis to inguinal lymph nodes.

Stage D_2: Metastasis to pelvic lymph nodes below the aortic bifurcation.

Stage D_3: Metastasis to distant organs.

Clinical Findings

A. Symptoms: Urethral bleeding or spotting is the most common complaint of women with urethral carcinoma. Hematuria, however, is uncommon. The patient's symptoms may mimic those of benign urethrovesical disease; complaints of dysuria, urinary frequency, perineal pain, and incontinence are common. Urinary retention has been reported in one-fourth to one-third of patients.

B. Signs: Neoplasms arising in the meatal or distal urethra may present as a papillary growth, a collarlike ring of induration, or a fleshy red or meaty mass protruding from the urethral meatus. Thickening and induration are usually demonstrable by palpation for lesions arising in the mid or proximal urethra.

C. Laboratory Findings: Pus and bacteria resulting from secondary infection of the tumor or urinary obstruction may be found in the urine. Microscopic hematuria is common, but gross hematuria is rare.

D. Instrumental Examination: Endoscopic findings can be misleading when intraluminal growth is minimal or when the tumor has little or no papillary component. In these situations, stripping the floor of the urethra by continuous upward and caudal pressure exerted by a finger in the vagina at the time of urethroscopy may force previously unrecognized disease into the lumen of the urethra. Rarely, a carcinoma may arise within a diverticulum.

Differential Diagnosis

Urethral carcinoma has occasionally been mistaken for a urethral caruncle. However, Marshall, Uson, and Melicow (1960) found only 9 instances of urethral carcinoma among 376 clinically diagnosed caruncles, an error of only 2%. The induration and thickening of the urethra associated with early tumors may be confused with chronic inflammatory changes associated with benign conditions. When erosion into the vagina occurs, usually late in the disease, the tumor may be difficult to distinguish from a primary vaginal tumor on the basis of physical findings alone.

Treatment

A. Specific Measures: Very small, exophytic,

well-differentiated lesions of the external meatus or distal urethra can sometimes be controlled exclusively by wide surgical excision. Most superficial tumors (stage 0 and A) are best managed with interstitial irradiation, used alone or as an adjunct to surgical excision (Johnson, O'Connell, and Delclos, 1983). Patients with invasive disease (stage B and C) are best treated using a combination of preoperative irradiation (5000 rads given in 25 fractions over 5 weeks) followed after 6 weeks' convalescence by radical cystourethrectomy and ileal conduit diversion (Johnson and O'Connell, 1983). Patients who refuse radical cystectomy are treated with either external-beam irradiation alone (6500 rads over 6½ weeks) or with external-beam irradiation followed by iridium implants. Groin dissection is suggested for regional nodal involvement (stage D_1) and systemic chemotherapy for stages D_2 and D_3.

Caution: Because of the significant morbidity rates associated with groin dissections and the observation that cancer of the urethra remains regionally localized for long periods of time, the surgeon should not use lymphadenectomy routinely or prophylactically in patients without proved lymphatic spread. Groin dissection should be restricted to patients who have inguinal lymph node metastases proved on sentinel lymph node biopsy (see pp 400). Prophylactic external-beam-irradiation to the nodes has not been successful in preventing future lymph node metastases.

B. Palliative Measures: When patients present with large fungating skin tumors resulting from extension of inguinal lymph node metastases, an approach combining surgical debulking, rotational skin flaps to cover the wound defect in the groin, and early postoperative irradiation is helpful in local tumor control (Johnson et al, 1975). Regional or systemic chemotherapy employing drug programs similar to those for bladder cancer may offer some palliation.

C. Follow-Up Care: Periodic examination is necessary for early diagnosis of local recurrences. Endoscopy is required at regular intervals for patients who had surgical excision or received radiotherapy as primary treatment.

Prognosis

The prognosis is fair, with 5-year disease-free survival rates ranging from 31 to 50%. The prognosis for patients with tumor located in the distal or meatal region is reportedly better than for those whose lesions involve the proximal or entire urethra.

TUMORS OF THE MALE URETHRA

Primary carcinoma of the male urethra is rare; fewer than 500 cases have been reported. It arises most frequently in the bulbomembranous area (58%) and less often in the penile urethra (36%) and prostatic urethra (6%). Although it has been diagnosed in males of all ages, it is seen predominantly in the sixth decade of life.

Pathogenesis & Pathology

Squamous cell carcinomas account for three-fourths of the tumors arising in the male urethra (Ray and Guinan, 1979). Less common histologic types include transitional cell carcinomas, adenocarcinomas, and undifferentiated or mixed carcinomas. Since adenocarcinomas occur only in the bulbomembranous urethra, this has raised the question as to whether they are truly primary in the urethra or arise instead from Cowper's glands or the periurethral glands of Littre. Squamous cell carcinomas are believed to arise from the columnar epithelium of the penile and bulbomembranous urethra through the process of metaplasia.

Carcinoma of the male urethra has an indolent growth rate, and despite the common findings of extensive local invasion, visceral metastases are infrequent. Most metastases occur by embolization through the lymphatics to the inguinal and pelvic lymph nodes. Hematogenous metastases occur occasionally, most commonly in the lungs, liver, kidney, adrenal glands, and pleura.

Tumor Staging

The rarity with which carcinoma of the male urethra is encountered has limited the usefulness of any staging system. At present, it is more important in planning therapy to categorize the lesions accurately according to location and the presence or absence of either regional lymph node or distant metastases.

Clinical Findings

A. Symptoms: Most patients (80%) complain of a urethral mass that is frequently tender. Urethrocutaneous fistulas or periurethral abscesses may be present.

B. Signs: The presence of urethral stricture disease and an associated acute and chronic inflammatory reaction may mask underlying urethral cancer. A urethral stricture that bleeds easily or profusely following minimal trauma or that requires increasingly frequent dilatation should immediately arouse suspicion about the possibility of urethral cancer. Any unusual urethral or periurethral mass warrants biopsy.

C. Instrumental Examination: Endoscopy usually reveals either a papillary, polypoid, or scirrhoid lesion whose unusual and suspicious appearance should make the wary endoscopist request histologic diagnosis. Tissue for histologic diagnosis is best obtained by either the resectoscope, cup biopsy forceps, or urethral curettage. Open biopsy can cause a malignant urethrocutaneous fistula that may compromise later definitive therapy.

D. Cytologic Examination: Cytologic examination of the urethral secretions, washings, or urine may help in establishing the correct diagnosis.

Differential Diagnosis

Carcinoma of the male urethra is frequently mistaken for sexually trasmitted disease or disease due to urethral stricture. Many patients have a history of sexually transmitted disease (40%) and urethral stricture

(20–80%). Not uncommonly, patients are treated for what is thought to be a recently developed urethral stricture that requires progressively more frequent dilatations.

Treatment

A. Specific Measures: Treatment depends largely on the location and anatomic extent of the disease. Penile urethral lesions are treated with either partial or total penectomy. Partial penectomy is recommended for distal penile lesions in cases in which the patient would still have sufficient penile length to stand and direct his urinary stream after at least a 2-cm surgical margin had been excised. Otherwise, a total penectomy, preserving sufficient length of the corpus spongiosum for perineal urethrostomy, is required. Tumors arising in the bulbomembranous region require radical exenterative surgery. Total penectomy with en bloc pubectomy, prostatoseminovesiculectomy, cystectomy, bilateral pelvic lymphadenectomy, and excision of the necessary perineal tissue is mandatory if local recurrences are to be eliminated and long-term cures obtained (Johnson, O'Connel, and Delclos, 1983). Frequently, gracilis myocutaneous flaps are required to close the perineal defect.

Tumor arising de novo in the prostatic urethra is rare. A superficial, noninvasive papillary tumor arising in the prostatic urethra can be successfully treated by transurethral resection. When the tumor involves the periurethral ducts or invades the prostatic stroma, radical cystectomy with en bloc urethrectomy is required.

Radiotherapy for carcinoma of the male urethra, regardless of site, has proved disappointing.

Note: See Caution on p 383.

B. Palliative Measures: About half of patients with posterior urethral tumors have disease too extensive for surgical removal. In such cases, palliative measures may include suprapubic urinary diversion, local irradiation, and neurosurgical procedures for control of pain. Patients who receive either no therapy or palliative treatment usually die within 3 months of diagnosis. No effective systemic chemotherapy programs have been identified.

C. Follow-Up Care: Periodic examination of the remaining urethra, pelvis, and inguinal regions is necessary for early diagnosis of local recurrence. Patients not treated by total exenteration should periodically undergo endoscopy and cytologic examination of urethral washings.

Prognosis

Five-year survival rates exceed 60% for patients with anterior urethral tumors. In the past, the survival rate was poor for patients with bulbomembranous urethral tumors, owing to the high local recurrence rate. The recent introduction of more radical exenterative surgery has markedly changed the outlook for these patients (Bracken, Henry, and Ordonez, 1980; Shuttleworth and Lloyd-Davies, 1969).

TUMORS OF THE SPERMATIC CORD & PARATESTICULAR TISSUES

Most tumors of the spermatic cord are benign and are composed of connective tissue elements (lipoma, fibroma, etc). Fewer than 200 cases of malignant tumors have been reported in the literature (Arlen, Grabstald, and Whitmore, 1969), including 19 types of sarcoma described by Banowsky and Schultz (1970).

The clinical diagnosis of a spermatic cord tumor may be difficult. The lesion is frequently confused with hernia, hydrocele, spermatocele, and testicular neoplasm. These tumors arise intrascrotally and, while separate and distinct from the testis, are located either adjacent or slightly superior to the testicle. Although the adult patient may describe the lesion as having been present for months to years, this fact should not alter the need for early surgical exploration.

The initial treatment should be inguinal exploration. The spermatic cord is occluded at the internal inguinal ring, after which the neoplasm and scrotal contents are delivered for examination and diagnosis of frozen sections. Wide local excision of the tissue immediately surrounding the neoplasm is mandatory to prevent local recurrence. Once the histologic diagnosis has been established, careful assessment for regional and distant spread should be undertaken in a fashion similar to that described for testicular cancer. In the absence of hematogenous metastases, a retroperitoneal lymphadenectomy should be considered. Its value has not been proved for liposarcoma, fibrosarcoma, or leiomyosarcoma (Johnson, Harris, and Ayala, 1978; Wertzner, 1973; Banowsky and Schultz, 1970), but the procedure is definitely indicated in patients with rhabdomyosarcoma. As many as 44–50% of these patients already have retroperitoneal lymph node involvement (Johnson, McHugh, and Jaffe, 1982; Raney et al, 1978).

The prognosis depends on both the histologic type and the stage of disease at presentation. An improved control rate has been reported following lymph node dissection, radiotherapy, and chemotherapy, particularly in children. Results from the Intergroup Rhabdomyosarcoma Study showed that, of 18 children who could be evaluated later, 16 were free of disease at a median of 23 months from diagnosis (Raney et al, 1978). Johnson, Harris, and Ayala (1978) reported 3 of 4 patients treated for liposarcoma of the spermatic cord alive longer than 5 years after treatment.

TUMORS OF THE TESTIS

Malignant tumors of the testis are relatively rare; only 2–3 new cases per 100,000 males occur in the USA each year (Mostofi and Price, 1973). Of these, 94% are germ cell tumors and the rest are tumors of the gonadal stroma and secondary tumors of the testis. In 1976, testicular cancer was the third leading cause of death due to malignant disease among males 15–34 years of age, exceeded only by leukemia and cancer of the brain or nervous system (*Cancer Facts and Figures,* 1979).

Although the tumors may occur at any age, most types have a predilection for patients of specific age groups. While teratomas and embryonal carcinomas (including yolk sac tumors) are characteristically seen in infants, seminomas and choriocarcinomas are not. All germ cell tumors occur in young adults but at somewhat different ages: choriocarcinoma at 24–26.3 years, teratocarcinoma (embryonal carcinoma plus teratoma) at 26.1–33 years, and seminoma at 33.7–41.9 years (Johnson, 1976). Finally, spermatocytic seminoma, malignant lymphoma, and other secondary tumors predominate in adults over 50 years of age.

Germ cell tumors of the testis occur infrequently in blacks, a consistent finding throughout the world. Testicular tumors occur slightly more often on the right side, as does cryptorchidism. Bilateral tumors (1–2% incidence) may occur simultaneously or asynchronously. Seminoma is the most common germ cell tumor to affect both sides, although malignant lymphoma is the most common bilateral testicular tumor. Testicular tumors have also been reported in members of the same family.

Although the cause of testicular tumor is unknown, several possible relationships have been suggested, the strongest of which is maldescent of the testes, or cryptorchidism. Various series report that 3.6–11.6% of testicular tumors arise in patients with a history of cryptorchidism, and as many as 20% are in the normally descended testes. The risk of malignant disease is approximately 1 in 20 for abdominal testes and 1 in 80 for inguinal testes. Orchiopexy does not necessarily prevent the subsequent development of malignant disease; it simply makes the tumor easier to diagnose. Mostofi (1973) has suggested 5 factors that may account for the incidence of tumor in cryptorchid testes—abnormal germ cells, elevated temperature, interference with blood supply, endocrine disturbances, and gonadal dysgenesis—but evidence is not conclusive. Carcinoma in situ is also known to be associated with cryptorchidism, even in the contralateral testis (Berthelsen et at, 1982), and has been found in association with all types of germ cell tumors (Klein, Melamed, and Whitmore, 1985). Furthermore, Muller et al (1984) reported one case in which atypical infantile germ cells progressed to adult carcinoma in

situ and, ultimately, to invasive germ cell carcinoma 10 years later. Although these reports support the hypothesis that germ cell tumors originate as intratubular neoplasms or so-called carcinoma in situ in the seminiferous tubules, the management of patients with carcinoma in situ remains controversial.

Although a history of trauma is frequently reported by patients with testicular tumor, no evidence supports a direct causal relationship. This is true despite several laboratory experiments in which intratesticular injection of chemicals or mechanical trauma appears to lead to tumor formation in rats and fowl. The occasional development of testicular tumor in an atrophic testis has suggested to some that an inductor substance may be liberated during the process of atrophy, that hormonal imbalance secondary to atrophy promotes malignant transformation, or that a viral infection triggers carcinogenesis.

The similar incidence of testicular tumors among blacks in Uganda and those in the USA, and likewise among whites in the 2 countries, suggests that differences in incidence rates are due to genetic rather than environmental factors (Templeton, 1972). Furthermore, concordance of tumor cell types was high (71%) for monozygotic twin pairs, although it was low for father-son pairs and nontwin siblings (Mills, Newell, and Johnson, 1984).

GERM CELL TUMORS OF THE TESTIS

A number of classifications for germ cell tumors have been proposed. Based on a review of 922 cases, Friedman and Moore (1946) proposed 5 groups: seminoma, teratoma, teratocarcinoma, embryonal carcinoma, and choriocarcinoma. This was modified 6 years later into the classification widely used today (Dixon and Moore, 1952):

Type I: Seminoma alone.

Type II: Embryonal carcinoma, alone or with seminoma.

Type III: Teratoma, alone or with seminoma.

Type IV: Teratoma with either embryonal carcinoma or choriocarcinoma or both, and with or without seminoma.

Type V: Choriocarcinoma, alone or with either embryonal carcinoma or seminoma or both.

Mostofi (1973) proposed to classify germ cell tumors by dividing them into those with one histologic type and those with more than one, and WHO adopted a classification based on this proposal (Mostofi and Sobin, 1977).

Pathogenesis & Pathology

A. Histogenesis: The origin of germ cell tumors is now generally conceded to be from primordial germ cells. Seminoma arises from the germinal epithelium of the seminiferous tubules, although the exact cell is not clearly established. An intratubular origin was first suggested because of the close resemblance of seminoma cells to spermatogonia and the frequent findings of seminoma within the seminiferous tubules. Because undifferentiated seminoma cells closely resemble primordial germ cells, spermatogonia, and spermatocytes, researchers suggest that seminomas may arise from any or all of the spermatocytic elements, depending on their relative availability and their responsiveness to carcinogenic stimuli (Pierce, 1963).

The cell of origin for germ cell tumors other than seminoma is more controversial. Willis (1967) postulated that all nonseminomas are teratomas descended from blastomeres that were displaced in early embryonic development and escaped organization. This concept is favored by Collins and Pugh (1964), who are responsible for the British classification of testicular tumors. However, the more widely accepted theory is that all nonseminomas originate from totipotential primordial germ cells (Melicow, 1965; Stevens, 1967). The primordial germ cell can develop along somatic lines (complete differentiation forms teratomatous elements, ie, ectoderm, endoderm, mesoderm) or trophoblastic lines (complete differentiation results in choriocarcinoma). Thus, embryonal carcinoma results from early differentiation. The arguments in favor of these tumors arising from primordial germ cells have been summarized previously (Johnson, 1976).

B. Pathology: A single cell pattern is seen in about 60% of germ cell tumors, while 40% show more than one cell type. Mostofi and Price (1973) have provided detailed descriptions of the various tumors.

1. Seminoma (35%)—Subtypes are classic (the most common), anaplastic, and spermatocytic. In 85% of men, the testis is enlarged, sometimes greatly. The cut surface shows grayish-white, lobulated, homogeneous tissue, usually without hemorrhage or necrosis. Although the tumor is not encapsulated, it is clearly different from normal testicular tissue. Microscopic examination reveals a monotonous sheet of distinct, uniform cells supported by a delicate connective tissue stroma. The cells have clear or slightly granular cytoplasm with a large centrally located hyperchromatic nucleus; mitoses are rare. Tumor giant cells, either syncytiotrophoblasts or foreign body giant cells, are common in the stroma. Lymphocytic infiltration is prominent in about 80% of seminomas, and granulomatous reaction (fibroblastic and histiocytic) is present in about half.

Some degree of anaplasia is present in many seminomas, and in about 10% the bulk of the tumor is anaplastic. No features are grossly distinctive, but the presence of 3 or more mitoses per high-power microscopic field justifies the designation of anaplastic seminoma. Stage for stage, anaplastic seminoma has no worse prognosis than classic seminoma (Johnson, Gomez, and Ayala, 1975).

Spermatocytic seminoma comprises 4–8% of all seminomas; over half of the reported patients are over age 50 (Rosai, Silber, and Khodadoust, 1969). The tumor is large, yellowish, soft, and slightly mucoid or slimy. Microscopically, the cells vary more in size, and the cytoplasm stains more deeply. The nuclei are round and contain coarsely granular condensed chromatin resembling the nuclei of spermatogonia and spermatocytes. Mitotic figures in giant cells are present, but stroma is scant, and lymphocytic infiltration and granulomatous reaction are absent. Ultrastructurally, spermatocytic seminoma cells contain a larger number of cytoplasmic organelles than do cells of classic seminoma, but the controversy as to whether they produce spermatocytes remains unsettled (Rosai, Khodadoust, and Silber, 1969; Talerman, Fu, and Okagaki, 1984). However, it is generally agreed that spermatocytic seminoma represents a better differentiated variant of seminoma than the classic type. The prognosis, based on the few reported patients, appears to be excellent.

2. Embryonal carcinoma (20%)—The adult type and the juvenile or infantile variant are common; the so-called polyembryoma is rare. Embryonal carcinoma grossly is the smallest germ cell tumor. Cut surfaces show a variegated appearance with grayish-white, smooth or granular, bulging soft tissue, little evidence of encapsulation, and extensive hemorrhage and necrosis. Histologically, the cells resemble malignant epithelial cells that vary considerably in size, shape, and arrangement. They may be large and pleomorphic without distinctive cell borders. Nuclei are also pleomorphic, and mitotic figures are common. Cells may be arranged in sheets, but frequently they are arranged in irregular glands, papillary structures, or both. More than one pattern is common.

The infantile variant is also known as orchioblastoma, yolk sac tumor, and endodermal sinus tumor. It is the most common testicular tumor seen in infants and children (about 75% of cases), but it also occurs in adults (Talerman, 1975; Teilum, 1978). Grossly, it is homogeneous, yellowish, and mucinous. Histologically, stellate endothelial cells form a loose, areolar, vacuolated network with wide meshes containing cystic spaces lined by flat mesothelioid cells. Schiller-Duval (embryoid) bodies are present, composed of perivascular endothelioid cells forming a mantle around a small cavity containing a central blood vessel.

3. Teratoma (5%)—Teratomas are complex tumors containing elements of more than one germ layer in various stages of maturation. They are found most often in patients during the first, second, and third decades of life. Grossly, the testis is usually enlarged, and the cut surface reveals cysts filled with clear, gelatinous, or mucinous material. Varying amounts of solid tissue, including muscle, cartilage, and bone, are interspersed between the cysts. Microscopically, ectoderm may be represented by squamous epithelium or neuronal tissue, endoderm by gastrointestinal and respiratory tissue and other mucous glands, and mesoderm by bone, cartilage, and muscle. In infants, teratomas behave clinically as benign neoplasms, but they should never be designated or treated as benign in adults.

4. Choriocarcinoma—Pure choriocarcinoma is extremely rare: only 18 cases were reported among 6000 testicular tumors in the American Testicular Registry at the Armed Forces Institute of Pathology. It is highly malignant, is generally confined to patients in the second and third decades of life, and is defined by the presence of 2 cells: cytotrophoblasts and syncytiotrophoblasts. Grossly, the testis commonly exhibits hemorrhage. Microscopically, the cytotrophoblasts are usually uniform, medium in size, and closely packed with clear cytoplasm; they have distinct cell borders and a single uniform nucleus. The typical syncytiotrophoblastic cells, which usually provide a cap to the cytotrophoblastic cells in a way that suggests villuslike formation, are large multinucleated cells with many hyperchromatic, irregular nuclei in a vacuolated eosinophilic cytoplasm. Syncytiotrophoblastic cells may occur in other germ cell tumors, but when cytotrophoblasts and syncytiotrophoblasts appear together, the diagnosis is choriocarcinoma.

5. Mixed cell types (40%)—The most frequently mixed cell types are embryonal carcinoma and teratoma (Dixon-Moore type IV), referred to as teratocarcinoma. Seminoma may also be present in another 6%. Small percentages of tumors show every other possible permutation of combinations.

C. Metastatic Spread: Testicular germ cell tumors almost always spread lymphatically first and hematogenously later; choriocarcinoma, the exception, metastasizes early and principally by the hematogenous route. Metastatic tumors are usually histologically the same as the primary tumor, but they may be different and may contain more than one cell type (Dixon and Moore, 1952).

Lymphatic metastases follow a stepwise, predictable pattern: from the right testis to the interaortocaval, precaval, preaortic, paracaval, right common iliac, and right external iliac lymph nodes, in that order; and from the left testis to the para-aortic, preaortic, left common iliac, and left external iliac lymph nodes (Rouvière, 1932). Solitary crossover metastases from right to left are fairly common, but they have not been reported from left to right. Nodes draining the testis extend from the level of T1 to L4, but they are concentrated near and just below the renal pedicles. Furthermore, in the absence of other lymph node involvement, isolated suprahilar lymph node involvement is exceedingly rare (Donohue, Zachary, and Maynard, 1982). The presence of metastatic nodal disease increases the incidence of affected contralateral, suprahilar, and iliac nodes because of obstruction and retrograde flow, collateral circulation, and lymphaticovenous anastomosis. Invasion of the epididymis or spermatic cord alters the primary drainage of the tumor and increases the likelihood of involving the distal external iliac and obturator lymph nodes. Inguinal metastases may occur if the tumor invades the tunica albuginea or if prior inguinal surgery has disrupted normal lymphatic drainage. Visceral metastases occur most commonly in the lung, liver, brain, kidney, gastrointestinal tract, bone, adrenal, peritoneum, and spleen, in that order (Johnson et al, 1976).

Tumor Staging

Numerous staging classifications have been developed, and many remain in use today. Most are modifications of one proposed by Boden and Gibb (1951), classifying stage A as tumor confined to the testicle with no spread through the capsule or to the spermatic cord, stage B as clinical or radiographic evidence of tumor extension beyond the testicle but not beyond regional lymph nodes, and stage C as disseminated disease.

A. Seminomas: For seminomas, for which the treatment is primarily radiotherapy, strictly clinical staging classifications were developed at the M.D. Anderson Hospital:

Stage I: Tumor confined to the testis.

Stage IIA: Tumor in the regional lymph nodes, with retroperitoneal nodal masses no greater than 10 cm in diameter.

Stage IIB: Tumor in the regional lymph nodes, with retroperitoneal nodal masses 10 cm or greater in diameter.

Stage IIIA: Tumor beyond the diaphragm, with involvement of the mediastinal or supraclavicular lymph nodes.

Stage IIIB: Tumor beyond the diaphragm, with extranodal disease.

B. Nonseminomatous Germ Cell Tumors: Staging systems for nonseminomatous germ cell tumors are diverse (Johnson, 1983), but most agree that stage I (or A) is tumor confined to the testis and that stage II (or B) shows spread to regional lymph nodes, with subcategories (eg, B_1, B_2, B_3) for the volume of disease. Clinically palpable abdominal disease is stage B_3 in some staging systems and stage III (or C) in others; either way it identifies advanced disease and helps physicians plan treatment, assess prognosis, and compare results. This has become especially important in comparing results of the plethora of treatment schedules in use today. Samuels et al (1976) devised the most precise classification for patients with stage III disease:

Stage IIIA: Disease in supraclavicular lymph nodes.

Stage IIIB-1: Gynecomastia, either unilateral or bilateral, with or without elevated levels of human chorionic gonadotropin (hCG). No detectable gross disease.

Stage IIIB-2: Minimal pulmonary disease. Up to 5 metastatic masses in each lung, the largest no greater than 2 cm in diameter.

Stage IIIB-3: Advanced pulmonary disease. Any mediastinal or hilar mass, neoplastic pleural effusion, or intrapulmonary mass greater than 2 cm in diameter.

Stage IIIB-4: Advanced abdominal disease. Any palpable mass, ureteral displacement by enlarged periaortic nodes, or obstructive uropathy.

Stage IIIB-5: Visceral disease (excluding lung), eg, liver, gastrointestinal tract, brain.

Clinical Findings

A painless testicular mass must be considered cancer until proved otherwise. Unfortunately, despite attempts to expand awareness among young men and to teach self-examination, delay in making an early correct diagnosis remains common. In 150 cases at Walter Reed Army Medical Center, the average delay from the time of initial detection to the time of treatment was 6 months (Borski, 1973).

A. Symptoms: By far the most common presenting complaint is a painless enlargement of the testis, which occurs in 65% of patients and is sometimes described as a sense of "heaviness." Pain, which in the collected experience of 9 series totaling almost 3000 patients varied in incidence between 13 and 49%, is rarely acute unless hemorrhage or infarction is present (Johnson, 1976). Abdominal pain in a patient with cryptorchidism can signify an intra-abdominal testicular tumor, which may undergo torsion, rupture, or infarction.

Since metastases are already present at diagnosis in 32% of patients (Dixon and Moore, 1952), up to 14% present with complaints secondary to the metastatic tumor (Johnson, 1976). The most common, back pain, is usually the result of enlarged retroperitoneal lymph nodes. Other symptoms are vague abdominal pain, anorexia, nausea, vomiting, and weight loss, probably the result of large tumor masses; cough and dyspnea, when present, may reflect large parenchymal pulmonary metastases or irritation of the tracheobronchial tree by nodal masses. Up to 8% of patients present with no symptoms at all, in which case the tumor may be discovered incidentally after trauma or during sexual activity.

B. Signs: A mass or swelling, the most common sign, has been reported in 74–91% of patients comprising 9 large series (Johnson, 1976). Enlargement is gradual. The generally firm mass is sometimes tender but usually painless. If a hydrocele is present (in 5–10% of patients) and interferes with adequate examination, the hydrocele must be aspirated and the testis reexamined immediately. Transillumination of the testicular tumor will reveal it to be solid, unlike a hydrocele.

Among the many signs secondary to metastatic tumor are hemoptysis, denoting advanced pulmonary disease; lymphatic metastases, which may be detectable in the supraclavicular region or even in the groin as a large mass; and a palpable flank mass, perhaps indicating a hydronephrotic kidney secondary to obstruction by retroperitoneal lymph nodes. Gynecomastia, although not pathognomonic for testicular tumor, is present in 2–4% of patients.

C. Laboratory Findings: Routine laboratory tests play a smaller role in the diagnosis and management of this disease than in many others. A complete blood count should be obtained, but anemia is unusual unless metastases are widespread. Serum multiple analysis (SMA-12) permits evaluation of liver function (abnormalities may suggest metastases or hepatitis, important information for the patient who might need chemotherapy) and renal function (creatinine levels may be elevated secondary to ureteral obstruction by large retroperitoneal nodal masses). The serum level of lactate dehydrogenase (LDH), particularly its isoenzyme LDH-1, may be elevated in patients with testicular cancer (Javadpour, 1980). Urinalysis may indicate infection. Abnormal tumor markers may be present (see below).

D. X-Ray Findings: Radiographic studies can accurately evaluate the 2 most common sites of metastasis, the retroperitoneum and the lungs. Routine posteroanterior and lateral chest x-rays are mandatory and detect 85–90% of pulmonary metastases. Whole-lung tomography and CT scanning (see below) detect even smaller nodules, although with decreased specificity, but their role in the clinical management of patients with testicular cancer is not yet defined.

Wallace et al (1961) first suggested that bilateral pedal lymphangiography be used to evaluate the retroperitoneal lymph nodes of patients with testicular cancer (Fig 19–23). Lymphangiography can detect very small intranodal disease. False-positive interpre-

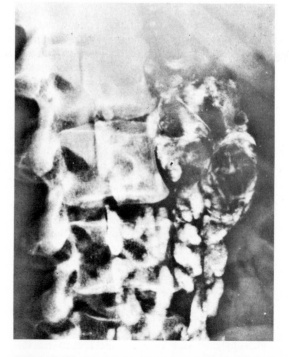

Figure 19–23. Carcinoma of the testis. Lymphangiogram demonstrates enlarged lumbar lymph nodes involved by metastatic tumor.

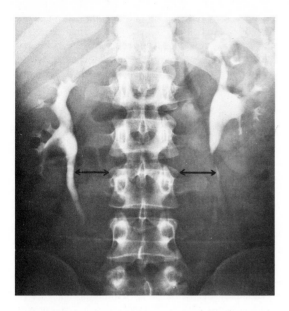

Figure 19–24. Carcinoma of the testis. Excretory urogram showing lateral displacement of both upper ureters by metastases to lumbar lymph nodes.

tations are rare if both the lymphatic and nodal phases are read and metastasis is strictly defined as a nodal defect not traversed by lymphatics. False-negative readings occur in 15–20% of patients, owing to small tumor deposits below the resolution of the test or to complete replacement of one or more lymph nodes by tumor so that the dye reveals no opacification at all. At least one group has shown that the accuracy of lymphangiography in demonstrating testicular cancer is good (79%) even when read by relatively inexperienced observers (Safer et al, 1975). Furthermore, if the lymph nodes are not removed surgically, prolonged retention of dye permits follow-up by a plain abdominal x-ray (kidney, ureter, and bladder film), and subtle changes not noted on the initial reading can be detected on subsequent examination.

Excretory urography is important in evaluating patients with testicular cancer, unless a CT scan is used to provide the same information. Either shows the location of the kidneys, particularly important in patients with seminomas, which are treated with radiotherapy. The radiotherapist needs to plan treatment portals to avoid injury to a horseshoe or ectopic kidney. Excretory urography is a safe and easy way to demonstrate ureteral deviation (Fig 19–24) or nonfunction secondary to bulky retroperitoneal nodal masses.

Inferior venacavography and skeletal surveys are rarely performed today.

E. Ultrasonography and CT Scanning: Although lymphangiography clearly detects intranodal disease, bulky nodal metastases are better demonstrated by ultrasonography or CT scanning, which are often more readily available than lymphangiography. CT scans are more accurate and specific, but they are difficult to interpret when patients have little or no retroperitoneal fat. Ultrasonography may then provide more information. Ultrasonography has also been used to help diagnose intrascrotal masses, reportedly with accuracy up to 96% (Valvo, Wilson, and Frank, 1983). CT scans should not replace lymphangiography but should be considered complementary to it.

F. Radionuclide Imaging: Liver function tests are more sensitive than liver scans in screening for liver disease (Belville et al, 1980). Scans with ^{67}Ga may demonstrate metastases, particularly of seminoma (Patterson, Peckham, and McCready, 1977). Radiolabeled antibodies to human chorionic gonadotropin (hCG) or alpha-fetoprotein (AFP) and total body scintiscanning remain experimental (Javadpour et al, 1981).

G. Biopsy: The correct "biopsy" for suspected testicular tumor is inguinal orchiectomy. Supraclavicular node biopsy should be restricted to those patients with suspicious nodes.

H. Tumor Markers: The recent development of highly sensitive and specific radioimmunoassays for hCG and AFP have dramatically improved the management of testicular cancer. The glycoprotein hCG has a molecular weight of about 38,000 and is composed of an alpha-subunit and a beta-subunit. The alpha-subunit is identical to that of luteinizing hormone (LH), while the unique beta-subunit conveys the protein biologic activity. Normal males do not have significant amounts of beta-hCG, but testicular tumors produce it; thus, it is a sensitive tumor marker (Braunstein et al, 1973). Javadpour (1980) reported that the serum levels of beta-hCG were elevated in 100% of patients with choriocarcinoma, 60% of those with embryonal carcinoma, 57% with teratocarcinoma, 25% with yolk sac tumor, and 7.7% with seminoma. Experience at the M.D. Anderson Hospital suggests that seminomas may produce elevated hCG levels in over 40% of patients.

The glycoprotein AFP has a molecular weight of about 70,000. It is present in high concentrations in the fetus and newborn but in concentrations of less than 16 ng/mL in normal adults (Waldmann and McIntire, 1974). Serum levels of AFP are elevated in patients with yolk sac tumor, embryonal carcinoma, and teratocarcinoma. Elevated levels have not been reported in patients with choriocarcinoma or seminoma. At present, a diagnosis of pure seminoma is untenable when the AFP level is elevated; nonseminomatous elements must account for the elevation.

The presence of these 2 proteins in significant concentration generally indicates tumor, although their absence does not rule out tumor. The half-life of hCG is about 24 hours, and that of AFP is 5 days; therefore, the level of either of these may be elevated in tumor-free patients because the protein has not yet been completely metabolized. Finally, because cross-reactivity between hCG and LH is possible, an apparent elevation of the hCG level may represent an elevation of the LH level as a result of orchiectomy or chemotherapy. Nonetheless, persistent elevated levels of hCG, AFP, or both after orchiectomy indicate metastatic disease. Experience has proved their indisputable value in staging, monitoring therapy, and surveillance.

The absence of tumor markers does not exclude malignant disease, since many tumors do not produce either protein. One series reported that 50% of patients with low-volume retroperitoneal disease (stage B_1) and 36% of those with moderate-volume retroperitoneal disease (stage B_2) had normal marker levels prior to therapy, and another group reported that 10% of patients with advanced metastatic disease still had normal protein levels (Lange, McIntire, and Waldmann, 1980). Chemotherapy may increase the false-negative responses.

Other markers that have been described for testicular tumor include placental proteins other than hCG and AFP, particularly pregnancy-specific B_1 glycoprotein (SP_1), human placental lactogen (hPL), and placental alkaline phosphatase (PLAP) (Javadpour, 1980; Lange et al, 1980; Jeppsson et al, 1983). Lactate dehydrogenase (LDH) is a nonspecific tumor marker that may be particularly helpful in monitoring patients with seminoma. Serum levels of another nonspecific marker, serum ferritin, also appear to correlate with disease activity.

Differential Diagnosis

The differential diagnosis of testicular carcinoma includes all conditions that produce an intrascrotal mass. The most common is epididymitis or epididymo-orchitis, which was the initial diagnosis in 16% of 510 cases of testicular tumor at Walter Reed Army Medical Center (Patton and Mallis, 1959). In epididymitis, the epididymis is usually tender and indurated, but the testis per se may be uninvolved. If the testis cannot be palpated well enough to exclude a testicular mass and if no signs or symptoms suggest urinary tract infection, the diagnosis of epididymitis should be made reluctantly. Epididymitis should respond promptly to a brief trial of antibiotics. If it does not improve within a week, surgical exploration is the conservative and recommended approach. Mumps orchitis without epididymitis can be diagnosed by the accompanying signs and symptoms of mumps. Tuberculosis affects the epididymis more often than the testis; the diagnosis is facilitated if the vas deferens is beaded.

The second most common mistaken diagnosis is hydrocele. Transillumination can distinguish tumor from hydrocele, since even cystic tumors do not transilluminate. Nonetheless, since 5–10% of testicular tumors have associated hydroceles, if the testis cannot be adequately palpated, the hydrocele fluid must be aspirated and the testis examined immediately. Testicular cancer has been misdiagnosed as an inguinal hernia, but careful physical examination of the scrotum and the inguinal areas should differentiate these 2 lesions.

Hematocele or hematoma may produce an intrascrotal mass that does not transilluminate; surgery is required, which permits the correct diagnosis. A spermatocele is a cystic mass that transilluminates and that lies above and behind the testis, permitting the careful examiner to palpate the testis separately. Varicoceles, which result from engorgement of the pampiniform plexus of veins of the spermatic cord, should collapse when the patient lies down.

Treatment

All intrascrotal masses should be considered malignant until proved otherwise. If malignant disease cannot be excluded by thorough examination, the surgeon should make an inguinal incision, cross-clamp the spermatic cord with a noncrushing clamp, and deliver the testis onto the carefully draped field for inspection and palpation. If testicular cancer cannot be excluded even then, the surgeon should perform a radical orchiectomy that includes the testis, epididymis, and spermatic cord up to the internal ring.

A. Specific Measures:

1. Seminomas– Standard therapy for seminoma is based on 2 principles: (1) Seminomas are very radiosensitive. (2) Lymphatic spread is orderly (retroperitoneum, supraclavicular region, mediastinum), and early hematogenous spread is rare. Irradiation is usually delivered to the area of nodal drainage one echelon higher than any clinically recognized tumor. Therefore, at the M.D. Anderson Hospital, clinical stage I seminoma is treated by delivering 2500 rads in 3 weeks (given in 15 fractions) to the ipsilateral iliac and periaortic areas to the level of the diaphragm. Prophylactic radiation therapy to the mediastinal and supraclavicular nodes is unnecessary.

Stage IIA seminoma is treated by delivering 2500 rads in 3 weeks to the same iliac and periaortic areas, plus giving a 500-rad boost through reduced fields to the initial tumor masses. Data from the Princess Margaret Hospital suggest that prophylactic radiation therapy above the diaphragm is not needed for patients whose retroperitoneal masses are not palpable (Thomas, 1985), and we have abandoned mediastinal fields.

Recommended treatment for stage IIB seminoma is in a state of flux. Traditionally, patients received only radiation therapy, but low postradiation disease-free rates and extremely high morbidity rates have been reported with this form of treatment. This consideration and the recent demonstration that cisplatin is so effective for treating seminoma have led some clinicians to treat bulky retroperitoneal seminoma in the same manner as stage III disease, with chemotherapy as primary therapy (Ball, Barrett, and Peckham, 1982; Vugrin and Whitmore, 1984; Friedman et al, 1985). Irradiation in relatively small doses delivered to substantially reduced fields can be used for residual nodal masses.

Radiotherapy for low-stage seminoma has been effective whether or not the serum level of hCG was elevated and even for anaplastic seminoma (Johnson, Gomez, and Ayala, 1975; Ball, Barrett, and Peckham, 1982; Swartz, Johnson, and Hussey, 1984). Elevation of the serum AFP level, however, is incompatible with the diagnosis of pure seminoma; therefore, irradiation should not be the primary therapy. Although retroperitoneal lymphadenectomy has been recommended for pure seminoma by a few surgeons, surgery should generally be considered only when masses do not respond to radiation therapy or when the AFP level is elevated.

2. Nonseminomatous germ cell tumors— Because the clinical staging of testicular tumors results in understaging in 15–20% of cases, patients with nonseminomatous germ cell tumors have traditionally been treated with radiotherapy, retroperitoneal lymphadenectomy, or chemotherapy after radical orchiectomy. Subclinical disease appears to respond to 4500–5000 rads and gross nodal disease to 5500 rads (Caldwell, 1978). This forms the basis for historically important postorchiectomy treatment plans that used either a "sandwich" technique of radiation therapy, retroperitoneal lymphadenectomy, and radiation therapy or prelymphadenectomy radiation therapy.

Today, radiotherapy without lymphadenectomy is still used extensively in Europe, with results comparable to those for lymphadenectomy alone in stage I and stage II disease (Babaian and Johnson, 1980). Patients with stage I disease seldom have relapses of disease within the irradiated area, but when retroperitoneal nodal masses are greater than 2 cm, only 33% of patients treated by irradiation remain disease-free (Tyrrell and Peckham, 1976). However, the high dose of radiation required to control the nonseminomatous tumors invites complications. Aggressive radiation therapy for testicular cancer has resulted in severe retroperitoneal fibrosis, bowel injury, nephritis with renal hypertension, and compromised bone marrow. Myelosuppression may delay chemotherapy or require dose adjustments, and radiation-induced secondary malignant tumors may occur.

Until recently, the most popular treatment in the USA for stage I and stage II nonseminomatous germ cell tumors has been retroperitoneal lymphadenectomy. The basic limits of dissection have traditionally been the renal vessels to the bifurcation of the common iliac arteries and ureter to ureter, although various modifications have been practiced. The operation can be performed through a variety of incisions, the most popular of which are thoracicoabdominal and upper midline transabdominal, and the procedure has been demonstrated to successfully remove all retroperitoneal nodal tissue (Kaswick, Bloomberg, and Skinner, 1976). Retroperitoneal lymphadenectomy has had a dual purpose: it has provided accurate postsurgical histopathologic staging, and it has been therapeutic in some patients. Recurrence is rare in the retroperitoneum after lymphadenectomy, but without additional treatment, distant metastases occur in 30–50% of patients, depending on the volume of tumor in the retroperitoneal nodes.

Because of the high recurrence rate for patients with stage II disease treated by retroperitoneal lymphadenectomy alone, chemotherapy is generally added to the treatment regimen. Chemotherapy was first given as adjuvant therapy following lymphadenectomy in which grossly positive nodes were found. Several authors have reported good results using a variety of chemotherapy programs, although it appears that full-dose aggressive programs are superior to "softer" programs (Vugrin et al, 1981). While there is little dispute that moderate- to high-volume disease in the retroperitoneum requires chemotherapy after lymphadenectomy, there is considerable controversy about the need for adjuvant therapy in patients whose lymph nodes are negative or contain microscopic or low-volume disease (Scardino, 1980; Donohue, Einhorn, and Williams, *Urol Clin North Am* 1980; Pizzocaro and Monfardini, 1984).

Today, when patients present with bulky disease in the retroperitoneum, they are treated in the same manner as patients who present with stage III disease, ie, they are given aggressive primary chemotherapy (Donohue and Rowland, 1984; Stoter et al, 1984). In fact, some investigators are now advocating primary chemotherapy for patients with moderate-volume stage II nonseminomatous germ cell tumors, especially those who would otherwise be at high risk for subsequent relapse distantly and who would require chemotherapy in any case (Logothetis et al, *J Urol* 1985; Peckham and Hendry, 1985; Vugrin and Whitmore, 1985). The results show that many of these patients achieved complete regression of the retroperitoneal masses and required no surgery, especially if the original testicular primary tumor contained no teratomatous elements. The rationale for this approach is not that the morbidity of intensive chemotherapy is less than that of a retroperitoneal lymphadenectomy, but that some patients may be successfully treated with chemotherapy alone and be spared double therapy.

For patients with either stage II or III initially, when pulmonary or other distant metastases have resolved and all biologic markers have returned to normal, the surgeon must remove any residual retroperitoneal masses. Donohue et al (1982) and Bracken et al (1983) have reported that viable malignant elements remain in about one-third of these patients, mature teratoma in one-third, and only scar or fibrous tissue in one-third. These authors noted that surgery was not successful if performed before chemotherapy had achieved complete stable control (markers normal even if residual masses were present). Likewise, histologic evidence of residual tumor (viable cancer) is an adverse prognostic feature (Tait et al, 1984; Kreuser et al, 1985). Postchemotherapy surgery is important, therefore, to indicate which patients need additional therapy and to remove teratomatous elements that may grow and create problems (Logothetis et al, 1982).

Two changes may reduce the incidence of residual tumor in future explorations. Logothetis et al (*J Clin Oncol* 1985) have reported that cyclic chemotherapy alternating 2 different combinations of drugs *and* giving 2 courses of chemotherapy after biomarkers have returned to normal and there has been maximum stable regression of the mass has reduced the incidence of viable tumor in the surgical specimen to nil in 24 cases.

Similarly, Freiha et al (1984) have reported an incidence of 2.5% in 40 patients by continuing their chemotherapy until tumor markers were normal and there was no further decrease in the size of radiographically apparent residual masses.

Complications of retroperitoneal lymphadenectomy have been reported in 7–15% of patients and consist of wound infection, pulmonary embolism and atelectasis, lymphocyst formation, chylous ascites, pancreatitis, and bowel obstruction (Babaian and Johnson, 1980). More important is the absence of ejaculate that causes infertility in a large percentage of men. Although erectile potency and orgasm have generally not been affected significantly, 82% of patients who underwent retroperitoneal lymphadenectomy at the M.D. Anderson Hospital had greatly reduced semen volume; 57% consistently had dry orgasms (Schover et al, 1985). This is a source of concern to these patients, who are usually young and have rarely completed, or even started, their families. Attempts to modify the operative technique by reducing its boundaries have been reported to preserve ejaculatory function in many patients (Javadpour and Moley, 1985; Pizzocaro, Salvíoni, and Zanoni, 1985; Richie and Garnick, 1985). It is not yet known, however, whether such modifications can maintain fertility effectively without compromising the intended staging goals.

Accordingly, and because a large number of patients with clinical stage I disease who undergo retroperitoneal lymphadenectomy have pathologically negative nodes (85–90%), several studies are examining whether orchiectomy alone is reasonable treatment for selected patients. Reports to date indicate that a "no-treatment" postorchiectomy policy is feasible (Johnson et al, 1984; Sogani et al, 1984; Pizzocaro et al, 1985; Hoskin et al, 1986). Relapse rates have been reported up to 29.5%. Embryonal carcinoma relapses at a higher rate than teratocarcinoma, and vascular or lymphatic invasion is a particularly adverse prognostic indicator (Moriyama et al, 1985). Relapses are as likely to occur outside the retroperitoneum as in the retroperitoneal nodes, and, with rare exceptions, all relapsing patients to date have been rendered disease-free by chemotherapy, surgery, or both.

Although technologic developments such as CT scanning and more sensitive biologic markers have permitted greater accuracy in clinical staging and although chemotherapy has developed to the point where we expect to control low-volume metastatic disease, surveillance programs at present are still controversial. Further data, best collected under a valid protocol, are required to define which patients might consistently benefit from this approach.

B. Follow-Up Care: All patients should be followed at regular intervals. Patients at the M.D. Anderson Hospital are usually followed at 3-month intervals for the first 3 years, then every 6 months until 5 years after treatment, and once a year thereafter. However, those in the hospital's experimental surveillance program are followed at 2-month intervals for the first year and are then seen at the same schedule as described above.

Since the incidence of bilateral disease is 1–2%, careful palpation of the remaining testis is mandatory. Likewise, palpation of the abdomen and supraclavicular areas will reveal any new lymph node metastases. Chest x-ray is needed routinely, and serum levels of AFP and beta-hCG should be determined on every visit. If the patient had a seminoma, any other previously elevated levels of marker proteins should be measured during routine follow-up. In patients with nonseminomatous germ cell tumors who have not undergone retroperitoneal lymphadenectomy, a plain abdominal x-ray (kidney, ureter, and bladder film) is taken at every clinic visit until no residual contrast material remains in the opacified lymph nodes (postlymphangiogram), and a CT scan is done at 6 and 12 months.

Prognosis

The prognosis for patients with testicular tumor has improved dramatically during the past few years, a direct result of improvements in the efficacy of chemotherapy. Although optimal programs (in terms of drug selection, dose, and frequency and duration of treatment) have not yet been defined, good results clearly can be obtained in most patients today even in the face of advanced disease. The survival rate for 544 patients with nonseminomatous germ cell tumors of all stages who were followed for 30 months between 1973 and 1976 was 65%, but the rate rose to 78% for 545 patients with corresponding conditions who were followed for 30 months between 1977 and 1979 (Li, Connelly, and Myers, 1982). For patients with distant nonseminomatous lesions, the 30-month survival rate rose from 22% (1973–1976) to 56% (1977–1979); 30-month survival rates (1977–1979) were 91% for patients with localized and nonseminomatous germ cell tumors, 79% for those with regional nonseminomatous germ cell tumors, and 92% for those with seminomas of all stages.

The M.D. Anderson Hospital 10-year experience (1970–1980) with 119 patients with seminoma reveals the following disease-free rates: stage I, 98%; stage IIA, 94%; stage IIB, 75%; stage IIIA, 71%; stage IIIB, 33%; and overall (all stages), 92%. These patients were followed for a variable period ranging from 10 months to 10 years.

For stage I nonseminomatous germ cell tumors, results of orchiectomy plus retroperitoneal lymphadenectomy or radiation therapy, with chemotherapy reserved for treatment failures, should today produce long-term survival rates of 90–100% (Whitmore, 1982). Results for stage II have to be interpreted in light of the volume of retroperitoneal disease—bulky abdominal disease is worse than gross nodal disease, and the latter is worse than microscopic disease. Thus, for microscopic or low-volume disease, the combination of surgery and chemotherapy should yield survival rates in excess of 90% (Williams and Einhorn, 1982; Vugrin et al, 1983). For bulky retroperitoneal disease, chemotherapy plus surgery should yield survival rates approaching 80–85% (Donohue, Einhorn, and Williams, *J Urol* 1980; Bracken et al, 1983). Finally, for patients who present with disseminated disease, survival rates depend on the site and volume of disease. Complete-response rates of up to 92% can be achieved with modern chemotherapy protocols (Vugrin, Whitmore, and Golbey, 1983; Logothetis et al, *J Clin Oncol* 1985).

Despite the overall success rate in treating testicular cancer, better results are obtained for less advanced disease and correlate with earlier diagnosis (Swanson, 1985). Furthermore, less therapy can be given for selected patients who present with early disease while maintaining a high cure rate.

With regards to long-term results, the late-relapse rate, the general refractoriness to additional chemotherapy in patients with residual cancer following surgical excision of retroperitoneal masses, and the induction of secondary malignant tumors all need to be more clearly defined before long-term survival or "cure" can be estimated for patients with advanced disease. At present, however, the patient with advanced metastatic disease has roughly a 50% chance of long-term survival, and patients with less ominous stage III presentations have a substantially better chance.

NON-GERM CELL TUMORS
OF THE TESTIS
(Tumors of the Gonadal Stroma)

About 6% of testicular tumors are categorized as tumors of the gonadal stroma (Mostofi and Price, 1973). These may be pure Leydig cell tumors, pure Sertoli cell tumors, undifferentiated tumors, or combinations of the above. The gonadoblastoma has a mixture of both germ cell and gonadal stromal elements.

Pathogenesis & Pathology
A. Leydig Cell (Interstitial Cell) Tumors:
These tumors constitute 1–3% of all testicular neoplasms (Mostofi and Price, 1973; Gallager, 1976; Kim, Young, and Scully, 1985). They occur at all ages but are most frequent between the ages of 30 and 50 years. Bilateral involvement is seen in 5–10% of cases. The involved testis, which may be diffusely enlarged or have one or more nodules, is generally soft but may be firm to hard. The cut surface of the tumor is yellow to brown. It can vary histologically, but the most common picture is a mosaiclike pattern of medium-sized hexagonal cells with indistinct cell borders and brightly eosinophilic, finely granular or vacuolated cytoplasm and bland normal nuclei. The pathognomonic feature of Leydig cells is the presence of Reinke's crystals, a cigar-shaped, faintly eosinophilic-staining cytoplasmic inclusion.

B. Sertoli Cell Tumors and Other Tumors of the Gonadal Stroma: Comprising fewer than 1% of

testicular neoplasms, these tumors may consist of pure Sertoli cells, pure granulosa cells, spindle fibroblastic thecalike cells, or a mixture. The gross appearance is highly variable. Microscopic examination reveals that tumors contain epithelial and stromal components, both of which vary in differentiation and arrangement. Sertoli cells are recognizable as hexagonal or tall columnar cells with a single large round or oval nucleus containing a fine chromatin network and solitary basophilic nucleolus. The cytoplasm contains large vacuoles, often filled with lipid.

C. Gonadoblastomas: These tumors are restricted almost exclusively to patients who have an underlying gonadal disorder associated with abnormal gonads and abnormal secondary sex characteristics. Microscopically, the characteristic picture is a distinct aggregate of proliferating germ cells, usually mixed in with Sertoli and granulosa cells, with Leydig cells also present. The germ cells are similar to seminoma cells (dysgerminoma). Other germ cell tumors may be present in the same testis.

Clinical Findings
A. Symptoms and Signs: All children with Leydig cell tumor show macrogenitosomia with enlarged penis, deep voice, pubic hair and hirsutism, precocious musculoskeletal development, and sexual precocity. Up to 36% of affected adults have gynecomastia, and teenagers may show both macrogenitosomia and gynecomastia. Other signs of feminization may be present.

About one-third of patients with Sertoli cell tumor and other tumors of the gonadal stroma present with gynecomastia. Some patients complain of decreased libido.

The clinical picture for gonadoblastomas is that of an underlying gonadal disorder.

B. Laboratory Findings: The typical laboratory findings peculiar to these non-germ cell tumors are abnormal results in endocrine studies (Pearson, 1981). With Leydig cell tumor, 17-ketosteroid levels are elevated in both blood and urine. Levels 3–6 times above normal occur with primary tumors, and levels 10–30 times above normal occur with metastatic tumors. Levels of estrogens and other steroidal products are also elevated. Usually all elevated levels fall after orchiectomy. When patients have Sertoli cell tumor or other tumors of the gonadal stroma, hormonal studies may reveal increased urinary excretion of androgens, estrogens, and pregnanediol, but normal levels of estrogens and androgens may also be present. Levels of 17-ketosteroid are usually normal.

Treatment & Prognosis
Treatment for all tumors of the gonadal stroma is radical orchiectomy. Partial or complete regression of secondary sex characteristics in children generally follows removal of the primary tumor, as does regression of gynecomastia in adults. About 10% of these tumors can be considered malignant. The most common sites for metastasis are lymph nodes, lung, liver, and bone,

but because of the extremely low incidence of metastatic disease, routine treatment is radical orchiectomy plus careful follow-up. Chemotherapy may be initiated if metastatic disease is discovered.

SECONDARY TUMORS OF THE TESTIS

Secondary (metastatic) tumors of the testis are rare. They are most commonly discovered incidentally at autopsy in patients who have died of widespread metastatic disease, although some are diagnosed clinically and may herald the primary malignant disease.

Malignant Lymphoma

The most common metastatic testicular tumor is malignant lymphoma (Johnson and Butler, 1976). Its incidence has been reported as 1–7% in various series, and M.D. Anderson Hospital has found an incidence of just under 3%. The tumor occurs most often in patients 55–75 years of age and is the most common type of testicular tumor in men over age 50 (Mostofi and Price, 1973). It may be bilateral, affects all races equally, and is not associated with cryptorchidism.

The usual presenting symptom is painless testicular enlargement, although pain may be present. About 25% of patients present with more generalized symptoms such as anorexia, weight loss, and weakness. Physical examination reveals the enlarged testis or testes and occasionally reveals cutaneous lymphomatous lesions elsewhere.

The cut surface of the tumor is bulging, firm, and pinkish gray, cream-colored, or buff-colored. The margins are ill-defined, and the tumor may extend outside the testis. Microscopically, the most common histologic pattern is that of diffuse histiocytic lymphoma, but other types of lymphoma have been reported (Turner, Colby, and MacKintosh, 1981). The correct diagnosis can be difficult to determine immediately. Malignant lymphoma of the testis has been incorrectly called granulomatous orchitis, embryonal carcinoma, and, most commonly, seminoma.

Initial treatment for testicular lumphoma is radical orchiectomy. A thorough investigation for other lymphomatous disease must then be performed. In most patients, the testicular lymphoma is the initial manifestation of occult disseminated disease (Turner, Colby, and MacKintosh, 1981), although malignant lymphoma limited to the testis has been well described. In such cases, radical orchiectomy alone has yielded survival times longer than 5 years, although some authors feel that adjuvant chemotherapy or radiation therapy should be given even if staging laparotomy yields negative results.

Most patients who have no evidence of extratesticular lymphoma at the time of orchiectomy go on to exhibit systemic disease. In fact, only 30% of patients in one series had disease-free intervals greater than 6 months postorchiectomy, and 90% of these patients died of generalized lymphoma within 2 years (Sussman et al, 1977).

Nonlymphomatous Tumors

Secondary testicular involvement from metastatic carcinoma is rare, with fewer than 200 cases reported prior to 1976 (Johnson and Ayala, 1976). The primary sites for carcinoma metastatic to the testis are the prostate (most frequent), lung, kidney, intestine, and stomach. Leukemia may involve the testis; results of routine bilateral testicular biopsy in children with acute lymphocytic leukemia who are otherwise disease-free and about to discontinue all therapy suggest that the testis may be a disease sanctuary (Forrest, Sabio, and Howards, 1982; Bowman et al, 1984). Nonetheless, routine testicular biopsy in patients completing chemotherapy for acute lymphocytic leukemia is currently being questioned (Hudson et al, 1985; Pui et al, 1985).

EXTRAGONADAL GERM CELL TUMORS

Extragonadal tumors are histologically identical to those originating in the testis (Luna, 1976). The vast majority occur in men during the third decade of life and arise in the anterior mediastinum or the retroperitoneum. Other less common sites of origin are the pineal gland, bladder, prostate, stomach, and thymus. These tumors constitute an estimated 1% of all germ cell tumors.

Despite earlier contention that extragonadal germ cell tumors arose from occult testicular primary sites or represented distant spread and regression of the primary tumor in the testis, substantial evidence now indicates that they represent a distinct clinical entity. Today, most authorities accept that extragonadal germ cell tumors arise from primordial germ cells displaced from their normal pathway (along the dorsal mesentery of the hindgut) from the yolk sac endoderm to the urogenital ridge (which embryologically extends from C6 to S2) and ultimately to the gonads.

The clinical presentation depends on the location and extent of tumor. Anterior mediastinal tumors may produce chest pain, cough, dyspnea, dysphagia, hoarseness, or even superior vena cava syndrome. They may be discovered on routine chest x-ray. Symptoms and signs of advanced disease (eg, weight loss) may be present, as may gynecomastia secondary to elevated serum hCG levels. The differential diagnosis of anterior mediastinal germ cell tumors should include lymphoma and thymoma.

Retroperitoneal tumors present as an abdominal mass with or without pain. Back pain, anorexia, weight loss, gastrointestinal symptoms, lower extremity edema, fever, and night sweats may occur (Buskirk et al, 1982).

Metastases are most frequently found in the regional lymph nodes, lungs, liver, bone, and brain. Therefore, the workup should include all of the tests used to evaluate the patient with a germ cell tumor of the testis, including lymphangiography, CT scanning of the abdomen, and determinations of serum levels of biologic markers such as beta-hCG and AFP. Careful palpation of the testes is mandatory. Ultrasonography of the testes is highly recommended.

Treatment of extragonadal germ cell tumors should parallel that for testicular tumors of similar histologic cell types. For low- or moderate-volume seminoma, radiation therapy alone is appropriate and has produced good results (Buskirk et al, 1982). Like advanced testicular seminoma, bulky extragonadal seminoma may benefit from primary chemotherapy, with or without subsequent radiation therapy (Jain et al, 1984; Logothetis et al, *J Clin Oncol* 1985). For nonseminomatous disease, chemotherapy followed by surgery for residual mass is currently recommended. If the diagnosis is established by exploratory laparotomy, no attempt should be made to debulk the tumor; primary therapy is chemotherapy. Prognosis also parallels, but is somewhat poorer than, that for testicular germ cell tumors (Israel et al, 1985; Logothetis et al, *J Clin Oncol* 1985).

Follow-up should always include careful palpation of the testes, since a primary tumor in the testis may not manifest itself until years after obvious metastasis (Meares and Briggs, 1972). Neither castration for serial section nor random biopsy should be performed, nor should the testes be routinely explored unless an abnormality is palpable (Luna, 1976).

TUMORS OF THE EPIDIDYMIS

Primary tumors of the epididymis are rare. The most common one is the adenomatoid tumor, a benign tumor of uncertain origin that has also been called adenofibroma and mesothelioma, among other names (Mostofi and Price, 1973). It arises in the lower pole 50% more frequently than in the upper pole. Most common in the third through fifth decades of life, it is virtually always asymptomatic. Physical examination reveals a small solid tumor, usually discrete, that does not transilluminate. Microscopically, these tumors reveal epithelioid cells and fibrous stroma. They are generally well circumscribed but occasionally extend into the interstitium of the rete testis and, rarely, into the adjacent parenchyma testis. If the tumor cannot be demarcated from the adjacent testis, surgical exploration is essential.

A second benign tumor is the cystadenoma, also called papillary adenoma and hamartoma (Mostofi and Price, 1973). Lesions are commonly bilateral and frequently occur in patients with von Hippel-Lindau disease. In fact, Mostofi and Price (1973) believe that the unilateral papillary cystadenoma of the epididymis may be regarded as a forme fruste of that disease. The tumor is characteristically asymptomatic, occurs most often in young adults, and is situated in or near the head of the epididymis. It is typically cystic owing to ectasia of the efferent ducts with papillary projections of epithelial cells. Differentiation from renal cell carcinoma can be difficult.

Malignant tumors of the epididymis have only rarely been reported, and their clinical behavior is hard to characterize based on so few cases (Farrel and Donnelly, 1980). If surgical exploration is undertaken, epididymectomy will suffice if frozen section establishes that the tumor is benign. If it is malignant, radical orchiectomy must be performed.

TUMORS OF THE PENIS

Penile cancer, although posing a significant world health problem, accounts for fewer than 0.4% of cases of cancer in men in the USA and causes fewer than 0.2% of cancer deaths. Its incidence, however, fluctuates widely among various geographic locations. During the past 25 years, the reported incidence (in number of cases per 100,000 males) has ranged from a low of 0.1 in Israel to a high of 5 in Puerto Rico, with intermediate rates reported as follows: 0.7 in Canada, Poland, Yugoslavia, Hungary, and Finland; 1–1.3 in England, Denmark, Sweden, Iceland, Norway, and the Netherlands; and 2.3 in Colombia. Previously, penile cancer accounted for 22%, 15%, 14%, 12%, and 7%, respectively, of male cancers in China, Burma, Ceylon, South Vietnam, and Thailand (Persky, 1977).

In 97% of cases, penile cancer is squamous cell in origin and resembles squamous cell carcinoma occurring elsewhere in the body. Sporadic cases of melanoma, Kaposi's sarcoma, and secondary deposits from other malignant disease have been reported.

Etiology

The causes of penile carcinoma are poorly understood. Phimosis, accompanied by accumulated smegma in the preputial sac and frequently associated with chronic inflammation, has long been thought to be the most probable etiologic factor. Recent experimental work suggests, however, that if human smegma has carcinogenic potential, its potential is weak and is influenced by genetic factors (Reddy and Baruah, 1963). Owing to the high incidence of sexually transmitted disease in patients with penile cancer, syphilis and gonorrhea have been implicated as causative factors, but continuing studies suggest that neither is a predisposing factor. A recent report by Cartwright and Sinson (1980) of 3 instances of penile carcinoma occurring over a 10-year period in residents living on the same street raises interesting speculation as to a possible viral origin. Two of the 3 patients, who were neighbors, had wives who died from cervical carcinoma. Although many studies have suggested a relationship between these 2 malignant diseases, no cluster of patients had been reported previously.

While one can only speculate about the roles that phimosis, chronic inflammation, smegma, trauma, and viruses play in inducing, promoting, and expressing penile cancer, there are no arguments against the statement that the disease can be effectively prevented by circumcision.

Pathogenesis & Pathology

Early malignant changes occurring within the dermis have been labeled by some as erythroplasia of Queyrat and by others as Bowen's disease. Erythroplasia presents as a small, bright red spot that slowly progresses into a sharply defined, glistening, velvety lesion, while Bowen's disease is usually drier in appearance and is often crusted and ulcerated. However, the 2 conditions have similar histopathologic findings and may be clinically indistinguishable. In both, thickened epidermis is replaced by atypical cells that form a plaquelike acanthosis. Hypokeratosis and fewer multinucleated and malignant dyskeratotic cells distinguish erythroplasia from Bowen's disease.

Squamous cell carcinoma of the penis occurs predominantly on the glans and the inner surface of the foreskin. The growth usually begins as a raised, red, firm plaque or as an ulcer. As it grows, it may be proliferative or ulcerative. Normal cellular maturation and polarity are lost, and excessive numbers of abnormal mitoses are present in all layers of the epidermis. The normal rete pegs are disrupted. A marked inflammatory infiltrate is universally present in the corneum and may mask areas of early invasion.

Metastases usually occur by embolization through the lymphatics to involve the superficial and deep inguinal lymph nodes. The iliac lymph nodes rarely, if ever, become involved until metastases have first reached the superficial inguinal nodes and subinguinal nodes. In spite of the rich blood supply of the penis and the many possible avenues of spread via the pelvic veins and paravertebral system, visceral metastases are rare. Death from penile cancer has usually resulted from uncontrolled regional lymphatic spread leading to skin necrosis, chronic infection, and resultant debilitation and sepsis. Distant metastases occur in fewer than 10% of patients; they appear most commonly in the lungs, liver, and bones.

Tumor Staging

There is no universally accepted staging system for penile carcinoma. Perhaps the most widely used is the one suggested by Jackson (1966):

Stage I: Lesion is limited to the glans or foreskin.

Stage II: Tumor involves the shaft of the penis.
Stage III: Inguinal lymph nodes are involved but operable.
Stage IV: Disease is disseminated.

Clinical Findings

A. Symptoms: The most common presenting complaint is the lesion itself, which may be nodular, ulcerative, or fungating in appearance. Other symptoms may include penile discharge, local pain, bleeding, and problems associated with urination (frequency, dysuria, urgency, or incontinence).

B. Signs: An ulcerative or fungating tumor may at times result in either partial or total loss of the penile shaft. Infrequently, the presence of phimosis prevents adequate visualization of the tumor, and the only sign is a firm, palpable lump in the region of the glans. Confirmation of the exact nature of the lesion should await a dorsal slit and adequate biopsies, performed in the controlled environment of an operating room.

Inguinal lymphadenopathy is present at the time of diagnosis in more than 50% of patients. However, in most instances, the lymph nodes are soft and rubbery in consistency and only represent an inflammatory response to the infected primary lesion. The lymph nodes occasionally are hard and matted together, indicative of metastatic disease. Rarely, the tumor is so advanced that it has ulcerated through the inguinal skin.

C. Laboratory Findings: Laboratory studies serve chiefly as ancillary studies, determining the extent of disease. Leukocytosis, a frequent finding, is usually secondary to local infection. Several instances of hypercalcemia, associated with localized carcinoma of the penis and cured by removal of the tumor, have been reported.

D. X-Ray Findings: Lymphangiography may identify metastases to the inguinal lymph nodes, but its applicability in this disease is limited by (1) the usually advanced age of the patient; (2) the frequent presence of enlarged, inflamed inguinal nodes that can be exacerbated by contrast medium, making subsequent clinical assessment difficult and causing severe edema of the lower extremities; and (3) the routine difficulties in evaluating inguinal lymph nodes for metastasis by lymphangiography.

E. CT Scanning: CT scanning is a less invasive and safer method than lymphangiography for assessing the pelvic and retroperitoneal areas of patients with this disease.

Differential Diagnosis

Syphilitic chancre may simulate a small ulcerating epithelioma. Darkfield examination should reveal *Treponema pallidum*. In case of doubt, biopsy is indicated.

Chancroid sometimes causes confusion in diagnosis. It is ordinarily a rapidly spreading, painful, ulcerative lesion. Complement fixation tests or findings of *Haemophilus ducreyi* on smears from the lesion are diagnostic.

Condylomata acuminata (see p 600) are soft, warty growths, caused by a virus that is usually transmitted sexually. They are usually not invasive. If any doubt exists, a biopsy should be performed.

Treatment

Treatment of patients with penile carcinoma is best carried out in stages. After the primary lesion has been treated and the patient has recovered, attention is directed toward control of the regional lymph nodes. Penile carcinoma usually spreads in an orderly, stepwise fashion by embolization through the lymphatics, not by lymphatic permeation or venous dissemination.

A. Local Lesion: The first step in treating penile cancer is obtaining adequate biopsies to establish a positive diagnosis of malignant disease. This is best done in the operating room, with the patient under either regional or general anesthesia. Sometimes it is difficult for the pathologist to differentiate between condyloma acuminatum and either a verrucous carcinoma or a well-differentiated squamous cell carcinoma. Deep biopsies usually make accurate diagnosis possible.

In selecting therapy for patients with penile carcinoma, the clinician must choose the form that is most likely to eradicate the primary lesion, prevent local recurrence, and preserve maximum usable penile length. Other factors, such as age and general medical condition of the patient, risks and side effects associated with the procedure, and overall cost-effectiveness, enter into the decision.

1. Carcinoma in situ–Squamous carcinoma in situ (Bowenoid papulosis, pigmented penile papules with carcinoma in situ changes, erythroplasia of Queyrat, Bowen's disease) is a readily recognized histologic picture of intraepithelial carcinoma, which usually requires only conservative local therapy. Topical chemotherapy (5% fluorouracil cream) is recommended for patients who can be trusted to apply the medication religiously and to return for the required frequent follow-up visits. Preliminary results with the neodymium:YAG laser (photoirradiation) have been encouraging. Although the necrosis produced by the laser may take 6–8 weeks to heal, long-term scars or defects have been minimal, and the results are usually cosmetically pleasing.

2. Verrucous carcinoma–This peculiarly slowly evolving but relentlessly expanding variant of squamous cell carcinoma accounts for 5–16% of penile carcinomas. Although this tumor has a wide disparity in clinical appearance, it is usually easily diagnosed by the histologic appearance: (1) a warty, densely keratinized surface; (2) a sharply circumscribed deep margin; (3) bulbous, well-oriented rete ridges composed of well-differentiated keratinizing squamous epithelium lacking anaplasia; (4) a pushing, rather than infiltrating, type of advancing margin; and (5) an associated inflammatory infiltrate in the adjacent stroma. Minute foci of invasive squamous carcinoma have been identified in about one-fourth of the tumors (Johnson et al, 1985). The preferred treatment

is wide surgical excision. Partial penectomy can be performed for cases involving the glans and distal shaft, provided the remaining penile length is sufficient to allow the patient to stand and direct his urinary stream. When the lesion occurs on the proximal shaft or base of the penis, or in an instance when the extent of disease precludes salvage of sufficient penile length to allow direction of the urinary stream while standing, total penectomy and perineal urethrostomy are required. As surgeons gain greater experience in using the neodymium:YAG laser, this modality may replace surgery as the preferred treatment.

3. Squamous carcinoma–Small lesions (< 3 cm) without evidence of metastasis can be destroyed by megavoltage x-ray (5000–5700 rads in 3–5½ weeks). Duncan and Jackson (1972) report that the primary lesion was cured at 3 years in 18 of the first 20 consecutive patients (90%). Delclos (1982) reported good results with either radium needles or iridium wire implants. However, even though results of radiotherapy have been satisfactory, the long interval of time required to deliver the therapy, the slow rate of regression of the tumor after treatment has been completed, and the weeks of discomfort while the radiation reaction is subsiding prove major disadvantages to the elderly, debilitated patient. Consequently, surgery is frequently the simplest, safest, most timesaving and cost-effective way to manage the primary tumor. Radiotherapy is best reserved for young patients with small lesions.

Wide excision, leaving tumor-free margins, is the guiding principle for treating the primary lesion. Circumcision alone can be performed safely when the lesion is noninvasive and limited to the foreskin. Attempts to locally excise a lesion confined to the glans should be avoided, because recurrence rates as high as 40% and a worsened prognosis have been reported. Partial amputation should be considered for all cases involving the glans and distal shaft when the remaining penile length is sufficient to allow the patient to stand and direct his urinary stream. Local recurrence is rare when amputation has been done at least 2 cm proximal to the tumor. Total penectomy and perineal urethrostomy are required in cases in which the malignant tumor occupies the proximal shaft or the base of the penis or in which the extent of disease precludes salvage of sufficient penile length to allow the patient to stand and direct his urinary stream.

B. Regional Lymph Nodes: Until recently, it was believed that penile carcinoma could, at times, bypass the inguinal lymph nodes and drain directly into the pelvic nodes. However, recent anatomic and clinical studies (Cabanas, 1977; Puras, Gonzales-Flores, and Rodriguez, 1977) have convincingly demonstrated that lymphatic channels do not lead directly from the penis to the pelvic nodes and that patients do not have iliac metastasis without inguinal-femoral lymph node involvement. Consequently, since the inguinal lymph nodes are the first barrier against lymphatic spread, attention must be focused on the groin areas as soon as the primary malignant lesion has been diagnosed and appropriately treated.

The significant morbidity (eg, delayed wound healing, lymphedema) associated with groin dissection and the excessive mortality rates resulting from a "wait-and-watch" policy (removing the inguinal lymph nodes only when they become palpably suspect [Johnson and Lo, 1984]) has created a treatment dilemma, which until recently had not been resolved. Today, a reasonable compromise is to perform a sentinel lymph node biopsy after the primary tumor has been eradicated and to follow it with a formal ilioinguinal lymph node dissection (Johnson and Ames, 1985) if metastatic disease is identified. The technique, as originally described by Cabanas (1977), requires a 5-cm incision to be made parallel to the inguinal ligament, 2 finger-breadths (4.5 cm) lateral and 2 finger-breadths distal to the pubic tubercle. The incision lies over the greater saphenofemoral junction. The sentinel lymph node is encountered by inserting a finger under the flap toward the pubic tubercle. The sentinel lymph node lies near the superficial epigastric vein.

In performing the sentinel lymph node biopsy, the surgeon should exercise extreme care to be sure to remove the correct nodes, and the pathologist should examine multiple histologic sections to reduce the possibility of overlooking micrometastasis. In the past, bilateral groin dissections were recommended for patients with unilateral nodal involvement because of the numerous lymphatic communications that exist between the base of the penis and both groins. Today, however, sentinel lymph node biopsies allow the lymphadenectomy to be performed only on the side harboring proved metastatic disease.

C. Systemic Disease: The number of reports describing the treatment of patients with systemic involvement is limited, owing to the infrequent occurrence of penile carcinoma and its rather peculiar natural history of remaining regionally localized until very late. To date, only 4 chemotherapeutic agents have shown distinct activity against penile carcinoma: bleomycin, methotrexate, cisplatin, and 5-fluorouracil. However, no long-term responders have been reported.

Prognosis

The 5-year survival rate for patients whose tumors are localized to the penis (stages I and II) is 65–90%. When inguinal lymph nodes are involved with metastases but the iliac nodes are not, 5-year survival rates range from 30 to 50%. The presence of iliac node involvement drops the 5-year survival rate to 20%, and when distant metastases are present, the cure rate is zero.

TUMORS OF THE SCROTUM

Tumors of the scrotal skin are rare. Although in the past the majority arose from occupational exposure to chimney soot, tars, paraffin, machine oil, and other petroleum products, recent reports (Ray and Whitmore, 1977; McDonald, 1982) suggest that industrial practices have changed, so that most cases today are the result of poor hygiene and chronic inflammation. Squamous cell carcinoma accounts for most of the tumors, but occasional cases of basal cell carcinoma, lymphoma, melanoma, leiomyosarcoma, liposarcoma, and Kaposi's sarcoma have been encountered.

A visible skin lesion noted as a sore papular area, a nonhealing abscess, a wart, or a chronic pruritic area should alert the physician to the possibility of scrotal cancer. There may be an additional history of other skin cancers or neoplasms arising in the digestive and respiratory tracts. Biospy is required to substantiate the correct histologic diagnosis.

Initial therapy consists of wide local excision of the scrotal lesion, with precautions taken to provide generous margins of both skin and subcutaneous tissue around the tumor.

Similarities in the anatomic, clinical, and pathologic data from patients with penile and scrotal carcinoma make indications for groin dissections for squamous carcinoma of the scrotum and extramammary Paget's disease (adenocarcinoma) similar to those for penile cancer. Both groins should be examined initially for possible metastatic disease by performing sentinel lymph node biopsies. In those patients and on the side where metastatic disease is demonstrated, ilioinguinal lymphadenectomy should be performed. In view of the low potential of basal cell carcinomas to metastasize, neither sentinel lymph node biopsy nor inguinal lymphadenectomy is required unless the histopathologic evidence places the patient at high risk for developing metastatic disease (lymphatic or vascular invasion).

The prognosis for patients with disease limited to the scrotum is good; over 60% are rendered free of disease. However, the cure rate is less than 25% when inguinal lymph node metastases occur, and there are few survivors when iliac nodes are found to contain tumor.

RETROPERITONEAL EXTRARENAL TUMORS

Although retroperitoneal extrarenal tumors and cysts are rare, they must be considered in the differential diagnosis of renal and suprarenal masses, since

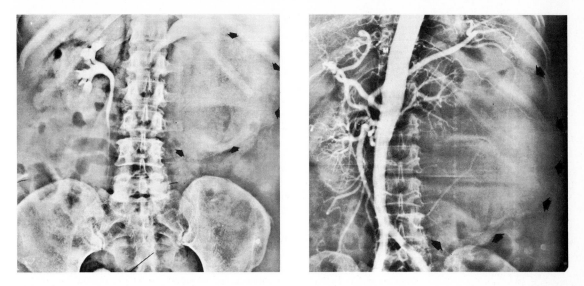

Figure 19–25. Retroperitoneal lipoma. *Left:* Excretory urogram showing large soft tissue mass (see arrows) in left upper quadrant displacing kidney superomedially. Right kidney is normal. *Right:* Renal angiogram, same patient, revealing large, relatively avascular mass in left abdomen. Left renal vasculature displaced medially and superiorly.

they present as masses in the flank. Most of these tumors arise from mesothelial tissues of the retroperitoneum and are therefore of connective tissue origin. They may be composed of a single type of cell (eg, lipoma, fibroma) but more commonly are mixed tumors (eg, chondrolipomyxoma). Many are malignant (eg, lipomyxorhabdomyosarcoma). Others, for the most part, arise from the mesonephros and its duct and from the gonads. The cystic tumors are benign; the solid growths may be benign but are more often malignant. Even if benign, however, they tend to grow to large size and to surround and displace adjacent organs.

The most common finding is a painless mass in the flank. Gastrointestinal symptoms caused by displacement or invasion of intraperitoneal organs may also be noted. Edema of the legs may occur if the vena cava is occluded. A plain film of the abdomen may show a large soft tissue mass in the upper abdomen. The kidney may be displaced, yet its caliceal system is not distorted; this is a cardinal sign of retroperitoneal extrarenal tumor (Fig 19–25). Hydronephrosis may develop from ureteral compression. Gastrointestinal studies may reveal displacement of the stomach or colon. Renal tumors or cysts cause distortion of the pelvis and calices; extrarenal tumors ordinarily do not. CT scanning and ultrasonography will show that the mass does not arise from the kidney but merely displaces it. A tumor will be more dense than a cyst. Angiography shows a relatively avascular mass whose blood supply is largely derived from the lumbar arteries.

Adrenal tumors are rarely large enough to be palpable. The x-ray findings are the same in both adrenal and retroperitoneal extrarenal tumors, but most adrenal tumors are associated with symptoms and signs of hyperfunction. Angiography, ultrasonography, or CT scanning will differentiate between the two.

An enlarged spleen may present as a mass in the left upper abdomen and at times can displace the kidney. Hematologic changes may accompany splenomegaly; findings elsewhere consistent with lymphoma may be helpful. Again, angiography, ultrasonography, or CT scanning will make the diagnosis.

The main complication is displacement, envelopment, or invasion of adjacent organs (eg, spleen, stomach, liver, ureter, kidney, vena cava, and aorta).

Surgical removal of the cyst or tumor is the only method of cure. The solid tumors are difficult to remove in toto because of their penchant for invading and surrounding vital structures. Though these tumors

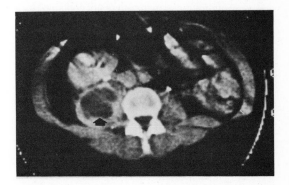

Figure 19–26. Right psoas abscess. CT scan shows massive enlargement of right psoas muscle with lobulated low-density center (*arrow*) characteristic of psoas abscess. Necrotic retroperitoneal neoplasm may present similar appearance.

are considered radioresistant, Duncan and Evans (1977) recommend radiation therapy following surgical excision. Binder, Katz, and Sheridan (1978) feel that if the tumor is large, preoperative irradiation might shrink it, making resection easier. In both cases, irradiation should be augmented by chemotherapy.

The prognosis after the excision of cysts is good. The recurrence rate after removal of the solid tumors is high even when the tumor is benign.

CHEMOTHERAPY OF UROLOGIC MALIGNANT DISEASES

Samuel D. Spivack, MD

The chemotherapy of urologic cancer exemplifies many of the recent advances in the field of oncology in general and also encompasses still unsolved problems. The number of effective chemotherapeutic agents has increased dramatically over the last 3 decades, and advances in supportive care have permitted more aggressive use of single agents and combinations. Interdisciplinary cooperative efforts among oncologists in the fields of surgery, radiotherapy, and chemotherapy are producing greater benefits than each discipline alone could offer. This discussion will consider current therapeutic approaches to urologic cancer.

CLASSIFICATION OF TUMORS

Although the term tumor originally denoted any mass or swelling, it is now generally synonymous with neoplasm (a new pathologic growth of tissue). A neoplasm may be characterized as benign or malignant depending upon its histologic, gross, and clinical features. Malignant neoplasms usually show imperfect differentiation and structure atypical of the tissue of origin, an infiltrative growth pattern not contained by a true capsule, and relatively frequent and abnormal mitotic figures. Growth rarely ceases, although the rate of growth may be irregular, and many malignant tumors have a propensity for metastasis. Benign tumors generally lack these features, although they may be fatal as a result of impingement on other structures and impairment of function.

Neoplasms are classified according to their tissue of origin. Those derived from mesenchyme (muscle, bone, tendon, cartilage, fat, vessels, lymphoid, and connective tissue) are called sarcomas. Malignant tumors of epithelial origin are carcinomas and may be further classified, according to their histologic appearance, as adenocarcinomas (glandular) or squamous (epidermoid), transitional, or undifferentiated carcinomas. Tumors may be composed of one neoplastic cell type (although also containing nonneoplastic stromal elements such as blood vessels); may contain several neoplastic cell types of common derivation from the same germ cell layer (mixed tumors); or may derive from more than one embryonic germ cell layer (teratomas).

ETIOLOGIC FACTORS IN TUMOR FORMATION

Immunologic Disease & Cancer

Cancer as a sequel to immunologic derangements has long been observed and is thought to represent a failure of immune surveillance or ineffective immune control. Neoplasms are more common when cell-mediated immunity is impaired, and some tumors have a distinctly better prognosis when lymphocytic infiltration of the tumor or regional nodes is noted histologically. Tumor-specific antigens are present in experimental animal tumors induced by chemicals and viruses. Human colon cancer contains carcinoembryonic antigens capable of eliciting an immunologic response. Recently, similar evidence has also been forthcoming for Burkitt's lymphoma, malignant melanoma, neuroblastoma, and osteosarcoma. Serum "blocking factors" that impair lymphocyte-mediated tumor inhibition have been demonstrated in patients with progressive, uncontrolled neuroblastoma and are absent in patients whose disease is controlled. Immunologic manipulations aimed at reconstituting host immune defenses are now being investigated, although no specific form of "immunotherapy" has yet been established as effective in the prevention or treatment of human neoplasms.

The most recent example of immunologic derangement associated with cancer, acquired immune deficiency syndrome (AIDS), appeared in the summer of 1981, when physicians noted an unexpected and dramatic increase in the incidence of Kaposi's sarcoma and *Pneumocystis carinii* pneumonia in young homosexual men, usually in large cities and often among users of "recreational" drugs. These patients are immunodeficient compromised hosts who have a high death rate from opportunistic infections.

Patients with AIDS-associated Kaposi's sarcoma were given a trial of biosynthetic recombinant interferon α-2b. High doses administered intravenously achieved an overall response rate of 40%. Only 20% of patients responded to lower doses given subcutaneously—about the same rate as can be achieved with vinblastine in low doses given weekly.

Preliminary data for a new virostatic agent, zidovudine (Retrovir), suggest improved overall survival rates and infection-free survival in patients with AIDS who have had *Pneumocystis* pneumonia.

Chemical Oncogenesis

One of the first documented associations between occupation and disease was made by Sir Percival Pott, who recognized that chimney sweeps were at increased risk of scrotal carcinoma induced by exposure to coal tar carcinogens. Chemical carcinogenesis induced by coal tars, aromatic amines, azo dyes, aflatoxins, or alkylators is a 2-stage phenomenon consisting of tumor initiation and subsequent neoplastic growth, with a variable but distinct latent period between these 2 stages. Carcinogenesis requires cell proliferation once the malignant initiation phase has occurred. Carcinogens are dose-dependent, additive, and irreversible. According to the Huebner hypothesis of oncogenesis, carcinogens may activate the "oncogene" or may modify host RNA in such a way that faulty "reserve transcription" occurs according to the Temin theory (see below).

Diet, Nutrition, & Cancer

Diet, among other environmental factors, may play a role in causing or promoting cancer in humans. Some investigators estimate that diet may be responsible for one-third to one-half of all human cancers. A recent publication by the Committee on Diet, Nutrition, and Cancer of the National Research Council (Grobstein, 1982) exhaustively cites evidence for the carcinogenicity of certain foods, pesticides, industrial chemicals, and environmental contaminants. The evidence reviewed by the committee suggests that cancers of most major sites are influenced by dietary patterns. However, data are not sufficient to estimate the effect of diet on overall cancer risk or to determine in what way dietary modifications might reduce risk. Interim dietary guidelines recommended by the committee include the following:

(1) Consumption of both saturated and unsaturated fats should be reduced in the average North American diet from 40% to 30% or less of total calories. This will probably decrease the incidence of breast and colon cancers.

(2) Citrus fruits, carotene-rich vegetables, and whole-grain cereal products should be included in the daily diet.

(3) The consumption of foods preserved by salt curing or smoking should be minimized. This may reduce the incidence of gastric and esophageal carcinomas in at least some parts of the world, especially China, Japan, and Iceland.

(4) The carcinogenicity of intentional additives and inadvertent contaminants should be determined so that safe levels in foods can be established.

(5) Further efforts should be made to identify mutagens in foods and test for their carcinogenicity. Where feasible, mutagens should be removed or decreased.

(6) Alcoholic beverage consumption, particularly when combined with cigarette smoking, has been associated with increased risk of upper gastrointestinal and respiratory tract cancers. Use of alcohol and cigarettes should be reduced or eliminated.

Radiation Oncogenesis

Radiation oncogenesis is a complex process that appears to involve irreversible injury to chromosomes. The incidence of the spontaneous human neoplasms is increased by radiation, probably in proportion to the incidence of the spontaneous tumor in the population at risk. Chronic myelocytic leukemia, all forms of acute leukemia, malignant lymphomas, osteosarcoma, breast and lung carcinoma, and pancreatic, pharyngeal, thyroid, and colon carcinomas—the neoplasms that account for 85% of human cancer morbidity and mortality—are increased in populations exposed to radiation above background levels.

Viral Oncogenesis

The contention that viruses may cause cancer in humans rests mainly on analogous reasoning from observations in other species, particularly laboratory animals. Of the oncogenic DNA viruses, a human herpesvirus of major interest is the Epstein-Barr (EB) virus, which was discovered by electron microscopy in cultured Burkitt's lymphoma cells and subsequently found in many isolates of Burkitt's lymphoma. EB virus has also been associated with nasopharyngeal carcinoma, but its causal role in that illness is far from certain. A herpesvirus has also been associated with cancer of the uterine cervix, since viral antibodies are present in more women with this cancer than in control populations.

Oncogenic RNA viruses (oncornaviruses) have recently been thought to cause some human cancers. An RNA tumor virus might produce a stable genetic trait if viral RNA served as the template for DNA synthesis and the DNA became integrated into the host genome, resulting in neoplastic transformation. This revolutionary concept challenged the classic Watson-Crick hypothesis that information flow was unidirectional from DNA to RNA to protein. This hypothesis became more tenable with the demonstration that "reverse transcriptase" existed in nearly all RNA viruses with oncogenic potential, in human lymphoblastic leukemia cells, and in viruslike C particles from human milk in patients with breast cancer and, to a lesser extent, in their seemingly normal relatives.

Oncogenes are small structural segments within DNA that encode for substances involved in normal cellular division. These products have been identified for many known oncogenes and include growth factors, protein kinases, membrane receptors, and DNA-binding proteins. Of the more than 30 known oncogenes, most have been localized to certain chromosomes; they are normal regulatory genes that cause uncontrolled cellular division when they are inappropriately activated. The factors that activate these genes are unknown, but chromosomal breaks are frequently observed near the activated oncogene site. For example, the 9:22 translocation (Philadelphia chromosome), which is associated with chronic myelocytic leukemia, occurs at the c-abl oncogene site on the 9 chromosome. Current research efforts are devoted to blocking oncogenic expression in hopes of inhibiting malignant growth.

VALUE OF GRADING & STAGING IN MALIGNANT DISEASE

For most curable neoplasms, the first therapeutic attempt must be definitive if cure is to be achieved; this means that initial therapy must be radical enough to encompass and extirpate or sterilize all existing foci of disease. An accurate delineation of the stage and extent of disease is thus an important initial step in determining the most appropriate treatment for the patient.

Grading and staging of neoplasms are attempts to describe the degree of malignancy and the extent of its dissemination. Histologic grading determines the degree of anaplasia of tumor cells, varying from grade I (very well differentiated) to grade IV (undifferentiated). Grading has prognostic value in some tumors (transitional cell carcinoma of bladder, astrocytoma, and chondrosarcoma) but is of little predictive value in others (melanoma or osteosarcoma). Staging of cancer is based upon the extent of its spread rather than on histologic appearance and has been standardized for many cancers by use of the TNM system. T refers to the degree of local extension at the primary site, N to the clinical findings in regional nodes, and M to the presence of distant metastases. Some cancers are staged by clinical examination alone (eg, squamous cell carcinoma of the cervix), whereas for others (eg, transitional cell carcinoma of the bladder and adenocarcinoma of the colon) the stage is determined on the basis of findings in the resected surgical specimen. In both instances, there is an excellent correlation of stage with prognosis.

For many neoplasms, both the histologic grading and the clinical staging are relevant to the choice of treatment and prognosis.

THERAPY OF MALIGNANT DISEASES

SURGERY

Surgical excision is the most effective means of removing the primary lesion of most neoplasms. It also provides palliation of symptoms, as by the relief of intestinal obstruction in tumors that may be unresectable or may have already metastasized. A number of highly malignant tumors have been found to respond favorably to limited surgical excision combined with radiation therapy and chemotherapy.

Solitary Metastasis

Even though more than 80% of apparently solitary metastases are eventually found to be multiple, an occasional cure results from their excision. In patients with a solitary lung metastasis, lobectomy gives 5-year survival rates of 15–60% depending upon the

tissue of origin, the histologic characteristics of the tumor, and the time of appearance of the metastasis. The best results have been achieved when the metastasis was discovered more than 2 years after treatment of the primary lesion. Surgery is much less successful for solitary brain metastases from lung tumors. The prognosis for solitary bony and liver metastases is poor, but occasional cures have followed removal of metastases from hypernephroma, testicular and gynecologic neoplasms, various sarcomas, and occasional intestinal tumors.

Long-term palliation sometimes follows radiation therapy for metastases from certain radiosensitive tumors such as Wilms' tumor, seminoma, neuroblastoma, and some sarcomas.

Radiotherapy has also produced long-term survival in patients with metastases in neck nodes from an occult primary lesion, presumably in the oropharynx or nasopharynx.

RADIATION THERAPY

Radiation therapy, alone or in conjunction with surgery or chemotherapy, may also serve as definitive treatment of certain malignant diseases. Local obstructions and inoperable masses are frequently and effectively controlled by radiation therapy.

CANCER IMMUNOLOGY & IMMUNOTHERAPY

Immunology and immunotherapy are emerging as contributory disciplines in multiagent therapy of cancer. Successful treatment of antigenic animal tumors in model systems and preliminary response data for human trials have identified promising regimens suitable for further development.

The search for tumor-associated antigens in humans has yielded the oncodevelopmental antigens: carcinoembryonic antigen (CEA), alpha-fetoprotein (AFP), and human chorionic gonadotropin (hCG). Antibodies (including monoclonal antibodies) to these antigens have been developed and are currently used to monitor patients whose tumors bear these markers. Research is under way to determine whether antibodies to these and other tumor-associated antigens can be used for imaging and immunotherapy. Theoretically, selective binding of these antibodies should allow high concentrations of radiotherapeutic or toxic agents to be delivered selectively to the tumors. Further research will include attempts to find other antigens with high expression on tumors and low expression on normal tissue and to eliminate nonspecific uptake of antibodies by the reticuloendothelial system.

Tumor-specific antigens—antigens unique to tumors—have been difficult to identify in humans. Preliminary work in melanoma has identified several candidate antigens. The use of whole tumor cell vaccines to augment the immune response is based on the premise that such antigens exist. Data from animal models support this approach for adjuvant therapy, and controlled clinical trials are now in progress.

Nonspecific immunostimulants were extensively tested during the 1970s. Despite early enthusiastic reports, controlled trials have demonstrated only limited effects. For BCG, regression was observed in about 50% of directly injected melanoma lesions, but there was little effect on noninjected lesions and none on distant visceral lesions.

Cytokines are cellular hormones that have a complex role in immunoregulation. Recombinant DNA technology has now been applied to the production of large quantities of pure cytokines for use in clinical trials. The cytokine interferon is produced by leukocytes (α), fibroblasts (β), and lymphocytes (γ). α-Interferon was the first to become available in large quantities. Early trials suggested that it had therapeutic benefit in a wide variety of tumors, but the results of subsequent controlled trials have been disappointing except for the treatment of hairy cell leukemia, where responses are seen in 90% of patients. γ-Interferon, recently available in large quantities, may have a more potent immunotherapeutic effect. Another cytokine, tumor necrosis factor (TNF), is currently entering clinical trials. Interleukin-2, a cytokine produced by "helper" lymphocytes, causes lymphocytes to expand in vitro and kill tumor cells. Preliminary results of clinical trials with this agent indicate activity for some cancers, specifically melanoma and renal cancer.

Transfer of activated immune cells (adoptive immunotherapy) also shows great promise in animal models. Clinical trials in humans have utilized cells that are activated by culturing in interleukin-2 (lymphokine-activated killer cells [LAK]). Preliminary results show activity in a variety of cancers. Current research is centered on increasing the response rate while decreasing the toxicity. Tumor-infiltrating lymphocytes (TIL) are MHC-restricted tumor-specific cytotoxic T lymphocytes (CTL) cultured directly from tumors. In animal models, TILs are highly effective in eradicating immunogenic tumors. The challenges to applications in humans are to demonstrate immunogenicity of the tumors and then to expand the range of specific CTLs.

Research is also going forward on ways of boosting the immune response, which is suppressed by the tumor itself and the major treatment methods: surgery, irradiation, and chemotherapy. Expanding knowledge of the immune system and its response to tumors presages a significant future role for immunologic methods in the treatment of cancer.

CHEMOTHERAPY

Scientific Basis of Chemotherapy

A. Selective Toxicity: The Qualitative Approach: A basic goal of cancer chemotherapy is the development of agents that have "selective toxicity"

against replicating tumor cells but at the same time spare replicating host tissues. Such an ideal drug has not yet been found, and only the hormones and asparaginase (and, to a lesser extent, mitotane [o,p'-DDD; Lysodren] and streptozocin) approach this goal. Although these drugs have important side effects, their toxicity is not primarily directed against normal replicating cells.

B. The Quantitative Kinetic Approach: Since in most instances qualitative metabolic differences between normal and neoplastic cells have not been discovered, the chemotherapist must plan according to quantitative differences in the proliferative kinetics of normal and neoplastic cell growth if tumor regression without major host toxicity is to be achieved. Early bacteriologists, in their study of germicidal agents, formulated the concept of "the logarithmic order of cell kill." According to this theory, any particular treatment will kill a certain fraction of cells *independently* of the total number of cells present (provided the growth rate is constant). Thus, "cure," in the sense of killing the last remaining tumor cells, is more readily achieved by drugs when the total tumor cell burden is small. For example, a drug that is 99% efficient kills 2 logs of cells regardless of the total number of cells present and will reduce a tumor cell population of 100 to a single remaining cell, whereas it will leave 10,000 remaining cells of an initial tumor cell number of 1 million.

The quantitative evaluation of drug effects on normal and neoplastic tissues was furthered by the development of an in vivo assay system to allow measurement of the dose-response relationship of a variety of agents against both neoplastic and normal hematopoietic stem cells. As a result of these experiments, at least 2 cell survival curves are generated. The first curve shows decimation of both normal and neoplastic cells to almost the same degree, whereas the other curve shows a much greater decimation of tumor cells than of normal stem cells. The selectivity of the agents in the second class was attributed to a differential effect of the agents, which attacked proliferating cells in the mitotic cycle while sparing resting cells not in mitotic division. Thus arose the classification of forms of therapy into (1) cell cycle-specific (CCS) agents, which attack only actively proliferating cells engaged in DNA synthesis and the mitotic cycle; and (2) cell cycle-nonspecific (CCNS) agents, which kill both normal and tumor cells regardless of their proliferative state.

The important implications of these data are borne out by evidence in experimental tumor systems and to some extent in humans: (1) Differences in sensitivity of normal hematopoietic precursors and neoplastic cells are a function of the difference in their proliferative states and not a result of any inherent qualitative biochemical differences between the 2 cell types. (2) Injured or "stimulated" marrow or normal tissue that is proliferating as rapidly as neoplastic tissue will be affected to the same extent as neoplastic tissue.

As a general rule, any tissue, normal or neoplastic,

manifests an early logarithmic phase of exponential growth during which most cells are in active mitosis. When a certain bulk is achieved, there is a transition to a later "steady-state" plateau phase of growth during which a lesser fraction of cells is in the proliferative cycle. To maximize the therapeutic effects of CCS antineoplastic agents, resting cells must be induced to enter the proliferative cycle without at the same time increasing normal tissue vulnerability. This implies a reduction of tumor bulk with a reentry from the plateau phase into the log phase of exponential growth. Methods of reducing tumor bulk presently include treatment by CCNS agents such as x-ray radiation or mechlorethamine and removal of gross tumor masses at surgery, but these stratagems all too often have attendant toxicities.

Utilizing these concepts, Schabel (1969) proposed an approach to "curative" sequential chemotherapy of advanced tumors using a CCNS agent followed by a CCS agent in repeated courses.

While this is an idealized approach to curative therapy, similar approaches have led to cure of laboratory-induced neoplasms, and such concepts form the basis for several successful new antileukemic regimens—particularly for childhood leukemia. Clearly, this approach will be furthered by a better understanding of human tumor cell kinetics in individual patients, by new knowledge about the dose, duration, and site of action of antitumor agents, by the development of new "marrow-sparing" agents, and by appropriately synergistic combinations of drugs as well as better means of measuring their effects on microscopic tumor deposits.

A new technique for growing tumor stem cells with clonogenic or colony-forming capability has recently been developed. The clonogenic cells are obtained from a fresh tumor biopsy specimen and can be grown in soft agar and tested against standard and new anticancer drugs for inhibition of clonogenicity. This technique may simplify the identification of clinically effective drugs. It is 99% accurate in predicting lack of clinical response, which suggests that the assay may be most useful in avoiding fruitless clinical trials. Further studies using the tumor stem cell assay will focus on the use of drug combinations. If the results of prospective studies follow the pattern predicted by this assay, the design of future trials and individual patient treatment will be radically altered from the present empiric approach.

Guidelines for the Institution of Cancer Chemotherapy

A. Establish the Diagnosis: A firm diagnosis of neoplastic disease must be made before treatment is started. This will usually (and preferably) include a histologic diagnosis, but in some instances the diagnosis may be based solely on analysis of exfoliative cytology. In rare instances, a biochemical parameter (eg, chorionic gonadotropin [hCG]) in a consistent clinical setting may constitute a rationale for institution of therapy, although tissue diagnosis is always preferable. In emergency situations (eg, superior vena cava syndrome), it may be necessary to institute appropriate therapy without histologic or biochemical documentation; in such cases, appropriate diagnostic pro-

---

Anticancer Drugs

Allopurinal (Zyloprim)
Aminoglutethimide (Cytadren)
Asparaginase (L-asparaginase, Elspar)
BCNU (see Carmustine)
Bleomycin (Blenoxane)
Busulfan (Myleran)
Carmustine (bischloroethylnitrosourea, BCNU)
CCNU (see Lomustine)
Chlorambucil (Leukeran)
Cisplatin (Platinol)
Cyclophosphamide (Cytoxan)
Cyproterone acetate*
Cytarabine (Ara-C, Cytosar-U)
Dacarbazine (dimethyltriazeno imidazole carboxamide, imidazole carboxamide)
Dactinomycin (actinomycin D, Cosmegen)
Daunorubicin (Cerubidine)
Doxorubicin (Adriamycin)
Estramustine phosphate (Emcyt)
Etoposide (VP-16-213, VePesid)
Fluorouracil (5-FU, Efudex)
Flutamide*
Hexamethylmelamine*
Hydroxyurea (Hydrea)
Interferon α-2a (Roferon-A), interferon α-2b (Intron A)
Leuprolide (Lupron)
Lomustine (cyclohexylchloroethylnitrosourea, CCNU)
Mechlorethamine (nitrogen mustard, HN2, Mustargen)
Melphalan (phenylalanine mustard, L-sarcolysin, Alkeran)
Mercaptopurine (6-MP, Purinethol)
Methotrexate (amethopterin)
Methyl-CCNU (methylcyclohexylchloroethylnitrosourea)
Mithramycin (Mithracin)
Mitomycin (Mutamycin)
Mitotane (o,p'-DDD, Lysodren)
Mitoxantrone* (Novantrone)
Natoxide*
Phenylalanine mustard (melphalan, Alkeran, L-sarcolysin)
Procarbazine (Matulane)
Streptozocin*
Tamoxifen (Nolvadex)
Thioguanine (6-TG)
Thiotepa (triethylenethiophosphoramide)
Vinblastine sulfate (Velban)
Vincristine sulfate (Oncovin)

*See Note to Reader, below.

Note to reader: Agents designated with an asterisk in the following discussion and in Table 19–3 are investigational and not generally available to the practicing physician. Further information concerning these agents may be obtained from the various regional or national cooperative cancer chemotherapy study groups or the National Cancer Institute.

cedures are required after clinical stabilization has been achieved.

B. Delineate the Stage and Extent of Disease: This can frequently be achieved by correlating symptoms and the known natural history of the neoplasm with appropriate radiologic, chemical, and surgical staging data. The lymphomas are staged according to the modified Ann Arbor classification; many solid tumors are best staged by the TNM system.

C. Establish the Goal of Therapy: The histologic diagnosis and extent of the disease frequently define the goal of therapy as either curative or palliative with or without likelihood for prolongation of survival, and they frequently determine the most appropriate treatment—surgery, radiotherapy, chemotherapy, or a combination of these.

Thus, the therapeutic objective should be based upon what can be accomplished by each mode of therapy. For example, the following disseminated cancers are curable by chemotherapy: most postgestational choriocarcinomas, many Wilms' tumors and seminomas, some childhood acute lymphoblastic leukemias, adult and childhood lymphomas, and some testicular carcinomas in young men. For other neoplasms, chemotherapy may afford significant palliation and prolongation of life, even in advanced stages of breast, endometrial, prostate, thyroid, and oat cell cancers and for acute leukemia, lymphomas, myeloma, and macroglobulinemia. Some patients with colon or gastric carcinoma, sarcomas, and head and neck tumors may be relieved of symptoms by chemotherapy, but survival cannot yet be prolonged. Most patients with disseminated melanoma and lung, renal, and pancreatic carcinoma are not objectively benefited by systemic chemotherapy.

D. Measure Antitumor Response: After treatment is started, serial observations of objectively measured parameters are essential to judge antitumor response (measurable mass, tumor product, or remote effect) and to monitor the toxicity of the treatment. For example, in the treatment of gestational trophoblastic disease, assay of chorionic gonadotropin (hCG) measures a tumor product that correlates directly with the numbers of neoplastic cells, and it also reveals subclinical amounts (10^6 cells or less) of tumor that require additional chemotherapy. The sensitivity of this assay is largely responsible for the 90% cure rate of trophoblastic disease. In contrast, a "complete clinical remission" of acute leukemia (a normal bone marrow) occurs with a tumor cell mass of 10^9; most solid tumors contain $10^{10} - 10^{11}$ (10–100 g) of tumor cells before the mass can be detected clinically.

Currently useful markers for testicular tumors include the beta-subunit of hCG, carcinoembryonic antigen (CEA), and alpha-fetoprotein (AFP). Serial measurements showing a rise in CEA titer may also predict in a nonquantitative manner the recurrence of progression of colonic carcinoma, and AFP may indicate the presence of a hepatocellular carcinoma. Other tumor products—such as monoclonal paraproteins (myeloma, macroglobulinemia, occasional lymphomas),

5-hydroxyindoleacetic acid (carcinoid), and acid phosphatase (prostatic cancer)—and ectopic hormone production (oat cell carcinomas) may correlate positively with the presence and proliferation of specific neoplasms. Estrogen and progesterone receptors should be measured in tissue from breast carcinoma, since the findings predict responsiveness to hormone manipulations for metastatic disease. Radionuclide, CT, and ultrasound scanning provide serial noninvasive measurements of tumor response to therapy. Only rarely should a "second look" laparotomy be necessary to determine the status of a previously treated abdominal neoplasm.

E. Establish the Acceptable Drug Toxicity: The degree of toxicity that is acceptable depends on the probability and risks of achieving the therapeutic goal, other clinical characteristics of the individual patient, and the availability of supportive facilities to manage the anticipated toxicity.

F. Evaluate the Status of the Patient: The patient's subjective and functional status must always be considered in formulating and instituting a therapeutic program. Subjective symptoms of disease usually parallel objective parameters of progression or regression of the neoplasm. When this is not so, other factors such as unrecognized drug toxicity, unreliable parameters of tumor response, and the masking of disease progression by certain forms of therapy (eg, corticosteroids) must be considered. The Karnofsky performance index (Table 19–2) is useful for following the functional status of the patient and must be considered at least as valuable as objectively measurable

Table 19–2. Karnofsky performance index.

	%	
Able to carry on normal activity. No special care is needed.	100	Normal. No complaints. No evidence of disease.
	90	Able to carry on normal activity. Minor signs or symptoms of disease.
	80	Normal activity with effort. Some signs or symptoms of disease.
Unable to work. Able to live at home and care for most personal needs. A varying amount of assistance is needed.	70	Cares for self. Unable to carry on normal activity or to do active work.
	60	Requires occasional assistance but is able to care for most personal needs.
	50	Requires considerable assistance and frequent medical care.
Unable to care for self. Requires equivalent of institutional or hospital care. Disease may be progressing rapidly.	40	Disabled. Requires special care and assistance.
	30	Severely disabled. Hospitalization is indicated, although death is not imminent.
	20	Very sick. Hospitalization necessary.
	10	Moribund. Fatal process progressing rapidly.
	0	Dead.

parameters, especially when the goal of treatment is palliation.

The above considerations apply generally to cancer chemotherapy. Use of experimental drugs or treatment protocols may be considered if all of the following criteria are met: (1) Proved methods of effective therapy have been exhausted. (2) Data collection and dissemination of the information obtained will contribute toward answering the questions asked in the protocol. (3) The patient's human rights are fully protected, and informed consent has been obtained. (4) There is a reasonable expectation that the treatment will do more good than harm.

●　　●　　●

CHEMOTHERAPEUTIC AGENTS

See Table 19–3.

Chemotherapeutic Agents With Selective Toxicity

Only the adrenocortical hormones, sex hormones, and asparaginase have demonstrated a predictable **selective killing power of tumor cells** based on metabolically exploitable differences between neoplastic and normal tissue.

A. Glucocorticoids: The glucocorticoids exert a "lympholytic" effect that can repeatedly induce remission of acute lymphoblastic leukemia, especially in combination with vincristine. This lympholytic effect, which does not depend on the mitotic activity of the tumor, is also useful in chronic lymphocytic leukemia, lymphomas, and myeloma.

The adrenal corticosteroids are also beneficial for certain hormonally sensitive tumors such as breast and prostatic cancer. They improve cerebral edema accompanying brain tumors, palliate hemolytic anemias associated with chronic lymphocytic leukemia and the lymphomas, and correct hypercalcemia associated with various neoplasms. Their antineoplastic effects are less if they are given on an intermittent schedule; large daily doses for the shortest time necessary to produce the desired effect are preferred. Toxicity may be metabolic (hyperglycemia, sodium retention, potassium wasting), gastrointestinal (peptic ulceration), or immunosuppressive (increased susceptibility to infection). Myopathies, psychosis, hypertension, and osteoporosis are important side effects of long-term administration.

B. Estrogens: The estrogenic steroids were used in the early 1940s for prostatic carcinoma and represented one of the first successful attempts at rational cancer chemotherapy. Shortly thereafter, estrogens were found useful in postmenopausal patients with breast cancer. Diethylstilbestrol, the most widely used estrogen, is potent, inexpensive, and effective when given orally but may cause gastrointestinal disturbance, fluid retention, feminization in males, and

uterine bleeding. Its administration may cause hypercalcemia and "tumor flare" of disseminated breast carcinoma.

C. Synthetic Progestational Agents: These drugs are useful in pharmacologic doses for disseminated or uncontrolled carcinoma of the endometrium and occasionally for hypernephroma and breast cancer.

D. Androgens: The androgens are used principally in the treatment of disseminated breast cancer, especially in pre- and perimenopausal (1–4 years) women. They also have a role in the stimulation of erythropoiesis in anemic patients with several neoplastic and myelophthisic diseases. The toxic effects of androgens include excessive virilization of women, prostatism in men, and fluid retention; tumor flare and hypercalcemia occur occasionally. The halogenated androgens, which are effective when given orally, can produce cholestatic jaundice. although the parenteral nonhalogenated compounds do not do so.

E. Antihormones: Antiestrogens (nafoxidine* and tamoxifen [Nolvadex]) are a new class of nonsteroidal agents that block estrogen receptor sites on tumor cells and antagonize estrogen stimulation of hormone-dependent tumors such as breast and possibly renal carcinoma. Nausea, hot flashes, and mild thrombocytopenia are toxicities of oral administration.

Antiandrogens include cyproterone acetate, a steroidal congener that possesses potent progestational actions; and flutamide,* a nonsteroidal anilide that acts by inhibiting androgen binding and tumor tissue. These drugs may be of benefit in advanced prostatic carcinoma no longer responsive to hormonal manipulations that were effective in the past. No major toxicities are reported in a few small trials.

Reactivation of tumors responsive to prior castration or estrogen therapy or failure to repond in 30–40% of patients may be due to persistent androgens of adrenal origin. Therefore, a new antihormonal strategy has been developed to achieve complete androgen blockage. A luteinizing hormone-releasing hormone (LHRH) agonist or surgical castration is used to block testicular androgens in association with a pure antiandrogen (flutamide*) in order to neutralize adrenal androgens.

Labrie believes that complete androgen blockade is the treatment of choice in an effort to achieve more complete remissions of longer duration for metastatic prostatic cancer and to minimize the appearance of androgen-resistant cell clones. Several randomized clinical trials currently in progress are comparing LHRH agonists alone with such treatment in combination with flutamide.* No results have yet been reported.

The discovery of gonadotropin-releasing hormone (GRH) and its analogs has allowed for the demonstrated ability to suppress Leydig cell function in humans. Efficacy in the treatment of prostatic cancer has

---

* See note to reader on p 404.

Table 19–3. Drugs useful in urologic malignancy.*

Agent	Route	Toxicity	Usual Adult Dose†	Specificity‡
Hormones				
Glucocorticoids	Orally. (IV and IM preparations also available.)	Sodium retention, potassium wasting, hyperglycemia, peptic ulcer, immunosuppression, hypertension, osteoporosis.	Prednisone: 1–2 mg/kg/d for brief intervals (<6 weeks if possible); then maintain at minimal required daily dosage.	CCNS
Estrogens	Orally	Sodium retention, feminization, uterine bleeding, nausea and vomiting.	Diethylstilbestrol: 2.5–5 mg/d for prostate. Ethinyl estradiol: 1 mg/d.	CCNS
Progestogens	Orally, IM	Sodium retention.	Hydroxyprogesterone: 1 g 2–3 times weekly IM. Medroxyprogesterone: 200–600 mg orally twice weekly.	CCNS
Androgens	Orally, IM	Sodium retention, masculinization; cholestatic jaundice with oral preparations.	Testosterone propionate: 100 mg 2–3 times weekly. Fluoxymesterone: 10–40 mg/d orally. Calusterone: 200 mg/d orally.	CCNS
Antihormones				
Antiestrogens Tamoxifen (Nolvadex)	Orally	Nausea, hot flashes.	20–60 mg/d.	CCNS
Nafoxidine*	Orally	Nausea, dermatitis; rarely, tumor flare.	60–180 mg/d.	CCNS
Antiandrogens Flutamide*	Orally	Gynecomastia; loss of male body hair.	750 mg–1.5 g/d	CCNS
Cyproterone acetate	Orally	Fluid retention.	200–300 mg/d.	CCNS
Hormone-alkylator complex Estramustine phosphate (Emcyt)	Orally	Nausea and vomiting, phlebitis, mild marrow depression.	15 mg/kg/d as single dose.	Not known
Alkylators				
Mechlorethamine (nitrogen mustard, HN2, Mustargen)	IV, intracavitary	Nausea and vomiting, marrow depression, ulcer if extravasated, hypogonadism, fetal anomalies, alopecia.	0.4 mg/kg IV as single dose every 4–6 weeks; 0.4 mg/kg by intracavitary injection.	CCNS
Cyclophosphamide (Cytoxan)	IV, orally	Nausea and vomiting, marrow depressioin, alopecia, hemorrhagic cystitis.	40–60 mg/kg IV every 3–5 weeks; 5 mg/kg/d orally for 10 days, then 1–3 mg/kg/d as maintenance.	(?)CCNS
Chlorambucil (Leukeran)	Orally	Marrow depression, gastroenteritis.	0.1–0.2 mg/kg/d.	CCNS
Melphalan (phenylalanine mustard, Alkeran)	Orally	Marrow depression (occasionally prolonged), gastroenteritis.	0.25 mg/kg/d orally for 4 days every 6 weeks; 2–4 mg/d as maintenance.	CCNS
Thiotepa	IV, intracavitary	Marrow depression.	0.8 mg/kg IV as single dose every 4–6 weeks; 0.8 mg/kg by intracavitary injection.	CCNS
Nitrosoureas				
Carmustine (BCNU), lomustine (CCNU), methyl-CCNU	BCNU, IV; CCNU and methyl-CCNU, orally	Nausea and vomiting, prolonged marrow depression, local phlebitis.	BCNU: 75–100 mg/m² IV daily for 2 days every 4–6 weeks. CCNU: 130 mg/m² orally every 6 weeks. Methyl-CCNU: 200 mg/m² orally every 6 weeks.	CCNS
Structural analogs				
Methotrexate (amethopterin)	Orally, IV intrathecally	Ulcerative mucositis, gastroenteritis, dermatitis, marrow depression, hepatitis, abortion.	20–40 mg IV twice weekly; 5–15 mg intrathecally weekly; 2.5–5 mg/d orally.	CCS

Table 19–3 (cont'd). Drugs useful in urologic malignancy.*

Agent	Route	Toxicity	Usual Adult Dose†	Specificity‡
Fluorouracil (5-FU, Adrucil)	IV	Atrophic dermatitis, gastroenteritis, mucositis, marrow depression, neuritis.	15–20 mg/kg IV weekly for at least 6 weeks.	CCS
Dacarbazine	IV	Gastroenteritis, marrow depression, hepatitis, phlebitis.	150–250 mg/m²/d IV for 5 days every 4–6 weeks.	Not known
Cytotoxic antibiotics Dactinomycin (actinomycin D, Cosmegen)	IV	Nausea and vomiting, stomatitis, gastroenteritis, proctitis, marrow depression, ulcer if extravasated, alopecia; radiation potentiator.	0.01 mg/kg/d for 5 days every 4–6 weeks.	CCS
Doxorubicin (Adriamycin)	IV	Alopecia, marrow depression, myocardiopathies, ulcer if extravasated; stomatitis.	1 mg/kg/wk; total cumulative dose should not exceed 550 mg/m².	CCNS
Mithramycin (Mithracin)	IV	Marrow depression, nausea and vomiting, complex coagulopathies, hepatotoxicity.	0.05 mg/kg IV every other day to toxicity or 8 doses per course.	Not known
Bleomycin (Blenoxane)	IV, IM, subcut	Allergic dermatitis, pulmonary fibrosis, fever, mucositis.	15 mg twice weekly; total cumulative dosage should not exceed 300 mg.	Not known
Vinca alkaloids Vinblastine (Velban)	IV	Marrow depression, alopecia, ulcer if extravasated, nausea and vomiting, neuropathy.	0.1–0.2 mg/kg IV weekly.	CCS
Vincristine (Oncovin)	IV	Alopecia, neuropathy (peripheral and autonomic), ulcer if extravasated; rarely, marrow depression.	1.5 mg/m² weekly or less. No individual dose should exceed 2 mg.	CCS
Miscellaneous agents Mitotane (o,p'-DDD, Lysodren)	Orally	Gastroenteritis, dermatitis, CNS abnormalities.	5–12 g/d orally.	Not known
Aminoglutethimide (Cytardren)	Orally	Gastroenteritis, dermatitis, somnolence.	1–1.5 g/d orally in 3–4 divided doses.	CCNS
Inorganic metallic salt Cisplatin (Platinol)	IV with mannitol diuresis	Nausea and vomiting, bone marrow depressioin, nephrotoxicity, ototoxicity.	1 mg/kg every 3 weeks IV, or 80 mg/m² IV every 3 weeks. Use lower dose when renal function is impaired.	CCNS
Podophyllotoxin derivative Etoposide (VP-16-213, VePesid)	IV, orally	Marrow depression, nausea and vomiting, hypotension, alopecia.	50–100 mg/m²/d IV for 5 days; orally at approximately double the IV dose.	CCS

*See Note to Reader on p 404.

†Modifications of drug dosages: If white count is >4500 and platelet count >150,000, give full dose; if white count is 3500–4500 and platelet count is 100,000–150,000, give 75% of full dose; if white count is 3000–3500 and platelet count is 75,000–100,000, give 50–75% of full dose; if white count is <3000 and platelet count is <75,000, give 0–25% of full dose.

‡CCS = cell cycle-specific. CCNS = cell cycle-nonspecific. See text.

been shown with LHRH agonists with the elimination of estrogenic side effects. Leuprolide (Lupron) is such an agonist; it is a synthetic nonapeptide that can achieve medical castration and appears to be as effective as DES with fewer side effects. Leuprolide is available at present only in an injectable form; an intranasal preparation is in development.

The Alkylators

The alkylators, whose prototype is mechlorethamine, react with nucleophilic substances within the cell to form cross-links at the guanine residues of parallel double DNA strands. With the possible exception of cyclophosphamide, the alkylators are cell cycle-nonspecific and affect both resting and dividing cells; both normal and malignant cells are injured.

Mechlorethamine (nitrogen mustard, HN2, Mustargen) is the alkylator of choice in the treatment of Hodgkin's disease, either singly or in combination with other drugs. For Burkitt's lymphoma, **cyclophosphamide** may be curative, and it is also the agent of choice for undifferentiated small cell carcinoma of the lung. Cyclophosphamide has a unique role in childhood acute leukemia, in which other alkylators are ineffective. For most purposes, however, equivalent doses of the various alkylators produce equivalent responses, and there is cross-resistance among the various alkylators except for the nitrosoureas (see below). The choice of alkylators thus rests upon the desired route and mode of administration and variations in toxicity.

Chlorambucil (Leukeran) has had its major use in chronic lymphocytic leukemia, Hodgkin's disease, and Waldenström's macroglobulinemia. Its major advantage is its narrow spectrum of toxicity (hematopoietic only) and ease of administration (oral). **Melphalan (phenylalanine mustard)** is usually given for multiple myeloma, but this may be merely traditional; **busulfan (Myleran)** is customarily used in chronic myelocytic leukemia and in polycythemia vera; all alkylators are equally effective against ovarian carcinoma.

Mechlorethamine is a vesicant if extravasated. **Cyclophosphamide (Cytoxan)** and **thiotepa** are much less irritating if applied directly to tissues, because they must first be metabolized to the active form. The immediate effects of intravenous alkylator administration are nausea and vomiting beginning within 30 minutes and persisting for 8–10 hours; premedication with phenothiazine is preventive. The important delayed effects of alkylators are principally on rapidly proliferating tissues (hematopoietic, gonadal, epithelial, and gastrointestinal), with bone marrow suppression being the most prominent. In the marrow, cell necrosis begins at 12 hours; the nadir of blood count depression is at 7–10 days; and marrow regeneration time limits the administration of mechlorethamine to intervals of 4–6 weeks.

Several of the alkylators cause relatively characteristic adverse reactions. Examples are alopecia and hemorrhagic cystitis associated with cyclophosphamide and melanosis and pulmonary fibrosis with busulfan. All alkylators can cause hypospermia, menstrual irregularities, and fetal anomalies.

Thiotepa is discussed in Table 19–3.

The Nitrosoureas

BCNU, CCNU, and methyl-CCNU are cell cycle-nonspecific synthetic chemicals that act much like the classic alkylators but have several unique and exploitable properties, including lipid solubility and delayed onset of marrow suppression compared to the alkylators (see above). Moreover, there appears to be no cross-resistance with other alkylators. These drugs are effective in Hodgkin's disease but less so in non-Hodgkin's lymphomas; they appear promising for metastatic and primary central nervous system neoplasms because of their lipid solubility. BCNU is administered intravenously; CCNU and methyl-CCNU are given orally.

Structural Analogs
(Antimetabolites)

The antimetabolites are specific cytotoxic agents closely related to substrates normally utilized by cells for metabolism and growth. The structural analogs interfere with nucleic acid synthesis to impair prolifera-

tion of normal and neoplastic cells. They are generally cell cycle-specific, with proliferating cells being more vulnerable to their effects than are resting cells.

A. Methotrexate: Methotrexate competitively inhibits dihydrofolate reductase; acquired resistance to methotrexate results from increased dihydrofolate reductase activity, since the rate of enzyme synthesis exceeds the rate of methotrexate uptake by resistant cells.

Methotrexate toxicity may be hematologic, gastrointestinal, hepatic, and dermatologic. These effects may be alleviated or prevented by the prompt (preferably within 1 hour, but no longer than several hours) administration of folinic acid (citrovorum factor). One treatment regimen has used folinic acid to "rescue" the marrow after administration of toxic doses, although it is not yet certain that the antitumor effect is more pronounced. Methotrexate may be administered orally, intramuscularly, intravenously, or intrathecally; it is bound to plasma protein and excreted in the urine. Hepatic or renal failure is a contraindication; leukopenia, thrombocytopenia, stomatitis, and gastroenteritis with diarrhea are the toxic side effects that may require reduction in dosage.

Methotrexate can cure most cases of gestational choriocarcinoma. It has been used extensively in the treatment of epithelial neoplasms of the head and neck and is useful in breast cancer, testicular tumors, lung cancer, medulloblastomas, and other brain tumors.

B. Fluorouracil: Fluorouracil (5-FU) is a thymine analog that in vivo interferes with thymidylate synthetase, an enzyme involved in the formation of thymidylic acid, a DNA precursor. The agent is first metabolized to 2'-deoxy-5-fluorouridine. This compound itself is now available (as floxuridine; FUDR) for use by perfusion, but it has not been shown to have a clear advantage over fluorouracil. Fluorouracil is metabolized principally in the liver. Its major toxicities include stomatitis, enteritis, and marrow suppression; significant atrophic dermatitis is occasionally reported; neurotoxicity is rare.

Fluorouracil has been most useful in breast and colonic adenocarcinoma, but it is also beneficial against pancreatic, gastric, ovarian, and prostatic cancer. The preferred schedule of administration is once weekly rather than the 4-day loading dose schedule initially advocated, since the latter is more toxic without being more effective. The dosage should be in the range of 15–20 mg/kg intravenously, weekly as tolerated.

Since antimetabolites such as methotrexate and fluorouracil act only on rapidly proliferating cells, they damage the cells of mucosal surfaces such as the gastrointestinal tract. Methotrexate has similar effects on the skin. These toxicities are at times more significant than those that have occurred in the bone marrow, and they should be looked for routinely when these agents are used.

Erythema of the buccal mucosa is an early sign of mucosal toxicity. If therapy is continued beyond this point, oral ulceration will develop. In general, it is wise to discontinue therapy if early oral ulceration appears. This symptom usually heralds the appearance of similar but potentially more serious ulceration at other sites lower in the gastrointestinal tract. Therapy can usually be reinstituted when the oral ulcer heals (within 1 week to 10 days). The dose of drug used may need to be modified downward at this point, with titration to an acceptable level of effect on the mucosa.

Cytotoxic Antibiotics

These agents, the first of which was dactinomycin, were isolated in the 1940s by Waksman from soil strains of bacteria of the *Streptomyces* class.

A. Dactinomycin: Dactinomycin (actinomycin D, Cosmegen) is an inhibitor of DNA-dependent synthesis of RNA by ribosomes. Its toxicities include hematopoietic suppression, ulcerative stomatitis, and gastroenteritis. It causes intense local tissue necrosis if extravasated. The drug is retained for a considerable time intracellularly, and acquired resistance is thought to correlate with poor cellular uptake or poor retention of the drug. The major use for dactinomycin is in sequential combination with radiation therapy for Wilms' tumor; "maintenance" long-term administration of the drug adds significantly to the salvage obtained with combinations of surgery, radiation therapy, and "adjuvant" short-term courses of the drug. Dactinomycin is of proved value in trophoblastic malignant disease, soft tissue sarcomas, and testicular carcinoma, especially in combination with alkylators and antimetabolites. The optimal scheduling and combination of drugs with dactinomycin is not known, but the most customary has been in courses of several days at dosages of 15 μg/kg/d intravenously, repeated after 2–4 weeks as toxicity allows.

B. Doxorubicin: Doxorubicin (Adriamycin) and daunorubicin are tumoricidal antibiotics that intercalate between adjacent base pairs of double-stranded DNA. Toxicity includes marrow suppression, alopecia, and mucositis. Severe local tissue necrosis occurs if the drug is extravasated. Doxorubicin is excreted mainly through the bile and must be used in reduced dosage in patients whose hepatic function is impaired. The anthracycline antibiotics doxorubicin and daunomycin both have a delayed cardiac toxicity. The problem is greater with doxorubicin, because this drug has a major role in the treatment of sarcomas, breast cancer, lymphomas, and certain other solid tumors; the use of daunorubicin is limited to the treatment of acute leukemias. Recent studies of left ventricular function indicate that some reversible changes in cardiac dynamics occur in most patients by the time they have received 300 mg/m^2. Serial echocardiographic measurements can detect these abnormalities. Echocardiographic measurement of left ventricular ejection fraction appears most useful in this regard. Alternatively, the left ventricular voltage can be measured serially on ECGs. Doxorubicin should not be used in elderly patients with significant intrinsic cardiac disease, and no patient should receive a total dose in excess of 550 mg/m^2. Patients who have had prior

chest or mediastinal radiotherapy may be more prone to develop doxorubicin heart disease. ECGs should be obtained serially. The appearance of a high resting pulse may herald the appearance of overt cardiac toxicity. Unfortunately, toxicity may be irreversible or fatal at high dosage levels. At lower dosages (eg, 350 mg/m^2), the symptoms and signs of cardiac failure generally respond well to digitalis, diuretics, and cessation of doxorubicin therapy.

A new anthracycline derivative, mitoxantrone* (Novantrone), has displayed a spectrum of antitumor efficacy similar to that of doxorubicin but with less cardiac toxicity and milder alopecia. The dose-limiting side effect is granulocytopenia when the drug is administered every 3 weeks; when lower daily doses are given for 5 consecutive days, mucositis is the major toxic effect. Mitoxantrone is currently an investigational agent for protocol use, but its release for clinical practice is expected soon.

C. Mithramycin: Mithramycin (Mithracin) is useful in the treatment of hypercalcemia resistant to hydration and corticosteroids, and the dosage may be less than that required for tumoricidal activity although still within the toxic range. Its major usefulness is in embryonal cell carcinoma and other testicular tumors, and its toxicity includes marrow suppression, hepatic and gastrointestinal injury, and complex coagulopathies.

D. Bleomycin (Blenoxane): Bleomycin is an antitumor antibiotic that in clinical use as an anticancer drug is a mixture of various fractions differing in the amine moiety. The principal mode of action appears to be scission of DNA strands or inhibition of ligase, thus impairing cell division. The most serious toxic effects are pulmonary interstitial pneumonitis and fibrosis, which may be fatal and are usually dose-related, occurring with a cumulative dosage greater than 150 units/m^2 or less if given in conjunction with prior pulmonary radiation. Generally, older patients or those with preexisting lung disease are most susceptible. Bleomycin hypersensitivity pneumonitis with eosinophilia may occur at any dosage and may respond favorably to corticosteroid administration—in contrast to fibrosing pneumonitis, for which steroids are not as effective.

Other bleomycin toxicities include anaphylactic and acute febrile reactions, stomatitis, and dermatitis with hyperpigmentation and desquamation of palms, soles, and pressure areas. The drug is marrow-sparing and may be administered by the intravenous, intramuscular, or subcutaneous routes, although the intravenous route is usual. Its major usefulness is in testicular neoplasms, squamous cell carcinomas, lymphomas, and cervical carcinoma.

E. Mitomycin: Mitomycin is a useful agent against gastric and pancreatic adenocarcinoma and shows promise against breast cancer.

---

* See note to reader on p 404.

The Plant Alkaloids

The plant alkaloids include the periwinkle (*Vinca rosea*) derivatives vincristine and vinblastine, 2 closely related compounds with widely different toxicities and somewhat different spectra of activity. Both *Vinca* alkaloids are bound to cytoplasmic precursors of the mitotic spindle in S phase, with polymerization of the microtubular proteins that comprise the mitotic spindle.

A. Vinblastine: Vinblastine sulfate (Velban) is a major agent against Hodgkin's disease and testicular carcinoma and has lesser efficacy in the non-Hodgkin's lymphomas. The toxicity of vinblastine is primarily marrow suppression, but gastroenteritis, neurotoxicity, and alopecia also occur—the latter much less commonly than with vincristine. The drug is usually given once a week. Severe local ulceration may occur if the drug extravasates into the subcutaneous tissues.

B. Vincristine: Vincristine sulfate (Oncovin) is primarily neurotoxic and may induce peripheral, autonomic, and, less commonly, cranial neuropathies. The peripheral neuropathy can be sensory, motor, autonomic, or a combination of these effects. In its mildest form it consists of paresthesias ("pins and needles") of the fingers and toes. Occasional patients develop acute jaw or throat pain after vincristine therapy. This may be a form of trigeminal neuralgia. With continued vincristine therapy, the paresthesias extend to the proximal interphalangeal joints, hyporeflexia appears in the lower extremities, and significant weakness develops in the quadriceps muscle group. At this point, it is wise to discontinue vincristine therapy until the neuropathy has subsided somewhat. Peroneal weakness should be avoided lest symptomatic footdrop and impairment of gait occur.

Constipation is the most common symptom of the autonomic neuropathy that occurs with vincristine therapy. This symptom should always be dealt with prophylactically, ie, patients receiving vincristine should be started on stool softeners and mild cathartics when therapy is instituted. If this potential complication is neglected, severe impaction may result in association with an atonic bowel.

More serious autonomic involvement can lead to acute intestinal obstruction with signs indistinguishable from those of an acute abdomen. Bladder neuropathies are uncommon but may be severe.

Alopecia occurs in 20% of patients, but hematologic suppression is unusual. The drug is extremely effective in inducing remissions in acute lymphoblastic leukemia, especially in combination with prednisone, and is quite active in all forms of lymphoma. It is one of the most effective agents against childhood tumors, choriocarcinoma, and various sarcomas. Because of its lack of significant overlapping toxicity with most other chemotherapeutic agents, vincristine is receiving wide use in combination with other agents. The optimal dosage and scheduling for this agent remain to be elucidated; weekly administration is customary but may not be the best regimen.

Miscellaneous Compounds

Mitotane (*o,p′*-DDD; Lysodren) is a DDT congener that may cause adrenocortical necrosis and therefore plays a useful role in reducing excessive steroid output in 70% of patients with adrenocortical carcinoma; in about 35%, an objective decrease in tumor mass is also recorded. Toxicities include dermatitis, gastroenteritis, and central nervous system abnormalities.

Aminoglutethimide (Cytadren) is a derivative of glutethimide, a sedative-hypnotic drug that causes adrenal insufficiency with chronic use. Aminoglutethimide blocks adrenal steroidogenesis by inhibiting the enzymatic conversion of cholesterol to pregnenolone, thus reducing mineralocorticoid, glucocorticoid, and sex steroid production. The "medical adrenalectomy" thus induced can be beneficial for breast and prostatic cancers, although the degree of benefit is not precisely defined as yet. Toxicities include somnolence, nausea and vomiting, and, occasionally, skin rash. Supplemental mineralocorticoids and glucocorticoids must be administered with aminoglutethimide.

Estramustine phosphate (Emcyt) is a promising new compound that combines an estradiol and an alkylator. It is not yet clear whether this complex will prove to be superior to either agent used alone, but the approach may lead to similar combinations in the future. Toxicities of oral administration include nausea and vomiting, thrombophlebitis, and mild hematopoietic suppression.

Dacarbazine is a synthetic derivative of the triazene class that has both antimetabolite and alkylator-like activity. Dacarbazine has significant activity against melanoma and, in combination with doxorubicin, against various sarcomas. Toxicities may include gastroenteritis, marrow depression, hepatitis, phlebitis, alopecia, ulcer if extravasated, and a flulike syndrome with myalgias.

Cisplatin (Platinol) is a member of a new class of heavy metal antitumor agents whose mechanism of action is unknown. Major acute toxicities may include severe vomiting and renal tubular necrosis, which may be minimized by careful hydration and mannitol administration to promote brisk diuresis during the infusion of cisplatin. Other toxicities include high-frequency ototoxicity and bone marrow suppression, with leukopenia, thrombocytopenia, and anemia. The drug is usually given as a 2-hour infusion in a covered bottle (because it is light-sensitive). Major uses include testicular, bladder, and ovarian carcinomas.

Etoposide (VP-16-213, VePesid), a podophyllotoxin derivative (an extract of mandrake root), was found to demonstrate cytolytic properties in the cure of venereal warts. Antimitotic effects are related to breakage in single-stranded DNA. The drug shows significant activity as a single agent against small cell lung cancer and lymphomas and is an important component of potentially curative "salvage therapy" combinations against testicular carcinoma. The principal toxicity of etoposide is hematopoietic suppression, predominantly leukopenia with a nadir in white blood count at 7–14 days and recovery by 21 days. Nausea, vomiting, alopecia, and (occasionally) peripheral neuropathy may also occur. Hypotension and anaphylactic reactions have been reported, especially with rapid intravenous administration. The drug should be given by slow intravenous infusion over 30–60 minutes. Oral administration is also effective with the dosage approximately double the intravenous dose.

Alpha-interferons. Clinical experience with alpha-interferons has shown marked therapeutic activity in patients with hairy cell leukemia. There is also a potential role for interferon in combination with cytotoxic drugs for the treatment of multiple myeloma, and interferon appears to be effective in cutaneous T cell lymphomas and chronic lymphocytic leukemia. It may also be effective in chronic myelocytic leukemia, and among the solid tumors, melanoma, renal carcinoma, and ovarian carcinoma have all shown modest benefit in early trials. Toxicity consists primarily of flulike symptoms (chills, fever, malaise), central nervous symptoms (somnolence, confusion), hypotension, and granulocytopenia—all dose-related and rapidly reversible with cessation of therapy.

SURGICAL ADJUVANT CHEMOTHERAPY

It has been suggested that surgical or radiotherapeutic (cell cycle-nonspecific) measures that reduce tumor bulk and increase the growth fraction of a tumor might increase tumor sensitivity to chemotherapeutic agents (cell cycle-specific) without increasing marrow sensitivity. Thus, chemotherapeutic agents given after operation might improve results when there is no clinical evidence of residual disease but recurrence is statistically likely.

Adjuvant chemotherapy has been of documented worth in Wilms' tumor and neuroblastoma and may be of benefit in stage II–IIIB Hodgkin's disease in conjunction with radiation therapy. Adjuvant chemotherapy with high-dose methotrexate therapy followed by citrovorum (folinic acid) "rescue" or with doxorubicin has been shown to prolong the disease-free interval in childhood osteosarcoma after appropriate control of the primary lesion. Among other tumors that seem promising candidates for controlled studies of adjuvant chemotherapy are ovarian carcinoma, testicular tumors, and certain other soft tissue sarcomas.

Rhabdomyosarcoma in children can now be treated effectively by wide local excision (avoiding amputation) followed by irradiation and repeated cyclic therapy with dactinomycin and vincristine.

Adjuvant chemotherapy after surgery for colon and breast carcinoma is under intensive study. Adjuvant chemotherapy for breast carcinoma is now a well-established regimen for premenopausal patients judged to be at high risk of recurrence (stage II); CMF (cyclophosphamide, methotrexate, and fluorouracil) is given for 6 months. Postmenopausal stage II patients who are hormone-receptor positive may be treated prophylactically with tamoxifen for at least 2 years.

LATE COMPLICATIONS OF CHEMOTHERAPY

The increasing effectiveness of chemotherapy in prolonging survival has meant that treated patients are often at increased risk of developing a second malignant growth. The most frequent second cancer is acute myelogenous leukemia; other second drug- or radiation-associated cancers are sporadic. Acute myelogenous leukemia has been observed in up to 2% of long-term survivors of Hodgkin's disease treated with radiotherapy and MOPP (mechlorethamine, vincristine, procarbazine, prednisone) and in patients with ovarian carcinoma or myeloma treated with melphalan. Despite this problem, the risk/benefit ratio is strongly in favor of the initial therapeutic regimen. However, the risks of adjuvant alkylator therapy of stage I breast carcinoma may exceed benefits if the incidence of leukemia surpasses 2%. There is evidence that certain drugs (melphalan, procarbazine) are more carcinogenic or leukemogenic than other alkylators, such as cyclophosphamide, and other classes of drugs, such as antimetabolites.

INFUSION & PERFUSION THERAPY

Selective arterial infusion has been used to deliver higher concentrations of drugs to the tumor than could be tolerated by systemic administration. One worker gave fluorouracil by hepatic arterial infusion to 200 patients with hepatic metastases, most of whom had failed to respond to intravenous fluorouracil. About 60% of the patients showed objective improvement and survived an average of 8.7 months; nonresponders lived an average of 2.5 months.

Regional perfusion is an experimental technique that has given promising results in the following situations: (1) melanoma of an extremity perfused with mechlorethamine, phenylalanine mustard, or dacarbazine; (2) head and neck tumors perfused through the carotid artery with alkylators, fluorouracil, or methotrexate; and (3) hepatomas and metastatic adenocarcinoma in the liver infused via the hepatic artery with fluorouracil and other drugs.

Recently, the development of a totally implanted drug delivery system for hepatic arterial chemotherapy has been shown to be safe and effective. A Silastic cannula is placed by laparotomy and a pump is implanted subcutaneously; the pump can be refilled percutaneously. In a small preliminary series, 11 of 13 patients responded to floxuridine (FUDR) via continuous infusion for a median time of 6 months. This implanted system should facilitate further investigation of regional hepatic chemotherapy.

Another intravascular approach to palliation of abdominal neoplasms is transcatheter occlusion by Gelfoam or coil embolization (see Chapter 7). This technique is used most often for renal cell carcinoma but is also useful for dearterializing hepatic tumors by embolic occlusion of the hepatic artery.

COMBINATION CHEMOTHERAPY

Combinations of drugs that block multiple biosynthetic pathways are given in an attempt to obtain a synergistic effect on the tumor. The drugs of a combination are selected to avoid overlapping toxicity. This approach has been of greatest value where no single agent is highly effective. Thus, vincristine plus prednisone or cytarabine plus thioguanine produces more complete remissions of acute leukemia than either agent alone, and toxicity is not enhanced. Survival is prolonged in proportion to the duration of remission, which documents the importance of achieving complete remission.

The treatment of testicular cancers is representative of an era of chemotherapeutic and radiotherapeutic progress since the development in 1960 by Li et al of combination chemotherapy (chlorambucil, methotrexate, and dactinomycin) for patients with disseminated disease. Nonseminomatous testicular carcinomas have recently been treated successfully with varying combinations of bleomycin, vinblastine, and cisplatin. Samuels (1975) reported an overall 75% response rate, with a 45% complete remission rate, to a regimen of vinblastine and bleomycin. Einhorn and Donohue (1977) treated 50 patients with a triple combination of bleomycin, vinblastine, and cisplatin, with 75% complete and 25% partial remissions. Toxicity was significant, but remissions lasted for 6 months to more than 30 months, with cure later established for most remissions longer than 2 years.

UNPROVED METHODS IN CANCER THERAPY

Unorthodox methods of therapy and unproved drugs for cancer have been represented by proponents as "nontoxic and more effective" alternatives to accepted and proved palliative and even curative chemotherapy in diseases such as acute lymphoblastic leukemia of childhood and testicular carcinoma. The most frequently used unproved drug is Laetrile (amygdalin), which is currently legal in 27 states to provide "freedom of choice," even though there is no scientific evidence for any efficacy whatever. A recent clinical trial of Laetrile in 178 patients not only showed no benefit but revealed important toxicity from high blood cyanide levels in some patients. Despite this evidence, patients often turn to unorthodox treatment methods if they feel that established therapies are hopeless. Therefore, when the physician explains the risks and benefits of rational chemotherapy, the patient should not be made to feel that the situation is hopeless, no matter what the statistical evidence shows. Statistics accurately define events for a population but not for individuals, and a desperate patient will sometimes seek the solace of a soothsayer rather than submit to a regimen of therapy that has a statistically poor outcome.

• • •

EVALUATION & MANAGEMENT OF PATIENTS WITH AN UNKNOWN PRIMARY CARCINOMA

About 15% of cancer patients present with metastatic tumor of unknown primary origin. The most common sources are pancreas and lung. If the presenting metastasis is a squamous cell carcinoma, the primary site is most often lung, but occasionally an occult nasal, oropharyngeal, or laryngeal primary lesion is found that may be treated with curative intent if evaluation reveals no dissemination beyond regional nodes.

For adenocarcinomas or undifferentiated carcinomas, an extensive search for the primary lesion may be unrevealing until late in the course of the illness. The objectives of care are to palliate symptoms from the metastases and diagnose the primary source, especially in the case of more treatable (often hormonally responsive) tumors such as those of the breast, prostate, uterus, and thyroid. Extensive radiologic and endoscopic evaluation is justified in the search for a primary source of a solitary metastasis, but it usually produces little benefit for patients with multiple sites of dissemination; palliative therapy of symptoms caused by the metastases is usually more important. Unusual sites of metastatic presentation include the skin (usually from a lung, colon, or kidney primary), intraocular structures (usually from a female breast primary), and the lower female genital tract (usually from an ovarian or uterine primary).

Several new tissue techniques are useful in making the pathologic diagnosis; these require forethought on the part of the surgeon submitting the specimen. Electron microscopy may be helpful in detecting melanosomes in melanoma or specific inclusion bodies of APUD (Amine Precursor Uptake and Decarboxylation) in endocrine tumors. Hormone receptor proteins may be of value in defining breast or endometrial carcinoma, and lymphocyte markers for T and B cells help to support a diagnosis of malignant lymphoma. Each of these techniques requires special fixation or handling of fresh tissue. Serum markers (carcinoembryonic antigen [CEA], alpha-fetoprotein [AFP], human chorionic gonadotropin [hCG], and acid phosphatase) may also be useful in suggesting the origin of cancers.

Unless the above data reveal a chemosensitive tumor, treatment of widely disseminated neoplasms of uncertain primary origin should be directed to symptomatic palliation. Chemotherapeutic combinations such as FAM (fluorouracil, Adriamycin, and mito-mycin) have not been particularly useful in these cases, but local surgical extirpation or radiotherapy of solitary nodal metastases can provide significant benefit, especially if the lesion is a well-differentiated squamous cell carcinoma located in the upper or mid cervical nodes. Improved survival can also be achieved by resection of solitary pulmonary and he-patic metastases, depending upon the site of origin of the primary tumor and the disease-free interval before the occurrence of the solitary lesion.

Several recent reports have described young men with poorly differentiated and rapidly growing neo-plasms, usually in a midline distribution (retroperi-toneal or mediastinal) and in most cases accompanied by findings of marker substances (beta-hCG or AFP) in serum or intracellularly by immunocytochemical methods. Whether these tumors arise from germ cell rests or by conversion of somatic cells to neoplasms expressing features of a germ cell tumor is currently unknown. It is, however, important to recognize that the extragonadal germ cell cancer syndrome is highly treatable by chemotherapeutic agents and shows a good response rate even when widely disseminated tu-mor is present.

THE PARANEOPLASTIC SYNDROMES

The paraneoplastic ("beyond tumor growth") syn-dromes (Table 19–4) may present bizarre signs and symptoms resembling primary endocrine, metabolic, hematologic, or neuromuscular disorders. These syn-dromes may be the first clue to the presence of certain tumors, the early diagnosis of which may favorably af-fect the prognosis. All too often, however, they are a manifestation of disseminated or advanced disease; even then, their palliation may provide more symp-tomatic relief than would reduction of tumor mass alone.

CHEMOTHERAPY OF SPECIFIC UROLOGIC CANCERS

Adrenal Cortical Carcinoma

In the past decade, mitotane (*o,p'*-DDD, Lyso-dren) has been used in the management of metastatic or functional adrenal cortical neoplasms. Mitotane produces a decrease in corticosteroid excretion in 70% of patients as a result of degeneration of the zona retic-ularis and zona fasciculata of the adrenal gland. Cush-ing's syndrome and virilism associated with hyper-adrenocorticism are often palliated after 3–4 weeks of therapy, and in 35% of patients so treated, tumor re-gression occurs as well.

Aminoglutethimide (Cytadren) has also been use-ful for control of hypersecretion of corticosteroids be-cause it inhibits adrenal synthesis through interference

Table 19–4. The paraneoplastic syndromes.

Syndrome	Usual Causes
Hypercalcemia	Breast, lung, renal, or prostatic carcinomas; multiple myeloma.
Cushing's syndrome	Lung, adrenal carcinomas.
Inappropriate ADH secre-tion	Lung carcinoma.
Hypoglycemia	Hepatoma, retroperitoneal sar-coma, insulinoma.
Hypertrophic osteoarthropathy	Bronchogenic carcinoma.
Erythrocytosis	Renal carcinoma.
Selective red cell aplasia of marrow	Thymoma.
Hyperthyroidism	Choriocarcinomas, teratocar-cinomas.
Fever	Hodgkin's and non-Hodgkin's lymphoma, hypernephroma, hepatoma.
Neuromyopathies	Lung, breast, thymus, and pros-tatic carcinomas.
Dermatomyositis	Lung, breast, and pancreatic carcinomas.
Coagulopathy and throm-bophlebitis	Prostatic, pancreatic, and breast carcinomas.
Immunodeficiency	Myeloma, lymphoma, thymoma.
Nonmetastatic hepatic dysfunction	Renal carcinoma.

with the conversion of cholesterol to pregnenolone The drug is beneficial when Cushing's syndrome is uncontrolled by mitotane or the toxicity of mitotane prohibits its use in doses large enough to be effective. However, aminoglutethimide is not cytotoxic against tumor tissue and does not reduce tumor bulk.

Neuroblastoma

Chemotherapy has not been very effective for this tumor but must be tried where disseminated disease makes surgical control impossible. Cyclophos-phamide (Cytoxan), vincristine (Oncovin), and dacar-bazine can be used. Recently, some success has been achieved where chemotherapy followed surgical exci-sion of the tumor. Evans et al (1980) report very good results in children who had widespread metastases (but not to bone).

Renal Cell Carcinoma (Hypernephroma)

Metastatic renal cell carcinoma is not highly sus-ceptible to cytotoxic chemotherapy, although favor-able responses are reported in the treatment of pul-monary metastases with vinblastine (Velban), 0.1–0.2 mg/kg intravenously weekly, and with nitro-soureas such as lomustine (CCNU), 130 mg/m² orally every 6 weeks. A 25% remission rate was reported in one study of 135 patients treated with vinblastine, whereas nitrosourea produced remissions in only 9%

of 79 patients. Other studies have shown little effectiveness for these agents.

Bloom (1973) suggests that hormonal therapy may be beneficial in renal cell carcinoma. He observed that stilbestrol implants in male hamsters sometimes produced renal carcinomas and adenomas and that removal of the pellets altered the growth of induced tumors, as did the administration of testosterone or progesterone. Clinically, fewer than 15% of patients so treated show an objective response to pharmacologic doses of progesterone (Depo-Provera, Megace) or testosterone, but individual very good responses and relatively mild toxicity make this treatment worthy of consideration when a 1- to 2-month trial administration can be evaluated. Antiestrogens (tamoxifen [Nolvadex], nafoxidine*) have not yet been definitively evaluated but may also be of benefit in some patients whose tumor tissue is assay-positive for estrogen or progesterone receptors. According to one recent study, a 15% response rate was obtained with antiestrogen therapy as compared to a 5% response rate with progestogens.

Alpha-interferon species clearly have induced tumor regression in patients with metastatic renal cell carcinoma more consistently than any other hormonal or chemotherapeutic agent studied thus far. The overall major response rate is on the order of 15%.

Although there are reports of rare instances of regression of pulmonary metastases after nephrectomy to remove the primary neoplasm, this procedure is not likely to be of significant benefit for disseminated disease. If symptoms referable to the primary tumor are present (eg, pain, hematuria), nephrectomy may be justified for local control.

The sometimes unusual clinical behavior of metastatic renal carcinoma suggests that host immune factors may be operative, but there is no documentation of significant benefit from any type of immunotherapy except in anecdotal cases.

Wilms' Tumor
(Nephroblastoma)

The treatment of Wilms' tumor is a singular example of the benefits of adjuvant chemotherapy and of multimodal forms of combined treatment, including sequential therapy with surgery, radiation therapy, and chemotherapy with curative intent, even where metastatic disease is present. Nephrectomy alone cures 20% of children with localized Wilms' tumor; the addition of radiation therapy to the tumor bed after nephrectomy increases the cure rate to 47%; and the addition of multiple courses of dactinomycin as adjuvant treatment has increased the overall cure rate to 80%. Furthermore, half of children who develop multiple pulmonary metastases may be curable by the use of bilateral whole lung radiation therapy combined with chemotherapy using dactinomycin and possibly vincristine. The combination of dactinomycin and vincristine may be more effective than either drug used alone in this previously fatal cancer. Doxorubicin is also a useful drug for patients who fail to respond to dactinomycin with or without vincristine. Metastases solely to the lungs appear to have a distinctly better prognosis than liver, brain, or bone metastases.

The optimum dosage schedules and duration of therapy are not known with certainty, but recommended regimens are as follows:

(1) Dactinomycin, 15 mg/kg intravenously daily for 5 days, or 600 μg/m^2 intravenously every other day for 4 doses, beginning as soon as the diagnosis is established and continuing within 24 hours after surgery, followed by multiple courses at 6 weeks and 3, 7, 9, 12, and 15 months thereafter.

(2) Vincristine, 1.5 mg/m^2 intravenously weekly for 6 weeks beginning postoperatively, followed by 2 doses (4 days apart) of 1.5 mg/m^2 intravenously, repeated every 3 months for 15 months. No single dose of vincristine should exceed 2 mg.

Transitional Cell Tumor

Tumors of the renal pelvis and ureter, which are uncommon, are biologically related to urothelial tumors arising in the bladder. Chemotherapy has not generally been effective for the palliation of such neoplasms, but newer drugs such as doxorubicin and cisplatin, reportedly useful for bladder carcinoma, may also be of some benefit for other urothelial cancers.

Bladder carcinomas are a histologically and biologically heterogeneous group whose aggressiveness and prognosis are related to the stage and grade of tumor. For a further discussion of staging and grading, see p 356.

Up to two-thirds of selected patients with multiple small superficial papillary tumors show a favorable response to thiotepa, 60 mg instilled into the bladder in 60 mL of sterile water and retained for 2 hours. One-third of patients may achieve a complete remission, which can be maintained with 30- to 60-mg instillations every 4–6 weeks. Adverse effects include marrow suppression and cystitis.

Doxorubicin is one of the most useful drugs for palliation of advanced bladder cancer. An overall response rate of 23% was reported in a study of 235 patients with objective regressions of skin, liver, lung, and nodal metastases occurring within 1 month and lasting up to 5 months. Fluorouracil is one of the most carefully studied drugs for treatment of bladder cancer, with an overall response rate of 35% in 74 patients. Cisplatin is also an active agent in the treatment of bladder cancer, with a response rate of 40%, and may be synergistic with concomitant radiation therapy. Mitomycin may also be a useful agent, especially when instilled intravesically.

Immunotherapy with alpha-interferon has been effective in some patients with bladder carcinoma.

Combined regimens of cyclophosphamide, doxorubicin, and cisplatin are more effective than single agents in small series, but the response rate in large numbers of patients is not yet determined.

---

* See note to reader on p 404.

Adjuvant chemotherapy of high-risk invasive bladder carcinoma has been proposed, and studies are under way; definitive results have not yet been reported from a randomized trial now being conducted.

Bladder Sarcoma

Bladder sarcomas may respond temporarily to combination chemotherapy with doxorubicin and dacarbazine in up to 40% of adults treated as follows: doxorubicin, 60 mg/m^2 intravenously on day 1, and dacarbazine, 250 mg/m^2 intravenously on days 1 through 5, with the cycle repeated every 22 days unless toxicity prohibits.

Childhood rhabdomyosarcomas of the lower urinary tract, bladder, and vagina can be controlled, with achievement of a 5-year remission in half of patients, by a cooperative effort with surgery, where feasible, in conjunction with radiation therapy and combination adjuvant chemotherapy consisting of dactinomycin and vincristine. Twenty percent of children with clinical evidence of metastases are curable by aggressive combined therapy with 3 drugs (dactinomycin, vincristine, and cyclophosphamide) in conjunction with radiation therapy. Drugs are given in 3-month cycles for 1–2 years, as in the following regimen: vincristine, 2 mg/m^2 intravenously weekly for 12 weeks (maximum, 2 mg/dose); dactinomycin, 0.075 mg/kg/course intravenously over 5 days (maximum, 0.5 mg/d) every 3 months for 5 courses; and cyclophosphamide, 2.5 mg/kg orally daily for 2 years.

Prostatic Carcinoma

Disseminated symptomatic or rapidly progressive prostatic carcinoma should be considered for palliative therapy even though no increase in survival can be documented by controlled studies. Eighty percent of patients receiving hormonal therapy or orchiectomy experienced both subjective and objective benefit of symptoms. The era of hormonal antineoplastic therapy began with the observation that patients with prostatic carcinoma improved following androgenic hormone suppression or treatment with estrogens. Hormonal therapy is discussed on p 377. The new GnRH agonist leuprolide is discussed on p 408.

Also noteworthy is the recent development of the antiandrogens (flutamide* and cyproterone acetate) and of the estradiol-alkylator complex estramustine phosphate (Emcyt). Estramustine has been extensively studied in Europe, where a response rate of 38% has been reported in over 200 patients with advanced prostatic carcinoma following intravenous administration. Oral estramustine is reported to yield a 22% response rate, according to Mittelman, Shukla, and Murphy (1976).

Chemotherapy of prostatic carcinoma that has not responded to endocrine therapy has been moderately effective, with responses of approximately 35% reported for fluorouracil, cyclophosphamide, and dox-

orubicin as single agents. Such therapy was superior to secondary palliative hormonal manipulations after failure of orchiectomy or estrogen therapy. Other effective single agents include cisplatin and dacarbazine in small series.

Patients who respond to chemotherapy fare better in terms of pain palliation, and their overall survival rate is 1 ½ times to twice that of nonresponders. Combinations of drugs may yield higher response rates, with doxorubicin plus cyclophosphamide or cisplatin apparently one of the most effective combinations; however, the numbers of patients so treated are too small and follow-up periods too brief to justify any statements about the duration of benefit. Full dosage of these cytotoxic agents is often not possible, because of extensive previous radiation therapy to marrow-bearing areas of bone or because of bone marrow infiltration by the tumor. Hypercalcemia is sometimes a complication of prostatic carcinoma with extensive bony involvement.

Testicular Neoplasm

The treatment of testicular cancers exemplifies the progress made in chemotherapy and radiotherapy since 1960, when Li et al developed combination chemotherapy (chlorambucil, methotrexate, and dactinomycin) for patients with disseminated disease. Friedman and Purkayastha (1960) showed that relatively low doses of radiation may be curative for seminoma when metastases to the neck and mediastinum are present.

Metastases contain pure seminomatous elements in two-thirds of cases, and these are usually radiosensitive; in one-fourth of cases, the metastatic tissue type is embryonal carcinoma, implying that apparently "pure" seminomas may in fact contain combinations of germ cell elements, including chorionic tissue in 9% and teratomatous elements in 4%. Alkylators such as melphalan and chlorambucil have been reported to be effective in 90% of cases; in instances where combined elements are documented, dactinomycin, cisplatin, vinblastine, and bleomycin in various combinations may be the drugs of choice.

The presence of nonseminomatous elements in a testicular tumor is suggested by finding AFP or beta-hCG tumor markers in serum as determined by radioimmunoassay or in tumor tissue as determined by immunocytochemical techniques.

The beta-subunit of hCG is unique and specific to the hCG molecule and does not give false-positive radioimmunoassays with elevated levels of luteinizing hormone (LH) or other stimulating hormones. Up to 60% of nonseminomatous germ cell tumors of the testis are associated with initially high serum hCG levels, which return to normal with effective therapy. A persistently elevated or rising level implies the presence of active disease.

An elevation in serum AFP indicates an element of embryonal carcinoma in a testicular tumor. In 70% of testicular neoplasms, AFP levels are elevated, as detected by sensitive radioimmunoassay techniques; per-

---

* See note to reader on p 404.

sistent elevation implies recurrent or progressive tumor. One or the other marker is elevated in as many as 90% of patients with nonseminomatous testicular tumors, whereas fewer than 10% of pure seminomas produce these markers. CEA (carcinoembryonic antigen) has also been reported to be a product of testicular germ cell neoplasms but is not as tissue-specific as hCG and AFP.

Nonseminomatous testicular carcinomas have recently been treated successfully with varying combinations of bleomycin, vinblastine, and cisplatin. Samuels (1975) reports an overall 75% response rate, with a 45% complete remission rate, to a regimen of vinblastine, 0.2 mg/kg intravenously daily on days 1 and 2; and bleomycin, 30 units infused in 1000 mL of 5% glucose and water over 24 hours on day 2 and for 5 additional days.

Courses are repeated every 3–4 weeks for 3 or 4 cycles depending upon the degree and duration of toxicity. Side effects include severe leukopenia (80%), thrombocytopenia (40%), and stomatitis (100%). Anemia and pneumonitis due to bleomycin occur in a lower percentage of patients. Median duration of response was 34 weeks.

The Memorial Sloan-Kettering program of therapy consists of continuous intravenous infusion of bleomycin, 0.5 unit/kg daily for 7 days, combined with cisplatin, 1 mg/kg intravenously on day 7. Responses were observed in 11 of 16 patients who were resistant to previous weekly bleomycin and vinblastine or dactinomycin therapy. Responses lasted 2–7 months, and toxicity was predominantly mucosal, with one-third of patients also having transient nephrotoxicity and ototoxicity due to platinum.

Einhorn, Furnas, and Powell (1976) used a triple combination of bleomycin, vinblastine, and cisplatin with 100% success in 20 patients, 15 of whom achieved complete remission with a median duration of 9 months (range 6–18 months). This regimen is as follows: vinblastine, 0.2 mg/kg intravenously on days 1 and 2 every 3 weeks; bleomycin, 30 units intravenously weekly for 12 weeks; and cisplatin, 20 mg/m² intravenously daily on days 1–5 every 3 weeks.

Williams and Einhorn (1982) have recently used combinations of bleomycin, doxorubicin, and cisplatin with etoposide to obtain a 50% rate of complete remission in patients who were refractory to initial therapy with cisplatin, vinblastine, and bleomycin.

If a complete remission is not achieved after 4 courses of combination chemotherapy, surgical excision of residual disease should be considered if feasible. This means wedge resection of a solitary pulmonary nodule or multiple nodules confined to a single lobe of the lung and resection of persistent abdominal masses detected by CT scanning or palpation. Occasionally, pathologic examination of resected tissue reveals only necrotic fibrous tissue or benign mature teratomas.

Aggressive chemotherapy should be undertaken only by a clinician experienced in the use of the drugs involved, since major toxicities may ensue and require

skillful supportive care. Cisplatin causes moderate to severe nausea and vomiting in nearly all patients and requires vigorous intravenous hydration before and during administration to avoid significant nephrotoxicity. In many patients, creatinine clearance is reduced to 25–50% of the baseline pretreatment value. Granulocytopenia with sepsis is a major manifestation of the hematologic toxicity of bleomycin, vinblastine, and cisplatin; the use of aminoglycoside antibiotics may cause further deterioration of renal function. Anemia and thrombocytopenia are frequently observed also, but they are usually less severe than granulocytopenia. Other toxicities include weight loss, high-frequency hearing loss, fever, alopecia, myalgias, and pulmonary manifestations of bleomycin toxicity.

Mithramycin has been useful as a single agent, with a 36% response rate when used in embryonal carcinoma, or in various combinations; and doxorubicin is also reportedly a useful agent, with a 20% response rate.

It is apparent that the use of these aggressive chemotherapeutic combination regimens can achieve significant disease control for relatively long durations and can be curative in some patients, but they may also carry the risk of major toxicity and must be given by knowledgeable clinicians experienced in their administration and in a setting where adequate supportive facilities are available.

Penile Carcinoma

Penile carcinoma with massive inguinal or pelvic nodal metastases refractory to radiation therapy and beyond the scope of surgery may, on occasion, be successfully treated with bleomycin with or without methotrexate, although the contributions of chemotherapy have not been well defined for this cancer.

PAIN PALLIATION IN CANCER

Malignant disease may cause pain by obstruction of a hollow viscus, by destruction of the supporting architecture of weight-bearing bones, by infiltration of nerve roots or plexuses by tumor, and by infiltrative growth within a closed compartment such as periosteum, fascia, or a visceral capsule. Pain can sometimes be controlled by decreasing tumor bulk with radiation therapy, surgery, and chemotherapy. Radiation therapy is most effective for bony metastases; surgery may bypass an obstruction of bowel or biliary tract; regional intra-arterial chemotherapy can reduce liver pain of hepatic metastases in 50–70% of selected patients.

All too often, however, these measures are only temporarily or partially effective, and nonspecific symptomatic treatment of pain is required. Aspirin and acetaminophen are the most effective nonnarcotics and, combined with codeine, are useful for ambulatory patients. Narcotic analgesics such as morphine or hydromorphone (Dilaudid) are often required in terminal cancer; the fear of producing drug addiction should never prevent their administration to such patients. In patients with persistent or recurrent pain, a regular schedule of administration at 3- to 4-hour intervals may afford better palliation than larger doses at less frequent intervals.

Neurosurgical and anesthetic measures are appropriate in patients who have not responded to other palliative measures or who have neuroanatomically localized pain that can be eradicated without producing major neurologic dysfunction. Dorsal rhizotomy is appropriate for segmental somatic pain of thoracicoabdominal dermatomes but would be a poor choice for pain in an extremity, because of the concomitant loss of sensory function resulting from the procedure. Percutaneous cordotomy is an effective procedure for unilateral pain located in segments lower than the upper thoracic area. Thalamotomy may be useful in control of head and facial pain, as may tractotomy (trigeminal or spinal thalamic). Somatic nerve and autonomic plexus blocks may be useful when a more effective surgical procedure is refused or otherwise unavailable.

PALLIATION OF EMESIS CAUSED BY CHEMOTHERAPY

Nausea and vomiting are among the most frequent and disabling toxicities of cancer chemotherapy. Protracted bouts of retching have caused some patients to withdraw from potentially curative therapy, especially regimens containing cisplatin. Phenothiazines are among the safest effective antiemetics for adults receiving moderately emetogenic drugs such as fluorouracil, methotrexate, and moderate doses of cyclophosphamide (Cytoxan). Prochlorperazine may be given in 10-mg doses orally or intramuscularly every 6 hours; absorption from suppositories is somewhat unpredictable. The major adverse reaction of phenothiazines is extrapyramidal reactions or agitation, which can usually be controlled by concomitant administration of diphenhydramine (Benadryl). For more potent emetogenic regimens such as cisplatin and high-dose cyclophosphamide, metoclopramide (Reglan), 2 mg/kg given slowly intravenously over a 10- to 30-minute period every 2 hours, is effective and well tolerated.

Marihuana derivatives such as tetrahydrocannabinol (THC) are about as effective as oral prochlorperazine but less effective than metoclopramide against strongly emetic drugs such as cisplatin. Tetrahydrocannabinol is available in the USA to oncologists working in institutions that have completed an investigative new drug application for protocol trials. This agent seems to be better tolerated and more effective in younger patients and is relatively contraindicated in elderly patients or those with cardiovascular or psychiatric disabilities.

Haloperidol is useful against strongly emetogenic drugs such as cisplatin, mechlorethamine, and doxorubicin. Cardiovascular side effects are fewer than with phenothiazines; sedation is the most common side effect. The usual dosage is 2 mg parenterally before chemotherapy is administered. Another agent

useful against strongly emetogenic drugs is lorazepam, 1–2 mg given slowly intravenously before administration of chemotherapeutic agents.

BACTERIAL SEPSIS IN CANCER PATIENTS

Infection is the cause of death in 60–75% of patients with leukemia or lymphoma and 40–50% of patients with solid tumors. In some instances, this is due to impaired host defense mechanisms (leukemia, lymphoma, myeloma); in others, it is due to the myelosuppressive and immunosuppressive effects of cancer therapy or progressive malignancy with cachexia.

In patients with acute leukemia or granulocytopenia (granulocyte count $< 600/\mu L$), infection is a medical emergency, and fever is virtually pathognomonic of infection, usually with gram-negative organisms, in these patients.

Appropriate cultures (eg, blood, sputum, urine, cerebrospinal fluid) should always be obtained before starting therapy; however, one usually cannot await the results of these studies before beginning bactericidal antibiotic therapy. Gram's stains may clearly demonstrate the presence of a predominant organism.

In the absence of granulocytopenia and in nonleukemic patients, the empiric combination of a cephalosporin type antibiotic and tobramycin has been very beneficial for patients with acute bacteremia. This therapy has a very broad spectrum, however, and therefore must be used judiciously and should always be replaced by the most appropriate antibiotics as soon as culture data become available. The combination of cephalosporin and kanamycin is ineffective against *Pseudomonas* infection. In the current era of intensive chemotherapy of cancer, *Pseudomonas* bacteremia is now the most frequent infection in granulocytopenic patients and is all too often fulminant and fatal within 72 hours. Prompt institution of combination therapy with tobramycin and ticarcillin may offer the best chance of cure. Because of drug interactions, these 2 compounds cannot be mixed but must be administered separately. This combination is less effective against *Escherichia coli* sepsis and should not be used for that purpose. Initial treatment of febrile patients with acute leukemia or granulocytopenia should consist of 3 drugs: cephalothin, tobramycin, and ticarcillin. If a causative organism is isolated, the combination is replaced with the best agent or agents; otherwise, the combination is continued until the infection has resolved.

Granulocyte transfusions have recently been proved to have significant value for granulocytopenic cancer patients with sepsis; however, until recently, complex procurement procedures limited their availability. Untreated patients with chronic myelogenous leukemia can serve as excellent granulocyte donors for cancer patients with granulocytopenia. Although collection is ideally carried out with a blood cell separator, simple leukapheresis techniques may also be of value with chronic myelogenous leukemia donors. Use of normal donors requires a blood cell separator or filtration-leukapheresis device. Optimal use of normal granulocyte transfusion appears to require at least 4 daily transfusions (in addition to antibiotics) to localize infection.

MANAGEMENT OF VESICANT DRUG EXTRAVASATIONS

Infiltration of chemotherapeutic agents may cause severe local tissue necrosis. The greatest problems occur with mechlorethamine, vincristine, vinblastine, dactinomycin, doxorubicin, daunorubicin, mithramycin, mitomycin, and dacarbazine. As soon as infiltration is suspected, intravenous administration should be discontinued and a record made of the approximate amount, volume, and extent of extravasation. No drug is injected locally. The patient is instructed to apply ice for 20 minutes 4 times a day for 72 hours. This causes local vasoconstriction and decreases fluid absorption in the initial hours after injury. Although initially the lesion may show only local induration and then superficial blistering, this may be misleading, as the ultimate extent may include chronic ulceration, painful fibrosis, and injury to muscles and tendons, which may impair hand function. Within 72 hours, the patient should be evaluated by a plastic surgeon, who should follow the patient closely. With this approach, only 12 of 50 patients have required surgery. If extreme pain or tissue necrosis is present, surgical excision of the area of infiltration, particularly of the subcutaneous tissues, should be performed promptly. For established ulcers with tissue fibrosis, however, adequate treatment usually requires a wide excision down to the level of healthy tissue. In the forearm or dorsum of the hand, removal of extensor tendons and immediate coverage with a meshed split-thickness skin graft may be required. The use of flaps is avoided whenever possible.

To avoid extravasation, a properly flowing intravenous infusion should be established before injection of the drug. A convenient route of vascular access in cancer patients is the Silastic catheter surgically placed in the cephalic or jugular vein and positioned in the superior vena cava with the distal end tunneled beneath the skin to an accessible exit point on the lower chest wall. The Dacron wool cuff becomes infiltrated by connective tissue, which secures the catheter position and forms a barrier to infection of the tunnel. Drugs, blood products, fluids, and parenteral nutrition solutions may be administered through the catheter. Blood may be withdrawn, which avoids the pain and complications of difficult venipunctures. These catheters may remain in place for prolonged periods with a low rate of infection, so that the problems of drug extravasation, phlebitis, and difficult venous access may be avoided.

A totally implantable system of intravenous access

has recently become available also (Porto-Cath, Infusa-Port).

PALLIATION OF LOCAL COMPLICATIONS OF NEOPLASMS

Effusions

At least half of all patients with lung or breast cancer will develop a pleural effusion at some time during their illness. Ascites is a common complication of ovarian carcinoma. Lymphomas may be associated with chylous or nonchylous effusion of either or both sites. One-fourth of all effusions are neoplastic in origin, and where pulmonary infarction is unlikely, most bloody effusions are from neoplasm. The diagnosis in malignant pleural effusions can be established by cytologic study of the fluid and pleural biopsy with the Cope needle.

Diuretics may be sufficient to control neoplastic ascitic effusions. However, when recurrent accumulations of fluid cause dyspnea, abdominal distention, or pericardial tamponade, palliative control should be attempted.

A. Pleural Effusions: Control of pleural effusions is best achieved by obliteration of the pleural space with sclerosing agents such as mechlorethamine, bleomycin, or tetracycline. Up to 90% of pleural effusions can be palliated with this technique. Criteria for obliteration and details of procedure should be decided upon by experienced personnel only.

B. Ascitic Effusions: Ascites is generally best treated by attempting to control the underlying disease, usually ovarian carcinoma or malignant lymphoma. Mechlorethamine frequently induces chemical peritonitis. Thiotepa and bleomycin do not have a vesicant action on tissues and are thus more gentle. For selected patients, the peritoneovenous shunt (LeVeen shunt) may control ascites.

C. Pericardial Effusions: Pericardial effusions are best treated by irradiation except when previous radiotherapy has included the proposed field or when the effusion is due to a radioresistant tumor. Impending tamponade must always be anticipated and treated by pericardiocentesis, creation of a pericardial window, or pericardiectomy. If needle pericardiocentesis is performed for a malignant effusion, thiotepa may be instilled into the pericardial cavity (in systemic doses) at the termination of the procedure. Mechlorethamine should not be used, since it induces too severe an inflammatory response.

Obstructions & Lytic Lesions of Bone

A. Caval Obstruction: Superior vena caval obstruction is a medical emergency that should be treated by a combination of chemotherapy and radiotherapy. It is characterized by venous congestion and distention of tributaries of the superior vena cava and thus presents clinically as edema of the face and arms—frequently associated with dyspnea and the hazard of cerebral venous thrombosis or cerebral edema. The syndrome may occur with various diseases affecting the mediastinum, but neoplastic disease—especially bronchogenic carcinoma and the malignant lymphomas—is by far the most common cause. Although a biopsy should be obtained whenever possible, this should not delay the start of therapy. Thoracic surgery or mediastinoscopy should not be performed, since such intervention increases morbidity and mortality rates. Treatment should be started as soon as the clinical syndrome is recognized and consists of diuretics, corticosteroids, and maintenance of the upright posture. An intravenous alkylator should be given through an unobstructed vein (eg, femoral vein) and radiotherapy begun immediately. Cyclophosphamide or thiotepa is preferable to mechlorethamine, since the former agents induce less vomiting. Venography or ^{99m}Tc sodium pertechnetate scanning will demonstrate large collateral veins and a block to the flow of contrast material into the right heart. Although the underlying carcinoma is usually incurable when this condition develops, emergency therapy may provide substantial palliation.

B. Bony Lytic Lesions: Palliation of metastases to weight-bearing bones is best achieved by irradiation. If pathologic fracture is impending, prophylactic fixation can minimize morbidity, especially in areas such as the femoral neck that are susceptible to considerable stress. Prolonged bed rest should be avoided whenever possible, for in addition to the usual complications, patients with bony disease are prone to develop hypercalcemia, and this tendency is accentuated by immobilization. Supportive bracing is often a useful adjunct for vertebral involvement.

Metabolic Complications of Neoplasms

A. Hypercalcemia Associated With Neoplastic Disease: Hypercalcemia occurs most commonly with myeloma, breast carcinoma, and lung carcinoma and is occasionally seen in patients with prostatic carcinoma, lymphomas, and leukemia. It has also been reported with a wide variety of metastatic or disseminated neoplasms. Symptoms include confusion, somnolence, nausea and vomiting, constipation, dehydration with polyuria, and general clinical deterioration that can easily be mistaken for progressive disease or direct neurologic involvement by tumor. The true nature of this metabolic complication may easily be overlooked, resulting in hypercalcemic death secondary to cardiac, neurologic, and renal toxicity. Hypercalcemia may be due to elaboration of a parathyroid hormone-like substance by tumor (lung carcinoma), to osteolytic sterols (as secreted by breast tumors), or to increased bone resorption by invasion and neoplastic destruction of bone (as in myeloma).

The mainstay of therapy to reduce calcium is hydration with isotonic saline (to promote a diuresis of 2–3 L/24 h) in addition to appropriate tumoricidal

therapy, mobilization of the bedridden, institution of a low-calcium diet devoid of dairy products, and appropriate treatment of bacterial infections. If the patient was receiving androgens or estrogens for breast carcinoma, they should be withdrawn. Chelating agents such as sodium citrate promote renal excretion of calcium, and potent diuretics such as furosemide or ethacrynic acid also inhibit calcium resorption by the renal tubule. These measures, however, may not be appropriate in patients with impaired renal function or congestive heart failure or may not be sufficient of themselves, and other measures such as glucocorticoids (prednisone, 60–100 mg/d) may be required. The corticosteroids appear to act by reducing calcium resorption from bone. Oral phosphate is often rapidly effective, but intravenous phosphates are too hazardous to be recommended. Mithramycin, 25 μg/kg intravenously, is a prompt and effective agent for marked hypercalcemia. It may be the drug of choice where vigorous hydration is not possible because of renal failure or fluid overload; preexisting pancytopenia is a relative contraindication. A rapid fall in serum calcium concentration will also be produced by salmon calcitonin, 4 MRC units/kg intramuscularly every 12 hours, when it is used in conjunction with other measures discussed above.

B. Hyperuricemia Associated With Neoplastic Disease: Hyperuricemia is a potentially lethal result of high nucleic acid turnover associated with some cancers—especially after effective cytotoxic therapy. Uric acid nephropathy is related to intraluminal precipitation of uric acid in the distal renal tubule and collecting duct, with progressive intrarenal obstruction and failure. This sequence of events can often be avoided by maintaining satisfactory hydration and alkalinization of the urine to pH 7.0 by oral sodium bicarbonate (6–12 g/d) or by giving acetazolamide (Diamox) (0.5–1 g/d). Although allopurinol does not replace these measures, the preventive use of this drug (300–800 mg/d) should be considered in patients with leukemia, lymphomas, and myeloproliferative disorders. If mercaptopurine is being given, the dose must be reduced to one-fourth to one-third of usual when allopurinol is started. In addition to the above measures, peritoneal dialysis or hemodialysis may be required to treat established urate uropathy.

NUTRITIONAL SUPPORT IN CANCER PATIENTS

Many patients with malignant disease eat and digest a normal diet but nevertheless continue to lose weight. Superimposed pain or therapeutic ministrations such as chemotherapy, radiation therapy, or surgery may lead to anorexia and inanition. The quickest and safest way to improve nutrition in the cachectic patient is by intravenous hyperalimentation, but this is appropriate only when the patient appears likely to benefit from further antineoplastic therapy.

PSYCHOLOGIC SUPPORT OF THE PATIENT WITH NEOPLASTIC DISEASE

The physician who undertakes primary management of a patient with neoplastic disease assumes an obligation that may extend from initial diagnosis to terminal care. Because of the wide variations in the clinical course of the disease, this period may be brief or extend over many years. During this time, the physician must coordinate various methods of therapy. However, among the major palliative benefits offered by the physician will be rapport with the patient and family based upon skillful treatment, effective and honest communication, and humane care and consideration. Such a relationship can support hope despite the statistical unlikelihood of long survival, because the patient's anxieties and fears are usually of abandonment, dependency, pain, and loss of individuality or of dignity rather than of impending death.

HOME CARE OF THE PATIENT WITH ADVANCED CANCER

Some patients with advanced cancer and their families may prefer that the terminal phase of illness be spent in the home, with its comforts and access to relatives and friends. Careful assessment of the patient's physical and emotional needs must be considered by the physician before discharge from the hospital. It is important to ensure a smooth transition to home care by obtaining in advance all required equipment and supportive assistance (Table 19–5). Home care is not appropriate for all patients but must be individually determined. The physician in charge should ideally be the coordinator of all supportive personnel—including visiting nurses, the dietitian, home health aides, priests and ministers, and medical social workers—rather than delegating this responsibility to others who do not have an established therapeutic relationship with the patient and family. In many instances, the guidance thus provided is more significant and more beneficial than the specialized technical therapies discussed throughout this chapter. Quality of care is best secured by acting upon the principle that much can yet be done for the patient even when little can be done against the neoplasm.

Table 19–5. Checklist of supplies and potential equipment needs for home care.

Bedroom
1. Adjustable electric bed with egg-crate mattress or sheepskin pad.
2. Bedside commode, bedpan, urinal, and catheter equipment.
3. Oxygen tank, valve, humidifier, and mask.
4. Oral suction equipment.
5. Rubber doughnut or foam pillow.

Bathroom
1. Shower stool or bath bench and grab bars.
2. Elevated toilet seat.
3. Ostomy care supplies and disposable enemas.

Mobility aids
1. Wheelchair (collapsible).
2. Four-point walker or cane.

Medications
1. Analgesics.
   a. Oral tablets or liquids (eg, morphine sulfate solution, Brompton's mixture, Schlesinger's solution).
   b. Parenteral premeasured narcotics in disposable syringes with needles and alcohol sponges (eg, Tubex).
   c. Suppositories (eg, hydromorphone [Dilaudid], 3 mg).
2. Antiemetics (eg, oral, parenteral, or suppository forms of phenothiazines).
3. Mouth care supplies (eg, hydrogen peroxide, viscous lidocaine, glycerin swabs, nystatin suspension or lozenges for candidiasis).
4. Nutritional liquid dietary supplements.

REFERENCES

Benign Tumors of the Renal Parenchyma

Bennington JL, Beckwith JB: *Tumors of the Kidney, Renal Pelvis, and Ureter.* Fascicle 12 of: *Atlas of Tumor Pathology,* 2nd series. Armed Forces Institute of Pathology, 1975.

Bissada NK et al: Tuberous sclerosis complex and renal angiomyolipoma. *Urology* 1975;**6:**105.

Dennis RL et al: Juxtaglomerular cell tumor of the kidney. *J Urol* 1985;**134:**334.

Dunnick NR et al: The radiology of juxtaglomerular tumors. *Radiology* 1983;**147:**321.

Farrow GM et al: Renal angiomyolipoma: A clinical pathological study of 32 patients. *Cancer* 1968;**22:**564.

Jardin A et al: Diagnosis and treatment of renal angiomyolipoma (based on 15 cases): Arguments in favor of conservative surgery (based on 8 cases). *Eur Urol* 1980;**6:**69.

Oesterling JE et al: Management of renal angiomyolipoma. *J Urol* 1986;**135:**1121.

Shapiro RA et al: Renal tumors associated with tuberous sclerosis: The case for aggressive surgical management. *J Urol* 1984;**132:**1170.

Squires JP et al: Juxtaglomerular cell tumor of the kidney. *Cancer* 1984;**53:**516.

Zerhouni EA et al: Management of bleeding renal angiomyolipomas by transcatheter embolization following CT diagnosis. *Urol Radiol* 1984;**6:**205.

Adenocarcinoma of the Kidney

Almgard LE et al: Treatment of renal adenocarcinoma by embolic occlusion of the renal circulation. *Br J Urol* 1973;**45:**474.

Altaffer LF III, Chenault OW Jr. Paraneoplastic endocrinopathies associated with renal tumors. *J Urol* 1979;**122:**573.

Babaian RJ, Swanson DA: Serum haptoglobin: A nonspecific tumor marker for renal cell carcinoma. *South Med J* 1982;**75:**145.

Balfe DM et al: Evaluation of renal masses considered indeterminant on computed tomography. *Radiology* 1982;**142:**421.

Bander NH: Comparison of antigen expression of human renal cancers in vivo and in vitro. *Cancer* 1984;**53:**1235.

Barnes CA, Beckman EN: Renal oncocytoma and its congeners. *Am J Clin Pathol* 1983;**79:**312.

Beahrs OH, Myers MH (editors): *Manual for Staging Cancer,* 2nd ed. Lippincott, 1983.

Bell ET: *Renal Diseases,* 2nd ed. Lea & Febiger, 1950.

Bennington JL, Beckwith JB: *Tumors of the Kidney, Renal Pelvis, and Ureter.* Armed Forces Institute of Pathology, 1975.

Bennington JL, Kradjian RM: *Renal Carcinoma.* Saunders, 1967.

Bennington JL, Laubscher FA: Epidemiologic studies on carcinoma of the kidney. 1. Association of renal adenocarcinoma with smoking. *Cancer* 1968;**21:**1069.

Bloom HJG: Hormone-induced and spontaneous regression of metastatic renal cancer. *Cancer* 1973;**32:**1066.

Bowers TA et al: Bone metastases from renal carcinoma: The preoperative use of transcatheter arterial occlusion. *J Bone Joint Surg [Am]* 1982;**64:**749.

Boxer RJ et al: Renal carcinoma: Computer analysis of 96 patients treated by nephrectomy. *J Urol* 1979;**122:**598.

Bracken RB et al: Secondary renal neoplasms: An autopsy study. *South Med J* 1979;**72:**806.

Brereton HD et al: Indomethacin-responsive hypercalcemia in a patient with a renal cell carcinoma. *N Engl J Med* 1974;**291:**83.

Bush WH Jr, Burnett LL, Gibbons RP: Needle tract seeding of renal cell carcinoma. *AJR* 1977;**129:**725.

Cherrie RJ et al: Prognostic implications of vena caval extension of renal cell carcinoma. *J Urol* 1982;**128:**910.

Cho C, Friedland GW, Swenson RS: Acquired renal cystic disease and renal neoplasms in hemodialysis patients. *Urol Radiol* 1984;**6:**153.

Chuang VP, Wallace S, Swanson DA: Technique and complications of renal carcinoma infarction. *Urol Radiol* 1981;**2:**223.

Chuang VP et al: Arterial occlusion in the management of pain from metastatic renal carcinoma. *Radiology* 1979;**133:**611.

Cockett ATK: Lymphatic network of the kidney. 1. Anatomic and physiologic considerations. *Urology* 1977;**9:**125.

Cohen AJ et al: Hereditary renal cell carcinoma associated with a chromosomal translocation. *N Engl J Med* 1979;**301:**592.

Cronan JJ, Zeman RK, Rosenfield AT: Comparison of computed tomography, ultrasound, and angiography in staging renal cell carcinoma. *J Urol* 1982;**127:**712.

Daniel WW JR et al: Calcified renal masses: A review of ten years' experience at the Mayo Clinic. *Radiology* 1972;**103:**503.

deKernion JB: Lymphadenectomy for renal cell carcinoma. *Urol Clin North Am* 1980;**7:**697.

deKernion JB, Berry D: The diagnosis and treatment of renal cell carcinoma. *Cancer* 1980;**44(Suppl):**1947.

deKernion JB, Ramming KP: The therapy of renal adenocarcinoma with immune RNA. *Invest Urol* 1980;**17:**378.

deKernion JB et al: The treatment of renal cell carcinoma with human leukocyte alpha-interferon. *J Urol* 1983;**130:**1063.

Engelmann U et al: Digital subtraction angiography in staging renal cell carcinoma: Comparison with computerized tomography and histopathology. *J Urol* 1984;**132:**1093.

Figlin RA et al: Treatment of renal cell carcinoma with alpha (human leukocyte) interferon and vinblastine in combination: A phase 1–11 trial. *Cancer Treat Rep* 1985;**69:**263.

Finstad CL et al: Specificity analysis of mouse monoclonal antibodies defining cell surface antigens of human renal cancer. *Proc Natl Acad Sci USA* 1985;**85:**2955.

Flocks RH, Kadesky MC: Malignant neoplasms of the kidney: An analysis of 353 patients followed 5 years or more. *J Urol* 1958;**79:**196.

Fossä SD et aL: Recombinant interferon α-2a with or without vinblastine in metastatic renal cell carcinoma. *Cancer* 1986;**57:**1700.

Freed SZ, Halperin JP, Gordon M: Idiopathic regression of metastases from renal cell carcinoma. *J Urol* 1977;**118:**538.

Gibbons RP et al: Manifestations of renal cell carcinoma. *Urology* 1976;**8:**201.

Goldberg MF et al: Renal adenocarcinoma containing a parathyroid hormone-like substance and associated with marked hypercalcemia. *Am J Med* 1964;**36:**805.

Golimbu M et al: Renal cell carcinoma: Survival and prognostic factors. *Urology* 1986;**27:**291.

Harris DT: Hormonal therapy and chemotherapy of renal-cell carcinoma. *Semin Oncol* 1983;**10:**422.

Hellekant C, Nyman CL: Routine celiac arteriography in patients with renal cell carcinoma. *J Urol* 1979;**122:**17.

Heney NM, Nocks BN: The influence of perinephric fat involvement on survival in patients with renal cell carcinoma extending into the inferior vena cava. *J Urol* 1982;**128:**18.

Hoehn W, Hermanek P: Invasion of veins in renal cell carcinoma: Frequency, correlation and prognosis. *Eur Urol* 1983;**9:**276.

Holland JM: Cancer of the kidney: Natural history and staging. *Cancer* 1973;**32:**1030.

Hop WCJ, van der Werf-Messing BHP: Prognostic indexes for renal cell carcinoma. *Eur J Cancer* 1980;**16:**833.

Horn L, Horn HL: An immunological approach to the therapy of cancer. *Lancet* 1971;**2:**466.

Horton WA, Wong V, Eldridge R: Von Hippel-Lindau disease: Clinical and pathological manifestations in nine families with 50 affected members. *Arch Intern Med* 1976;**136:**769.

Hricak H et al: Magnetic resonance imaging in the diagnosis and staging of renal and perirenal neoplasms. *Radiology* 1985;**154:**709.

Hrushesky WJ, Murphy GP: Current status of the therapy of advanced renal carcinoma. *J Surg Oncol* 1977;**9:**277.

Hughson MD, Buchwald D, Fox M: Renal neoplasia and acquired cystic kidney disease in patients receiving long-term dialysis. *Arch pathol Lab Med* 1986;**110:**592.

Hulten L et al: Occurrence and localization in lymph node metastases in renal carcinoma. *Scand J Urol Nephrol* 1969;**3:**129.

Jacobs SC, Berg SI, Lawson RK: Synchronous bilateral renal cell carcinoma: Surgical excision. *Cancer* 1980;**46:**2341.

Johnson DE, von Eschenbach AC, Sternberg J: Bilateral renal cell carcinoma. *J Urol* 1978;**119:**23.

Kato T et al: Transcatheter arterial chemoembolization of renal cell carcinoma with microencapsulated mitomycin C. *J Urol* 1981;**125:**19.

Kearney GP et al: Results of inferior vena cava resection for renal cell carcinoma. *J Urol* 1981;**125:**769.

Kirkman H: Estrogen-induced tumors of the kidney. *Natl Cancer Inst Monogr* 1959;**1:**1.

Klein MJ, Valensi QJ: Proximal tubular adenocarcinoma of the kidney with so-called oncocytic features: A clinical pathologic study of 13 cases of a rarely reported neoplasm. *Cancer* 1976;**38**:906.

Krane RJ et al: Removal of renal cell carcinoma extending into the right atrium using cardiopulmonary bypass, profound hypothermia and circulatory arrest. *J Urol* 1984;**131**:945.

Krown SE et al: Treatment of advanced renal cell carcinoma (RCC) with recombinant leukocyte A interferon (rIFN-A). (Abstract.) *Am Soc Clin Oncol* 1983;**2**:58.

Lang ED: Arteriography in the diagnosis and staging of hypernephromas. *Cancer* 1973;**32**:1043.

Lang EK: Comparison of dynamic and conventional computed tomography, angiography, and ultrasonography in the staging of renal cell carcinoma. *Cancer* 1984;**54**:2205.

Lang EK, Sullivan J, deKernion JB: Work in progress: Transcatheter embolization of renal cell carcinoma with radioactive infarct particles. *Radiology* 1983;**147**:413.

Levine E et al: CT of acquired cystic kidney disease and renal tumors in long-term dialysis patients. *AJR* 1984;**142**:125.

Lieber MM, Tomera KM, Farrow GM: Renal oncocytoma. *J Urol* 1981;**125**:481.

Lieber MM et al: Renal adenocarcinoma in young adults: Survival and variables affecting prognosis. *J Urol* 1981;**125**:164.

Ljungberg B et al: Prognostic significance of DNA content in renal cell carcinoma. *J Urol* 1986;**135**:422.

Lytton B, Rosof B, Evans JS: Parathyroid hormone-like activity in a renal carcinoma producing hypercalcemia. *J Urol* 1965;**93**:127.

Maldazys JD, deKernion JB: Prognostic factors in metastatic renal carcinoma. *J Urol* 1986;**136**:376.

Malek RS, Utz DC, Culp OS: Hypernephroma in the solitary kidney: Experience with 20 cases and review of the literature. *J Urol* 1976;**116**:553.

Marshall FF, Reitz BA, Diamond DA: A new technique for management of renal cell carcinoma involving the right atrium: Hypothermia and cardiac arrest. *J Urol* 1984;**131**:103.

McCune Cs, Schapira DV, Henshaw EC: Specific immunotherapy of advanced renal carcinoma: Evidence for the polyclonality of metastases. *Cancer* 1981;**47**:1984.

McDonald JR, Priestly JT: Malignant tumors of the kidney: Surgical and prognostic significance of tumor thrombosis of the renal vein. *Surg Gynecol Obstet* 1943;**77**:295.

McDonald MW: Current therapy for renal carcinoma. *J Urol* 1982;**127**:211.

McNichols DW, Segura JW, DeWeerd JH: Renal cell carcinoma: Long-term survival and late recurrence. *J Urol* 1981;**126**:17.

Morales A et al: Cytoreductive surgery and systemic bacille Calmette-Guérin therapy in metastatic renal cancer: A phase II trial. *J Urol* 1982;**127**:230.

Morlock CG, Horton BT: Variations in systolic blood pressure in renal tumors: A study of 491 cases. *Am J Med Sci* 1936;**191**:647.

Murphy JB, Marshall FF: Renal cyst versus tumor: A continuing dilemma. *J Urol* 1980;**123**:566.

Neidhart JA: Interferon therapy for the treatment of renal cancer. *Cancer* 1986;**57(8 Suppl)**:1696.

Neidhart JA et al: Active specific immunotherapy of stage IV renal carcinoma with aggregated tumor antigen adjuvant. *Cancer* 1980;**46**:1128.

Neidhart JA et al: Interferon-alpha therapy of renal cancer. *Cancer Res* 1984;**44**:4140.

Novick AC et al: Partial nephrectomy in the treatment of renal adenocarcinoma. *J Urol* 1977;**118**:932.

Novick AC et al: Surgical enucleation for renal cell carcinoma. *J Urol* 1986;**135**:235.

Oberling C, Riviere M, Haguenau F: Ultrastructure of the clear cells in renal cell carcinoma and its importance for the demonstration of their renal origin. *Nature* 1960;**186**:402.

O'Dea MJ et al: The treatment of renal cell carcinoma with solitary metastasis. *J Urol* 1978;**120**:540.

Otto U et al: Tumor cell deoxyribonucleic acid content and prognosis in human renal cell carcinoma. *J Urol* 1984;**132**:237.

Parienty RA et al: Local recurrence after nephrectomy for primary renal cancer: Computerized tomography recognition. *J Urol* 1984;**132**:246.

Petersson S et al: Diagnostic value of lipid content in cyst fluid. Pages 433–434 in: *Renal Tumors: Proceedings of the First International Symposium on Kidney Tumors.* Kuss R et al (editors). A. R. Liss, 1982.

Petkovic S: Le stade anatomique dans l'appréciation du prognostique des tumeurs rénales. *Urologia* 1956;**23**:125.

Petkovic S: The value of tumor tissue penetration into the renal veins and lymph nodes as an anatomical classification in kidney tumor prognostic parameters. *Eur Urol* 1980;**6**:289.

Pritchett TR, Lieskovsky G, Skinner DG: Extension of renal cell carcinoma into vena cava: Clinical review and surgical approach. *J Urol* 1986;**135**:460.

Quesada JR, Swanson DA, Gutterman JU: Phase II study of interferon alpha in metastatic renal-cell carcinoma: A progress report. *J Clin Oncol* 1985;**3**:1086.

Quesada JR et al: Antitumor activity of recombinant-derived interferon alpha in metastatic renal cell carcinoma. *J Clin Oncol* 1985;**3**:1522.

Riches EW, Griffiths IH, Thackray AC: New growths of the kidney and ureter. *Br J Urol* 1951;**23**:297.

Richie JP et al: Computerized tomography scan for diagnosis and staging of renal cell carcinoma. *J Urol* 1983;**129**:1114.

Richie JP et al: Current treatment of metastatic renal cell carcinoma with xenogeneic immune ribonucleic acid. *J Urol* 1984;**131**:236.

Robey EL, Schellhammer PF: Adrenal gland and renal cell carcinoma: Is ipsilateral adrenalectomy a necessary component of radical nephrectomy? *J Urol* 1986;**135**:453.

Robson CJ, Churchill B, Anderson W: Radical nephrectomy for renal cell carcinoma. *J Urol* 1969;**101**:297.

Rosenberg SA et al: Observations on the systemic administration of autologous lymphokine-activated killer cells and recombinant interleukin-2 to patients with metastatic cancer. *N Engl J Med* 1985;**313**:1485.

Rouvière H: *Anatomy of the Human Lymphatic System.* Tobias MJ (translator). Edwards Brothers, 1938.

Schaner EG et al: Comparison of computed and conventional whole lung tomography in detecting pulmonary nodules: A prospective radiologic-pathologic study. *AJR* 1978; **131**:51.

Spiessl B, Scheibe O, Wagner G (editors): *TNM-Atlas: Illustrated Guide to the Classification of Malignant Tumors.* Springer-Verlag, 1982.

Stauffer MH: Nephrogenic hepatosplenomegaly. *Gastroenterology* 1961;**40**:694.

Sufrin G et al: Hormones in renal cancer. *J Urol* 1977;**117**:433.

Swanson DA: Management of stage IV renal cancer. In: *Principles and Management of Urologic Cancer,* 2nd ed. Javadpour N (editor). Williams & Wilkins, 1983.

Swanson Da: Transabdominal radical nephrectomy. Pages

321–335 in: *Genitourinary Tumors: Fundamental Principles and Surgical Techniques*. Johnson DE, Boileau MA (editors). Grune & Stratton, 1982.

Swanson DA, Bernardino ME: "Silent" osseous metastases in renal cell carcinoma: Value of CT. *Urology* 1982;**20**:208.

Swanson DA, Liles A: Bladder metastasis: A rare cause of hematuria in renal carcinoma. *J Surg Oncol* 1982;**20**:80.

Swanson DA et al: Angioinfarction and nephrectomy for metastatic renal cell carcinoma: An update. *J Urol* 1983;**130**:449.

Swanson DA et al: Osseous metastases secondary to renal cell carcinoma. *Urology* 1981;**18**:556.

Tallberg T et al: Active specific immunotherapy with supportive measures in the treatment of palliatively nephrectomized, renal adenocarcinoma patients: A thirteen-year follow-up study. *Eur Urol* 1985;**11**:233.

Topley M, Novick AC, Montie JE: Long-term results following partial nephrectomy for localized renal adenocarcinoma. *J Urol* 1984;**131**:1050.

van der Werf-Messing B, van der Heul RO, Ledeboer RC: Renal cell carcinoma trial. *Cancer Clin Trials* 1978;**1**:13.

Vickers M Jr: Serum haptoglobins: A preoperative detector of metastatic renal carcinoma. *J Urol* 1974;**112**:310.

Wallace AC, Nairn RC: Renal tubular antigens in kidney tumors. *Cancer* 1972;**29**:977.

Warren MM, Kelalis PT, Utz DL: The changing concept of hypernephroma. *J Urol* 1970:104:376.

Wehle MJ, Grabstald H: Contraindications to needle aspiration of solid renal mass: Tumor dissemination by renal needle aspiration. *J Urol* 1986;**136**:446.

Williams RD, Hricak H: Magnetic resonance imaging in urology. *J Urol* 1984;**132**:641.

Wynder EL, Mabuchi K, Whitmore WF Jr: Epidemiology of adenocarcinoma of the kidney. *J Natl Cancer Inst* 1974;**53**:16.

Zabbo A et al: Digital subtraction angiography for evaluating patients with renal carcinoma. *J Urol* 1985;**134**:252.

Zincke H et al: Treatment of renal cell carcinoma by in situ partial nephrectomy and extracorporeal operation with autotransplantation. *Mayo Clin Proc* 1985;**60**:651.

Nephroblastoma

Beckwith JB, Palmer NF: Histopathology and prognosis of Wilms' tumor. *Cancer* 1978;**41**:1937.

Bennington JL, Beckwith JB: *Tumors of the Kidney, Renal Pelvis, and Ureter*. Armed Forces Institute of Pathology, 1975.

Bishop HC et al: Survival in bilateral Wilms' tumor: Review of 30 National Wilms' Tumor Study cases. *J Pediatr Surg* 1977;**12**:631.

Bolande RP, Brough AJ, Izant RJ Jr: Congenital mesoblastic nephroma of infancy: A report of 8 cases and the relationship to Wilms' tumor. *Pediatrics* 1967;**40**:272.

Bove KE, McAdams AJ: The nephroblastomatosis complex and its relationship to Wilms' tumor: A clinical pathologic treatise. *Perspect Pediatr Pathol* 1976;**3**:185.

Bracken RB et al: Preoperative chemotherapy for Wilms' tumor. *Urology* 1982;**19**:55.

Breslow NE, Beckwith JB: Epidemiological features of Wilms' tumor: Results of the National Wilms' Tumor Study. *J Natl Cancer Inst* 1982;**68**:429.

Breslow NE et al: Prognosis for Wilms' tumor patients with nonmetastatic disease of diagnosis: Results of the second National Wilms' Tumor Study. *J Clin Oncol* 1985;**3**:521.

Clouse JW et al: The changing management of Wilms' tumor over a 30-year period: 1949–1978. *Cancer* 1985;**56**:1484.

D'Angio GJ et al: The treatment of Wilms' tumor: Results of the National Wilms' Tumor Study. *Cancer* 1976;**38**:633.

D'Angio GJ et al: The treatment of Wilms' tumor: Results of the Second National Wilms' Tumor Study. *Cancer* 1981;**47**:2302.

D'Angio GJ et al: Wilms' tumor: Genetic aspects and etiology: A report of the National Wilms' Tumor Study (NWTS) Committee of the NWTS Group. Pages 43–57 in: *Renal Tumors: Proceedings of the First International Symposium on Kidney Tumors*. Kuss R et al (editors). A.R. Liss, 1982.

D'Angio GJ et al: Wilms' tumor: An update. *Cancer* 1980;**45**:1791.

deKraker J et al: Preoperative chemotherapy in Wilms' tumour: Results of clinical trials and studies on nephroblastomas conducted by the International Society of Paediatric Oncology (SIOP). Pages 131–194 in: *Renal Tumors: Proceedings of the First International Symposium on Kidney Tumors*. Kuss R et al (editors). A.R. Liss, 1982.

Farewell VT et al: Retrospective validation of a new staging system for Wilms' tumor. *Cancer Clin Trials* 1981;**4**:167.

Hartman DS et al: Mesoblastic nephroma: Radiologic, pathologic correlation of 20 cases. *AJR* 1981;**136**:69.

Jaffe N et al: Childhood urologic cancer therapy related sequelae and their impact on management. *Cancer* 1980;**45**:1815.

Kay R, Tank E: Current management of bilateral Wilms' tumor. *J Urol* 1986;**135**:983.

Knudson Ag Jr, Strong LC: Mutation in cancer: A model for Wilms' tumor of the kidney. *J Natl Cancer Inst* 1972;**48**:313.

Leape LL: Diagnosis and management of Wilms' tumor and neuroblastomas. Pages 179–199 in: *Genitourinary Cancer*. Skinner DG, deKernion JB (editors). Saunders, 1978.

Leape LL, Breslow NE, Bishop HC: The surgical treatment of Wilms' tumor: Results of the National Wilms' Tumor Study. *Ann Surg* 1978;**187**:351.

Lemierle J: The treatment of Wilms' tumor in 1982: The status of the art. Pages 167–171 in: *Renal Tumors: Proceedings of the First International Symposium on Kidney Tumors*. Kuss R et al (editors). A.R. Liss, 1982.

Lemerle J et al: Effectiveness of preoperative chemotherapy in Wilms' tumor: Results of an International Society of Paediatric Oncology (SIOP) clinical trial. *J Clin Oncol* 1983;**1**:604.

Lemerle J et al: Wilms' tumor: Natural history and prognostic factors: A retrospective study of 248 cases treated at the Institute Gustave-Roussy 1952–1967. *Cancer* 1976;**36**:2557.

Pendergrass TW: Congenital anomalies in children with Wilms' tumor. *Cancer* 1976;**37**:403.

Rous SN et al: Nodular renal blastema, nephroblastomatosis, and Wilms' tumor: Different points on the same disease spectrum. *Urology* 1976;**8**:599.

Yunis JJ, Ramsay NKC: Familial occurrence of the aniridia-Wilms' tumor syndrome with deletion 11. *J Pediatr* 1980;**96**:1027.

Sarcoma of the Kidney

Bennington JL, Beckwith JB: *Tumors of the Kidney, Renal Pelvis, and Ureter*. Armed Forces Institute of Pathology, 1975.

Farrow GM et al: Sarcomas and sarcomatoid and mixed malignant tumors of the kidney in adults. *Cancer* 1968; **22:**545.

Srinivas V et al: Sarcomas of the kidney. *J Urol* 1984;**132:**13.

Tumors of the Renal Pelvis

Almgard LE et al: Thorotrast-induced renal tumors after retrograde pyelograms. *Eur Urol* 1977;**3:**69.

Batata MA et al: Primary carcinoma of the ureter: A prognostic study. *Cancer* 1975;**35:**1626.

Boijsen E, Falin J: Angiography in carcinoma of the renal pelvis. *Acta Radiol [Diagn] (Stockh)* 1961;**56:**81.

Brookland RK, Richter MP: The postoperative irradiation of transitional cell carcinoma of the renal pelvis and ureter. *J Urol* 1985;**133:**952.

Grabstald H, Whitmore WF, Melamed MR: Renal pelvic tumors. *JAMA* 1971;**281:**845.

Johansson S, Wahlqvist L: A prognostic study of urothelial renal pelvic tumors: Comparison between the prognosis of patients treated with intrafascial nephrectomy and perifascial nephroureterectomy. *Cancer* 1979;**43:**2525.

Melicow MM: Tumor of the urinary drainage tract: Urothelial tumors. *J Urol* 1945;**54:**186.

Mitty HA, Baron MG, Fuler M: Infiltrating carcinoma of the renal pelvis: Angiographic features. *Radiology* 1969;**92:**994.

Toppercer A: Fibroepithelial tumor of the renal pelvis. *Can J Surg* 1980;**23:**269.

Tumors of the Ureter

Arger PH et al: Ultrasonic assessment of renal transitional cell carcinoma: Preliminary report. *AJR* 1979;**132:**407.

Babaian RJ, Johnson DE, Chan RC: Combination nephroureterectomy and postoperative radiotherapy for infiltrative ureteral carcinomas. *Int J Radiat Oncol Biol Phys* 1980;**6:**1229.

Batata MA et al: Primary carcinoma of the ureter: A prognostic study. *Cancer* 1975;**35:**1626.

Gill WB, Lu CT, Bibbo M: Retrograde ureteral brushing. *Urology* 1978;**12:**279.

Huffman JL et al: Endoscopic diagnosis and treatment of upper-tract urothelial tumors: A preliminary report. *Cancer* 1985;**55:**1422.

Johnson DE, Babaian RJ: Conservative surgical management for noninvasive distal ureteral carcinoma. *Urology* 1979;**13:**365.

Kiriyama T, Hironaka H, Fukuda K: Six years of experience with retrograde biopsy of intraureteral carcinoma using the Dormia stone basket. *J Urol* 1976;**116:**308.

Schmauz R, Cole P: Epidemiology of cancer of the renal pelvis and ureter. *J Natl Cancer Inst* 1974;**52:**1431.

Tumors of the Bladder

Anderstrom C et al: A prospective randomized study of preoperative irradiation with cystectomy or cystectomy alone for invasive bladder carcinoma. *Eur Urol* 1983;**9:**142.

Babaian RJ et al: Metastases from transitional cell carcinoma of urinary bladder. *Urology* 1980;**16:**142.

Benson RC Jr: Treatment of diffuse transitional cell carcinoma in situ by whole bladder hematoporphyrin derivative photodynamic therapy. *J Urol* 1985;**134:**675.

Boileau MA et al: Bladder carcinoma: Results with preoperative radiotherapy and radical cystectomy. *Urology* 1980;**16:**569.

Botto H et al: Treatment of malignant bladder tumors by iridium-192 wiring. *Urology* 1980;**16:**467.

Bracken RB, McDonald MW, Johnson DE: Cystectomy for

superficial bladder tumors. *Urology* 1981;**18:**459

Brosman SA: The use of bacillus Calmette-Guérin in the therapy of bladder carcinoma in situ. *J Urol* 1985;**134:**36.

Burnand KG et al: Single dose intravesical thiotepa as an adjuvant to cystodiathermy in the treatment of transitional cell bladder carcinoma. *Br J Urol* 1976;**48:**55.

Byar D, Blackard C: Veterans Administration Cooperative Urological Research Group: Comparisons of placebo, pyridoxine, and topical thiotepa in preventing recurrence of stage I bladder cancer. *Urology* 1977;**10:**556.

Chan RC, Bracken RB, Johnson DE: Single dose whole pelvis megavoltage irradiation for palliative control of hematuria or ureteral obstruction. *J Urol* 1979;**122:**750.

Cole P, Hoover R, Fridell GH: Occupation and cancer of the lower urinary tract. *Cancer* 1972;**29:**1250.

Collan Y, Makinen J, Heikkinen A: Histological grading of transitional cell tumours of the bladder: Value of histological grading (WHO) in prognosis. *Eur Urol* 1979;**5:**311.

Connolly JG et al: Relationship between the use of artificial sweeteners and bladder cancer. (Correspondence.) *Can Med Assoc J* 1978;**119:**408.

Cummings KB et al: Segmental resection in the management of bladder carcinoma. *J Urol* 1978;**119:**56.

Dart RO: Grading of epithelial tumors of urinary bladder. *J Urol* 1936;**36:**651.

deKernion JB et al: The management of superficial bladder tumors and carcinoma in situ with intravesical bacillus Calmette-Guérin. *J Urol* 1985;**133:**598.

Dretler SP, Ragsdale BD, Leadbetter WF: The value of pelvic lymphadenectomy in the surgical treatment of bladder cancer. *J Urol* 1973;**109:**414.

England HR et al: Evaluation of Helmstein's distention method for carcinoma of the bladder. *Br J Urol* 1973;**45:**593.

Falor WH, Ward RM: Prognosis in early carcinoma of the bladder based on chromosomal analysis. *J Urol* 1978;**119:**44.

Falor WH, Ward RM: Prognosis in well-differentiated noninvasive carcinoma of the bladder based on chromosomal analysis. *Surg Gynecol Obstet* 1977;**144:**515.

Fisher MR, Hricak H, Tanagho EA: Urinary bladder MR imaging. 2. Neoplasm. *Radiology* 1985;**157:**471.

Glashan RW: Treatment of carcinoma in situ of the bladder with doxorubicin (Adriamycin). *Cancer Chemother Pharmacol* 1983;**II (Suppl):**S35.

Hall RR: Intravesical hyperthermia for transitional cell carcinoma of the bladder. Pages 267–270 in: *Bladder Tumors and Other Topics in Urological Oncology*. Vol 1. Pavone-Macaluso M, Smith PH, Edsmyr F (editors). Plenum Press, 1980.

Hatch TR, Barry JM: Value of excretory urography in staging bladder cancer. *J Urol* 1986; **135:**49.

Heney NM: First-line chemotherapy of superficial bladder cancer: Mitomycin vs thiotepa. *Urology* 1985; **26 (Suppl):**27.

Herr HW et al: Long-term effect of intravesical bacillus Calmette-Guérin on flat carcinoma in situ of bladder. *J Urol* 1986;**135:**265.

Hewitt CB, Babiszewski JF, Antunez AR: Update on intracavitary radiation in the treatment of bladder tumors. *J Urol* 1981;**126:**323.

Hicks RM: Multistage carcinogenesis in the urinary bladder. *Br Med Bull* 1980;**36:**39.

Hicks RM, Chowaniec J, Wakefield J: Experimental induction of bladder tumors by a two-stage system. Pages 475–489 in: *Carcinogenesis: Mechanisms of Tumor Pro-*

motion and Cocarcinogenesis. Vol 2. Slaga TJ, Sivak A, Boutwell RK (editors). Raven, 1978.

Hope-Stone HF et al: T3 bladder cancer: Salvage rather than elective cystectomy after radiotherapy. *Urology* 1984; **24**:315.

International Union Against Cancer: *TNM Classification of Malignant Tumors,* 3rd ed. International Union Against Cancer, 1978.

Itzchak Y, Singer D, Fischelavitch Y: Ultrasonographic assessment of bladder tumors. 1. Tumor detection. *J Urol* 1981;**126**:31.

Jakse G, Hofstädter F, Marberger H: Topical doxorubicin hydrochloride therapy for carcinoma in situ of the bladder: A follow-up. *J Urol* 1984;**131**:41.

Javadpour N: Current status of biological markers in bladder and testis cancer. Lesson 13 in: *American Urological Association Update Series.* Vol 1. American Urological Association, 1982.

Jewett HJ, Strong GH: Infiltrating carcinoma of the bladder: Relation of depth of penetration of the bladder wall to incidence of local extension and metastasis. *J Urol* 1946;**55**:366.

Johnson DE: Surgery for carcinoma of the urinary bladder. *Cancer Treat Rev* 1974;**1**:271.

Klein FA et al: Flow cytometry of normal and nonneoplastic diseases of the bladder: An estimate of the false-positive rates. *J Urol* 1982;**127**:946.

Koss LG: *Tumors of the Urinary Bladder.* Fascicle II of: *Atlas of Tumor Pathology,* 2nd series. Armed Forces Institute of Pathology, 1975.

Lamm DL: Bacillus Calmette-Guérin immunotherapy for bladder cancer. *J Urol* 1985;**134**:40.

Lamm DL et al: Complications of bacillus Calmette-Guérin immunotherapy in 1,278 patients with bladder cancer. *J Urol* 1986;**135**:272.

LaPlante M, Brice M II: The upper limits of hopeful application of radical cystectomy for vesical carcinoma: Does nodal metastasis always indicate incurability? *J Urol* 1973;**109**:261.

Lerman RI, Hutter RVP, Whitmore WF Jr: Papilloma of the urinary bladder. *Cancer* 1970;**25**:333.

Logothetis CJ et al: Cyclophosphamide, doxorubicin and cis-platin chemotherapy for patients with locally advanced urothelial tumors with or without nodal metastases. *J Urol* 1985;**134**:460.

Marshall VF: The relation of the preoperative estimate to the pathologic demonstration of the extent of vesical neoplasms. *J Urol* 1952;**68**:714.

Martínez-Piñeiro JA: BCG vaccine in superficial bladder tumors: Eight years later. *Eur Urol* 1984;**10**:93.

Masina F: Segmental resection for tumours of the urinary bladder: Ten year follow-up. *Br J Surg* 1965;**52**:279.

Mathur VK, Krahn HP, Ramsey EW: Total cystectomy for bladder cancer. *J Urol* 1981;**125**:784.

McAninch JW, Kiesling VJ, Beck PN: Diagnostic biopsies of bladder and urethra in outpatients. Page 19 in: *Proceedings of the Kimbrough Urological Seminar.* Vol 12. Brodock Press, 1978.

Meyers FJ et al: Fate of bladder in patients with metastatic bladder cancer treated with cisplatin, methotrexate and vinblastine: Northern California oncology group study. *J Urol* 1985;**134**:1118.

Miller LS, Johnson DE: Megavoltage irradiation for bladder cancer: Alone, postoperative, or preoperative. Pages 771–782 in: *Seventh National Cancer Conference Proceedings.* Lippincott, 1973.

Montie JE, Straffon RA, Stewart BH: Radical cystectomy without radiation therapy for carcinoma of the bladder. *J Urol* 1984;**131**:477.

Morrison AS, Buring JE: Artificial sweeteners and cancer of the lower urinary tract. *N Engl J Med* 1980;**302**:537.

Mostofi FK: Pathology and staging of bladder cancer. Pages 213–218 in: *Advances in Medical Oncology, Research and Education.* Vol 11: *Clinical Cancer: Principal Sites 2.* Wilkinson PM (editor). Pergamon, 1979.

Mostofi FK, Sobin LH, Torlini H: *Histological Typing of Urinary Bladder Tumours.* World Health Organization, 1973.

Newell GR, Hoover RN, Kolbye AC: Status report on saccharin in humans. *J Natl Cancer Inst* 1978;**61**:275.

Nseyo UO et al: Whole bladder photodynamic therapy for transitional cell carcinoma of bladder. *Urology* 1985; **26**:274.

Ojeda L, Johnson DE: Partial cystectomy: Can it be incorporated into an integrated program? *Urology* 1983;**12**:115.

Periss JA, Waterhouse K, Cole AT: Complications of partial cystectomy in patients with high grade bladder carcinoma. *J Urol* 1977;**118**:761.

Pinsky CM et al: Intravesical administration of bacillus Calmette-Guérin in patients with recurrent superficial carcinoma of the urinary bladder: Report of a prospective, randomized trial. *Cancer Treat Rep* 1985;**69**:47.

Purtilo DT et al: Familial urinary bladder cancer. *Semin Oncol* 1979;**6**:254.

Resnick MI, Kursh ED: Transurethral ultrasonograpy in bladder cancer. *J Urol* 1986;**135**:253.

Resnick MI, O'Conor VJ Jr: Segmental resection for carcinoma of the bladder: Review of 102 patients. *J Urol* 1973;**109**:1007.

Rider WD, Evans DH: Radiotherapy in the treatment of recurrent bladder cancer. *Br J Urol* 1976;**48**:595.

Sandberg AA: Chromosome studies in bladder cancer. Pages 127–141 in: *Carcinoma of the Bladder.* Connolly JG (editor). Raven, 1981.

Schellhammer PF, Ladaga LE, Fillion MB: Bacillus Calmette-Guérin for superficial transitional cell carcinoma of bladder. *J Urol* 1986;**135**:261.

Shipley WU, Rose MA: Bladder cancer: The selection of patients for treatment by full-dose irradiation. *Cancer* 1985;**55**:2278.

Silverberg E: Cancer statistics, 1981. *CA* 1981;**31**:13.

Soloway MS: Treatment of superficial bladder cancer with intravesical mitomycin C: Analysis of immediate and long-term response in 70 patients. *J Urol* 1985;**134**:1107.

Stein BS et al: Specific red cell adherence: Immunologic evaluation of random mucosal biopsies in carcinoma of the bladder. *J Urol* 1981;**126**:37.

Sternberg CN et al: Preliminary results of M-VAC (methotrexate, vinblastine, doxorubicin, and cisplatin) for transitional cell carcinoma of the urothelium. *J Urol* 1985;**133**:403.

Utz DC, Farrow GM: Management of carcinoma in situ of the bladder: The case for surgical management. *Urol Clin North Am* 1980;**7**:533.

Utz DC et al: A clinicopathologic evaluation of partial cystectomy for carcinoma of the urinary bladder. *Cancer* 1973;**32**:1075.

van der Werf-Messing B: Cancer of the urinary bladder treated by interstitial radium implant. *Int J Radiat Oncol Biol Phys* 1978;**4**:373.

van der Werf-Messing B: Carcinoma of the bladder $T_3N_2M_0$ treated by preoperative irradiation followed by cystectomy: Third report of the Rotterdam Radio-Therapy Institute. *Cancer* 1975;**36**:718.

Veenema RJ et al: Bladder carcinoma treated by direct instillation of thiotepa. *J Urol* 1962;**88:**60.

Veenema RJ et al: Thiotepa bladder instillations: Therapy and prophylaxis for superficial bladder tumors. *J Urol* 1969;**101:**711.

Wallace DM, Bloom HJG: The management of deeply infiltrating (T₃) bladder carcinoma: Controlled trial of radical radiotherapy versus preoperative radiotherapy and radical cystectomy. *Br J Urol* 1976;**48:**587.

Whitmore WF Jr: Integrated irradiation and cystectomy for bladder cancer. *Br J Urol* 1980;**52:**1.

Wigle DT: Bladder cancer: Possible new high-risk occupation. *Lancet* 1977;**2:**83.

Wynder EL, Goldsmith K: The epidemiology of bladder cancer: A second look. *Cancer* 1977;**40:**1246.

Zincke H et al: Pelvic lymphadenectomy and radical cystectomy for transitional cell carcinoma of the bladder with pelvic nodal disease. *Br J Urol* 1985;**57:**156.

Tumors of the Prostate Gland

Armenian HK et al: Relationship between benign prostatic hyperplasia and cancer of the prostate. *Lancet* 1974;**2:**115.

Franks LM: Benign nodular hyperplasia of the prostate: A review. *Ann R Coll Surg Engl* 1954;**14:**92.

Geraghty JT: Treatment of malignant disease of the prostate and bladder. *J Urol* 1922;**7:**33.

Greenwald P et al: Cancer of the prostate among men with benign prostatic hyperplasia. *J Natl Cancer Inst* 1974;**53:**335.

Hodges CV, Wan ST: The relationship between benign prostatic hyperplasia and prostatic carcinoma. Pages 167–173 in: *Benign Prostatic Hypertrophy.* Hinman F Jr (editor). Springer-Verlag, 1983.

Lowsley OS: The development of the human prostate gland with reference to the development of the other structures at the neck of the urinary bladder. *Am J Anat* 1912;**13:**299.

McNeil JE: Regional morphology and pathology of the prostate. *Prostate* 1981;**2:**35.

Benign Prostatic Hyperplasia (Hypertrophy)

Andersen JT, Nordling J: Prostatism. 1. The correlation between symptoms: Cystometric and urodynamic findings. *Scand J Urol Nephrol* 1979;**13:**229.

Cabot AT: The question of castration for enlarged prostate. *Ann Surg* 1896;**24:**265.

Caine M, Perlberg S, Gordon R: The treatment of benign prostatic hypertrophy with flutamide (SCH 13521): A placebo-controlled study. *J Urol* 1975;**114:**564.

Caine M, Perlberg S, Meretyk S: A placebo-controlled double-blind study of the effect of phenoxybenzamine in benign prostatic obstruction. *Br J Urol* 1978;**50:**551.

Donkervoort TK et al: Megestrol acetate in treatment of benign prostatic hypertrophy. *Urology* 1975;**6:**580.

Geller J et al: Effect of megestrol acetate on uroflow rates in patients with benign prostatic hypertrophy. *Urology* 1979;**14:**467.

Huggins C, Stevens RA: The effect of castration on benign hypertrophy of the prostate in man. *J Urol* 1940;**43:**705.

Lytton B, Emery JM, Harvard BM: The incidence of benign prostatic obstruction. *J Urol* 1968;**99:**639.

Mebust WK, Valk WL: Transurethral prostatectomy. Pages 829–846 in: *Benign Prostatic Hypertrophy.* Hinman F Jr (editor). Springer-Verlag, 1983.

Melchior J et al: Transurethral prostatectomy: Computerized

analysis of 2,223 consecutive cases. *J Urol* 1974;**112:**634.

Melchior J et al: Transurethral prostatectomy in the azotemic patient. *J Urol* 1974;**112:**643.

Neubauer DL: Endocrine and cellular inductive factors in the development of human benign prostatic hypertrophy. Pages 179–192 in: *Benign Prostatic Hypertrophy.* Hinman F Jr (editor). Springer-Verlag, 1983.

Scott WW, Wade JC: Medical treatment of benign nodular prostatic hyperplasia with cyproterone acetate. *J Urol* 1969;**101:**81.

Walsh A et al: Indications for prostatectomy: Mandatory and optional. Pages 771–775 in: *Benign Prostatic Hypertrophy.* Hinman F Jr (editor). Springer-Verlag, 1983.

Walsh PC, Hutchins GM, Ewing LL: Tissue content of dehydrotestosterone in human prostatic hyperplasia is not supranormal. *J Clin Invest* 1983;**72:**1772.

White JW: The results of double castration in hypertrophy of the prostate. *Ann Surg* 1895;**22:**1.

Carcinoma of the Prostate

Bagshaw MA: Radiotherapy of prostatic cancer: Stanford University experience. *Prog Clin Biol Res* 1984;**153:**493.

Bass RB Jr, Barrett DM: Radical retropubic prostatectomy after transurethral prostatic resection. *J Urol* 1980;**124:**495.

Bonar RA: Carcinogenesis in urogenital tissues in genitourinary cancer. In: *Cancer Treatment and Research.* Vol 6. Paulson DF (editor). Martinus Nijhoff, 1982.

Braeckman J, Denis L: The practice and pitfalls of ultrasonography in the lower urinary tract. *Eur Urol* 1983;**9:**193.

Brawn PN et al: Histologic grading study of prostatic adenocarcinoma: The development of a new system and comparison with other methods. A preliminary study. *Cancer* 1982;**49:**525.

Bridges CH et al: Stage A prostatic carcinoma and repeat transurethral resection: A reappraisal 5 years later. *J Urol* 1983;**129:**307.

Broder AC: Carcinoma grading and practical applications. *Arch Pathol* 1926;**2:**376.

Byar DP: Survival of patients with incidentally found microscopic cancer of the prostate: Results of a clinical trial of conservative treatment. *J Urol* 1972;**108:**908.

Byar DP, Mostofi FK, Veterans Administration Cooperative Urological Research Group: Carcinoma of the prostate: Prognostic evaluation of certain pathologic features in 208 radical prostatectomies. *Cancer* 1972;**30:**5.

Catalona WJ, Stein AJ: Accuracy of frozen section detection of lymph node metastases in prostatic carcinoma. *J Urol* 1982;**127:**460.

Clark P, Houghton L: Subcapsular orchidectomy for carcinoma of the prostate. *Br J Urol* 1977;**49:**419.

Cox JD, Stoffel TJ: The significance of needle biopsy after irradiation for stage C adenocarcinoma of the prostate. *Cancer* 1977;**40:**156.

Foti AG et al: The detection of prostatic cancer by solid phase radioimmunoassay of serum prostatic acid phosphatase. *N Engl J Med* 1977;**297:**1357.

Franks LM: Latent carcinoma of the prostate. *J Urol Pathol Bacteriol* 1954;**68:**603.

Freiha FS, Bagshaw MA: Carcinoma of the prostate: Results of postirradiation biopsy. *Prostate* 1984;**5:**19.

Freiha FS, Pistenma DA, Bagshaw MA: Pelvic lymphadenectomy for staging prostatic carcinoma: Is it always necessary? *J Urol* 1979;**122:**176.

Gagnon JD, Moss WT, Stevens KR: Preestrogen breast irradiation for patients with carcinoma of the prostate: A critical review. *J Urol* 1979;**121**:182.

Gleason DF, Mellinger GT: Veterans Administration Cooperative Urologic Research Group: Prediction of prognosis for prostatic adenocarcinoma by combined histological grading and clinical staging. *J Urol* 1974;**111**:58.

Guerriero WG, Carlton CE Jr, Hudgins PT: Combined interstitial and external radiotherapy in the definitive management of carcinoma of the prostate. *Cancer* 1980;**45**:1922.

Hanash KA et al: Carcinoma of the prostate: A 15 year follow-up. *J Urol* 1972;**107**:450.

Herr HW: Complication of pelvic lymphadenectomy and retropubic prostatic ^{125}I implantation. *Urology* 1979; **14**:226.

Hirayama T: Epidemiology of prostate cancer with special reference to the role of diet. *Natl Cancer Inst Monogr* 1979;**53**:149.

Jacobs SC: Spread of prostatic cancer to bone. *Urology* 1983;**21**:337.

Jewett HJ: The present status of radical prostatectomy for stages A and B prostatic cancer. *Urol Clin North Am* 1975;**2**:105.

Johnson DE, von Eschenbach AC: Prostatic carcinoma: A trilogy of expressions. *South Med J* 1980;**73**:1304.

Johnson DE, von Eschenbach AC: Role of lymphangiography and pelvic lymphadenectomy in staging prostatic carcinoma. *J Urol* 1981;**17(Suppl)**:66.

Jordan WP Jr, Blackard CE, Byar DP: Reconsideration of orchiectomy in the treatment of advanced prostatic carcinoma. *South Med J* 1977;**70**:1411.

Kuriyama M et al: Multiple marker evaluation in human prostate cancer with the use of tissue-specific antigens. *J Natl Cancer Inst* 1982;**68**:99.

Labrie F et al: New approach in the treatment of prostate cancer: Complete instead of partial withdrawal of androgens. *Prostate* 1983;**4**:579.

Lee F et al: Transrectal ultrasound in the diagnosis of prostate carcinoma: Location, echogenicity, histopathology, staging. *Prostate* 1985;**7**:117.

Leuprolide Study Group: Leuprolide versus diethylstilbestrol for metastatic prostate cancer. *N Engl J Med* 1984; **311**:1281.

Logothetis CJ et al: Doxorubicin, mitomycin C, and 5-fluorouracil (DMF) in the treatment of metastatic hormonal-refractory adenocarcinoma of the prostate, with a note on the staging of metastatic cancer. *J Clin Oncol* 1983;**1**:368.

McLaughlin AP et al: Prostatic carcinoma: Incidence and location of unsuspected lymphatic metastases. *J Urol* 1976;**115**:89.

McMillen SM, Wettlaufer JN: The role of repeat transurethral biopsy in stage A carcinoma of the prostate. *J Urol* 1976;**116**:759.

Middleton RG, Smith JA Jr: Radical prostatectomy for stage B2 prostatic cancer. *J Urol* 1982;**127**:702.

Mostofi FK: Grading of prostatic carcinoma. *Cancer Chemother Res* 1975;**59**:111.

Murphy GP: Chemotherapy of advanced prostatic cancer. *Rev Surg* 1977;**34**:75.

Nesbitt RM, Baum WC: Endocrine control of prostatic carcinoma. *JAMA* 1950;**143**:1317.

Nichols RT, Barry JM, Hodges CV: The morbidity of radical prostatectomy for multifocal stage I prostatic adenocarcinoma. *J Urol* 1977;**117**:83.

Paulson DF, Urologic Oncology Research Group: The impact of current staging procedures in assessing disease extent of prostatic carcinoma. *J Urol* 1979;**121**:300.

Rich AR: On the frequency of occurrence of occult carcinoma of the prostate. *J Urol* 1935;**33**:215.

Rotkin ID: Epidemiologic studies in prostatic cancer. *Cancer Treat Rep* 1977;**61**:173.

Schroeder FH, Belt E: Carcinoma of the prostate: A study of 213 patients with stage C tumors treated by total perineal prostatectomy. *J Urol* 1975;**114**:257.

Seamonds B et al: Evaluation of prostate-specific antigen and prostatic acid phosphatase as prostate cancer markers. *Urology* 1986;**28**:472.

Sheldon CA et al: Incidental carcinoma of the prostate: A review of the literature and critical appraisal of classification. *J Urol* 1980;**124**:626.

Veterans Administration Cooperative Urological Research Group: Carcinoma of the prostate: A continuing cooperative study. *J Urol* 1964;**91**:590.

Walsh PC: Physiologic basis for hormonal therapy in carcinoma of the prostate. *Urol Clin North Am* 1975;**2**:125.

Walsh PC, Donker PJ: Impotence following radical prostatectomy. *J Urol* 1982;**128**:492.

Walsh PC, Jewett HJ: Radical surgery for prostatic cancer. *Cancer* 1980;**45(Suppl 7)**:1906.

Whitmore WF Jr: Hormone therapy in prostatic cancer. *Am J Med* 1956;**21**:697.

Whitmore WF Jr: The natural history of prostatic cancer. *Cancer* 1973;**32**:1104.

Whitmore WF Jr, Hilaris B, Grabstald H: Retropubic implantation of iodine 125 in the treatment of prostatic cancer. *J Urol* 1972;**109**:918.

Winkelstein W Jr, Ernster VL: Epidemiology and etiology in prostatic cancer. Page 1 in: *Prostatic Cancer*. Murphy GP (editor). PSG Publishing, 1979.

Zincke H et al: Radical retropubic prostatectomy and pelvic lymphadenectomy for high-stage cancer of the prostate. *Cancer* 1981;**47**:1901.

Tumors of the Prostatic Ducts

Dube VE, Farrow GM, Greene LF: Prostatic adenocarcinoma of ductal origin. *Cancer* 1973;**32**:402.

Greene LF et al: Prostatic adenocarcinoma of ductal origin. *J Urol* 1979;**121**:303.

Tumors of the Seminal Vesicles

Lathem JE: Carcinoma of seminal vesicle. *South Med J* 1975;**68**:473.

Tumors of the Urethra

Bracken RB, Henry R, Ordonez N: Primary carcinoma of the male urethra. *South Med J* 1980;**73**:1003.

Grabstald H et al: Cancer of the female urethra. *JAMA* 1966;**197**:835.

Johnson DE, O'Connell JR: Primary carcinoma of the female urethra. *Urology* 1983;**12**:115.

Johnson DE, O'Connell JR, Delclos L: Cancer of the urethra. In: *Principles and Management of Urologic Cancer*, 2nd ed. Javadpour N (editor). Williams & Wilkins, 1983.

Johnson DE et al: Rotational skin flaps to cover wound defect in groin. *Urology* 1975;**6**:461.

Marshall FC, Uson AC, Melicow MM: Neoplasms and caruncles of the female urethra. *Surg Gynecol Obstet* 1960;**110**:723.

Ray B, Guinan PD: Primary carcinoma of the urethra. In: *Principles and Management of Urologic Cancer*. Javadpour N (editor). Williams & Wilkins, 1979.

Shuttleworth KED, Lloyd-Davies RW: Radical resection for tumors invading the posterior urethra. *Br J Urol* 1969; **41**:739.

Zeigerman JH, Gordon SF: Cancer of the female urethra: A curable disease. *Obstet Gynecol* 1970;**36**:785.

Tumors of the Spermatic Cord & Paratesticular Tissues

Adrien M, Grabstald H, Whitmore WF Jr: Malignant tumors of the spermatic cord. *Cancer* 1969;**23**:525.

Banowsky LH, Schultz GN: Sarcoma of the spermatic cord and tunica: Review of the literature, case report and discussion of the role of retroperitoneal lymph node dissection. *J Urol* 1970;**103**:628.

Johnson DE, Harris JD, Ayala AG: Liposarcoma of spermatic cord *Urology* 1978;**11**:190.

Johnson DE, McHugh T, Jaffe N: Paratesticular rhabdomyosarcoma in childhood. *J Urol* 1982;**128**:1275.

Raney RB Jr et al: Paratesticular rhabdomyosarcoma in childhood. *Cancer* 1978;**42**:729.

Wertzner S: Leiomyosarcoma of the spermatic cord and uteroperitoneal lymph node dissection. *Am Surg* 1973; **39**:352.

Tumors of the Testis

Babaian RJ, Johnson DE: Management of stage I and II nonseminomatous germ cell tumors of the testis. *Cancer* 1980;**45**:1775.

Ball D, Barrett A, Peckham MJ: The management of metastatic seminoma testis. *Cancer* 1982;**50**:2289.

Belville WD et al: The liver scan in urologic oncology. *J Urol* 1980;**123**:901.

Berthelsen JG et al: Screening for carcinoma in situ of the contralateral testis in patients with germinal testicular cancer. *Br Med J* 1982;**285**:1683.

Boden G, Gibb R: Radiotherapy in testicular neoplasms. *Lancet* 1951;**2**:1195.

Borski AA: Diagnosis, staging and natural history of testicular tumor. *Cancer* 1973;**32**:1202.

Bowman WP et al: Isolated testicular relapse in acute lymphocytic leukemia of childhood: Categories and influence on survival. *J Clin Oncol* 1984;**2**:924.

Bracken RB et al: The role of surgery following chemotherapy in stage III germ cell neoplasms. *J Urol* 1983;**129**:39.

Braunstein GD et al: Ectopic production of human chorionic gonadotropin by neoplasms. *Ann Intern Med* 1973;**78**:39.

Caldwell WL: Why retroperitoneal lymphadenectomy for testicular tumors? *J Urol* 1978;**119**:754.

Cancer Facts and Figures, 1979, American Cancer Society, 1978.

Collins DH, Pugh RCB: Classification and frequency of testicular tumors. *Br J Urol* 1964;**36(Suppl)**:1.

Dixon FH, Moore RA: *Tumors of the Male Sex Organs,* Armed Forces Institute of Pathology, 1952.

Donohue JP, Rowland RG: The role of surgery in advanced testicular cancer. *Cancer* 1984;**54**:2716.

Donohue JP, Einhorn LH, Williams SD: Cytoreductive surgery for metastatic testis cancer: Considerations of timing and extent. *J Urol* 1980;**123**:876.

Donohue JP, Einhorn LH, Williams SD: Is adjuvant chemotherapy following retroperitoneal lymph node dissection for nonseminomatous testicular cancer necessary? *Urol Clin North Am* 1980;**7**:747.

Donohue JP, Zachary JM, Maynard BR: Distribution of total metastases in nonseminomatous testis cancer. *J Urol* 1982;**128**:315.

Donohue JP et al: Cytoreductive surgery for metastatic testicular cancer: Analysis of retroperitoneal masses after chemotherapy. *J Urol* 1982;**127**:1111.

Forrest JB, Sabio H, Howards SS: Testicular relapse in acute childhood leukemia. *J Surg Oncol* 1982;**21**:132.

Freiha FS et al: The extent of surgery after chemotherapy for advanced germ cell tumors. *J Urol* 1984;**132**:915.

Friedman EL et al: Therapeutic guidelines and results in advanced seminoma. *J Clin Oncol* 1985;**3**:1325.

Friedman NB, Moore RA: Tumors of the testis: A report of 922 cases. *Milit Med* 1946;**99**:573.

Gallager HS: Pathology of testicular and peritesticular neoplasms. Pages 1–30 in: *Testicular Tumors,* 2nd ed. Johnson DE (editor). Med Exam Pub, 1976.

Hoskin P et al: Prognostic factors in stage I nonseminomatous germ-cell testicular tumors managed by orchiectomy and surveillance: Implications for adjuvant chemotherapy. *J Clin Oncol* 1986;**4**:1031.

Hudson MM et al: Diagnostic value of surgical testicular biopsy after therapy for acute lymphocytic leukemia. *J Pediatr* 1985;**107**:50.

Javadpour N: Tumor markers in urologic cancer. *Urology* 1980;**16**:127.

Javadpour N, Moley J: Alternative to retroperitoneal lymphadenectomy with preservation of ejaculation and fertility in stage I nonseminomatous testicular cancer: A prospective study. *Cancer* 1985;**55**:1604.

Javadpour N et al: The role of radioimmunodetection in the management of testicular cancer. *JAMA* 1981;**246**:45.

Jeppsson A et al: A clinical evaluation of serum placental alkaline phosphatase in seminoma patients. *Br J Urol* 1983;**55**:73.

Johnson DE: Clinical staging. Pages 131–144 in: *Testis Tumors.* Donohue JP (editor). Williams & Wilkins, 1983.

Johnson DE: Epidemiology. Pages 37–46 in: *Testicular Tumors,* 2nd ed. Johnson DE (editor). Med Exam Pub, 1976.

Johnson DE, Ayala AG: Secondary neoplasms of the testis. Pages 249–260 in: *Testicular Tumors,* 2nd ed. Johnson DE (editor). Med Exam Pub, 1976.

Johnson DE, Bracken RB, Blight EM: Prognosis for pathologic stage I nonseminomatous germ cell tumors of the testis managed by retroperitoneal lymphadenectomy. *J Urol* 1976;**116**:63.

Johnson DE, Butler JJ: Malignant lymphoma of the testis. Pages 234–248 in: *Testicular Tumors,* 2nd ed. Johnson DE (editor). Med Exam Pub, 1976.

Johnson DE, Gomez JJ, Ayala AG: Anaplastic seminoma. *J Urol* 1975;**114**:80.

Johnson DE et al: Metastases from testicular carcinoma: Study of 78 autopsied cases. *Urology* 1976;**8**:234.

Johnson DE et al: Surveillance alone for patients with clinical stage I nonseminomatous germ cell tumors of the testis: Preliminary results. *J Urol* 1984;**131**:491.

Kaswick JA, Bloomberg SD, Skinner DG: Radical retroperitoneal lymph node dissection: How effective is removal of all retroperitoneal nodes? *J Urol* 1976;**115**:70.

Kim I, Young RH, Scully RE: Leydig cell tumors of the testis: A clinicopathological analysis of 40 cases and review of the literature. *Am J Surg Pathol* 1985;**9**:177.

Klein FA, Melamed MR, Whitmore WF Jr: Intratubular malignant germ cells (carcinoma in situ) accompanying invasive testicular germ cell tumors. *J Urol* 1985;**133**:413.

Kreuser ED et al: Bulky germinal tumors: Comparison of different induction regimens and significance of residual disease. *Eur Urol* 1985;**11**:163.

Lange PH et al: Is SP-1 a marker for testicular cancer? *Urology* 1980;**15**:251.

Li SP, Connelly RR, Myers M: Improved survival rates among testicular cancer patients in the US. *JAMA* 1982;**247**:825.

Logothetis CJ et al: The growing teratoma syndrome. *Cancer* 1982;**50:**1629.

Logothetis CJ et al: Improved survival with cyclic chemotherapy for nonseminomatous germ cell tumors of the testis. *J Clin Oncol* 1985;**3:**326.

Logothetis CJ et al: Primary chemotherapy followed by a selective retroperitoneal lymphadenectomy in the management of clinical stage II testicular carcinoma: A preliminary report. *J Urol* 1985;**134:**1127.

Melicow MM: New British classification of testicular tumors: A correlation, analysis and critique. *J Urol* 1965;**94:**64.

Mills PK, Newell GR, Johnson DE: Familial patterns of testicular cancer. *Urology* 1984;**24:**1.

Moriyama N et al: Vascular invasion as a prognosticator of metastatic disease in nonseminomatous germ cell tumors of the testis: Importance in "surveillance only" protocols. *Cancer* 1985;**56:**2492.

Mostofi SK: Testicular tumors: Epidemiologic, etiologic, and pathologic features. *Cancer* 1973;**32:**1186.

Mostofi SK, Price EB Jr: *Tumors of the Male Genital System.* Armed Forces Institute of Pathology, 1973.

Mostofi SK, Sobin LH: *International Histologic Classification of Tumors. No. 16. Histological Typing of Testis Tumors.* World Health Organization, 1977.

Müller J et al: Cryptorchidism and testis cancer: Atypical infantile germ cells followed by carcinoma in situ and invasive carcinoma in adulthood. *Cancer* 1984;**54:**629.

Patterson AHG, Peckham MJ, McCready VR: Value of gallium-scanning in seminoma of the testis. *Br Med J* 1977;**1:**1118.

Patton JF, Mallis N: Tumors of the testis. *J Urol* 1959;**81:**457.

Pearson JC: Endocrinology of testicular neoplasms. *Urology* 1981;**17:**119.

Peckham MJ, Hendry WF: Clinical stage II nonseminomatous germ cell testicular tumours: Results of management by primary chemotherapy. *Br J Urol* 1985;**57:**763.

Pierce GB: Ultrastructure of human testicular cancer. *Cancer* 1966;**19:**1963.

Pizzocaro G, Monfardini S: No adjuvant chemotherapy in selected patients with pathologic stage II nonseminomatous germ cell tumors of the testis. *J Urol* 1984;**131:**677.

Pizzocaro G, Salvioni R, Zanoni F: Unilateral lymphadenectomy in intraoperative stage I nonseminomatous germinal testis cancer. *J Urol* 1985;**134:**485.

Pizzocaro G et al: Surveillance or lymph node dissection in clinical stage I nonseminomatous germinal testis cancer? *Br J Urol* 1985;**57:**759.

Pui CH et al: Elective testicular biopsy during chemotherapy for childhood leukaemia is of no clinical value. *Lancet* 1985;**2:**410.

Richie JP, Garnick MB: Limited retroperitoneal lymphadenectomy for patients with clinical stage I testicular tumor. (Abstract.) *Proc Am Soc Clin Oncol* 1985;**4:**110.

Rosai J, Silber I, Khodadoust K: Spermatocytic seminoma. 1. Clinicopathologic study of six cases and review of the literature. *Cancer* 1969;**24:**92.

Rosai J, Khodadoust K, Silber I: Spermatocytic seminoma. 2. Ultrastructural study. *Cancer* 1969;**24:**103.

Rouviere H: *Anatomie de lymphatiques de l'homme.* Maison et Cie, 1932.

Safer ML et al: Lymphangiographic accuracy in the staging of testicular tumors. *Cancer* 1975;**35:**1603.

Samuels ML et al: Combination chemotherapy in germinal tumors. *Cancer Treat Rev* 1976;**3:**185.

Scardino PT: Adjuvant chemotherapy is of value following retroperitoneal lymph node dissection for nonseminomatous testicular tumors. *Urol Clin North Am* 1980;**7:**735.

Schover LR, von Eschenbach AC: Sexual and marital relationships after treatment for nonseminomatous testicular cancer. *Urology* 1985;**25:**251.

Sogani PC et al: Orchiectomy alone in the treatment of clinical stage I nonseminomatous germ cell tumor of the testis. *J Clin Oncol* 1984;**2:**267.

Stevens LC: Origin of testicular teratoma from primordial germ cells in mice. *J Natl Cancer Inst* 1967;**138:**549.

Stoter G et al: Five-year survival of patients with disseminated nonseminomatous testicular cancer treated with cisplatin, vinblastine, and bleomycin. *Cancer* 1984;**54:**1521.

Sussman EB et al: Malignant lymphoma of the testis: A clinical pathologic study of 37 cases. *J Urol* 1977;**17:**1004.

Swanson DA: Benefits of early diagnosis of testis cancer. *Cancer Bull* 1985;**37:**291.

Swartz DA, Johnson DE, Hussey DH: Should an elevated human chorionic gonadotropin titer alter therapy for seminoma? *J Urol* 1984;**131:**63.

Tait D et al: Postchemotherapy surgery in advanced nonseminomatous germ-cell testicular tumours: The significance of histology with particular reference to differentiated (mature) teratoma. *Br J Cancer* 1984;**50:**601.

Talerman A: The incidence of yolk sac tumor (endodermal sinus tumor) elements in germ cell tumors of the testis in adults. *Cancer* 1975;**33:**211.

Talerman A, Fu YS, Okagaki T: Spermatocytic seminoma: Ultrastructural and microspectrophotometric observations. *Lab Invest* 1984;**51:**343.

Teilum G: The concept of endodermal sinus (yolk sac) tumor. *Scand J Immunol* 1978;**8(Suppl):**75.

Templeton AC: Testicular neoplasms in Ugandan Africans. *Afr J Med Sci* 1972;**3:**157.

Thomas GM: Controversies in the management of testicular seminoma. *Cancer* 1985;**55(9 Suppl):**2296.

Thomas GM et al: Seminoma of the testis: Results of treatment and patterns of failure after radiation therapy. *Int J Radiat Oncol Biol Phys* 1982;**8:**165.

Turner RR, Colby TV, MacKintosh FR: Testicular lymphomas: A clinical pathologic study of 35 cases. *Cancer* 1981;**48:**2095.

Tyrrell CJ, Peckham MJ: The response of lymph node metastases of testicular teratoma to radiation therapy. *Br J Urol* 1976;**48:**363.

Valvo JR, Wilson P, Frank IN: Ultrasonic examination of scrotum: Review of 108 cases. *Urology* 1983;**22:**78.

Vugrin D, Whitmore WF Jr: The role of chemotherapy and surgery in the treatment of retroperitoneal metastases in advanced nonseminomatous testis cancer. *Cancer* 1985;**55:**1874.

Vugrin D, Whitmore WF Jr: The VAB-6 regimen in the treatment of metastatic seminoma. *Cancer* 1984;**53:**2422.

Vugrin D et al: Adjuvant chemotherapy in non-seminomatous testis cancer: "Mini-VAB" regimen. Long-term follow-up. *J Urol* 1981;**126:**49.

Vugrin D et al: VAB-6 combination chemotherapy in resected II-B testicular cancer. *Cancer* 1983;**51:**5.

Waldmann TA, McIntire KR: The use of radioimmunoassay for alpha-fetoprotein in the diagnosis of malignancy. *Cancer* 1974;**34:**1510.

Wallace S et al: Lymphangiograms: Their diagnostic and therapeutic potential. *Radiology* 1961;**76:**179.

Whitmore WF Jr: Surgical treatment of clinical stage I nonseminomatous germ cell tumors of the testis. *Cancer*

Treat Rep 1982;**66**:5.

Williams SD, Einhorn LH: Clinical stage I testis tumor: The medical oncologist's view. *Cancer Treat Rep* 1982;**66**:15.

Willis RA: *Pathology of Tumors*. Appleton-Century-Crofts, 1967.

Extragonadal Germ Cell Tumors

Buskirk SJ et al: Primary retroperitoneal seminomas. *Cancer* 1982;**49**:1934.

Israel A et al: The results of chemotherapy for extragonadal germ-cell tumors in the cisplatin era: The Memorial Sloan-Kettering Cancer Center experience (1975 to 1982). *J Clin Oncol* 1985;**3**:1073.

Jain KK et al: The treatment of extragonadal seminoma. *J Clin Oncol* 1984;**2**:820.

Logothetis CJ et al: Chemotherapy of extragonadal germ cell tumors. *J Clin Oncol* 1985;**3**:316.

Luna MA: Extragonadal germ cell tumors. Pages 261–265 in: *Testicular Tumors*, 2nd ed. Johnson DE (editor). Med Exam Pub, 1976.

Meares EM Jr, Briggs EM: Occult seminoma masquerading as primary extragonadal germinal neoplasms. *Cancer* 1972;**30**:300.

Tumors of the Epididymis

Farrell MA, Donnelly BJ: Malignant smooth muscle tumors of the epididymis. *J Urol* 1980;**124**:151.

Mostofi FK, Price EB Jr: *Tumors of the Male Genital System*. Armed Forces Institute of Pathology, 1973.

Tumors of the Penis

Cabanas RM: An approach for the treatment of penile carcinoma. *Cancer* 1977;**39**:456.

Cartwright RA, Sinson JD: Carcinoma of the penis and cervix. *Lancet* 1980;**1**:97.

Delclos L: Interstitial irradiation of the penis. Pages 219–225 in: *Genitourinary Tumors: Fundamental Principles and Surgical Techniques*. Johnson DE, Boileau MA (editors). Grune & Stratton, 1982.

Duncan W, Jackson SM: The treatment of early cancer of the penis with megavoltage x-rays. *Clin Radiol* 1972;**23**:246.

Jackson SM: The treatment of carcinoma of the penis. *Br J Surg* 1966;**53**:33.

Johnson DE, Ames FC: *Groin Dissection*. Doody DJ (editor). Year Book, 1985.

Johnson DE, Lo RK: Complications of groin dissection in penile cancer: Experience with 101 lymphadenectomies. *Urology* 1984;**24**:312.

Johnson DE, Lo RK: Management of regional lymph nodes in penile carcinoma: Five-year results following therapeutic groin dissections. *Urology* 1984;**24**:308.

Johnson DE et al: Verrucous carcinoma of the penis. *J Urol* 1985;**133**:216.

Persky L: Epidemiology of the penis. Pages 97–109 in: *Tumors of the Male Genital System*. Grundmann E, Vahlensieck W (editors). Springer, 1977.

Puras A, Gonzalez-Flores B, Rodriguez R: Treatment of carcinoma of the penis. Pages 143–152 in: *Proceedings of the Kimbrough Urological Seminar*. Stevenson HG (editor). Brodock Press, 1977.

Reddy DG, Baruah IKSM: Carcinogenic action of human smegma. *Arch Pathol* 1963;**75**:414.

Tumors of the Scrotum

McDonald MW: Carcinoma of the scrotum. *Urology* 1982;**19**:269.

Ray B, Whitmore WF Jr: Experience with carcinoma of the scrotum. *J Urol* 1977;**117**:741.

Retroperitoneal Extrarenal Tumors

Binder SC, Katz B, Sheridan B: Reproperitoneal liposarcoma. *Ann Surg* 1978;**187**:257.

Damascelli B et al: Angiography of retroperitoneal tumors: A review. *Am J Roentgenol* 1975;**124**:565.

Duncan RE, Evans AT: Diagnosis of primary retroperitoneal tumors. *J Urol* 1977;**117**:19.

Kinne DW et al: Treatment of primary and recurrent retroperitoneal liposarcoma: Twenty-five year experience at Memorial Hospital. *Cancer* 1973;**31**:53.

Polsky MS et al: Retrovesical liposarcoma. *Urology* 1974;**3**:226.

Sadoughi N et al: Retroperitoneal xanthogranuloma. *Urology* 1973;**1**:470.

Smith EH, Bartum RJ Jr: Ultrasonic evaluation of pararenal masses. *JAMA* 1975;**231**:51.

Stephens DH et al: Computed tomography of the retroperitoneal space. *Radiol Clin North Am* 1977;**15**:377.

Stephens DH et al: Diagnosis and evaluation of retroperitoneal tumors by computed tomography. *AJR* 1977;**129**:395.

CHEMOTHERAPY OF UROLOGIC MALIGNANT DISEASES

General References

Bagshawe KD (editor): *Medical Oncology*. Blackwell, 1975.

Bodansky O: *Biochemistry of Human Cancer*. Academic Press, 1975.

Brodsky I, Kahn SB, Moyer JH: *Cancer Chemotherapy: Basic and Clinical Applications*. (Twenty-Second Hahnemann Symposium.) Grune & Stratton, 1972.

Carter SK et al: *Chemotherapy of Cancer*. Wiley, 1977.

Cline MJ, Haskell CM III: *Cancer Chemotherapy*, 3rd ed. Saunders, 1980.

Criss WE, Ono T, Sabine JR (editors): *Control Mechanisms in Cancer*. Raven Press, 1976.

DeVita VT Jr, Hellman S, Rosenberg S: *Cancer: Principles and Practice of Oncology*. Lippincott, 1982.

Dunphy JE: On caring for the patient with cancer. *N Engl J Med* 1976;**295**:313.

Haskell CM: *Cancer Treatment*. Saunders, 1980.

Holland JF, Frei E III (editors): *Cancer Medicine*. Lea & Febiger, 1973.

Horton J, Hill GJ II (editors): *Clinical Oncology*. Saunders, 1977.

Jones SE, Salmon SE (editors): *Adjuvant Therapy of Cancer II*. Grune & Stratton, 1977.

Krakoff IH: Cancer chemotherapeutic agents. *CA* 1977;**27**:130.

Krakoff IH (editor): Symposium on medical aspects of cancer. *Med Clin North Am* 1971;**55**:525. [Entire issue.]

Lawrence W Jr, Terz JJ (editors): *Cancer Management*. Grune & Stratton, 1977.

Moss WT, Brand WN, Battifora H: *Radiation Oncology*. Mosby, 1979.

Munster AM (editor): *Surgical Immunology*. Grune & Stratton, 1976.

Nealon TF Jr (editor): *Management of the Patient With Cancer*, 2nd ed. Saunders, 1976.

Noskell CM: *Cancer Treatment*. Saunders, 1980.

Salmon SE: Cancer chemotherapy. Chap 45, pp 477–513, in: *Review of Medical Pharmacology*, 7th ed. Lange, 1980.

Salmon SE, Jones SE (editors): *Adjuvant Therapy of Cancer*. Vol 3. Grune & Stratton, 1981.

Van Der Veer LD Jr, Balini JA: Chemotherapy of gastrointestinal malignancy. *Am J Gastroenterol* 1980;**74**:40.

Veidenheimer MC (editor): Symposium on the care and treatment of the cancer patient. *Surg Clin North Am* 1967;**47**:557.

Etiologic Factors in Tumor Formation

Allen DW et al: Viruses and human cancer. *N Engl J Med* 1972;**286**:70.

American Cancer Society: Second National Conference on Diet, Nutrition, and Cancer. *Cancer* 1986;**59(Suppl)**: 1791.

Bast RC Jr et al: BCG and cancer. (2 parts.) *N Engl J Med* 1974;**290**:1413.

Bootwell R: Tumor promoters in human carcinogenesis. Pages 16–27 in: *Important Advances in Oncology 1985*. DeVita VT, Hellman S, Rosenberg SA (editors). Lippincott, 1985.

Durack DT: Opportunistic infections and Kaposi's sarcoma in homosexual men. (Editorial.) *N Engl J Med* 1981; **305**:1465.

Farber E: Chemical carcinogenesis. *N Engl J Med* 1981; **305**:1379.

Gallo RC: RNA-dependent DNA polymerase in viruses and cells. *Blood* 1972;**39**:117.

Gofman JW, Tamplin AR: Radiation, cancer, and environmental health. *Hosp Pract* (Oct) 1970;**5**:91.

Greenwald P, Ershow AG, Novelli WD (editors): *Cancer Diet, and Nutrition: A Comprehensive Sourcebook*. Who's Who, Inc., 1985.

Grobstein C (editor): *Diet, Nutrition and Cancer*. National Academy Press, 1982.

Ryser HJP: Chemical carcinogenesis. *N Engl J Med* 1971;**285**:721.

Smith RT: Possibilities and problems of immunologic intervention in cancer. *N Engl J Med* 1972;**287**:439.

Zamcheck N et al: Immunologic evaluation of human digestive tract cancer: Carcinoembryonic antigens. *N Engl J Med* 1972;**286**:83.

AIDS

Allen JR: Epidemiology of the acquired immunodeficiency syndrome (AIDS) in the United States. *Semin Oncol* 1984;**11**:4.

Gallo RC et al: T cell malignancies and human T cell leukemia virus. *Semin Oncol* 1984;**11**:12.

Volberding P: Therapy of Kaposi's sarcoma in AIDS. *Semin Oncol* 1984;**11**:60.

Oncogenes

Gordon H: Oncogenes. *Mayo Clin Proc* 1985;**60**:697.

Green AR, Wyke JA: Anti-oncogenes: A subset of regulatory genes involved in carcinogenesis? *Lancet* 1985;**2**:475.

Solitary Metastasis

Adkins PC et al: Thoracotomy on the patient with previous malignancy: Metastasis or new primary? *J Thorac Cardiovasc Surg* 1968;**56**:361.

Rubin P, Green J: *Solitary Metastases*. Thomas, 1968.

Immunotherapy

Beutler B, Cerami A: Cachectin and tumour necrosis factor as two sides of the same biological coin. *Nature* 1986;**320**:584.

Gutterman JU et al: Leukocyte interferon-induced tumor regression in human metastatic breast cancer, multiple myeloma, and malignant lymphoma. *Ann Intern Med* 1980;**93**:399.

Lotze MT et al: Monoclonal antibody imaging of human melanoma: Radioimmunodetection by subcutaneous or systemic injection. *Ann Surg* 1986;**204**:223.

Munster AM (editor): *Surgical Immunology*. Grune & Stratton, 1976.

Pinsky CM et al: Biological response modifiers. *Semin Oncol* 1986;**13**:131 [Entire issue.].

Rosenberg SA, Speiss P, La Freniere R: A new approach to the adoptive immunotherapy of cancer with tumor-infiltrating lymphocytes. *Science* 1986;**233**:1318.

Rosenberg SA et al: Observations on the systemic administration of autologous lymphokine-activated killer cells and recombinant interleukin-2 to patients with metastatic cancer. *N Engl J Med* 1985;**313**:1485.

Smith RT: Possibilities and problems of immunologic intervention in cancer. *N Engl J Med* 1972;**287**:437.

Terry WD (editor): Symposium on immunotherapy in malignant disease. *Med Clin North Am* 1976;**60**:387. [Entire issue.]

Terry WD, Windhorst D (editors): *Immunotherapy of Cancer: Present Status of Trials in Man*. Vol 6 of: *Progress in Cancer Research and Therapy*. Raven Press, 1978. [Entire volume.]

Vadhan-Raj S et al: Phase I trial of recombinant interferon gamma in cancer patients. *J Clin Oncol* 1986;**4**:137.

Chemotherapy

Alberts DS: In-vitro clonogenic assay for predicting response of ovarian cancer to chemotherapy. *Lancet* 1980;**2**:340.

Bergevin PR, Tormey DC, Blom J: Guide to the use of cancer chemotherapeutic agents. *Mod Treat* 1972;**9**:185.

Bergsagel DE: New perspectives in chemotherapy: Focus on Novantrone. *Semin Oncol* 1984;**11(Suppl 1)**:1. [Entire issue.]

Borgmann V et al: Treatment of prostatic cancer with LH-RH analogues. *Prostate* 1983;**4**:553.

Bruce WR et al: Comparison of the sensitivity of normal hematopoietic and transplanted lymphoma colony-forming cells to chemotherapeutic agents administered in vivo. *J Natl Cancer Inst* 1966;**37**:233.

The choice of therapy in the treatment of malignancy. *Med Lett Drugs Ther* 1973;**15**:9.

DeVita VT: Cell kinetics and the chemotherapy of cancer. *Cancer Chemother Rep* 1971;**2**:23.

DeVita VT, Schein PS: The use of drugs in combination for the treatment of cancer. *N Engl J Med* 1973;**288**:988.

Holland JF: Karnofsky Memorial Lecture: Breaking the cure barrier. *J Clin Oncol* 1983;**1**:75.

Labrie F et al: New approach in the treatment of prostate cancer: Complete instead of partial withdrawal of androgens. *Prostate* 1983;**4**:579.

Livingston RB, Carter SK: *Single Agents in Cancer Chemotherapy*. Plenum Press, 1970.

Phillips NC, Lauper RD: Review of etoposide. *Clin Pharm* 1983;**2**:112.

Pinedo HM, Chabner BA (editors): *Cancer Chemotherapy Annual*. Elsevier, 1984.

Rall DP (chairman): Design of more selective antitumor agents. *Cancer Res* 1969;**29**:2384.

Salmon SE (editor): Clinical correlation of drug sensitivity. Pages 265–285 in: *Cloning of Human Tumor Stem-Cells*. Liss, 1980.

Salmon SE et al: Quantitation of differential sensitivities of human-tumor stem-cells to anti-cancer drugs. *N Engl J Med* 1978;**298:**1231.

Santen RJ et al: Long-term effects of administration of a gonadotropin-releasing hormone superagonist analog in men with prostatic carcinoma. *J Clin Endocrinol Metab* 1984;**58:**397.

Schabel FM: The use of tumor growth kinetics in planning "curative" chemotherapy of advanced solid tumors. *Cancer Res* 1969;**29:**2384.

Skipper HE et al: Implications of biochemical, cytokinetic, pharmacologic, and toxicologic relationships in the design of optimal therapeutic schedules. *Cancer Chemother Rep* 1970;**54:**431.

Spiegel RJ: Intron A (interferon α-2b): Clinical overview and future directions. *Semin Oncol* 1986;**13(Suppl 2):**89.

Valeriote FA, Edelstein MB: The role of cell kinetics in cancer chemotherapy. *Semin Oncol* 1977;**4:**217.

Surgical Adjuvant Chemotherapy

Bonnadonna G et al: Combination chemotherapy as an adjuvant treatment in operable breast cancer. *N Engl J Med* 1976;**294:**405.

Fisher B et al: L-Phenylalanine mustard (L-PAM) in the management of primary breast cancer: A report of early findings. *N Engl J Med* 1975;**292:**117.

Fisher F et al: Surgical adjuvant chemotherapy in cancer of the breast: Results of a decade of cooperative investigation. *Ann Surg* 1968;**168:**337.

Jones SE, Salmon SE (editors): *Adjuvant Therapy of Cancer II.* Grune & Stratton, 1977.

Li MC et al: Chemoprophylaxis for patients with colorectal cancer. *JAMA* 1976;**235:**2825.

Mackman S, Curreri AR, Ansfield FS: Second look operation for colon cacinoma after fluorouracil therapy. *Arch Surg* 1970;**100:**527.

Infusion & Perfusion Therapy

Ansfield FJ et al: Intrahepatic arterial infusion with 5-fluorouracil. *Cancer* 1971;**28:**1147.

Ensminger W et al: Totally implanted drug delivery system for hepatic arterial chemotherapy. *Cancer Treat Rep* 1981;**65:**393.

Freckman HA: Chemotherapy for metastatic colorectal liver carcinoma by intra-aortic infusion. *Cancer* 1971;**28:**1152.

Goldstein HM et al: Transcatheter occlusion of abdominal tumors. *Radiology* 1976;**120:**539.

Krementz ET, Creech O Jr, Ryan RF: Evaluation of chemotherapy of cancer by regional perfusion. *Cancer* 1967;**20:**834.

Combination Chemotherapy

Carbone PP, Davis TE: Medical treatment for advanced breast cancer. *Semin Oncol* 1978;**5:**417.

DeVita VT Jr, Serpick AA, Carbone PP: Combination chemotherapy in the treatment of advanced Hodgkin's disease. *Ann Intern Med* 1970;**73:**881.

DeVita VT Jr et al: Combination versus single agent chemotherapy: A review of the basis for selection of drug treatment of cancer. *Cancer* 1975;**35:**98.

Einhorn LH, Donohue J: Cis-diamminedichloroplatinum, vinblastine, and bleomycin combination chemotherapy in disseminated testicular cancer. *Ann Intern Med* 1977;**87:**293.

Greenspan EM: Combination cytotoxic chemotherapy in advanced disseminated breast carcinoma. *Mt Sinai J Med NY* 1966;**33:**1.

Li MC et al: Effects of combined drug therapy on metastatic cancer of the testis. *JAMA* 1960;**174:**1291.

Luce JK: Chemotherapy for lymphomas: Current status. Page 295 in: *Leukemia-Lymphoma.* Year Book, 1969.

Samuels ML: Continuous intravenous bleomycin therapy with vinblastine in testicular and extragonadal germinal tumors. (Abstract.) *Proc Am Assoc Cancer Res* 1975;**16:**112.

Unproved Methods in Cancer Therapy

Herbert V: Unproven (questionable) dietary and nutritional methods in cancer prevention and treatment. *Cancer* 1986;**58(8 Suppl):**1930.

Moertel CG et al: A clinical trial of amygdalin (Laetrile) in the treatment of human cancer. *N Engl J Med* 1982;**306:**201.

Evaluation & Management of Patients With an Unknown Primary Carcinoma

Altman E, Cadman E: An analysis of 1539 patients with cancer of unknown primary site. *Cancer* 1986;**57:**120.

Brady LW et al: Unusual sites of metastases. *Semin Oncol* 1977;**4:**59.

Didolkar MS et al: Metastatic carcinomas from occult primary tumors: A study of 254 patients. *Ann Surg* 1977;**186:**625.

Greco FA, Oldham RK, Fer MF: The extragonadal germ cell cancer syndrome. *Semin Oncol* 1982;**9:**448.

Grosbach AB: Carcinoma of unknown primary site: A clinical enigma. *Arch Intern Med* 1982;**142:**357.

Karsell PR, Sheedy PF II, O'Connell MJ: Computed tomography in search of cancer of unknown origin. *JAMA* 1982;**248:**340.

Nystrom JS et al: Identifying the primary site in metastatic cancer of unknown origin: Inadequacy of roentgenographic procedures. *JAMA* 1979;**241:**381.

Nystrom JS et al: Metastatic and histologic presentations in unknown primary cancer. *Semin Oncol* 1977;**4:**53.

Osteen RT, Kopf G, Wilson RE: In pursuit of the unknown primary. *Am J Surg* 1978;**135:**494.

Woods RL et al: Metastatic adenocarcinomas of unknown primary site: A randomized study of two combination-chemotherapy regimens. *N Engl J Med* 1980;**303:**87.

Paraneoplastic Syndromes

Hall TC (editor): Paraneoplastic syndromes. *Ann NY Acad Sci* 1974;**230:**1. [Entire issue.]

Waldenström JG: *Paraneoplasia.* Wiley, 1978.

Neuroblastoma

Evans AE et al: A review of 17IV-S neuroblastoma patients at the Children's Hospital of Philadelphia. *Cancer* 1980;**45:**833.

Renal Cell Carcinoma

Bloom HJG: Proceedings: Hormone-induced and spontaneous regression of metastatic renal cancer. *Cancer* 1973;**32:**1066.

Klippel KF, Altwein JE: Palliative Therapiemoglichkeiten beim metastasierten Hypernephrom. *Dtsch Med Wochenschr* 1979;**104:**28.

Krown SE: Therapeutic options in renal-cell carcinoma. *Semin Oncol* 1985;**12(Suppl 5):**13.

Lokich JJ, Harrison JH: Renal cell carcinoma: Natural history and chemotherapeutic experience. *J Urol* 1975;**114:**371.

Talley RW: Proceedings: Chemotherapy of adenocarcinoma of the kidney. *Cancer* 1973;**32**:1062.

Wilms' Tumor

Green DM, Jaffe N: Wilms' tumor: Model of a curable pediatric malignant solid tumor. *Cancer Treat Rev* (Sept) 1978;**5**:143.

Transitional Cell Tumor

Carter SK: Chemotherapy and genitourinary oncology. 1. Bladder cancer. *Cancer Treat Rev* (June) 1978;**5**:85.

Hahn RG: Bladder cancer treatment considerations for metastatic disease. *Semin Oncol* 1979;**6**:236.

Koontz WW Jr: Intravesical chemotherapy and chemoprevention of superficial, low grade, low stage bladder carcinoma. *Semin Oncol* 1979;**6**:217.

Prostatic Carcinoma

Mittelman A, Shukla SK, Murphy GP: Extended therapy of stage D carcinoma of the prostate with oral estramustine phosphate. *J Urol* 1976;**115**:409.

Torti FM, Carter SK: The chemotherapy of prostatic adenocarcinoma. *Ann Intern Med* 1980;**92**:681.

Testicular Neoplasm

Cvitkovic E et al: Bleomycin (BLEO) infusion with cisplatinum diammine dichloride (CPDD) as secondary chemotherapy for germinal cell tumors. (Abstract.) *Proc Am Assoc Cancer Res* 1975;**16**:273.

Einhorn LH, Donohue JP: Combination chemotherapy in disseminated testicular cancer. *Semin Oncol* 1979;**6**:87.

Einhorn LH, Furnas BE, Powell N: Combination chemotherapy of disseminated testicular carcinoma with cis-platinum diammine chloride (CPDD), vinblastine (VLB), and bleomycin (BLEO). (Abstract.) *Proc Am Assoc Cancer Res* 1976;**17**:240.

Friedman M, Purkayastha MC: Recurrent seminoma: The management of late metastasis, recurrence, or a second primary tumor. *Am J Roentgenol* 1960;**83**:25.

Golbey RB, Reynolds TF, Vugrin D: The chemotherapy of metastatic germ cell tumors. *Semin Oncol* 1979;**6**:82.

Javadpour N: The value of biologic markers in the diagnosis and treatment of testicular carcinoma. *Semin Oncol* 1979;**6**:37.

Li MC et al: Effects of combined drug therapy on metastatic cancer of the testis. *JAMA* 1960;**174**:1291.

Samuels ML: Continuous intravenous bleomycin therapy with vinblastine in testicular and extragonadal germinal tumors. (Abstract.) *Proc Am Assoc Cancer Res* 1975;**16**:112.

Williams SD, Einhorn LH: Etoposide salvage therapy for refractory germ cell tumors: An update. *Cancer Treat Rev* 1982;**9(Suppl A)**:67.

Pain Palliation in Cancer

Brechner VL, Ferrer-Brechner T, Allen GD: Anaesthetic measures in management of pain associated with malignancy. *Semin Oncol* 1977;**4**:99.

Catalano RB: The medical approach to management of pain caused by cancer. *Semin Oncol* 1975;**2**:379.

Palliation of Emesis Caused by Chemotherapy

Frytak S, Moertel CG: Management of nausea and vomiting in the cancer patient. *JAMA* 1981;**245**:393.

Frytak S et al: Delta-9-tetrahydrocannabinol as an antiemetic for patients receiving cancer chemotherapy: A comparison with prochlorperazine and a placebo. *Ann Intern Med* 1979;**91**:825.

Gralla RJ et al: Antiemetic efficacy of high-dose metoclopramide: Randomized trials with placebo and prochlorperazine in patients with chemotherapy-induced nausea and vomiting. *N Engl J Med* 1981;**305**:905.

Siegel LJ, Longo DL: The control of chemotherapy-induced emesis. *Ann Intern Med* 1981;**95**:352.

Bacterial Sepsis in Cancer Patients

Alavi JB et al: Randomized clinical trial of granulocyte transfusions and infection in acute leukemia. *N Engl J Med* 1977;**296**:706.

Dilworth JA, Mandell GL: Infections in patients with cancer. *Semin Oncol* 1975;**2**:349.

Herzig R et al: Successful granulocyte transfusion therapy for gram-negative septicemia: A prospectively randomized controlled study. *N Engl J Med* 1977;**296**:701.

Ketchel SJ, Rodriguez V: Acute infections in cancer patients. *Semin Oncol* 1978;**5**:167.

Wiernik PH: The management of infection in the cancer patient. *JAMA* 1980;**244**:185.

Management of Vesicant Drug Extravasations

Blacklock HA et al: Use of modified subcutaneous right-atrial catheter for venous access in leukaemic patients. *Lancet* 1980;**1**:993.

Larson DL: Treatment of tissue extravasation by antitumor agents. *Cancer* 1982;**49**:1796.

Palliation of Local Complications of Neoplasia

Davenport D et al: Radiation therapy in the treatment of superior vena caval obstruction. *Cancer* 1978;**42**:2600.

Lambert CJ: Treatment of malignant pleural effusions by closed trocar tube drainage. *Ann Thorac Surg* 1967;**3**:1.

Lenhard RE Jr (editor): Clinical case records in chemotherapy: The management of hypercalcemia complicating cancer. *Cancer Chemother Rep* 1971;**55**:509.

Levitt SH et al: Treatment of malignant superior vena caval obstruction. *Cancer* 1969;**24**:447.

Millburn L, Hibbs GG, Hendrickson FR: Treatment of spinal cord compression from metastatic carcinoma. *Cancer* 1968;**21**:447.

Perez CA, Bradfield JS, Morgan HC: Management of pathologic fractures. *Cancer* 1972;**29**:684.

Rubin P et al: Superior vena caval syndrome: Slow low dose versus rapid high dose schedule. *Radiology* 1963;**81**:388.

Nutritional Support in Cancer Patients

Copeland EM, Dudrick SJ: Cancer: Nutritional concepts. *Semin Oncol* 1975;**2**:329.

DeWys WD: Nutritional care of the cancer patient. *JAMA* 1980;**244**:374.

Psychologic Support of the Patient With Neoplastic Disease

Dunphy JE: Caring for the patient with cancer. *N Engl J Med* 1976;**295**:313.

Home Care of the Patient With Advanced Cancer

Rosenbaum EH: Principles of home care for the patient with advanced cancer. *JAMA* 1980;**244**:1484.

Neuropathic Bladder Disorders

20

Emil A. Tanagho, MD, & Richard A. Schmidt, MD, FACS

Virtually every neuropathic disease process can, and often does, cause changes in bladder function. This is evidence of the complex neural regulation of the bladder. Modern methods of tracing neural pathways within the central nervous system and careful evaluation of patients with electrophysiologic techniques have shown that most levels of the nervous system are in some way involved in regulation of the bladder. Just how this is accomplished or why it is that 2 patients with identical neuropathic disorders may have completely different types of bladder dysfunction remains to be understood.

Some common disorders associated with bladder dysfunction are multiple sclerosis, spinal injury, cerebrovascular disease, Parkinson's disease, diabetes mellitus, meningomyelocele, and amyotropic lateral sclerosis. Other causes of neuropathic bladder include pelvic operation, which can partially or completely disrupt the motor nerves to the bladder (eg, hysterectomy or abdominal perineal resection), spinal operation, or herniation of an intervertebral disk.

Significant bladder dysfunction can evolve for reasons not readily clear, possibly because of poor voiding habits developed in childhood or because of degenerative changes in peripheral tissues caused by aging, inflammation, or anxiety disorders. All can disrupt efficient reflex coordination between sphincter and bladder, and with time, this leads to symptomatic dysfunction.

NORMAL VESICAL FUNCTION

ANATOMY

Detrusor Muscle

The bladder wall is composed of a mesh of muscle fibers running in every direction except near the internal meatus, where they form 3 definite layers: inner longitudinal, middle circular, and outer longitudinal. The outer layer extends down the entire length of the female urethra and to the distal end of the prostate but is circular and spirally oriented; thus, it functions as the major involuntary sphincter. The middle circular layer ends at the internal meatus of the bladder and is most developed anteriorly. The inner layer remains longitudinal and reaches the distal end of the urethra in females and the end of the prostate in males. These converging fibers cause a thickening that forms the so-called vesical neck, but anatomically there is no true sphincter at this point.

External Sphincter

An external sphincter muscle composed of striated muscle fibers and under voluntary control lies between the fascial layers of the urogenital diaphragm. In females, it is maximally condensed around the distal third of the urethra (external to the outer layer of urethral musculature), while in males, these fibers surround the distal portion of the prostate and the membranous urethra. The striated muscles of the pelvic floor (eg, levator ani) act as an indirect sphincter and contribute to sphincteric function.

Diaphragm & Abdominal Muscles

These play only secondary roles in micturition. Their contraction may further increase intravesical pressure.

Nerve Supply

The distal portion of the spinal cord widens slightly to accommodate important centers of muscle control. This region of the cord is known as the lumbar intumescence. The distal half of this region, at vertebral levels T11–L1, is the center for micturition control. This region correlates with nerve levels S2–S4. Trauma to this level of the cord is more likely to result in a flaccid neurogenic bladder. Lesions of the cord, however, are often incomplete, and mixed patterns of spasticity and flaccidity often result. Trauma to the cord occurring above T12 most commonly results in a spastic neurogenic bladder, but, again, variable degrees of spasticity will be seen among patients with similar lesions.

A. Motor Innervation:

1. To the detrusor–The peripheral innervation of the detrusor is part of the parasympathetic nervous system. Motor nerves arise within the mediolateral gray matter of the spinal cord and reach the bladder via the sacral and pelvic nerves. Motor control in humans is concentrated at the S3 level, with some minor overlap at the S4 level. The S3 nerve would seem to be the principal source of parasympathetic innervation for the pelvic organs.

The trigonal portion of the bladder (because of its different embryology) receives its innervation from the sympathetic outflow of the spinal cord. The bladder neck, along with the seminal vesicles, ampula of the vas, and vas deferens, also receives sympathetic nerves from the thoracolumbar outflow (ie, T11–L2 spinal nerves). Damage to the sympathetic nerves to the pelvis will disturb the function of the trigone, bladder neck, and seminal vesicles. As a result, seminal emission and bladder neck closure do not occur with ejaculation.

2. To the external sphincter–The motor nerves to the striated musculature of the perineum originate within spinal nerves S2–S4. The pudendal nerve is composed of fibers arising from a nucleus of cells in the ventral gray matter referred to as the pudendal nucleus, or nucleus onuf. The external urethral innervation arises principally from the S2 and, to a lesser but still significant degree, the S3 nerves. The pelvic floor (ie, the levators) receives its innervation from the S3 and, to a lesser degree, the S4 nerves. Damage to the S2 nerve will weaken the external urethral sphincter but leave the detrusor innervation intact. Damage to the S3 nerve will preserve sphincter tone but result in a flaccid detrusor.

B. Sensory Innervation: Horseradish peroxidase (HRP) tracing techniques have been used to outline the afferent (and efferent) projections to the cord from perineal striated muscle, the detrusor body, the bladder neck, and the trigone. HRP applied to either the detrusor wall or the cut end of the pelvic nerve will be deposited in the dorsal laminations of the cord at levels 1–10, with heavy deposits in Lissauer's tract, the dorsal columns, and the mediolateral spinal gray matter at levels 5–7. The pattern of deposits is consistent with other observations of neurostimulation, ie, that the bladder is controlled by the S3–4 nerves. HRP applied to the cut end of the pudendal nerve will be distributed in the same dorsal areas as HRP transported along the pelvic nerve, with additional transport to the nucleus onuf. Similar studies have been used to trace spinal pathways to the dorsal tegmental nucleus in the cervical cord, and the results support the theory that there are important reflex connections to the bladder from centers in the cervical cord.

Peripheral sensation can be divided into exteroceptive (pain, temperature, and touch) and proprioceptive (response to stretch). All detrusor nerve endings are free and nonspecific. Afferents from the region of the bladder neck and trigone will travel via the sympathetic trunk to spinal cord segments T11–L2. Afferents from the detrusor wall will travel to the cord via the pelvic nerve.

Urethral sensory innervation is somewhat more specialized. Muscle spindles are found in the periurethral striated muscle but in relatively sparse distribution to those found in the remainder of the pelvic floor.

URODYNAMIC STUDIES
(See also Chapter 21.)

Urodynamic studies are techniques used to obtain graphic recordings of activity in the urinary bladder, urethral sphincter, and pelvic musculature. The 3 current methods are use of gas or water to transfer pressure to a transducer housed near a polygraph or use of a transducer-tipped catheter to transfer pressure recordings directly to a polygraph. All the techniques have limitations, with gas being the least reliable of the three. Pressure recordings may be complemented by electromyography of the perineal musculature, ultrasound, or radiography (Fig 20–1).

Uroflowmetry

Uroflowmetry is without doubt the most useful of all the urodynamic tests. It is the study of the flow of urine from the urethra. It is best performed separate from all other tests and, wherever possible, as a standard office screening or monitoring procedure. The normal flow rate for males is 20–25 mL/sec and for females 20–30 mL/sec. Lower flow rates suggest outlet obstruction or a weak detrusor; higher flow rates suggest bladder spasticity or excessive use of abdominal muscles to assist voiding. Intermittent flow patterns generally reflect spasticity of the sphincter or straining to overcome resistance in the urethra. The test can be very informative in assessing the functional state of the lower urinary tract. It is useful both as a diagnostic and a monitoring tool.

There are a number of electronic devices for recording the flow rate. However, a patient can record the flow rate simply by averaging the volume voided over time. A maximum or peak flow can be measured by timing only the middle portion of the void, when the flow is strongest.

Cystometry

Cystometry is the urodynamic evaluation of the reservoir function of the lower urinary tract. Both gas and water cystometers have been used. Gas cystometers originally became popular because they were simpler and faster to use, but they have proved less reliable and less informative than water cystometers. Gas cystometers should be used only for initial screening; if any abnormalities are found, they should be confirmed by water cystometry.

Cystometric evaluations are performed to ascertain total bladder **capacity;** intravesical pressure during filling, up to the point at which voiding occurs (**accommodation);** bladder pressure during voiding; ability of the bladder to **contract** and sustain a contraction; the presence of premature or **"unstable"** bladder activity; the ability to perceive **fullness;** the ability to **inhibit** or **initiate** voiding; and the presence of **residual** urine after voiding. Cystometry is most informative when combined with studies of the external urethral sphincter and pelvic floor.

Normal bladder capacity is 400–500 mL. Bladder pressure during filling should remain constant up to the point of voiding. The first desire to void is generally felt when the volume reaches 150–250 mL, but detrusor filling pressure should remain unchanged until there is a definite sense of fullness at 350–450 mL, the true capacity of the bladder. Detrusor contractions before this point are considered abnormal and the result of hyperreflexic or uninhibited behavior. Normal voiding pressures in the bladder should not rise above

30 cm of water pressure. With normal voiding there should not be any residual urine, and voiding should be accomplished without straining.

Urethral Pressure Recordings

Bladder function should be focused on expelling urine rather than overcoming abnormal resistance in the urethra. High pressures in the bladder during voiding reflect abnormal resistance in the urethral outlet. Increased outlet resistance can result from benign prostatic hypertrophy, urethral stricture, bladder neck stricture, or spasm of the external urethral sphincter. Low resistance in the urethral outlet generally reflects compromised function of the sphincter mechanism. Recording of urethral pressures with the bladder at rest as well as during contraction helps determine the presence of functional or anatomic disorders. It also helps assess the sphincteric integrity of the urethral musculature.

Electromyography

With electromyography, the activity of the striated urethral muscles can be monitored without obstructing the urethral lumen. In the normal urethra, activity will increase slightly as the bladder fills and will then fall precipitously just before voiding begins. Denervation results in an overall decrease in activity as well as production of denervation potentials. An overall increase in activity reflects a state of hyperreflexia. The disadvantages of the technique are dependence on accurate needle position and a tendency to record artifacts. The technique does provide a sensitive study of urethral and pelvic muscle behavior.

NEUROPHYSIOLOGY

Detrusor Muscle

The urinary bladder has 2 primary functions, storage and evacuation of urine. Both functions are accomplished with low pressure so as to protect the integrity of the kidneys. Neural regulation is accomplished via peripheral and central reflexes, which coordinate detrusor behavior with sphincter activity.

Pudendal afferents can either facilitate or inhibit the detrusor through peripheral reflexes. Normally, to promote urine storage, the inhibitory pathway dominates. Also, voluntary tightening of the sphincter is used to suppress inappropriate urge to void. Detrusor hyperreflexia (facilitation) may result from pathologic conditions affecting the urethra, eg, prostatitis or urethritis.

Two types of central reflex control have been identified. One involves a lengthy routing of afferent information to the brain stem (dorsolateral tegmental nucleus of the pons), and the other involves a short routing of afferent information to the detrusor nucleus in the spinal segments S3–S4. The latter pathway is believed to become significant only after spinal cord transection. The brain stem is felt to be a significant center for the regulation of bladder function. Stimula-

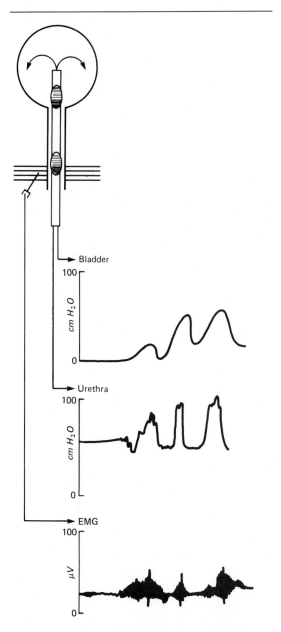

Figure 20–1. Simultaneous recording of bladder and urethral pressure as well as electromyographic recording of the external sphincter. Note the dyssynergic response. With bladder contraction there is increased activity in the external sphincter and pelvic floor, as recorded by the intraurethral pressure and EMG tracings.

tion of the region results in bladder contraction, and ablation results in permanent urinary retention. This may help explain why irritation of cervical systems (eg, burning or tingling of the palms or stiffness in the neck area) is found occasionally in patients with symptomatic urethral irritation.

Other regions of the brain are known to have regulatory influence on the bladder because of changes in detrusor behavior in certain disease states. Detrusor hyperreflexia is common in Parkinson's disease (implicating the basal ganglia in detrusor regulation) as well as in cerebrovascular lesions in the cerebral motor cortex. Areas in the prefrontal cortex and within the limbic system have been linked to neural regulation of the bladder. Emotional behavior has long been felt to be a factor in some voiding disturbances. These regions, for the most part, remain inaccessible for study in humans, and defining their role in neural regulation of the bladder is understandably difficult. Evoked potential studies have been somewhat helpful in the study of cortical influences on the bladder.

Urethra

Both periurethral and urethral striated muscle are present in the external sphincter. Striated muscle fibers are of 2 varieties. Fibers within the wall of the urethra are smaller and thinner than those located periurethrally and are slow twitch in character. The periurethral muscle is a mix of slow- and fast-twitch fibers. Slow-twitch muscle has a rich mitochondrial population and is resistant to fatigue. It is believed to be important in maintaining continence at rest. Fast-twitch fibers are characterized by a high glycogen content and easy fatigability. They are thought to help maintain continence during stress, eg, coughing or running.

Little is known about the neural regulation of these muscle fibers. Afferent feedback, which is inhibitory to the bladder, is associated with sustained resting tonus in the sphincter, and relaxation of the urethra always precedes a detrusor contraction. Detrusor inhibition can therefore be equated with tonus in the slow-twitch muscles. Spastic urethral behavior is often seen in association with detrusor hyperreflexia. Thus, fast-twitch muscle activity may equate with detrusor facilitation. These are observations consistent with peripheral afferent influence on the detrusor nucleus in the conus medullaris. Little is known of the suprasegmental regulation of the urethra save that areas of regulation for the urethra are similar to those for the detrusor.

Detrusor stretch will reflexly produce an increase in urethral tone to a point beyond which inhibition of urethral activity takes place. The influence of detrusor stretch can be a purely segmental reflex but is probably modulated by input from suprasegmental centers.

PHYSIOLOGY

Urinary control results largely from a simple peripheral reflex arc centered in the sacral segments of the spinal cord. This, in turn, is under the control of higher midbrain and cortical centers. The normal bladder is able to distend gradually to normal capacity (400 mL) without appreciable increase in intravesical pressure. At this point, sensations of fullness are transmitted to the sacral cord; if voluntary (cerebral) control is lacking (as in infants), the motor side of the reflex arc will effect a powerful, sustained detrusor contraction with spontaneous involuntary urination. As myelinization and training of the young child progress, cerebral inhibitory functions suppress the sacral reflex, and the individual voids when it is convenient to do so.

The urinary bladder is the only part of the urinary tract that is totally dependent on intact innervation to perform its function. It is made up of 3 main units that serve its functions.

Reservoir

The principal storage features of the bladder include (1) a normal capacity of 400–500 mL; (2) a sense of distention; (3) the ability to accommodate various volumes without a change in intraluminal pressure; (4) the ability to initiate and sustain a contraction until the bladder is empty; and (5) voluntary initiation or inhibition of voiding despite the involuntary nature of the organ.

Sphincteric Mechanism

In both males and females there are 2 sphincteric elements: (1) an internal involuntary smooth muscle sphincter at the bladder neck and (2) a voluntary skeletal sphincter located at the level of the membranous urethra. The bladder neck sphincter is a concentration of smooth muscle of the detrusor. It has the same parasympathetic nerve supply and shares the contractile properties of the bladder. In addition, there is a concentration of sympathetic nerve fibers in the area. In the relaxed filling state, the bladder neck will remain closed, providing a continence mechanism. With either spontaneous contraction or stimulation of the motor nerves to the bladder, the bladder neck opens. This suggests that the bladder neck can be actively opened by the pull of the contracting detrusor longitudinal muscle rather than it being an active relaxation. Active contraction of the bladder neck region occurs simultaneously with seminal emission, just prior to ejaculation.

The voluntary sphincter maintains a constant tonus that is the primary continence mechanism. While the resting tone is involuntary, it can be voluntarily increased to prevent or abolish voiding. Relaxation of the sphincter is mostly a voluntary act without which voiding is normally inhibited. Failure to initiate relaxation of the sphincter is a mechanism of urinary retention (a syndrome seen in young adult females).

The influence of higher centers in the regulation of micturition is evident in the development of infants and young children. In infancy, the detrusor behaves in an uninhibited fashion, but as the central nervous system matures, cerebral inhibition suppresses the peripheral reflex. Much of the learning process by which micturition is controlled is accomplished through voluntary regulation of the pelvic musculature.

The levator muscles contribute directly to the periurethral musculature and thus are actively involved in sphincter function. They also contribute indirectly through support of the bladder base. Weakness of the pelvic floor may therefore lessen the closure efficiency of these 2 otherwise normal units.

Ureterovesical Junction

The function of the ureterovesical junction is to prevent backflow of urine from the bladder to the upper urinary tract (reflux). Proper function will permit urine to flow freely from the ureter to the bladder but never in the reverse direction. Longitudinal muscle from the ureters contributes to the makeup of the trigone. Stretching the trigone has an occlusive effect on the ureteral openings. During normal detrusor contraction, the increased pull on the ureters prevents reflux of urine. The combination of detrusor hypertrophy and trigonal stretch due to residual urine can significantly obstruct the flow of urine from the ureters into the bladder.

Micturition

Micturition is completely under voluntary control. Detrusor response to stretch can be inhibited, permitting the bladder to accommodate larger volumes, or detrusor contraction can be initiated whether or not the bladder is full. Detrusor contraction is usually preceded by relaxation of the pelvic floor musculature, including the voluntary sphincter around the urethra. This appreciably reduces the efficiency of urethral closure and also leads to a drop in the vesical base, further minimizing urethral resistance.

Next, the trigone contracts, exerting increased pull on the ureterovesical junction and thus increasing ureteral occlusion. This prevents vesicoureteral reflux during the high intravesical pressure that develops with voiding. It also pulls the posterior portion of the bladder neck open, leading to its funneling. Only then do the detrusor fibers of the bladder contract, and intravesical pressure begins to rise. Because the vesical longitudinal muscles insert into the urethra, their contraction along with that of the trigone tends to pull the internal meatus of the bladder open, further contributing to funneling of the vesical outlet. The increased hydrostatic pressure (30–40 cm of water) exerted by the detrusor is directed down the urethra. The urethral counterpressure drops reciprocally, and voiding ensues. The detrusor maintains its contraction until the bladder is completely empty.

When the bladder is empty, the detrusor muscle relaxes, and the bladder neck is allowed to close; urethral and perineal muscle tone then return to normal. Finally, the trigone resumes its normal tone. The urinary stream can also be interrupted by voluntary contraction of the external sphincter. Detrusor muscle spasm then relaxes by reciprocal reflex action, and the bladder neck closes.

ABNORMAL VESICAL FUNCTION

CLASSIFICATION OF NEUROPATHIC BLADDER

Attempts have been made over the years to classify bladder dysfunction due to neural injury. The traditional classification was according to neurologic deficit. Thus, the terms motor, spastic, upper motor neuron, reflexic, and uninhibited were used to describe dysfunction found with injury above the spinal cord micturition center. Coordination between the bladder and the sphincter was then either balanced or unbalanced. The terms flaccid, atonic, areflexic, and sensory were used to describe loss of ability of the bladder to contract owing to injury of the pelvic nerves or the spinal micturition center. Dysfunction with both types of features was described as mixed.

Descriptions of neuromuscular dysfunction of the lower urinary tract should be individualized because no 2 neural injuries (no matter how similar) will predictably result in the same type of dysfunction. The standardization committee for the International Continence Society has attempted to create a functional classification that is easy to understand and provides a simple basis for therapy (Table 20–1).

Table 20–1. Various classifications of neuropathic bladder.

International Continence Society
  Detrusor: Normal (N), hyperreflexic (+), hyporeflexic (−)
  Striated sphincter: Normal (N), hyperactive (+),
    incompetent (−)
  Sensation: Normal (N), hypersensitive (+), hyposensitive
    (−)
Bors and Comarr
  Sensory neuron lesion
  Motor neuron lesion (balanced or unbalanced)
  Sensory-motor neuron lesion
    Upper motor neuron lesion
    Lower motor neuron lesion
    Mixed upper and lower motor neuron lesion
Nesbit, Lapides, and Baum
  Sensory neuron lesion
  Motor neuron lesion
  Uninhibited bladder
  Reflex bladder
  Autonomous bladder
Krane
  Detrusor hyperreflexia
    Coordinated sphincters
    Striated muscle dyssynergia
    Smooth muscle dyssynergia
  Detrusor areflexia
    Coordinated sphincters
    Nonrelaxing striated sphincter
    Denervated striated sphincter
    Nonrelaxing smooth sphincter
Wain, Benson, and Raezer
  Failure to empty
  Failure to store

1. NEUROPATHIC BLADDER DUE TO LESIONS ABOVE THE MICTURITION CENTER

Most lesions above the level of the cord where the micturition center is located will cause bladder spasticity. Sacral reflex arcs remain intact, but loss of inhibition from higher centers results in spastic bladder and sphincter behavior on the segmental level. The degree of spasticity will vary between the bladder and sphincter, from lesion to lesion, and from patient to patient with similar lesions. Common lesions found above the brain stem that affect voiding include dementia, vascular accidents, multiple sclerosis, tumors, and inflammatory disorders such as encephalitis or meningitis. These lesions can produce a wide range of functional changes, including precipitate urge, frequency, residual urine, retention of urine, recurrent urinary tract infections, or gross incontinence. Symptoms range from mild to disabling. Obviously, incontinence is especially troublesome. Leakage may occur because the need to void cannot be felt or because the sphincter becomes more relaxed and can no longer inhibit spontaneous voiding.

Lesions of the internal capsule include vascular accidents and Parkinson's disease. Both spastic and semiflaccid voiding disorders are found with these lesions.

Spinal cord injury can be the result of trauma, herniated intervertebral disk, vascular lesions, multiple sclerosis, tumor, syringomyelia, or myelitis or may be iatrogenic. Traumatic spinal cord lesions are of greatest clinical concern. Partial or complete injuries may cause equally severe genitourinary dysfunction. Sphincter spasticity and voiding dyssynergia can lead to detrusor hypertrophy, high voiding pressures, ureteral reflux, or ureteral obstruction. With time, renal function may become compromised. If infection is combined with back pressure on the kidney, loss of renal function can be particularly rapid.

Spinal cord injuries at the cervical level are often associated with a condition known as **autonomic dysreflexia.** Because the lesions occur above the sympathetic outflow from the cord, hypertensive blood pressure fluctuations, bradycardia, and sweating can be triggered by insertion of a catheter, mild overdistention of the bladder with filling, or dyssynergic voiding.

In summary, the spastic neuropathic bladder is typified by (1) reduced capacity, (2) involuntary detrusor contractions, (3) high intravesical voiding pressures, (4) marked hypertrophy of the bladder wall, (5) spasticity of the pelvic striated muscle, and (6) autonomic dysreflexia in cervical cord lesions.

2. NEUROPATHIC BLADDER DUE TO LESIONS AT OR BELOW THE MICTURITION CENTER

Injury to the Detrusor Motor Nucleus

The most common cause of flaccid neuropathic bladder is injury to the spinal cord at the micturition center, S3–4. Other causes of anterior horn cell damage include infection due to poliovirus or herpes zoster and iatrogenic factors such as radiation or surgery. Herniated disks can injure the micturition center but more commonly affect the cauda equina or sacral nerve roots. Myelodysplasias could also be grouped here, but the mechanism is actually failure in the development or organization of the anterior horn cells. Lesions in this region of the cord are often incomplete, with the result often being a mixture of spastic behavior with weakened muscle contractility. Mild trabeculation of the bladder may occur. External sphincter and perineal muscle tone are diminished. Urinary incontinence usually does not occur in these cases because of the compensatory increase in bladder storage. Because pressure in the bladder is low, little outlet resistance is needed to provide continence. Evacuation of the bladder may be accomplished by straining, but with variable success.

Injury to the Afferent Feedback Pathways

Flaccid neuropathic bladder also results from a variety of neuropathies, including diabetes mellitus, tabes dorsalis, pernicious anemia, and posterior spinal cord lesions. Here the mechanism is not injury of the detrusor motor nucleus but a loss of sensory input to the detrusor nucleus or a change in motor behavior due to loss of neurotransmission in the dorsal horns of the cord. The end result is the same. Loss of perception of bladder filling permits overstretching of the detrusor. Atony of the detrusor results in weak, inefficient contractility. Capacity is increased and residual urine significant.

In summary, the flaccid neuropathic bladder is typified by (1) large capacity, (2) no voluntary detrusor contractions, (3) low intravesical pressure, (4) mild trabeculation (hypertrophy) of the bladder wall, and (5) decreased tone of the external sphincter.

Injury Causing Poor Detrusor Distensibility

Another cause of atonic neuropathic bladder is peripheral nerve injury. This category includes injury caused by radical surgical procedures such as low anterior resection of the colon or Wertheim hysterectomy. This type of dysfunction has been referred to as autonomous because the smooth muscle remains active but there is no central reflex to organize muscle activity. The end result is a bladder that stores poorly owing to failure to accommodate with filling. There is a rather steep pressure rise in the bladder with filling due to hypertonicity in the detrusor wall.

Radiation can result in denervation of the detrusor or the sphincter. More commonly, it will damage the detrusor, resulting in fibrosis and loss of distensibility. Other inflammatory causes of injury to the detrusor include chronic infection, interstitial cystitis, or carcinoma in situ. These lesions produce a fibrotic bladder wall that, for obvious reasons, distends poorly.

Selective Injury to the External Sphincter

Pelvic fracture often tears the nerves to the external sphincter. Selective denervation of the external sphincter muscle, with incontinence, can follow if the bladder neck is not sufficiently competent. Radical surgery in the perineum is highly unlikely to damage the pundendal innervation to the urethra.

SPINAL SHOCK & RECOVERY OF VESICAL FUNCTION AFTER SPINAL CORD INJURY

Immediately following severe injury to the spinal cord or conus medullaris, regardless of level, there is a stage of flaccid paralysis, with numbness below the level of the injury. The smooth muscle of the detrusor and rectum is affected. The result is detrusor overfilling to the point of overflow incontinence and rectal impaction.

Spinal shock may last a few weeks to 6 months (usually 2–3 months). Reflex behavior in striated muscle is usually present from the time of injury but is suppressed. With time, the reflex excitability of striated muscle progresses until a spastic state is achieved. Smooth muscle is much slower to evolve this hyperreflex activity, and unlike striated muscle, does not demonstrate spontaneous behavior early in the injury. Urinary retention is therefore the rule in the early months following injury.

Urodynamic studies are indicated periodically to monitor the progressive return of reflex behavior. In the early recovery stages, a few weak contractions of the bladder may be found. Later, in injuries above the micturition center, more significant reflex activity will be found. Low pressure storage can be managed via intermittent catheterization. High pressure storage should be addressed early to avoid problems with the upper urinary tract.

A seldom used but valuable test is instillation of ice water. A strong detrusor contraction in response to filling with cold saline (3.3 °C [38 °F]) is one of the first indications of return of detrusor reflex activity. This test is of value in differentiating upper from lower motor neuron lesions early in the recovery phase.

Activity of the bladder after the spinal shock phase depends upon the site of injury and extent of the neural lesion. With upper motor neuron (suprasegmental) lesion, there is obvious evidence of spasticity toward the end of the spinal shock phase (eg, spontaneous spasms in the extremities, spontaneous leakage of urine or stool, and, possibly, the return of some sensation). A

plan of management can be made at this time. A few patients will retain the ability to empty the bladder reflexly by using trigger techniques, ie, by tapping or scratching the skin above the pubis. More often, detrusor hyperreflexia must be suppressed by anticholinergic medication to prevent incontinence. Evacuation of urine can then be accomplished by intermittent catheterization. Although incomplete lesions are more amenable to this approach than complete lesions, 70% of complete lesions can ultimately be managed using this program. Patients who cannot be managed in this way can be evaluated for sphincterotomy, rhizotomy, diversion, augmentation, or a pacemaker procedure.

In cases of lower motor neuron (segmental or infrasegmental) lesions, it is difficult to distinguish spinal shock from the end result of the injury. Spontaneous detrusor activity cannot be elicited on urodynamic evaluation. If the bladder is allowed to fill, overflow incontinence will occur. Striated muscle reflexes will be suppressed or absent. The bladder may be partially emptied by the Credé maneuver, ie, by manually pushing on the abdomen above the pubic symphysis.

DIAGNOSIS OF NEUROPATHIC BLADDER

The diagnosis of a neuropathic bladder disorder depends on a complete history and physical (including neurologic) examination, as well as use of radiologic studies (urethrography, cystography, excretory urography, CT scanning, MR imaging, where necessary); urologic studies (cystoscopy, ultrasound); urodynamic studies (cystometry, urethral pressure recordings, uroflowmetry); and neurologic studies (electromyography, evoked potentials). Patients should be reevaluated often as recovery progresses.

1. SPASTIC NEUROPATHIC BLADDER

Spastic neuropathic bladder results from partial or extensive neural damage above the conus medullaris (T12). The bladder functions on the level of segmental reflexes, without efficient regulation from higher brain centers.

Clinical Findings

A. Symptoms: The severity of symptoms depends on the site and extent of the lesion as well as the length of time from injury. Symptoms include involuntary urination, which is often frequent, spontaneous, scant, and triggered by spasms in the lower extremities. A true sensation of fullness is lacking, though vague lower abdominal sensations due to stretch of the overlying peritoneum may be felt. The major nonurologic symptoms are those of spastic paralysis and objective sensory deficits.

B. Signs: A complete neurologic examination is

most important. The sensory level of the injury needs to be established, followed by assessment of the renal, bulbocavernosal, knee, ankle, and toe reflexes. These reflexes will vary in degree of hyperreflexia on a scale of 1–4. Levator muscle tone and anal tone should be gauged separately, also on a scale of 1–4. Bladder volumes in established lesions are usually less than 300 mL (not infrequently, < 150 mL) and cannot be detected by abdominal percussion. Ultrasound can be a useful, rapid means of determining detrusor capacity. Voiding often can be triggered by stimulation of the skin of the abdomen, thigh, or genitalia, often with spasm of the lower extremities.

With high thoracic and cervical lesions, distention of the bladder (due to a plugged catheter or during cystometry or cystoscopy) can trigger a series of responses, including hypertension, bradycardia, headache, piloerection, and sweating. This phenomenon is known as **autonomic dysreflexia.** It is triggered by pelvic autonomic afferent activity (overdistention of bowel or bladder, erection) and somatic afferent activity (ejaculation, spasm of lower extremities, insertion of a catheter, dilation of the external urethral sphincter). The headache can be severe and the hypertension life-threatening. Treatment must be immediate. Inserting a catheter and leaving the catheter on open drainage will usually quickly reverse the dysreflexia. Prophylaxis against troublesome dysreflexic tendencies can be achieved by giving procardia orally or chlorpromazine intramuscularly immediately before catheterization or by long-term therapy with an alpha blocker (eg, phenoxybenzamine, clonidine, minipress). Spinal anesthesia or administration of ganglionic or postganglionic blocker is rarely necessary unless a surgical procedure is to be performed.

C. Laboratory Findings: Virtually all patients will experience one or more urinary tract infections during the recovery phase of spinal shock. This is due to the necessity of catheter drainage, either intermittent or continuous. Urinary stasis, prolonged immobilization, and urinary tract infections predispose to stone formation. Renal function may be normal or impaired, depending on the efficacy of treatment and the absence of complications (hydronephrosis, pyelone-

phritis, calculosis). Red cells in the urine may reflect a number of abnormalities. Uremia will result if complications are not addressed appropriately and the patient is not checked at regular intervals. In this era of medicine and with this group of patients, renal failure should not occur.

D. X-Ray Findings: Periodic excretory urograms and retrograde cystograms are essential because complications are common. A trabeculated bladder of small capacity is typical of this type of neuropathic dysfunction. The bladder neck may be dilated. The kidneys may show evidence of pyelonephritic scarring, hydronephrosis, or stone disease. The ureters may be dilated from obstruction or reflux. A voiding film often will clearly outline a narrowed zone created by the spastic sphincter but may also identify a strictured segment of the urethra. Most, if not all, of these features can be detected with ultrasound. MR imaging is especially useful for the sagittal view it offers of the bladder neck and posterior urethral zones.

E. Instrumental Examination: Cystoscopy and panendoscopy help assess the integrity of the urethra and identify stricture sites. The bladder will show variable degrees of trabeculation, occasionally with diverticulas. Bladder capacity, stones, competency of the ureteral orifices, changes secondary to chronic infection or indwelling catheters, and the integrity of the bladder neck and external urethral sphincter can be assessed.

F. Urodynamic Studies: Combined recording of bladder and urethral sphincter activity during filling will reveal a low-volume bladder with spastic dyssynergy of the external sphincter (Fig 20–2). High voiding pressures in the bladder are not unusual. Ureteral reflux or obstruction is more likely if voiding pressures exceed 40 cm of water. A high resting pressure is noted in the external sphincter on the urethral pressure profile, and labile spastic behavior is noted during filling and voiding. Various auras replace a true sense of bladder filling, eg, sweating, vague abdominal discomfort, spasm of the lower extremities. Movement of a catheter in the urethra can trigger detrusor contraction and voiding.

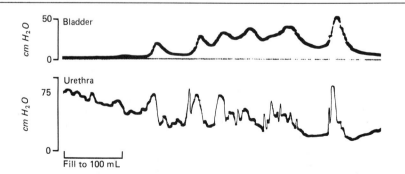

Figure 20–2. Spinal cord injury at T12. Simultaneous recording of intravesical and urethral pressure with bladder filling. Note the rise in intravesical pressure associated with unstable activity of the external sphincter, as reflected on the urethral pressure tracing.

2. MILDLY SPASTIC NEUROMUSCULAR DYSFUNCTION

Incomplete lesions of the cerebral cortex, pyramidal tracts, or spinal cord may weaken, but not abolish, cerebral restraint. The patient may have frequency and nocturia or urinary incontinence due to precipitous urge or voiding. Common causes include brain tumors, Parkinson's disease, multiple sclerosis, dementias, cerebrovascular accidents, prolapsed disks, or partial spinal injury.

In many cases, the cause is unclear. The hyperreflexic behavior often seems to be associated with a peripheral abnormality (eg, prostatitis, benign prostatic hypertrophy, urethritis) or follows pelvic surgery (eg, anterior colporraphy, anteroposterior tumor resection). Symptoms are commonly associated with psychologic factors.

Clinical Findings

A. Symptoms: Frequency, nocturia, and urgency are the principal symptoms. Hesitancy, intermittency, double voiding, and residual urine are also common. Incontinence may vary from pre- or postvoiding dribbling to complete voiding that the patient does not recognize or cannot inhibit once started.

B. Signs: The degree of voiding dysfunction does not parallel neurologic deficits. Slight physical disabilities can be associated with gross disturbances in bladder function, and the reverse is also true. However, it is always important to check lower extremity and perineal reflexes for evidence of hyperreflexia. Sensory or motor deficits may also be detected in the lumbar or sacral segments.

C. X-Ray Findings: For the most part, radiologically evident change is minimal in both the lower and upper urinary tracts. Low bladder volume and mild trabeculation of the bladder are usually evident.

D. Instrumental Examination: Cystoscopy and urethroscopy are generally unremarkable. Mild detrusor and sphincter irritability and diminished capacity can be demonstrated.

E. Urodynamic Studies: The behavior patterns of the sphincter and bladder are similar to those of the previous group but on a milder scale. Uninhibited detrusor activity evident urodynamically may not be associated with the same symptom pattern on the clinical level. The patient occasionally perceives a sense of urgency and the need to void. However, these sensations may not be present, and the patient may complain of the actual leakage as the main inconvenience. Morphologic changes in the bladder will be slight, with changes in the upper urinary tract occurring rarely because of lower pressures in the bladder.

3. FLACCID (ATONIC) BLADDER

Direct injury to the peripheral innervation of the bladder or sacral cord segments S3–4 will result in flaccid paralysis of the urinary bladder. Characteristically, the capacity is large, intravesical pressure low, and involuntary contractions absent. Because smooth muscle is intrinsically active, fine trabeculations in the bladder may be seen. Common causes of this type of bladder behavior are trauma, tumors, tabes dorsalis, and congenital anomalies (eg, spina bifida, meningomyelocele).

Clinical Findings

A. Symptoms: The patient experiences flaccid paralysis and loss of sensation affecting the muscles and dermatomes below the level of injury. The principal urinary symptom is retention with overflow incontinence. Male patients lose their erections. Surprisingly, despite weakness in the striated sphincter, neither bowel nor urinary incontinence is a major factor. Storage pressures within the bladder remain below the outlet resistance.

B. Signs: Neurologic changes are typically lower motor neuron. Extremity reflexes are hypoactive or absent. Sensation is diminished or absent. It is important to check sensation over the penis (S2) and perianal region (S2–3) for evidence of a mixed or partial injury. Anal tone (S2) should be compared with levator tone (S3–4), again for evidence of a mixed injury.

Similarly, sensation over the outside of the foot (S2), sole of the foot (S2–3), and large toe (S3) should be compared for evidence of mixed injury. Occasionally, extremity findings will not parallel those of the perineum, with the pattern being absent sensation and tone in the feet but partial tone or sensation in the perineum. This is especially true in spina bifida and meningomyelocele patients.

C. Laboratory Findings: Repeated urinalysis at regular intervals is no less important in this group than in others. Infection with white blood cells and bacteria may occur because of the need for bladder catheterization. Advanced renal change is unusual because bladder storage is under low pressure, but chronic renal failure secondary to pyelonephritis, hydronephrosis, or calculus formation is still possible. The PSP (phenosulfonphthalein) test, if performed, should be done with a catheter in place because of the large volume of residual urine. The papaverine test for potency is usually negative but may be positive in partial injuries in which some spontaneous reflex turgescence of the penis remains.

D. X-Ray Findings: A plain film of the abdomen may reveal fracture of the lumbar spine or extensive spina bifida. Calcific shadows compatible with urinary stone may be seen. Excretory urograms should be performed initially to check for calculus, hydronephrosis, pyelonephritic scarring, or ureteral obstruction secondary to an overdistended bladder. A cystogram will check on morphologic changes in the detrusor (it is usually large and thin-walled). Checks on the integrity of both the lower and upper urinary tracts can subsequently be made using ultrasound.

E. Instrumental Examination: Visual inspection is performed to rule out pathologic changes (eg, bladder stones, urethral stricture, or ureteral reflux or obstruction).

Cystoscopy and urethroscopy performed some months or weeks after the injury will confirm the laxity and areflexia of the sphincter and pelvic floor; the bladder neck should be intact, as sympathetic tone is preserved, and the bladder should be large and smooth-walled. The integrity of the ureteral orifices should be normal. Fine trabeculation may be evident.

F. Urodynamic Studies: The urethral pressure profile reflects low smooth and striated sphincter tone, bladder filling pressures are low, detrusor contractions are weak or absent, voiding is accomplished by straining or by the Credé maneuver, if at all, and there is a large volume of residual urine. Awareness of filling is markedly diminished and usually results from stretch on the peritoneum or abdominal distention.

G. Penodynamic Studies: Papaverine injection into the corpora cavernosa results in turgescence of the penis but poor rigidity. Ultrasound measurement of blood flow reflects only moderate change in arterial diameter, and venous leakage may be found on cavernosography.

H. Denervation Hypersensitivity: This test is classically performed by giving urecholine subcutaneously. A cystometrogram is performed after 20 minutes and compared with the findings before giving the urecholine. If positive, a rise in filling pressure of more than 15 cm of water is noted, with a shift in the filling curve to the left; ie, the same behavior in the bladder is noted only at a lower filling volume and slightly higher pressure. No change on filling reflects myogenic damage to the detrusor. A more physiologic way to perform the test is to fill the bladder to about half its capacity, administer urecholine, and monitor for change in storage pressure. The ice water test also checks for detrusor hypersensitivity.

Urecholine does not facilitate a detrusor contraction; it can only increase tone in the detrusor wall, which in turn might trigger the voiding reflex. The test is *not* a check on the integrity of the voiding reflex and should not be confused as such.

The test is not applicable in patients with reduced bladder capacity, decreased compliance (ie, sharp rise in detrusor filling pressure), or forceful contractions of the detrusor.

DIFFERENTIAL DIAGNOSIS OF NEUROPATHIC BLADDER

The diagnosis of neurogenic bladder is usually obvious from the history and physical examination. Neural impairment is evidenced by abnormal sacral reflex activity and decreased perineal sensation. Some disorders with which neuropathic bladder may be confused are cystitis, chronic urethritis, vesical irritation secondary to psychic disturbance, interstitial cystitis, cystocele, and infravesical obstruction.

Cystitis

Inflammation of the bladder, both nonspecific and

tuberculous, causes frequency of urination and urgency, even to the point of incontinence. Infections secondary to residual urine caused by neuropathic behavioral disturbance should be ruled out.

The urodynamics of the inflamed bladder are similar to those of the uninhibited neuropathic bladder. However, with inflammation, symptoms will disappear after definitive antibiotic therapy, and the urodynamic behavior will revert to normal. If symptoms persist or infections return repeatedly, a neuropathic behavioral abnormality should be considered (eg, multiple sclerosis or even idiopathic detrusor/sphincter dysfunction).

Chronic Urethritis

Symptoms of frequency, nocturia, and burning on urination may be due to chronic inflammation of the urethra not necessarily associated with infection. Urethroscopy will reveal signs of urethral inflammation most prominently in the region of the external sphincter. The urodynamics will show an irritable urethral sphincter zone with labile, spastic tendencies. The cause is unknown but is thought to be long-standing inefficiency of the sphincter, perhaps complicated by superimposed serious acute infection.

Vesical Irritation Secondary to Psychic Disturbance

Anxious, tense individuals or those with pathologic psychologic fixation on the perineum may present a long history of periodic bouts of urinary frequency or perineal or pelvic pain. The clinical picture and urodynamic findings are similar to those described above for chronic urethritis. Often, however, if the patient's anxieties can be allayed, the symptoms will subside. The underlying problem is one of excessive pelvic muscle tension and inefficient sphincter behavior.

Interstitial Cystitis

This condition is poorly understood and commonly overdiagnosed and may be confused with chronic urethritis. The typical patient is over 40 years of age, with symptoms of frequency, nocturia, urgency, and suprapubic pain. The symptoms are brought on by bladder distention. Capacity is limited (often < 100 mL in the most symptomatic and disabled patients). Urinalysis is normal, and there is no residual urine. Urodynamic studies show a hypertonic, poorly compliant bladder. Distention of the bladder with cystoscopy produces a typical bleeding from petechial hemorrhages and fissuring in the mucosa. The condition represents an end stage inflammatory process of unknown cause in the detrusor. Severe symptoms are usually relieved only through bladder augmentation.

Cystocele

Relaxation of the pelvic floor following childbirth may cause some frequency, nocturia, and stress incontinence. Residual urine may be present and predispose to infection. Loss of urine occurs with lifting, standing, or coughing.

Pelvic examination usually reveals relaxation of the anterior vaginal wall and descent of the urethra and bladder when the patient strains to void. Cystoscopy shows similar findings. Urodynamic studies will show definite improvement in sphincter tone when the bladder is held in the proper supported position, as compared with the nonsupported position.

Infravesical Obstruction

Urethral strictures, benign or malignant enlargement of the prostate gland, and congenital urethral valves can all produce significant obstruction of the urinary outlet. Hypertrophy (ie, trabeculation) of the detrusor develops, and residual urine can accumulate. Uninhibited detrusor activity is often found at this stage and resembles that of the spastic neuropathic bladder.

If decompensation occurs, the vesical wall becomes attenuated and atonic, and capacity may be markedly increased. Overflow incontinence may develop. The behavior of the bladder is similar to that of the flaccid neuropathic bladder.

If the difficulty is nonneuropathic, the anal sphincter tone is normal and the bulbocavernosus reflex intact. Peripheral sensation, voluntary muscle contraction, and limb reflexes should also be normal. Cystoscopy and urethroscopy will reveal the local lesion causing obstruction. Once the obstruction is relieved, bladder function will improve but may never return to normal.

COMPLICATIONS OF NEUROPATHIC BLADDER

The principal complications of the neuropathic bladder are recurrent urinary tract infection, hydronephrosis secondary to ureteral reflux or obstruction, and stone formation. The primary factors contributing to these complications are the presence of residual urine, sustained high intravesical pressures, and immobilization, respectively.

Incontinence in neuropathic disorders may be passive, as in flaccid lesions where outlet resistance is compromised, or may be the result of uninhibited detrusor contractions, as in spastic lesions.

Infection

Infection is virtually inevitable with the neuropathic bladder state. During the stage of spinal shock that follows cord injury, the bladder must be emptied by catheterization. Sterile (or clean) intermittent catheterization is recommended at this stage, but for practical purposes or for the sake of convenience, a Foley catheter is often left indwelling. Chronic catheter drainage will guarantee infection regardless of any preventive measures taken.

The upper urinary tract is usually protected from infection by the integrity of the ureterovesical junction. If this becomes incompetent, infected urine will reflux up to the kidneys. Decompensation of the ureterovesical junction results from the high intravesical pressures generated by the spastic bladder. It is most important that these cases be treated aggressively with an intensive program of self-catheterization and anticholinergic medication. The Credé maneuver should not be used.

A number of infective complications can result from the presence of a chronically indwelling Foley catheter. These include cystitis and periurethritis resulting from mechanical irritation. A periurethral abscess may follow, with formation of a fistula via eventual rupture of the abscess through the perineal skin. Drainage may also take place through the urethra, with the end result being a urethral diverticulum. Infection may travel up into the prostatic ducts (prostatitis) or seminal vesicles (seminal vesiculitis) or along the vas into the epididymes (epididymitis) and testes (orchitis).

Hydronephrosis

Two mechanisms lead to back pressure on the kidney. Early, the effect of trigonal stretch secondary to residual urine and detrusor hypertonicity becomes compounded by evolving trigonal hypertrophy. The combination causes abnormal pull upon the ureterovesical junction, with increased resistance to the passage of urine. A "functional" obstruction results, which leads to progressive ureteral dilatation and back pressure on the kidney. At this stage, this condition can be relieved by continuous catheter drainage or by combined intermittent catheter drainage and use of anticholinergics.

A more delayed consequence of trigonal hypertrophy and detrusor spasticity is reflux due to decompensation of the ureterovesical junction. The causative factor appears to be a combination of high intravesical pressure and trabeculation of the bladder wall. The increased stiffness of the ureterovesical junction weakens its valvelike function, slowly eroding its ability to prevent reflux of urine during forceful bladder contractions.

Calculus

A number of factors contribute to stone formation in the bladder and kidneys. Bed rest and inactivity cause demineralization of the skeleton, mobilization of calcium, and subsequent hypercalciuria. Recumbency and inadequate fluid intake both contribute to urinary stasis, possibly with increased concentration of urinary calcium. Catheterization of the neurogenic bladder may introduce bacteria. Subsequent infection is usually due to a urea-splitting organism, which causes the urine to become alkaline, with reduced solubility of calcium and phosphate.

Renal Amyloidosis

Secondary amyloidosis of the kidney is a common cause of death in patients with neuropathic bladder. It is a result of chronic debilitation in patients with difficult decubitus ulcers and poorly controlled infection. Fortunately, due to better medical care, this is an uncommon finding today.

Sexual Dysfunction

Men who have suffered traumatic cord or cauda equina lesions experience varying degrees of sexual dysfunction. Those with upper motor lesions fare well, with the majority having reflexogenic erectile capability. Dangerous elevations in blood pressure can occur with erections in patients with high thoracic or cervical lesions. Problems of quality of erection or premature detumescence are found with all levels of injury. Patients with lower motor lesions are, as a rule, impotent, unless the lesion is incomplete. There is a high degree of variability in the sexual capabilities of patients with all levels of spinal injury. Fortunately, impotence need not be permanent, as sexual function can be restored to most patients following implantation of a penile prosthesis.

Often, patients with spinal injury lose the ability to ejaculate even with preservation of functional erections. This is a result of lost coordination between reflexes normally synchronized through higher center regulation. Patients may have the capability to ejaculate after an erection but are either unable to trigger this sexual event or are unable to trigger it in proper sequence. Techniques using electrical stimulation are now being developed to accomplish semen collection in patients with "functional infertility."

Autonomic Dysreflexia

Autonomic dysreflexia is sympathetically mediated reflex behavior triggered by excessive sacral afferent feedback to the spinal cord. The phenomenon is seen in patients with cord lesions above the sympathetic outflow from the cord. As a rule, it occurs in rather spastic lesions above T1 but on occasion in lesions of mild spasticity or those as low as T5. Symptoms include dramatic elevations in systolic or diastolic blood pressure (or both), increased pulse pressure, sweating, bradycardia, headache, and piloerection. Symptoms are brought on by overdistention of the bladder or spasm of the bladder against a closed sphincter. Immediate catheterization is indicated and will usually bring about prompt lowering of blood pressure. This observation has led to the use of sphincterotomy to prevent recurring problems with autonomic dysreflexia. Peripheral rhizotomy may be equally effective in eliminating somatic afferent feedback responsible for dysreflexia.

TREATMENT OF NEUROPATHIC BLADDER

The treatment of any form of neuropathic bladder is guided by the need to restore low pressure activity to the bladder. In doing so, renal function will be preserved, continence restored, and infection more readily controlled. Reflex evacuation may develop if detrusor integrity is protected and trigger techniques are practiced.

1. SPINAL SHOCK

Following severe injury to the spinal cord, the bladder becomes atonic. With most spinal injuries, it will gradually recover its contractile capabilities within months. A spastic state will evolve the degree of which will vary from patient to patient according to level of injury. Injuries to the sacral cord, if complete enough, may leave the bladder permanently flaccid. More often, however, these lesions are partial, and a mixed degree of detrusor/sphincter spasticity is found along with a variable degree of weakness. Lesions of the cervical cord tend to produce hypertonic, and less dynamically spastic, bladders than do injuries of the thoracic cord.

During the spinal shock stage, some type of bladder drainage must be instituted immediately and maintained. Chronic overdistention can damage the detrusor smooth muscle and limit functional recovery of the bladder. Intermittent catheterization using strict aseptic technique has proved to be the best form of management. This avoids urinary tract infection as well as the complications of an indwelling catheter (eg, urethral stricture, abscess, erosions, stones).

If a Foley catheter becomes necessary, a few principles need to be followed. The catheter should not be larger than 16F and should preferably be made of silicon, and it should be taped to the abdomen. Taping the catheter to the leg puts unnecessary stress on the penoscrotal junction and bulbous urethra (ie, the curves in the urethra), and this can lead to stricture formation. The catheter should be changed with sterile procedure every 2–3 weeks.

Some urologists advocate the use of suprapubic cystostomy rather than a urethral catheter to avoid the risks associated with permanent indwelling catheters. Certainly, whenever catheter-related complications occur, the physician should not hesitate in resorting to cystostomy drainage.

Irrigation of the bladder with antibiotic solutions, use of systemic antibiotics, or covering the tip of the meatus with antibiotic creams does not significantly lower the long-term risk of bladder infection. Keeping the meatus lubricated will, however, help avoid meatal stricturing.

As peripheral reflex excitability gradually returns, urodynamic evaluation should be performed. A cystogram is needed to rule out reflux. The urodynamic study should be repeated periodically as long as spasticity is improving and then annually to check for complications of the upper urinary tract.

In order to control infection, a fluid intake of at least 2–3 L/D should be maintained (100–200 mL/h) if at all possible. This reduces stasis and decreases the concentration of calcium in the urine. Renal and ureteral drainage are enhanced by moving the patient frequently, with ambulation in a wheelchair as soon as possible, and even by raising the head of the bed. These measures improve ureteral transport of urine, reduce stasis, and lower the risk of infection.

Additional measures will aid in prophylaxis for calculus formation (eg, reduction of intake of calcium and oxalate and elimination of vitamin D in the diet).

2. SPECIFIC TYPES OF NEUROPATHIC BLADDER

Once a neuropathic voiding disorder is established, regardless of cause, the following steps should be taken to attain optimum function.

Spastic Neuropathic Bladder

A. Patient With Reasonable Bladder Capacity: To successfully rehabilitate a bladder to a functional state, a patient should be able to go 2–3 hours between voiding and not be incontinent during this interval. Voiding is initiated using trigger techniques—tapping the abdomen suprapubically, tugging on the pubic hair, squeezing the penis, or scratching the skin of the lower abdomen, genitalia, or thighs. Patients can accomplish this on their own unless they are high quadriplegics with no upper limb function.

Some patients in this category will empty the bladder completely but are incontinent due to inconvenient triggering of the voiding reflex. They may be helped by low-dose anticholinergic medication or by placing an electrode on the pudendal nerve to effect chronic stimulation of the urethral sphincter.

B. Patient With Markedly Diminished Functional Vesical Capacity: If the functional capacity of the bladder is under 100 mL, involuntary voiding can occur as often as every 15 minutes. Satisfactory training of the bladder cannot be achieved, and alternative measures must be taken. These choices include the following:

1. The possibility that reduced functional bladder capacity is due to a large residual volume of urine must be ruled out. One of the following treatment regimens can then be administered.

2. A permanent indwelling catheter with or without anticholinergic medication.

3. A condom catheter and a leg bag in males. Residual urine should not be a concern, and the patient should not have bladder pressures above 40 cm of water on urodynamic evaluation. If either of these parameters is found, the upper urinary tract is considered at risk from obstruction or reflux.

4. Performance of a sphincterotomy in males. It is possible to turn the bladder into a urinary conduit by surgically eliminating all outlet resistance from the bladder. This option should be used only when other options have failed, as it is irreversible. Patients having this procedure are usually suffering from more serious sequelas of a highly spastic bladder (ie, upper urinary tract dilatation, recurrent urinary tract infections, or marked autonomic dysreflexia).

5. The spastic bladder could be converted to a flaccid bladder through sacral rhizotomy. Complete surgical section or percutaneous heat fulguration of the S3 and S4 roots would be necessary. Chemical rhizotomy is unreliable, as spasticity usually returns after 6–9 months. These procedures may cause loss of reflex erections, and the decision to perform them should be weighed accordingly. They can relieve spasticity, lower intravesical pressures, increase bladder storage, and decrease the risk of damage to the upper urinary tract. The bladder would then be managed as a flaccid bladder (see below).

6. Neurostimulation of the sacral nerve roots to accomplish bladder evacuation (see below).

7. Urinary diversion for irreversible, progressive upper urinary tract deterioration. A variety of procedures are available, including the standard ileal conduit, cutaneous ureterostomies, transureteroureterostomy, or nonrefluxing urinary diversions (eg, Mainz pouch, Koch pouch, or one of several other imaginative and useful diversions designed to protect the upper urinary tract and kidneys).

8. In females with a spastic bladder, one does not have the option of performing a sphincterotomy as in males. If pharmacologic methods are unsuccessful, surgical conversion to a flaccid, low-pressure system or a urinary diversion should be considered.

C. Parasympatholytic Drugs: Because of the chronic nature of the neuropathic bladder, patients are not always willing to tolerate the side effects of parasympatholytic drugs. Two drugs in this category can be given alternatively to reduce individual side effects. They also may be useful when given with skeletal muscle relaxants. Dosages must be individualized. Commonly used drugs and dosages are as follows: oxybutynin chloride (Ditropan), 5 mg 2–3 times daily; dicyclomine hydrochloride (Bentyl), 80 mg in 4 equally divided doses daily; methantheline bromide (Banthine), 50–100 mg every 6 hours; propantheline bromide (Pro-Banthine), 15 mg 30 minutes before meals and 30 mg at bedtime. These drugs may not be effective if incontinence is the result of uninhibited sphincter relaxation or compliance changes in the bladder wall.

D. Neurostimulation (Bladder Pacemaker): Neuroprosthetics are becoming an established alternative to managing selective neuropathic bladder disorders. Patients are evaluated for a bladder pacemaker primarily by urodynamic monitoring of bladder and sphincter responses to trial stimulation of the various sacral nerve roots. Selective blocks are then prepared to the right and left pudendal nerves. If voiding is produced, patients are considered suitable for a neuroprosthesis. Other factors such as detrusor storage capability, sphincter competence, age, kidney function, and overall neurologic and psychologic status are also taken into consideration.

Electrodes are implanted on the motor (ventral) nerve roots of those sacral nerves that will produce detrusor contraction on stimulation (always S3, occasionally S4) (Fig 20–3). Steps are then taken to reduce sphincter hyperreflexia by selectively dividing the sensory (dorsal) component of these same sacral nerve roots and selective branches of the pudendal nerves. The electrodes are connected to a subcutaneous receiver that can be controlled from outside the body.

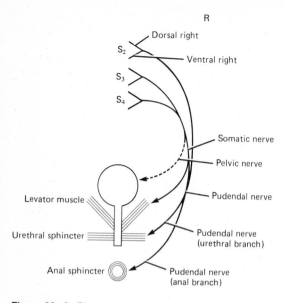

Figure 20–3. Diagrammatic representation of various elements involved in the innervation of the lower urinary tract and pelvic floor, with identification of potential sites for elective stimulation or selective neurotomy.

Bladder or bowel evacuation or continence can then be controlled selectively by the external transmitter.

There are 3 overall goals in the management of the bladder in spastic upper motor neuron lesions—preservation of renal function, continence, and evacuation. The first 2 are accomplished by reducing intravesical pressures. This step will protect the integrity of the upper urinary tract and restore continence by increasing storage capacity. Both can be achieved by combining neurostimulation of the sphincter with selective sacral neurotomies. This approach preserves sphincter integrity and avoids the need for drugs. Other options include complete bladder denervation or bladder augmentation.

The third goal, restoration of controlled evacuation, eliminates the need for catheters and associated risk of infection. This is the most difficult goal to achieve, and patients need to be carefully evaluated for their suitability.

Flaccid Neuropathic Bladder

If the neurologic lesion completely destroys the micturition center, volitional voiding cannot be accomplished without manual suprapubic pressure, ie, the Credé maneuver. Bladder evacuation can be accomplished by straining, using the abdominal and diaphragmatic muscles to raise intra-abdominal pressures. Partial injuries to the lower spinal cord (T10–11) result in a spastic bladder and a weak or weakly spastic sphincter. Incontinence can then result from spontaneous detrusor contraction.

A. Bladder Training and Care: In partial lower motor neuron injury, voiding should be tried every 2 hours by the clock to avoid embarrassing leakage.

This will help protect the bladder from overdistention due to a buildup of residual urine.

B. Intermittent Catheterization: Any patient with adequate bladder capacity can benefit from regular intermittent catheter drainage every 3–6 hours. This technique eliminates residual urine, helps prevent infection, avoids incontinence, and protects against damage to the upper urinary tract. It simulates normal voiding and is easily learned and adapted by patients. It is an extremely satisfactory solution to the problems of the flaccid neuropathic bladder. A clean technique is used rather than the inconvenient, expensive sterile technique. Urinary tract infections are infrequent, but if they occur, a prophylactic antibiotic can be given once daily. It is contraindicated if ureteral reflux is present, unless the reflux is mild and the bladder emptied frequently. Otherwise, patients are better managed with an indwelling Foley catheter, at least until the reflux is corrected.

C. Surgery: Transurethral resection is indicated for hypertrophy of the bladder neck or an enlarged prostate, either of which may cause obstruction of the bladder outlet and retention of residual urine. It may also be performed in some male patients to weaken the outlet resistance of the bladder to permit voiding by the Credé maneuver or abdominal straining.

Complete urinary incontinence due to sphincter incompetence can be managed by implanting an artificial sphincter. Bladder pressure should be low, however, for this to be successful. Bladder neck reconstruction may also be considered as a way to increase outlet resistance.

Incontinence in this group of patients can be treated by drugs or neurostimulation if it results from mild bladder spasticity.

D. Parasympathomimetic Drugs: The stable derivatives of acetylcholine are at times of value in assisting the evacuation of the bladder. Although they *do not* initiate or effect bladder contractions, they do provide increased bladder tonus. They may be helpful in symptomatic treatment of the milder types of flaccid neuropathic bladder. Drugs may be tried empirically, but usefulness is best gauged during urodynamic evaluation. If filling pressures or resting tonus is increased after urecholine is administered, evacuation of the bladder through trigger reflexes or straining should be more effective. The drug then should be clinically helpful.

Bethanechol chloride (Urecholine) is the drug of choice. It is given orally, 25–50 mg every 6–8 hours. In special situations (eg, urodynamic study or immediately following operation), it may be given subcutaneously, 5–10 mg every 6–8 hours.

Neuropathic Bladder Associated With Spina Bifida

Spina bifida is incomplete formation of the neural arch at various levels of the spine. The defect is recognized at birth and closed immediately to prevent infection. The scarring that results can entrap and tether nerves in the cauda equina. With failure of the neural arch to close, there is failure of anterior horn cell development and organization. The end result is a mixed type of neuropathic defect. Roughly two-thirds of patients will have a spastic bladder with weakness in the feet and toes. About one-third will have a flaccid bladder. Often, there is a greater degree of flaccidity in the pelvic floor than in the detrusor.

The goals of therapy are to control incontinence and preserve renal function.

A. Conservative Treatment: Clean intermittent catheterization is the best management. Parents can be taught to do this for the child, and eventually the child can take over this function. Frequency should be determined by the storage capacity of the bladder and the fluid intake, usually every 3–6 hours. An anticholinergic drug may be required to mediate bladder spasticity and improve storage function in order to control incontinence.

1. Mild symptoms–If there is occasional dribbling or some residual urine associated with lack of desire to void, the patient should try to void every 2 hours when awake. Manual suprapubic pressure will enhance the efficiency of emptying. An external condom catheter or a small pad can be worn to protect against small-volume urine losses.

2. More severe symptoms–If urinary incontinence is associated with residual urine or if ureteral reflux is found, the following steps should be taken:

a. Hypotonic bladder–If reflux has been demonstrated, intermittent self-catheterization 4–6 times a day may protect the upper urinary tract from deterioration and the consequences of pyelonephritis. Ureteral reimplantation can be considered for bilateral reflux or a transureteroureterostomy for single-sided reflux if all other considerations are favorable. Intermittent catheterization should then be reinstituted.

b. Hypertonic bladder–The problem with patients in this category is more serious because the bladder is spastic with reduced capacity and the sphincter is hypotonic. Virtually constant dribbling can result. The cystogram will reveal heavy trabeculation of the bladder, often with reflux and advanced hydroureteronephrosis. Anticholinergic medication should be given, and an indwelling catheter should be inserted for several months. Once upper urinary tract dilatation has improved and the bladder has been restored to a more spherical shape, intermittent catheterization may be reinstituted. With time and care, many of these children develop a more balanced type of bladder behavior. Continence may be gained without compromising the upper urinary tract.

Most of these patients will not require urinary diversion if they are carefully followed and if the parents actively participate in their care.

B. Surgical Treatment: If the bladder is of the spastic type with diminished capacity, there are several surgical options short of actual urinary diversion. Sacral nerve block during urodynamic evaluation will help in determining whether sacral nerve root section would be beneficial. This will help in cases of spastic bladder but not in cases of poorly compliant, fibrotic bladder. Sectioning the S3 nerves will reduce intravesical pressures, improve storage, and reduce the risk of reflux or obstruction of the ureters. A selective pudendal neurectomy might accomplish a similar goal, but, again, the effect should be tested urodynamically before operation is performed.

For the patient with a mildly spastic bladder and reasonable storage capacity (> 200 mL), urinary incontinence might be controlled via electrostimulation of the pelvic floor. Many of these patients have intact nerves to the sphincter. These can be stimulated to enhance sphincter tone and inhibit voiding.

If the refluxing patient suffers recurrent fever (equivalent to pyelonephritis) despite the presence of an indwelling catheter or if incontinence cannot be controlled because of poor detrusor compliance, then urinary diversion must be considered. Nonrefluxing diversions offer the most favorable long-term outlook for preservation of the upper urinary tract.

3. CONTROL OF URINARY INCONTINENCE

In the Hospital

Urinary incontinence is one of the most distressing aspects of neurovesical dysfunction, especially when the bladder has otherwise adequate function. The problem is minimized in men who are hospitalized because supervision is available, bathrooms are nearby, and a bedside urinal is always available. Women have a greater problem because they must use a bedpan or may require an indwelling catheter. Catheters have associated risks and do not always control leakage associated with spastic bladder. No simple, satisfactory solution to this problem has been devised for females.

After Discharge

After discharge from the hospital, most men with spastic bladders will rely on a condom catheter for protection against leakage and for practical urine collection. The only exception will be patients who are predictably dry between catheterizations. The condom catheter attaches to the penis without pressure and has a conduit to a leg bag. The adhesives are nonirritating and long-lasting. Problems involved in keeping these catheters in place are limited to noncircumcised patients and those with large suprapubic fat pads that shorten the length of the shaft of the penis. Circumcision or placement of a penile prosthesis will correct for these limitations.

Urethral compression by means of a Cunningham clamp is occasionally preferred by patients. This protects only against low-pressure leakage, however, and if it is applied too tightly, a urethral diverticulum may develop.

Other types of external collection devices are available (McGuire urinal, Texas catheter), but with advancements in adhesive glues for condom catheters and use of penile prostheses, these other methods are being used less frequently.

Recent Developments

Extensive research continues to be conducted on methods of restoring complete voluntary control over the storage and evacuation functions of the bladder. Sacral and pudendal nerve anatomy has been determined, so that surgical exposure of these nerves and their branches is possible. An electrode can be placed for selective stimulation of the bladder, levator, and urethral or anal sphincters. A number of possibilities exist for neurostimulation or rhizotomy, but only a few are practical. Urodynamic evaluation of bladder function following a nerve block or during neurostimulation can help determine the therapeutic value of these treatments.

Single or multiple electrodes can be placed on selected nerves and then coupled to a subcutaneous receiver. The desired function (continence or evacuation) can be selected. Usually, one or the other is needed in any one patient. Much will change in this approach as technologic advances become adapted to the increased understanding of bladder physiology. Striking successes are also being seen with electro-evacuation in highly selected patients.

TREATMENT OF COMPLICATIONS OF NEUROPATHIC BLADDER

The most common and significant complications can be discovered by cystography, cystoscopy, urography, ultrasound, and urodynamic studies. Patients should be evaluated once a year for changes in lower urinary tract behavior, ureteral reflux or obstruction, and deterioration of the renal integrity.

Infection

A. Pyelonephritis: Episodic renal infection should be treated aggressively and quickly to prevent progressive renal loss. Appropriate antibiotics should be administered and the source or cause of infection addressed.

B. Epididymitis: This is a complication of dyssynergic voiding patterns. High voiding pressures in the prostatic urethra due to a spastic external sphincter predispose to reflux of urine into the prostatic ducts and vas deferens. Infected urine eventually backwashes into the dilated ductal system, causing inflammation in the prostate, seminal vesicles, and epididymis. Indwelling catheters can predispose to these conditions because they are irritating in themselves, and, as foreign bodies, they increase the bacterial concentration throughout the urethra.

Treatment follows the usual regimen of appropriate antibiotics, bed rest, and scrotal elevation. If possible, an indwelling catheter should be removed or replaced with a suprapubic catheter. Preferred long-term management would be to place the patient on an intermittent self-catheterization program with prophylactic antibiotics. Rarely, ligation of the vas is required.

Hydronephrosis

Ureteral reflux, as shown by cystography, is an indication to radically adjust previous methods of bladder care. An indwelling catheter will manage the problem over the short term. If, despite prolonged drainage, reflux persists, vesicoureteroplasty must be considered. An additional procedure may also be needed to reduce high pressures in the bladder (augmentation of the bladder, sacral rhizotomy, transurethral resection [TUR] of the bladder outlet). Progressive hydronephrosis may require nephrostomy drainage to be lifesaving. Urinary diversion is a last-resort measure that should be avoidable if a patient is followed regularly.

Calculus

A. Bladder Stones: Vesical stones, diagnosed by x-ray or cystoscopy, are usually composed of calcium phosphate. They result from the presence of residual urine, which has a raised pH due to chronic infection. They are generally soft, are crushed or broken easily, and can be washed out through a rigid cystoscope sheath. Occasionally, they are large and must be removed via suprapubic cystotomy.

B. Ureteral Stones: Ureteral stones can be suspected on a KUB of the abdomen, but intravenous urography is needed to diagnose stones in the urinary tract. If no radiopaque fluid is excreted, cystoscopy must be performed, with passage of a ureteral catheter and retrograde injection of contrast medium. Virtually all ureteral stones are now removed using antegrade or retrograde techniques of retrieval (see Chapter 16). Operative removal is occasionally necessary when direct ureteroscopy is unsuccessful.

C. Renal Stones: The diagnosis of renal stones is made by radiography. Ultrasound is increasingly valuable in screening patients for calculus in the renal pelvis. If the stone is obstructive, it must be removed; if not, the patient can be followed for a time. Stones in the renal pelvis can now be removed using extracorporeal shock-wave lithotripsy (ESWL). Due to its non-surgical approach, stones in the renal pelvis do not have to be tolerated for long periods. Kidney stones in a patient with neurogenic bladder generally are the result of urinary tract infection and also serve as sources for recurring infection and subsequent sequellae (eg, pyelonephritis, pyonephrosis, renal abscess and renal failure). Stones are therefore a source of potential trouble, and removing them can minimize risks to the kidneys.

PROGNOSIS

The greatest threat to the patient with a neuropathic bladder is progressive renal damage (pyelonephritis, calculosis, and hydronephrosis). Advances in the management of the neuropathic bladder, together with better follow-up of patients at regular intervals, have substantially improved the outlook for long-term survival.

REFERENCES

Applebaum ML et al: Unmyelinated fibers in the sacral 3 and caudal 1 ventral roots of the cat. *J Physiol* 1976;**256**:557.

Barrington FJF: The component reflexes of micturition in the cat. *Brain* 1941;**64**:239.

Barrington FJF: The component reflexes of micturition in the cat. (2 parts.) *Brain* 1931;**54**:177.

Bazeed MA et al: Histochemical study of urethral striated musculature in the dog. *J Urol* 1982;**128**:406.

Bradley WE: Cerebrocortical innervation of the urinary bladder. *Tohoku J Exp Med* 1980;**131**:7.

Bradley WE, Conway CJ: Bladder representation in the pontine mesencephalic reticular formation. *Exp Neurol* 1966;**16**:237.

Bradley WE, Teague CT: Cerebellar regulation of the micturition reflex. *J Urol* 1969;**101**:396.

Bradley WE, Teague CT: Spinal cord organization of micturition reflex afferents. *Exp Neurol* 1968;**22**:504.

DeGroat WC, Booth AM: Inhibition and facilitation in parasympathetic ganglia of the urinary bladder. *Fed Proc* 1980;**39**:2990.

DeGroat WC et al: Organization of the sacral parasympathetic reflex pathways to the urinary bladder and large intestine. *J Auton Nerv Syst* 1981;**3**:135.

DeGroat WC et al: Parasympathetic preganglionic neurons in the sacral spinal cord. *J Auton Nerv Syst* 1982;**5**:23.

Donker PJ, Droes JT, VanUlden BM: Anatomy of the musculature and innervation of the bladder and the urethra. In: *Scientific Foundations of Urology*. Williams DI, Chisolm GD (editors). Year Book, 1976.

Enhorning G: Simultaneous recording of intraurethral and intravesical pressure. *Acta Chir Scand [Suppl]* 1961;**276**:1.

Gosling J: The structure of the bladder and urethra in relation to function. *Urol Clin North Am* 1979;**6**:31.

Gosling JA, Dixon JS: Sensory nerves in the mammalian urinary tract: An evaluation using light and electron microscopy. *J Anat* 1974;**117**:133.

Gosling JA, Dixon JS, Lendon RG: The autonomic innervation of the human male and female bladder neck and proximal urethra. *J Urol* 1977;**118**:302.

Gosling JA et al: A comparative study of the human external sphincter and periurethral levator ani muscles. *Br J Urol* 1981;**53**:35.

Hackler RH: A 25-year prospective mortality study in the spinal cord injured patient: Comparison with the long-term living paraplegic. *J Urol* 1977;**117**:486.

Klück P: The autonomic innervation of the human urinary bladder, bladder neck and urethra: A histochemical study. *Anat Rec* 1980;**198**:439.

Krane RJ, Siroky MB: Classification of neurourologic disorders. In: *Clinical Neurourology*. Krane RJ, Siroky MB (editors). Little, Brown, 1979.

Kuru M: Nervous control of micturition. *Physiol Rev* 1965;**45**:425.

Léger L, Hernandez-Nicaise ML: The cat locus coeruleus: Light and electron microscopic study of the neuronal somata. *Anat Embryol* 1980;**159**:181.

Lewin RJ, Porter RW: Inhibition of spontaneous bladder activity by stimulation of the globus pallidus. *Neurology* 1965;**15**:1049.

Mackel R: Segmental and descending control of the external urethral and anal sphincters in the cat. *J Physiol* 1979;**294**:105.

McGuire EJ, Rossier AB: Treatment of acute autonomic dysreflexia. *J Urol* 1983;**129**:1185.

McGuire EJ, Savastano JA: Long-term follow-up of spinal cord injury patients managed by intermittent catheterization. *J Urol* 1983;**129**:775.

Millard RJ, Oldenburg BF: Symptomatic, urodynamic and psychodynamic results of bladder re-education programs. *J Urol* 1983;**130**:715.

Morgan CW, Nadelhaft I, DeGroat WC: The distribution of visceral primary afferents from the pelvic nerve to Lissauer's tract and the spinal gray matter and its relationship to the sacral parasympathetic nucleus. *J Comp Neurol* 1981;**201**:415.

Morgan CW, Nadelhaft I, DeGroat WC: Location of bladder preganglionic neurons in the parasympathetic nucleus of the cat. *Neurosci Lett* 1979;**14**:189.

Murnaghan GF: Neurogenic disorders of the bladder in parkinsonism. *Br J Urol* 1961;**33**:403.

Pengelly A: Effect of prolonged bladder distention on detrusor function. *Urol Clin North Am* 1979;**6**:279.

Rhame FS, Perkash I: Urinary tract infections occurring in recent spinal cord injury patients on intermittent catheterization. *J Urol* 1979;**122**:669.

Ryall RW, Piercy MF: Visceral afferent and efferent fibers in sacral ventral roots in cats. *Brain Res* 1970;**23**:57.

Satoh K: Descending projection of the nucleus tegmentis laterodorsalis to the spinal cord. *Neurosci Lett* 1978;**8**:9.

Satoh K: Localization of the micturition center at dorsolateral pontine tegmentum of the rat. *Neurosci Lett* 1978;**8**:27.

Schmidt RA: Advances in genitourinary neurostimulation. *Neurosurgery* 1986;**19**:1041.

Schmidt RA: Neural prostheses and bladder control. *Engineering in Biology and Medicine* 1983;**2**:31.

Snyder SH: Brain peptides as neurotransmitters. *Science* 1980;**209**:976.

Sundin T et al: The sympathetic innervation and adrenoreceptor function of the human lower urinary tract in the normal state and after parasympathetic denervation. *Invest Urol* 1977;**14**:322.

Thomas TM, Karran OD, Meade TW: Management of urinary incontinence in patients with multiple sclerosis. *J R Coll Gen Pract* 1981;**31**:296.

Tohyama M et al: Organization and projections of the neurons in the dorsal tegmental area of the rat. *J Hirnforsch* 1978;**19**:165.

Torrens MJ, Griffith HB: Management of the uninhibited bladder by selective sacral neurectomy. *J Neurosurg* 1976;**44**:176.

Twiddy DAS, Downie JW, Awad SA: Response of the bladder to bethanechol after acute spinal cord transection in cats. *J Pharmacol Exp Ther* 1980;**215**:500.

Woodside JR, McGuire EJ: Detrusor hypertonicity as a late complication of a Wertheim hysterectomy. *J Urol* 1982;**127**:1143.

21

Urodynamic Studies

Emil A. Tanagho, MD

Urodynamic study is becoming an important part of the evaluation of patients with voiding dysfunctions—dysuria, urinary incontinence, neuropathic disorders, etc. Formerly, the examiner simply observed the act of voiding, noting the strength of the urinary stream and drawing inferences about the possibility of obstruction of the bladder outlet. In the 1950s, it became possible to observe the lower urinary tract by fluoroscopy during the act of voiding; and in the 1960s, the principles of hydrodynamics were applied to lower urinary tract physiology. The field of urodynamics now has clinical applications in evaluating voiding problems resulting from lower urinary tract disease.

The nomenclature of the tests used in urodynamic studies is not yet settled, and the meanings of urodynamic terms are sometimes overlapping or confusing. In spite of these difficulties, however, urodynamic tests are extremely valuable. Symptoms elicited by the history or by physical, endoscopic, or even radiographic examination must often be further investigated by urodynamic tests so that therapy can be devised that is based on an understanding of the altered physiology of the lower urinary tract.

As is true of many high-technology testing procedures (eg, electrocardiography, electroencephalography), urodynamic tests have greatest clinical validity when their interpretation is left to the treating physician, who should either supervise the study or be responsible for correlating all of the findings with personal clinical observations.

FUNCTIONS RELEVANT TO URODYNAMICS & TESTS APPLICABLE TO EACH

Urodynamic study of the lower urinary tract can provide useful clinical information about the function of the urinary bladder, the sphincteric mechanism, and the voiding pattern itself.

Bladder function has been classically studied by cystography and active motion fluoroscopy. Urodynamic studies utilize cystometry. Conventional radiographic studies and urodynamic studies can of course be usefully combined.

Sphincteric function depends upon 2 elements: the smooth muscle sphincter and the voluntary sphincter. The activity of both elements can be recorded urodynamically by pressure measurements; the activity of

the voluntary sphincter can be recorded by electromyography.

The act of voiding is a function of the interaction between bladder and sphincter, and the result is the **flow rate.** The flow rate is one major aspect of the total function of the lower urinary tract: It is generally recorded in milliliters per second as well as by total urine volume voided. The simultaneous recording of bladder activity (by intraluminal pressure measurements), sphincteric activity (by electromyography or pressure measurements), and flow rate will reveal interrelationships between the 3 elements. Each measurement may give useful information about the normality or abnormality of one specific aspect of lower urinary tract function. A more complete picture is provided by integrating all 3 lower tract elements in a simultaneously recorded comparative manner. This comprehensive approach may involve synchronous recordings of variable pressures, flow rate, volume voided, and electrical activity of skeletal musculature around the urinary sphincter (electromyography), along with fluoroscopic imaging of the lower urinary tract. The multiple pressures to be recorded are quite variable and usually include intravesical pressure, intraurethral pressure at several levels, intra-abdominal pressure, and anal sphincter pressure as a function of muscular activity of the pelvic floor.

The techniques of urodynamic study must be tailored to the needs of specific patients. Each method has advantages and limitations depending upon the requirements of each study. In one patient, results of a single test might be sufficient to establish the diagnosis and suggest appropriate therapy; in another, many more studies might be necessary.

PHYSIOLOGIC & HYDRODYNAMIC CONSIDERATIONS

URINARY FLOW RATE

Because urinary flow rate is the product of detrusor action against outlet resistance, a variation from the normal flow rate might reflect dysfunction of either.

The normal flow rate from a full bladder is about 20–25 mL/s in men and 25–30 mL/s in women. These variations are directly related to the volume voided and the subject's age. Obstruction should be suspected in any adult voiding with a full bladder at a rate of less than 15 mL/s. A flow rate less than 10 mL/s is considered definite evidence of obstruction. Occasionally, one encounters "supervoiders" with flow rates far above the normal range. This may signify low outlet resistance but is of less concern clinically than obstruction.

Outlet Resistance

Outlet resistance is the primary determinant of flow rate and varies according to mechanical or functional factors. Functionally, outlet resistance is primarily related to sphincteric activity, which is controlled by both the smooth sphincter and the voluntary sphincter. The smooth sphincter is rarely overactive in women; we have never seen an example of it in any of our urodynamic evaluations. Overactivity of the smooth sphincter is rarely seen in men but may occur in association with hypertrophy of the bladder neck due to neurogenic dysfunction or distal obstruction. However, such cases must be critically evaluated before this conclusion is reached.

Increased voluntary sphincter activity is not uncommon. It is often neglected as a primary underlying cause of increased sphincteric resistance. It is manifested either as lack of relaxation or as actual overactivity during voiding. The normal voluntary sphincter provides adequate resistance, along with the smooth sphincter, to prevent escape of urine from the bladder; if the voluntary sphincter does not relax during detrusor contraction, partial functional obstruction occurs. Overactivity of the sphincter, resulting in increased outlet resistance, is usually a neuropathic phenomenon. However, it can also be functional, resulting from irritative phenomena such as infection or other factors—chemical, bacterial, hormonal, or, even more commonly and often not appreciated, psychologic.

Mechanical Factors

Mechanical factors resulting in obstruction to urine flow are the easiest to identify by conventional methods. In women, they may take the form of cystoceles, urethral kinks, or, most commonly, iatrogenic scarring, fibrosis, and compression from previous vaginal or periurethral operative procedures. Mechanical factors in men are well known to all urologists; the classic form is benign prostatic hypertrophy. Urethral stricture due to various causes and posterior urethral valves are other common causes of urinary obstruction in males, and there are many others.

Normal voiding with a normal flow rate is the product of both detrusor activity and outlet resistance. A high intravesical pressure resulting from detrusor contraction is not necessary to initiate voiding, because outlet resistance has usually dropped to a minimum. Sphincteric relaxation usually precedes detrusor contraction by a few seconds, and when relaxation is maximal, detrusor activity starts and is sustained until the bladder is empty.

Variations in Normal Flow Rate

The sequence just described is not essential for normal flow rates. The flow rate may be normal in the absence of any detrusor contraction if sphincteric relaxation is assisted by increased intra-abdominal pressure from straining. Persons with weak outlet resistance and weak sphincteric control can achieve a normal flow rate by complete voluntary sphincteric relaxation without detrusor contraction or straining. A normal flow rate can be achieved in spite of increased sphincteric activity or lack of complete relaxation if detrusor contraction is increased to overcome outlet resistance.

Because a normal flow rate can be achieved in spite of abnormalities of one or more of the mechanisms involved, recording the flow rate alone does not provide insight into the precise mechanisms by which it occurs. Distinction between patterns of flow can be difficult. For practical purposes, if the flow rate is adequate and the recorded pattern and configuration of the flow curve are normal, these variations may not be clinically significant except in rare cases.

Nomenclature

The study of urinary flow rate itself is usually called **uroflowmetry.** The flow rate is generally identified as **maximum flow rate, average flow rate, flow time, maximum flow time** (the time elapsed before maximum flow rate is reached), and **total flow time** (the aggregate of flow time if the flow has been interrupted by periods of no voiding) (Fig 21–1). The **flow rate pattern** is characterized as continuous or intermittent, etc.

Pattern Measurement of Flow Rate

A normal flow pattern is represented by a bell-shaped curve (Fig 21–1). However, the curve is rarely completely smooth; it may vary within certain limits and still be normal. Flow rate can be determined by measuring a 5-second collection at the peak of flow and dividing the amount obtained by 5 to arrive at the average rate per second. This rough estimate is useful, especially if the flow rate is normal and the values are above 20 mL/s. Peak urine flow can also be measured quite easily with a Peakometer—a device employing a color indicator strip that, when impregnated with urine, shows maximum flow rate by changes in color against a predetermined scale. The Drake uroflowmeter is a plastic container with several chambers into which the patient voids; the maximum flow rate is determined by noting how many chambers contain urine.

In modern practice, the flow rate is more often recorded electronically: The patient voids into a container on top of a measuring device that is connected to a transducer, the weight being converted to volume and recorded on a chart in mL/s. Fig 21–2 is an example of such a recording from a normal man. The general bell-shaped curve is quite clear, and the tracing

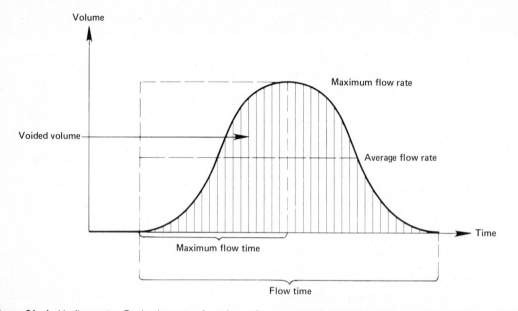

Figure 21–1. Uroflowmetry. Basic elements of maximum flow, average flow, total flow time, and total volume voided.

shows all of the values discussed above: total flow time, maximum flow time, maximum flow rate, average flow rate, and total volume voided. Occasional "supervoiders" can exceed the limits of the chart, but this is usually not of clinical concern (Fig 21–3). A possible variation in the bell appearance is seen in Fig 21–4.

The overall appearance of the flow curve may disclose unsuspected abnormalities. In Fig 21–5, for example, flow time is greatly prolonged. Maximum flow rate may not be low, but the average flow rate is very low—though the maximum flow rate is at one time within the normal range. Such fluctuation in flow rate is most commonly related to variations in voluntary sphincter activity. In Fig 21–6, this pattern is extreme: Maximum flow rate never exceeds 15 mL/s and

average flow rate is about 10 mL/s, which is indicative of obstruction. (Again, this fluctuation in pattern probably reflects sphincteric hyperactivity.)

The flow rate pattern reveals a great deal about the forces involved. For example, if the patient is voiding without the aid of detrusor contractions—primarily by straining—this can be easily deduced from the pattern of the flow rate. Fig 21–7 shows an example of intermittent voiding, primarily by straining, with no detrusor activity and at a rate that sometimes does not reach the usual peaks. With experience, one becomes expert at detecting the mechanism underlying abnormalities in flow rate. For example, in Fig 21–5, the maximum flow rate is in the normal range, the average flow rate is slightly low, and the curve has a general bell pattern, yet brief partial intermittent obstructions to flow can

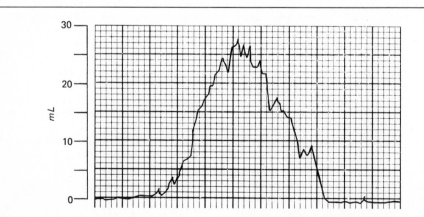

Figure 21–2. Classic normal flow rate, with peak of about 30 mL/s and average of about 20 mL/s. On the horizontal scale, one large square equals 5 seconds.

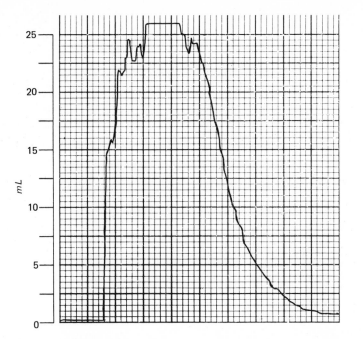

Figure 21–3. Flow rate of "supervoider." Maximum flow rate exceeds limits of chart. Tracing shows fast build-up and complete bladder emptying of large volume of urine in very short period. On the horizontal scale, one large square equals 5 seconds.

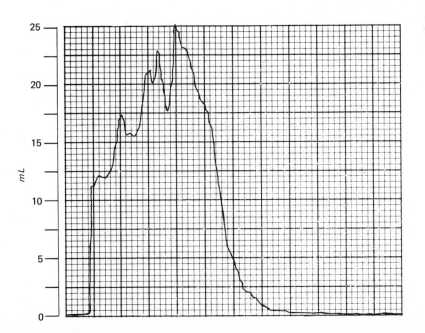

Figure 21–4. Normal flow rate but with some variation in appearance of curve. Note rapid pressure rise but progressive increase to maximum, then a sharp drop. There is also fluctuation in ascending limb of tracing. On the horizontal scale, one large square equals 5 seconds.

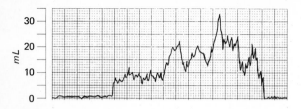

Figure 21–5. Rather low flow rate (not exceeding 10 mL/s), yet at one point the peak reaches 30–32 mL/s. Note again fluctuation in flow. On the horizontal scale, one large square equals 5 seconds.

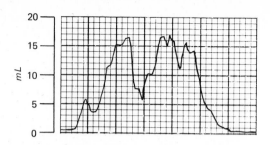

Figure 21–6. Very low flow rate of short duration and small volume. Note that maximum flow is not above 15 mL/s; however, flow average is less than 10 mL/s, and flow is almost completely interrupted in middle. On the horizontal scale, one large square equals 5 seconds.

be readily interpreted as due to overactivity of the voluntary sphincter, a mild form of detrusor/sphincter dyssynergia (see below).

Flow rates in mechanical obstruction are totally different, classically in the range of 5–6 mL/s; flow time is greatly prolonged, and there is sustained low flow with minimal variation (Fig 21–8). Fig 21–9 shows a striking example of a patient with benign prostatic hypertrophy. No simultaneous studies are needed with such a pattern, since the pattern is obviously one of mechanical obstruction.

Reduced flow rate in the absence of mechanical obstruction is due to some impairment of sphincteric or detrusor activity. This is seen in a variety of conditions, eg, normal detrusor contraction with no associated sphincteric relaxation and normal detrusor contraction with sphincteric overactivity, which is more serious. These 2 entities are commonly referred to as **detrusor/sphincter dyssynergia.** If, with detrusor contraction, the sphincter does not relax and open up or (worse) if it becomes overactive, urine flow is obstructed, ie, flow rate is reduced and of abnormal pattern. Reduced flow rate may occur even with increased detrusor activity if the latter is not adequate to overcome sphincteric resistance.

So many variations are possible in the shape of the flow curve—no matter how accurately the flow is recorded or how often the study is repeated to confirm abnormal findings—that it is beneficial to relate it to simultaneous recordings, such as of bladder pressure, pelvic floor electromyography, urethral pressure

profile, or simply cinefluoroscopy. Nevertheless, by itself it can be one of the most valuable urodynamic studies undertaken to evaluate a specific type of voiding dysfunction. Flowmetry not only is of diagnostic value but is also valuable in follow-up studies and in deciding on treatment. In some cases, however, flowmetry alone does not provide enough data about the abnormality in the voiding mechanism. More information must then be obtained by evaluation of bladder function.

BLADDER FUNCTION

The basic factors of normal bladder function are bladder capacity, sensation, accommodation, contractility, voluntary control, and response to drugs. All of them can be evaluated by cystometry. If all are within the normal range, bladder physiology can be assumed to be normal. Every evaluation of every factor has its own implication and, before a definitive conclusion is reached, must be examined in the light of associated manifestations and findings.

Capacity, Accommodation, & Sensation

Cystometry can be done by either of 2 basic methods: (1) allowing physiologic filling of the bladder

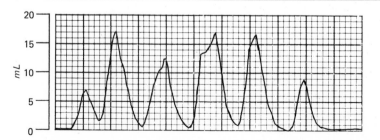

Figure 21–7. Classic flow rate due to abdominal straining with no detrusor activity. See effect of spurts of urine with complete interruption between them, since patient cannot sustain increased intra-abdominal pressure. On the horizontal scale, one large square equals 5 seconds.

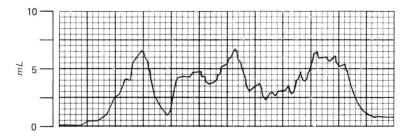

Figure 21–8. Flow rate in a case of urinary obstruction showing very low average flow rate (not above 5 or 6 mL/s). Prolonged duration of flow is associated with incomplete emptying. On the horizontal scale, one large square equals 5 seconds.

with secreted urine and continuously recording the intravesical pressure throughout a voiding cycle (starting the recording when the patient's bladder is empty and continuing it until the bladder has been filled—at which time the patient is asked to urinate—and voiding begins); or (2) by filling the bladder with water and recording the intravesical pressure against the volume of water introduced into the bladder. (Gas cystometry is now being used in some laboratories as a substitute for water cystometry. However, the results are so unreliable that the technique should be used only for preliminary screening. If gas cystometry reveals any abnormality, the results must be confirmed by water cystometry.)

With the first (physiologic filling) method, the assessment of bladder function is based on voided volume (assuming that the presence of residual urine has been ruled out). The second method permits accurate determination of the volume distending the bladder and of the pressures at each particular level of filling, yet it has inherent defects: Fluid is introduced rather than naturally secreted, and bladder filling occurs more rapidly than normal.

The cystometrogram (Fig 21–10) is obtained during the phase of bladder filling; the volume of fluid in the bladder is plotted against the intravesical pressure to show bladder wall compliance to filling. The normal cystometric curve shows a fairly constant low intravesical pressure until the bladder nears capacity, then a moderate rise until capacity is reached, and then a sharp rise as voiding is initiated. Normally, the sensation of fullness is first perceived when the bladder contains 100–200 mL of fluid and strongly felt as the bladder nears capacity; the desire to void occurs when the bladder is full (normal capacity, 400–500 mL). However, the bladder has a power of accommodation, ie, it can maintain an almost constant intraluminal pressure throughout its filling phase regardless of the volume of fluid present, and this directly influences compliance. As the bladder progressively accommodates larger volumes with no change in intraluminal pressure, the compliance values become higher (Compliance = Volume ÷ Pressure) (Fig 21–10).

Contractility & Voluntary Control

The bladder normally shows no evidence of contractility or activity during the filling phase. However, once it is filled to capacity and the subject perceives the desire to urinate and consciously allows urination to proceed, strong bladder contractions will occur and will be sustained until the bladder is empty. The individual can of course consciously inhibit detrusor contraction. Both of these aspects of voluntary detrusor control must be assessed during cystometric study in order to rule out uninhibited bladder activity and to determine whether the patient can inhibit urination with a full bladder and initiate urination when asked to do so. The latter is occasionally difficult to verify clinically because of conscious inhibition by a patient who may be embarrassed by the unnatural circumstances.

Responses to Drugs

Drugs are being used with increasing frequency in the evaluation of detrusor function. They can help to

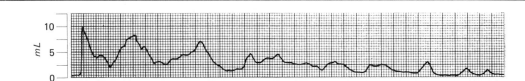

Figure 21–9. Classic low flow rate of bladder outlet obstruction (benign prostatic hypertrophy), markedly prolonged flow time, and fluctuation due to attempt at improving flow by increasing intra-abdominal pressure. On the horizontal scale, one large square equals 5 seconds.

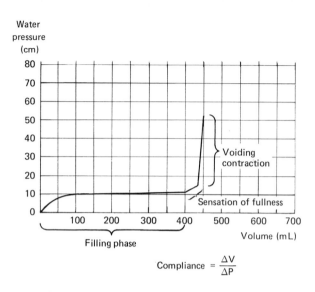

Figure 21–10. Cystometrogram of patient with normal bladder capacity. Note stable intravesical pressure during filling phase; slight rise at end of filling phase, indicating bladder capacity perceived as sense of fullness; and sharp rise at end (voiding contraction).

diagnose underlying neuropathy and to determine whether drug treatment might be of value in individual cases. Study of the relationship of bladder capacity in a given patient to intravesical pressure and bladder contractility gives a rough evaluation of the patient's bladder function. Low intravesical pressure with normal bladder capacity might not be significant, whereas low pressure with a very large capacity might imply sensory loss or flaccid lower motor neuron lesion, a chronically distended bladder, or a large bladder due to myogenic damage. High pressure (usually associated with reduced capacity) that rises rapidly with bladder filling is most commonly due to inflammation, enuresis, or reduced bladder capacity. However, uninhibited bladder activity during this high-pressure filling phase might indicate neuropathic bladder or an upper motor neuron lesion.

The parasympathetic drug bethanechol chloride (Urecholine) is often used to assess bladder muscle function in patients with low bladder pressure associated with lack of detrusor contraction. No response to bethanechol suggests myogenic damage; a normal response indicates a bladder of large capacity with normal musculature; and an exaggerated response indicates a lower motor neuron lesion. The test has so many variables that it must be done meticulously to give reliable results.

Testing with anticholinergic drugs or muscle depressants may be helpful in the evaluation of uninhibited detrusor contraction or increased bladder tonus and low compliance. The information thus obtained can be useful in choosing drugs for treatment.

Recording of Intravesical Pressure

Intravesical pressure can be measured directly from the vesical cavity, either by a suprapubic approach or via a transurethral catheter. The pressure inside the bladder is actually a function of both intra-abdominal and intravesical pressure. Thus, true detrusor pressure is the pressure recorded from the bladder cavity (intravesical pressure) minus intra-abdominal pressure. The point is important because variations in intra-abdominal pressure may alter the recorded intravesical pressure, and if the recorded intravesical pressure is mistakenly considered to reflect only detrusor pressure and not increased intra-abdominal pressure due to straining as well, erroneous conclusions may be reached.

In clinical practice, it is not necessary to measure intra-abdominal pressure, since abdominal wall contraction can be observed during the course of cystometry. A notation in the patient's chart will serve to distinguish true detrusor contraction from possible overlap or increase in intra-abdominal pressure. When necessary—ie, in case of uncertainty and in order to be absolutely accurate—intra-abdominal pressure should be recorded simultaneously with intravesical pressure, since there is no other way to determine the true detrusor pressure. Intra-abdominal pressure is usually recorded by a small balloon catheter inserted high in the rectum and connected to a separate transducer.

The most valuable part of the cystometric study is the determination of voiding activity or voiding contraction. The characteristics of intravesical pressure can be quite significant. Normally, voiding contractions are not high (20–40 cm of water); this magnitude of intravesical pressure is generally adequate to deliver a normal flow rate of 20–30 mL/s and completely empty the bladder if it is well sustained. A higher voiding pressure is indicative of possible increase in outlet resistance yet denotes an overactive, healthy detrusor musculature. Fig 21–11 shows a normal flow rate associated with normal detrusor contraction at a magnitude of 20 cm of water that is well sus-

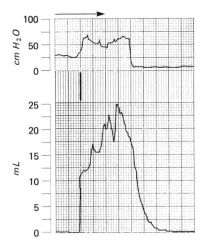

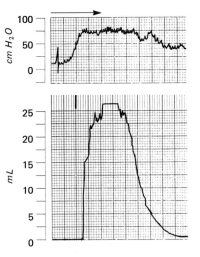

Figure 21–11. Simultaneous recording of voiding contraction and resulting flow rate. Note normal range of intravesical pressure during voiding phase as well as adequate normal flow rate (shown in Fig 21–4). On the horizontal scale, one large square equals 5 seconds.

Figure 21–12. Recording of bladder pressure simultaneously with flow rate. Note slightly higher intravesical pressure with high flow rate which, at its maximum, is that of a supervoider (see Fig 21–3). On the horizontal scale, one large square equals 5 seconds.

tained and of short duration and results in complete bladder emptying.

The quality of bladder pressure can also be informative, even without simultaneous recording of flow rate. However, in such cases, it is preferable to record flow rate under normal circumstances. A well-sustained detrusor contraction, high at initiation and then well sustained at normal values, is seen in Fig 21–12. In Fig 21–13, the voiding pressure is too high—there is an element of sphincter dyssynergia triggering variations in voiding pressures and flow rate. Simultaneous recording of bladder and intra-abdominal pressures would provide more information. As suggested above, recording the intravesical pressure alone does not give as much information as may be required, and increased intra-abdominal pressure might be mistaken for detrusor action. This is illustrated in Fig 21–14: The bladder pressure appears to indicate good detrusor function; nevertheless, simultaneous recording of intra-abdominal pressure makes it clear that all of the apparent changes in vesical intraluminal pressure in fact represent variations in intra-abdominal pressure.

Fig 21–15 shows the 2 pressures recorded on the same chart, on the same channel, by having the writ-

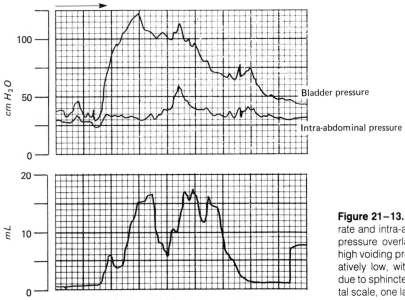

Figure 21–13. Simultaneous recording of flow rate and intra-abdominal pressure; intravesical pressure overlap in top recording. Note very high voiding pressure. However, flow rate is relatively low, with some interruption most likely due to sphincteric over-activity. On the horizontal scale, one large square equals 5 seconds.

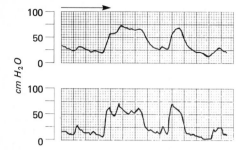

Figure 21–14. Simultaneous recording of intra-abdominal and intravesical pressures. If one considers only intravesical pressure (top recording), one might assume adequate detrusor contraction. Comparison with intra-abdominal pressure (lower recording) shows that they are almost identical and that there is no detrusor contraction at all.

ing pen share the time between 2 transducers—one recording intra-abdominal pressure; the other, intravesical pressure.

A. Pathologic Changes in Bladder Capacity: The bladder capacity is normally 400–500 mL, but it can be reduced or increased in a variety of disorders and lesions (Table 21–1). Some common causes of reduced bladder capacity are enuresis, urinary tract infection, contracted bladder, upper motor neuron lesion, and defunctionalized bladder. Reduced capacity also occurs in association with some cases of incontinence and in postsurgical bladder. Increased bladder capacity is not uncommon in women who have trained themselves to retain large volumes of urine. Bladder capacity is increased also in sensory neuropathic disorders, lower motor neuron lesions, and chronic obstruction from myogenic damage. It is important to relate bladder capacity to the intravesical pressure (Table 21–2). Slight variations in bladder capacity with no change in bladder pressure might be of less significance than the reverse. What is usually of greatest significance is the bladder with reduced capacity associated with normal pressure or, more importantly, with increased pressure, or the bladder with large capacity associated with decreased pressure.

Table 21–1. Causes of reduced or increased bladder capacity. (Normal capacity in adults is 400–500 mL.)

Causes of reduced bladder capacity
Enuresis or incontinence
Bladder infections
Bladder contracture due to fibrosis (from tuberculosis, interstitial cystitis, etc)
Upper motor neuron lesions
Defunctionalized bladder
Postsurgical bladder
Causes of increased bladder capacity
Sensory neuropathic disorders
Lower motor neuron lesions
Megacystis (congenital)
Chronic urinary tract obstruction

B. Pathologic Changes in Accommodation: Accommodation reflects intravesical pressure in response to filling. In a bladder with normal power of accommodation—in which case the micturition center of the spinal cord is controlled by the central nervous system—intravesical pressure will not vary with progressive bladder filling until capacity is reached—or, in other words, when compliance is reduced—there will be progressive increase in intravesical pressure and loss of accommodation; this usually occurs at smaller volumes and with reduced capacity. The patient being studied by cystometry can always note the presence or absence of a sensation of fullness. One normally does not sense volumes in the bladder but only changes in pressure.

C. Pathologic Changes in Sensation: A slight rise in intravesical pressure on cystometry signifies that the bladder is full to normal capacity and that the patient is perceiving it. This sign is usually absent in pure sensory neuropathy and in mixed sensory and motor loss. (Other sensations can be tested for in different ways; see Chapter 20.)

D. Pathologic Changes in Contractility: The bladder is normally capable of sustaining contraction until it is empty. Absence of residual urine after voiding usually denotes well-sustained contractions. Neuropathic dysfunction is usually associated with residual urine of variable amount depending on the type of dysfunction. Significant outlet resistance—mechanical or functional—is also a cause of residual urine.

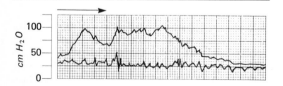

Figure 21–15. Simultaneous recording of 2 measurements—intravesical pressure (*top*) and intra-abdominal pressure (*bottom*)—on a single channel. The difference between the 2 can be clearly seen as pure detrusor contraction.

Table 21–2. Relationship between intravesical pressure and capacity in various diseases.

Low intravesical pressure
Normal capacity
Large capacity
Sensory deficits (diabetes mellitus, tabes dorsalis)
Flaccid lower motor neuron lesions
Large bladder (due to repeated stretching)
High intravesical pressure
Rapidly rising
Reduced capacity
Inflammation
Enuresis
Uninhibited contraction
Uninhibited neurogenic bladder
Upper motor neuron lesions

Table 21–3. Variations in detrusor contractility in various diseases.

Normal contractions
Normal volume
Well-sustained contractions
Absent or weak contractions
Sensory neuropathic disorders
Conscious inhibition of contractions
Lower motor neuron lesions
Uninhibited contractions
Upper motor neuron lesions
Cerebrovascular lesions

Cystometric study may disclose complete absence of detrusor contractility due to motor or sensory deficits or conscious inhibition of detrusor activity (Table 21–3). Detrusor hyperactivity is shown as uninhibited activity, usually due to interruption of the neural connection between spinal cord centers and the higher midbrain and cortical centers.

An integrated picture of bladder capacity, intravesical pressure, and contractility is useful for general assessment of the basic physiologic mechanisms of the bladder. Low intravesical pressure in a patient with normal bladder capacity may have no clinical significance, whereas low pressure with a very large capacity may signify sensory loss or a flaccid lower motor neuron lesion, a chronically distended bladder, or a large bladder due to myogenic damage. High pressure (usually associated with reduced capacity) that rises rapidly with bladder filling is most commonly associated with inflammation, enuresis, or actually reduced bladder capacity. However, uninhibited activity during the interval of rising pressure that occurs with bladder filling may indicate a neurogenic bladder or an upper motor neuron lesion.

SPHINCTERIC FUNCTION

Urinary sphincteric function can be evaluated either by recording the electromyographic activity of the voluntary component of the sphincteric mechanism or by recording the activity of both smooth and voluntary components by measuring the intraurethral pressure of the sphincteric unit. The latter method is called pressure profile measurement (profilometry).

Profilometry

The urethral pressure profile is determined by recording the pressure in the urethra at every level of the sphincteric unit from the internal meatus to the end of the sphincteric segment. Profilometry has been performed by gas or water perfusion techniques, but these methods have serious limitations. Gas profilometry requires a very high flow rate (120–150 mL/min) and is neither accurate, consistent, nor sensitive; it should no longer be used. Water profilometry, which requires a flow rate of about 2 mL/min, gives fairly accurate results. It may be used for screening patients with incontinence or functional obstruction, but it is not very sensitive and only provides information about total urethral pressure. The membrane catheter and microtransducer techniques of profilometry described below provide much more accurate and detailed information.

A. Membrane Catheter Technique: Membrane catheters used for recording pressure profiles usually have several channels, so that several measurements can be obtained simultaneously. Our current membrane catheter has 4 lumens and an outside diameter of 7F. Two of the 4 lumens are open at the end, one for bladder filling and the other for recording bladder pressure; the other 2 lumens, which are respectively situated 7 and 8 cm from the catheter tip, are covered by a thin membrane with a small chamber underneath (Fig 21–16). The space under the membrane and the lumen connected to it are filled with fluid, free of any gas, and connected to a pressure transducer. The pressure under this membrane should be zero at the level of the transducer, so it can register any pressure applied to the membrane whatever its level at any particular time. The catheter also has radiopaque markers at 1-cm intervals starting at the tip, with a heavier marker every 5 cm; it also has a special marker showing the site of each membrane. The markers permit fluoroscopic visualization of the catheter and the membrane levels during the entire study.

B. Microtransducer Technique: The results of

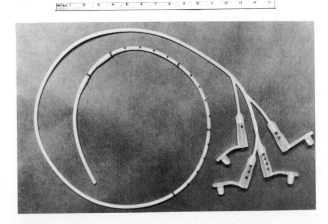

Figure 21–16. Membrane catheter showing radiopaque markers. Note 2 membrane chambers for urethral pressure measurements and 4 separate channels—2 channels for urethral pressure recording, one for bladder pressure recording, and one for bladder filling—each of which is connected to a separate ending. (Reproduced, with permission, from Tanagho EA, Jonas U: Membrane catheter: Effective for recording pressure in lower urinary tract. *Urology* 1977;**10**:173.)

microtransducer profilometry are as accurate as those obtained with the membrane catheter. Two microtransducers can be counted on the same catheter, one at the tip for recording of bladder pressure and the other about 5–7 cm from the tip to record the urethral pressure profile as the catheter is gradually withdrawn from the bladder cavity to below the sphincteric segment.

Electromyographic Study of Sphincteric Function

Electromyography alone gives useful information about sphincteric function, but it is most valuable when done in conjunction with cystometry. There are several techniques for electromyographic studies of the urinary sphincter—essentially by surface electrodes or by needle electrodes. Surface electrode recordings can be obtained either from the lumen of the urethra in the region of the voluntary sphincter or, preferably, from the anal sphincter by using an anal plug electrode. Recording via needle electrodes can be obtained from the anal sphincter, from the bulk of the musculature of the pelvic floor, or from the external sphincter itself, though in the latter case the placement is difficult and the accuracy of the results is questionable.

Direct needle electromyography of the urethral sphincter provides the most accurate information. However, because the technique is difficult, simpler approaches are generally used. The anal sphincter is readily accessible for electromyographic testing, and testing of any area of the pelvic floor musculature will generally reflect the overall electrical activity of the pelvic floor, including the external sphincter. Electromyography is not simple, and the assistance of an experienced electromyographer is probably essential. Electromyographic study makes use of the electrical activity that is constantly present within the pelvic floor and external urinary sphincter at rest and that increases progressively with bladder filling. If the bladder contracts for voiding, electrical activity ceases completely, permitting free flow of urine, and is resumed at the termination of detrusor contraction to se-

cure closure of the bladder outlet (Fig 21–17). Electromyography is important in showing this effect and, along with bladder pressure measurement, can pinpoint the exact time of detrusor contraction. Persistence of electromyographic activity during the phase of detrusor contraction for voiding—or, even worse, its overactivity during that phase—interferes with the voiding mechanism and leads to incoordination between detrusor and sphincter (**detrusor/sphincter dyssynergia**). During the interval of detrusor contraction, increased electromyographic activity interferes with the free flow of urine, as can be shown by simultaneous recording of flow rate.

Electromyographic recording shows only the activity of the voluntary component of the urinary sphincteric mechanism and the overall activity of the pelvic floor. More information is gained when the electromyogram is recorded simultaneously with detrusor pressure or flow rate. However, it gives no information about the smooth component of the urinary sphincter.

Pressure Measurement for Evaluation of Sphincteric Function

Perfusion profilometry, usually performed with the patient supine and with an empty bladder, provides a simple pressure profile that allows determination of the maximum pressure within the urethra. This is adequate for screening patients with incontinence or functional obstruction. However, in order to determine the maximum closure pressure (see below), the bladder pressure must be recorded simultaneously with the urethral pressure profile. Such simultaneous recording is not possible with perfusion profilometry. The membrane catheter and microtransducer techniques of profilometry, because they utilize multichannel recording, routinely provide much more detailed information; at least 4 distinct sets of measurements can be obtained from the simplest pressure profile made using the membrane catheter or microtransducer (Fig 21–18): (1) the maximum pressure exerted around the sphincteric segment, (2) the net closure pressure of the

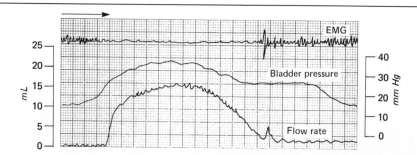

Figure 21–17. Simultaneous recording of bladder pressure, flow rate, and electromyography of anal sphincter. With rise in bladder pressure for voiding, start of flow rate has a smooth, continuous, bell-shaped curve. Note also complete absence of electromyographic activity of the anal sphincter throughout the voiding act. On the horizontal scale, one large square equals 5 seconds.

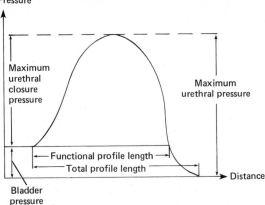

Figure 21–18. Urethral pressure profile and its components. Note functional length, anatomic length, and the shape of the profile, with maximum closure pressure in the middle segment of the urethra rather than at the level of the internal meatus. (Reproduced, with permission, from Bradley W: Cystometry and sphincter electromyography. *Mayo Clin Proc* 1976;**329**:335.)

urethra, (3) the distribution of this closure pressure along the entire length of the sphincter, and (4) the exact functional length of the sphincteric unit and its relation to the anatomic length.

A. Total Pressure: The urethral pressure profile recording shows the pressure directly recorded within the urethral lumen along the entire length of the urethra from internal to external meatus. From this, the maximum pressure exerted around the sphincteric segment can be determined.

B. Closure Pressure: The urethral closure pressure is the difference between intravesical pressure (bladder pressure) and urethral pressure, ie, the net closure pressure. The **maximum closure pressure** is the most important measurement in evaluating the activity of the sphincteric unit and its responses to various factors.

C. Distribution of Closure Pressure: As the catheter is withdrawn down the urethra, the closure pressure at various levels along the entire length of the sphincteric segment will be recorded.

D. Functional Length of the Sphincteric Unit: The functional length of the sphincteric unit is that portion with positive closure pressure, ie, where urethral pressure is greater than bladder pressure. The distinction between anatomic length and functional length is important. Regardless of the anatomic length, the effectiveness of the urethral sphincter may be limited to a shorter segment. In women, the pressure is normally rather low at the level of the internal meatus but builds up gradually until it reaches its maximum in the mid urethra, where the voluntary sphincter is concentrated; it slowly drops until it is at its lowest at the external meatus. On the basis of these measurements, it is clear that the anatomic and functional lengths of the normal urethra in women are

about the same and that the maximum closure pressure is at about the center of the urethra—not at the level of the internal meatus. In men, the pressure profile is slightly different: The functional length is longer, and the maximum closure pressure builds up in the prostatic segment, reaches a peak in the membranous urethra, and drops as it reaches the level of the bulbous urethra (Fig 21–19). The entire functional length in men is about 6–7 cm; in women, it is about 4 cm.

Dynamic Changes in Pressure Profile

The usefulness of the pressure profile is enhanced if the examiner notes the sphincteric responses to various physiologic stimuli: (1) postural changes (supine, sitting, standing), (2) changes in intra-abdominal pressure (sharp increase with coughing; sustained increase with bearing down), (3) voluntary contractions of the pelvic floor musculature to assess activity of the voluntary sphincter, and (4) bladder filling. The latter test consists of making baseline recordings with both an empty bladder and a full bladder and comparing these recordings with recordings made under conditions of stress (coughing, bearing down) and during voluntary contraction with an empty bladder and a full bladder.

A simple pressure profile is informative but does not provide data that will delineate and identify specific sites of sphincteric dysfunction. The advantage of using a membrane catheter or microtransducer

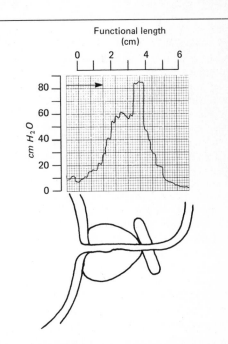

Figure 21–19. Normal male urethral pressure profile showing progressive rise throughout prostatic segment and peak being reached in membranous urethra. (Reproduced, with permission, from Tanagho EA: Membrane and microtransducer catheters: Their effectiveness for profilometry of the lower urinary tract. *Urol Clin North Am* 1979; 6:110.)

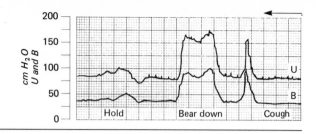

Figure 21-20. Simultaneous recording of intraurethral (U) and intravesical (B) pressures and their responses to coughing and bearing down. Rise in intravesical pressure as a result of increase in intra-abdominal pressure is associated with simultaneous rise in intraurethral pressure, maintaining a constant closure pressure.

is that the pressure profile can be expanded by slowing the rate of withdrawal of the catheter and speeding up the motion of the recording paper. Since the catheter can be held at different levels for any length of time, other tests can be made and their effects monitored. Response to stress (particularly when standing), response to bladder distention, response to changes in position, the effects of drugs, and the effects of nerve stimulation can all be evaluated if needed. Bladder filling normally leads to increase in tonus of the sphincteric element, with some rise in closure pressure, especially when bladder filling approaches maximum capacity. Stress from coughing or straining also normally results in sustained or increased closure pressure (Fig 21-20). When the patient stands up, closure pressure is usually substantially increased (Fig 21-21). Testing for activity of the voluntary sphincter by the hold maneuver (asking the patient to actively contract the perineal muscles) produces a significant rise in urethral pressure (Fig 21-22). When the effects of all of these responses are recorded concomitantly with intravesical pressure, the data can be interrelated and the exact closure pressure at any given time can be ascertained.

The response to stress with the patient standing should usually be recorded also. Especially in cases of stress incontinence, weakness of the sphincteric mechanism may not be apparent with the patient sitting or supine but becomes clear when the patient stands up.

The effectiveness of drugs in increasing or reducing the urethral pressure profile can be tested also. For example, phenoxybenzamine (Regitine) can be administered and then the urethral pressure profile recorded: A drop in pressure indicates that alpha blockers may be an effective means of decreasing urethral resistance, with obvious implications for the

management of urinary obstruction. Anticholinergic drugs such as propantheline bromide can be tested for possible use as detrusor depressants. Detrusor activity can be investigated by administering bethanechol chloride (Urecholine) and simultaneously recording bladder and urethral pressures.

Characteristics of the Normal Pressure Profile (Fig 21-23)

The basic features of the ideal pressure profile are not easily defined. In women, the normal urethral pressure profile has a peak of 100-120 cm of water, and the closure pressure is in the range of 90-100 cm of water. Closure pressure is lowest at the level of the internal meatus, gradually builds up in the proximal 0.5 cm, and reaches its maximum about 1 cm below the internal meatus. It is sustained for another 2 cm and then starts to drop in the distal urethra. The functional length of a normal adult female urethra is about 4 cm. The response to stress with coughing and bearing down is sustained or augmented closure pressure. Standing up also increases this pressure, with maximum rise in the mid segment. Nervous stimulation is rarely tested in normal subjects, but sacral root stimulation can reveal the closure pressure in the voluntary element of the sphincteric segment of the urethra.

Pressure Profile in Certain Pathologic Entities

A. Urinary Stress Incontinence: The classic pressure changes noted in this type of incontinence are as follows:

1. Low urethral closure pressure.

2. Short urethral functional length at the expense of the proximal segment.

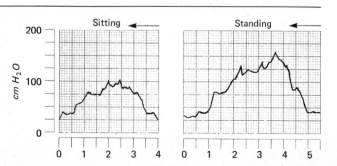

Figure 21-21. Urethral pressure profile of normal woman in sitting and standing positions. Note marked improvement in closure pressure (in both functional length and magnitude) when patient stands up. (Reproduced, with permission, from Tanagho EA: Urodynamics of female urinary incontinence with emphasis on stress incontinence. *J Urol* 1979;**122**:200.)

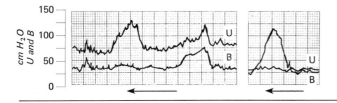

Figure 21–22. *Right:* Urethral pressure profile in normal range. U = urethra, B = bladder. *Left:* Main point of effect of hold maneuver is significant increase in closure pressure of urethra (U) without change in bladder pressure (B)—act of voluntary sphincter.

3. Weak responses to stress.

4. Loss of urethral closure pressure with bladder filling.

5. Fall in closure pressure upon assuming the upright position.

6. Weak responses to stress in the upright position.

B. Urinary Urge Incontinence: The most pertinent pressure changes in this type of incontinence are normal or high closure pressures with normal responses to stress, normal responses to bladder filling, and normal responses when the patient stands up. Urge incontinence can result from any of the following mechanisms (Fig 21–24):

1. Detrusor hyperirritability, with active detrusor contractions overcoming urethral resistance and leading to urine leakage.

2. The exact reverse, ie, a constant detrusor pressure with no evidence of detrusor instability, but urethral instability in that urethral pressure becomes less than bladder pressure, so that urine leakage occurs without any detrusor contraction.

3. A combination of the above (the most common form), ie, some drop in closure pressure and some rise in bladder pressure. In such cases, the drop in urethral pressure is often the initiating factor.

C. Combination of Stress and Urge Incontinence: In this common clinical condition, profilometry is used to determine the magnitude of each component, ie, whether the incontinence is primarily urge, primarily stress, or both equally. As a guide to treatment, profilometric studies sometimes show that stress incontinence precipitates urge incontinence. The stress elements initiate urine leakage in the proximal urethra, exciting detrusor response and sphincteric relaxation and ending with complete urine leakage. Once the stress components are corrected, the urge element disappears. This combination cannot be detected clinically.

D. Postprostatectomy Incontinence: After prostatectomy, there is usually no positive pressure in the entire prostatic fossa, minimal closure pressure at the apex of the prostate, and normal or greater than normal pressure within the voluntary sphincteric segment of the membranous urethra. It is the functional length of the sphincteric segment above the genitourinary diaphragm that determines the degree of incontinence; the magnitude of closure pressure in the voluntary sphincteric segment has no bearing on the patient's symptoms. High pressure is almost always recorded within the voluntary sphincter, despite the common belief that what someone termed "iatrogenically induced incontinence" is due to damage to the voluntary sphincter—which is definitely not the case.

E. Detrusor/Sphincter Dyssynergia: In this situation, findings of cystometric studies are normal at the filling phase, with possible closure pressure above average. However, the pathologic entity becomes clear when the patient attempts to void: Detrusor contraction is associated with a simultaneous increase in urethral closure pressure instead of a drop in pressure. This is a direct effect of overactivity of the voluntary component, leading to obstructive voiding or low flow rate and frequent interruption of voiding. This phenomenon is commonly seen in patients with supraspinal lesions. It can be encountered in several other conditions as well.

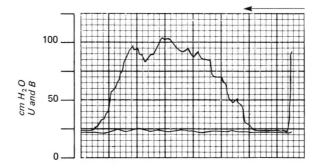

Figure 21–23. Recording of normal female urethral pressure profile, showing basic features and actual values, including anatomic as well as functional length. U = urethra, B = bladder. (Reproduced, with permission, from Tanagho EA: Membrane and microtransducer cathters: Their effectiveness for profilometry of the lower urinary tract. *Urol Clin North Am* 1979;6:110.)

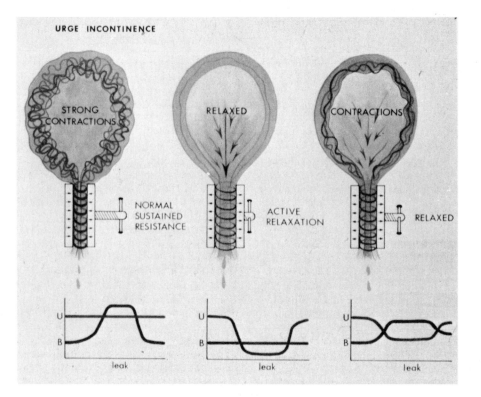

Figure 21–24. Three mechanisms of urinary urge incontinence. *Left:* Normal sphincter activity exceeded by hyperactive detrusor. *Center:* Normal detrusor, without any overactivity, yet unstable urethra with marked drop in urethral pressure leading to leakage. *Right:* Most common combination—some rise in intravesical pressure due to detrusor hyperirritability associated with drop in urethral pressure due to sphincteric relaxation. U = urethra, B = bladder.

VALUE OF SIMULTANEOUS RECORDINGS

Measurement of each of the physiologic variables described above gives useful clinical information. A rise in intravesical pressure has greater significance when related to intra-abdominal pressure. The urine flow rate is more significant if recorded in conjunction with the total volume voided as well as with evidence of detrusor contraction. The urethral pressure profile is more significant when related to bladder pressure and to variations in intra-abdominal pressure and voluntary muscular activity. And for greatest clinical usefulness, all data must be recorded simultaneously, so that the investigator can analyze the activity involved in each sequence.

At a minimum, a proper urodynamic study should include recordings of intravesical pressure and intra-abdominal pressure (true detrusor pressure is intravesical pressure minus intra-abdominal pressure), urethral pressure or electromyography, flow rate, and, if possible, voided volume. For a complete study, the following are necessary: intra-abdominal pressure, intravesical pressure, urethral sphincteric pressure at various (usually 2) levels, flow rate, voided volume, anal sphincter pressure (as a function of pelvic floor activity), and electromyography of the anal or urethral

striated sphincter. These physiologic data are recorded with the patient quiet as well as during activity (ie, voluntary increase in intra-abdominal pressure, changes in the state of bladder filling, voluntary contraction of perineal muscles, or—more comprehensively—an entire voiding act starting from an empty bladder and continuing through complete filling of the bladder, initiation of voiding, and until the bladder is empty).

The data derived from urodynamic studies are descriptive of urinary tract function. Simultaneous visualization of the lower urinary tract as multiple recordings are made gives more precise information about the pathologic changes underlying the symptoms. By means of cinefluoroscopy, the examiner can observe the configuration of the bladder, bladder base, and bladder outlet during bladder filling (usually with radiopaque medium). The information obtained can then be correlated with the level of catheters, with pressure recordings, and with changes in pelvic floor support during voiding. Combined cinefluoroscopy and pressure measurements thus represent the ultimate in urodynamic studies.

A model of such a urodynamic laboratory has been developed at the University of California School of Medicine (San Francisco). As shown in Fig 21–25, the patient sits in a specially designed toilet chair over a device for collecting urine and measuring flow rate.

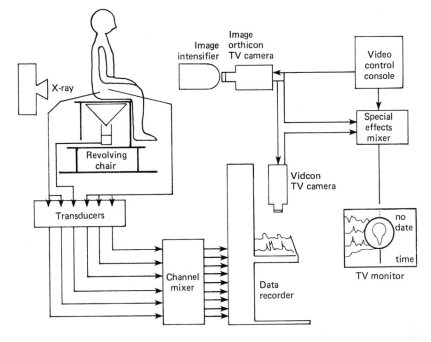

Figure 21–25. Urodynamic laboratory with specially designed toilet chair where patient sits between x-ray tube and image intensifier. A television camera records the fluoroscopic image, and a second camera picks up recordings from a polygraph machine to be projected onto one television monitor, photographed, and recorded on videotape.

The patient faces the x-ray tube that receives the image of the bladder and bladder outlet, to be projected on a fluoroscopic screen. The pressure-recording catheters are connected to a set of transducers that are in turn connected to a polygraph recording machine, on top of which a television camera is mounted. On a separate television monitor, the image of the pressure recording is combined with the image from the fluoroscopic monitor. A permanent record can be obtained on videotape or motion picture film.

Such studies are recorded on a polygraph chart as well as on motion picture film or videotape. Sound can usually be added to the film or videotape to provide the history as well as the examiner's observations and instructions during the study and a spoken version of pressure measurements so they can be followed from outside the examination room.

Several machines are available for recording urodynamic studies. Some of them are simple, limited to one or 2 channels; more complex machines may have as many as 8 channels. Each type is designed to meet a particular need of the investigator or institution. The needs in private practice are quite different from those of a large institution or referral center for complex urologic problems, especially neuropathic dysfunctions. In our laboratory, we have developed a series of pressure-recording units ranging from a single-channel instrument to a 4-channel instrument. Every channel is

capable of recording 2 sets of measurements, so that the single-channel machine represents in reality 2 channels and the 4-channel machine represents 8 channels. Pressure recordings are obtained with an 8-channel machine (Fig 21–26). Six such channels are used to record bladder pressure, 2 urethral pressures, rectal pressure, flow rate, and total volume voided; and 2 additional channels are used to record anal sphincter pressure and electromyogram (not shown). Because every channel can be used to record 2 sets of measurements simultaneously, the investigator can record intra-abdominal pressure and bladder pressure overlapped (so that the net detrusor pressure is recorded) and anal sphincteric pressure and midurethral pressure in such a way that the reflection of each on the other is also readily seen (Fig 21–27).

The complete recording machine contains 4 data-transmission channels attached to transducers; plotters to record the volume infused into the bladder, the volume voided, and the flow rate; devices for visual and auditory monitoring of data; and a variable-speed pump for infusing fluids into the bladder, with an automatic control for limiting the total volume infused (between 25 and 1000 mL, depending on the patient's age and bladder capacity). The recording machine is portable, ie, it can be rolled anywhere; and it can be attached to the cinefluoroscopic machine if this is desired.

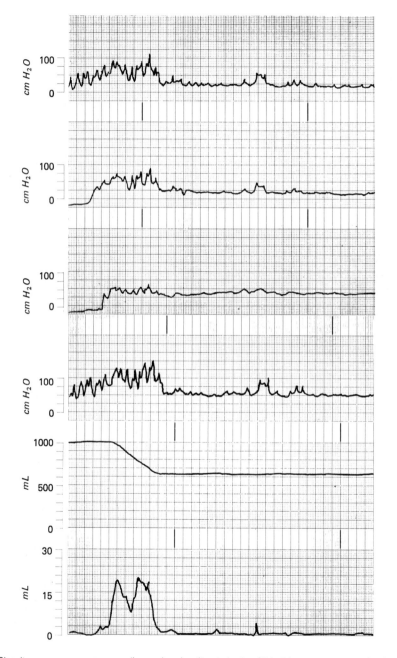

Figure 21–26. Simultaneous pressure recordings, showing (top to bottom) bladder pressure, proximal urethral pressure, midurethral pressure, intra-abdominal pressure, total volume voided, and flow rate. On the horizontal scale, one large square equals 5 seconds.

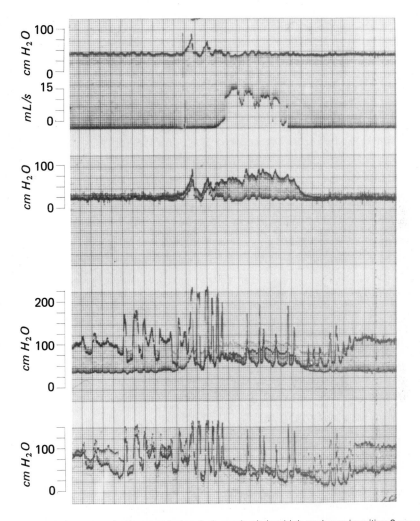

Figure 21–27. Eight sets of measurements recorded on 4-channel unit, in which each pen is writing 2 records. *Top channel:* Flow rate and intra-abdominal pressure. *Second channel:* Combination of bladder pressure and intra-abdominal pressure, the difference between the 2 showing true detrusor contraction pressure. *Third channel:* Combination of bladder pressure and maximum urethral pressure, the difference between the 2 showing urethral closure pressure. *Bottom channel:* Anal sphincter pressure and midurethral pressure as a function of overall perineal activity. Any combination can be set on such a machine.

REFERENCES

Urethra & Bladder

Abrams PH: Perfusion urethral profilometry. *Urol Clin North Am* 1979;**6:**103.

Abrams PH, Martin S, Griffiths DJ: The measurement and interpretation of urethral pressures obtained by the method of Brown and Wickham. *Br J Urol* 1978;**50:**33.

Andersen JT, Bradley WE: Urethral pressure profilometry: Assessment of urethral function by combined intraurethral pressure and EMG recording. *Urol Int* 1978;**33:**40.

Attenburrow AA, Stanley TV, Holland RPC: Nocturnal enuresis: A study. *Practitioner* 1984;**228:**99.

Awad SA et al: Urethral pressure profile in female stress incontinence. *J Urol* 1978;**120:**475.

Bazeed MA et al: Histochemical study of urethral striated musculature in the dog. *J Urol* 1982;**128:**406.

Bruschini H, Schmidt RA, Tanagho EA: Effect of urethral stretch on urethral pressure profile. *Invest Urol* 1977;**15:**107.

Bruschini H, Schmidt RA, Tanagho EA: The male genitourinary sphincter mechanism in the dog. *Invest Urol* 1978;**15:**288.

Bruskewitz R, Raz S: Urethral pressure profile using microtip catheter in females. *Urology* 1979;**14:**303.

Coolsaet B: Bladder compliance and detrusor activity during the collection phase. *Neurourol Urodynam* 1985;**4:**263.

Desai P: Bladder pressure studies combined with micturating cystourethrography. *Radiography* 1985;**51:**2.

Drutz HP, Mandel F: Urodynamic analysis of urinary incontinence symptoms in women. *Am J Obstet Gynecol* 1979;**134:**789.

Eastwood HDH: Provocative cystometry in the elderly patient with urinary incontinence. *Proc Int Continence Soc* 1985;**15:**129.

Erlandson B-E, Fall M: Urethral pressure profile studies by two different microtip transducers and an open catheter system. *Urol Int* 1978;**33:**79.

Finkbeiner AE: Is bethanechol chloride clinically effective in promoting bladder emptying? A literature review. *J Urol* 1985;**134:**443.

Gershon CR, Diokno AC: Urodynamic evaluation of female stress urinary incontinence. *J Urol* 1978;**119:**787.

Gilmour RF et al: Analysis of the urethral pressure profile using a mechanical model. *Invest Urol* 1980;**18:**54.

Glen ES, Eadie A, Rowan D: Urethral closure pressure profile measurements in female urinary incontinence. *Acta Urol Belg* 1984;**52:**174.

Gosling JA et al: A comparative study of the human external sphincter and periurethral levator ani muscles. *Br J Urol* 1981;**53:**35.

Graber P, Laurent G, Tanagho EA: Effect of abdominal pressure rise on the urethral profile: An experimental study on dogs. *Invest Urol* 1974;**12:**57.

Henriksson L, Andersson K-E, Ulmsten U: The urethral pressure profiles in continence and stress-incontinent women. *Scand J Urol Nephrol* 1979;**13:**5.

Henriksson L, Aspelin P, Ulmsten U: Combined urethrocystometry and cineflurography in continent and incontinent women. *Radiology* 1979;**130:**607.

Hurt WG, Fantl JA: Direct electronic urethrocystometry. *Clin Obstet Gynecol* 1978;**21:**695.

Jonas U, Hohenfellner R: Which anatomical structures in fact achieve urinary continence? *Urol Int* 1978;**33:**199.

Jonas U, Klotter HJ: Study of three urethral pressure recording devices: Theoretical considerations. *Urol Res* 1978;**6:**119.

Jones KW, Schoenberg HW: Comparison of the incidence of bladder hyperreflexia in patients with benign prostatic hypertrophy and age-matched female controls. *J Urol* 1985;**133:**425.

Khan Z, Mieza M, Leiter E: Role of detrusor hyperreflexia (bladder instability in primary enuresis). *Proc Int Continence Soc* 1984;**14:**107.

Koefoot RB Jr, Webster GD: Urodynamic evaluation in women with frequency, urgency symptoms. *Urology* 1983;**21:**648.

Lindstrom K, Ulmsten U: Some methodological aspects on the measurement of intraluminal pressures in the female urogenital tract in vivo. *Acta Obstet Gynecol Scand* 1978;**57:**63.

Mayo ME, Ansell JS: Urodynamic assessment of incontinence after prostatectomy. *J Urol* 1979;**122:**60.

McGuire EJ, Brady S: Detrusor-sphincter dyssynergia. *J Urol* 1979;**121:**774.

Meunier P, Mollard P: Urethral pressure profile in children: A comparison between perfused catheters and microtransducers, and a study of the usefulness of urethral pressure profile measurements in children. *J Urol* 1978;**120:**207.

Nørgaard JP, Djurhuus JC: Detrusor activity at rest in patients with idiopathic detrusor hyperreflexia. *Urol Res* 1984;**12:**209.

Parnell JP II, Marshall VF, Vaughan ED Jr: Primary management of urinary stress incontinence by the Marshall-Marchetti-Krantz vesicourethropexy. *J Urol* 1982;**127:**679.

Robertson JR: Gynecologic urology. 2. Gas urethroscopy with pressure studies. *Clin Obstet Gynaecol* 1978;**5:**39.

Rossier AB et al: Urodynamics in spinal shock patients. *J Urol* 1979;**122:**783.

Schmidt RA, Tanagho EA: Urethral syndrome or urinary tract infection? *Urology* 1981;**18:**424.

Schmidt RA, Witherow R, Tanagho EA: Recording urethral pressure profile. *Urology* 1977;**10:**390.

Schmidt RA et al: Urethral pressure profilometry with membrane catheter compared with perfusion catheter systems. *Urol Int* 1978;**33:**345.

Tanagho EA: Interpretation of the physiology of micturition. Pages 18–45 in: *Hydrodynamics.* Hinman F Jr (editor). Thomas, 1971.

Tanagho EA: Membrane and microtransducer catheters: Their effectiveness for profilometry of the lower urinary tract. *Urol Clin North Am* 1979;**6:**110.

Tanagho EA: Neurophysiology of urinary incontinence. Pages 31–60 in: *Female Urinary Stress Incontinence.* Cantor EB (editor). Thomas, 1979.

Tanagho EA: Urinary stress incontinence. *Urol Arch (Belgrade)* 1977;**8:**17.

Tanagho EA: Urodynamics of female urinary stress incontinence with emphasis on stress incontinence. *J Urol* 1979;**122:**200.

Tanagho EA: Vesicourethral dynamics. Pages 215–236 in: *Urodynamics.* Lutzeyer W, Melchior H (editors). Springer-Verlag, 1974.

Tanagho EA, Jones U: Membrane catheter: Effective for recording pressure in lower urinary tract. *Urology* 1977;**10:**173.

Tanagho EA, Meyers FH, Smith DR: Urethral resistance: Its components and implications. 2. Striated muscle component. *Invest Urol* 1969;**7:**136.

Tanagho EA, Miller ER: Functional considerations of urethral sphincteric dynamics. *J Urol* 1973;**109:**273.

Teague CT, Merrill DC: Comparative study of air and water measurements of peak and stabilized static urethral pressures. *Urology* 1978;**12:**481.

Teague CT, Merrill DC: Laboratory comparison of urethral profilometry techniques. *Urology* 1979;**13:**221.

Ulmsten U, Hok B, Lindstrom K: Aspects of present and future possibilities for intraluminal pressure recordings in the urogenital tract. *Acta Pharmacol Toxicol* 1978;**43:**41.

Woodside JR, McGuire EJ: A simple inexpensive urodynamic catheter. *J Urol* 1979;**122:**788.

Yalla SV et al: Striated sphincter participation in distal passive urinary continence mechanisms: Studies in male subjects deprived of proximal sphicter mechanism. *J Urol* 1979;**122:**655.

Urinary Flow

Abrams P, Torrens M: Urine flow studies. *Urol Clin North Am* 1979;**6:**71.

Drach GW, Ignatoff J, Layton T: Peak urinary flow rate: Observation in female subjects and comparison to male subjects. *J Urol* 1979;**122:**215.

Gleason DM, Bottaccini MR: Urodynamic norms in female voiding. 2. Flow modulation zone and voiding dysfunction. *J Urol* 1982;**127:**495.

Jensen KM-E, Jørgensen JB, Mogensen P: Relationship between uroflowmetry and prostatism. *Proc Int Continence Soc* 1985;**15:**134.

Jørgensen JB, Jensen KM-E, Mogensen P: Uroflowmetry in asymptomatic elderly males. *Proc Int Continence Soc* 1985;**15:**136.

Kondo A, Mitsuya H, Torii H: Computer analysis of micturition parameters and accuracy of uroflowmeter. *Urol Int* 1978;**33:**337.

Nyman CR, Boman J, Gidlof A: Von Garrelts' uroflowmeter: A technical evaluation. *Urol Int* 1979;**34:**184.

Siroky MB, Olsson CA, Krane RJ: The flow rate nomogram. 1. Development. *J Urol* 1979;**122:**665.

Siroky MB, Olsson CA, Krane RJ: The flow rate nomogram. 2. Clinical correlation. *J Urol* 1980;**23:**208.

Stubbs AJ, Resnic MI: Office uroflowmetry using maximum flow rate purge meter. *J Urol* 1979;**122:**62.

Tanagho EA, McCurry E: Pressure and flow rate as related to lumen caliber and entrance configuration. *J Urol* 1971;**105:**583.

Electromyography

Colstrup H et al: Urethral sphincter EMG activity registered with surface electrodes in the vagina. *Neurourol Urodynam* 1985;**4:**15.

DiBenedetto M, Yalla SV: Electrodiagnosis of striated urethral sphincter dysfunction. *J Urol* 1979;**122:**361.

Girard R et al: Anal and urethral sphincter electromyography in spinal cord injured patients. *Paraplegia* 1978;**16:**244.

King DG: Anal stimulating electrodes in electromyography. *Urology* 1979;**13:**345.

King DG, Teague CT: Choice of electrode in electromyography of external urethral and anal sphincter. *J Urol* 1980;**124:**75.

Koyanagi T et al: Experience with electromyography of the external urethral sphincter in spinal cord injury patients. *J Urol* 1982;**127:**272.

Nielsen KK et al: A comparative study of various electrodes in electromyography of the striated urethral and anal sphincter in children. *Br J Urol* 1985;**57:**557.

Urodynamic Testing

Barrent DM, Wein AJ: Flow evaluation and simultaneous external sphincter electromyography in clinical urodynamics. *J Urol* 1981;**125:**538.

Bauer SB et al: Predictive value of urodynamic evaluation in newborns with myelodysplasia. *JAMA* 1984;**252:**650.

Blaivas JG: Multichannel urodynamic studies. *Urology* 1984;**23:**421.

Blaivas JG: Urodynamics: Second generation. *J Urol* 1983;**129:**783.

Blaivas JG, Fischer DM: Combined radiographic and urodynamic monitoring: Advances in technique. *J Urol* 1981;**125:**693.

Blaivas JG, Salinas JM, Katz GP: The role of urodynamic testing in the evaluation of subtle neurologic lesions. *Neurourol Urodynam* 1985;**4:**211.

Blaivas JG et al: Cystometric response to propantheline in detrusor hyperreflexia: Therapeutic implications. *J Urol* 1980;**124:**259.

Bratt CG et al: Intrapelvic pressure and urinary flow rate in obstructed and nonobstructed human kidneys. *J Urol* 1982;**127:**1136.

Giacobini S et al: To the ICS committee for standardization of the terminology in urodynamics: A possible contribution to define urethral functionality. *Proc Int Continence Soc* 1985;**15:**201.

Hinman F Jr: Electronic or clinical urodynamic testing. Pages 75–78 in: *Current and Future Trends in Urology*. Miranda SI, de Voogt HJ (editors). Bunge Scientific Publishers, 1979.

Hinman F Jr: Urodynamic testing: Alternatives to electronics. *J Urol* 1980;**121:**256.

Layton TN, Drach GW: Selectivity of peak versus average male urinary flow rates. *J Urol* 1981;**125:**839.

Massey A, Abrams P: Urodynamics of the female lower urinary tract. *Urol Clin North Am* 1985;**12:**231.

McGuire EJ: Observations of part-time urodynamicist. *J Urol* 1983;**129:**102.

McGuire EJ, Woodside JR: Diagnostic advantages of fluoroscopic monitoring during urodynamic evaluation. *J Urol* 1981;**125:**830.

Penders L, De Leval J: Simultaneous urethrocystometry and hyperactive bladders: A manometric differential diagnosis. *Neurourol Urodynam* 1985;**4:**89.

Plevnik S, Janez J: Urethral pressure variations. *Urology* 1983;**21:**207.

Resnick NM, Yalla SV, Reilly CH: Detrusor hyperreflexia with impaired contractility: A previously uncharacterized, distinct and common cause of incontinence in frail elderly. *Proc Int Continence Soc* 1985;**15:**53.

Ryall R, Marshall VR: Laws of urodynamics. *Urology* 1982;**20:**106.

Ryall RL, Marshall VR: Office method for calibrating uroflowmeter. *J Urol* 1982;**127:**482.

Sand PK, Bowen LW, Ostergaard DR: Uninhibited urethral relaxation: An unusual cause of incontinence. *Proc Int Continence Soc* 1985;**15:**117.

Schafer W: Urethral resistance? Urodynamic concepts of physiological and pathological bladder outlet function during voiding. *Neurourol Urodynam* 1985;**4:**161.

Schmidt RA: Urethrovesical reflexes and their inhibition. Pages 589–596 in: *Benign Prostatic Hypertrophy*. Hinman F Jr (editor). Springer-Verlag, 1983.

Shulman Y, Brown J: Pressure flow-analysis of micturition: A reappraisal. *Urology* 1982;**19:**450.

Siroky MB: Urodynamic assessment of detrusor denervation and areflexia. *World J Urol* 1984;**2:**181.

Sutherst JR, Brown MC: Comparison of single and multi-channel cystometry in diagnosing bladder instability. *Br Med J* 1984;**288:**1720.

Tanagho EA: Membrane and microtransducer catheters: Their effectiveness for profilometry of the lower urinary tract. *Urol Clin North Am* 1979;**6:**110.

Tanagho EA: Urodynamics of female urinary incontinence with emphasis on stress incontinence. *J Urol* 1979; **122:**200.

Thüroff JW: Mechanism of urinary continence: Animal model to study urethral responses to stress conditions. *J Urol* 1982;**127:**1202.

Toguri AG, Bee DE, Bunce H III: Variability of water urethral closure pressure profiles. *J Urol* 1980;**124:**407.

Turner-Warwick R, Brown AD: A urodynamic evaluation of urinary incontinence in the female and its treatment. *Urol Clin North Am* 1979;**6:**203.

Turner-Warwick R, Milroy E: A reappraisal of the value of routine urological procedures in the assessment of urodynamic function. *Urol Clin North Am* 1979;**6:**63.

Vardi Y, Ginesin Y, Levin DR: Preoperative evaluation of prostatic size by urethral pressure profilometry. *Eur Urol* 1985;**11:**257.

Webster GD, Older RA: Video urodynamics. *Urology* 1980; **16:**106.

Wein AJ et al: Effects of bethanechol chloride on urodynamic parameters in normal women and in women with significant residual urine volumes. *J Urol* 1980;**124:**397.

Winter CC: Peripubic urethropexy for urinary stress incontinence in women. *Urology* 1982;**20:**408.

Zinner NR: Progress in urodynamics. (Editorial.) *J Urol* 1980;**124:**683.

Disorders of the Adrenal Glands

22

Peter H. Forsham, MD

Diseases of the adrenal glands are accompanied by characteristic physical changes secondary to hormonal alterations or by abdominal pressure or pain due to the size of the diseased glands. Diagnosis can be made by appropriate hormonal and localizing determinations (Fig 22–1).

There are, in addition to functioning tumors and hyperplasias of the adrenal cortex and medulla and nonfunctioning malignant tumors, other, often benign types of involvement of the adrenal glands. These enter into the differential diagnosis of adrenal lesions.

ADRENAL HEMORRHAGE IN THE NEWBORN

Adrenal hemorrhage is not an unusual result of trauma during childbirth (Khuri et al, 1980). It may be unilateral or bilateral. An upper abdominal mass is present as well as jaundice and anemia. In a few patients, adrenal insufficiency may supervene. An association between adrenal hemorrhage and renal vein thrombosis has been reported (Lebowitz and Belman, 1983). Excretory urography, sonography, or CT scan shows downward displacement of the ipsilateral kidney. The blood is revealed as a mixed lucent pattern. Because the surrounding fascia affords a tamponade effect, conservative treatment is indicated unless exsanguination is threatened despite blood replacement. The retroperitoneal blood is gradually absorbed. Replacement therapy may be required for adrenal insufficiency. The adrenals often undergo later calcification. The prognosis must be guarded.

ADRENAL CYST

Adrenal cysts are ordinarily asymptomatic, but displacement of adjacent organs by large cysts may cause discomfort. Adrenal cysts are usually discovered on examination of other organs. The mass may be outlined on excretory urograms, and the ipsilateral kidney may be displaced. Both sonography and CT scan will reveal the cystic nature of the mass. Its capsule often contains curvilinear calcification. A few cases have been reported in the pediatric age group and 13 in newborns (Zivković et al, 1983).

Because of the adhesions to vital organs, surgical resection of adrenal cysts can be difficult. Small and asymptomatic cysts are best left alone. Large sympto-

matic cysts can usually be cured by percutaneous aspiration under ultrasonic control (Nosher et al, 1982). Spontaneous infection of cysts has been reported (Okafo, Nickel, and Morales, 1983).

METASTASES FROM OTHER ORGANS

Metastases from malignant tumors of other organs are common. At autopsy, such adrenal metastases are noted in 20% of cancer patients. The primary tumor is most commonly in the breast, lung, or lymphatics (Cedermark and Ohlsén, 1981). CT scans are thought to be the best method for detecting metastatic adrenal tumors. Needle biopsy can be done if necessary (Zornoza et al, 1981).

MYELOLIPOMA

Myelolipoma is a rather rare benign adrenal tumor. On sonography and CT scan, it appears as a lucent mass that contains bone. It appears avascular on adrenal angiography (Ishikawa et al, 1981).

DISEASES OF THE ADRENAL CORTEX

CUSHING'S SYNDROME

Cushing's syndrome or Cushing's disease is caused by overproduction of cortisol (hydrocortisone). Most cases (85%) are due to bilateral adrenocortical hyperplasia stimulated by overproduction of pituitary adrenocorticotropic hormone (corticotropin, ACTH). A few cases are due to an undifferentiated ectopic ACTH-producing tumor that may be found (in decreasing order of incidence) in the lungs, the bronchial tree, the kidneys, the islets of the pancreas, or the thymus. Adrenal adenoma is the cause in 10% of cases and adenocarcinoma in 5%. In children, tumors are the most common cause.

Pathophysiology

Overproduction of cortisol or closely related glucocorticoids by adrenocortical tissue leads to a protein catabolic state. This causes liberation of amino acids from muscle tissue; the acids are transformed into glucose and glycogen in the liver by gluconeogenesis. The resulting weakened protein structures (muscle and elastic tissue) cause a protuberant abdomen and poor wound healing, generalized muscle weakness, and marked osteoporosis, which is made worse by excessive loss of calcium in the urine and is nearly irreversible in adults.

The protein catabolic state leads to a variety of secondary changes. Excess glucose is transformed largely into fat and appears in characteristic sites such as the abdomen, supraclavicular fat pads, and cheeks. There is a tendency to diabetes, with an elevated fasting plasma glucose level in 20% of cases and diabetic glucose tolerance curve in 80%, yet with insulinoplethora in the majority of cases.

Destruction of most of the lymphoid tissue leads to impairment of the immune mechanisms, which makes these patients susceptible to repeated infection. Inhibition of fibroplasia by excess cortisol further interferes with wound healing and host defenses against infection.

Hypertension is present in 99% of cases. Although the aldosterone level is not usually elevated, cortisol itself exerts a hypertensive effect when present in excessive amounts, as does 11-deoxycorticosterone, which is elevated in most forms of Cushing's syndrome.

The moderate rise in serum sodium with a marked fall in serum potassium is due to an excess of cortisol and of the primary mineralocorticoid 11-deoxycorticosterone. The plasma bicarbonate level is often ele-

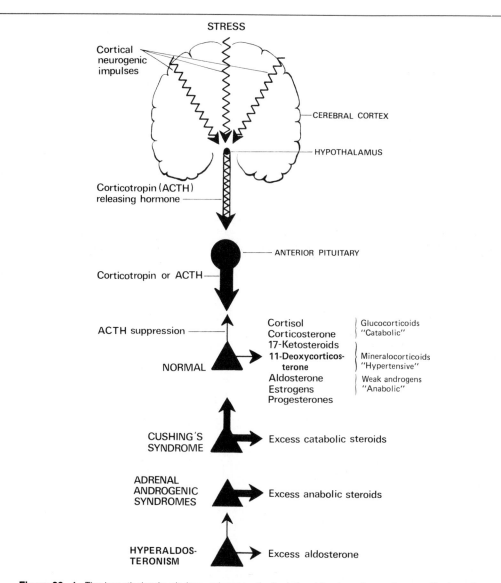

Figure 22–1. The hypothalamic-pituitary-adrenocortical relationships in various adrenocortical syndromes.

vated as a consequence of the low serum potassium level.

An adrenal adenoma is stimulated to grow by the administration of ACTH in the same way as are hyperplastic adrenals. Adenocarcinoma of an adrenal gland, on the other hand, is independent of pituitary influence and does not respond to the administration of exogenous ACTH.

Pathology

The cells in adrenal hyperplasia resemble those of the zona fasciculata of the normal adrenal cortex. Frank adenocarcinoma reveals pleomorphism and invasion of the capsule, the vascular system, or both (Fig 22–2). Local invasion may occur, and functional metastases are common to the liver, lungs, bone, or brain. Differentiation between adenoma and adenocarcinoma is sometimes difficult. The former is stimulated by the administration of exogenous ACTH, as reflected in an increased urinary or plasma level of hydroxycorticosteroids; this does not usually occur with adenocarcinoma.

In the presence of adenoma or malignant tumor, atrophy of the cortices of both adrenals occurs because the main secretory product of the tumor is cortisol, which inhibits the pituitary secretion of ACTH. Thus, although the tumor continues to grow, the contralateral adrenal cortex undergoes atrophy.

Clinical Findings

A. Symptoms and Signs: (Figs 22–3 and 22–4.) The presence of at least 3 of the following strongly suggests Cushing's syndrome:

1. Marked weakness, especially in the quadriceps femoris, making unaided rising from a chair difficult.

2. Obesity (with sparing of the extremities), moon face, and fat pads over the clavicles and the seventh cervical vertebra (buffalo hump). The abnormal distribution of fat is more characteristic of the disease than any rise in body weight, which rarely exceeds 100 kg (220 lb).

3. Striae (red and depressed) over the abdomen and thighs. Festering ulcers of the skin may be present.

4. Irritability, difficulty in sleeping, and sometimes psychotic personality.

5. Hypertension (almost always present).

6. Osteoporosis (common), with back pain from compression fractures of the lumbar vertebrae as well as rib fractures.

7. In 80% of cases, a diabetic glucose tolerance curve is present, and in 20% there is an elevated fasting plasma glucose level.

8. To a variable extent, there are features of the adrenogenital syndrome in cases of Cushing's syndrome—least marked in the case of adenoma, most severe with carcinoma, and to an intermediate degree with bilateral adrenocortical hyperplasia. They consist of recession of the hairline, hirsutism, small breasts, and generalized muscular overdevelopment, with lowering of the voice. These relate to the excess of ketosteroids in general.

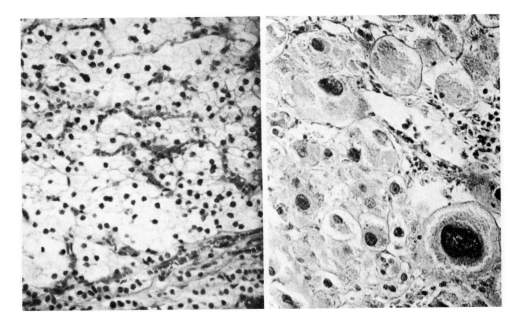

Figure 22–2. *Left:* Histologic appearance of a typical benign adenoma of the adrenal cortex made up of a large number of identical cells from the zona fasciculata removed from a 39-year-old woman with Cushing's syndrome. *Right:* Section of an adenocarcinoma removed from a 36-year-old woman with metastatic adenocarcinoma showing significant pleomorphism of the cells. Invasion of a large vein is not shown in this micrograph. Note that benign adenomas will occasionally have this appearance but without invasion of the bloodstream. (Reproduced, with permission, from Forsham PH: The adrenal cortex. In: *Textbook of Endocrinology,* 4th ed. Williams RH [editor]. Saunders, 1968.)

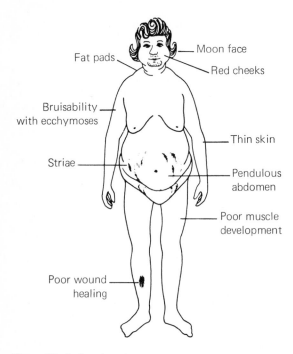

Figure 22–3. Drawing of a typical case of Cushing's syndrome showing the principal clinical features. (Reproduced, with permission, from Forsham PH: The adrenal cortex. In: *Textbook of Endocrinology,* 4th ed. Williams RH [editor]. Saunders, 1968.)

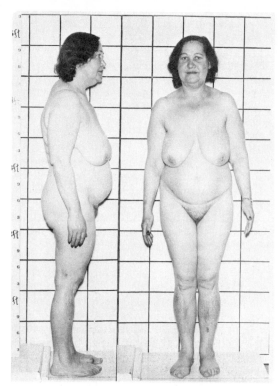

Figure 22–4. A case of Cushing's syndrome due to bilateral hyperplasia. Note the red moon face, receding hairline, buffalo hump over the seventh vertebra, protuberant abdomen, and inappropriately thin arms and legs. The combined adrenal weight was 20 g (as opposed to normal weight of 10 g).

On the basis of the foregoing clinical findings alone, it is not possible to differentiate between bilateral adrenocortical hyperplasia, unilateral adenoma, and adenocarcinoma.

The most rapid onset is noted in cases caused by ectopic ACTH-producing tumor with high glucocorticoid output or those due to adrenal adenocarcinoma. In the case of adenoma or adenocarcinoma, the tumor may be palpable above the kidneys.

B. Laboratory Findings: The white count is elevated to the range of 12,000–20,000/μL, usually with fewer than 20% lymphocytes. Eosinophils are few in number or absent. Polycythemia is present in over half of cases, with the hemoglobin ranging from 14 to 16 g/dL. Anemia, however, is found in association with ectopic ACTH-producing tumors in the lungs, pancreas, kidney, thymus, and other organs.

Blood chemical analyses are apt to show an increase in serum Na^+ and CO_2 levels and a decrease in serum K^+ levels (metabolic alkalosis). A diabetic glucose tolerance curve is usually found.

1. Specific tests for Cushing's syndrome– The following tests are performed to determine whether the patient has Cushing's syndrome or is an anxious individual with elevated plasma levels of cortisol.

a. 24-Hour urinary free cortisol level–Measurement of the urinary free cortisol level in a 24-hour specimen of urine is the most specific and reliable single test for Cushing's syndrome. To make certain that the urine specimen is a complete 24-hour specimen, creatinine levels should also be determined. If the urinary creatinine level is 800–1500 mg, the specimen is complete; if it is not, another specimen should be taken. A urinary free cortisol level above 120 μg in an adequate specimen establishes the diagnosis of Cushing's syndrome with near certainty. Obesity or hyperthyroidism does not raise the level of urinary free cortisol above normal.

b. Suppression of ACTH and plasma cortisol by dexamethasone–In normal individuals, the ACTH level is twice as high at night as in the late afternoon (Fig 22–5). In patients with cortical hyperplasia, this diurnal variation does not occur. In those with cortical tumors producing hydrocortisone, production of ACTH is suppressed. If dexamethasone is given at 11 PM, ACTH is suppressed in normal persons but not in those with Cushing's syndrome. Dexamethasone is useful because it has 30 times the potency of hydrocortisone as an ACTH suppressant. It therefore can be used in such a small amount that it will have no effect upon the determination of circulating 17-hydroxycorticosteroids.

The procedure is to give 1–2 mg of dexamethasone by mouth at 11 PM with 0.2 g of pentobarbital to allay anxiety that might stimulate adrenocortical activity.

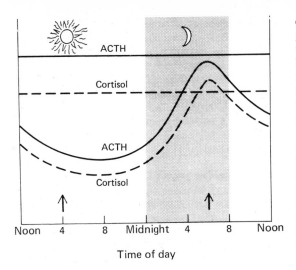

Figure 22–5. The circadian rhythm of ACTH and cortisol secretion that forms the basis of the dexamethasone suppression test for Cushing's syndrome.

Draw blood in the morning for measurement of plasma cortisol. If the level is below 5 μg/dL (normal is 5–20 μg/dL), Cushing's syndrome can be ruled out. If the value is above 10 μg/dL, Cushing's syndrome is present (Fig 22–6). A level in the range of 5–10 μg/dL is equivocal, and the test should be repeated.

Women taking birth control pills will have high plasma cortisol levels because, as in pregnancy, the estrogen stimulates production of the cortisol-binding globulin. The pills must be withheld for at least 3 weeks before the dexamethasone suppression test, or a baseline plasma cortisol level must be obtained one morning shortly before the test. Normally, a greater than 50% suppression is observed, whereas in Cushing's syndrome a significantly smaller suppression is noted.

c. 24-Hour urinary 17-hydroxycorticosteroid and 17-ketosteroid levels–These levels must be determined in a specimen collected for exactly 24 hours for comparison with normal levels (Table 22–1). This procedure, while not as diagnostic as the 2 tests discussed above, does reveal the degree of androgenic excess in comparison with glucocorticoids by comparing their urinary excretory products. In Cushing's syndrome, levels of both 17-hydroxycorticosteroids and 17-ketosteroids are elevated if adrenal hyperplasia or adenocarcinoma is present; with adenoma, 17-ketosteroid levels remain normal or low. Since 17-hydroxycorticosteroid levels vary with body weight, a high level in an obese patient is significant only if the value (in mg) exceeds the body weight in pounds × 0.06. In hyperthyroidism, high levels are noted in the presence of normal plasma levels.

2. Specific tests for differentiation of causes of Cushing's syndrome–The various causes of Cushing's syndrome can be determined today with great accuracy (95% of cases).

a. Plasma ACTH level–If the diagnosis of Cushing's syndrome has been established, this test will differentiate between adrenal hyperplasia and tumor (Fig 22–7). Draw blood in the morning in a plastic heparinized syringe (glass absorbs ACTH). The blood must be stored in ice. (New methods for deter-

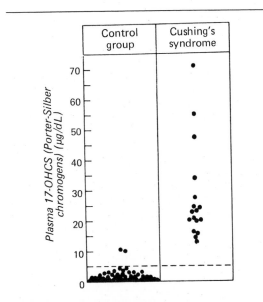

Figure 22–6. Results of the dexamethasone suppression test in obese individuals and patients with Cushing's syndrome. See text for procedure. 17-OHCS = 17-hydroxycorticosteroids. (Reproduced, with permission, from Pavlatos FC, Smilo RP, Forsham PH: A rapid screening test for Cushing's syndrome. *JAMA* 1975;**193**:720.)

Table 22–1. Normal "steroid" levels in plasma and urine.*

	Children	Adult Males	Adult Females
Plasma			
17-Hydroxycorticosteroids (μg/dL as cortisol)	5–20	5–20	5–20
Testosterone (ng/dL)	<10	300–1200	30–120
Urine (mg/24 h as cortisol or dehydroepiandrosterone†)			
17-Hydroxycorticosteroids (per kg body weight)	0.02–0.04	6–10	4–8
17-Ketogenic steroids‡	0.03–0.05	8–12	6–10
Cortisol (free)	1 μg/kg	20–120	20–120
17-Ketosteroids	Low, but rises to normal adult levels during puberty	8–20	5–15
Pregnanetriol		0.5–3	0.5–2.5

*There may be wide variations with different techniques and as done by different laboratories.
†Except as noted in the case of cortisol in second column.
‡This artificially derived entity is used in many laboratories in lieu of 17-hydroxycorticosteroids.

mining pro-ACTH, which is more stable than ACTH, will make refrigeration of the blood specimen unnecessary.) The normal range for ACTH is 20–100 pg/mL. A higher value indicates hyperplasia; a lower level means that tumor is present. The highest levels are found in ectopic ACTH syndromes. Administration of corticotropin-releasing hormone will produce an increase in the plasma ACTH level in patients with pituitary ACTH tumors but not in patients with ectopic ACTH-producing tumors, eg, in the lung or the pancreas.

b. ACTH administration—Give ACTH (eg, Cortrosyn), 0.25–0.5 mg subcutaneously to characterize tumors of the adrenal causing Cushing's syndrome. Collect blood at 1 and 2 hours for plasma hydroxycorticosteroid determinations. With adenoma, there is usually a rise; with carcinoma, there is not.

c. 11-Deoxycortisol level—A marked increase in the concentration of 11-deoxycortisol in the urine suggests adenocarcinoma.

C. X-Ray Findings and Special Examinations:

1. Localization of source of ACTH excess—When tests suggest bilateral adrenal cortical overactivity and an elevated plasma level of ACTH is present, the source of ACTH must be identified. A possible source is a microadenoma of the pituitary gland. Rarely, an adenoma produces no radiologic findings. If an adenoma of the pituitary is not identified, a search should be made for an ectopic source of ACTH.

2. Localization of a tumor—Following good catharsis but without enemas, a CT scan of the suprarenal area may reveal a mass on one side and adrenal atrophy on the other (Fig 22–8). This finding is typical of an adrenal tumor. With bilateral hyper-

plasia, 2 enlarged adrenal shadows are seen. However, this finding is not diagnostic, since perirenal fat may simulate adrenal enlargement.

A CT scan or, preferably, magnetic resonance imaging (MRI) of the sella turcica may reveal a small low-density defect against the contrast medium and the blood surrounding the sella, which is highly suggestive of a pituitary microadenoma. The ACTH tumors are usually only 3–5 mm in diameter, and large tumors are rare.

Differential Diagnosis

An adrenal cyst presenting as a suprarenal mass with displacement of the kidney can be reliably differentiated by ultrasonography. There is often some curvilinear calcification in its capsule (Ghandur-Mnaymneh, Slim, and Muakassa, 1979), and it is devoid of endocrinologic function.

A tumor or cyst of the upper pole of the kidney may appear to be a suprarenal mass, but excretory urograms will reveal the caliceal distortion of a space-occupying lesion, while renal angiography will show its intrinsic nature.

Fluid in the cardiac end of the stomach may appear as a round opacity in the left suprarenal area on a plain film of the abdomen. It disappears on an upright film. CT scans are also conclusive. Rarely, the splenic shadow will simulate a left adrenal mass.

Enlargement of the liver or spleen may displace the kidney downward; this will be revealed by physical examination and CT scanning.

Complications

Hypertension may lead to cardiac failure or stroke. Diabetes may be a problem but is usually mild. Intractable skin or systemic infections are common. Compression fractures of osteoporotic vertebrae and rib fractures (often remarkably painless) may develop. Renal stones are not uncommon as a result of leaching of calcium from the bones. Gastric (stress) ulcer may become a problem. Psychosis is not uncommon; it usually subsides after successful surgery.

Treatment

A. Bilateral Adrenocortical Hyperplasia: Pituitary microadenoma, which is the most common cause of bilateral adrenocortical hyperplasia, must be located and removed surgically. **Transsphenoidal resection** performed by an experienced neurosurgeon is the method of choice. Success is reported in over 90% of cases, and in most instances the endocrine functions of the pituitary gland are preserved.

Total bilateral adrenalectomy is indicated in patients with pituitary tumor or ectopic carcinoma in whom the source of excess ACTH cannot be removed and in most cases in which no pituitary adenoma is found at operation. In general, total removal of the adrenocortical mass is preferred to subtotal procedures because of the invariable and unpredictable regrowth of adrenal tissue. In 5% of cases treated by total adrenalectomy, ectopic adrenocortical tissue will lead

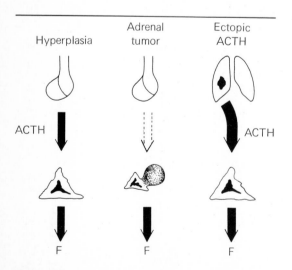

Figure 22–7. Schematic presentation of the pituitary-adrenal interrelationship in cases of hyperplasia, functional adrenocortical tumors, and ectopic ACTH syndrome. (Reproduced, with permission, from Forsham PH: The adrenal cortex. In: *Textbook of Endocrinology*, 4th ed. Williams RH [editor]. Saunders, 1968.)

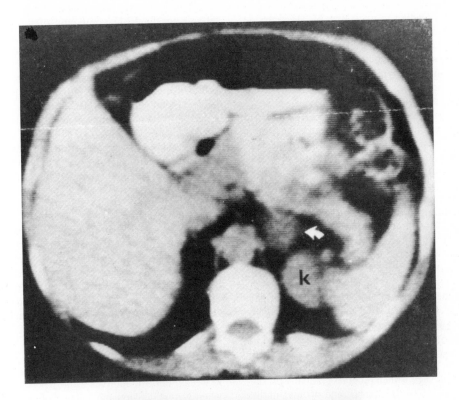

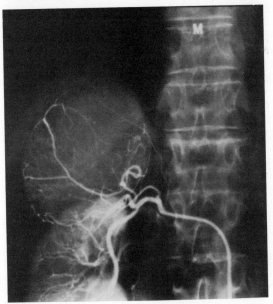

Figure 22–8. Localization of adrenal lesions. *Top:* CT scan of a 3-cm left adrenal adenoma (*white arrow*) anteromedial to the left kidney (k). (Reproduced, with permission, from Korobkin MT et al: *AJR* 1979;**132**:231.) *Bottom:* Selective arteriogram showing large right adrenal adenoma above the upper pole of the right kidney.

to recrudescence of Cushing's disease. An undesirable consequence of total adrenalectomy is the rapid growth of chromophobe pituitary adenomas in up to 25% of cases, leading to excessive ACTH secretion (Nelson's syndrome). These tumors may be treated by irradiation of the pituitary or surgery (or both), but they may become malignant and are difficult to eradicate. **Total anterior hypophysectomy** is justified in patients no longer of child-bearing age.

1. Preoperative preparation–Because removal of the source of excessive cortisol will inevitably lead to temporary or permanent adrenal insufficiency, it is of the utmost importance to administer cortisol preoperatively and to continue substitution therapy after surgery to control Addison's disease. In the post-operative period, the dose is tapered downward until oral medication provides sufficient control.

2. Postoperative status–The patient feels moderately well following removal of the source of excess ACTH or adrenalectomy or while receiving a high dose of hydrocortisone in excess of the usual daily output of approximately 20 mg. When dosage approaches the maximum normal physiologic output, the patient may complain of nausea, abdominal pain resembling that of pancreatitis (which in fact may occur), and extreme weakness with the adrenocortical withdrawal syndrome. Thus, it is important to reduce the steroid substitution gradually over a period of several days. On the day of operation, 200 mg of cortisol is given; the dosage is then reduced gradually on successive days (150, 100, 80, 60, and 40 mg) until a maintenance dosage of 20–30 mg cortisol combined with 0.1 mg fludrocortisone is reached.

3. Follow-up–The status of adrenocortical secretion cannot be determined during substitution therapy, since one-third of administered cortisol appears in the urine. In order to obtain a valid measurement of 24-hour urinary 17-hydroxycorticosteroid levels, it is necessary to stop the usual cortisol replacement and give 1 mg of dexamethasone daily for 2 days while covering with additional sodium chloride.

Urinary 17-hydroxycorticosteroids or 17-ketogenic steroid levels should be measured at intervals of 3–6 months. The patient should cease taking cortisol temporarily and should be given 1 mg of dexamethasone orally on the day before and the day of the urine collection, along with a high sodium intake. This will reveal any reactivation of residual adrenal cortical tissue.

If Nelson's syndrome develops postoperatively, plasma ACTH measurements, which are usually somewhat elevated when the patient is on standard adrenocortical replacement therapy, will become progressively higher. The skin color of patients will turn significantly darker. A CT scan of the sella turcica, when compared with preoperative scans, will reveal an expanding chromophobe tumor. This study should be done every 6 months until the patient has remained asymptomatic for 1 year, especially if increased melanin pigmentation occurs due to excess ACTH secretion.

B. Adrenal Adenoma and Adenocarcinoma: Depending on the size of the tumor and the patient's body habitus, the lesion can be approached through the flank with resection of the eleventh or twelfth rib. For large tumors, a transthoracic transdiaphragmatic incision provides ideal exposure of the mass.

1. Preoperative preparation–This is the same as for bilateral hyperplasia, because removal of one adrenal gland and the invariable atrophy of the contralateral gland almost always result in immediate hypoadrenalism.

2. Postoperative treatment and follow-up–Because of atrophy of the contralateral adrenal, postoperative substitution therapy must encourage return of function of the atrophic gland. Hydrocortisone is given orally in a dosage of 10 mg 3 times daily initially and reduced within 2–3 weeks to 10 mg daily given at 7 or 8 AM. Substitution therapy may be necessary for 1 month to 2 years depending on the rate of recovery of the residual gland. Sodium supplementation is rarely necessary, since the atrophic adrenal usually produces sufficient aldosterone. Serial determinations of urinary cortisol, 17-hydroxycorticosteroid, and 17-ketosteroid levels can be used as tumor markers.

Prognosis

Treatment of hypercortisolism usually leads to disappearance of symptoms and many signs within days to weeks, but osteoporosis usually persists in adults, whereas hypertension and diabetes often improve. Bilateral hyperplasia treated by pituitary adenomectomy has an excellent early prognosis, and long-term follow-up shows a recurrence rate of about 10%. Removal of an adrenal adenoma offers an excellent prognosis.

The outlook for patients with adenocarcinoma is poor. The antineoplastic drug mitotane (o,p'-DDD; Lysodren) given in doses of up to 30 g orally daily reduces the symptoms and signs of Cushing's syndrome but does little to prolong survival, and nausea is usually troublesome. This drug in combination with fluorouracil has recently been shown to arrest metastases.

ADRENAL ANDROGENIC SYNDROMES

These conditions are more common in females. Congenital bilateral adrenal hyperplasia and tumors, both benign and malignant, may be observed. They all represent excessive or abnormal levels of androgen. In contrast to Cushing's syndrome, which is protein catabolic, the androgenic syndromes are strongly anabolic. In untreated cases, there is a marked recession of the hairline, increased beard growth, and excessive growth of pubic and sexual hair in general in both sexes. In males, there is enlargement of the penis, usually with atrophic testes; in females, enlargement of the clitoris occurs, with atrophy of the breasts and amenorrhea (Fig 22–9). Muscle mass increases and fat content decreases, leading to a powerful but trim figure. The voice becomes deeper, particularly in females; this condition is irreversible, since it is due to enlargement of the larynx. The psyche of these patients is often deranged. In both sexes there is increased physical aggressiveness and libido.

1. CONGENITAL BILATERAL ADRENAL ANDROGENIC HYPERPLASIA

Pathophysiology

A congenital defect in certain adrenal enzymes results in the production of abnormal steroids (Fig 22–10), causing **pseudohermaphroditism** in females and **macrogenitosomia** in males. The enzyme defect is associated with excess androgen production in utero. In females, the müllerian duct structures (eg, ovaries, uterus, and vagina) will develop normally, but the excess androgen exerts a masculinizing effect on the urogenital sinus and genital tubercle, so that the vagina is connected to the urethra, which, in turn, opens at the base of an enlarged clitoris. The labia are often hypertrophied. Externally, the appearance is that of severe hypospadias with cryptorchidism.

The adrenal cortex secretes mostly anabolic and androgenic steroids, leading to various degrees of cortisol deficiency depending on the nature of the enzyme block. This increases the secretion of ACTH, which causes hyperplasia of both adrenal cortices. The cortices continue to secrete large amounts of inappropriate anabolic, androgenic, or hypertensive steroids. Absence or severe reduction of the usual tissue concentration of various enzymes—oxidases, hydrogenases, isomerases, or desmolases—accounts for blocks in the adrenocortical synthetic pathways (Fig 22–10).

A block at C_{20} with absence of 20,22-desmolase leads to the rare congenital lipoid adrenal hyperplasia with complete absence of any steroidal hormone production; the infant will die at an early age unless full substitution therapy is given for life.

A block at C_3 with lack of 3β-hydroxydehydrogenase and isomerase prevents formation of progesterone, aldosterone, and cortisol. Dehydroepiandrosterone is produced in excess. This uncommon syndrome is characterized by hypotension, hypoglycemia, and male pseudohermaphroditism, with females showing unusual sexual development with hirsutism. There is variable melanin pigmentation.

A block at C_{21} with deficiency or absence of 21-hydroxylase does not allow for the transformation of 17α-hydroxyprogesterone to cortisol. This more com-

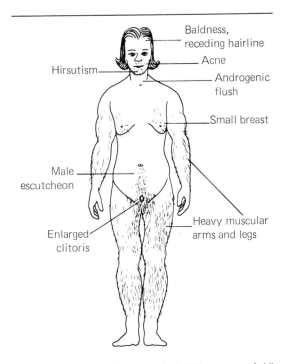

Figure 22–9. Clinical features of a full-blown case of virilism in a female with adrenogenital syndrome. (Reproduced, with permission, from Forsham PH: The adrenal cortex. In: *Textbook of Endocrinology,* 4th ed. Williams RH [editor]. Saunder, 1968.)

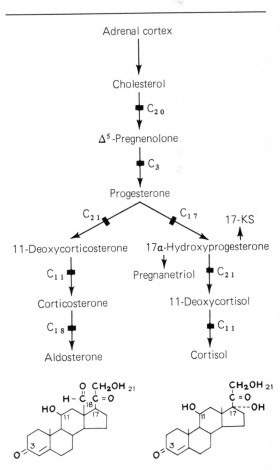

Figure 22–10. Deficiencies in hydroxylases and related enzymes in the adrenal cortex, giving rise to typical cases of adrenogenital syndrome.

mon deficiency occurs in 2 forms: the salt-losing variety, with low to absent aldosterone, and the more frequent non-salt-losing type. Hirsutism, virilism, hypotension, and melanin pigmentation are common.

A **block at C_{17}** with lack of 17-hydroxylase occurs mostly in females and may not be discovered until adulthood. Findings include low cortisol levels with high ACTH levels, primary amenorrhea, and sexual infantilism, as neither the glucocorticoids nor the sex steroids are produced in adequate amounts. Rarely, there is male pseudohermaphroditism. Hypertension due to excess mineralocorticoids, notably 11-deoxy-corticosterone, is characteristically present.

A **block at C_{11}** with lack of 11-hydroxylase prevents formation of cortisol and corticosterone and thus leads to a marked excess of ACTH, with deep melanin pigmentation. Unlike Addison's disease, there is hypertension due to excess 11-deoxycorticosterone. There are no marked sexual abnormalities.

A **block at C_{18}** with lack of an oxidase is exceedingly rare; 11-deoxycorticosterone will take over from aldosterone as the essential mineralocorticoid.

Increased androgenicity manifested by hirsutism and amenorrhea only rarely develops after puberty and seldom leads to virilism in middle age. This acquired mild enzyme abnormality of the adrenals is known as **benign androgenic overactivity of the adrenal cortices.**

Clinical Findings

A. Symptoms and Signs: In newborn girls, the appearance of the external genitalia resembles severe hypospadias with cryptorchidism. Infant boys may appear quite normal at birth. The earlier in intrauterine life the fetus has been exposed to excess androgen, the more marked the anomalies.

In untreated cases, hirsutism, excess muscle mass, and, eventually, amenorrhea are the rule. Breast development is poor. In males, growth of the phallus is excessive. The testes are often atrophic because of inhibition of gonadotropin secretion by the elevated androgens. On rare occasions, hyperplastic adrenocortical rests in the testes make them large and firm. In most instances, there is aspermia after puberty.

In both males and females with androgenic hyperplasia, the growth rate is initially increased, so that they are taller than their classmates. At about age 9–10 years, premature fusion of the epiphyses caused by excess androgen causes termination of growth, so that these patients are short as adults. In both sexes, there is increased aggressiveness and libido that can cause social and disciplinary problems, particularly in some boys.

B. Laboratory Findings: Urinary 17-ketosteroid levels are higher than normal for sex and age (Table 22–1). Urinary pregnanetriol levels are elevated early (this is a more sensitive test than measurement of 17-ketosteroid levels, since pregnanetriol is the precursor of the androgenic steroids). The most sensitive indicator of androgenic activity is elevation of plasma 17-hydroxyprogesterone levels, and this test

is particularly useful in children. The buccal smear is positive for Barr bodies in females. Chromosome studies are normal.

C. X-Ray Findings: X-rays will show acceleration of bone age. A lateral cystourethrogram may show the vagina as well as the urethra and bladder (Fig 22–11).

D. CT Scans: Scans will usually show the hypertrophied adrenals.

E. Instrumental Examination: Urethroscopy may permit visualization of the point at which the vagina opens into the posterior wall of the urethra. The vaginal tract can often be entered and the cervix seen.

Differential Diagnosis

A number of congenital anomalies that affect the development of the external genitalia resemble adrenal androgenic syndrome. These include (1) severe hypospadias with cryptorchidism, (2) female pseudohermaphroditism of the nonadrenal type (caused by administration of androgens or progestational compounds during the pregnancy), (3) male pseudohermaphroditism, and (4) true hermaphroditism. These children show no hormonal abnormalities, and bone age and maturation are not accelerated.

Treatment

It is imperative to make the diagnosis early. Treatment of the underlying cause is medical, with the goal of suppressing excessive ACTH secretion, thus minimizing excess androgenicity. This is accomplished by giving the long-acting glucocorticoid dexamethasone,

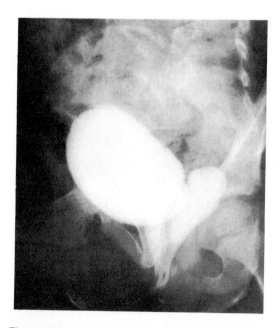

Figure 22–11. Urogenital sinus in congenital virilizing cortical hyperplasia. Oblique urethrogram showing connection of vagina with distal urethra. (Courtesy of F Hinman, Jr.)

0.5–1.5 mg orally at 11 PM every night, so that the adrenal cortex is suppressed at the time of its greatest activity, ie, 2–8 AM. In a severe case of salt-losing syndrome, fludrocortisone (0.05–0.3 mg, depending on severity and age) together with good salt intake is necessary to stabilize blood pressure and body weight.

After puberty, the vaginal opening can be surgically separated from the urethra and opened in the normal position on the perineum. If frequent clitoral erections occur, resection or, preferably, recession of the clitoris should be considered (Parrott, Scheflan, and Hester, 1980). Judicious administration of estrogens or birth control pills will feminize the figure in pseudohermaphrodites and improve their psyche considerably.

Prognosis

If the condition is recognized early and ACTH suppression is begun even before surgical repair of the genital anomaly, the outlook for normal linear growth and development is excellent. Delay in treatment will inevitably result in stunted growth and a propensity to coronary artery disease, with early death due to myocardial infarction. In some female pseudohermaphrodites, menses begin after treatment, and conception and childbirth can occur when the anatomic abnormalities are minimal or have been surgically repaired.

2. ADRENOCORTICAL TUMORS

The **dexamethasone suppression test** is used to differentiate between hyperplasia (a medical problem) and adrenocortical tumor (a surgical problem). A number of methods are now available for determining dexamethasone suppression of plasma levels of 17-hydroxyprogesterone, dehydroepiandrosterone, or androstenedione. The most common dexamethasone suppression test employs measurement of urinary 17-ketosteroids. The procedure is as follows: A 24-hour urine specimen is collected and 17-ketosteroids measured. An adult patient is then given dexamethasone, 2 mg orally 4 times a day. On the second day, a 24-hour urine specimen is taken again and the concentration of 17-ketosteroids measured. If the second specimen contains less than half the 17-ketosteroids found in the first specimen, adrenal activity is suppressible and the condition is due to hyperplasia. Suppression does not occur when adrenal overactivity is due to tumor. Zaitoon and Mackie (1978) have reviewed the literature on adrenal cortical tumors in children.

The tumor can be located by CT scans (Fig 22–8). In these cases, there is no atrophy of the contralateral adrenal because there is no marked elevation of 17-hydroxycorticosteroid levels. Therefore, preoperative cortisol medication can be minimal, eg, 50 mg of cortisol phosphate given intramuscularly just before induction of anesthesia. The tumor can readily be removed through the flank. In contrast to patients with Cushing's syndrome, hemostasis is easy to obtain and wound healing is normal.

Adenocarcinoma is a highly malignant tumor that metastasizes to the liver, lungs, and brain. Successive determinations of urinary 17-ketosteroids as a tumor marker will reveal the completeness of the resection and the presence or later development of metastases. When metastases have occurred, hyperandrogenicity can be combated by giving up to 30 g of mitotane (*o,p'*-DDD; Lysodren) orally daily. Unfortunately, this drug only temporarily halts tumor growth, and fluorouracil (5-FU; Adrucil) is not successful either. X-ray treatment in large doses may postpone the inevitable death of these patients, and mitotane combined with fluorouracil may offer some help.

THE HYPERTENSIVE, HYPOKALEMIC SYNDROME (Primary Aldosteronism)

Excessive production of aldosterone, due mostly to aldosteronoma or to spontaneous bilateral nodular hyperplasia of the zona glomerulosa of the adrenal cortex, leads to the combination of hypertension, hypokalemia, nocturia, and, rarely, diabetes insipidus. Rarer causes for these are an adrenocortical aldosterone-producing carcinoma, a glucocorticoid-remediable ACTH excess syndrome, and indeterminate aldosteronism that in part appears to be due to an adenoma hyperplasia. The low serum potassium level may lead to muscular weakness with fully conscious collapse and postural hypotension due to baroreceptor paralysis, leading to syncope. A syndrome resembling diabetes insipidus may occur as a result of reversible damage to the renal collecting tubules. The alkalosis may produce tetany.

Pathophysiology

Excessive aldosterone, acting on most cell membranes in the body, produces typical changes in the distal renal tubule and the small bowel that lead to urinary potassium loss together with increased renal sodium reabsorption and hydrogen ion secretion. This results in potassium depletion, metabolic alkalosis, increased plasma sodium concentration, and hypervolemia. Potassium depletion affects baroreceptors, so that postural fall in blood pressure no longer results in reflex tachycardia. With low serum levels of potassium, the concentrating ability of the kidney is lowered and the tubules no longer respond to the administration of vasopressin by increased reabsorption of water. Finally, impairment of insulin release secondary to potassium depletion increases carbohydrate intolerance in about 50% of cases.

Plasma renin and, secondarily, plasma angiotensin are depressed by excess aldosterone, presumably as a result of blood volume expansion (Fig 22–12). Early in the course of excess aldosterone production, there may be hypertension with a normal serum potassium level. Later, the potassium level will be low as well, and this suggests the diagnosis.

Clinical Findings

A. Symptoms and Signs: Whereas adenoma predominates in females, bilateral nodular adrenal hyperplasia occurs predominantly in young males. Headaches are common, nocturia is invariably present, and rare episodes of paralysis occur with very low serum potassium levels. Numbness and tingling of the extremities are related to alkalosis that may lead to tetany. Hypertension is of varying severity. Orthostatic hypotension is common. Inappropriate control of vasomotor tone is usually demonstrable. Feel the pulse while the patient is standing. Then have the patient crouch and straighten up and take the pulse again. In a normal person, the pulse will be slower the second time; with hyperaldosteronism, it is not.

Ophthalmoscopic examination usually shows normal vessels inconsistent with the degree of hypertension. Unless acute heart failure is present, there is no edema. The Chvostek sign is often positive.

B. Laboratory Findings: Before the tests outlined below are done, one must ascertain that the patient is not taking oral contraceptives or other estrogen preparations, since these may increase renin and angiotensin levels and therefore aldosterone levels, thus raising the blood pressure artificially. Withdrawal of these medications for 1 week is mandatory. Diuretics must also be discontinued, since they lower blood volume and induce secondary aldosteronism and hypokalemia. Also, if the patient is taking a salt-restricted diet, aldosterone is normally elevated.

Before serum electrolytes are measured, the patient receives a loading dose of 6 g of salt for at least 2 days. This will furnish exchangeable sodium in the distal tubule and allow potassium to exchange with sodium, thus clearly revealing the low serum potassium level

and electrolyte imbalance. Later, serum potassium must also be replenished, because a very low level of this ion may artificially decrease the secretory rate of aldosterone.

In true aldosterone excess, serum sodium will be slightly elevated and CO_2 increased, whereas serum potassium will be very low, eg, 3 meq/L or less. Urine and serum potassium determinations while the patient is receiving good sodium replacement provide a screening test. Potassium wasting is considered to be established if the urinary potassium level is greater than 30 meq/L/24 h but the serum potassium level is low (3 meq/L or less).

Definitive diagnosis rests on demonstration of an elevated urine or plasma aldosterone level or a positive desoxycorticosterone acetate test (Table 22–2). Before aldosterone is measured, the patient should be loaded with salt (6 g/d) to avoid a decrease in plasma volume, which by itself raises the aldosterone level. In hyperaldosteronism, urinary aldosterone is more than 10 μg/d after suppression with desoxycorticosterone acetate or fludrocortisone.

C. Localization: Tomograms do not usually reveal small adenomas ranging from 1 to 2 cm in diameter (Fig 22–13). CT scans may locate the tumor. [131]I-19-iodocholesterol scan (Fig 22–8) is the noninvasive method of choice.

Differential Diagnosis

Secondary hyperaldosteronism may accompany renovascular hypertension. An abdominal bruit will suggest this condition initially. This too is associated with hypokalemic alkalosis. Differentiation requires estimation of blood volume and serum sodium. In primary aldosteronism, both tend to be elevated. In the secondary form, both may be low.

Essential hypertension does not cause changes in the electrolyte pattern. Definitive tests for hyperaldosteronism show negative results.

The diagnosis of pheochromocytoma (see below) is based on catecholamine measurements, which in pa-

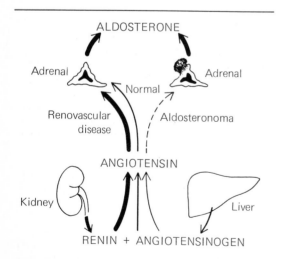

Figure 22–12. The angiotensin-aldosterone relationships in a case of aldosteronoma and hypertension due to renal vascular disease. (Reproduced, with permission, from Forsham PH: The adrenal cortex. In: *Textbook of Endocrinology,* 4th ed. Williams RH [editor]. Saunders, 1968.)

Table 22–2. Desoxycorticosterone acetate test for primary aldosteronism.

Patient preparation
  (1) Withdraw all hypotensive drugs for 1 week.
  (2) Give 6+ g of salt for 3 days.
  (3) Give 100 meq (7 g) of potassium chloride for 3 days.
Test procedure
  (1) Collect 24-hour urine sample for aldosterone determination.
  (2) Give 5 mg of desoxycorticosterone acetate (eg, Percorten Acetate) IM daily for 3 days or 1 mg fludrocortisone orally twice daily for 3 days.
  (3) On third day, repeat 24-hour urine test for aldosterone.
Result (aldosterone concentration in urine, μg/d)

	Normal	Primary Aldosteronism	Secondary Aldosteronism
Control day	9	18	25
Third day of suppression	3	17	9

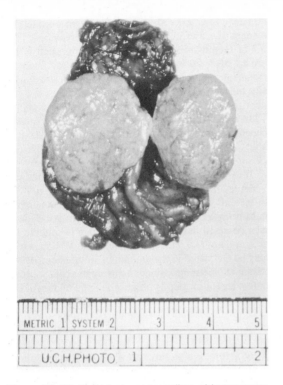

Figure 22–13. A typical canary-yellow aldosteronoma associated with the syndrome of hypertension, hyperkalemia, and alkalosis. Note the relatively small size of this tumor compared to other types of adrenocortical tumors.

tients suffering from paroxysmal hypertension are not elevated during normotensive intervals. Careful administration of glucagon, 1 mg intravenously, will cause a rise in both blood pressure and catecholamine levels. Aldosterone levels remain normal.

Cushing's syndrome is associated with hypertension, but physical examination and appropriate hormonal assays will establish the diagnosis.

Treatment

A. Aldosteronoma: If the site of the tumor has been established, only the affected adrenal need be removed. A flank incision with resection of the eleventh or twelfth rib will provide good exposure. Two-thirds of adenomas are in the left adrenal. They are almost never bilateral.

B. Bilateral Nodular Hyperplasia: Most authorities do not recommend resection of both adrenals, since the fall in blood pressure is only temporary and electrolyte imbalance may continue. Medical treatment is recommended.

C. Medical Treatment: If surgery must be postponed, if the hypertension is mild in an older person, or if bilateral hyperplasia is the cause, one may treat medically with spironolactone (Aldactone), 25–50 mg orally 4 times daily.

Prognosis

In rare cases, hypotension may persist for as long as 2 years after removal of the adenoma; this can be controlled by increased sodium intake. Following removal of an adenomatous adrenal, 60% of patients become normotensive and 40% show some lowering of hypertension. Bilateral nodular hyperplasia is not amenable to surgical treatment, and the results of medical treatment are only fair.

DISEASES OF THE ADRENAL MEDULLA

PHEOCHROMOCYTOMA

Pheochromocytoma, derived from the neural crest, is one of the surgically curable hypertensive syndromes. There is no sex predilection. Pheochromocytoma accounts for fewer than 1% of cases of hypertension, but it is readily diagnosed if the possibility is kept in mind. It usually occurs spontaneously but may result from a familial disease known as multiple endocrine neoplasia type 2, which is inherited as an autosomal dominant trait. In up to 5% of patients, pheochromocytoma occurs as part of a pluriglandular syndrome including medullary carcinoma of the thyroid, hyperparathyroidism (adenoma or hyperplasia), Cushing's syndrome with excess ACTH, and oral mucosal neuromas with neuroectodermal dysplasia, including neurofibromatosis. The tumor is bilateral or extra-adrenal in 5% of cases in adults and in an even greater percentage in children and is then most often familial.

Clinical Findings

A. Symptoms and Signs: Hypertension is both systolic and diastolic. The appearance of the retinal vessels on ophthalmoscopic examination is commensurate with the severity of the hypertension and the duration of the disease state. Hypertension may be either sustained and indistinguishable from ordinary blood pressure elevation, or paroxysmal, coming on for variable lengths of time and then subsiding to normal levels. Such attacks are usually precipitated by trigger mechanisms of various sorts, eg, emotional upsets or straining at stool.

Headache is a frequent complaint and is commensurate in severity with the degree of hypertension. Increased sweating without appropriate causes such as exertion or environmental heat resembles the phenomenon seen during menopause and may be accompanied by flushing or blanching. Tachycardia with palpitations occurs mainly as a consequence of epinephrine rather than norepinephrine excess. Postural hypotension is a frequent finding, partly as a result of diminished plasma volume and ganglionic blocking of normal pressor pathways by excess catecholamines.

Profound weakness may occur after an attack of hypertension. Weight loss is common, partly because of the anorexia that results from elevated blood glucose and fatty acid levels—the former caused by increased glycogenolysis and the latter by the increased lipolysis induced by elevated catecholamine levels.

Decreased gastrointestinal motility occurs, leading to nausea and vomiting, especially in children, and constipation. This effect is a direct pharmacologic consequence of excessive circulating catecholamines. Episodes of psychic instability verging on hysteria are frequent and are probably due to increased concentrations of catecholamines and other neurotransmitters in the brain, although circulating catecholamines, unlike some of their precursors, penetrate the blood-brain barrier to only a limited extent.

In the 5% of patients with associated neuroectodermal disease, café au lait spots are found with smooth outlines ("coast of California") rather than the ragged ones ("coast of Maine") that occur only with the unrelated fibrous dysplasia of bone. Telangiectasia and, rarely, cerebellar involvement may coexist in neuroectodermal disease.

In a very few patients, the tumor is palpable. Even if it is not palpable, pressure over the site of the tumor may cause an exacerbation of hypertension. Thus, if a tumor is embedded in the bladder, the blood pressure rises with micturition (Flanigan et al, 1980).

B. Laboratory Findings: The hematocrit is usually elevated, and the white cell count is high, with few lymphocytes. Serum protein levels are elevated. The fasting plasma glucose level is often elevated and accompanied by a diabetic glucose tolerance curve.

Urinary catecholamine levels must be measured. The patient must discontinue all medication except diuretics, digitalis, and barbiturates for at least 2 days. An exact 24-hour urine collection, in a bottle containing 15 mL of 6 N hydrochloric acid, is then obtained. The test must be performed within 48 hours. The normal limits are shown in Table 22–3.

In individual cases, epinephrine or norepinephrine (or both) may be elevated, but elevation of only epinephrine suggests that the tumor is in the adrenal medulla, in ectopic medullary tissue, or in the organ of Zuckerkandl, since the methylating enzyme necessary for transforming norepinephrine to epinephrine is present only in medullary tissue.

Urinary normetanephrine, metanephrine, and vanilmandelic acid (VMA) are breakdown products of epinephrine and norepinephrine. Whereas less than 5% of secreted catecholamines appear as such in the urine, over 50% appear as metabolites, such as metanephrine or normetanephrine, and these are usually independent of any medication taken by the patient. Before collection of urine for measurement of VMA, the patient must have no vanilla ice cream, chocolate, coffee, tea, or citrus fruits for at least 48 hours. The range of normal values is shown in Table 22–3.

If estimations of both urinary catecholamines and VMA are performed, the diagnostic accuracy is 98%. In patients with paroxysmal hypertension, the urine must be collected during an attack. A spot urine specimen obtained during a brief paroxysm is suitable for determination of catecholamines and VMA, which may be compared to the amount of simultaneously determined creatinine. Since the average urinary excretion of creatinine per 24 hours is 1.4 g, a finding of 0.2 g of creatinine in the aliquot means that the amount of catecholamines and VMA should be multiplied by 7 to obtain a rough estimate of the 24-hour excretion of these substances.

As a rule, a high ratio of VMA to catecholamines indicates a large tumor; a low ratio indicates a small one (Farndon et al, 1980).

Glucagon test. If pheochromocytoma is suspected as a cause of hypertension in a patient who may be in a period of remission (normotensive), give 1 mg of glucagon intravenously. If pheochromocytoma is present, both blood pressure and catecholamine levels will rise markedly within 2 minutes. A hormonal assay can then be done. It is also advisable to determine plasma calcitonin, which will be elevated in cases of concurrent medullary carcinoma of the thyroid.

C. X-Ray Findings: Preoperative localization by x-ray can be attempted but is of limited importance, since up to 7% of the tumors are multiple and 13% are extra-adrenal and require direct exploration. Since the tumors are often quite large (Fig 22–14), tomograms with or without excretory urograms will often reveal the tumor (Fig 22–15, left). CT scans may reveal more than one tumor (Laursen and Damgaard-Pedersen, 1980).

A retrograde arteriogram (Fig 22–15, right) or venogram will reveal small or multiple tumors. Determination of plasma catecholamine concentrations at different levels during catheterization of the vena cava is quite helpful as a means of localizing ectopic tumors (Modlin et al, 1979).

Radioactive iodine-labeled metaiodobenzylguanidine (MIBG) has proved useful in both structural and functional localization of pheochromocytomas and their metastases, particularly since it is not taken up by normal adrenal medullary tissue.

Differential Diagnosis

Thyrotoxicosis may be suggested because of the marked hypermetabolism, nervousness, and weight loss. However, normal thyroid indices, constipation

---

Table 22–3. Catecholamines in urine and plasma.*

Urine
  Norepinephrine: 10–100 μg/24 h
  Epinephrine: Up to 20 μg/24 h
  Normetanephrine and metanephrine:<1.5 mg/24 h
  Vanilmandelic acid (VMA): 2–9 mg/24 h
Plasma
  Norepinephrine: 100–200 pg/mL
  Epinephrine: 30–50 pg/mL

*The values listed represent the means of the normal ranges, which vary for each laboratory.

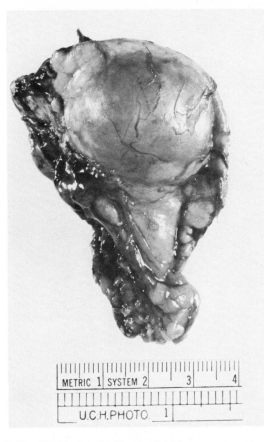

Figure 22–14. A typical large pheochromocytoma. Removal was followed by complete remission of hypertension.

rather than diarrhea, and a low rather than high blood lymphocyte count (as seen with pheochromocytoma) rule out a diagnosis of thyrotoxicosis.

Diabetes mellitus must always be suspected because of the elevated fasting plasma glucose level. With pheochromocytoma, epinephrine directly inhibits insulin secretion from the B cells while transforming liver glycogen to glucose by stimulating the process of glycogenolysis. Only persistent hyperglycemia after removal of the pheochromocytoma shows whether permanent diabetes mellitus exists.

In many patients with pheochromocytoma, organic heart disease is suggested by findings of hypertension, cardiac murmurs, and ventricular hypertrophy. These features resolve in most patients following correction of catecholamine excess; their persistence will establish a definite diagnosis of primary cardiac disease.

Treatment

The sooner hypertension can be cured, the better for the patient. Vascular accidents are common, and the longer the disease exists the more likely the hypertension is to become irreversible.

A. Preoperative Management: Hypovolemia has been noted in up to 80% of cases and may cause fatal postoperative vascular collapse. Blood and plasma volumes must be checked and normal volumes restored before surgery. Oral administration of an α-adrenergic blocking agent such as phenoxybenzamine (Dibenzylene), 40–200 mg/d in 2 divided doses, will control the blood pressure. If this can be started at least 3 weeks before surgery, the hypovolemia can be corrected. For fine adjustment of blood pressure before and during induction of anesthesia, when the danger of development of hypertensive crisis is greatest, the α-adrenergic blocking agent phentolamine (Regitine), 5 mg in 200 mL of 5% dextrose in water, can be infused intravenously at a rate that will maintain the blood pressure at nearly normal level.

B. Anesthetic Management: Thiopental (Pentothal) sodium and nitrous oxide combined are used with curare or other muscle relaxants as necessary for muscle relaxation, since they do not raise catecholamine secretion as some other agents do.

C. Surgical Treatment: Since 10% of tumors (even more in children) are multiple and ectopic, a transperitoneal approach is recommended. An anterior transverse (subcostal) incision provides the best exposure. When an adrenal tumor is found, early ligation of the adrenal vein should be performed to avoid sudden blood pressure elevation from handling the tumor. Intravenous phentolamine during surgery will control blood pressure. After removal of the tumor, there is always a fall in systemic blood pressure of variable severity and duration. This can be minimized by preoperative restoration of blood volume (as discussed above). Hypotension should be treated by infusion of norepinephrine or related pressor agents. If hypotension still persists, hydrocortisone phosphate, 100 mg intravenously, may reestablish the pressure or response. Only when both adrenals are removed is there an absolute need for cortisol replacement.

D. Immediate Postoperative Care: Two to 3 days following surgery, a 24-hour urinary VMA level should be obtained. If it is normal, similar tests every 6 months need be done only in patients with a family history of pheochromocytoma. If the VMA value is still elevated immediately after surgery, another site of pheochromocytoma exists. Malignancies (and, therefore, functional metastases) are very rare.

E. Medical Treatment: Although often effective in decreasing catecholamine production, drugs such as metyrosine (Demser) that limit the production of catecholamines are not in general use because they do not prevent tumor growth and because numerous side effects, including anxiety, sedation, diarrhea, lactation, and tremor, are reported. Antineoplastic drugs to inhibit the growth of metastases have been only moderately successful.

Prognosis

In general, the prognosis is good. With better understanding of the disease, surgical deaths are now rare. Blood pressure will fall to normal levels in about 70% of patients. In most of the remainder, blood pres-

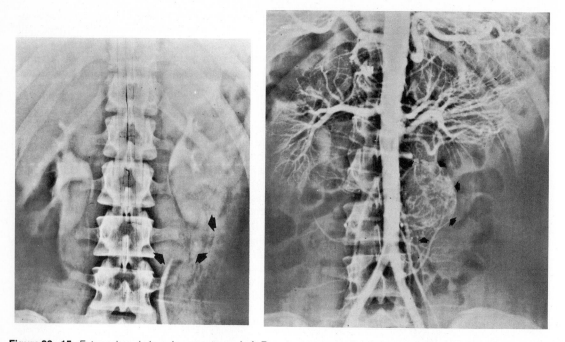

Figure 22–15. Extra-adrenal pheochromocytoma. *Left:* Excretory urogram showing normal kidneys but a soft tissue mass just below and medial to the left kidney. *Right:* Angiogram, same patient. Vascular mass below left renal arteries.

sure will remain elevated. In rare cases, the patient will become worse as a consequence of secondary vascular changes that have irreversibly activated various pressure systems. Although this persistent hypertension can be controlled with antihypertensive therapy, it is preferable to avoid the problem by early diagnosis and operation.

NEUROBLASTOMA

Neuroblastoma (Fig 22–16) is of neural crest origin and may therefore develop from any portion of the sympathetic chain. Most arise in the retroperitoneum, and 45% involve the adrenal gland. The latter offer the poorest prognosis. In childhood, neuroblastoma is the third most common neoplastic disease after leukemia and brain tumors. Most are encountered in the first 2 ½ years of life, but a few are seen as late as the sixth decade, when they seem to be less aggressive (Rowe, Oram, and Scott, 1979). Most of these patients have lymphocytes that are cytotoxic to neuroblastoma cells in tissue culture. Most members of the patient's family show the same lymphocytic reaction. It has been observed that the more lymphocytes found in the peripheral blood or the tumor, the better the prognosis (Bill, 1971). Mancini et al (1982) found 24 examples of more than one case of neuroblastoma in a family. In 5 cases, bilateral tumors were discovered in identical twins, which suggests the hereditary nature of the disease. Abnormalities of muscle and heart and hemihypertrophy have been observed in association with neuroblastoma.

Metastases spread through both the bloodstream and lymphatics. Common sites in children include the skull and long bones, regional lymph nodes, liver, and lungs (Holland et al, 1980). Local invasion is common. In infants, who enjoy the best prognosis, metastases are usually limited to the liver and subcutaneous fat.

Evans, D'Angio, and Randolph (1971) evolved the following staging of neuroblastoma:

Stage A: Tumors confined to the structure of origin.

Stage B: Tumors extending in continuity beyond the organ but not crossing the midline. Ipsilateral lymph nodes may be involved.

Stage C: Tumors extending in continuity beyond the midline. Regional lymph nodes may be involved.

Stage D: Remote disease involving skeletal organs, soft tissues, and distant lymph node groups.

Stage E: Stage A or B tumors locally but with distant metastases.

Clinical Findings
A. Symptoms: An abdominal mass is usually noted by parents, the physician, or the patient. About 70% of patients have metastases when first seen. Symptoms relating to metastases include fever, malaise, bone pain, failure to thrive, and constipation or diarrhea.

B. Signs: A flank mass is usually palpable and may even be visible; it often extends across the mid-

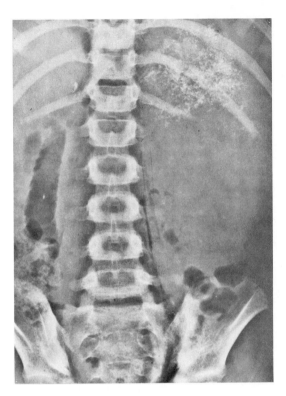

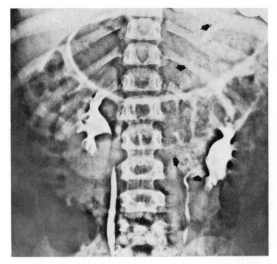

Figure 22–16. Neuroblastoma of adrenal gland. *Left:* Plain film, child age 7 years, showing large mass occupying left flank. Punctate calcification in upper portion is typical of neuroblastoma. *Right:* Excretory urogram, child age 4 years, revealing lateral and downward displacement and rotation of left kidney by suprarenal mass. No caliceal deformity; calcific areas in mass are compatible with neuroblastoma.

line. The tumor is usually nodular and fixed, since it tends to be locally invasive. Evidence of metastases may be noted: ocular proptosis from metastases to the skull, enlarged nodular liver, or a mass in bone. Hypertension is often found.

C. Laboratory Findings: Anemia is common. Urinalysis and renal function are normal. Because 70% of neuroblastomas elaborate increased levels of norepinephrine and epinephrine, urinary vanilmandelic acid (VMA) and homovanillic acid (HVA) levels should be measured. Serial estimations of these substances during definitive treatment can be used as tumor markers. A return to normal levels is encouraging, while rising levels imply residual tumor. Bone marrow aspiration may reveal tumor cells.

Hann et al (1981) noted a marked difference in prognosis in those patients with advanced local disease and widespread metastases. The incidence of spontaneous regression was high in those without bone involvement but not in those with metastases to bone. They found that serum ferritin levels were elevated in almost all of the patients with bone metastases but normal in those without osseous metastases. E rosette-inhibiting factor was also studied in both groups; it was present in most patients with metastases to bone but absent in the other group. These tests seem to have some value in judging prognosis.

Reynolds et al (1981) noted some difficulty in differentiating some neuroblastomas from Ewing's sarcoma, acute lymphoid leukemia, and lymphoma. They devised a rapid catecholamine fluorescence test and subjected biopsy specimens to tissue culture. With

neuroblastomas, the fluorescence test was positive for catecholamines and the tissue cultures revealed neuritic outgrowth; small round cell tumors did not so respond.

D. X-Ray Findings: Excretory urography usually reveals a large area of grayness in one of the upper abdominal quadrants. At least 50% of these tumors contain punctate calcific deposits. Intestinal gas is displaced by the mass, and the ipsilateral kidney, which usually functions normally, is also displaced by the suprarenal mass (Fig 22–16).

An inferior venacavogram may show occlusion from tumor invasion. Such a finding indicates the need for radiotherapy before surgical excision is attempted. Other necessary tests include a chest film, a complete bone survey, a total body bone scan (Howman-Giles, Gilday, and Ash, 1979), and a liver scan.

CT scans will not only delineate the tumor but may also yield information about invasion of adjacent tissues or organs.

Differential Diagnosis

Nephroblastoma (Wilms' tumor) is also a disease of childhood. Intravenous urograms show the caliceal distortion characteristic of an intrinsic renal tumor; no such distortion is shown in neuroblastoma, which merely displaces the kidney. Urinary catecholamines are normal with Wilms' tumor but are usually elevated in neuroblastoma. Urinary lactic dehydrogenase may be increased with Wilms' tumor but is normal with neuroblastoma. An aortogram will reveal the site of the lesion. Sonography and CT scans are also helpful.

Hydronephrosis may also occur as a flank mass but is ordinarily neither hard nor nodular. Evidence of urinary infection is common. Hydronephrosis is often bilateral, in which case renal function is depressed. Excretory urograms will reveal the dilated pelvis and calices and the site of obstruction.

Polycystic renal disease usually presents with palpable masses in both flanks. Renal function is impaired, and urograms, renal scan, or angiography will establish the diagnosis.

Neonatal adrenal hemorrhage may be confused with neuroblastoma (Smith and Middleton, 1980). These infants have a palpable upper quadrant mass, are apt to be jaundiced, and have increased serum bilirubin and a low hematocrit. Excretory urograms show grayness in the area with displacement of bowel gas. The ipsilateral kidney is displaced downward. The mass is sonolucent on ultrasound (Mittelstaedt et al, 1979). Neuroblastomas cause the excretion of large amounts of catecholamines (eg, vanilmandelic acid).

Treatment

Surgical excision of a tumor should be followed by radiotherapy to the tumor bed. If the tumor is very large or is deemed unresectable, preoperative x-ray therapy should be given, followed by surgical excision. In disseminated disease, chemotherapy must be given. Useful drugs include cyclophosphamide (Cytoxan), vincristine (Oncovin), and dacarbazine. In the past there has been little enthusiasm for chemotherapy, but Lopez, Karakousis, and Rao (1980) treated 4 adults with chemotherapy following surgical excision of the tumor. Later study showed complete maturation of the metastases in one of them. Evans et al (1980) noted very good results in children who had widespread metastases (but not to bone).

Prognosis

About 90% of patients who die of the disease do so within 14 months following initiation of treatment. Infants have the best prognosis; their 2-year survival rate approaches 60%, and if the tumor is confined to the primary site with or without adjacent regional spread, the cure rate is about 80%. Less than 10% of children age 2 or older are cured. When the disease is disseminated, few cures are obtained.

In a few infants, spontaneous maturation of neuroblastoma to ganglioneuroma has been observed. It is thought by some that x-ray and chemotherapy can also accomplish this.

Serial estimation of urinary catecholamines following therapy will usually indicate the presence of residual tumor.

REFERENCES

General

Goldman SM, Siegelman SS: Computerized tomography in the scheme of things. *J Urol* 1982;**127**:724.

Siekavizza JL, Bernardino ME, Samaan NA: Suprarenal mass and its differential diagnosis. *Urology* 1981;**18**:625.

Stewart BH: Adrenal surgery: Current state of the art. *J Urol* 1983;**129**:1.

Yeh H-C: Sonography of the adrenal glands: Normal glands and small masses. *AJR* 1980;**135**:1167.

Adrenal Hemorrhage in the Newborn

Khuri FJ et al: Adrenal hemorrhage in neonates: Report of 5 cases and review of the literature. *J Urol* 1980;**124**:684.

Lebowitz JM, Belman AB: Simultaneous idiopathic adrenal hemorrhage and renal vein thrombosis in the newborn. *J Urol* 1983;**129**:574.

Adrenal Cyst

Cheema P, Cartgena R, Staubitz W: Adrenal cysts: Diagnosis and treatment. *J Urol* 1981;**126**:396.

Nosher JL et al: Fine needle aspiration of the kidney and adrenal gland. *J Urol* 1982;**128**:895.

Okafo BA, Nickel C, Morales A: Pyogenic cyst of the adrenal gland. *Urology* 1983;**21**:619.

Zivokvić SM et al: Adrenal cysts in the newborn. *J Urol* 1983;**129**:1031.

Metastases From Other Organs

Cedermark BJ, Ohlsén H: Computed tomography in the diagnosis of metastases of the adrenal gland. *Surg Genecol Obstet* 1981;**152**:13.

Zornoza J et al: Percutaneous biopsy of adrenal tumors. *Urology* 1981;**18**:412.

Myelolipoma

Ishikawa H et al: Myelolipoma of the adrenal gland. *J Urol* 1981;**126**:777.

Cushing's Syndrome & Adrenocortical Tumors

Aron DC et al: Cushing's syndrome: Problems in management. *Endocr Rev* 1981;**3**:229.

Baxter JD, Tyrrell JB: The adrenal cortex. In: *Endocrinology and Metabolism*. Felig P et al (editors). McGraw-Hill, 1981.

Burke CW, Beardwell CG: Cushing's syndrome: An evaluation of the clinical usefulness of urinary free cortisol and other urinary steroid measurements in diagnosis. *Q J Med* 1972;**42**:175.

Chandur-Mnaymneh L, Slim M, Muakassa K: Adrenal cyst: Pathogenesis and histologic identification with report of 6 cases. *J Urol* 1979;**122**:87.

Chrousos GP et al: The corticotropin-releasing factor stimulation test: An aid in the evaluation of patients with Cushing's syndrome. *N Engl J Med* 1984;**310**:622.

Crapo L: Cushing's syndrome: A review of diagnostic tests. *Metabolism* 1979;**28**:955.

Cushing H: The basophil adenomas of the pituitary body and their clinical manifestations (pituitary basophilism). *Bull Johns Hopkins Hosp* 1932;**50**:137.

Findling JW et al: Selective venous sampling for ACTH in Cushing's syndrome. *Ann Intern Med* 1981;**94**:647.

Fitzgerald PA et al: Cushing's disease: Transient secondary adrenal insufficiency after selective removal of pituitary microadenomas: Evidence for a pituitary origin. *J Clin Endocrinol Metab* 1982;**54**:413.

Flint LD: Surgical exposures for adrenal endocrinopathies. *Surg Clin North Am* 1973;**53**:445.

Herwig KR, Sonda LP III: Usefulness of adrenal venography and iodocholesterol scan in adrenal surgery. *J Urol* 1979;**122**:7.

Krieger DT: Physiopathology of Cushing's disease. *Endocr Rev* 1983;**4**:22.

McKeever PE et al: Refractory Cushing's disease caused by multinodular ACTH-cell hyperplasia. *J Neuropathol Exp Neurol* 1982;**41**:490.

Nelson DH et al: ACTH-producing tumor of the pituitary gland. *N Engl J Med* 1958;**259**:161.

Singer W et al: Ectopic ACTH syndrome: Clinicopathological correlations. *J Clin Pathol* 1978;**31**:591.

Wilson CB et al: Cushing's disease: Surgical management. Pages 199–208 in: *Hormone-Secreting Pituitary Tumors.* Year Book, 1982.

Wilson JM, Woodhead DM, Smith RB: Adrenal cysts: Diagnosis and management. *Urology* 1974;**4**:248.

Zaitoon MM, Mackie GG: Adrenal cortical tumors in children. *Urology* 1978;**12**:645.

Adrenogenital Syndromes

Biglieri EG, Herron MA, Brust N: 17-Hydroxylation deficiency in man. *J Clin Invest* 1966;**45**:1946.

Bongiovanni AM et al: Disorders of adrenal steroid biogenesis. *Recent Prog Horm Res* 1967;**23**:375.

Felig P et al (editors): Hirsutism and virilism. Pages 488–496 in: *Endocrinology and Metabolism.* Felig P et al (editors). McGraw-Hill, 1981.

Givens JR: Hirsutism and hyperandrogenism. *Adv Intern Med* 1976;**21**:221.

Goldzieher JW: Polycystic ovarian disease. *Fertil Steril* 1981;**35**:39.

Gooding GA: Ultrasonic spectrum of adrenal masses. *Urology* 1979;**13**:211.

Hajjar RA, Hickey RC, Samaan NA: Adrenal cortical carcinoma: A study of 32 patients. *Cancer* 1975;**35**:549.

Harrison JH, Mahoney E, Bennett AH: Tumors of the adrenal cortex. *Cancer* 1973;**32**:1227.

Hoffman DL, Mattox VR: Treatment of adrenocortical carcinoma with o,p'-DDD. *Med Clin North Am* 1972; **56**:999.

Maroulis GB: Evaluation of hirsutism and hyperandrogenemia. *Fertil Steril* 1981;**36**:273.

New MI et al: Congenital adrenal hyperplasia and related conditions. Chap 47, pp 973–1000, in: *The Metabolic Basis of Inherited Disease,* 5th ed. Stanbury JB et al (editors). McGraw-Hill, 1983.

Parrott TS, Scheflan M, Hester TR: Reduction clitoroplasty and vaginal construction in a single operation. *Urology* 1980;**16**:367.

Shons AR, Gamble WG: Nonfunctioning carcinoma of the adrenal cortex. *Surg Gynecol Obstet* 1974;**138**:705.

Tang CM, Gray GF: Adrenocortical neoplasms: Prognosis and morphology. *Urology* 1975;**5**:691.

Zaitoon MM, Mackie GG: Adrenal cortical tumors in children. *Urology* 1978;**12**:645.

Hyperaldosteronism

Conn JW et al: Normokalemic primary aldosteronism. *JAMA* 1966;**195**:21.

Horton R, Finck E: Diagnosis and localization in primary aldosteronism. *Ann Intern Med* 1972;**76**:885.

Hunt TK, Schambelan M, Biglieri EG: Selection of patients and operative approach in primary aldosteronism. *Ann Surg* 1975;**182**:353.

Liddle GW: The adrenal cortex. Pages 233–283 in: *Textbook of Endocrinology,* 5th ed. Williams RH (editor). Saunders, 1974.

Tarazi RC et al: Hemodynamic characteristics of primary aldosteronism. *N Engl J Med* 1973;**289**:1330.

Weinberger MH, Donohue JP: Aldosterone updated. *J Urol* 1973;**110**:1.

White EA et al: Use of computed tomography in diagnosing the cause of primary aldosteronism. *N Engl J Med* 1980;**303**:1503.

Pheochromocytomas & Related Tumors

Bravo EL et al: Pheochromocytoma: Diagnosis, localization and management. *N Engl J Med* 1984;**311**:1298.

Farndon JR et al: VMA excretion in patients with pheochromocytoma. *Ann Surg* 1980;**191**:259.

Flanigan RC et al: Malignant pheochromocytoma of urinary bladder. *Urology* 1980;**16**:386.

Freier DT, Tank ES, Harrison TS: Pediatric and adult pheochromocytomas: A biochemical and clinical comparison. *Arch Surg* 1973;**107**:252.

Funyu T et al: Familial pheochromocytoma: Case report and review of the literature. *J Urol* 1973;**110**:151.

Himathongkam T et al: Pheochromocytoma: Medical emergency management. *JAMA* 1974;**230**:1692.

Laursen K, Damgaard-Pedersen K: CT for pheochromocytoma diagnosis. *AJR* 1980;**134**:277.

Mahoney EM, Harrison JH: Malignant pheochromocytoma: Clinical course and treatment. *J Urol* 1977;**118**:225.

Melmon KL: Catecholamines and the adrenal medulla. Pages 283–322 in: *Textbook of Endocrinology,* 5th ed. Williams RH (editor). Saunders, 1974.

Modlin IM et al: Phaeochromocytoma in 72 patients: Clinical and diagnostic features, treatment and long term results. *Br J Surg* 1979;**66**:456.

Pont A: Multiple endocrine neoplasia syndromes. *West J Med* 1980;**59**:100.

Swensen T et al: Use of ^{131}I-MIBG scintigraphy in the evaluation of suspected pheochromocytoma. *Mayo Clin Proc* 1985;**60**:299.

Neuroblastoma

Bill AH: Immune aspects of neuroblastoma: Current information. *Am J Surg* 1971;**122**:142.

D'Angio GJ, Evans AE, Koop CE: Special pattern of widespread neuroblastoma with favorable prognosis. *Lancet* 1971;**1**:1046.

Evans AE, D'Angio GJ, Randolph J: A proposed staging for children with neuroblastoma. *Cancer* 1979;**27**:374.

Evans AE et al: A review of 17 IV-S neuroblastoma patients at the Children's Hospital of Philadelphia. *Cancer* 1980; **45**:833.

Gitlow SE et al: Diagnosis of neuroblastoma by qualitative and quantitative determination of catecholamine metabolites in urine. *Cancer* 1970;**25**:1377.

Green AA, Hayes FA, Hustu HO: Sequential cyclophosphamide and doxorubin for induction of complete remission in children with disseminated neuroblastoma. *Cancer* 1981;**48**:2310.

Hann H-WL et al: Biologic differences between neuroblastoma stages IV-S and IV: Measurement of serum ferritin and E-rosette inhibition in 30 children. *N Engl J Med* 1981;**305**:425.

Harrison J et al: Results of combination chemotherapy, surgery, and radiotherapy in children with neuroblastoma. *Cancer* 1974;**34:**485.

Hayes FA et al: Clinical evaluation of sequentially scheduled cisplatin and VM26 in neuroblastoma. *Cancer* 1981; **48:**1715.

Holland T et al: The current management of neuroblastoma. *J Urol* 1980;**124:**579.

Howman-Giles RB, Gilday DL, Ash JM: Radionuclide skeletal survey in neuroblastoma. *Radiology* 1979; **131:**497.

Liebner EJ: Serial catecholamines in the radiation management of children with neuroblastoma. *Cancer* 1973; **32:**623.

Lopez R, Karakousis C, Rao U: Treatment of adult neuroblastoma. *Cancer* 1980;**45:**840.

Mancini AF et al: Neuroblastoma in a pair of identical twins. *Med Pediatr Oncol* 1982;**10:**45.

Mittelstaedt CA et al: The sonographic diagnosis of neonatal adrenal hemorrhage. *Radiology* 1979;**131:**453.

Ninane J, Pritchard J, Malpas JS: Chemotherapy of advanced neuroblastoma: Does Adriamycin contribute? *Arch Dis Child* 1981;**56:**544.

Reynolds CP et al: Catecholamine fluorescence and tissue culture morphology: Technics in the diagnosis of neuroblastoma. *Am J Clin Pathol* 1981;**75:**275.

Rogers LE, Lyon GM Jr, Porter FS: Spot test for vanillylmandelic acid and other guaiacols in urine of patients with neuroblastoma. *Am J Clin Pathol* 1972;**58:**383.

Rowe PH, Oram JJ, Scott GW: Neuroblastoma in adults. *Postgrad Med J* 1979;**55:**579.

Smith JA Jr, Middleton RG: Neonatal adrenal hemorrhage. *J Urol* 1980;**122:**674.

Varkarakis MJ et al: Current status of prognostic criteria in neuroblastoma. *J Urol* 1973;**109:**94.

Wilson LMK, Draper GJ: Neuroblastoma, its natural history and prognosis: A study of 487 cases. *Br Med J* 1974;**3:**301.

Disorders of the Kidneys

23

Jack W. McAninch, MD

CONGENITAL ANOMALIES OF THE KIDNEYS

Congenital anomalies occur more frequently in the kidney than in any other organ. Some cause no difficulty, but many (eg, hypoplasia, polycystic kidneys) cause impairment of renal function. It has been noted that children with a gross deformity of an external ear associated with ipsilateral maldevelopment of the facial bones are apt to have a congenital abnormality of the kidney (eg, ectopy, hypoplasia) on the same side as the visible deformity. Lateral displacement of the nipples has been observed in association with bilateral renal hypoplasia.

A significant incidence of renal agenesis, ectopy, malrotation, and duplication has been observed in association with congenital scoliosis and kyphosis. Unilateral agenesis, hypoplasia, and dysplasia are often seen in association with supralevator imperforate anus. (See General References at end of chapter.)

For a better understanding of these congenital abnormalities, see the discussion of the embryology and development of the kidney in Chapter 2.

AGENESIS

Bilateral renal agenesis is extremely rare; no more than 400 cases have been reported. The children do not survive. The condition does not appear to have any predisposing factors. Prenatal suspicion of the anomaly exists when oligohydramnios is present on fetal ultrasound examination. Pulmonary hypoplasia and facial deformities (Potter facies) are usually present. Abdominal ultrasound examination will usually establish the diagnosis.

One kidney may be absent. This in some cases is probably because the ureteral bud (from the wolffian duct) failed to develop or, if it did develop, did not reach the metanephros (adult kidney). Without a drainage system, the metanephric mass undergoes atrophy. The ureter is absent on the side of the unformed kidney in 50% of cases, although a blind ureteral duct may be found. (See Chapter 2.)

Renal agenesis causes no symptoms; it is usually found by accident on urography. It is not an easy diagnosis to establish even though on inspection of the

bladder the ureteral ridge is absent and no orifice is visualized, for the kidney could be present but be drained by a ureter whose opening is ectopic (into the urethra, seminal vesicle, or vagina). If definitive diagnosis seems essential, midstream angiography, renal venography, isotope studies, ultrasonography, and CT scans should establish the diagnosis (Cope and Trickey, 1982).

There appears to be an increased incidence of infection, hydronephrosis, and stones in the contralateral organ. Other congenital anomalies associated with this defect include cardiac, vertebral column, and anal anomalies as well as anomalies of the long bones, hands, and genitalia.

HYPOPLASIA

Hypoplasia implies a small kidney. The total renal mass may be divided in an unequal manner, in which case one kidney is small and the other correspondingly larger than normal. Some of these congenitally small kidneys prove, on pathologic examination, to be dysplastic. Qazi et al (1979) have observed unilateral or bilateral hypoplasia in infants suffering from fetal alcohol syndrome.

Differentiation from acquired atrophy is difficult. Atrophic pyelonephritis usually reveals typical distortion of the calices. Vesicoureteral reflux in the infant may cause a dwarfed kidney even in the absence of infection. Stenosis of the renal artery leads to shrinkage of the kidney.

Cha, Kandzari, and Khoury (1972) noted that such kidneys have small renal arteries and branches and are associated with hypertension, which is relieved by nephrectomy. Selective renal venography is helpful in differentiating between a congenitally absent kidney and one that is small and nonvisualized. A major side effect of the administration of cisplatin is shrinkage of the kidneys as revealed by serial radioisotope scans.

SUPERNUMERARY KIDNEYS

The presence of a third kidney is very rare; the presence of 4 separate kidneys in one individual has only been reported once. The anomaly must not be confused with duplication (or triplication) of the renal pelvis in one kidney, which is not uncommon (N'Guessan and Stephens, 1983).

DYSPLASIA & MULTICYSTIC KIDNEY

Renal dysplasia presents protean manifestations. Multicystic kidney of the newborn is usually unilateral, nonhereditary, and characterized by an irregularly lobulated mass of cysts; the ureter is usually absent or atretic. It may develop because of faulty union of the nephron and the collecting system. At most, only a few embryonic glomeruli and tubules are observed. The only finding is the discovery of an irregular mass in the flank. Nothing is shown on urography, but in an occasional case, some radiopaque fluid may be noted (Warshawsky, Miller, and Kaplan, 1977). Bloom and Brosman (1978) noted that if the cystic kidney is large, its mate is usually normal. However, when the cystic organ is small, the contralateral kidney is apt to be abnormal. The cystic nature of the lesion may be revealed by sonography. Friedberg, Mitnick, and Davis (1979) were able to establish the diagnosis by ultrasonography in utero. If the physician feels that the proper diagnosis has been made, no treatment is necessary (Bloom and Brosman, 1978). If there is doubt about the diagnosis, nephrectomy is considered the procedure of choice.

Multicystic kidney is often associated with contralateral renal and ureteral abnormalities. Contralateral ureteropelvic junction obstruction is one of the common problems noted. Diagnostic evaluation of both kidneys is required to establish the overall status of anomalous development.

Dysplasia of the renal parenchyma is also seen in association with ureteral obstruction or reflux that was probably present early in pregnancy. It is relatively common as a segmental renal lesion involving the upper pole of a duplicated kidney whose ureter is obstructed by a congenital ureterocele. It may also be found in urinary tracts severely obstructed by posterior urethral valves; in this instance, the lesion may be bilateral.

Microscopically, the renal parenchyma is "disorganized." Tubular and glomerular cysts may be noted; these elements are fetal in type. Islands of metaplastic cartilage are often seen. The common denominator seems to be fetal obstruction (Fisher and Smith, 1975).

ADULT POLYCYSTIC KIDNEYS
(See also p 522.)

Adult polycystic kidney disease is an autosomal dominant hereditary condition and almost always bilateral (95% of cases). Lee, McClennan, and Kissane (1978) discussed one case of unilateral polycystic disease, but it is not clear that their patient did not have multiple renal cysts or congenital multicystic kidney disease. The disease encountered in infants is different from that seen in adults, although Kaye and Lewy (1974) reported from the literature 4 cases of infants with the adult type. The former is an autosomal recessive disease in which life expectancy is short, whereas

that diagnosed in adulthood is autosomal dominant; symptoms ordinarily do not appear until after age 40. Cysts of the liver, spleen, and pancreas may be noted in association with both forms. The kidneys are larger than normal and are studded with cysts of various sizes.

Etiology & Pathogenesis

The evidence suggests that the cysts occur because of defects in the development of the collecting and uriniferous tubules and in the mechanism of their joining. Blind secretory tubules that are connected to functioning glomeruli become cystic. As the cysts enlarge, they compress adjacent parenchyma, destroy it by ischemia, and occlude normal tubules. The result is progressive functional impairment.

Pathology

Grossly, the kidneys are usually much enlarged. Their surfaces are studded with cysts of various sizes (Fig 23-1). On section, the cysts are found to be scattered throughout the parenchyma. Calcification is rare. The fluid in the cyst is usually amber-colored but may be hemorrhagic.

Microscopically, the lining of the cysts consists of a single layer of cells. The renal parenchyma may show peritubular fibrosis and evidence of secondary infection. There appears to be a reduction in the num-

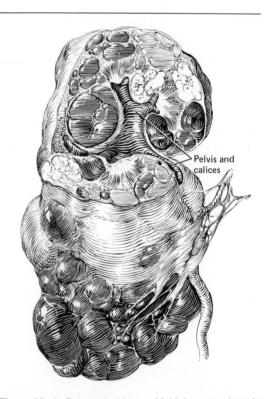

Figure 23-1. Polycystic kidney. Multiple cysts deep in the parenchyma and on the surface. Note distortion of the calices by the cysts.

ber of glomeruli, some of which may be hyalinized. Renal arteriolar thickening is a prominent finding in adults.

Clinical Findings

A. Symptoms: Pain over one or both kidneys may occur because of the drag on the vascular pedicles by the heavy kidneys, from obstruction or infection, or from hemorrhage into a cyst. Gross or microscopic total hematuria is not uncommon and may be severe; the cause for this is not clear. Colic may occur if blood clots or stones are passed. The patient may notice an abdominal mass (Segal, Spataro, and Barbaric, 1977).

Infection (chills, fever, renal pain) commonly complicates polycystic disease. Symptoms of vesical irritability may be the first complaint. When renal insufficiency ensues, headache, nausea and vomiting, weakness, and loss of weight occur.

B. Signs: One or both kidneys are usually palpable. They may feel nodular. If infected, they may be tender. Hypertension is found in 60–70% of these patients. Evidence of cardiac enlargement is then noted.

Fever may be present if pyelonephritis exists or if cysts have become infected. In the stage of uremia, anemia and loss of weight may be evident. Ophthalmoscopic examination may show changes typical of moderate or severe hypertension.

C. Laboratory Findings: Anemia may be noted, caused either by chronic loss of blood or, more commonly, by the hematopoietic depression accompanying uremia. Proteinuria and microscopic (if not gross) hematuria are the rule. Pyuria and bacteriuria are common.

Progressive loss of concentrating power occurs. Renal clearance tests will show varying degrees of renal impairment. About a third of patients with polycystic kidney disease are uremic when first seen.

D. X-Ray Findings: Both renal shadows are usually enlarged on a plain film of the abdomen, even as much as 5 times normal size. Kidneys more than 16 cm in length are suspect.

Excretory infusion urograms with tomography are helpful to establish the diagnosis. Tomography will reveal multiple lucencies representing cysts. On tomograms or on retrograde urograms, the renal masses are usually enlarged and the caliceal pattern is quite bizarre (spider deformity). The calices are broadened and flattened, enlarged, and often curved, as they tend to hug the periphery of adjacent cysts (Fig 23–2). Often the changes are only slight or may even be absent on one side, leading to the erroneous diagnosis of tumor of the other kidney.

If cysts are infected, perinephritis may obscure the renal and even the psoas shadows.

Angiography will reveal bending of small vessels around the cysts and the "negative" shadows (nonvascular) of the cysts (Fig 23–2).

E. CT Scanning: CT scanning is an excellent noninvasive technique used to establish the diagnosis of polycystic disease. The multiple thin-walled cysts filled with fluid and the large renal size make this imaging modality extremely accurate (95%) for diagnosis.

F. Isotope Studies: Photoscans (see Chapter 9) will reveal multiple "cold" avascular spots in large renal shadows.

G. Ultrasonography: Sonography appears to be superior to both excretory urography and isotope scanning in diagnosis of polycystic disorders (Adult polycystic disease of the kidneys, 1981).

H. Instrumental Examination: Cystoscopy may show evidence of cystitis, in which case the urine will contain abnormal elements. Bleeding from a ureteral orifice may be noted.

Ureteral catheterization and retrograde urograms are rarely indicated.

Differential Diagnosis

Bilateral hydronephrosis (on the basis of congenital or acquired ureteral obstruction) may present bilateral flank masses and signs of impairment of renal function, but urography and ultrasonography will show changes quite different from those of the polycystic kidney.

Bilateral renal tumor is rare but may mimic polycystic kidney disease perfectly on urography. Differentiation of a unilateral tumor may be quite difficult if one of the polycystic kidneys shows little or no distortion on urography. However, tumors are usually localized to one portion of the kidney, whereas cysts are quite diffusely distributed. The total renal function should be normal with unilateral tumor but is usually depressed in patients with polycystic kidney disease. Computed tomography or renal angiography may be needed at times to differentiate between the 2 conditions (Fig 23–2). Photoscans or sonograms may also prove helpful in differentiation.

In **von Hippel-Lindau disease** (angiomatous cerebellar cyst, angiomatosis of the retina, and tumors or cysts of the pancreas), multiple bilateral cysts or adenocarcinomas of both kidneys may develop. Urograms or nephrotomograms may suggest polycystic kidney disease. The presence of other stigmas should make the diagnosis. CT Scanning, angiography, sonography, or scintiphotography should be definitive (Lamiell, Stor, and Hsia, 1980; Sandle, Raval, and David, 1985).

Tuberous sclerosis (convulsive seizures, mental retardation, and adenoma sebaceum) is typified by hamartomatous tumors often involving the skin, brain, retinas, bones, liver, heart, and kidneys (see p 331). The renal lesions are usually multiple and bilateral and microscopically are angiomyolipomas. Urograms obtained during the stage of uremia are apt to suggest polycystic disease; the presence of other stigmas and use of CT scanning or sonography should make the differentiation.

Simple cyst (see below) is usually unilateral and single; total renal function should be normal. Urograms usually show a single lesion (Fig 23–3), whereas polycystic kidney disease is bilateral and has multiple filling defects.

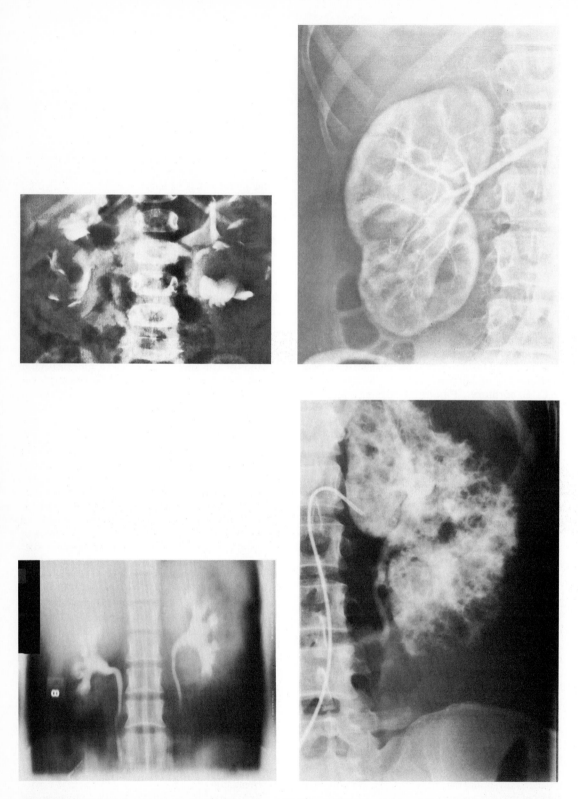

Figure 23–2. Polycystic kidneys. *Upper left:* Excretory urogram in a child, showing elongation, broadening, and bending of the calices around cysts. Good renal function. *Upper right:* Angiogram of right kidney, showing "negative" shadows of cysts. *Lower left:* Angionephrotomogram showing kidneys of essentially normal size. All infundibula on left and infundibulum of right upper calix are widened, suggesting polycystic kidneys. *Lower right:* Nephrogram phase of left selective angiogram (same patient) showing multiple small regative shadows representing the cysts.

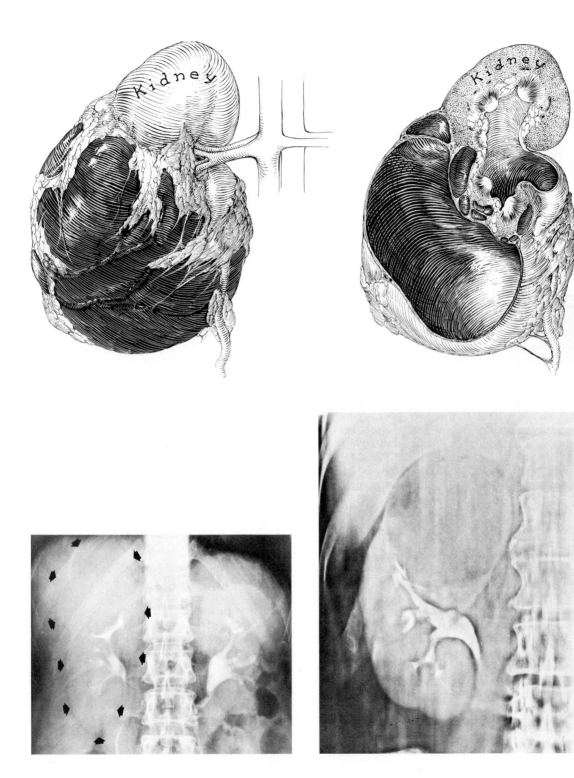

Figure 23–3. Simple cyst. *Upper left:* Large cyst displacing lower pole laterally. *Upper right:* Section of kidney showing one large and a few small cysts. *Lower left:* Excretory urogram showing soft tissue mass in upper pole of right kidney. Elongation and distortion of upper calices by cyst. *Lower right:* Infusion nephrotomogram showing large cyst in upper renal pole distorting upper calices and dislocating upper portion of kidney laterally.

Complications

For reasons that are not clear, pyelonephritis is a common complication of polycystic kidney disease. It may be asymptomatic; pus cells in the urine may be few or absent. Stained smears or quantitative cultures make the diagnosis. A gallium-67 citrate scan will definitely reveal the sites of infection, including abscess.

Infection of cysts will be associated with pain and tenderness over the kidney and a febrile response. The differential diagnosis between infection of cysts and pyelonephritis may be difficult, but here again a gallium scan will prove helpful.

In rare instances, gross hematuria may be so brisk and persistent as to endanger life.

Treatment

Except for unusual complications, the treatment is conservative and supportive.

A. General Measures: Place the patient on a low-protein diet (0.5–0.75 g/kg/d of protein) and force fluids to 3000 mL or more per day. Physical activity may be permitted within reason, but strenuous overexercise is contraindicated. When the patient is in the state of absolute renal insufficiency, treat as for uremia from any cause. Hypertension should be controlled. Hemodialysis may be indicated.

B. Surgery: There is no evidence that excision or decompression of cysts improves renal function. If a large cyst is found to be compressing the upper ureter, causing obstruction and further embarrassing renal function, it should be resected or aspirated. When the degree of renal insufficiency becomes life-threatening, chronic dialysis or renal transplantation should be considered (Pechan et al, 1981).

C. Treatment of Complications: Pyelonephritis must be rigorously treated to prevent further renal damage. Infection of cysts requires surgical drainage. If bleeding from one kidney is so severe as to threaten exsanguination, nephrectomy or embolization of the renal or, preferably, the segmental artery must be considered as a lifesaving measure.

Concomitant diseases (eg, tumor, obstructing stone) may require definitive surgical treatment.

Prognosis

When the disease affects children, it has a very poor prognosis. The large group presenting clinical signs and symptoms after age 35–40 years has a somewhat more favorable prognosis. Although there is wide variation, these patients usually do not live longer than 5 or 10 years after the diagnosis is made unless dialysis is made available or renal transplantation is done.

SIMPLE (SOLITARY) CYST

Simple cyst (Figs 23–3 and 23–4) of the kidney is usually unilateral and single but may be multiple and multilocular and, more rarely, bilateral. It differs from polycystic kidneys both clinically and pathologically.

Etiology & Pathogenesis

Whether simple cyst is congenital or acquired is not clear. Its origin may be similar to that of polycystic kidneys, ie, the difference may be merely one of degree. On the other hand, simple cysts have been produced in animals by causing tubular obstruction and local ischemia; this suggests that the lesion can be acquired.

As a simple cyst grows, it compresses and thereby may destroy renal parenchyma, but rarely does it destroy so much renal tissue that renal function is impaired (Roth and Roberts, 1980). A solitary cyst may be placed in such a position as to compress the ureter, causing progressive hydronephrosis. Infection may then complicate the picture.

Feiner, Katz, and Gallo (1981) have noticed that acquired cystic disease of the kidney is commonly observed as an effect of chronic dialysis. Kessel and Tynes (1981) have observed the spontaneous regression of cysts in 2 cases.

Pathology

Simple cysts usually involve the lower pole of the kidney. Those that produce symptoms average about 10 cm in diameter, but a few are large enough to fill the entire flank. They usually contain a clear amber fluid. Their walls are quite thin, and the cysts are "blue-domed" in appearance. Calcification of the sac is occasionally seen. About 5% contain hemorrhagic fluid, and possibly one-half of these have papillary cancers on their walls.

Simple cysts are usually superficial but may be deeply situated. When a cyst is situated deep in the kidney, the cyst wall is adjacent to the epithelial lining of the pelvis or calices, from which it may be separated only with great difficulty. Cysts do not communicate with the renal pelvis (Fig 23–3). Microscopic examination of the cyst wall shows heavy fibrosis and hyalinization; areas of calcification may be seen. The adjacent renal tissue is compressed and fibrosed. A number of cases of simple cysts have been reported in children (Bartholomew et al, 1980). However, large cysts are rare in children; the presence of cancer must therefore be ruled out.

Multilocular renal cysts may be confused with tumor on urography. Sonography usually makes the diagnosis (Banner, 1981).

Clinical Findings

A. Symptoms: Pain in the flank or back, usually intermittent and dull, is not uncommon. If bleeding suddenly distends the cyst wall, pain may come on abruptly and be severe. Gastrointestinal symptoms are occasionally noted and may suggest peptic ulcer or gallbladder disease. The patient may discover a mass in the abdomen, although cysts of this size are unusual. If the cyst becomes infected, the patient usually complains of pain in the flank, malaise, and fever.

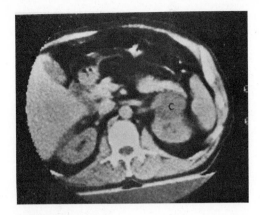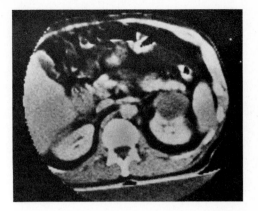

Figure 23–4. Left renal cyst. *Left:* CT scan shows a homogeneous low-density mass (C) arising from anterior border of left kidney just posterior to tail of the pancreas. The CT attenuation value was similar to that of water, indicating a simple renal cyst. *Right:* After intravenous injection of contrast material, the mass did not increase in attenuation value, adding further confirmatory evidence of its benign cystic nature.

B. Signs: Physical examination is usually normal, although occasionally a mass in the region of the kidney may be palpated or percussed. Tenderness in the flank may be noted if the cyst becomes infected.

C. Laboratory Findings: Urinalysis is usually normal. Microscopic hematuria is rare. Renal function tests are normal unless the cysts are multiple and bilateral (rare). Even in the face of extensive destruction of one kidney, compensatory hypertrophy of the other kidney will maintain normal total function.

D. X-Ray Findings: An expansion of a portion of the kidney shadow or a mass superimposed upon it can usually be seen on a plain film of the abdomen. The axis of the kidney may be abnormal because of rotation due to the weight or position of the cyst. Streaks of calcium can sometimes be seen in the border of the mass.

Excretory urograms establish the presumptive diagnosis of cyst. On a film taken 1–2 minutes after infusion of radiopaque fluid, the vascularized parenchyma becomes white while the space-occupying cyst does not because it is avascular. The urographic series will show changes compatible with a mass. One or more calices or the renal pelvis will usually be indented or bent around the cyst; these are often broadened and flattened or even obliterated (Figs 23–3 and 23–5). Oblique and lateral films may prove helpful. If a mass occupies the lower pole of the kidney, the upper part of the ureter may be displaced toward the spine. The kidney itself may be rotated. The psoas muscle may be seen through the radiolucent cyst fluid.

If the routine urogram fails to significantly opacify the parenchyma, infusion nephrotomography should be done to increase the contrast between vascular renal tissue and the cyst (Fig 23–3). Occasionally, a renal parenchymal tumor may be relatively avascular and thus be confused with a cyst. In a few instances, carcinoma may grow on the cyst wall (Ambrose et al, 1977; Sufrin et al, 1975; Varma et al, 1974). Because of these phenomena, further steps in differential diagnosis should be performed.

E. CT Scanning: CT scan appears to be the most accurate means of differentiating renal cyst and tumor (Fig 23–4) (Sagel et al, 1977). Cysts have an attenuation approximating that of water, whereas the density of tumors is similar to that of normal parenchyma (Fig 19–8). Parenchyma is made more dense with the intravenous injection of radiopaque fluid, but a cyst remains unaffected. The wall of a cyst is sharply demarcated from the renal parenchyma; a tumor is not. The wall of a cyst is thin; that of a tumor is not. CT scanning may well supplant cyst puncture in the differentiation of cyst and tumor in many cases.

F. Renal Ultrasonography: Renal ultrasonography is a noninvasive diagnostic technique that in a high percentage of cases differentiates between a cyst and a solid mass (Bartholomew et al, 1980). If findings on ultrasonography are also compatible with cyst, a needle can be introduced into the cyst under ultrasonographic control and the cyst can be aspirated.

G. Isotope Scanning: A rectilinear scan will clearly delineate the mass but does not differentiate cyst from tumor. The technetium scan, made with the camera, will reveal that the mass is indeed avascular (see Chapter 9).

H. Percutaneous Cyst Aspiration With Cystography: If the above studies leave some doubt about the differentiation between cyst and tumor, aspiration should be done. (See Treatment, below, and p 111.)

Differential Diagnosis

Carcinoma of the kidney also occupies space but tends to lie more deeply in the organ and therefore causes more distortion of the calices. Hematuria is common with tumor, rare with cyst. If a solid tumor overlies the psoas muscle, the edge of the muscle is obliterated on the plain film; it can be seen through a

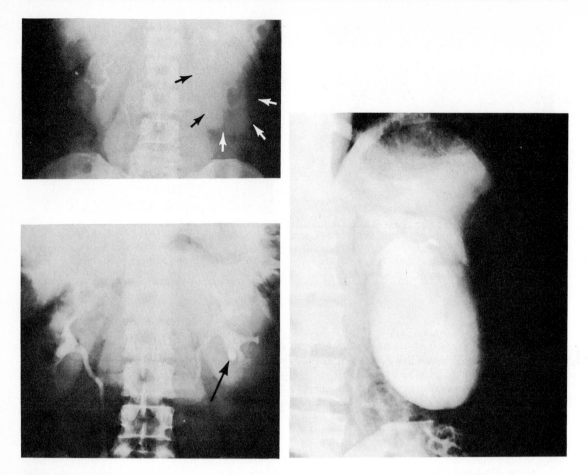

Figure 23 – 5. *Upper left:* Excretory urogram showing large smooth mass in lower pole of left kidney with distortion of calices. *Right:* Cyst punctured and radiopaque fluid instilled. Cyst is smooth-walled, lophendylate then instilled. *Lower left:* Excretory urogram 3 months later, lophendylate occupies what is left of cyst in the lower medial calix (*arrow*). Urogram normal.

cyst, however. Evidence of metastases (ie, loss of weight and strength, palpable supraclavicular nodes, chest film showing metastatic nodules), erythrocytosis, hypercalcemia, elevated levels of CEA in plasma or urine, and increased sedimentation rate suggest cancer. It must be remembered, however, that the walls of a simple cyst may undergo cancerous degeneration. If the renal vein is occluded by cancer, the excretory urogram may be visualized only faintly or not at all. Sonography or CT scan should be almost definitive in differential diagnosis. Angiography (Fig 19–5) or nephrotomography (Fig 19–4) may reveal "pooling" of the medium in the highly vascularized tumor, whereas the density of a cyst is not affected (Fig 23–6). It is wise to assume that all space-occupying lesions of the kidneys are cancers until proved otherwise.

Polycystic kidney disease is almost always bilateral, as shown by urography (Fig 23–2). Diffuse caliceal and pelvic distortion is the rule. Simple cyst is usually solitary and unilateral. Polycystic kidney disease is usually accompanied by impaired renal function and hypertension; simple cyst is not.

Renal carbuncle is a rare disease. A history of skin infection a few weeks before the onset of fever and local pain may be obtained. Urograms may show changes similar to cyst or tumor, but the renal outline as well as the edge of the psoas muscle may be obscured because of perinephritis. The kidney may be fixed; this can be demonstrated by comparing the position of the kidney when the patient is supine and upright. Angiography will demonstrate an avascular lesion (Fig 19–8). A gallium-67 scan will demonstrate the inflammatory nature of the lesion, but an infected simple cyst might have a similar appearance.

Hydronephrosis may present the same symptoms and signs as simple cyst, but the urograms are quite different. Cyst causes caliceal distortion; with hydronephrosis, dilatation of the calices and pelvis due to an obstruction is present. Acute or subacute hydronephrosis usually produces more local pain because of increased intrapelvic pressure and is more apt to be complicated by infection.

Extrarenal tumor (eg, adrenal, mixed retroperitoneal sarcoma) may displace a kidney, but rarely does it invade it and distort its calices.

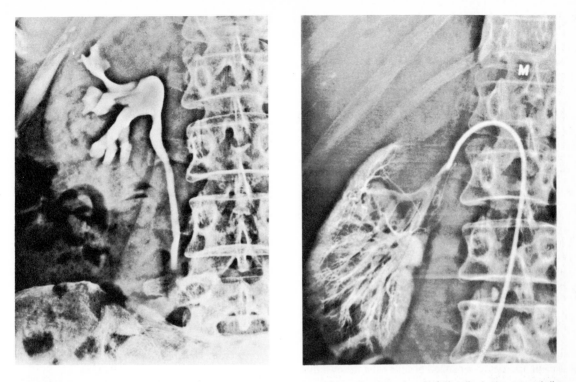

Figure 23–6. Diagnosis of simple renal cyst. *Left:* Excretory urogram showing lateral and inferior displacement and distortion of upper calix, right kidney. Differential diagnosis: Cyst versus tumor. *Right:* Same patient. Selective femoral angiogram showing a completely avascular mass typical of cyst.

If an echinococcal cyst of the kidney does not communicate with the renal pelvis, it may be difficult to differentiate from solitary cyst, for no scoleces or hooklets will be present in the urine. The wall of a hydatid cyst often reveals calcification on x-ray examination (Fig 14–5). A skin sensitivity test (Casoni) for hydatid disease may prove helpful.

Complications
(Rare)

Spontaneous infection in a simple cyst is rare, but when it occurs, it is difficult to differentiate from carbuncle. Hemorrhage into the cyst sometimes occurs. If sudden, it causes severe pain. The bleeding may come from a complicating carcinoma arising on the wall of the cyst.

Hydronephrosis may develop if a cyst of the lower pole impinges upon the ureter. This in itself may cause pain from back pressure of urine in the renal pelvis. This obstruction may lead to renal infection.

Treatment

A. Specific Measures:

1. If excretory urography, nephrotomograms, sonograms, and CT scan do not lead to a definitive diagnosis, renal angiography might be necessary, but percutaneous needle aspiration of the cyst (see p 111) should probably be the next step. This may be done under either fluoroscopic or sonographic control (Gross, 1979). The recovery of clear fluid is an encouraging sign, but the fluid must be examined cytologically. Its fat content should be estimated. Increased fat levels are compatible with tumor. The cyst is then drained, and cyst fluid is replaced with a radiopaque fluid. Films are taken in various positions to prove that the cyst wall is smooth and that there are no excrescences that might represent tumor. Before the radiopaque fluid is removed, 3 mL of iophendylate (Pantopaque) should be instilled into the cavity. This will decrease the chances for reaccumulation of fluid (Fig 23–5) (Wettlaufer and Modarelli, 1978). Bean (1981) recommends the injection of 95% ethanol into an emptied cyst; with this method, only one recurrence was noted in 29 patients. If simple aspiration alone is utilized, most cysts will refill (Raskin et al, 1975).

If the aspirate contains blood, immediate nephrectomy should be considered, because the chances are great that the growth is cancerous.

2. If the diagnosis can be clearly established, one should consider leaving the cyst alone, since it is rare for a cyst to harm the kidney.

3. Surgical exploration should be considered if the diagnosis is still in doubt. Ambrose et al (1977) prefer exploration in most cases diagnosed as cysts. Of the 55 cases they explored, 5 proved to be cancer (9%). Usually only the extrarenal portion of the cyst is excised. If the kidney is badly damaged, nephrectomy may be indicated, but this is rare.

B. Treatment of Complications: If the cyst becomes infected, intensive antimicrobial therapy should be instituted, although Muther and Bennett (1980) found that antimicrobial drugs attained very low concentrations in the cyst fluid. Therefore, surgical drainage is often required. Surgical excision of the extrarenal portion of the cyst wall and drainage will prove curative.

If, on exploration, the cyst appears to contain blood (and the other kidney is normal), immediate nephrectomy should be strongly urged without preliminary incision into the cyst, because cancer is likely to be present. Drainage of the contents of a cancerous cyst, by either incision or needle, invites growth of carcinoma in the wound.

If hydronephrosis is present, excision of the obstructing cyst will relieve the ureteral obstruction (Hinman, 1978).

Pyelonephritis in the involved kidney should suggest urinary stasis secondary to impaired ureteral drainage. Removal of the cyst and consequent relief of urinary back pressure will make antimicrobial therapy more effective.

Prognosis

Simple cysts can be diagnosed with great accuracy utilizing sonography and CT scan. Yearly sonography is recommended as a method of following the cyst for changes in size, configuration, and internal consistency. CT scan may be done if changes suggest carcinoma, and aspiration may then be performed if necessary to establish a diagnosis. Most cysts cause little difficulty.

RENAL FUSION

About one in 1000 individuals has some type of renal fusion, the most common being the horseshoe kidney. The fused renal mass almost always contains 2 excretory systems and therefore 2 ureters. The renal tissue may be divided equally between the 2 flanks, or the entire mass may be on one side. Even in the latter case, the 2 ureters open at their proper places in the bladder.

Etiology & Pathogenesis

It appears that this fusion of the 2 metanephroi occurs early in embryologic life, when the kidneys lie low in the pelvis. For this reason, they seldom ascend to the high position that normal kidneys assume. They may even remain in the true pelvis. Under these circumstances, such a kidney may derive its blood supply from many vessels in the area (eg, aorta, iliacs).

In patients with both ectopia and fusion, 78% will have extraurologic anomalies and 65% will exhibit other genitourinary defects.

Pathology
(Fig 23–7)

Because the renal masses fuse early, normal rotation cannot occur; therefore, each pelvis lies on the anterior surface of its organ. Thus, the ureter must ride over the isthmus of a horseshoe kidney or traverse the anterior surface of the fused kidney. Some degree of ureteral compression may arise from this or from obstruction by one or more aberrant blood vessels. The incidence of hydronephrosis and, therefore, infection is high. Vesicoureteral reflux has frequently been noted in association with fusion.

In horseshoe kidney, the isthmus usually joins the lower poles of each kidney; each renal mass lies lower than normal. The axes of these masses are vertical, whereas the axes of normal kidneys are oblique to the spine, because they lie along the edges of the psoas muscles.

On rare occasions, the 2 nephric masses are fused into one mass containing 2 pelves and 2 ureters. The mass may lie in the midline in order to open into the bladder at the proper point (crossed renal ectopy with fusion).

Clinical Findings

A. Symptoms: Most patients with fused kidneys have no symptoms. Some, however, develop ureteral obstruction. Gastrointestinal symptoms (renodigestive reflex) mimicking peptic ulcer, cholelithiasis, or appendicitis may be noted. Infection is apt to occur if ureteral obstruction and hydronephrosis or calculus develop.

B. Signs: Physical examination is usually negative unless the abnormally placed renal mass can be felt. With horseshoe kidney, it may be possible to palpate a mass over the lower lumber spine (the isthmus). In the case of crossed ectopy, a mass may be felt in the flank or lower abdomen.

C. Laboratory Findings: Urinalysis is normal unless there is infection. Renal function is normal unless disease coexists in each of the fused renal masses.

D. X-Ray Findings: In the case of horseshoe kidney, the axes of the 2 kidneys, if visible on a plain film, are parallel to the spine. At times the isthmus can be identified. The plain film may also reveal a large soft tissue mass in one flank yet not show a renal shadow on the other side (Fig 23–8).

Excretory urograms establish the diagnosis if the renal parenchyma has maintained good function. The increased density of the renal tissue may make the position or configuration of the kidney more distinct. Urograms will also visualize the pelvis and ureters.

1. With horseshoe kidney, the renal pelves lie on the anterior surfaces of their respective kidney masses, whereas the normal kidney has its pelvis lying mesial to it. The most valuable clue to the diagnosis of horseshow kidney is the presence of calices in the region of the lower pole that point medially and lie medial to the ureter (Figs 23–7 and 23–8).

2. Crossed renal ectopy with fusion shows 2 pelves and 2 ureters. One ureter must cross the midline in order to empty into the bladder at the proper point (Figs 23–7 and 23–8).

3. A cake or lump kidney may lie in the pelvis (fused pelvis kidney), but again its ureters and pelves will be shown (Figs 23–7 and 23–8). It may compress the dome of the bladder.

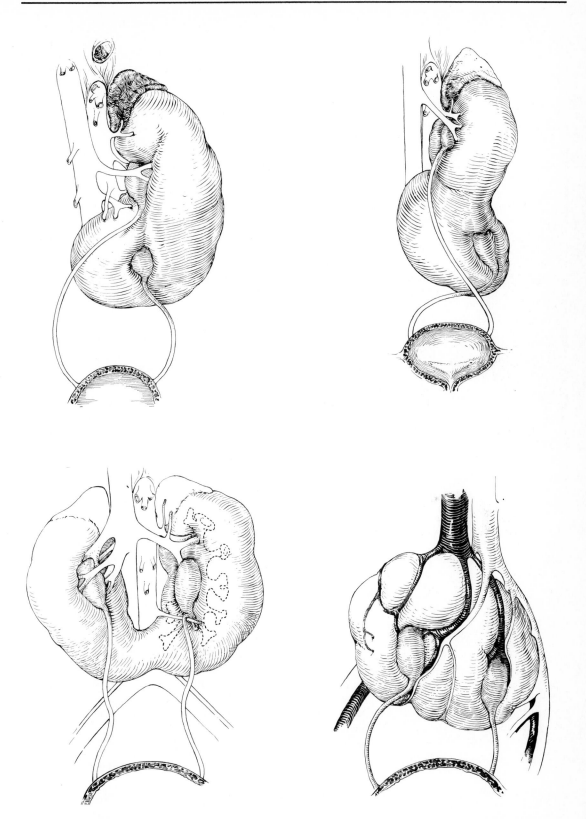

Figure 23–7. Renal fusion. *Upper left:* Crossed renal ectopy with fusion. The renal mass lies in the left flank. The right ureter must cross over the midline. *Upper right:* Example of "sigmoid" kidney. *Lower left:* Horseshoe kidney. Pelves are anterior. Note aberrant artery obstructing left ureter and the low position of renal mass. *Lower right:* Pelvic kidney. Pelves are placed anteriorly. Note aberrant blood supply.

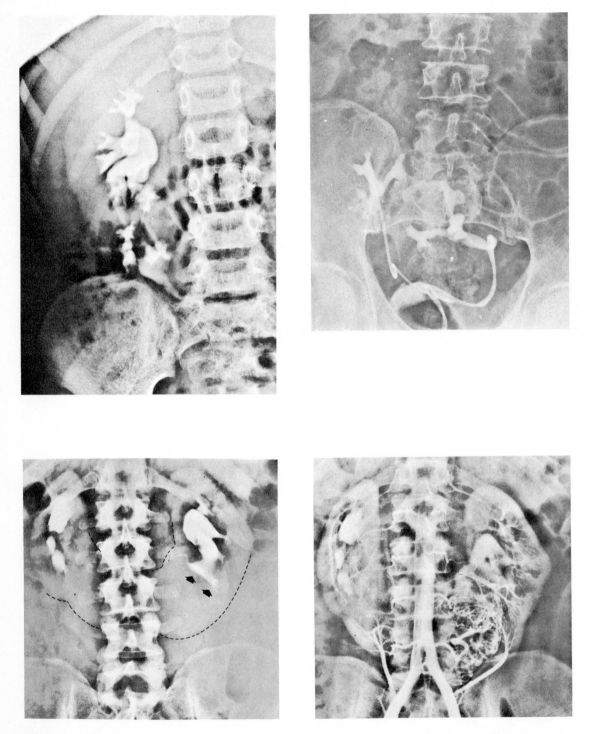

Figure 23–8. Renal fusion. *Upper left:* Excretory urogram showing fused renal masses on the right side. Both kidneys are normal. Crossed renal ectopy. *Upper right:* Retrograde urogram showing pelvic kidney. *Lower left:* Excretory urogram showing horseshoe kidney with expansion of left side of isthmus and compression of lower left caliceal system. *Lower right:* Angiogram on same patient. Hypervascular mass in left side of isthmus typical of adenocarcinoma.

CT scans will clearly outline the renal mass but are seldom necessary for diagnosis.

With pelvic fused kidney or one lying in the flank, the plain film taken with ureteral catheters in place will give the first hint of the diagnosis. Retrograde urograms will show the position of the pelves and demonstrate changes compatible with infection or obstruction (Fig 23–9). Renal scanning will delineate the renal mass and its contour (see Chapter 9), as will sonography.

Differential Diagnosis

Separate kidneys that fail to undergo normal rotation may be confused with horseshoe kidney. They lie along the edges of the psoas muscles, whereas the poles of a horseshoe kidney lie parallel to the spine and the lower poles are placed on the psoas muscles. The calices in the region of the isthmus of a horseshoe kidney point medially and lie close to the spine.

The diagnosis of fused or lump kidney may be missed on excretory urograms if one of the ureters is markedly obstructed so that a portion of the kidney and pelvis and ureter fail to visualize. Infusion urograms or retrograde urograms will demonstrate both excretory tracts in the renal mass.

Complications

Fused kidneys are prone to ureteral obstruction because of a high incidence of aberrant renal vessels and the necessity for one or both ureters to arch around or over the renal tissue. Hydronephrosis, stone, and infection therefore are common.

A large fused kidney occupying the concavity of the sacrum may cause dystocia.

Treatment

No treatment is necessary unless obstruction or infection is present. Drainage of a horseshoe kidney may be improved by dividing its isthmus. If one pole of a horseshoe is badly damaged, it may require surgical resection.

Prognosis

In most cases, the outlook is excellent. If ureteral obstruction and infection occur, renal drainage must be improved by surgical means so that antimicrobial therapy will be effective.

ECTOPIC KIDNEY

Congenital ectopic kidney usually causes no symptoms unless complications such as ureteral obstruction or infection develop.

Simple Ectopy

Simple congenital ectopy is usually a low kidney on the proper side that failed to ascend normally. It may lie over the pelvic brim or in the pelvis. Rarely, it may be found in the chest (Fig 23–9) (Kirshenbaum, Puri, and Rao, 1981). It takes its blood supply from adjacent vessels, and its ureter is short. It is prone to ureteral obstruction and infection, which may lead to pain or fever. At times such a kidney may be palpable, leading to an erroneous presumptive diagnosis (eg, cancer of the bowel, appendiceal abscess).

Excretory urograms (Fig 23–9) will reveal the true position of the kidney. Hydronephrosis, if present, will be evident. There is no redundancy of the ureter, as is the case with nephroptosis or acquired ectopy (eg, displacement by large suprarenal tumor).

Obstruction and infection may complicate simple ectopy and should be treated by appropriate means.

Crossed Ectopy Without Fusion

In crossed ectopy without fusion, the kidney lies on the opposite side of the body but is not attached to its normally placed mate. Unless 2 distinct renal shadows can be seen, it may be difficult to differentiate this condition from crossed ectopy with fusion (Fig 23–7). Sonography, angiography, or CT scan should make the distinction.

ABNORMAL ROTATION

Normally, when the kidney ascends to the lumbar region, the pelvis lies on its anterior surface. Later, the pelvis comes to lie mesially. Such rotation may fail to occur, although this seldom leads to renal disease. Urography demonstrates the abnormal position.

MEDULLARY SPONGE KIDNEY (Cystic Dilatation of the Renal Collecting Tubules)

Medullary sponge kidney is a congenital autosomal recessive defect characterized by widening of the distal collecting tubules. It is usually bilateral, affecting all of the papillae, but it may be unilateral. At times, only one papilla is involved. Cystic dilatation of the tubules is often present also. Infection and calculi are occasionally seen as a result of urinary stasis in the tubules. It is believed that medullary sponge kidney is related to polycystic kidney disease. Its occasional association with hemihypertrophy of the body has been noted.

The only symptoms are those arising from infection and stone formation. The diagnosis is made on the basis of excretory urograms (Fig 23–10). The pelvis and calices are normal, but dilated (streaked) tubules are seen just lateral to them; many of the dilated tubules contain round masses of radiopaque material (the cystic dilatation). If stones are present, a plain film will reveal small, round calculi in the pyramidal regions just beyond the calices. Retrograde urograms often do not reveal the lesion unless the mouths of the collecting ducts are widely dilated.

The differential diagnosis includes tuberculosis, healed papillary necrosis, and nephrocalcinosis. Tuberculosis is usually unilateral, and urography shows

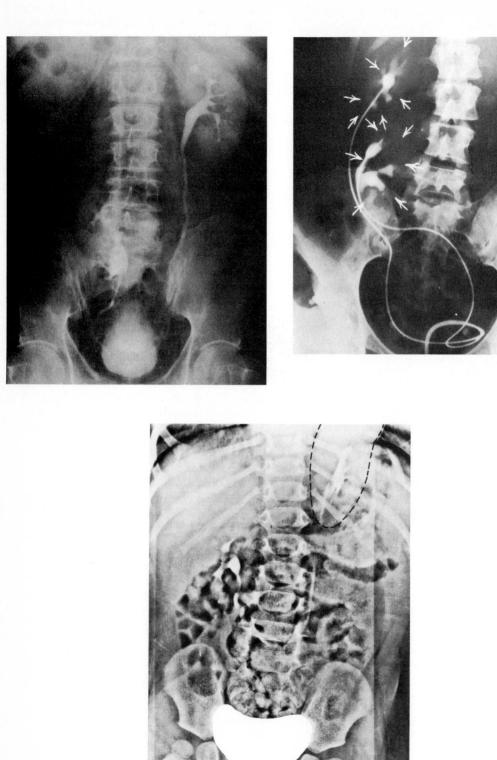

Figure 23–9. Renal ectopy. *Upper left:* Excretory urogram showing congenital ectopy, right kidney. *Upper right:* Retrograde urogram showing crossed renal ectopy. In this film, the differentiation between fusion and nonfusion cannot be made. *Bottom:* Left kidney, ectopic in the chest.

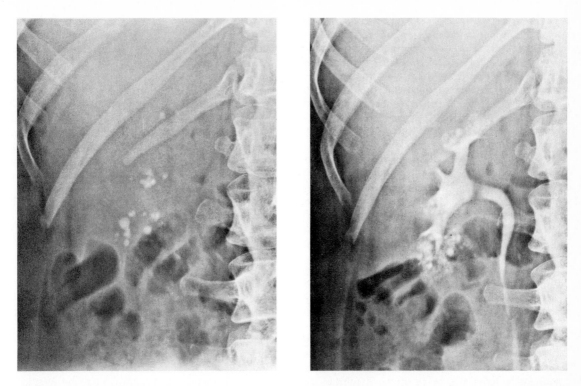

Figure 23–10. Medullary sponge kidneys. *Left:* Plain film of right kidney showing multiple small stones in its mid portion. *Right:* Excretory urogram showing relationship of calculi to calices. Typically, the calices are large; the stones are located in the dilated collecting tubules.

ulceration of calices; tubercle bacilli are found on bacteriologic study. Papillary necrosis may be complicated by calcification in the healed stage but may be distinguished by its typical caliceal deformity, the presence of infection and, usually, impaired renal function (Figs 13–5 and 13–6). The tubular and parenchymal calcification seen in nephrocalcinosis is more diffuse than that seen with sponge kidney (Fig 16–7); the symptoms and signs of primary hyperparathyroidism or renal tubular acidosis may be found.

There is no treatment for medullary sponge kidney. Therapy is directed toward the complications (eg, pyelonephritis and renal calculi). Only a small percentage of people with sponge kidney develop complications. The overall prognosis is good. A few patients may pass small stones occasionally.

ABNORMALITIES OF RENAL VESSELS

A single renal artery is noted in 75–85% of individuals and a single renal vein in an even higher percentage. Aberrant veins and, especially, arteries occur. An aberrant artery passing to the lower pole of the kidney or crossing an infundibulum can cause obstruction and hydronephrosis. These causes of obstruction can be diagnosed on angiography.

ACQUIRED LESIONS OF THE KIDNEYS

ANEURYSM OF THE RENAL ARTERY

Aneurysm of the renal artery usually results from degenerative arterial disease that weakens the wall of the artery so that intravascular pressure may balloon it out. It is most commonly caused by arteriosclerosis or polyarteritis nodosa (Fisher, 1981), but it may develop secondary to trauma or syphilis. Well over 300 cases have been reported. Congenital aneurysm has been recorded. Most cases represent an incidental finding on angiography (Hageman et al, 1978).

Aneurysmal dilatation has no deleterious effect upon the kidney unless the mass compresses the renal artery, in which case some renal ischemia and, therefore, atrophy are to be expected. A true aneurysm may rupture, producing a false aneurysm. This is especially likely to occur during pregnancy. The extravasated blood in the retroperitoneal space finally becomes encapsulated by a fibrous covering as organization occurs. An aneurysm may involve a small artery within the renal parenchyma. It may rupture into the renal pelvis or a calix.

Most aneurysms cause no symptoms unless they rupture, in which case there may be severe flank pain and even shock. If an aneurysm ruptures into the renal pelvis, marked hematuria occurs. The common cause of death is severe hemorrhage from rupture of the aneurysm. Hypertension is not usually present. A bruit should be sought over the costovertebral angle or over the renal artery anteriorly. If spontaneous or traumatic rupture has occurred, a mass may be palpated in the flank.

A plain film of the abdomen may show an intrarenal or extrarenal ringlike calcification (Fig 23–11). Urograms may be normal or reveal renal atrophy. Some impairment of renal function may be noted if compression or partial obstruction of the renal artery has developed. Aortography will delineate the aneurysm. Sonography and CT scanning may prove helpful.

The differential diagnosis of rupture of an aneurysm and injury to the kidney is difficult unless a history or evidence of trauma is obtained. A hydronephrotic kidney may present a mass, but urography will clarify the issue.

Because a significant number of noncalcified and large calcified aneurysms rupture spontaneously, the presence of such a lesion is an indication for operation particularly during pregnancy (Love, Robinette, and Vernon, 1981). The repair of extrarenal aneurysms may be considered, but complications (eg, thrombosis) are not uncommon. If an intrarenal aneurysm is situated in one pole, heminephrectomy may be feasible. If, however, it is in the center of the organ, nephrectomy will be required. Therapeutic occlusion

of an aneurysm by intra-arterial injection of autologous muscle tissue has been reported. Those few patients with hypertension may become normotensive following definitive surgery.

RENAL INFARCTS

Renal infarcts are caused by arterial occlusion. The major causes are subacute infective endocarditis, atrial of ventricular thrombi, arteriosclerosis, polyarteritis nodosa, and trauma. A thrombotic process in the abdominal aorta may gradually extend upward to occlude the renal artery. Renal infarcts may be unilateral or bilateral.

If smaller arteries or arterioles become obstructed, the tissue receiving blood from such a vessel will first become swollen and then undergo necrosis and fibrosis. Multiple infarcts are the rule. If the main renal artery becomes occluded, the entire kidney will react in kind. The kidney may therefore become functionless and atrophic as it undergoes necrosis and fibrosis.

Partial renal infarction is usually a silent disease. Sudden and complete infarction may cause renal or chest pain and at times gross or microscopic hematuria. Proteinuria and leukocytosis are found. Warner, Tessler, and Andronaco (1982) have noted "epitheluria" that represents sloughing of renal tubular cells. Tenderness over the flank may be elicited. The kidney is not significantly enlarged by arterial occlusion. Serum aspartate aminotransferase (glutamic-oxaloacetic transaminase, SGOT) and lactate dehydro-

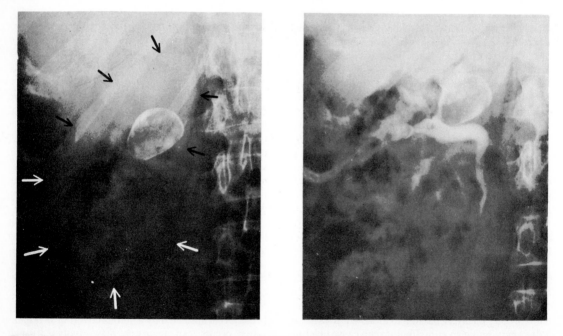

Figure 23–11. Intrarenal aneurysm of renal artery. *Left:* Plain film showing calcified structure over right renal shadow. *Right:* Excretory urogram relating calcific mass to pelvis and upper calix. (Courtesy of CD King.)

genase levels will be elevated for 1 or 2 days after the incident.

Excretory urograms may fail to visualize a portion of the kidney with partial infarction; with complete infarction, none of the radiopaque fluid is excreted. If complete renal infarction is suspected, a radioisotope renogram should be performed. A completely infarcted kidney will show little or no radioactivity. A similar picture will be seen on CT scans performed after injection of radiopaque contrast medium. Even though complete loss of measurable function has occurred, renal circulation may be restored spontaneously in some instances.

Renal angiography makes the definitive diagnosis. A dynamic technetium scan will reveal no perfusion of the affected renal vasculature.

During the acute phase, infarction may mimic ureteral stone. With stone the excretory urogram may also show lack of renal function, but even so there is usually enough medium in the tubules so that a "nephrogram" is obtained (Fig 16–3). This will not occur with complete infarction. Evidence of a cardiac or vascular lesion is helpful in arriving at a proper diagnosis.

The complications are related to those arising from the primary cardiovascular disease, including emboli to other organs. In a few cases, hypertension may develop a few days or weeks after the infarction. It may later subside.

While emergency surgical intervention has been done, it has become clear that anticoagulation therapy is the treatment of choice. Recently, it has been shown that an infusion of streptokinase may dissolve the embolus (Rudy et al, 1982; Fischer et al, 1981). Renal function returns in most cases.

grams may then show notching of the upper ureter caused by dilated collateral veins.

Ultrasonography shows the thrombus in the vena cava in 50% of cases. The involved organ is enlarged (Fowler and Paciulli, 1977; Braun, Welleman, and Welgand, 1981). CT scan is also a valuable diagnostic tool; visualization of the thrombus can be noted in a high percentage of cases. Renal angiography reveals stretching and bowing of small arterioles. In the nephrographic phase, the pyramids may become quite dense. Late films may show venous collaterals. Venacavography or, preferably, selective renal venography will demonstrate the thrombus in the renal vein (Fig 23–12) and, at times, in the vena cava. If washout from the vein gives poor filling, filling may be enhanced by an injection of epinephrine into the renal artery.

The symptoms and signs resemble obstruction from a ureteral calculus. The presence of a stone in the ureter should be obvious; some degree of dilatation of the ureter and pelvis should then also be expected. Clot obstruction in the ureter must be differentiated from an obstructing calculus.

While thrombectomy and even nephrectomy have been recommended in the past, it has become increasingly clear that medical treatment is usually efficacious. The use of heparin anticoagulation in the acute phase and warfarin chronically offers satisfactory resolution of the problems in most patients. In infants and children, it is essential to correct fluid and electrolyte problems and administer anticoagulants. Renal function is usually fully recovered.

THROMBOSIS OF THE RENAL VEIN

Thrombosis of renal vein is rare in adults. It is frequently unilateral and usually associated with membranous glomerulonephritis and nephrotic syndrome. Invasion of the renal vein by tumor or retroperitoneal disease can be the cause. Thrombosis of the renal vein may occur as a complicaton of severe dehydration and hemoconcentration in children with severe diarrhea from ileocolitis. The thrombosis may extend from the vena cava into the peripheral venules or may originate in the peripheral veins and propagate to the main renal vein. The severe passive congestion that develops causes the kidney to swell and become engorged. Degeneration of the nephrons ensues. There is usually flank pain, and hematuria may be noted. A large, tender mass is often felt in the flank. Thrombocytopenia may be noted. The urine contains albumin and red cells. In the acute stage, urograms show poor or absent secretion of the radiopaque material in a large kidney. Stretching and thinning of the caliceal infundibula may be noted. Clots in the pelvis may cause filling defects. Later, the kidney may undergo atrophy. Uro-

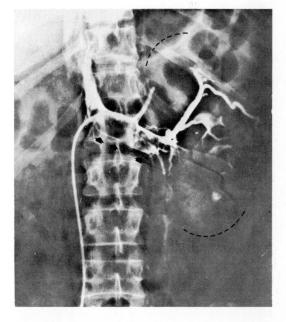

Figure 23–12. Thrombosis of renal vein. Selective left renal venogram showing almost complete occlusion of vein. Veins to lower pole failed to fill. Note large size of kidney.

ARTERIOVENOUS FISTULA

Arteriovenous fistula may be congenital (25%) or acquired. A number of these fistulas have been reported following needle biopsy of the kidney or trauma to the kidney. A few have occurred following nephrectomy secondary to suture or ligature occlusion of the pedicle. These require surgical repair. A few have been recognized in association with adenocarcinoma of the kidney.

A thrill can often be palpated and a murmur heard both anteriorly and posteriorly. In cases with a wide communication, the systolic blood pressure is elevated and a widened pulse pressure is noted. Renal angiography or isotopic scan establishes the diagnosis. CT scan and sonography are particularly helpful. Arteriovenous fistula involving the renal artery and vein requires surgical repair of nephrectomy. Most, however, can be occluded by embolization, balloon, or steel coil. Those that develop secondary to renal biopsy tend to heal spontaneously.

ARTERIOVENOUS ANEURYSM

About 100 instances of this lesion have been reported (Fig 23–13). Most follow trauma. Hypertension is to be expected and is associated with high-output cardiac failure. A bruit is usually present.

Nephrectomy is usually indicated.

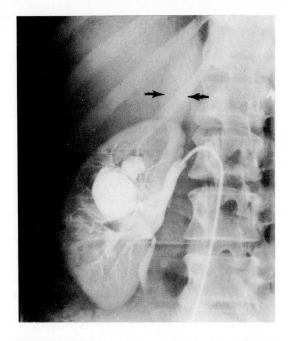

Figure 23–13. Arteriovenous aneurysm. Selective renal angiogram. Note aneurysm in center of kidney, with prompt filling of the vena cava (shown by arrows).

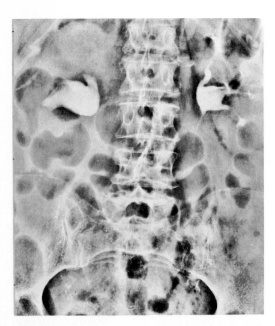

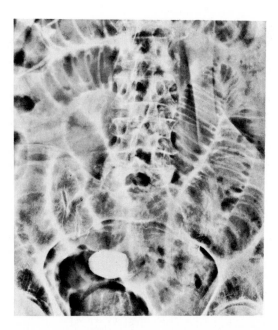

Figure 23–14. Nephroduodenal fistula and small bowel obstruction from renal staghorn calculus. *Left:* Excretory urogram showing nonfunction of right kidney; staghorn stone. *Right:* Patient presented with symptoms and signs of bowel obstruction 4 years later. Plain film showing dilated loops of small bowel down to a point just proximal to ileocecal valve. Obstruction due to stone extruded into duodenum. (Courtesy of CD King.)

RENOALIMENTARY FISTULA

Over 100 instances of renoalimentary fistula have been reported. They usually involve the stomach, duodenum, or adjacent colon, although fistula formation with the esophagus, small bowel, appendix, and rectum has been reported.

The underlying cause is usually a pyonephrotic kidney that becomes adherent to a portion of the alimentary tract and then ruptures spontaneously, thus creating a fistula (Fig 23–14). A few cases following trauma have been reported. The patient is apt to suffer symptoms and signs of acute pyelonephritis. Urography may show radiopaque material escaping into the gastrointestinal tract. Gastrointestinal series may also reveal the connection with the kidney. The treatment is nephrectomy with closure of the opening into the gut.

RENOBRONCHIAL FISTULA

Nephrobronchial fistulas are rare. They are caused by rupture of an infected, calculous kidney through the diaphragm. Rubin and Morettin (1982) have observed 2 such cases and cite 67 others from the literature.

REFERENCES

CONGENITAL ANOMALIES

General

Belman AB, King LR: Urinary tract abnormalities associated with imperforate anus. *J Urol* 1972;**108**:823.

Fleisher DS: Lateral displacement of the nipples, a sign of bilateral renal hypoplasia. *J Pediatr* 1966;**69**:806.

Kaplan MR: Inherited renal disease and genetic counseling. *Clin Exp Dial Apheresis* 1981;**5**:213.

Taylor WC: Deformity of ears and kidneys. *Can Med Assoc J* 1965;**93**:107.

Vitko RJ, Cass AS, Winter RB: Anomalies of the genitourinary tract associated with congenital scoliosis and congenital kyphosis. *J Urol* 1972;**108**:655.

Agenesis

Cain DR et al: Familial renal agenesis and total dysplasia. *Am J Dis Child* 1974;**128**:377.

Cope JR, Trickey SE: Congenital absence of the kidney: Problems in diagnosis and management. *J Urol* 1982;**127**:10.

Emanuel B et al: Congenital solitary kidney: A review of 74 cases. *J Urol* 1974;**111**:394.

Kohn G, Borns PF: The association of bilateral and unilateral renal aplasia in the same family. *J Pediatr* 1973;**83**:95.

Potter EL: Bilateral absence of kidneys and ureters: A report of 50 cases. *Obstet Gynecol* 1965;**25**:3.

Hypoplasia

Cha EM, Kandzari S, Khoury GH: Congenital renal hypoplasia: Angiographic study. *Am J Roentgenol* 1972;**114**:710.

Kanasawa M et al: Dwarfed kidneys in children. *Am J Dis Child* 1965;**109**:130.

Supernumerary Kidneys

N'Guessan GH, Stephens FD: Supernumerary kidney. *J Urol* 1983;**130**:649.

Dysplasia & Multicystic Kidney

Abt AB, Demers LM, Shochat SJ: Cystic nephroma: An ultrastructural and biochemical study. *J Urol* 1979;**122**:539.

Azimi F, Kodroff MB: Congenital renal dysplasia: Osathanondh-Potter type II polycystic kidneys. *Urology* 1976;**7**:550.

Bloom DA, Brosman S: The multicystic kidney. *J Urol* 1978;**120**:211.

De Klerk DP, Marshall FF, Jeffs RD: Multicystic dysplastic kidney. *J Urol* 1977;**118**:306.

Fisher C, Smith JF: Renal dysplasia in nephrectomy specimens from adolescents and adults. *J Clin Pathol* 1975;**28**:879.

Friedberg JE, Mitnick JS, Davis DA: Antipartum ultrasonic detection of multicystic kidney. *Radiology* 1979;**131**:198.

Hattery RR: Computed tomography of renal abnormalities. *Radiol Clin North Am* 1977;**15**:401.

Stecker JF Jr, Rose JG, Gillenwater JT: Dysplastic kidneys associated with vesicoureteral reflux. *J Urol* 1973;**110**:341.

Warshawsky AB, Miller KE, Kaplan GW: Urographic visualization of multicystic kidneys. *J Urol* 1977;**117**:94.

Polycystic Kidneys

Adult polycystic disease of kidneys. (Leading article.) *Br Med J* 1981;**282**:1097.

Bernstein J: Heritable cystic disorders of the kidney: The mythology of polycystic disease. *Pediatr Clin North Am* 1971;**18**:435.

Kaye C, Lewy PR: Congenital appearance of adult-type (autosomal dominant) polycystic kidney disease. *J Pediatr* 1974;**85**:807.

Kendall AR, Pollack HM, Karafin L: Congenital cystic disease of kidney: Classification and manifestations. *Urology* 1974;**4**:635.

Lamiell JM, Stor RA, Hsia YE: Von Hippel-Lindau disease simulating polycystic kidney diseases. *Urology* 1980;**15**:287.

Lee JKT, McClennan BL, Kissane JM: Unilateral polycystic kidney disease. *AJR* 1978;**130**:1165.

Levine E et al: Computed tomography in the diagnosis of renal carcinoma complicating Hippel-Lindau syndrome. *Radiology* 1979;**130**:703.

Lufkin EG et al: Polycystic kidney disease: Earlier diagnosis using ultrasound. *Urology* 1974;**4**:5.

Pechan W et al: Management of end stage polycystic kidney disease with renal transplantation. *J Urol* 1981;**125**:622.

Qazi Q et al: Renal anomalies in fetal alcohol syndrome. *Pediatrics* 1979;**63**:886.

Sagel SS et al: Computed tomography of the kidney. *Radiology* 1977;**124**:359.

Segal AJ, Spataro EF, Barbaric ZL: Adult polycystic kidney disease: A review of 100 cases. *J Urol* 1977;**118**:711.

Simple Cyst

Ambrose SS et al: Unsuspected renal tumors associated with renal cysts. *J Urol* 1977;**117**:704.

Androulakakis PA, Kirayiannis B, DeLiveliotis A: The parapelvic cyst: A report of 8 cases with particular emphasis on diagnosis and management. *Br J Urol* 1980;**52**:342.

Banner MP: Multilocular renal cysts: Radiologic-pathologic correlation. *AJR* 1981;**136**:239.

Bartholomew TH et al: The sonographic evaluation and management of simple renal cysts in children. *J Urol* 1980;**123**:732.

Bean WJ: Renal cysts: Treatment with alcohol. *Radiology* 1981;**138**:329.

Feiner HD, Katz LA, Gallo GR: Acquired cystic disease of kidney in chronic dialysis patients. *Urology* 1981;**17**:260.

Gross DM: Diagnostic renal cyst puncture and percutaneous nephrostomy. *Urol Clin North Am* 1979;**6**:409.

Harris RD, Goergen TG, Talner LB: The bloody cyst aspirate: A diagnostic dilemma. *J Urol* 1975;**114**:832.

Hattery RR: Computed tomography of renal abnormalities. *Radiol Clin North Am* 1977;**15**:401.

Hinman F Jr: Obstructive renal cysts. *J Urol* 1978;**119**:681.

Kessel HC, Tynes WV II: Spontaneous regression of renal cysts. *Urology* 1981;**17**:356.

Lang EK et al: Assessment of avascular renal mass lesions: The use of nephrotomography, arteriography, cyst puncture, double contrast study and histochemical and histopathologic examination. *South Med J* 1972;**65**:1.

Mullin EM, Paulson DF: Renal cystic disease. *Urology* 1976;**8**:5.

Muther RS, Bennett WM: Concentration of antibiotics in simple renal cysts. *J Urol* 1980;**124**:596.

Norfray JF et al: Carcinoma in a renal cyst: Computed tomography diagnosis. *J Urol* 1981;**125**:102.

Raskin MM et al: Percutaneous management of renal cysts: Results of a four-year study. *Radiology* 1975;**115**:551.

Roth JK Jr, Roberts JA: Benign renal cysts and renal function. *J Urol* 1980;**123**:625.

Sagel SS et al: Computed tomography of the kidney. *Radiology* 1977;**124**:359.

Sandler CM, Raval B, David CL: Computed tomography of the kidney. *Urol Clin North Am* 1985;**12**:657.

Stables DP, Jackson RS: Management of an infected simple renal cyst. *Br J Radiol* 1974;**47**:290.

Sufrin G et al: Hypernephroma arising in wall of simple renal cyst. *Urology* 1975;**6**:507.

Varma KR et al: Papillary carcinoma in wall of simple renal cyst. *Urology* 1974;**3**:762.

Wettlaufer JN, Modarelli RO: Triple contrast percutaneous nephrocystography and analysis of cyst aspirate. *Urology* 1978;**12**:373.

Renal Fusion

Connelly TL et al: Abdominal aortic surgery and horseshoe kidney. *Arch Surg* 1980;**115**:1459.

Fishman M, Borden S: Crossed fused renal ectopia with single crossed ectopic ureterocele. *J Urol* 1982;**127**:117.

Friedland GW, de Vries P: Renal ectopia and fusion: Embryologic basis. *Urology* 1975;**5**:698.

Hendron WH, Donahoe PK, Pfister RC: Crossed renal ectopia in children. *Urology* 1976;**7**:135.

Kvarstein B, Mathisen W: Surgical treatment of horseshoe kidney: A follow-up study. *Scand J Urol Nephrol* 1974;**8**:10.

Pitts WR Jr, Muecke EC: Horseshoe kidneys: A 40-year experience. *J Urol* 1975;**113**:743.

Ectopic Kidney

Hertz M et al: Crossed renal ectopia: Clinical and radiological findings in 22 cases. *Clin Radiol* 1977;**28**:339.

Hildreth TA, Cass AS: Crossed renal ectopia with familial occurrence. *Urology* 1978;**12**:59.

Kirshenbaum AS, Puri HC, Rao BR: Congenital intrathoracic kidney. *J Urol* 1981;**125**:412.

Marshall FF: Freedman MT: Crossed renal ectopia. *J Urol* 1978;**119**:188.

Medullary Sponge Kidney

Eisenberg RL, Pfister RC: Medullary sponge kidney associated with congenital hemihypertrophy (asymmetry): A case report and survey of the literature. *Am J Roentgenol* 1972;**116**:773.

Hayt DB et al: Direct magnification intravenous pyelography in re-evaluation of medullary sponge kidney. *Am J Roentgenol* 1973;**119**:701.

Spence HM, Singleton R: What is sponge kidney disease and where does it fit in the spectrum of cystic disorders? *J Urol* 1972;**107**:176.

Swenson RS, Kempson RL, Friedland GW: Cystic disease of the renal medulla in the elderly. *JAMA* 1974;**228**:1404.

ACQUIRED LESIONS

Aneurysm of the Renal Artery

Altebarmakian VK et al: Renal artery aneurysm. *Urology* 1979;**13**:257.

Carron J et al: Renal artery aneurysm: Polyaneurysmal lesion of kidney. *Urology* 1975;**5**:1.

Clouse ME, Levin DC, Desautels RE: Transcatheter embolotherapy for congenital arteriovenous malformations. *Urology* 1983;**22**:360.

DuBrow RA, Patel SK: Mycotic aneurysm of the renal artery. *Radiology* 1981;**138**:577.

Fisher RG: Renal artery aneurysms in polyarteritis nodosa: A multiepisodic phenomenon. *AJR* 1981;**136**:983.

Hageman JH et al: Aneurysms of the renal artery: Problems of prognosis and surgical management. *Surgery* 1978;**84**:563.

Love WK, Robinette MA, Vernon CP: Renal artery aneurysm rupture in pregnancy. *J Urol* 1981;**126**:809.

Poutasse EF: Renal artery aneurysms. *J Urol* 1975;**113**:443.

Renal Infarcts

Chehval MJ, Mehan DJ: Nonoperative management of renal artery embolus. *Urology* 1979;**14**:569.

Fay R et al: Renal artery thrombosis: A successful revascularization by autotransplantation. *J Urol* 1974;**111**:572.

Fergus JN, Jones NF, Thomas ML: Kidney function after arterial embolism. *Br Med J* 1969;**4**:587.

Fischer CP et al: Renal artery embolism: Therapy with intraarterial streptokinase infusion. *J Urol* 1981;**125**:402.

Frank PH et al: The cortical rim sign of renal infarction. *Br J Radiol* 1974;**47**:875.

Grablowsky OM et al: Renal artery thrombosis following blunt trauma: Report of four cases. *Surgery* 1970;**67**:895.

Harris RD, Dorros S: Computed tomographic diagnosis of renal infarction. *Urology* 1981;**17**:287.

Lessman RK et al: Renal artery embolism: Clinical features and long-term follow-up of 17 cases. *Ann Intern Med* 1978;**89**:477.

Mounger EJ: Hypertension resulting from segmental renal artery infarction. *Urology* 1973;**1**:189.

Rudy DC et al: Segmental renal artery emboli treated with low-dose intra-arterial streptokinase. *Urology* 1982; **19**:410.

Schramek A et al: Survival following late renal embolectomy in a patient with a single functioning kidney. *J Urol* 1973;**109**:342.

Smith SP Jr et al: Occlusion of the artery to a solitary kidney: Restoration of renal function after prolonged anuria. *JAMA* 1974;**230**:1306.

Warner RS, Tessler AN, Andronaco RB: Epitheliuria and early diagnosis or renal artery embolus. *Urology* 1982;**19**:628.

Thrombosis of the Renal Vein

Baum NH, Moriel E, Carlton CE Jr: Renal vein thrombosis. *J Urol* 1978;**119**:443.

Belman AB: Renal vein thrombosis in infancy and childhood: A contemporary survey. *Clin Pediatr* 1976; **15**:1033.

Braun B, Welleman LS, Welgand W: Ultrasonic demonstration of renal vein thrombosis. *Radiology* 1981;**138**:157.

Cade R et al: Chronic renal vein thrombosis. *Am J Med* 1977;**63**:387.

Chugh KS et al: Renal vein thrombosis in nephrotic syndrome: A prospective study and review. *Postgrad Med J* 1981;**57**:566.

Clark RA, Wyatt GM, Colley DP: Renal vein thrombosis: An underdiagnosed complication of multiple renal abnormalities. *Radiology* 1979;**132**:43.

Fowler JE Jr, Paciulli J: Renal vein thrombosis: Diagnosis by B-scan ultrasonography. *J Urol* 1977;**118**:849.

Kiruluta HG et al: The protean manifestations of renal vein thrombosis in the adult. *J Urol* 1976;**115**:634.

Llach F, Papper S, Massrey SG: The clinical spectrum of renal vein thrombosis: Acute and chronic. *Am J Med* 1980;**69**:819.

Rosenberg ER et al: Ultrasonic diagnosis of renal vein thrombosis in neonates. *AJR* 1980;**134**:35.

Thompson IM, Schneider R, Lababidi Z: Thrombectomy for neonatal renal vein thrombosis. *J Urol* 1975;**113**:396.

Arteriovenous Fistula

Hart PL, Ingram DW, Peckham GB: Postnephrectomy arteriovenous fistula causing "stroke" and congestive heart failure. *Can Med Assoc J* 1973;**108**:1400.

Hawkins IF, Garin EH: Therapeutic renal embolization in children. *J Pediatr* 1979;**94**:415.

Lisbona R et al: Radionuclide detection of iatrogenic arteriovenous fistulas of the genitourinary system. *Radiology* 1980;**134**:201.

Marshall FF et al: Treatment of traumatic renal arteriovenous fistulas by detachable silicone balloon embolization. *J Urol* 1979;**122**:237.

Tepper JP et al: Renal arteriovenous fistula: Angiographic and sonographic correlation. *J Urol* 1982;**127**:106.

Tucci P, Doctor D, Diagonale A: Embolization of post-traumatic renal arteriovenous fistula. *Urology* 1979;**13**:192.

Wallace S et al: Intrarenal arteriovenous fistulas: Transcatheter steel coil occlusion. *J Urol* 1978;**120**:282.

Arteriovenous Aneurysm

Merrit BA, Middleton RG: Repair of a huge renal arteriovenous aneurysm with preservation of the kidney. *J Urol* 1972;**107**:521.

O'Donnel KF, Pais VM: Arteriovenous aneurysm of kidney after open renal biopsy. *Urology* 1976;**7**:305.

Renoalimentary Fistulas

Bissada NK, Cole AT, Fried FA: Reno-alimentary fistula: An unusual urological problem. *J Urol* 1973;**110**:273.

Dunn M, Kirk D: Renogastric fistula: Case report and review of the literature. *J Urol* 1973;**109**:785.

Greene JE, Bucy JG, Wise L: Spontaneous pyeloduodenal and renocolic fistulas. *South Med J* 1975;**68**:641.

Newman JH, Jeans WD: Reno-colic fistula demonstrated by antegrade pyelography. *Br J Urol* 1972;**44**:692.

Schwartz DT et al: Pyeloduodenal fistula due to tuberculosis. *J Urol* 1970;**104**:373.

Renobronchial Fistulas

Rubin SA, Morettin LB: Nephrobronchial fistula: An uncommon manifestation of inflammatory renal disease. *J Urol* 1982;**127**:103.

24

Diagnosis of
Medical Renal Diseases

Marcus A. Krupp, MD

The medical renal diseases are those that involve principally the parenchyma of the kidneys. Many of the symptoms and signs of urinary tract disease are common to both medical and surgical diseases of the kidneys and other urologic organs. Hematuria, proteinuria, pyuria, oliguria, polyuria, pain, renal insufficiency with azotemia, acidosis, anemia, electrolyte abnormalities, hypertension, headache, and ocular involvement may occur in a wide variety of disorders affecting any portion of the parenchyma of the kidney, its blood vessels, or the excretory tract.

Every effort must be made to rule out nonsurgical disease of the urinary tract before resorting to diagnostic or therapeutic procedures that may prove to be unnecessary or dangerous.

A complete medical history and physical examination, a thorough examination of the urine, and blood chemistry examinations as indicated are essential initial steps in the workup of any patient.

History

A. Family History: The family history may reveal disease of genetic origin, eg, tubular metabolic anomalies, polycystic kidneys, unusual types of nephritis, or vascular or coagulation defects that may be essential clues to the diagnosis.

B. Past History: The past history should cover infections, injuries, and exposure to toxic agents, anticoagulants, or drugs that may produce toxic or sensitivity reactions, including blood dyscrasias. A history of diabetes, hypertensive disease, and autoimmune disease may be obtained. The inquiry must also elicit symptoms of uremia, debilitation, and the vascular complications of chronic renal disease.

Physical Examination

One must look for such physical signs as pallor, edema, hypertension, retinopathy, and the stigmas of congenital and hereditary disease (eg, enlarged kidneys with polycystic disease).

Urinalysis

Examination of the urine is the essential part of the investigation.

A. Proteinuria: Proteinuria of any significant degree (2–4+) is suggestive of "medical" renal disease (parenchymal involvement). Proteinuria should be in-

terpreted with consideration of the urine specific gravity, since a proteinuria of 1+ in a dilute urine may indicate a significantly great protein loss. Formed elements present in the urine usually establish the diagnosis. Only after careful examination of the patient and suitable urine specimens, as well as analysis of the chemical constituents of the blood, is urography or cystoscopy justified.

1. "Pathologic" proteinurias– Significant proteinuria is present in such disorders as glomerulonephritis, subacute or chronic nephritis, nephrotic syndrome, autoimmune disease, diabetic nephropathy, myeloma of the kidney, amyloid kidney, and polycystic kidney disease.

2. "Nonpathologic" proteinurias– When investigating causes, one must be careful not to overlook mild cases of glomerulonephritis or other parenchymal disease.

a. "Physiologic" proteinuria– Following vigorous exercise or protracted physical effort, protein, erythrocytes, casts, and tubule cells may appear transiently in urine samples. Repeat examination of the urine after a period of rest usually shows normal urine.

b. Orthostatic proteinuria– Some persons have proteinuria when they are up and about but not while recumbent. In any patient with proteinuria, the degree of proteinuria is usually more pronounced when the patient is upright, and especially when the patient is active. Absence of proteinuria when the patient is supine during the period of urine formation confirms the diagnosis of orthostatic proteinuria.

B. Red Cell Casts: Although red cells in the urine indicate extravasation of blood anywhere along the urinary tract, the occurrence of red cells in casts proves the renal origin of the bleeding. Formation of typical red cell casts by erythrocytes is indicative of glomerulitis.

C. Fatty Casts and Oval Fat Bodies: Tubule cells showing fatty changes occur in degenerative diseases of the kidney (nephrosis, glomerulonephritis, autoimmune disease, amyloidosis, and damage due to such toxins as mercury).

D. Other Findings: The presence of abnormal urinary chemical constituents may be the only indication of metabolic disorders involving the kidneys. These include diabetes mellitus, renal glycosuria, aminoacidurias (including cystinuria), oxaluria, gout, hyperparathyroidism, hemochromatosis, hemoglobinuria, and myoglobinuria.

Examination of the Kidneys & Urinary Tract

Roentgenographic, sonographic, and radioisotope studies provide information about the size, structure, blood supply, and function of the kidneys and urinary tract.

Renal Biopsy

Renal biopsy is a valuable diagnostic procedure that also serves as a guide to rational treatment. The technique has become well established, frequently providing sufficient tissue for light and electron microscopy and for immunofluorescence examination. Absolute contraindications include anatomic presence of only one kidney; severe malfunction of one kidney even though function is adequate in the other; bleeding diathesis; the presence of hemangioma, tumor, or large cysts; abscess or infection; hydronephrosis; and an uncooperative patient. Relative contraindications are the presence of serious hypertension, uremia, severe arteriosclerosis, and unusual difficulty in doing a biopsy due to obesity, anasarca, or inability of the patient to lie flat.

Clinical indications for renal biopsy, in addition to the necessity for establishing a diagnosis, include the need to determine prognosis, to follow progression of a lesion and response to treatment, to confirm the presence of a generalized disease (autoimmune disorder, amyloidosis, sarcoidosis), and to follow rejection response in a transplanted kidney.

GLOMERULONEPHRITIS

Information obtained from experimentally induced glomerular disease in animals and from correlations with evidence derived by modern methods of examination of tissue obtained by biopsy and at necropsy has provided a new concept of glomerulonephritis.

The clinical manifestations of renal disease are apt to consist only of varying degrees of hematuria, excretion of characteristic formed elements in the urine, proteinuria, and renal insufficiency and its complications. Alterations in glomerular architecture as observed in tissue examined by light microscopy are also apt to be minimal and difficult to interpret. For these reasons, attempts to correlate clinical syndromes with histologic features of renal tissue have failed to provide a satisfactory basis for precise diagnosis, treatment, and prognosis.

Immunologic techniques for demonstrating a variety of antigens, antibodies, and complement fractions have led to new concepts of the origins and pathogenesis of glomerular disease. Electron microscopy has complemented the immunologic methods.

Glomerular disease resulting from immunologic reactions may be divided into 2 groups:

(1) Immune complex disease, in which soluble

Table 24–1. Common patterns of abnormal urine composition in disease.*

Disease	Specific Gravity	Protein†	Red Cells†	Casts†	Microscopic (Casts and Cells) and Other Findings
Normal	1.003–1.030	0 to trace (up to 0.05 g)	0 to occ	0 to occ	Hyaline casts (urine must be acid and fresh or preserved).
Diseases with high fevers	Increased	Trace or +	0	0 to few	Hyaline casts, tubule cells.
Congestive heart failure	High; varies with renal function	1–2+	0 to +	+	Hyaline and granular casts.
Eclampsia	Increased	3–4+	0 to +	3–4+	Hyaline casts.
Diabetic coma	High	+	0	0 to +	Hyaline casts, glucose, ketone bodies.
Acute glomerulonephritis‡	Increased	2–4+	1–4+	2–4+	Blood, cellular, granular, hyaline casts; renal tubule epithelium.
Degenerative phase glomerulonephritis	Normal or increased	4+	1–2+	4+	Granular, waxy, hyaline, fatty casts; fatty tubule cells.
Terminal phase glomerulonephritis	Low, fixed	1–2+	Trace to +	1–3+	Granular, hyaline, fatty, broad casts.
Lipoid nephrosis	Very high	4+	0 to trace	4+	Hyaline, granular, fatty, waxy casts; fatty tubule cells.
Collagen diseases	Normal or decreased	1–4+	1–4+	1–4+	Blood, cellular, granular, hyaline, waxy, fatty, broad casts, fatty tubule cells.
Pyelonephritis	Normal or decreased	0 to +	0 to +	0 to +	Leukocyte and hyaline casts, pus cells, bacteria.
Benign hypertension (late)	Normal or low	0 to +	0 to trace	0 to +	Hyaline and granular casts.
Malignant hypertension	Low, fixed	1–2+	Trace to +	1–2+	Hyaline and granular casts.

*Modified from Krupp MA et al: *Physician's Handbook,* 21st ed. Lange, 1985.
†Scale of 0–4+.
‡May be anuric, or have low, fixed specific gravity.

antigen-antibody complexes in the circulation are trapped in the glomeruli. The antigens are not derived from glomerular components; they may be exogenous (bacterial, viral, chemical) or endogenous (circulating native DNA, thyroglobulin). Factors in the pathogenic potential of the antigen include its origin, quantity, and route of entry and the host's duration of exposure to it. The immune response to the antigen depends on the severity of inflammation or infection and the host's capacity to respond (immunocompetency).

In the presence of antigen excess, antigen-antibody complexes form in the circulation and are trapped in the glomeruli as they are filtered through capillaries rendered permeable by the action of vasoactive amines. The antigen-antibody complexes bind components of complement, particularly C3. Activated complement provides chemoactive factors that attract leukocytes whose lysosomal enzymes incite the injury to the glomerulus.

On electron microscopy and with immuno-fluorescence methods, these complexes appear as lumpy deposits between the epithelial cells and the glomerular basement membrane. IgG, IgM, occasionally IgA, β1C, and C3 are demonstrable.

(2) Anti-GBM (glomerular basement membrane) disease, in which antibodies are generated against the glomerular basement membrane of the kidney and often against lung basement membrane, which appears to be antigenically similar to GBM. The autoantibodies may be stimulated by autologous GBM altered in some way or combined with an exogenous agent. The reaction of antibody with GBM is accompanied by activation of complement, the attraction of leukocytes, and the release of lysosomal enzymes. The presence of thrombi in glomerular capillaries is often accompanied by leakage of fibrinogen and precipitation of fibrin in Bowman's space, with subsequent development of epithelial "crescents" in the space.

Immunofluorescence techniques and electron microscopy show the anti-GBM complexes as linear deposits outlining the GBM. IgG and C3 are usually demonstrable.

The current classification of glomerulonephritis is based on the immunologic concepts described above. However, the discussions in the following pages will be organized according to traditional clinical categories.

I. **Immunologic Mechanisms Likely**
   A. **Immune Complex Disease:**
     Glomerulonephritis associated with infectious agents, including streptococci, staphylococci, pneumococci, infective endocarditis, secondary syphilis, malaria, viruses of hepatitis (HBAg) and measles
     Lupus erythematosus
     Glomerulonephritis associated with other systemic (?autoimmune) diseases such as polyarteritis nodosa, scleroderma, and idiopathic cryglobulinemia

Membranous glomerulonephritis, cause unknown
Membranoproliferative glomerulonephritis, cause unknown
Focal glomerulonephritis
Rapidly progressive glomerulonephritis (some cases)
   B. **Anti-GBM Disease**
     Goodpasture's syndrome
     Rapidly progressive glomerulonephritis (some cases)
II. **Immunologic Mechanisms Not Clearly Demonstrated**
     Lipoid nephrosis
     Focal glomerulonephritis (some cases)
     Chronic sclerosing glomerulonephritis
     Diabetic glomerulosclerosis
     Amyloidosis
     Hemolytic-uremic syndrome and thrombotic thrombocytopenic purpura
     Wegener's granulomatosis
     Alport's syndrome
     Sickle cell disease

1. POSTSTREPTOCOCCAL GLOMERULONEPHRITIS

Essentials of Diagnosis

- History of preceding streptococcal infection.
- Malaise, headache, anorexia, low-grade fever.
- Mild generalized edema, mild hypertension, retinal hemorrhages.
- Gross hematuria; protein, red cell casts, granular and hyaline casts, white cells, and renal epithelial cells in urine.
- Elevated antistreptolysin O titer, variable nitrogen retention.

General Considerations

Glomerulonephritis is a disease affecting both kidneys. In most cases, recovery from the acute stage is complete; but progressive involvement may destroy renal tissue, and renal insufficiency results. Acute glomerulonephritis is most common in children age 3–10 years, although 5% or more of initial attacks occur in adults over age 50. By far the most common cause is an antecedent infection of the pharynx and tonsils or of the skin with group A β-hemolytic streptococci, certain strains of which are nephritogenic. Nephritis occurs in 10–15% of children and young adults who have clinically evident infection with a nephritogenic strain. In children under age 6, pyoderma (impetigo) is the most common antecedent; in older children and young adults, pharyngitis is a common and skin infection a rare antecedent. Rarely, nephritis may follow infection due to pneumococci, staphylococci, some bacilli and viruses, or *Plasmodium malariae* and exposure to some drugs. *Rhus* dermatitis and reactions to venom or chemical agents may be associated with renal disease clinically indistinguishable from glomerulonephritis.

The pathogenesis of the glomerular lesion has been further elucidated by the use of new immunologic techniques (immunofluorescence) and electron microscopy. A likely sequel to infection by nephritogenic strains of β-hemolytic streptococci is injury to the mesangial cells in the intercapillary space. The glomerulus may then become more easily damaged by antigen-antibody complexes developing from the immune response to the streptococcal infection. β1C globulin of complement is deposited in association with IgG or alone in a granular pattern on the epithelial side of the basement membrane and occasionally in subendothelial sites as well.

Gross examination of the involved kidney shows only punctate hemorrhages throughout the cortex. Microscopically, the primary alteration is in the glomeruli, which show proliferation and swelling of the mesangial and endothelial cells of the capillary tuft. The proliferation of capsular epithelium produces a thickened crescent about the tuft, and in the space between the capsule and the tuft there are collections of leukocytes, red cells, and exudate. Edema of the interstitial tissue and cloudy swelling of the tubule epithelium are common. As the disease progresses, the kidneys may enlarge. The typical histologic findings in glomerulitis are enlarging crescents that become hyalinized and converted into scar tissue and obstruct the circulation through the glomerulus. Degenerative changes occur in the tubules, with fatty degeneration and necrosis and ultimate scarring of the nephron. Arteriolar thickening and obliteration become prominent.

Clinical Findings

A. Symptoms and Signs: Often the disease is very mild, and there may be no reason to suspect renal involvement unless the urine is examined. In severe cases, about 2 weeks following the acute streptococcal infection, the patient develops headache, malaise, mild fever, puffiness around the eyes and face, flank pain, and oliguria. Hematuria is usually noted as "bloody" or, if the urine is acid, as "brown" or "coffee-colored." Respiratory difficulty with shortness of breath may occur as a result of salt and water retention and circulatory congestion. There may be moderate tachycardia and moderate to marked elevation of blood pressure. Tenderness in the costovertebral angle is common.

B. Laboratory Findings: The diagnosis is confirmed by examination of the urine, which may be grossly bloody or coffee-colored (acid hematin) or may show only microscopic hematuria. In addition, the urine contains protein (1–3+) and casts. Hyaline and granular casts are commonly found in large numbers, but the classic sign of glomerulitis, the erythrocyte cast (blood cast), may be found only occasionally in the urinary sediment. The erythrocyte cast resembles a blood clot formed in the lumen of a renal tubule; it is usually of small caliber, intensely orange or red, and under high power with proper lighting may show the mosaic pattern of the packed red cells held together by the clot of fibrin and plasma protein.

With the impairment of renal function (decrease in GFR and blood flow) and with oliguria, plasma or serum urea nitrogen and creatinine become elevated, the levels varying with the severity of the renal lesion. The sedimentation rate is rapid. A mild normochromic anemia may result from fluid retention and dilution. Infection of the throat with nephritogenic streptococci is frequently followed by increasing antistreptolysin O (ASO) titers in the serum, whereas high titers are usually not demonstrable following skin infections. Production of antibody against streptococcal deoxyribonuclease B (anti-DNase B) is more regularly observed following both throat and skin infections. Serum complement levels are usually low.

Confirmation of diagnosis is made by examination of the urine, although the history and clinical findings in typical cases leave little doubt. The finding of erythrocytes in a cast is proof that erythrocytes were present in the renal tubules and did not arise from elsewhere in the genitourinary tract.

Differential Diagnosis

Although erythrocyte casts are considered to be the hallmark of glomerulonephritis, they also occur along with other abnormal elements in any disease in which glomerular inflammation and tubule damage are present, eg, polyarteritis nodosa, disseminated lupus erythematosus, dermatomyositis, sarcoidosis, subacute infective endocarditis, "focal" nephritis, Goodpasture's syndrome, Henoch's purpura, or poisoning with chemicals toxic to the kidney.

Treatment

There is no specific treatment. Eradication of infection, prevention of overhydration and hypertension, and prompt treatment of complications such as hypertensive encephalopathy and heart failure require careful observation and management.

Prognosis

Most patients with the acute disease recover completely within 1–2 years; 5–20% show progressive renal damage. If oliguria, heart failure, or hypertensive encephalopathy is severe, death may occur during the acute attack. Even with severe acute disease, however, recovery is the rule, particularly in children.

2. CHRONIC GLOMERULONEPHRITIS

Progressive destruction of the kidney may continue for many years in a clinically latent or subacute form. The subacute form is similar to the latent form (see below) except that symptoms occur—malaise, mild fever, and sometimes flank pain and oliguria. Treatment is as for the acute attack. Exacerbations may appear from time to time, reflecting the stage of evolution of the disease.

3. LATENT GLOMERULONEPHRITIS

If acute glomerulonephritis does not heal within 1–2 years, the vascular and glomerular lesions continue to progress, and tubular changes occur. In the presence of smoldering, active nephritis, the patient is usually asymptomatic, and the evidence of disease consists only of the excretion of abnormal urinary elements.

The urinary excretion of protein, red cells, white cells, epithelial cells, and casts (including erythrocyte casts, granular casts, and hyaline and waxy casts) continues at levels above normal. As renal impairment progresses, signs of renal insufficiency appear (see below).

The differential diagnosis is the same as that for acute glomerulonephritis. Recent studies of tissue obtained by renal biopsy in cases of recurrent or persistent hematuria indicate a high incidence of mesangial deposition of immune complexes made up of IgM or IgA (rarely IgG) and fractions of complement.

Prevention

Treat intercurrent infections promptly and vigorously as indicated. Avoid unnecessary immunizations.

Prognosis

Worsening of the urinary findings may occur with infection, trauma, or fatigue. Exacerbations may resemble the acute attack and may be associated with intercurrent infection or trauma. Other exacerbations may be typical of the nephrotic syndrome (see below). Death in uremia is the usual outcome, but the course is variable, and the patient may live a reasonably normal life for 20–30 years.

4. IgA NEPHROPATHY
(Idiopathic Benign Hematuria; Primary Hematuria)

Primary hematuria (idiopathic benign and recurrent hematuria, Berger's disease) is now known to be an immune complex glomerulopathy in which deposition of IgA and occasionally IgG with C3 and fibrin-related antigens occurs in a granular pattern in the mesangium of the glomerulus.

Recurrent macroscopic and microscopic hematuria and mild proteinuria are usually the only manifestations of renal disease. Usually, there is progression of the glomerular disease with destruction of glomeruli and loss of renal function, often with hypertension. Exacerbations have occurred with upper respiratory tract infections. Progression is usually slow, extending over decades.

Diagnosis is made by renal biopsy and demonstra-

tion of the mesangial immune complex deposits. Similar deposits may be seen in disseminated lupus erythematosus, eclampsia, Henoch-Schönlein purpura, membranous glomerulonephritis, acute postinfectious glomerulonephritis, and other rare causes of glomerulopathy. The urine sediment resembles that of any latent glomerulonephritis, with protein, red cells, and casts, including erythrocyte casts. The paucity of clinical manifestations and slow progress may be the determinative diagnostic features of the history.

No specific treatment is available for this indolent disease.

5. ANTI-GLOMERULAR BASEMENT MEMBRANE NEPHRITIS (Goodpasture's Syndrome)

The patient usually gives a history of recent hemoptysis and often of malaise, anorexia, and headache. The clinical syndrome is that of a severe acute glomerulonephritis which may be accompanied by diffuse hemorrhagic inflammation of the lungs. The urine shows gross or microscopic hematuria, and laboratory findings of severely suppressed renal function are usually evident. Biopsy shows glomerular crescents, glomerular adhesions, and inflammatory infiltration interstitially. Electron microscopic examination shows an increase in basement membrane material and deposition of fibrin beneath the capillary endothelium. In some cases, circulating antibody against glomerular basement membrane can be identified. IgG, C3, and, often, other components of the classic complement pathway can be demonstrated as linear deposits on the basement membranes of the glomeruli and the lung. Anti-glomerular basement membrane antibody also reacts with lung basement membrane.

Only rare cases of survival have been documented. Large doses of corticosteroids in combination with immunosuppressive therapy may be useful. Plasmapheresis to remove circulating antibody has been reported to be effective in some patients. Hemodialysis and nephrectomy with renal transplantation may offer the only hope for rescue. Transplantation should be delayed until circulating anti-glomerular basement antibodies have disappeared.

Occasionally, acute renal disease with a similar clinical and immunologic pattern may occur without associated lung disease. Termed **idiopathic rapidly progressive glomerulonephritis,** it characteristically progresses to severe renal insufficiency in a few weeks.

NEPHROTIC SYNDROME

Essentials of Diagnosis

- Massive edema.
- Proteinuria > 3.5 g/d.
- Hypoalbuminemia < 3 g/dL.
- Hyperlipidemia: Cholesterol > 300 mg/dL.
- Lipiduria: Free fat, oval fat bodies, fatty casts.

General Considerations

Because treatment and prognosis vary with the cause of nephrotic syndrome (nephrosis), renal biopsy and appropriate examination of an adequate tissue specimen are important. Light microscopy, electron microscopy, and immunofluorescence identification of immune mechanisms provide critical information for identification of most of the causes of nephrosis.

Glomerular diseases associated with nephrosis include the following:

A. Minimal Glomerular Lesions: Lipoid nephrosis accounts for about 20% of cases of nephrosis in adults. No abnormality is visible by examination of biopsy material with the light microscope. With the electron microscope, alterations of the glomerular basement membrane, with swelling and vacuolization and loss of organization of foot processes of the epithelial cells (foot process disease), are evident. There is no evidence of immune disease by immunofluorescence studies. The response to treatment with corticosteroids is satisfactory. Renal function remains good.

B. Membranous Glomerulonephritis: (About 25–27% of cases.) Examination of biopsy material with the light microscope shows thickening of the glomerular capillary walls and some swelling of mesangial cells but no cellular proliferation. With the electron microscope, irregular lumpy deposits appear between the basement membrane and the epithelial cells, and new basement membrane material protrudes from the glomerular basement membrane as spikes or domes. Immunofluorescence studies show diffuse granular deposits of immunoglobulins (especially IgG) and complement (C3 component). As the membrane thickens, glomeruli become sclerosed and hyalinized.

This form of disease does not respond to any form of therapy. It usually progresses to renal failure in the course of a few to 10 years.

C. Membranoproliferative (Hypocomplementemic) Glomerulonephritis: (About 5% of cases.) Light microscopy shows thickening of glomerular capillaries, accompanied by mesangial proliferation and obliteration of glomeruli. With the electron microscope, subendothelial deposits and growth of mesangium into capillary walls are demonstrable. Immunofluorescence studies show the presence of the C3 component of complement and, rarely, the presence of immunoglobulins. There is no known treatment.

D. Proliferative Glomerulonephritis: (About 5% of cases.) This is considered to be a stage in the course of poststreptococcal nephritis.

E. Miscellaneous Diseases: A large number of metabolic, autoimmune, infectious, and neoplastic diseases and reactions to drugs and other toxic substances can produce glomerular disease. These include diabetic glomerulopathy, systemic lupus erythematosus, polyarteritis, Wegener's granulomatosis, amyloid disease, multiple myeloma, lymphomas, carcinomas, syphilis, reaction to toxins (bee venom, *Rhus* antigen), reaction to drugs (trimethadione, etc), and exposure to heavy metals.

Clinical Findings

A. Symptoms and Signs: Edema may appear insidiously and increase slowly; often it appears suddenly and accumulates rapidly. As fluid collects in the serous cavities, the abdomen becomes protuberant, and the patient may complain of anorexia and become short of breath. Symptoms other than those related to the mechanical effects of edema and serous sac fluid accumulation are not remarkable.

On physical examination, massive edema is apparent. Signs of hydrothorax and ascites are common. Pallor is often accentuated by the edema, and striae commonly appear in the stretched skin of the extremities. Hypertension, changes in the retina and retinal vessels, and cardiac and cerebral signs of hypertension may occur more often when collagen disease, diabetes mellitus, or renal insufficiency is present.

B. Laboratory Findings: The urine contains large amounts of protein, 4–10 g or more/24 h. The sediment contains casts, including the characteristic fatty and waxy varieties; renal tubule cells, some of which contain fatty droplets (oval fat bodies); and variable numbers of erythrocytes. A mild normochromic anemia is common, but anemia may be more severe if renal damage is great. Nitrogen retention varies with the severity of impairment of renal function. The plasma is often lipemic, and the blood cholesterol is usually greatly elevated. Plasma protein is greatly reduced. The albumin fraction may fall to less than 2 g or even below 1 g/dL. Some reduction of gamma globulin occurs in pure nephrosis, whereas in systemic lupus erythematosus, the protein of the γ fraction may be greatly elevated. Serum complement is usually low in active disease. The serum electrolyte concentrations are often normal, although the serum sodium may be slightly low; total serum calcium may be low, in keeping with the degree of hypoalbuminemia and decrease in the protein-bound calcium moiety. During edema-forming periods, urinary sodium excretion is very low and urinary aldosterone excretion elevated. If renal insufficiency (see above) is present, the blood and urine findings are usually altered accordingly.

Renal biopsy is essential to confirm the diagnosis and to indicate prognosis.

Differential Diagnosis

The nephrotic syndrome (nephrosis) may be associated with a variety of renal diseases, including glomerulonephritis (membranous and proliferative), collagen diseases (disseminated lupus erythematosus, polyarteritis, etc), amyloid disease, thrombosis of the renal vein, diabetic nephropathy, myxedema, multiple myeloma, malaria, syphilis, reaction to toxins such as bee venom, *Rhus* antigen, or heavy metals, drugs such as trimethadione, and constrictive pericarditis. In small children, nephrosis may occur without clear evidence of any cause.

Treatment

An adequate diet with restricted sodium intake (0.5–1 g/d) and prompt treatment of intercurrent infection are the basis of therapy. Other measures may be added as required.

The corticosteroids have been shown to be of value in treating nephrotic syndrome in children and in adults when the underlying disease is the minimal glomerular lesion (lipoid nephrosis), systemic lupus erythematosus, proliferative glomerulonephritis, or idiosyncratic reaction to toxin or venom. These drugs are less often effective in the treatment of membranous disease and membranoproliferative lesions of the glomerulus. They are of little or no value in amyloidosis or renal vein thrombosis and are contraindicated in diabetic nephropathy.

Diuretics may be given but are often ineffective. The most useful are the thiazide derivatives, eg, hydrochlorothiazide, 50–100 mg every 12 hours; other thiazides, chlorthalidone, and other diuretics may be employed at comparable effective dose levels. Spironolactone may be helpful when employed concurrently with thiazides. Salt-free albumin, dextran, and other oncotic agents are of little help, and their effects are transient.

Immunosuppressive drugs (aklylating agents, cyclophosphamide, mercaptopurine, azathioprine, etc) have been used in the treatment of nephrotic syndrome. Combination therapy with corticosteroids is similar to that employed in reversing rejection of homotransplants in humans. Encouraging early results have been reported in children and adults with proliferative or membranous lesions and with systemic lupus erythrmatosus. Those with minimal lesions refractory to corticosteroid therapy did no better when immunosuppressive agents were added. Improvement was noted in the glomerular changes and renal function in many patients responding well to treatment. It is not known what percentage of patients can be expected to benefit from these drugs.

Both the corticosteroids and the cytotoxic agents are commonly associated with serious side effects. At present, this form of therapy should be employed only by those experienced in treating nephrotic syndrome in patients who have proved refractory to well-established treatment regimens.

For renal vein thrombosis, treatment with heparin and long-term use of coumarin drugs is directed against progress of thrombus formation.

Prognosis

The course and prognosis depend upon the basic disease responsible for nephrotic syndrome. In about 50% of cases of childhood nephrosis, the disease appears to run a rather benign course when properly treated and to leave insignificant sequelae. Of the others, most go inexorably into the terminal state with renal insufficiency. Adults with nephrosis fare less well, particularly when the fundamental disease is glomerulonephritis, systemic lupus erythematosus, amyloidosis, or diabetic nephropathy. In those with minimal lesions, remissions, either spontaneous or following corticosteroid therapy, are common. Treatment is more often unsuccessful or only ameliorative when other glomerular lesions are present. Hypertension and nitrogen retention are serious signs.

RENAL INVOLVEMENT IN COLLAGEN DISEASES

The collagen diseases often produce symptoms and signs of renal disease indistinguishable from acute or chronic glomerulonephritis, nephrosis, renal vein thrombosis, and renal infarction. Although it may not be accurate to classify all of these disorders as collagen diseases, acute disseminated lupus erythematosus, polyarteritis nodosa, scleroderma, dermatomyositis, Wegener's granulomatosis, and thrombotic thrombocytopenic purpura have been implicated in producing a syndrome resembling glomerulonephritis. In about one-third to one-half of cases, the urine sediment is diagnostic, containing red blood cells and red blood cell casts; renal tubule cells, including some filled with fat droplets; and waxy and granular broad casts. The presence of these formed elements is indicative of active glomerular and tubular disease with extensive focal destruction of nephrons. The symptoms and signs of the primary disease and a variety of new tests of autoimmune disease help to differentiate the form of collagen disease present. When collagen disease involves the kidneys, complete recovery from the disease is not likely to occur, although steroid and immunosuppressive drugs (alone or in combination) may be effective for long-term amelioration.

DISEASES OF THE RENAL TUBULES & INTERSTITIUM

1. INTERSTITIAL NEPHRITIS

Acute interstitial disease may be due to systemic infections such as syphilis and sensitivity to drugs, including antibiotics (penicillins, colistin, sulfonamides), phenindione, and phenytoin. Recovery may be complete.

Chronic interstitial nephritis is characterized by focal or diffuse interstitial fibrosis accompanied by infiltration with inflammatory cells ultimately associated with extensive atrophy of renal tubules. It represents a nonspecific reaction to a variety of causes: analgesic abuse, lead and cadmium toxicity, nephrocalcinosis, urate nephropathy, radiation nephritis, sarcoidosis, Balkan nephritis, and some instances of obstructive uropathy. There are a few cases in which antitubule basement membrane antibodies have been identified.

2. ANALGESIC NEPHROPATHY

Long-term ingestion of nonsteroidal analgesic and anti-inflammatory drugs and fulminating urinary tract infection in the presence of diabetes mellitus are the 2 principal causes of renal papillary necrosis. Analgesic nephropathy typically occurs in a middle-aged woman with chronic and recurrent headaches or a patient with chronic arthritis who habitually consumes large amounts of the drugs. Phenacetin was implicated initially, but even with elimination of phenacetin from the mixtures, the incidence of analgesic nephropathy has not decreased. The ensuing damage to the kidneys usually is detected late, after renal insufficiency has developed.

The kidney lesion is pathologically nonspecific, consisting of peritubular and perivascular inflammation with degenerative changes of the tubule cells (chronic interstitial nephritis). There are no glomerular changes. Renal papillary necrosis extending into the medulla may involve many papillae.

Hematuria is a common presenting complaint. Renal colic occurs when necrotic renal papillae slough away. Polyuria may be prominent. Signs of acidosis (hyperpnea), dehydration, and pallor of anemia are common. Infection is a frequent complication. The history of excessive use of analgesics may be concealed by the patient.

The urine usually is remarkable only for the presence of blood and small amounts of protein. Hemolytic anemia is usually evident. Elevated blood urea nitrogen and creatinine and the electrolyte changes characteristic of renal failure are typically present.

Urograms show typical cavities and ring shadows of areas of destruction of papillae.

Treatment consists of withholding analgesics containing phenacetin and aspirin. Renal failure and infection are treated as outlined elsewhere in this chapter.

3. URIC ACID NEPHROPATHY

Crystals of urate produce an interstitial inflammatory reaction. Urate may precipitate out in acid urine in the calices to form uric acid stones. Patients with myeloproliferative disease under treatment may develop hyperuricemia and are subject to occlusion of the upper urinary tract by uric acid crystals. Alkalinization of the urine and a liberal fluid intake will help prevent crystal formation. Allopurinol is a useful drug to prevent hyperuricemia and hyperuricosuria.

4. OBSTRUCTIVE UROPATHY

Interstitial nephritis due to obstruction may not be associated with infection. Tubular conservation of salt and water is impaired. Following relief of obstruction, diuresis may be massive and may require vigorous but judicious replacement of water and electrolytes.

5. MYELOMATOSIS

Features of myelomatosis that contribute to renal disease include proteinuria (including filtrable Bence Jones protein and κ and λ chains) with precipitation in the tubules leading to accumulation of abnormal proteins in the tubule cells, hypercalcemia, and occasionally an increase in viscosity of the blood associated with macroglobulinemia. A Fanconi-like syndrome may develop.

Plugging of tubules, giant cell reaction around tubules, tubular atrophy, and, occasionally, the accumulation of amyloid are evident on examination of renal tissue.

Renal failure may occur acutely or develop slowly. Hemodialysis may rescue the patient during efforts to control the myeloma with chemical agents.

HEREDITARY RENAL DISEASES

The importance of inheritance and the familial incidence of disease warrants inclusion of a classification of hereditary renal diseases. Although relatively uncommon in the population at large, hereditary renal disease must be recognized to permit early diagnosis and treatment in other family members and to prepare the way for genetic counseling.

1. HEREDITARY CHRONIC NEPHRITIS

Evidence of the disease usually appears in childhood, with episodes of hematuria often following an upper respiratory infection. Renal insufficiency commonly develops in males but only rarely in females. Survival beyond age 40 is rare.

In many families, deafness and abnormalities of the eyes accompany the renal disease. Another form of the disease is accompanied by polyneuropathy. Infection of the urinary tract is a common complication.

The anatomic features in some cases resemble proliferative glomerulonephritis; in others, there is thickening of the glomerular basement membrane or podocyte proliferation and thickening of Bowman's capsule. In a few cases there are fat-filled cells (foam cells) in the interstitial tissue or in the glomeruli.

Laboratory findings are commensurate with existing renal function.

Treatment is symptomatic.

2. CYSTIC DISEASES OF THE KIDNEY

Congenital structural anomalies of the kidney must always be considered in any patient with hypertension, pyelonephritis, or renal insufficiency. The manifestations of structural renal abnormalities are related to the superimposed disease, but management and prognosis are modified by the structural anomaly.

Polycystic Kidneys

Polycystic kidney disease is familial and often involves not only the kidney but the liver and pancreas as well.

The formation of cysts in the cortex of the kidney is thought to result from failure of union of the collecting tubules and convoluted tubules of some nephrons. New cysts do not form, but those present enlarge and, by exerting pressure, cause destruction of ajacent tissue. Cysts may be found in the liver and pancreas. The incidence of cerebral vessel aneurysms is higher than normal.

Cases of polycystic disease are discovered during the investigation of hypertension, by diagnostic study in patients presenting with pyelonephritis or hematuria, or by investigation of families of patients with polycystic disease. At times, flank pain due to hemorrhage into a cyst will call attention to a kidney disorder. Otherwise the symptoms and signs are those commonly seen in hypertension or renal insufficiency. On physical examination, the enlarged, irregular kidneys are easily palpable.

The urine may contain leukocytes and red cells. With bleeding into the cysts, there may also be bleeding into the urinary tract. The blood chemical findings reflect the degree of renal insufficiency. Examination by echography or x-ray shows the enlarged kidneys, and urography demonstrates the classic elongated calices and renal pelves stretched over the surface of the cysts.

No specific therapy is available, and surgical interference is contraindicated unless ureteral obstruction is produced by an adjacent cyst. Hypertension, infection, and uremia are treated in the conventional manner.

Because persons with polycystic kidneys may live in reasonable comfort with slowly advancing uremia, it is difficult to determine when renal transplantation is in order. Hemodialysis can extend the life of the patient, but recurrent bleeding and continuous pain indicate the need for a transplant.

Although the disease may become symptomatic in childhood or in early adult life, it usually is discovered in the fourth or fifth decade. Unless fatal complications of hypertension or urinary tract infection are present, uremia develops very slowly, and patients live longer than with other causes of renal insufficiency.

Cystic Disease of the Renal Medulla

Two syndromes have been recognized with increasing frequency as their diagnostic features have become better known.

Medullary cystic disease is a familial disease that may become symptomatic during adolescence. Anemia is usually the initial manifestation, but azotemia, acidosis, and hyperphosphatemia soon become evident. Hypertension may develop. The urine is not remarkable, although there is often an inability to produce a concentrated urine. Many small cysts are scattered through the renal medulla. Renal transplantation is indicated by the usual criteria for the operation.

Sponge kidney is asymptomatic and is discovered by the characteristic appearance of the urogram. Enlargement of the papillae and calices and small cavities within the pyramids are demonstrated by the contrast media in the excretory urogram. Many small calculi often occupy the cysts, and infection may be troublesome. Life expectancy is not affected, and only symptomatic therapy for ureteral impaction of a stone or for infection is required.

3. ANOMALIES OF THE PROXIMAL TUBULE

Defects of Amino Acid Reabsorption

A. Congenital Cystinuria: Increased excretion of cystine results in the formation of cystine calculi in the urinary tract. Ornithine, arginine, and lysine are also excreted in abnormally large quantities. There is also a defect in absorption of these amino acids in the jejunum. Nonopaque stones should be examined chemically to provide a specific diagnosis.

Maintain a high urine volume by giving a large fluid intake. Maintain the urine pH above 7.0 by giving sodium bicarbonate and sodium citrate plus acetazolamide at bedtime to ensure an alkaline night urine. In refractory cases, a low-methionine (cystine precursor) diet may be necessary. Penicillamine has proved useful in some cases.

B. Aminoaciduria: Many amino acids may be poorly absorbed, resulting in unusual losses. Failure to thrive and the presence of other tubular deficits suggest the diagnosis.

There is no treatment.

C. Hepatolenticular Degeneration: In this congenital familial disease, aminoaciduria is associated with cirrhosis of the liver and neurologic manifestations. Hepatomegaly, evidence of impaired liver function, spasticity, athetosis, emotional disturbances, and Kayser-Fleischer rings around the cornea constitute a unique syndrome. There is a decrease in synthesis of ceruloplasmin, with a deficit of plasma ceruloplasmin and an increase in free copper that may be etiologically specific.

Give penicillamine to chelate and remove excess copper. Edathamil (EDTA) may also be used to remove copper.

Multiple Defects of Tubular Function (De Toni-Fanconi-Debré Syndrome)

Aminoaciduria, phosphaturia, glycosuria, and a variable degree of renal tubular acidosis characterize this syndrome. Osteomalacia is a prominent clinical feature; other clinical and laboratory manifestations are associated with specific tubular defects described separately above.

The proximal segment of the renal tubule is replaced by a thin tubular structure constituting the "swan neck" deformity. The proximal segment also is shortened to less than half the normal length.

Treatment consists of replacing cation deficits (especially potassium), correcting acidosis with bicarbonate or citrate, replacing phosphate loss with isotonic neutral phosphate (mono- and disodium salts) solution, and a liberal calcium intake. Vitamin D is usually useful, but the dose used must be controlled by monitoring serum calcium and phosphate.

Defects of Phosphorus & Calcium Absorption

A. Vitamin D-Resistant Rickets: Excessive loss of phosphorus and calcium results in rickets or osteomalacia that responds poorly to vitamin D therapy. Treatment consists of giving large doses of vitamin D and calcium supplementation of the diet.

B. Pseudohypoparathyroidism: As a result of excessive reabsorption of phosphorus, hyperphosphatemia and hypocalcemia occur. Symptoms include muscle cramps, fatigue, weakness, tetany, and mental retardation. The signs are those of hypocalcemia; in addition, the patients are short, round-faced, and characteristically have short fourth and fifth metacarpal and metatarsal bones. The serum phosphorus is high, serum calcium low, and serum alkaline phosphatase normal. There is no response to parathyroid hormone.

Vitamin D therapy and calcium supplementation may prevent tetany.

Defects of Glucose Absorption (Renal Glycosuria)

This results from an abnormally low ability to reabsorb glucose, so that glycosuria is present when blood glucose levels are normal. Ketosis is not present. The glucose tolerance response is usually normal. In some instances, renal glycosuria may precede the onset of true diabetes mellitus.

There is no treatment for renal glycosuria.

Defects of Glucose & Phosphate Absorption (Glycosuric Rickets)

The symptoms and signs are those of rickets or osteomalacia, with weakness, pain, or discomfort of the legs and spine and tetany. The bones become deformed, with bowing of the weight-bearing long bones, kyphoscoliosis, and, in children, signs of rickets. X-ray shows markedly decreased density of the bone, with pseudofracture lines and other deformities. Nephrocalcinosis may occur with excessive phosphaturia, and renal insufficiency may follow. Urinary calcium and phosphorus are increased and glycosuria is present. Serum glucose is normal, serum calcium is normal or low, serum phosphorus is low, and serum alkaline phosphatase is elevated.

Treatment consists of giving large doses of vitamin D and calcium supplementation of the diet.

Defects of Bicarbonate Reabsorption

Proximal renal tubular acidosis (RTA, type II) is due to a deficiency in the production of H^+ in the proximal tubule, with resultant loss of bicarbonate in the urine and decreased bicarbonate concentration in extracellular fluid. Accompanying the limitation of H^+ secretion are increased K^+ secretion into the urine and retrieval of Cl^- instead of HCO_3^-. The acidosis is therefore associated with hypokalemia and hyperchloremia. Transport of glucose, amino acids, phosphate, and urate may be deficient as well and may result in Fanconi's syndrome.

4. ANOMALIES OF THE DISTAL TUBULE

Defects of Hydrogen Ion Secretion & Bicarbonate Reabsorption (Classic Renal Tubular Acidosis, Type I)

Failure to secrete hydrogen ion and to form ammonium ion results in loss of "fixed base": sodium, potassium, and calcium. There is also a high rate of excretion of phosphate. Vomiting, poor growth, and symptoms and signs of chronic metabolic acidosis are accompanied by weakness due to potassium deficit and bone discomfort due to osteomalacia. Nephrocalcinosis, with calcification in the medullary portions of the kidney, occurs in about half of cases. The urine is alkaline and contains larger than normal quantities of sodium, potassium, calcium, and phosphate. The blood chemical findings are those of metabolic acidosis (low HCO_3^- or CO_2) with hyperchloremia, low serum calcium and phosphorus, low serum potassium, and, occasionally, low serum sodium.

Treatment consists of replacing deficits and increasing the intake of sodium, potassium, calcium, and phosphorus. Sodium and potassium should be given as bicarbonate or citrate. Additional vitamin D may be required.

Excess Potassium Secretion (Potassium "Wastage" Syndrome)

Excessive renal secretion or loss of potassium may occur in 4 situations: (1) chronic renal insufficiency with diminished H^+ secretion; (2) renal tubular acidosis and the De Toni-Fanconi syndrome, with cation loss resulting from diminished H^+ and NH_4^+ secretion; (3) hyperaldosteronism and hyperadrenocorticism; and (4) tubular secretion of potassium, the cause of which is as yet unknown. Hypokalemia indicates that the deficit is severe. Muscle weakness, metabolic alkalosis, and polyuria with dilute urine are signs attributable to hypokalemia.

Treatment consists of correcting the primary disease and giving supplementary potassium.

Defects of Water Absorption (Renal Diabetes Insipidus)

Nephrogenic diabetes insipidus occurs more frequently in males. Unresponsiveness to antidiuretic hormone is the key to differentiation from pituitary diabetes insipidus.

In addition to congenital refractoriness to antidiuretic hormone, obstructive uropathy, lithium, methoxyflurane, and demeclocycline may also render the tubule refractory.

Symptoms are related to an inability to reabsorb water, with resultant polyuria and polydipsia. The urine volume approaches 12 L/d, and osmolality and specific gravity are low. Mental retardation, atonic bladder, and hydronephrosis occur frequently.

Treatment consists primarily of an adequate water intake. Chlorothiazide may ameliorate the diabetes; the mechanism of action is unknown, but the drug may act by increasing isosmotic reabsorption in the proximal segment of the tubule.

5. UNSPECIFIED RENAL TUBULAR ABNORMALITIES

In **idiopathic hypercalciuria,** decreased reabsorption of calcium predisposes to the formation of renal calculi. Serum calcium and phosphorus are normal. Urine calcium excretion is high; urine phosphorus excretion is low.

See treatment of urinary stones containing calcium.

REFERENCES

General

Anaemia of chronic renal failure. (Editorial.) *Lancet* 1983;**1:**965.

Anderson RJ, Schrier RW: *Clinical Uses of Drugs in Patients With Kidney and Liver Disease.* Saunders, 1981.

Bennett WM et al: Drug prescribing in renal failure: Dosing guidelines for adults. *Am J Kidney Dis* 1983;**3:**155.

Brenner BM, Rector FC Jr: *The Kidney,* 3rd ed. Saunders, 1986.

Carvalho AC: Bleeding in a uremia: A clinical challenge. (Editorial.) *N Engl J Med* 1983;**308:**38.

Heptinstall RH: *Pathology of the Kidney,* 3rd ed. Little, Brown, 1983.

Klahr S: Pathophysiology of obstructive nephropathy. *Kidney Int* 1983;**23:**414.

Krupp MA: Genitourinary tract. Chapter 15 in: *Current Medical Diagnosis & Treatment 1987.* Krupp MA, Tierney LM Jr, Schroeder SA (editors). Appleton & Lange, 1987.

Massry SG, Glasscock RJ: *Textbook of Nephrology.* Williams & Wilkins, 1983.

Nephrology: An annotated bibliography of recent literature. *Ann Intern Med* 1983;**98:**563.

Schrier RW (editor): *Renal and Electrolyte Disorders,* 2nd ed. Little, Brown, 1980.

Urinalysis

Haber MH: *Urine Casts: Their Microscopy and Clinical Significance.* American Society of Clinical Pathologists, 1975.

Hauglustaine D et al: Detection of glomerular bleeding using a simple staining method for light microscopy. *Lancet* 1982;**2:**761.

Stamey TA, Kindrachuk RW: *Urinary Sediment and Urinalysis: A Practical Guide for the Health Professional.* Saunders, 1985.

Sternheimer R: A supravital cytodiagnostic stain for urinary sediments. *JAMA* 1975;**231:**826.

Glomerulonephritis

Baldwin DS: Chronic glomerulonephritis: Nonimmunologic mechanisms of progressive glomerular damage. *Kidney Int* 1982;**21:**109.

Carpenter CB: Immunologic aspects of renal disease. *Annu Rev Med* 1970;**21:**1.

Couser WG: Mesangial IgA nephropathies: Steady progress. (Editorial.) *West J Med* 1984;**140:**89.

Couser WG: What are circulating immune complexes doing in glomerulonephritis? (Editorial.) *N Engl J Med* 1981;**304:**1230.

Culpepper RM, Andreoli TE: The pathophysiology of the glomerulopathies. *Adv Intern Med* 1983;**28:**161.

Hood SA et al: IgA-IgG nephropathy: Predictive indices of progressive disease. *Clin Nephrol* 1981;**16:**55.

Seymour AE: Glomerulonephritis: Approach to classification. *Pathology* 1985;**17:**219.

Wilson CB: Immunological mechanisms of glomerulonephritis. *Calif Med* (March) 1972;**116:**56.

Nephrotic Syndrome

Cogan MG: Nephrotic syndrome. *West J Med* 1982;**136:**411.

Glasscock RJ et al: Primary glomerular disease. Page 955 in: *The Kidney,* 3rd ed. Brenner BM, Rector FC Jr (editors). Saunders, 1986.

Harrington JT: Thrombolytic therapy in renal vein thrombosis. (Editorial.) *Arch Intern Med* 1984;**144:**33.

Kaplan BS, Klassen J, Gault MH: Glomerular injury in patients with neoplasia. *Annu Rev Med* 1976;**27:**117.

Ponticelli C: Prognosis and treatment of membranous nephropathy. *Kidney Int* 1986;**29:**927.

Interstitial Nephritis

Blackshear JL, Davidman M, Stillman MT: Identification of risk for renal insufficiency from nonsteroidal anti-inflammatory drugs. *Arch Intern Med* 1983;**143:**1130.

Carmichael J, Shankel SW: Effects of nonsteroidal anti-inflammatory drugs on prostaglandins and renal function. *AM J Med* 1985;**78:**992.

Clive DM, Stoff JS: Renal syndromes associated with nonsteroidal anti-inflammatory drugs. *N Engl J Med* 1984;**310:**563.

Eknoyan G et al: Renal papillary necrosis: An update. *Medicine* 1982;**61:**55.

Garella S, Matarese RA: Renal effects of prostaglandins and clinical adverse effects of nonsteroidal anti-inflammatory agents. *Medicine* 1984;**63:**165.

Hartman GW et al: Analgesic-associated nephropathy: Pathophysiological and radiological correlation. *JAMA* 1984;**251:**1734.

Cystic Disease

Gardner KD Jr (editor): *Cystic Diseases of the Kidney.* Wiley, 1976.

Hatfield PM, Pfister RC: Adult polycystic disease of the kidneys (Potter type 3). *JAMA* 1972;**222:**1527.

Wahlqvist L: Cystic disorders of kidney: Review of pathogenesis and classification. *J Urol* 1967;**97:**1.

Tubule Disorders

Brenner RJ et al: Incidence of radiographically evident bone disease, nephrocalcinosis, and nephrolithiasis in various types of renal tubular acidosis. *N Engl J Med* 1982; **307:**217.

Chan JC, Alon U: Tubular disorders of acid-base and phosphate metabolism. *Nephron* 1985;**40:**257.

Hruska KA, Ban D, Avioli LV: Renal tubular acidosis. *Arch Intern Med* 1982;**142:**1909.

Mattern WD: Renal tubular acidosis. *Kidney* 1982;**15:**11.

Morris RC Jr: Renal tubular acidosis. (Editorial.) *N Engl J Med* 1981;**304:**418.

Morris RC Jr, Sebastian A: Disorders of renal tubules that cause disorders of fluid, acid-base, and electrolyte metabolism. In: *Clinical Disorders of Fluid and Electrolyte Metabolism,* 3rd ed. Maxwell MH, Kleeman CR (editors). McGraw-Hill, 1980.

Segal S: Disorders of renal amino acid transport. *N Engl J Med* 1976;**294:**1044.

Stanbury JB et al (editors): *The Metabolic Basis of Inherited Disease,* 5th ed. McGraw-Hill, 1983.

25 Oliguria; Acute Renal Failure

William J.C. Amend, Jr., MD, & Flavio G. Vincenti, MD

Oliguria literally means "too little" urine volume in response to the body's excretory needs. Oliguria is present when the daily urine volume is not sufficient to remove the endogenous solute loads that are the end products of metabolism. No precise figure for 24-hour urine volume can be used in defining oliguria, since urine volumes normally vary with fluid intake and the concentrating ability of the kidney. If the kidney can concentrate urine in a normal fashion to a specific gravity of 1.035, oliguria is present at urine volumes under 400 mL/d. On the other hand, if the kidney concentration is impaired and the patient can achieve a specific gravity of only 1.010, oliguria is present at urine volumes under 1000–1500 mL/d.

Acute renal failure is a condition in which the glomerular filtration rate is abruptly reduced, causing a sudden retention of endogenous metabolites (urea, potassium, phosphate, sulfate, creatinine) that are normally cleared by the kidneys. The urine volume is usually low (under 400 mL/d). However, if renal concentrating mechanisms are impaired (see above), the daily urine volume may be normal or even high ("high-output" or "nonoliguric" renal failure). Rarely, there is no urine output at all (anuria) in acute renal failure.

The causes of acute renal failure are listed in Table 25–1. Prompt differentiation of the cause is important in determining appropriate therapy. Prerenal renal failure is reversible if treated promptly, but a delay in therapy may allow it to progress into a fixed, nonspecific form of intrinsic renal failure (eg, acute tubular necrosis). The other causes of acute renal failure are classified on the basis of their involvement with vascular lesions, intrarenal disorders, or postrenal disorders.

PRERENAL RENAL FAILURE

The term prerenal denotes inadequate renal perfusion because of inadequate or ineffective intravascular volume. The most common cause of this form of acute renal failure is dehydration due to renal or extrarenal fluid losses from diarrhea, vomiting, excessive use of diuretics, etc. Less common causes are septic shock and excessive use of antihypertensive drugs, which cause relative or absolute depletion of intravascular fluid volume. Heart failure with reduced cardiac output can also reduce effective renal blood flow. Careful clinical assessment may identify the primary condition responsible for prerenal renal failure.

Clinical Findings

A. Symptoms and Signs: Except for rare cases with associated cardiac or "pump" failure, patients usually complain of thirst or of dizziness in the upright posture (orthostatic dizziness). There may be a history of overt fluid loss. Sudden weight loss usually reflects the degree of dehydration.

Physical examination frequently reveals poor skin turgor, collapsed neck veins, dry mucous membranes and axillas, and, most importantly, orthostatic or postural changes in blood pressure and pulse.

B. Laboratory Findings:

1. Urine– The urine volume is usually low. Accurate assessment may require bladder catheterization followed by hourly output measurements (which will also rule out lower urinary tract obstruction; see below). High urine specific gravity (> 1.025) and urine osmolality (> 600 mosm/kg) also are noted in this

Table 25–1. Etiology of acute renal failure.

I. Prerenal renal failure:
1. Dehydration.
2. Vascular collapse due to sepsis, antihypertensive drug therapy.
3. Reduced cardiac output.
4. Antihypertensive drugs (eg, captopril) interfering with autoregulation.

II. Vascular:
1. Atheroembolism.
2. Dissecting arterial aneurysms.
3. Malignant hypertension.

III. Parenchymal (intrarenal):
1. Specific:
   a. Glomerulonephritis.
   b. Interstitial nephritis.
   c. Toxin, dye-induced.
2. Nonspecific:
   a. Acute tubular necrosis.
   b. Acute cortical necrosis.

IV. Functional-hemodynamic:
1. Captopril.
2. Nonsteroidal anti-inflammatory drugs.
3. Cyclosporine.

V. Postrenal:
1. Calculus in patients with solitary kidney.
2. Bilateral ureteral obstruction.
3. Outlet obstruction.
4. Leak, posttraumatic.

form of acute renal failure. Routine urinalysis is generally not helpful.

2. Urine and blood chemistries—The blood urea nitrogen/creatinine ratio, normally 10:1, is usually increased with prerenal renal failure. Other findings are set forth in Table 25–2. Because mannitol and other diuretics affect the delivery and tubular handling of urea, sodium, and creatinine, urine and blood chemistry tests performed after these agents have been given will produce misleading results.

3. Central venous pressure—A low central venous pressure indicates hypovolemia, which may be due to blood loss or dehydration. If severe cardiac failure is the principal cause of prerenal renal failure (it is rarely the sole cause), reduced cardiac output and high central venous pressure will be apparent.

4. Fluid challenge—An increase in urine output in response to a carefully administered fluid challenge is both diagnostic and therapeutic in prerenal renal failure. Rapid intravenous administration of 300–500 mL of physiologic saline or 125 mL of 20% mannitol (25 g/125 mL) is the usual initial treatment. Urine output is measured over the subsequent 1–3 hours. A urine volume of more than 50 mL/h is considered a favorable response that warrants continued intravenous infusion with physiologic solutions to restore plasma volume and correct dehydration. If the urine volume does not increase, the physician should carefully review the results of blood and urine chemistry tests, reassess the patient's fluid status, and repeat the physical examination to determine if an additional fluid challenge (with or without furosemide) might be worthwhile.

Treatment

In states of dehydration, measured and estimated fluid losses must be rapidly corrected to treat oliguria of prerenal origin. Inadequate fluid management may cause further renal hemodynamic deterioration and eventual renal tubular degeneration (fixed acute tubular necrosis; see below). If oliguria persists in a well-hydrated patient, vasopressor drugs are indicated in an effort to correct the hypotension associated with sepsis or cardiogenic shock. Pressor agents that restore systemic blood pressure while maintaining renal blood

flow and renal function (eg, dopamine, 1–5 μg/kg/min) are most useful. Discontinuance of antihypertensive medications or diuretics can, by itself, cure the apparent acute renal failure resulting from prerenal causes.

VASCULAR RENAL FAILURE

Common causes of acute renal failure due to vascular disease include atheroembolic disease, dissecting arterial aneurysms, and malignant hypertension. Atheroembolic disease is rare before age 60 and in patients who have not undergone vascular procedures or angiographic studies. Dissecting arterial aneurysms and malignant hypertension are usually clinically evident. Acute renal venous thrombosis, unless it affects both kidneys, has no deleterious effect on renal clearance function.

Rapid assessment of the arterial blood supply to the kidney requires arteriography. The cause of malignant hypertension may be identified on physical examination (scleroderma, etc). Primary management of the vascular process is necessary to affect any renal failure.

INTRARENAL DISEASE STATES; INTRARENAL ACUTE RENAL FAILURE

Diseases in this category can be divided into specific and nonspecific parenchymal processes.

1. SPECIFIC INTRARENAL DISEASE STATES

The most common causes of intrarenal acute renal failure are acute or rapidly progressive glomerulonephritis, acute interstitial nephritis, and toxic nephropathies.

Clinical Findings

A. Symptoms and Signs: Usually the history shows some salient data such as sore throat or upper respiratory infection, use of antibiotics, or intravenous use of drugs (often illicit types). Bilateral back pain, at times severe, is occasionally noted. Gross hematuria may be present. It is unusual for pyelonephritis to present as acute renal failure unless there is (1) associated sepsis or dehydration, (2) obstruction, or (3) involvement of a solitary kidney. Systemic diseases in which acute renal failure occurs include Henoch-Schönlein purpura, thrombotic thrombocytopenic purpura, systemic lupus erythematosus, and scleroderma.

B. Laboratory Findings:

1. Urine—Urinalysis discloses many red and white cells and multiple types of cellular and granular casts ("telescopic urine"). In allergic interstitial nephritis, eosinophils may be noted. The urine sodium concentration may range from 10 to 40 meq/L.

Table 25–2. Acute renal failure versus prerenal azotemia.

	Acute Renal Failure	Prerenal Azotemia
Urine osmolality (mosm/L)	< 350	> 500
Urine/plasma urea	< 10	> 20
Urine/plasma creatinine	< 20	> 40
Urine Na (meq/L)	> 40	< 20
Renal failure index = $\dfrac{U_{Na}}{U/P_{Cr}}$	> 1	< 1
*FE_{Na} = $\dfrac{U/P_{Na}}{U/P_{Cr}}$ X 100	> 1	< 1

*Excreted fraction of filtered sodium. See Espinel CH: *JAMA* 1976;**236**:579; and Miller TR et al: *Ann Intern Med* 1978; **89**:47.

2. Serum—Components of serum complement are often diminished during deposition of immune complexes. In a few laboratories, circulating immune complexes can be identified. Other tests may disclose systemic diseases such as lupus erythematosus and thrombotic thrombocytopenic purpura.

3. Renal biopsy—Biopsy examination will show characteristic changes of acute interstitial nephritis or glomerulonephritis. There may be extensive crescents involving Browman's space.

C. X-Ray Findings: Poor visualization on intravenous urography or radionuclide renal scans is characteristic. Routine intravenous urography should be avoided because of the risk of dye-induced renal injury. For this reason, sonography is preferable.

Treatment

Therapy is directed toward eradication of infection, removal of antigen, elimination of toxic materials and drugs, suppression of autoimmune mechanisms, removal of autoimmune antibodies, or a reduction in effector-inflammatory responses. Immunotherapy may involve drugs, anticoagulants, or the temporary use of plasmapheresis.

2. NONSPECIFIC INTRARENAL STATES

These include acute tubular necrosis and acute cortical necrosis. The latter presents with anuria and associated intrarenal intravascular coagulation and has a generally poorer prognosis than the former.

Acute tubular necrosis was initially described by Lücke in World War II in patients suffering crush injuries and shock. Degenerative changes of the more distal tubules (lower nephron nephrosis) were believed to be due to ischemia. When dialysis became available, most of these patients recovered—sometimes completely—provided that intrarenal intravascular coagulation and cortical necrosis had not occurred.

Elderly patients are more prone to develop this form of oliguric acute renal failure following hypotensive episodes. It appears that exposure to certain drugs (eg, prostaglandin inhibitors such as nonsteroidal anti-inflammatory agents) may predispose patients to a greater risk of acute tubular necrosis. Although the classic picture of lower nephron nephrosis may not develop, a similar nonspecific acute renal failure is noted in some cases of mercury (especially mercuric chloride) poisoning and following exposure to radiocontrast agents in patients with diabetes mellitus or myeloma.

Clinical Findings

A. Symptoms and Signs: Usually the clinical picture is that of the associated clinical state. Dehydration and shock may be present concurrently but fail to improve following administration of intravenous fluids as with prerenal renal failure (see above). There may be only signs of excessive fluid retention in post-radiocontrast cases of acute renal failure. Symptoms

of uremia per se (ie, altered mentation or gastrointestinal symptoms) are unusual in acute renal failure (in contrast to patients with chronic renal failure).

B. Laboratory Findings: (See also Table 25-2.)

1. Urine—Although the specific gravity may be high immediately after the acute event, it usually becomes low or fixed in the 1.005–1.015 range. Urine osmolality is also low (< 450 mosm/kg and U/P osmolal ratio $< 1.5:1$). Urinalysis often discloses tubular cells and granular casts; the urine may be muddy brown. If the test for occult blood is positive, one must be concerned about the presence of myoglobin as well as hemoglobin. Tests for differentiating myoglobin pigment are available.

2. Central venous pressure—This is usually normal to slightly elevated.

3. Fluid challenges—There is no increase in urine volume following intravenous administration of mannitol or physiologic saline. Occasionally following the use of furosemide, a low urine output will be converted to a high fixed urine output (low-output renal failure to high-output renal failure), but there is no change in the rate of increase of blood urea nitrogen or creatinine.

Treatment

If there is no response to the initial fluid or mannitol challenge, the volume of administered fluid must be sharply curtailed and the amount given related to the measured urine volume. An early assessment of the rate of rise of serum creatinine and blood urea nitrogen and of the concentrations of electrolytes is necessary to provide criteria for possible use of dialysis therapy. There is some evidence that early use of hyperalimentation might be beneficial in reducing both the need for dialysis and morbidity and mortality rates. With appropriate regulation of the volume of fluid administered, solutions of glucose and essential amino acids to provide 30–35 kcal/kg may be used to correct or reduce the severity of the catabolic state accompanying acute tubular necrosis.

Serum or plasma potassium must be closely monitored and serial ECGs done to ensure early recognition of hyperkalemia. This condition can be treated with (1) intravenous sodium bicarbonate administration, (2) Kayexalate, 25–50 g (with sorbital) orally or by enema, (3) intravenous glucose and insulin, and (4) intravenous calcium preparations to prevent cardiac irritability. Peritoneal dialysis or hemodialysis should be used as necessary to avoid or correct uremia, hypokalemia, or fluid overload.

Prognosis

Most cases are reversible within 7–14 days. Residual renal damage may be noted, particularly in elderly patients.

POSTRENAL ACUTE RENAL FAILURE

The conditions listed in Table 25–1 involve primarily urologic diagnostic and therapeutic interventions. Following lower abdominal surgery, urethral or ureteral obstruction should be considered as a cause of acute renal failure. The causes of bilateral ureteral obstruction are (1) peritoneal or retroperitoneal neoplastic involvement, with masses or nodes; (2) retroperitoneal fibrosis; (3) calculous disease; or (4) postsurgical or traumatic interruption. With a solitary kidney, ureteral stones can produce total urinary tract obstruction and acute renal failure. Urethral or bladder neck obstruction is a frequent cause of renal failure, especially in elderly men. Posttraumatic urethral tears are discussed in Chapter 17.

Clinical Findings

A. Symptoms and Signs: Renal pain and renal tenderness may often be present. If there has been an operative ureteral injury with associated urine extravasation, urine may leak through a wound. Edema from overhydration may be noted. Ileus is often present along with associated abdominal distention and vomiting.

B. Laboratory Findings: Urinalysis is usually not helpful. A large volume of urine obtained by catheterization may be both diagnostic and therapeutic for lower tract obstruction.

C. X-Ray Findings: Poor visualization on intravenous urography is characteristic. Radionuclide renal scans may show a urine leak or, in cases of obstruction, retention of the isotope in the renal pelvis. Renal scans are helpful in acute but not in chronic obstruction. Ultrasound examination will often reveal a dilated upper collecting system with deformities characteristic of hydronephrosis.

D. Instrumental Examination: Cystoscopy and retrograde ureteral catheterization will demonstrate ureteral obstruction.

Treatment

For further discussion of ureteral injuries, see Chapter 17.

REFERENCES

Abel RM et al: Improved survival from acute renal failure after treatment with intravenous essential L-amino acids and glucose: Results of a prospective, double-blind study. *N Engl J Med* 1973;**288:**695.

Anderson RJ et al: Nonoliguric acute renal failure. *N Engl J Med* 1977;**296:**1134.

Cohn HE, Capelli JP: The diagnosis and management of oliguria in the postoperative period. *Surg Clin North Am* 1967; **47:**1187.

Davis BB Jr, Knox FG: Current concepts of the regulation of urinary sodium excretion: A review. *Am J Med Sci* 1970; **259:**373.

Figueroa JE: Acute renal failure: Its unusual causes and manifestations. *Med Clin North Am* 1967;**51:**995.

Hall JW et al: Immediate and long-term prognosis in acute renal failure. *Ann Intern Med* 1970;**73:**515.

Harrington JT, Cohen JJ: Acute oliguria. *N Engl J Med* 1975;**292:**89.

Lewers DJ et al: Long-term follow up of renal function and histology after acute tubular necrosis. *Ann Intern Med* 1970; **73:**523.

Lyon RP: Nonobstructive oliguria: Differential diagnosis. *Calif Med* 1963;**99:**83.

McMurray SD et al: Prevailing patterns and predictor values in patients with acute tubular necrosis. *Arch Intern Med* 1978;**138:**950.

Miller TR et al: Urinary diagnostic indices in acute renal failure: A prospective study. *Ann Intern Med* 1978;**89:**47.

Myers BD, Moran SM: Hemodynamically mediated acute renal failure. *N Engl J Med* 1986;**314:**97.

Schrier RW: Nephrology forum: Acute renal failure. *Kidney Int* 1979;**15:**205.

Tan SY, Shapiro R, Kish MA: Reversible acute renal failure induced by indomethacin. *JAMA* 1979;**241:**2732.

Wilkes BM, Mailloux LU: Acute renal failure: Pathogenesis and prevention. *Am J Med* 1986;**80:**1129.

26

Chronic Renal Failure & Dialysis

William J.C. Amend, Jr., MD, & Flavio G. Vincenti, MD

In chronic renal failure, reduced clearance of certain solutes principally excreted by the kidney results in their retention in the body fluids. The solutes are end products of the metabolism of substances of exogenous origin (eg, food) or endogenous origin (eg, catabolism of tissue). The most commonly used indicators of renal failure are blood urea nitrogen and serum creatinine. However, marked elevation of blood urea nitrogen can be due to nonrenal causes such as prerenal azotemia, gastrointestinal hemorrhage, or high protein intake. The clearance of creatinine can be used as a reasonable measure of glomerular filtration rate (GFR).

Renal failure may be classified as acute or chronic depending on the rapidity of onset and the subsequent course of azotemia. An analysis of the acute or chronic development of renal failure is important in understanding physiologic adaptations, disease mechanisms, and ultimate therapy. In individual cases, it is often difficult to establish the duration of renal failure. Historic clues such as preceding hypertension or radiologic findings such as small, shrunken kidneys tend to indicate a more chronic process. Certain forms of acute renal failure tend to progress to irreversible chronic renal failure.

For a discussion of acute renal failure, see Chapter 25.

The general incidence of chronic renal failure in the USA, defined as "people who can benefit from hemodialysis or renal transplantation," is 50 per million population per year. The medical acceptance criteria are strict. All age groups are affected. The severity and the rapidity of development of uremia are hard to predict. The use of dialysis and transplantation is expanding rapidly worldwide. Ninety thousand patients are currently being treated with either dialysis or transplantation, and it is estimated that 95,000 patients will be treated each year by 1988.

A trend of increasingly older patients has been noted in both treatment modality groups.

Historical Background

There are various causes of progressive renal dysfunction leading to end stage or terminal renal failure. In the 1800s, Bright described several cases that presented with edema, hematuria, and proteinuria and ended in death. Early chemical analyses of patients' sera drew attention to retained nonprotein nitrogen

(NPN) compounds, and an association was made between this and the clinical findings of uremia. Although the pathologic state of uremia was well described in the intervening years, long-term survival rates were not achieved in substantial numbers of patients until chronic renal dialysis and renal transplantation became available.

Etiology

A variety of disorders are associated with end stage renal disease. Either a primary renal process (eg, glomerulonephritis, pyelonephritis, congenital hypoplasia) or a secondary one (eg, a kidney affected by a systemic process such as diabetes mellitus or lupus erythematosus) may be responsible. Minor physiologic alterations secondary to dehydration, infection, or hypertension often "tip the scale" and put a borderline patient into uncompensated clinical uremia.

Clinical Findings

A. Symptoms and Signs: Symptoms such as pruritus, generalized malaise, lassitude, forgetfulness, loss of libido, nausea, and altered behavior patterns are subtle complaints in this chronic disorder. There is often a strong family history of renal disease. Growth failure is a primary complaint in preadolescent patients. Symptoms of a multisystem disorder (eg, arthritis in lupus erythematosus) may be present coincidentally. Most patients with renal failure have elevated blood pressure secondary to volume overload and overhydration. Occasionally, hyperreninemic conditions may be present. However, the blood pressure may be normal or low if patients are on a very low sodium diet or have marked salt-losing tendencies (eg, medullary cystic disease). The pulse and respiratory rates are rapid as manifestations of anemia and metabolic acidosis. Clinical findings of uremic fetor, pericarditis, neurologic findings of asterixis, reduced mentation, and peripheral neuropathy are often present. Palpable kidneys suggest polycystic disease. Ophthalmoscopic examination may show hypertensive or diabetic retinopathy. Alterations involving the cornea have been associated with metabolic disease (eg, Fabry's disease, cystinosis).

B. Laboratory Findings:

1. Urine composition–The urine volume varies depending on the severity and type of renal disease. Quantitatively normal amounts of water and salt losses in urine can be associated with polycystic and interstitial forms of disease. Usually, however, urine volumes are quite low when the GFR falls below 5% of normal. Daily salt losses become more fixed, and, if low, a state of sodium retention occurs soon after. Proteinuria may be variable but often is not excessive when the GFR is severely reduced.

2. Blood studies–Anemia is the rule, but the hematocrit may be normal in polycystic disease. Platelet dysfunction or thrombasthenia is characterized by abnormal bleeding times. Platelet counts and prothrombin content are normal.

Several abnormalities in serum electrolytes and mineral metabolism become manifest when the GFR drops below 30 mL/min. Progressive reduction of body buffer stores and an inability to excrete titrable acids results in progressive acidosis characterized by reduced serum bicarbonate and compensatory respiratory hyperventilation. The metabolic acidosis of uremia is associated with a normal anion gap, hyperchloremia, and normokalemia. Hyperkalemia is not usually seen unless the GFR is below 5 mL/min or conditions are present that predispose to an increase in serum potassium (ie, intercurrent illness associated with increased catabolism or acute acidosis). Patients with interstitial renal diseases, gouty nephropathy, and diabetic nephropathy may develop hyperchloremic metabolic acidosis with hyperkalemia (renal tubular acidosis, type IV) even when the GFR is over 30 mL/min. The acidosis and hyperkalemia are out of proportion to the degree of renal failure and are related to a decrease in renin and aldosterone secretion. Multiple factors lead to an increase in serum phosphate and a decrease in serum calcium. Uremic patients have a reduced appetite and thus ingest less calcium. In addition, vitamin D activity is diminished because of reduced conversion of vitamin D_2 to active vitamin D_3 in the kidney. The hyperphosphatemia develops as a consequence of reduced phosphate clearance by the kidney. These alterations lead to secondary hyperparathyroidism with skeletal changes of both osteomalacia and osteitis fibrosa cystica. Uric acid levels are frequently elevated secondary to reduced renal excretion but rarely lead to calculi or gout.

C. X-Ray Findings: Infusion nephrotomograms are required if the serum creatinine is 3 mg/dL or more. They will usually reveal small kidneys, congenital hypoplasia, polycystic disease, or some other structural disorder. Bone x-rays may show retarded growth, osteomalacia (renal rickets), or osteitis fibrosa. Soft tissue calcification may be present.

Renal sonograms are helpful in determining renal size and cortical thickness and in localizing tissue for percutaneous renal biopsy.

D. Renal Biopsy: Renal biopsies may not reveal much except end stage scarring and glomerulosclerosis. There may be pronounced vascular changes consisting of thickening of the media, fragmentation of elastic fibers, and intimal proliferation, which may be secondary to uremic hypertension or due to primary arteriolar nephrosclerosis. Percutaneous or open biopsies of end stage shrunken kidneys are associated with a high morbidity rate, particularly bleeding. However, if kidney size is still normal, a renal biopsy may be diagnostic. Appropriate examination by light microscopy, immunofluorescence, and electron microscopy is also indicated.

Treatment

Management should be conservative until it becomes impossible for patients to continue their customary life-styles. Conservative management includes restriction of dietary protein (0.5 g/kg/d), potassium, and phosphorus, as well as close sodium balance in the diet so that patients do not retain sodium or become sodium depleted. Use of bicarbonate can be helpful when moderate acidemia occurs. Transfusions may be helpful, but fresh blood should be used to avoid excessive release of potassium. Prevention of possible uremic osteodystrophy requires close attention to calcium and phosphorus balance; phosphate-retaining antacids and administration of calcium or vitamin D may be needed to maintain the balance. Extreme care must be paid to this management, however, because if the Ca × P product is greater than 65 mg/dL, metastatic calcifications can occur.

A. Chronic Peritoneal Dialysis: Chronic peritoneal dialysis is used electively or when circumstances (ie, no available vascular access) prohibit chronic hemodialysis. Improved soft catheters (Tenckhoff) can be used repeatedly. In comparison to hemodialysis, small molecules (such as creatinine and urea) are cleared less effectively than larger molecules (vitamin B_{12}), but excellent treatment can be accomplished. Either intermittent thrice-weekly treatment (IPPD) or chronic ambulatory peritoneal dialysis (CAPD) is possible. With the latter, the patient performs 3–5 daily exchanges using 1–2 L of dialysate at each exchange. Bacterial contamination and peritonitis are becoming less common with improvements in technology.

B. Chronic Hemodialysis: Chronic hemodialysis using semipermeable dialysis membranes is now widely performed. Access to the vascular system is by means of Scribner shunts, arteriovenous fistulas, and grafts. The actual dialyzers may be of a parallel plate, coil, or hollow fiber type. Body solutes and excessive body fluids can be easily cleared by using dialysate fluids of known chemical composition. Newer high-efficiency membranes are serving to reduce dialysis treatment time.

Treatment is intermittent—usually 3–5 hours 3 times weekly. It may be given in a kidney center, a satellite unit, or the home. Very ill patients or those who for any reason cannot be trained in the use of the equipment with an assistant require treatment in a dialysis center. Home dialysis is optimal because it provides greater scheduling flexibility and is generally more comfortable and convenient for the patient, but only 30% of dialysis patients meet the medical and training requirements for this type of therapy.

More widespread use of dialytic techniques has

permitted greater patient mobility. Treatment on vacations and business trips can be provided by prior arrangement.

Common problems with either type of chronic dialysis include infection, bone symptoms, technical accidents, persistent anemia, and psychologic disorders. The morbidity associated with atherosclerosis often occurs with long-term treatment. Bilateral nephrectomy should be avoided, because it increases the transfusion requirements of dialysis patients as well as the attendant morbidity and mortality risk from the procedure. Nephrectomy in dialysis patients should be performed in cases of refractory hypertension, reflux, and polycystic disease with recurrent bleeding and pain.

Yearly costs range from an average of $15,000 for patients who receive dialysis at home to as much as $30,000–$50,000 for patients treated at dialysis centers, but much of this is absorbed under HR-1 (Medicare) legislation. The mortality rates are 8–10% per year once maintenance dialysis therapy is instituted. Despite these medical, psychologic, social, and financial difficulties, most patients lead productive lives while receiving dialysis treatments.

C. Renal Transplantation: After immunosuppression techniques and genetic matching were developed, renal homotransplantation became an acceptable alternative to maintenance hemodialysis. Improved transplantation results are now noted due to the development of newer immunosuppressant drugs (cyclosporine and antilymphocyte preparations). The great advantage of transplantation is reestablishment of nearly normal constant body physiology and chemistry without intermittent dialysis. Diet can be less restrictive. The disadvantages include bone marrow suppression, susceptibility to infection, cushingoid body habitus, and the psychologic uncertainty of the homograft's future. Most of the disadvantages of transplantation are related to the medicines (azathioprine and corticosteroids) given to counteract the rejection. Later problems with transplantation include recurrent disease in the transplanted kidney. Genitourinary infection appears to be of minor importance if structural urologic complications (eg, leaks) do not occur.

Nephrology centers, with close cooperation between medical and surgical staff, attempt to use these treatment alternatives of dialysis and transplantation in an integrated fashion.

For a more detailed review, see Chapter 27.

REFERENCES

Bell PRF, Calman KC: *Surgical Aspects of Hemodialysis.* Churchill Livingstone, 1974.

Bricker NS: Adaptations in chronic uremia: Pathophysiologic "trade-offs." *Hosp Pract* (July) 1974;**9**:119.

Dunham C, Mattern WD, McGaghie WC: Preferences of nephrologists among end-stage renal disease treatment options. *Am J Nephrol* 1985;**5**:470.

Evans RW et al: The quality of life of patients with end-stage renal disease. *N Engl J Med* 1985;**312**:553.

Freeman RB: Treatment of chronic renal failure: An update. (Editorial.) *N Engl J Med* 1985;**312**:577.

Friedman E et al: Pragmatic realities in uremia therapy. *N Engl J Med* 1978;**298**:368.

Hampers CL, Schupak E: *Long-Term Hemodialysis,* 2nd ed. Grune & Stratton, 1973.

Laouari D, Kleinknecht C: The role of nutritional factors in the course of experimental renal failure. *Am J Kid Dis* 1985;**5**:147.

Lazarus JM: Complications in hemodialysis: An overview. *Kidney Int* 1980;**18**:783.

Merrill JP, Hampers CL: Uremia. (2 parts.) *N Engl J Med* 1970;**282**:953, 1014.

Nolph KD et al: Continuous ambulatory peritoneal dialysis in the United States: A three-year study. *Kidney Int* 1985;**28**:198.

Novick AC: Progress in renal transplantation. (Editorial.) *J Urol* 1985;**133**:439.

Proceedings of a conference on adequacy of dialysis: Eighth Scientific Conference of the Artificial Kidney-Chronic Uremia Program. *Kidney Int* 1975;**7 (Suppl 2)**:S1–S265. [Entire issue.]

Rubin J et al: Peritonitis during continuous ambulatory peritoneal dialysis. *Ann Intern Med* 1980;**92**:7.

Strange PD, Sumner AT: Predicting treatment costs and life expectancy in end stage renal disease. *N Engl J Med* 1978;**298**:372.

Renal Transplantation

27

Oscar Salvatierra, Jr., MD, & Nicholas J. Feduska, MD

Renal transplantation is an effective form of therapy for patients with end stage renal disease. More than 2800 renal transplants have been performed at the University of California, San Francisco (UCSF), and many of the conclusions in this chapter are based on that experience. Although the immunologic problems of rejection remain unchanged, technical complications and patient mortality rates have been significantly reduced by detailed attention to cadaver organ recovery and preservation, surgical techniques, and elimination of prolonged use of corticosteroids in high doses. Graft survival has been significantly improved by use of donor-specific blood transfusions before transplantation from a living related donor and by use of the new immunosuppressive agent cyclosporine, particularly in cadaver transplantation.

Selection & Preparation of Recipients

The principal indication for renal transplantation is end stage renal failure. According to the last report of the Human Renal Transplant Registry, the following are the most common diseases treated by renal transplantation: chronic glomerulonephritis (54%), chronic pyelonephritis (12%), polycystic kidney disease (5%), and malignant nephrosclerosis (6%). Other diseases, including hereditary nephritis, account for 23% of cases.

A. Exclusions: Patients with active infections, as well as those whose end stage renal failure is due to primary oxalosis, are generally not accepted for transplantation. Patients with systemic diseases such as juvenile diabetes mellitus and lupus erythematosus, however, are acceptable.

B. Preliminary Nephrectomy: Approximately 90% of all patients now receive transplants with their own kidneys left in situ. The indications for preliminary nephrectomy are as follows:

1. Anatomic abnormalities of the urinary tract with or without infection, eg, hydronephrosis or a moderate degree of ureteral reflux. In patients with reflux or ureteral abnormalities, nephroureterectomy should be performed.

2. Severe hypertension uncontrolled by medications or dialysis. This is currently a rare indication for nephrectomy.

3. Some cases of polycystic renal disease. If the patient has pyelonephritis or a history of hematuria re-

quiring blood transfusions, preparation by nephrectomy is a prerequisite to transplantation. In the absence of these factors, transplantation without nephrectomy is preferred and has proved to be safe. The size of the polycystic kidneys is not an indication for preliminary nephrectomy in our experience.

C. Splenectomy: Some transplant centers have performed splenectomy before transplantation, but there is still no clear evidence that it modifies the immunologic reaction. In addition, there is evidence that patients (particularly children) who have undergone splenectomy are predisposed to pneumococcal and other infections.

Donor Selection

The kidney to be transplanted can be obtained from either a living related donor or a cadaver donor.

A. Living Related Donor: Living related donors currently accepted are usually siblings or parents, but in some cases, more distant relatives may be accepted.

1. Donor-recipient matching—Histocompatibility is assessed by determination of human leukocyte antigens (HLA) to establish the inheritance pattern in a family group. The best donor-recipient combinations are siblings who share all HLA antigens (HLA-identical) and whose lymphocytes are nonstimulating in the mixed lymphocyte culture. The prognosis for long-term graft survival in this case is about 90%.

2. Donor-specific blood transfusions (DST)—In 1978, at UCSF, a pretransplantation protocol was introduced in order to alter the immune response in living, related, HLA-nonidentical (either 1 or 0 haplotype match) potential transplant recipients. Three donor-specific blood transfusions from the potential kidney donor are administered to the recipient according to a uniform protocol, and serial immunologic monitoring for T-warm and B-warm cytotoxic antibodies (directed against T and B lymphocytes) is performed during and following the transfusion period. The transplant is performed no earlier than 4 weeks after the third transfusion and only if the recipient does not become sensitized to the donor. More than 300 patients have undergone transplantation from blood donors following DST. Graft survival with this new method is 95% at 1 year and 77% at 7 years. Donor-specific blood transfusions have also led to good results for poorly matched transplants in patients with juvenile-onset diabetes mellitus. In addition, patients who do show evidence of sensitization following donor-specific blood transfusions do not appear to have difficulty in receiving cadaver transplants. The prospective transplant recipient with the least chance of sensitization is a candidate who (1) is receiving a transplant for the first time and (2) demonstrates less than 10% antibodies to a selected panel of 40 donor cells.

B. Cadaver Donor: If a suitable living related donor is not available, patients with end stage renal disease must depend upon cadaver organs for transplantation.

1. Unacceptable cadaver donors—Cadaver kidneys are unacceptable in the following circumstances:

a. Kidneys from newborns and those over age 55. Early thrombosis and poor function is the fate of most newborn kidneys. Kidneys from donors over age 55 do not appear to give results comparable to those achieved with kidneys from younger donors. Kidneys from children age 10 months and older have provided an excellent source of grafts, as renal hypertrophy occurs rapidly after transplantation.

b. History of generalized or intra-abdominal sepsis.

c. Preexisting disease that imposes a risk of renal involvement, such as hypertension, diabetes, or lupus erythematosus.

d. History of malignant neoplastic disease, except in the case of some types of brain tumors, because of the risk of transplanting tumor cells with the renal graft.

2. Donor-recipient matching—

a. No correlation between the quality of the HLA match at the conventional A and B loci on the major histocompatibility complex (located on chromosome 6) and cadaver graft survival was observed with more than 1800 cadaver transplants at UCSF. We have also shown that sensitive cross-matching is especially important for recipients with preformed cytotoxic antibodies. Cross-matching is the incubation of recipient serum with donor lymphocytes. At UCSF, there has been no evidence of impaired graft survival in recipients with high levels of preformed cytotoxic antibodies, where all pretransplant antibody-reactive sera are tested.

b. Currently, efforts are under way at many centers to determine if matching at the HLA-DR locus may influence cadaver graft survival. Reports at this time are mixed.

c. It is now evident that blood transfusions prior to transplantation enhance graft survival. Transfusions were formerly withheld from patients on dialysis, but the poorer graft survival in those who had not received transfusions has led to a more favorable assessment of the possible beneficial effects of transfusions. A beneficial transfusion effect has been well accepted where conventional immunosuppression is used but may not be as pronounced with cyclosporine immunosuppression.

Organ Preservation

Preservation of the cadaver kidney prior to transplantation can be accomplished in 2 ways: by simple hypothermic storage or by pulsatile perfusion. The method of preservation does not influence graft survival provided that transplantation is carried out within the limitations of the storage method.

A. Hypothermic Storage: In simple hypothermic storage, the kidneys are removed from the cadaver donor and then rapidly cooled, usually by a combination of a flush-out solution and external cooling to reduce the core temperature. The kidneys are stored in a simple container immersed in another container packed with crushed ice. The disadvantages of this method are that preservation is not consistently reliable after 24 hours have passed, especially if warm ischemia has occurred at the time of organ recovery, and that it provides no clues to the viability or physiologic quality of the kidney. There is experience with transplantation after more extended periods of storage, but the requirement for postoperative dialysis is high.

B. Pulsatile Perfusion: The perfusate for continuous pulsatile perfusion is currently a modified albumin solution. The 2 major advantages of continuous pulsatile perfusion are that no kidneys need be discarded because of the time limitations of the storage method and that if there is a sudden influx of several cadaver organs to a single transplant center, they can be satisfactorily transplanted by a small team. Kidneys have been transplanted after storage periods of up to 3 days. Continuous perfusion also allows viability testing to be performed after donor nephrectomy and before transplantation. Viability testing is essential if donors are accepted who have been in prolonged shock or had abnormal renal function prior to death. The 3 criteria for organ viability are a warm ischemia time of less than 1 hour, adequate perfusion characteristics, and a donor serum creatinine level that is less than twice normal at the time of nephrectomy. These criteria are fully reliable if perfusion preservation is started immediately after donor nephrectomy but insufficient if the kidney has also been subjected to a period of simple cold storage prior to perfusion preservation.

When perfusion preservation was started immediately after donor nephrectomy, the postoperative dialysis rate following transplantation has been 20%, and an average of only 2 or 3 dialysis treatments was required for each patient.

The incidence of renal dysfunction is currently of extreme importance because of the greater prevalence of cyclosprine nephrotoxicity in the presence of post-transplant acute tubular necrosis.

Donor Nephrectomy

Strict adherence to technical detail during donor nephrectomy is of the utmost importance.

A. Technique of Donor Nephrectomy: Donor nephrectomy in both cadaver and living related donors must be performed so that the blood supply to the ureter from the renal vessels is preserved. Although the blood supply of the ureter in situ has multiple origins, the ureter of the transplanted kidney receives its blood supply only from renal vessel branches that course in hilar and upper periureteral fat. Thus, no dissection should be performed in the area of the renal pelvis or the hilus of the kidney. Because the ureteral blood supply courses in the adventitia, the ureter must also be meticulously removed with adequate surrounding tissue. For maximum assurance of preservation of the ureteral blood supply, hilar and periureteral fatty tissue is removed en bloc with the kidney and ureter.

B. Management of Multiple Vessels: If multiple vessels are found in a cadaver kidney, the kidney is removed en bloc with the aorta, so that it can be perfused through the aorta. Subsequently, the kidney can be transplanted with a Carrel patch of aorta including the multiple vessels. If the vessels are in close proximity to each other, a single Carrel patch will suffice, but if the vessels are some distance apart, 2 Carrel patches are preferable. Since all living related donors have preoperative arteriograms, the presence of multiple arteries is determined prior to transplantation. Most donors have a single artery to at least one of their kidneys. Sometimes, a living related donor kidney with multiple arteries must be used but without a Carrel patch, because removal of a portion of the donor aorta would involve increased donor risk.

C. Treatment of Living Related Donor: Anesthesia is not started in the donor until intravenous hydration has resulted in excellent diuresis. If anesthesia is induced prior to diuresis, the ADH (antidiuretic hormone, vasopressin) effect will make it difficult to obtain diuresis after induction of anesthesia. In donor nephrectomy, it is also important to avoid traction on the pedicle and to feel the kidney frequently during manipulation in order to be certain that it is well perfused. It is stimulation of the nerve supply to the kidney during dissection that produces vasospasm and causes the kidney to become soft, with no urine output. If the kidney becomes soft, dissection should be discontinued until the kidney has again become firm. Mannitol is given in divided doses during dissection of the renal pedicle. It is imperative that the kidney be firm and that urine be spurting from the ureter prior to division of the renal vessels. By using this approach to donor nephrectomy, postoperative dialysis is rarely necessary in living related transplants.

D. Treatment of the Cadaver Donor: The potential cadaver donor is often hypovolemic and receiving vasopressors, so that rapid infusion of intravenous fluids is initially necessary to readjust the contracted blood volume. Subsequently, alpha-adrenergic blocking agents such as phenoxybenzamine (Dibenzyline) and phentolamine (Regitine) are given to prevent renal vasospasm. These agents are especially important when kidneys are removed after cardiac arrest. Once renal vasospasm is established, it will persist during preservation, resulting in inadequate tissue perfusion and organ damage.

Technique of Renal Transplantation

The surgical technique of renal transplantation involves vascular anastomoses and establishment of urinary tract continuity. Specific considerations may be outlined as follows:

In adults, the kidney is placed through an oblique lower abdominal incision and the common iliac and internal iliac (hypogastric) arteries are mobilized. The iliac veins are similarly mobilized so that an end-to-side renal vein-to-iliac vein anastomosis can be performed. An end-to-end renal artery-to-internal iliac artery anastomosis (Fig 27–1) is usually accomplished unless the internal iliac artery is unsuitable because of arteriosclerotic changes, in which case the renal artery is transplanted end-to-side to the common iliac artery.

When multiple arteries are present in cadaver donors, the kidneys are transplanted with anastomosis of a Carrel patch of aorta to the common iliac artery.

In small children, a midline abdominal incision is used and the cecum and ascending colon are mobilized, exposing the aorta and vena cava. An end-to-side anastomosis of the renal vessels to the vena cava and aorta is then easily accomplished, following which the kidney is placed retroperitoneally by repositioning the previously mobilized right colon.

When small pediatric cadaver kidneys are used, donor nephrectomy is carried out en bloc with the aorta and vena cava. The kidneys are then stored by

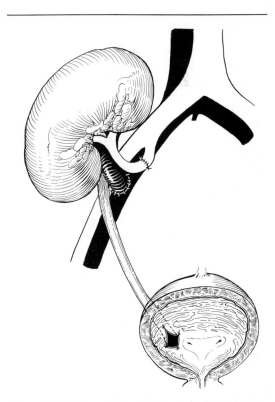

Figure 27–1. Renal transplantation (anastomoses to internal iliac artery, iliac vein, and bladder).

hypothermic pulsatile perfusion through the aorta. Subsequently, pediatric kidneys are transplanted as single units, with each donor providing kidneys for 2 recipients. Arterial anastomosis is performed by using a Carrel patch of donor aorta, and whenever possible, a Carrel patch of the vena is used for the venous anastomosis. If a Carrel patch of vena cava is not used, interrupted sutures for the venous anastomosis are used instead. Arterial and venous anastomoses are usually carried out on the iliac vessels, and the aorta and vena cava are utilized only in very small children.

Urinary tract continuity can be established by pyeloureterostomy, ureteroureterostomy, or ureteroneocystostomy. Ureteroneocystostomy by a modified Politano-Leadbetter technique is used at UCSF. The incidence of primary ureteral leaks with this method has been less than 1%.

Immediate Posttransplant Care

Postoperative management does not differ essentially from that of other surgical patients except that emphasis is placed upon the following:

Foley catheter drainage is maintained for 1 week, because of the impaired wound healing associated with immunosuppressive therapy. This method has essentially eliminated urinary leakage from the bladder. If bacteriuria develops, it is detected by appropriate urinary cultures and specifically treated.

Intravenous fluids are given immediately after the operation at a rate to maintain a good diuresis. The urinary output in the immediate posttransplant patient may be abundant, and this volume must be considered in determining the rate of administration of replacement fluids.

Renal scintiphotography is useful in the immediate posttransplant period to establish a baseline for future comparative studies and to evaluate the patency of vascular and ureteral anastomoses. Good isotope uptake in the renal cortex indicates adequate perfusion, while normal drainage of urine confirms patency of the ureteral anastomosis. Renal scintiphotography with excretion of 131 I-orthoiodohippurate is the principal method used to evaluate the graft and to complement clinical impressions and chemical determinations.

The differential diagnosis of renal failure following transplantation can be extremely difficult in 2 situations: (1) when urinary output suddenly decreases shortly after transplantation, and (2) when rejection is superimposed upon acute tubular necrosis. Our experience with scintiphotographic studies in renal transplant patients has shown these studies to be of great value in the evaluation of the structure, function, and viability of the transplanted kidney. The study causes no discomfort or harm to the patient. Furthermore, good renal visualization is possible in patients with oliguria or anuria.

Renal ultrasonography is of great benefit in the initial differentiation of acute rejection from cyclosporine nephrotoxicity.

Rejection

Hyperacute rejection is mediated by humoral antibodies. It occurs in patients who have preexisting circulating cytotoxic antibodies that react with the donor kidney. The classic picture of hyperacute rejection is seen when, after release of the vascular clamps following vascular anastomoses, the kidney appears normal but very rapidly turns into a bluish-black, nonviable organ. The only treatment is immediate nephrectomy. Subliminal sensitization can also occur; in this case, irreversible renal failure and graft nonviability take several days to become completely established. This is called accelerated rejection.

Acute rejection generally presents during the first several months following transplantation. This type of rejection is usually characterized by fever, oliguria, weight gain, tenderness and enlargement of the graft, hypertension, and chemical evidence of renal functional impairment. Treatment has traditionally been by increasing the dosage of corticosteroids, but the use of antithymocyte globulin or monoclonal antibodies has also proved very effective in reversing rejection. The advantage of the latter methods is that use of intermittent doses of steroid drugs is avoided.

Chronic rejection is a late cause of renal deterioration. Chronic rejection is most often diagnosed by evidence of slowly decreasing renal function in association with proteinuria and hypertension. This type of rejection is resistant to standard methods of corticosteroid rejection treatment, and graft loss will eventually occur, though at times not for several years after the inception of impaired renal function.

Immunosuppressive Therapy

The principal drugs used in conventional immunosuppression are prednisone and azathioprine (Imuran)—an antimetabolite—used in combination. A major disadvantage of conventional immunosuppression has been that its lack of specificity causes concomitant depression of multiple organ systems and immunologic responses rather than selective inhibition of the response to donor histocompatibility antigens. The use of conventional immunosuppression is primarily limited to living related transplantation after DST pretreatment where long-term, low-dose steroids can be expected as maintenance medication. However, major progress has been achieved in cadaver transplantation with cyclosporine, a new immunosuppressive agent. The potent immunosuppressive properties of cyclosporine were first reported by Borel in 1976. Besides its being responsible for improvements in graft survival, the major advantage of cyclosporine is its ability to inhibit only a few discrete processes in the immune response, thereby sparing host resistance. Its principal side effect is nephrotoxicity, particularly in cases where its use is coincident with acute tubular necrosis. One-year cadaver graft survival rates of greater than 80% are regularly achieved—a 25% improvement over previous cadaver graft survival with conventional immunosuppression alone.

Complications

A. Urologic: The urologic complication rate, including bladder leaks, ureteral obstruction, and ureteral leaks, is less than 2% in our center.

B. Vascular: Renal artery stenosis has occurred in 17 of our patients, an incidence of less than 1%. Stenosis has been of 2 types: (1) that limited to the suture line and secondary to reaction to the suture material, and (2) generalized stenosis of the main renal artery to its bifurcation due to extensive periadventitial cicatricial formation, probably a part of the generalized reaction to the graft. Renal artery stenosis is most often corrected surgically, but transluminal angioplasty may be useful in selected cases.

C. Infection: The primary wound infection rate is 0.7%. Topical use of antibiotics, strict adherence to careful surgical technique, and omission of wound drainage are mainly responsible for this low incidence.

D. Complications Secondary to Immunosuppressive Therapy: These complications, such as infection and sepsis, can be kept to a minimum by emphasizing low-dose immunosuppressive therapy.

Results

A. Patient Survival: After a policy of low-dose immunosuppressive therapy was adopted in 1972, the cumulative patient mortality rate has been reduced to 2% at 1 year and 3% at 2 years for living related transplants and 4% and 6% for cadaver transplants.

B. Graft Survival:

a. Living related transplantation, whether with an HLA-identical sibling combination or after the donor-specific blood transfusion protocol in nonidentical pairs, should achieve greater than 90% graft survival at 2 years with conventional immunosuppression.

b. The survival rate of cadaver grafts has been about 60% at 1 year and 55% at 2 years with conventional immunosuppression. Recent refinements in immunosuppressive therapy, particularly the use of cyclosporine, have improved cadaver graft survival rates to approximately 80% at 1 year and 75% at 2 years.

REFERENCES

Advisory Committee to the Renal Transplant Registry: The 13th Report of the Human Renal Transplant Registry. *Transplant Proc* 1977;**9**:9.

Belzer FO, Southard JH: The future of kidney preservation. *Transplantation* 1980;**30**:161.

Borel JF et al: Biologic effects of cyclosporin A: A new antilymphocytic agent. *Agents Actions* 1976;**6**:468.

Burlingham WJ et al: Improved renal allograft survival following donor-specific transfusions. *Transplantation* 1987;**43**:41.

Carpenter CB: HLA and renal transplantation. *N Engl J Med* 1980;**302**:860.

Casimi AB et al: Use of monoclonal antibodies to T-cell subsets for immunologic monitoring and treatment in recipients of renal allografts. *N Engl J Med* 1981;**305**:308.

Feduska NJ et al: Do blood transfusions enhance the possibility of a compatible transplant? *Transplantation* 1979;**27**:35.

Feduska NJ et al: Graft survival with high levels of cytotoxic antibodies. *Transplant Proc* 1981;**13**:73.

Ferguson RM et al: Cyclosporin A in renal transplantation: A prospective randomized trial. *Surgery* 1982;**92**:175.

Flechner SA et al: The effect of cyclosporine on early graft function in human renal transplantation. *Transplantation* 1983; **36**:268.

Melzer JS et al: The beneficial effect of pretransplant blood transfusions in cyclosporine-treated cadaver renal allograft recipients. *Transplantation* 1987;**43**:61.

Morris PJ: *Kidney Transplantation: Principles and Practice.* Grune & Stratton, 1984.

Najarian JS, Simmons RL: *Transplantation.* Lea & Febiger, 1972.

Salvatierra O: Renal transplantation. Pages 359–367 in: *Urologic Surgery.* Glenn JF (editor). Lippincott, 1983.

Salvatierra O et al: The advantages of 131 I-orthoiodohippurate scintiphotography in the management of patients after renal transplantation. *Ann Surg* 1974;**180**:336.

Salvatierra O et al: Deliberate donor-specific blood transfusions prior to living related renal transplantation. *Ann Surg* 1980;**192**:543.

Salvatierra O et al: Donor-specific blood transfusions versus cyclosporine—the DST story. *Transplant Proc* 1987;**19**:160.

Salvatierra O et al: End-stage polycystic kidney disease: Management by renal transplantation and selective use of preliminary nephrectomy. *J Urol* 1976;**115**:5.

Salvatierra O et al: Improved patient survival in renal transplantation. *Surgery* 1976;**79**:166.

Salvatierra O et al: Procurement of cadaver kidneys. *Urol Clin North Am* 1976;**3**:457.

Salvatierra O et al: The role of blood transfusions in renal transplantation. *Urol Clin North Am* 1983;**10**:243.

Salvatierra O et al: Urological complications of renal transplantation can be prevented or controlled. *J Urol* 1977;**117**:421.

Strom TB: The improving utility of transplantation in the management of end-stage renal disease. *Am J Med* 1982;**73**:105.

Terasaki PI: *Clinical Transplants 1986.* UCLA Tissue Typing Laboratory, 1986.

Terasaki PI et al: Microdroplet testing for HLA-A, -B, -C, and -D antigens. The Phillip Levine Award Lecture. *Am J Clin Pathol* 1978;**69**:103.

Disorders of the Ureter & Ureteropelvic Junction

Barry A. Kogan, MD

The ureter functions as a conduit carrying urine from the kidneys to the bladder. Any pathologic process that interferes with this activity can cause renal abnormalities, the most common sequels being hydronephrosis (see pp 172–175) and infection. Disorders of the ureter can be classified as congenital or acquired.

CONGENITAL ANOMALIES OF THE URETER

Congenital ureteral malformations are common and range from complete absence to duplication or triplication of the ureter. They may cause severe obstruction requiring urgent attention, or they may be asymptomatic and of no clinical significance. The nomenclature can be confusing and has recently been standardized to prevent ambiguity (Glassberg et al, 1984).

URETERAL ATRESIA

The ureter may be entirely absent, or it may end blindly after extending only part way to the flank. The anomaly is caused during embryologic development, either by failure of the ureteral bud to form from the mesonephric duct or by an arrest in its development before it comes in contact with the metanephric blastema. The end result is an absent or multicystic kidney. When bilateral, this condition presents as Potter's syndrome and is incompatible with life. When unilateral, it is usually asymptomatic and of no clinical significance, although it can be associated with hypertension (Javadpour et al, 1970) or infection (Yoshida and Sakamoto, 1986). The diagnosis can be confusing (Rubenstein and Brenner, 1985).

DUPLICATION OF THE URETER

Complete or incomplete duplication of the ureter is one of the most common congenital malformations of the urinary tract. Nation (1944) found some form of duplication of the ureter in 0.9% of a series of autopsies. The condition occurs more frequently in females than in males and is often bilateral. The mode of inheritance is autosomal dominant, although the gene is of incomplete penetrance (Atwell et al, 1974).

The incomplete (Y) type of duplication is caused by branching of the ureteral bud before it reaches the metanephric blastema. In most cases, this anomaly is associated with no clinical abnormality. However, disorders of peristalsis may occur near the point of union (Fig 28–1) (O'Reilly et al, 1984). In such cases, one segment may be obstructed or dilated owing to ureteroureteral reflux. If there is vesicoureteral reflux, both the upper and lower portions of the kidney are involved.

In complete duplication of the ureter, the presence of 2 ureteral buds leads to the formation of 2 totally separate ureters and 2 separate renal pelves. Because the ureter to the upper segment arises from a cephalad position on the mesonephric duct, it remains attached to the mesonephric duct longer and consequently migrates farther, ending medial and inferior to the ureter

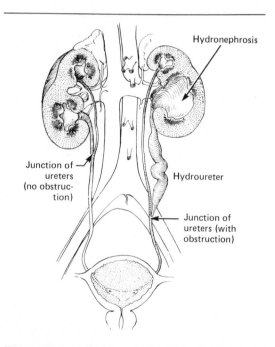

Figure 28–1. Duplication of the ureter. Incomplete (Y) type with hydronephrosis of lower pole of left kidney.

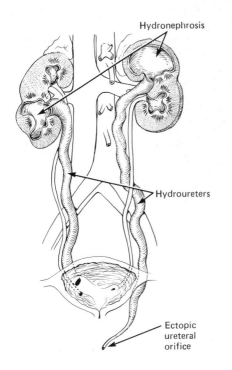

Figure 28–2. Duplication of the ureter. Complete duplication with reflux to lower pole of right kidney and chronic pyelonephritic scarring. Upper-pole ureter of left kidney is ectopic, and its associated renal parenchyma is dysplastic.

draining the lower segment (Weigert-Meyer law). Thus, the ureter draining the upper segment may migrate too far caudally and become ectopic and obstructed, while the ureter draining the lower segment may end laterally and have a short intravesical tunnel, which leads to vesicoureteral reflux (Fig 28–2) (Kaplan, Nasrallah, and King, 1978; Tanagho, 1976). The same general principle is noted in rare ureteral triplication (Zaontz and Maizels, 1985).

Although some patients with duplication of the ureter are asymptomatic, many present with persistent or recurrent infections. In females, the ureter to the upper pole may be ectopic, with an opening distal to the external sphincter or even outside the urinary tract. Such patients have classic symptoms: incontinence characterized by constant dribbling, but a normal pattern of voiding. In males, the ectopic ureter is always proximal to the external sphincter, and this type of incontinence does not occur.

Excretory urography and voiding cystourethrography should be performed. The excretory urogram will show the duplication in most cases. Occasionally, one segment of the ureter functions so poorly that it may not be visualized. In such cases, the diagnosis can be inferred from the displacement of the visualized calices or ureter or from the discrepancy between the amount of renal parenchyma and the relatively small number of visualized calices. The excretory urogram will also demonstrate any pyelonephritic scarring. The

voiding cystourethrogram will disclose vesicoureteral reflux and may demonstrate the presence of a ureterocele. Renal scanning (especially with ^{99m}Tc-dimercaptosuccinic acid) is helpful for estimating the degree of renal function in each kidney and renal segment (Fig 28–3).

The treatment of reflux alone should not be influenced by the presence of ureteral duplication. Lower grades of reflux are generally treated medically and higher grades of reflux surgically. If upper-pole obstruction or ectopy is present, surgery is almost always required. Numerous operative approaches have been recommended (Belman, Filmer, and King, 1974). If renal function in one segment is very poor, heminephrectomy is the most appropriate procedure (Barrett, Malek, and Kelalis, 1975). In an effort to preserve renal parenchyma, treatment by pyeloureterostomy, ureteroureterostomy, or ureteral reimplantation is feasible (Amar, 1970; Amar, 1978; Bockrath, Maizels, and Firlit, 1983).

URETEROCELE

A ureterocele is a sacculation of the terminal portion of the ureter (Fig 28–4). It may be either intravesical or ectopic; in the latter case, some portion is located at the bladder neck or in the urethra. Intravesical ureteroceles are generally associated with single ureters, whereas ectopic ureteroceles most often involve the upper-pole ureter of duplicated ureters. Ectopic ureteroceles are 4 times more common than intravesical ureteroceles (Snyder and Johnston, 1978). Ureterocele occurs 7 times more often in girls than in boys, and about 10% of cases are bilateral. Mild forms of ureterocele are occasionally found in adults examined for unrelated reasons.

Ureterocele has been attributed to delayed or incomplete canalization of the ureteral bud leading to an early prenatal obstruction and expansion of the ureteral bud prior to its absorption into the urogenital sinus (Tanagho, 1976). The cystic dilatation forms between the superficial and deep muscle layers of the trigone. Large ureteroceles may displace the other orifices, interfere with the muscular backing of the bladder, or even obstruct the bladder outlet. There is often significant hydroureteronephrosis, and a dysplastic segment of the upper pole of the kidney is not uncommonly found in association with a ureterocele. Recently, it has been shown that the dysplastic segment may contain nodular renal blastema and hence may be prone to neoplasia (Cromie, Engelstein, and Duckett, 1980).

Clinical findings vary considerably. Patients commonly present with infection, but bladder outlet obstruction or incontinence may be the initial complaint. Occasionally, a ureterocele may prolapse through the female urethra (Ahmed, 1984). Calculi can develop secondary to urinary stasis and are often seen in the distal ureter. Excretory urography (Figs 28–3 and 28–5) is usually diagnostic and may show a cystic dilatation or a filling defect in the bladder. The urogram

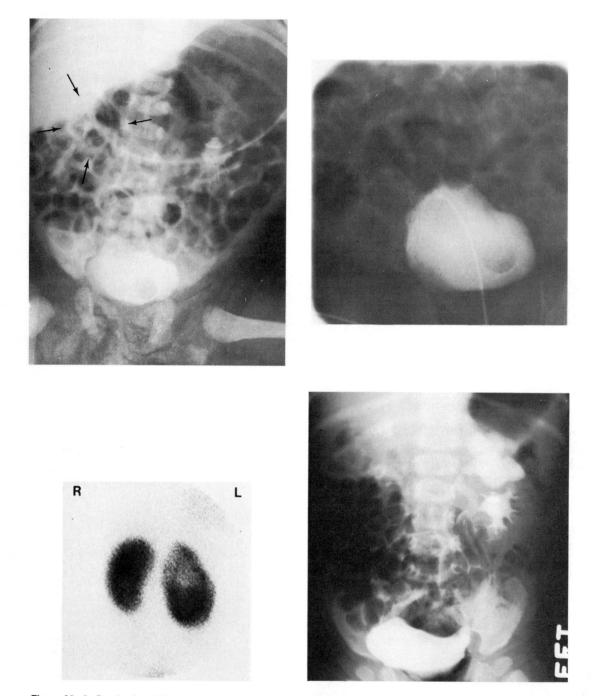

Figure 28–3. Duplication of the ureter and the ureterocele. *Upper left:* Excretory urogram shows duplication of right kidney and visualization of only lower pole of left kidney. There is a filling defect on the left side of the bladder. *Upper right:* Cystogram confirms the filling defect. There is no reflux. *Lower left:* Renal scan with ^{99m}Tc-dimercaptosuccinic acid shows some functioning parenchyma in upper pole to left kidney. *Lower right:* After excision of ureterocele and reimplantation of both ureters on left, repeat excretory urogram shows improved excretion of contrast medium from upper pole of left kidney.

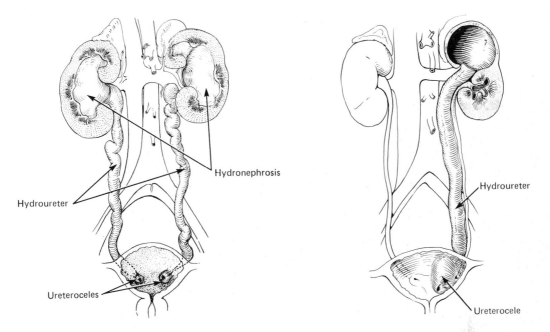

Figure 28–4. Ureterocele.*Left:* Orthotopic ureterocele associated with a single ureter. *Right:* Ureterocele associated with ureteral duplication and poor function of upper pole of kidney.

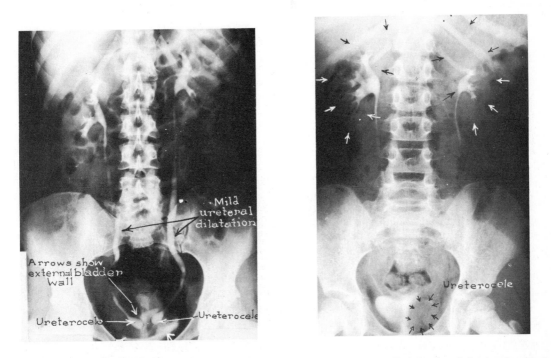

Figure 28–5. Ureterocele. *Left:* Excretory urogram in a woman shows "cobra head" deformity of distal ends of both ureters, bilateral ureteroceles causing minimal obstruction, and pressure on the bladder from the uterus. No treatment is indicated. *Right:* Excretory urogram in an 8-year-old girl shows a space-occupying lesion (left side of bladder) caused by ureterocele. Absence of caliceal system in upper portion of left kidney implies duplication of ureters and renal pelves and a nonfunctioning upper pole (advanced hydronephrosis); the dilated ureter from that pole drains into an obstructing ureterocele and displaces the visualized ureter laterally just below the kidney.

will also indicate the degree of hydronephrosis and may reveal a duplicated kidney. Voiding cystourethrography should be done (Bauer and Retik, 1978). It may demonstrate reflux, particularly into a lower-pole ureter, and occasionally shows eversion of the ureterocele during urination, in which case the ureterocele has the appearance of a diverticulum. Renal scanning is helpful for estimating renal function (Geringer et al, 1983).

Treatment must be individualized. Transurethral incision can be used in preparation for a later reconstructive procedure or in a very ill child with pyohydronephrosis; however, it is generally avoided, since vesicoureteral reflux frequently results (Tank, 1986). When surgery is justified, the procedure must be chosen on the basis of the anatomic location of the ureteral meatus, the position of the ureterocele, and the degree of hydroureteronephrosis and impairment of renal function. In general, choices range from heminephrectomy and ureterectomy to excision of the ureterocele, vesical reconstruction, and ureteral reimplantation. Often, a second procedure will be necessary (Caldamone, Snyder, and Duckett, 1984).

ECTOPIC URETERAL ORIFICE

Although an ectopic ureteral orifice most commonly occurs in association with ureterocele and duplication of the ureter (see above), single ectopic ureters do occur (Gotoh et al, 1983). They are caused by a delay or failure of separation of the ureteral bud from the mesonephric duct during embryologic development. The initial anomaly may be an abnormally located ureteral bud, which explains the high incidence of dysplastic kidneys associated with single ectopic ureters.

The clinical picture varies according to the sex of the patient and the position of the ureteral opening. Boys usually do not present with incontinence, but many are seen because of epididymitis. In these cases, the ureter drains directly into the vas deferens or seminal vesicle (Umeyama et al, 1985). In girls, the ureteral orifice may be in the urethra, vagina, or perineum. Although infection may be present, particularly when the ectopic ureter allows reflux, incontinence is the rule. Continual dribbling despite normal voiding is pathognomonic. Urgency and urge incontinence may confound the diagnosis. Genital tract anomalies are often present in patients with ectopic ureteral orifices (Johnson and Perlmutter, 1980).

Excretory urography and voiding cystourethrography will help delineate the problem; however, in the case of a single ectopic ureter, the entire kidney will be involved, and there may be no excretion of contrast medium. Ultrasonography is helpful in delineating a cystic mass. During cystoscopy, the ectopic orifice in boys may be visualized directly or demonstrated by retrograde catheterization of the ejaculatory duct (Fig 28–6). The presence of a hemitrigone plus a cystic mass in the flank is presumptive evidence of an ectopic ureter. In girls, the orifice can sometimes be visualized

next to the urethra by cystoscopy or by vaginoscopy. If so, a retrograde ureterogram may demonstrate anatomic abnormalities (Fig 28–7). Renal scanning is also helpful in delineating the structures and estimating the degree of renal function.

As in ureteroceles and duplication of the ureter, the clinical picture and the degree of renal function dictate the therapeutic approach. Surgical treatment usually involves their ureteral reimplantation or nephroureterectomy. Unlike most ureteral duplications, it is occasionally possible to reimplant only the ectopic ureter (Marshall, 1986).

ABNORMALITIES OF URETERAL POSITION

Retrocaval ureter (also called circumcaval ureter and postcaval ureter) is a rare condition in which an embryologically normal ureter becomes entrapped behind the vena cava because of abnormal development of the abdominal blood vessels. Persistence of the right subcardinal vein, as opposed to the supracardinal vein, forces the right ureter to encircle the vena cava from behind. There are 2 anatomic types of retrocaval ureter (Kenawi and Williams, 1976). In one, the upper ureter and renal pelvis are almost horizontal as they pass behind the vena cava; there is generally no obstruction, and no therapy is needed. In the other type, the ureter descends normally to approximately the level of L3, where it curves back upward in the shape of a reverse J to pass behind and around the vena cava. Obstruction generally results.

The diagnosis of retrocaval ureter can usually be made by excretory urography. If there is poor visualization, a retrograde ureterogram will show the abnormality quite clearly. A simultaneous venacavogram can be obtained but is usually not necessary (Fig 28–8).

Surgical repair for retrocaval ureter, when indicated, consists of dividing the ureter (preferably across the dilated portion) and then bringing the distal ureter from behind the vena cava and reanastomosing it to the proximal end. If the retrocaval part of the ureter is fibrotic or stenotic, the infracaval ureter is used for the anastomosis (Kumar and Bhandari, 1985).

A number of other rare anomalies of ureteral position occur. Brooks (1962) reported a retrocaval left ureter in a patient with situs inversus. Several cases of retroiliac ureter have been reported (Hanna, 1972). Treatment is similar to that described above.

OBSTRUCTION OF THE URETEROPELVIC JUNCTION

In children, primary obstruction of the ureter usually occurs at the ureteropelvic junction or the ureterovesical junction (Fig 28–9). Obstruction of the ureteropelvic junction is probably the most common congenital abnormality of the ureter. It is seen more

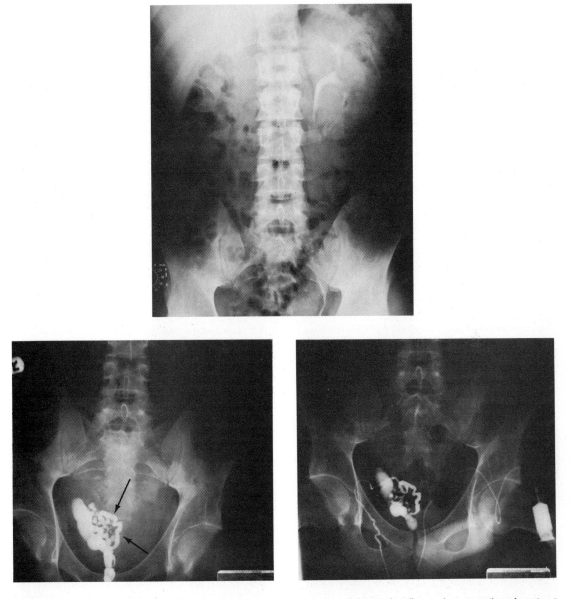

Figure 28–6. Ectopic ureter. *Top:* Excretory urogram demonstrates no right renal outline and no excretion of contrast medium on right. *Lower left:* Endoscopic injection of contrast medium into ejaculatory duct demonstrates seminal vesicle and stump of ectopic ureter. *Lower right:* Same anatomy visualized on a vasogram. (Courtesy of DW Ferguson.)

often in boys than in girls (5:2 ratio) and, in unilateral cases, more often on the left than on the right side (5:2 ratio). Bilateral obstruction occurs in 10–15% of cases and is especially common in infants (Johnson et al, 1977). The abnormality may occur in several members of the same family, but it shows no clear genetic pattern.

The exact cause of obstruction of the ureteropelvic junction is not often clear. Ureteral polyps and valves have been reported but are very rare (Punjani, 1983; Sant, Barbalias, and Klauber, 1985). There is almost always an angulation and kink at the junction of the dilated renal pelvis and ureter. This can in itself cause obstruction, but it is often unclear if this is primary or

merely secondary to another obstructive lesion. True stenosis is rarely found; however, a thin-walled, hypoplastic proximal ureter is frequently observed. Characteristic histologic and ultrastructural changes are observed in this area and could account for abnormal peristalsis through the ureteropelvic junction and consequent interference with pelvic emptying (Hanna et al, 1976). Two other findings sometimes seen at operation are a high origin of the ureter from the renal pelvis and an abnormal relationship of the proximal ureter to a lower-pole renal artery. It is debatable whether these findings are the result or the cause of pelvic dilatation, but Stephens (1982) has presented data suggesting that abnormal rotation of the renal

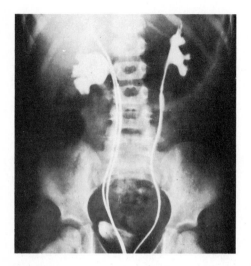 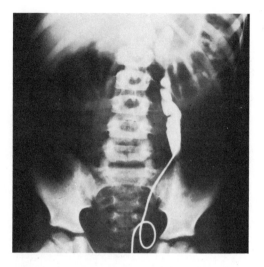

Figure 28–7. Ectopic ureter. *Left:* Cystoscopy in a 6-year-old girl with a lifelong history of urinary incontinence revealed 2 ureteral orifices on the right and one on the left; these were catheterized and urograms obtained. *Right:* Same patient. An ectopic ureteral orifice near the urethral meatus was catheterized. Retrograde urogram demonstrates second hydronephrotic renal pelvis on left. Resection of upper pole and ureter cured incontinence.

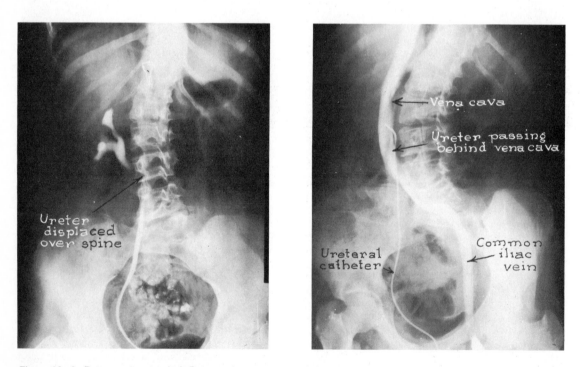

Figure 28–8. Retrocaval ureter. *Left:* Retrograde ureterogram shows upper ureter displaced onto vertebral bodies, suggesting retrocaval ureter. Note congenital deformity of spine. *Right:* Femoral venacavogram (right oblique view) shows ureter in retrocaval position.

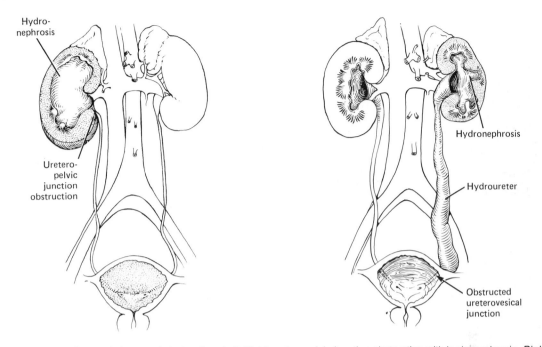

Hydro-
nephrosis

Uretero-
pelvic
junction
obstruction

Hydronephrosis

Hydroureter

Obstructed
ureterovesical
junction

Figure 28–9. Congenital ureteral obstruction. *Left:* Right ureteropelvic junction obstruction with hydronephrosis. *Right:* Left ureterovesical junction obstruction (obstructed megaureter) with hydroureteronephrosis.

pelvis allows the ureter to become entrapped in the blood vessels of the lower pole of the kidney, ultimately leading to obstruction. Using careful studies at the time of operation, it is possible to define whether the lesion is intrinsic or extrinsic (Koff et al, 1986; Johnston, 1969).

Clinical findings vary depending on the patient's age at diagnosis. Recent improvements in prenatal ultrasonography allow increasing numbers of cases to be diagnosed in utero. In infants, the most frequent finding is an abdominal mass. In children, pain and vomiting are the most common symptoms; however, hematuria and urinary infection may also be seen. A few patients have complications such as calculi (Fig 28–10), trauma to the enlarged kidney, or (rarely) hypertension. Some are completely asymptomatic.

The diagnosis is made by excretory urography. In equivocal cases, however, diuretic renography or antegrade urography with pressure flow studies is helpful (Thrall, Koff, and Keyes, 1981; Whitaker, 1973). Some surgeons consider a voiding cystourethrogram a routine part of the preoperative workup, since radiographic findings in vesicoureteral reflux may be similar to those in ureteropelvic junction obstruction. This is especially relevant when the ureter is well seen or dilated (or both) below the ureteropelvic junction (Maizels, Smith, and Firlit, 1984).

Obstruction of the ureteropelvic junction must be treated surgically. Because of anatomic variations, no single procedure is sufficient for all situations (Smart, 1979). Regardless of the technique used, all successful repairs have in common the creation of a dependent and funnel-shaped ureteropelvic junction of adequate

caliber. Although preservation of the intact ureteropelvic junction is feasible in some circumstances (Perlberg and Pfau, 1984), when the obstruction appears to be caused by a dyskinetic segment of proximal ureter the most popular operation is a dismembered pyeloureteroplasty (Anderson, 1963). Dismembered pyeloureteroplasty is also favored when the proximal ureter is hooked over a lower-pole blood vessel. When there is a dilated extrarenal renal pelvis, dismembered pyeloureteroplasty can be combined with a Foley Y–V plasty to create a more funnel-shaped ureteropelvic junction (Foley, 1937). Pelvic flap procedure (Culp and DeWeerd, 1951; Scardino and Prince, 1953) are ideally suited to cases in which the ureteropelvic junction has remained in a dependent position despite significant pelvic dilatation. They also have the advantage of interfering less with the ureteral blood supply; this is particularly relevant when distal ureteral surgery (eg, ureteral reimplantation) is contemplated in the future. Both the Y–V plasty and flap techniques are useful in managing ureteropelvic junction obstructions in horseshoe or pelvic kidneys, where the anatomy may prevent creation of a dependent ureteropelvic junction if a dismembered technique is attempted. The use of stenting catheters and proximal diversion at the time of pyeloplasty has been the subject of debate, and the issue has not been resolved. Excellent results have been reported both with and without stents and diversions (Bejjani and Belman, 1982; Perlmutter, Kroovand, and Lai, 1980; King et al, 1984;**132:**725).

The prognosis is generally good, since the disease is usually unilateral and since one side is nearly always

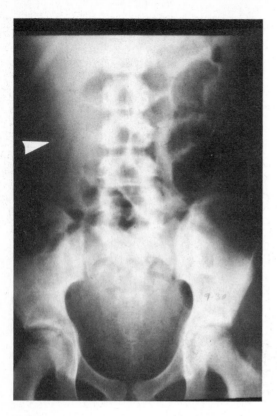

Figure 28–10. Ureteropelvic junction obstruction with calculi. *Top:* Plain film of abdomen shows radiopacities in region of right kidney. *Lower left:* Early film from excretory urogram demonstrates dilatation of calices on right and layering of calculi in large right renal pelvis. *Lower right:* Delayed film from excretory urogram shows a typical right ureteropelvic junction obstruction.

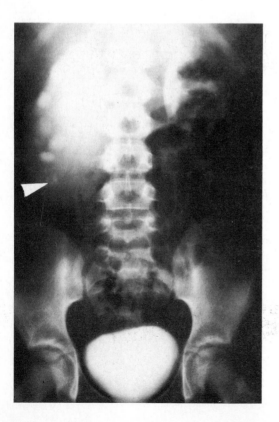

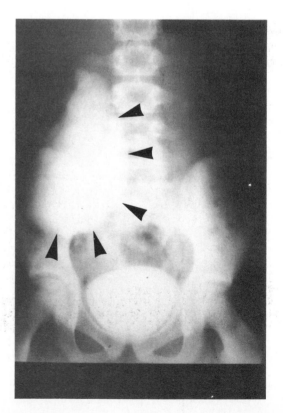

less involved in cases of bilateral disease. In several large series, the reported reoperation rate has been only 2–4%, but the postoperative radiographic appearance of the area is usually disappointing. There can be marked improvement when a large extrarenal renal pelvis has prevented massive caliceal distortion; however, in most cases, considerable deformity persists despite adequate drainage of the kidney.

The recent explosion in endourology as a subspecialty of urology has encouraged use of percutaneous techniques for the repair of ureteropelvic junction obstruction (Ramsay et al, 1984; Badlani, Eshghi, and Smith, 1986). The technique is similar to that reported by Davis (1943) but is done entirely endoscopically. Although early success rates range from 50% to 80%, much longer follow-up is necessary before the true efficacy of this approach is known. At present it seems appropriate to try the technique in patients in whom percutaneous stone removal will be done anyway or who have failed previous open pyeloplasty (King et al, 1984;**131:**1167).

OBSTRUCTED MEGAURETER

Obstruction at the ureterovesical junction is 4 times more common in boys than in girls. It is often bilateral but usually asymmetric. The left ureter is slightly more often involved than the right. Of more consequence is the observation that the contralateral kidney is either absent or dysplastic in 10–15% of cases (Tiburcio and Lima, 1978).

The embryogenesis of the lesion is uncertain. It is clear that in most cases there is no stricture at the ureterovesical junction. At operation, a retrograde catheter or probe can usually be passed through the area of obstruction. Close observation either at operation or by fluoroscopy reveals a failure of the distal ureter to transmit the normal peristaltic wave, resulting in a functional obstruction. Histologic findings include an excess of circular muscle fibers and collagen in the distal ureter, which may account for the problem (Tanagho, Smith, and Guthrie, 1970). Ultrastructural studies show that this obstruction is similar in appearance to obstruction of the ureteropelvic junction.

Common symptoms are infection, fever, and abdominal pain. Hematuria is frequent and may be seen even in the absence of infection. This is presumably due to disruption of mucosal vessels in the ureter secondary to ureteral distention. Hematuria may also be a sign of calculus formation secondary to urinary stasis. The excretory urogram usually shows the pathognomonic configuration of a dilated distal ureter, a less dilated proximal ureter, relatively normal appearing renal pelvis, and blunted calices (Fig 28–11). In some cases, retrograde or antegrade urograms are necessary to delineate the lesion. A diuretic renogram or perfusion study may be helpful.

Surgery is indicated in most cases. Ureteral reimplantation with excision of the distal ureter is curative. Because of the excessive dilatation of the ureter,

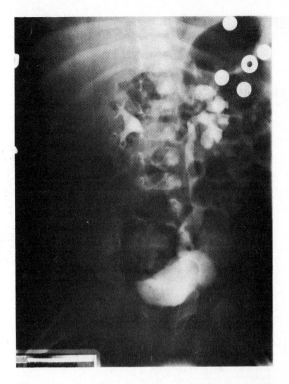

Figure 28–11. Obstructive megaureter. Follow-up study in a 9-month-old boy with unilateral hydronephrosis detected by ultrasonography in utero. Excretory urogram shows the classic configuration of a dilated distal ureter, a less dilated proximal ureter, and blunted calices.

ureteral tapering is frequently necessary. This is usually done by excision of a portion of the ureteral wall along the antimesenteric border (Hendren, 1969); however, there are recent reports of good results obtained by folding the ureter onto itself (Hanna, 1982; Ehrlich, 1985).

UPPER URINARY TRACT DILATATION WITHOUT OBSTRUCTION

It should not be assumed that every dilated upper urinary tract is obstructed. A voiding cystourethrogram is an essential part of the evaluation, not only to rule out reflux but also to ensure that no abnormality of the lower urinary tract is responsible for the upper urinary tract dilatation. Other cases in which diagnosis may be difficult include residual dilatation in a previously obstructed system, dilatation associated with bacterial infection (presumably related to a direct effect of endotoxin on the ureteral musculature), neonatal hydronephrosis (Homsy, Williot, and Danais, 1986), and prolonged polyuria in patients with diabetes insipidus.

In such cases, the usual investigations may not provide sufficient information. A radionuclide diuretic renogram is especially helpful in distinguishing nonobstructive from obstructive dilatation (Fig

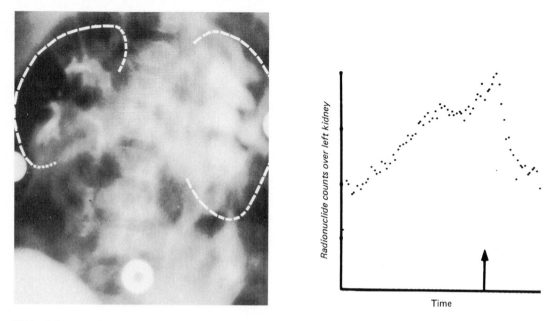

Figure 28–12. Upper urinary tract dilatation. *Left:* Three months after resection of posterior urethral valves, hydronephrosis in the right kidney has completely resolved. The left collecting system remains dilated. (Dashed lines outline kidneys.) *Right:* Radionuclide diuretic renography was performed to determine if there was secondary ureteropelvic or ureterovesical obstruction. Renogram demonstrates clear-cut "washout" of radionuclide following injection of furosemide *(arrow)*. There is no significant obstruction.

28–12) (Thrall, Koff, and Keyes, 1981). Use of percutaneous renal puncture is increasing; in the dilated system, it carries minimal risk, making antegrade urography and pressure flow studies feasible in selected cases. Measurement of the renal pelvic pressure during infusion of saline into the renal pelvis at high rates (10 mL/min) (the Whitaker test; see p 113) appears to be an excellent method for differentiating nonobstructive from obstructive dilatation (Wolk and Whitaker, 1982). Unfortunately, there is no true "gold standard," and these studies do not always agree; clinical judgment is the final arbiter (Lupton et al, 1985).

ACQUIRED DISEASES OF THE URETER

Nearly all acquired diseases of the ureter are obstructive in nature. They are frequently seen, but their actual incidence is uncertain. Their clinical manifestations, effects on the kidney, complications, and treatment are similar to those described above. The lesions can be broadly categorized as either intrinsic or extrinsic.

Intrinsic Ureteral Obstruction

The most common causes of intrinsic ureteral obstruction are as follows:

(1) Ureteral stones (see Chapter 16).

(2) Transitional cell tumors of the ureter (see Chapter 19).

(3) Chronic inflammatory changes of the ureteral wall (usually due to tuberculosis or schistosomiasis) leading to contracture or insufficient peristalsis (see Chapter 14 and Figs 14–2 and 14–4).

Extrinsic Ureteral Obstruction

The following are frequent causes of extrinsic ureteral obstruction:

(1) Severe constipation, sometimes with bladder obstruction, seen primarily in children but in adult women as well.

(2) Secondary obstruction due to kinks or fibrosis around redundant ureters. The primary process is either distal obstruction or massive reflux.

(3) Benign gynecologic disorders such as endometriosis or right ovarian vein syndrome (Gourdie and Rogers, 1986).

(4) Local neoplastic infiltration associated with carcinoma of the cervix, bladder, or prostate (Richie, Withers, and Ehrlich, 1979).

(5) Pelvic lymphadenopathy associated with metastatic tumors.

(6) Iatrogenic ureteral injuries, primarily after extensive pelvic surgery (Fig 28–13) and also after extensive radiotherapy.

(7) Retroperitoneal fibrosis.

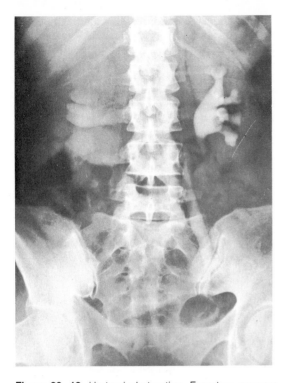

Figure 28–13. Ureteral obstruction. Excretory urogram obtained 2 weeks after Wertheim operation shows bilateral ureteral obstruction and advanced hydronephrosis on right.

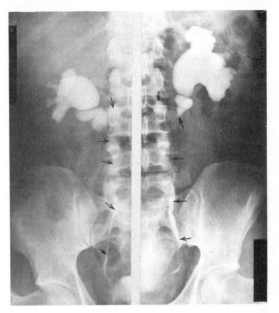

Figure 28–14. Retroperitoneal fibrosis. Right and left kidneys of same patient as shown by excretory urography. Note medial deviation of upper portions of ureters (*arrows*) with marked obstruction. (Courtesy of JA Hutch.)

RETROPERITONEAL FIBROSIS (Retroperitoneal Fasciitis, Chronic Retroperitoneal Fibroplasia, Ormond's Disease)

One or both ureters may be compressed by a chronic inflammatory process that involves the retroperitoneal tissues over the lower lumbar vertebrae. This occurs primarily in adults but may be seen in children (Chan, Johnson, and McLoughlin, 1979). There are numerous causes of retroperitoneal fibrosis. Malignant diseases (most commonly Hodgkin's disease, carcinoma of the breast, and carcinoma of the colon) should always be suspected and must be ruled out. Some medications have been implicated, most notably methysergide (Sansert), an ergot derivative used to treat migraine headaches. Rarely, inflammatory bowel disease (Siminovitch and Fazio, 1980) or an aortic aneurysm (Brock and Soloway, 1980; Peters and Cowie, 1978) is responsible. The remainder of cases are idiopathic, and these are sometimes referred to as Ormond's disease.

The symptoms are nonspecific and include low back pain, malaise, anorexia, weight loss, and, in severe cases, uremia. Infection is uncommon. The diagnosis is usually made by excretory urography (Fig 28–14). There is medial deviation of the ureters with proximal dilatation. A long segment of ureter is usually involved, and some cases have a pipe-stem ap-

malignant disease was at one time a terminal event. However, since therapy for malignant diseases has improved, urinary diversion is more frequently indicated in such cases. Diversion will usually be necessary for pearance caused by aperistalsis related to the fibrosis. A retrograde ureterogram is necessary when renal function is poor and, in any case, helps to delineate the length of the affected segment of ureter. Ultrasonography is useful, not only for diagnosis but also for monitoring the response to therapy. CT scanning or MRI is essential for evaluating the retroperitoneum itself, as well as for imaging the ureters (Hricak, Higgins, and Williams, 1983).

Treatment is usually surgical, although a course of corticosteroids may be tried first if the hydronephrosis is mild (Moody and Vaughan, 1979). When the response to corticosteroids is poor or the obstruction is severe, the ureter must be surgically dissected from the fibrous plaque. After it is freed, it should either be placed intraperitoneally or wrapped in omentum in an attempt to prevent recurrence (Lepor and Walsh, 1979). Rarely, autotransplantation is necessary (Deane, Gingell, and Pentlow, 1983). Numerous biopsies of the fibrous tissue should be obtained at the time of operation to determine whether there is a malignant tumor. Corticosteroids are sometimes used postoperatively; however, their efficacy is uncertain.

URETERAL OBSTRUCTION SECONDARY TO MALIGNANT DISEASE

Ureteral obstruction associated with widespread

malignant disease was at one time a terminal event. However, since therapy for malignant diseases has improved, urinary diversion is more frequently indicated in such cases. Diversion will usually be necessary for relatively short periods of time; either the tumor will be progressive, or, if therapy is effective, the obstruction will resolve. Thus, the goal of treatment is to leave the urinary tract intact and effect as little morbid-ity as possible. This can be accomplished with indwelling stents passed either retrogradely during cystoscopy (Hepperlen, Mardis, and Kammandel, 1979) or antegradely using percutaneous techniques (Elyaderani et al, 1982). Temporary percutaneous nephrostomy is a reasonable alternative, although indwelling stents are preferable for the patient (Ball et al, 1983; Andriole et al, 1984).

REFERENCES

CONGENITAL ANOMALIES

General

Glassberg KI et al: Suggested terminology for duplex systems, ectopic ureters and ureteroceles. *J Urol* 1984;**132**:1153.

Ureteral Atresia

Javadpour N et al: Hypertension in a child caused by a multi-cystic kidney. *J Urol* 1970;**104**:918.

Rubenstein DJ, Brenner RJ: Misleading features of blind-ending bifid ureter on computerized tomography examination. *J Urol* 1985;**134**:342.

Yoshida T, Sakamoto K: Bilateral blind-ending duplex ureters. *Br J Urol* 1986;**58**:459.

Duplication of the Ureter

Amar AD: Ipsilateral ureteroureterostomy for single ureteral disease in patients with ureteral duplication: A review of 8 years of experience with 16 patients. *J Urol* 1978;**119**:472.

Amar AD: Ureteropyelostomy for relief of single ureteral obstruction in cases of ureteral duplication. *Arch Surg* 1970;**101**:379.

Atwell JD et al: Familial incidence of bifid and double ureters. *Arch Dis Child* 1974;**49**:390.

Barrett DM, Malek RS, Kelalis PP: Problems and solutions in surgical treatment of 100 consecutive ureteral duplications in children. *J Urol* 1975;**114**:126.

Belman AB, Filmer RB, King LR: Surgical management of duplication of the collecting system. *J Urol* 1974;**112**:316.

Bockrath JM, Maizels M, Firlit CF: The use of lower ipsilateral ureteroureterostomy to treat vesicoureteral reflux or obstruction in children with duplex ureters. *J Urol* 1983;**129**:543.

Kaplan WE, Nasrallah P, King LR: Reflux in complete duplication in children. *J Urol* 1978;**120**:220.

Nation EF: Duplication of the kidney and ureter: A statistical study of 230 new cases. *J Urol* 1944;**51**:456.

O'Reilly PH et al: Ureteroureteric reflux: Pathologic entity or physiological phenomenon? *Br J Urol* 1984;**56**:159.

Tanagho EA: Embryologic basis for lower ureteral anomalies: A hypothesis. *Urology* 1976;**7**:451.

Zaontz MR, Maizels M: Type I ureteral triplication: An extension of the Weigert-Meyer law. *J Urol* 1985;**134**:949.

Ureterocele

Ahmed S: Prolapsed single system ureterocele in a girl. *J Urol* 1984;**132**:1180.

Bauer SB, Retik AB: The non-obstructive ectopic uterocele. *J Urol* 1978;**119**:804.

Caldamone AA, Snyder HM 3rd, Duckett JW: Ureteroceles in children: Follow-up of management with upper tract approach. *J Urol* 1984;**131**:1130.

Cromie WJ, Engelstein MS, Duckett JW Jr: Nodular renal blastema, renal dysplasia and duplicated collecting systems. *J Urol* 1980;**123**:100.

Geringer AM et al: The diagnostic approach to ectopic uterocele and the renal duplication complex. *J Urol* 1983;**129**:539.

Snyder HM, Johnston JH: Orthotopic ureteroceles in children. *J Urol* 1978;**119**:543.

Tanagho EA: Embryologic basis for lower ureteral anomalies: A hypothesis. *Urology* 1976;**7**:451.

Tank ES: Experience with endoscopic incision and open unroofing of ureteroceles. *J Urol* 1986;**136**:241.

Ectopic Ureteral Orifice

Gotoh T et al: Single ectopic ureter. *J Urol* 1983;**129**:271.

Johnson DK, Perlmutter S: Single system ectopic ureteroceles. *J Urol* 1980;**123**:81.

Marshall S: Reimplantation of the dilated ectopic ureter of the duplex system as a separate unit. *J Urol* 1986;**135**:574.

Umeyama T et al: Ectopic ureter presenting with epididymitis in childhood: Report of 5 cases. *J Urol* 1985;**134**:131.

Abnormalities of Ureteral Position

Brooks RJ: Left retrocaval ureter associated with situs inversus. *J Urol* 1962;**88**:484.

Hanna MK: Bilateral retroiliac artery ureters. *Br J Urol* 1972;**44**:339.

Kenawi MM, Williams DI: Circumcaval ureter: A report of 4 cases in children with a review of the literature and a new classification. *Br J Urol* 1976;**48**:183.

Kumar S, Bhandari M: Selection of operative procedure for circumcaval ureter (type I): A rational approach. *Br J Urol* 1985;**57**:399.

Obstruction of the Ureteropelvic Junction

Anderson JC: *Hydronephrosis*. Heinemann, 1963.

Badlani G, Eshghi M, Smith AD: Percutaneous surgery for ureteropelvic junction obstruction (endopyelotomy): Technique and early results. *J Urol* 1986;**135**:26.

Bejjani B, Belman AB: Ureteropelvic junction obstruction in newborns and infants. *J Urol* 1982;**128**:770.

Culp OS, DeWeerd JH: A pelvic flap operation for certain types of ureteropelvic obstruction. *Mayo Clin Proc* 1951;**26**:483.

Davis DM: Intubated ureterotomy: A new operation for ureteral and ureteropelvic strictures. *Surg Gynecol Obstet* 1943;**76**:513.

Foley FEB: A new plastic operation for stricture at the ureteropelvic junction. *J Urol* 1937;**38**:643.

Hanna MK et al: Ureteral structure and ultrastructure. 1. The normal human ureter. 2. Congenital ureteropelvic junction obstruction and primary obstructive megaureter. *J Urol* 1976;**116**:718, 725.

Johnston JH: The pathogenesis of hydronephrosis in children. *Br J Urol* 1969;**41**:724.

Johnston JH et al: Pelvic hydronephrosis in children: A review of 219 personal cases. *J Urol* 1977;**117**:97.

King LR et al: The case for immediate pyeloplasty in the neonate with ureteropelvic junction obstruction. *J Urol* 1984;**132**:725.

King LR et al: Initial experiences with percutaneous and transurethral ablation of postoperative ureteral strictures in children. *J Urol* 1984;**131**:1167.

Koff SA et al: Pathophysiology of ureteropelvic junction obstruction: Experimental and clinical observations. *J Urol* 1986;**136**:336.

Maizels M, Smith CK, Firlit CF: The management of children with vesicoureteral reflux and ureteropelvic junction obstruction. *J Urol* 1984;**131**:722.

Perlberg S, Pfau A: Management of ureteropelvic junction obstruction associated with lower polar vessels. *Urology* 1984;**23**:13.

Perlmutter AD, Kroovand RL, Lai Y-W: Management of ureteropelvic obstruction in the first year of life. *J Urol* 1980;**123**:535.

Punjani HM: Transitional cell papilloma of the ureter causing hydronephrosis in a child. *Br J Urol* 1983;**55**:572.

Ramsay JWA et al: Percutaneous pyelolysis: Indications, complications and results. *Br J Urol* 1984;**56**:586.

Sant GR, Barbalias GA, Klauber GT: Congenital ureteral valves: An abnormality of ureteral embryogenesis? *J Urol* 1985;**133**:427.

Scardino PL, Prince CL: Vertical flap ureteropelvioplasty. *South Med J* 1953;**46**:325.

Smart WR: Surgical correction of hydronephrosis. Page 2047 in: *Campbell's Urology*. Vol 3. Harrison JH et al (editors). Saunders, 1979.

Stephens FD: Ureterovascular hydronephrosis and the "aberrant" renal vessels. *J Urol* 1982;**128**:984.

Thrall JH, Koff SA, Keyes JW Jr: Diuretic radionuclide renography and scintigraphy in the differential diagnosis of hydroureteronephrosis. *Semin Nucl Med* 1981;**11**:89.

Whitaker RH: Methods of assessing obstruction in dilated ureters. *Br J Urol* 1973;**45**:15.

Obstructed Megaureter

Ehrlich RM: The ureteral folding technique for megaureter surgery. *J Urol* 1985;**134**:668.

Hanna MK: Recent advances and further experience with surgical techniques for one-stage total remodeling of massively dilated ureters. *Urology* 1982;**19**:495.

Hendren WH: Operative repair of megaureter in children. *J Urol* 1969;**101**:491.

Tanagho EA, Smith DR, Guthrie TH: Pathophysiology of functional ureteral obstruction. *J Urol* 1970;**104**:73.

Tiburcio MA, Lima SVC: Functionally obstructed megaureter. *Braz J Urol* 1978;**4**:36.

Upper Urinary Tract Dilatation Without Obstruction

Homsy YL, Williot P, Danais S: Transitional neonatal hydronephrosis: Fact or fantasy? *J Urol* 1986;**136**:339.

Lupton EW et al: A comparison of diuresis renography, the Whitaker test and renal pelvic morphology in idiopathic hydronephrosis. *Br J Urol* 1985;**57**:119.

Thrall JH, Koff SA, Keyes JW Jr: Diuretic radionuclide renography and scintigraphy in the differential diagnosis of hydroureteronephrosis. *Semin Nucl Med* 1981;**11**:89.

Wolk FN, Whitaker RH: Late follow-up of dynamic evaluation of upper urinary tract obstruction. *J Urol* 1982;**128**:346.

ACQUIRED DISEASES

General

Gourdie RW, Rogers ACN: Bilateral ureteric obstruction due to endometriosis presenting with hypertension and cyclical oliguria. *Br J Urol* 1986;**58**:244.

Richie JP, Withers G, Ehrlich RM: Ureteral obstruction secondary to metastatic tumors. *Surg Gynecol Obstet* 1979;**148**:355.

Retroperitoneal Fibrosis

Brock J, Soloway MS: Retroperitoneal fibrosis and aortic aneurysm. *Urology* 1980;**15**:14.

Chan SL, Johnson HW, McLoughlin MG: Idiopathic retroperitoneal fibrosis in children. *J Urol* 1979;**122**:103.

Deane AM, Gingell JC, Pentlow BD: Idiopathic retroperitoneal fibrosis: The role of autotransplantation. *Br J Urol* 1983;**55**:254.

Hricak H, Higgins CB, Williams RD: Nuclear magnetic resonance imaging in retroperitoneal fibrosis. *AJR* 1983; **141**:35.

Lepor H, Walsh PC: Idiopathic retroperitoneal fibrosis. *J Urol* 1979;**122**:1.

Elyaderani MK et al: Facilitation of difficult percutaneous ureteral stent insertion. *J Urol* 1982;**128**:1173.

Hepperlen TW, Mardis HK, Kammandel H: The pigtail ureteral stent in the cancer patient. *J Urol* 1979;**121**:17.

Moody TE, Vaughan ED Jr: Steroids in the treatment of retroperitoneal fibrosis. *J Urol* 1979;**121**:109.

Peters JL, Cowie AG: Ureteric involvement with abdominal aortic aneurysm. *Br J Urol* 1978;**50**:313.

Siminovitch JM, Fazio VW: Ureteral obstruction secondary to Crohn's disease: A need for ureterolysis? *Am J Surg* 1980;**139**:95.

Ureteral Obstruction Secondary to Malignant Disease

Andriole GL et al: Indwelling double-J ureteral stents for temporary and permanent urinary drainage: Experience with 87 patients. *J Urol* 1984;**131**:239.

Ball AJ et al: The indwelling ureteric stent: The Bristol experience. *Br J Urol* 1983;**55**:622.

Elyaderani MK et al: Facilitation of difficult percutaneous ureteral stent insertion. *J Urol* 1982;**128**:1173.

Hepperlen TW, Mardis HK, Kammandel H: The pigtail ureteral stent in the cancer patient. *J Urol* 1979;**121**:17.

29

Disorders of the Bladder, Prostate, & Seminal Vesicles

Emil A. Tanagho, MD

CONGENITAL ANOMALIES OF THE BLADDER*

EXSTROPHY

Exstrophy of the bladder is a complete ventral defect of the urogenital sinus and the overlying skeletal system (see Chapter 2). Other congenital anomalies are frequently associated with it. The lower central abdomen is occupied by the inner surface of the posterior wall of the bladder, whose mucosal edges are fused with the skin. Urine spurts onto the abdominal wall from the ureteral orifices.

The rami of the pubic bones are widely separated. The pelvic ring thus lacks rigidity, the femurs are rotated externally, and the child "waddles like a duck." Since the rectus muscles insert on the rami, they are widely separated from each other inferiorly. A hernia, made up of the exstrophic bladder and surrounding skin, is therefore present. Epispadias almost always accompanies it.

Many untreated exstrophic bladders reveal fibrosis, derangement of the muscularis mucosae, and chronic infection (Rudin, Tannenbaum, and Lattimer, 1972). These changes tend to defeat efforts to form a bladder of proper capacity. About 60 instances of adenocarcinoma developing in such bladders have been reported.

Renal infection is common, and hydronephrosis caused by ureterovesical obstruction may be found on urography. These films also reveal separation of the pubic bones.

During the last few years, there have been very encouraging reports of complete reconstruction of this defect. Earlier, urinary diversion and resection of the bladder, with later repair of the epispadiac penis, was usually accomplished. Now, however, with improved techniques and early surgery before the bladder deteriorates, good results are being obtained with complete reconstruction. Lattimer et al (1978), pioneers in this field, followed their 17 patients with reconstructed

bladders for as long as 20 years. They reported that the quality of life of these patients was good.

Ansel (1979) performed reconstruction in 28 patients in the neonatal period in an attempt to protect the bladder from later serious changes. Half of these patients did well, and most were continent. De Maria et al (1980) found the renal function and urine cultures of their patients to be normal. Eight of their patients had complete continence, while 12 suffered from enuresis. Toguri et al (1978) reported that all of their 23 patients were continent.

Lima et al (1981) reconstructed the bladder with human dura mater to increase vesical capacity; they were successful in 8 cases. They perform osteotomy as part of the first stage and recommend that the surgery be performed when patients are 3–18 months old. Mollard (1980) recommends the following steps for satisfactory repair of bladder exstrophy: (1) bladder closure with sacral osteotomy in order to close the pelvic ring at the pubic symphysis, plus lengthening of the penis; (2) anti-ureteral reflux procedure and bladder neck reconstruction; and (3) repair of the epispadiac penis. He completed 16 such 3-step procedures, with satisfactory results in 11. In 1983, Jeffs reported results of staged reconstruction: 19 of 22 patients who underwent primary repair were continent (86%), and renal function was preserved in approximately 90%. Urethral and genital reconstruction have been equally successful. These are the best reported results.

When the bladder is small, fibrotic, and inelastic, functional closure becomes inadvisable, and urinary diversion with cystectomy is the treatment of choice. Some physicians perform ureteroileocutaneous anastomosis, while others prefer to use the colon for the diversion. Continent diversion is a current consideration. Spence, Hoffman, and Pate (1975) employ ureterosigmoidostomy. Turner, Ransley, and Williams (1980) noted that, although untreated newborns have normal upper urinary tracts, urinary diversion often causes hydronephrosis or pyelonephritis in these patients.

Boyce (1972) and Gregoire and Schulman (1978) perform vesicorectal anastomosis after closure of the bladder; proximal colostomy is necessary.

The common complication of total reconstruction is urinary incontinence, but Light and Scott (1983) reported on the implantation of an artificial sphincter in

---

* Congenital vesicorectal fistulas are discussed with urethrorectal fistulas on p 572.

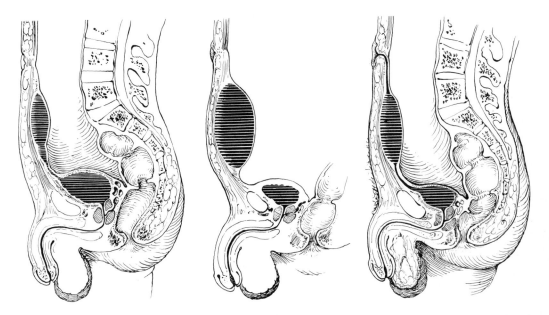

Figure 29–1. Types of persistent urachus. *Left:* Communicating urachus continuous with the bladder. This is a "pseudodiverticulum" and usually causes no symptoms. *Center:* Urachal cyst; usually causes no symptoms or signs unless it becomes larger or infected. *Right:* Patent urachus. There is constant drainage of urine from the umbilicus.

11 patients who were still incontinent after total reconstruction. They claimed 10 perfect results. Ikeme (1981) reported on 2 patients who became pregnant after repair of bladder exstrophy; one woman had 3 successful pregnancies, and the other had one.

PERSISTENT URACHUS

Embryologically, the allantois connects the urogenital sinus with the umbilicus. Normally, the allantois is obliterated and is represented by a fibrous cord (urachus) extending from the dome of the bladder to the navel (see Chapter 2). Urachal formation is directly related to bladder descent. Lack of descent is more commonly associated with patent urachus (more than with bladder outlet obstruction).

Incomplete obliteration sometimes occurs. If obliteration is complete except at the superior end, a draining umbilical sinus may be noted. If it becomes infected, the drainage will be purulent. If the inferior end remains open, it will communicate with the bladder, but this does not usually produce symptoms. Rarely, the entire tract remains patent, in which case urine drains constantly from the umbilicus. This is apt to become obvious within a few days of birth. If only the ends of the urachus seal off, a cyst of that body may form and may become quite large, presenting a low midline mass (Fig 29–1). If the cyst becomes infected, signs of general and local sepsis will develop.

Adenocarcinoma may occur in a urachal cyst, particularly at its vesical extremity, and will tend to invade the tissues beneath the anterior abdominal wall.

It may be seen cystoscopically. Stones may develop in a cyst of the urachus. These can be identified on a plain x-ray film.

Treatment consists of excision of the urachus, which lies on the peritoneal surface. If adenocarcinoma is present, radical resection is required.

Unless other serious congenital anomalies are present, the prognosis is good. The complication of adenocarcinoma offers a poor prognosis.

CONTRACTURE OF THE BLADDER NECK

There is considerable debate about the incidence of congenital narrowing of the bladder neck. Some feel that its presence is a common cause of vesicoureteral reflux, vesical diverticula, a bladder of large capacity, and the syndrome of irritable bladder associated with enuresis. A few observers consider this contracture a rare phenomenon and believe that the diagnosis is purely presumptive. The diagnosis is based upon endoscopic observation, which is an unreliable method. Voiding cystourethrography has been used to depict such narrowing, but interpretation of the films varies from urologist to urologist and radiologist to radiologist.

Nunn (1965) studied the intravesical and urethral pressures during voiding in cases with the signs mentioned above and found no evidence of bladder neck obstruction. The 2 recorded pressures were essentially equal. It appears that the bladder neck would have to be extremely stenotic to truly obstruct urine flow. It is becoming increasingly clear that, in little girls, the obstructive lesion is spasm of the periurethral striated muscle which develops secondary to distal urethral stenosis (see Chapter 31).

Empirical treatment is often employed; this consists of suprapubic bladder neck revision or transurethral resection. Making the bladder neck incompetent in young boys may later cause retrograde ejaculation and, therefore, infertility. Revision of the bladder neck in females may cause urinary incontinence. The diagnosis must therefore be made with caution.

Genuine functional bladder neck obstruction can only be detected in the presence of already high voiding pressures combined with lower resistance in the external sphincteric segment associated with a low flow rate. This condition is highly suggestive of functional bladder neck obstruction, although not 100% diagnostic.

ACQUIRED DISEASES OF THE BLADDER

INTERSTITIAL CYSTITIS
(Hunner's Ulcer, Submucous Fibrosis)

Interstitial cystitis is primarily a disease of middle-aged women. It is characterized by fibrosis of the vesical wall, with consequent loss of bladder capacity. Frequency, urgency, and pelvic pain with bladder distention are the principal symptoms.

Pathogenesis & Pathology

Infection does not appear to be the cause of fibrosis of the bladder wall, because the urine is usually normal. It has been postulated that the fibrosis is due to obstruction of the vesical lymphatics secondary to pelvic surgery or infection, but many of these patients fail to give such a history. It may be secondary to thrombophlebitis complicating acute infections of the bladder or pelvic organs or may be the result of prolonged intrinsic arteriolar spasm secondary to vasculitis or psychogenic impulses or could also be of neuropathic origin. Endocrinologic factors are also suggested.

Recently, however, evidence has been adduced which suggests that interstitial cystitis is an autoimmune collagen disease. Oravisto, Alfthan, and Jokinen (1970) studied 54 women afflicted with this disease. Antinuclear antibodies were found in 85%. A significant number had allergy of the reagin type or hypersensitivity to drugs. Jacobo, Stamler, and Culp (1974) and Gordon et al (1973) have confirmed these findings. An allergic cause would explain the favorable responses to corticosteroids.

The primary change is fibrosis in the deeper layers of the bladder. The capacity of the organ is decreased, sometimes markedly. The mucosa is thinned, espe-

cially where mobility is greatest as the bladder fills and empties (ie, over the dome), and small ulcers or cracks in the mucous membrane may be seen in this area. In the most severe cases, the normal mechanism of the ureterovesical junctions is destroyed, leading to vesicoureteral reflux. Hydroureteronephrosis and pyelonephritis may then ensue.

Microscopically, the mucosa may be thinned or even denuded. The capillaries of the tunica propria are often engorged, and signs of inflammation are apparent. The muscle is replaced by varying amounts of fibrous tissue, which is often quite avascular. The lymphatics may be engorged. Increased mast cells and lymphocytic infiltration are seen (Jacobo, Stamler, and Culp, 1974).

Clinical Findings

Interstitial cystitis should be considered when a middle-aged woman with clear urine complains of severe frequency and nocturia and suprapubic pain on vesical distention.

A. Symptoms: There is a long history of slowly progressive frequency and nocturia, both of which may be severe. The history does not suggest infection (burning on urination, cloudy urine). Suprapubic pain is usually marked when the bladder is full. Pain may also be experienced in the urethra or perineum. It is relieved on voiding. Gross hematuria is occasionally noted, usually when urination has had to be postponed (ie, following vesical overdistention). The patient is tense and anxious. Whether this is secondary to the prolonged and severe symptoms or is the primary cause of the vesical changes is not clear (see Chapter 36). A history of allergy may be obtained.

B. Signs: Physical examination is usually normal. Some tenderness in the suprapubic area may be noted. There may be some tenderness in the region of the bladder when it is palpated through the vagina.

C. Laboratory Findings: If the patient has had no previous treatment (eg, instrumentation), the urine is almost always free of infection. Microscopic hematuria may be noted. Results of renal function tests are normal except in the occasional patient in whom vesical fibrosis has led to vesicoureteral reflux or obstruction.

D. X-Ray Findings: Excretory urograms are usually normal unless reflux has occurred, in which case hydronephrosis is found. The accompanying cystogram will reveal a bladder of small capacity; reflux into a dilated upper tract may be noted on cystography.

E. Instrumental Examination: Cystoscopy is usually diagnostic. As the bladder fills, increasing suprapubic pain is experienced. The vesical capacity may be as low as 60 mL. In a patient not previously treated (by fulguration or hydraulic overdistention), the bladder lining may look fairly normal. However, if a second distention is done (Messing and Stamey, 1978), punctate hemorrhagic areas may appear over the most distensible portion of the wall. With further distention, an arcuate split in the mucosa will occur and may bleed profusely.

Lapides (1975) believes this disease is common in young women whose only complaint is frequency due to a small bladder capacity. However, he has found no vesical lesion in such cases.

Differential Diagnosis

Tuberculosis of the bladder may cause true ulceration but is most apt to involve the region of the ureteral orifice that drains the tuberculous kidney. Typical tubercles may be identified, pyuria is present, and tubercle bacilli can usually be found. Furthermore, urograms will often show the typical lesion of renal tuberculosis.

Vesical ulcers due to schistosomiasis will cause symptoms similar to those of interstitial cystitis. The diagnosis will be suggested if the patient lives in an area in which schistosomiasis is endemic. Most patients are males. The typical ova found in the urine and pathognomonic appearance of the bladder make the diagnosis.

Nonspecific vesical infection seldom causes ulceration. Pus and bacteria will be found in the urine. Antimicrobial treatment will be effective.

Utz and Zinke (1974) observed that 20% of their male patients who had been diagnosed as having interstitial cystitis actually had carcinoma. They stress the need for cytologic study and transurethral biopsy.

Complications

Gradual ureteral stenosis or reflux and its sequelae (eg, hydronephrosis) may develop.

Treatment

A. Specific Measures: There appears to be no definitive treatment for interstitial cystitis. The therapy usually employed frequently affords partial relief, but it may be completely ineffective.

Hydraulic overdistention, with or without anesthesia, sometimes gradually improves the bladder capacity. Vesical lavage with increasing strengths of silver nitrate (1:5000–1:100) may have the same effect. Superficial (transcystoscopic) electrocoagulation of the split mucosa is commonly performed and may afford temporary relief of pain. Greenberg et al (1974) believe that transurethral resection of the lesion affords better results than fulguration.

Stewart and Shirley (1976) report good symptomatic relief following the instillation of 50 mL of 50% dimethyl sulfoxide (DMSO) into the bladder every 2 weeks. It is left in for 15 minutes. Fowler (1981) reports similar success with this regimen.

Messing and Stamey (1978) claim their best results were obtained with vesical irrigations of 0.4% oxychlorosene sodium (Clorpactin WCS-90). At 10 cm of water pressure, the bladder is repeatedly filled to capacity until 1 L has been used. This must be done under anesthesia. Cystography should be done before instituting this therapy. The presence of vesicoureteral reflux has caused ureteral fibrosis (Messing and Freiha, 1979).

Parsons, Schmidt, and Pollen (1983) observed the results obtained in patients who failed to respond to hydraulic distention or the instillation of DMSO. They found that the bladder mucosa needs a layer of sulfonated glycosaminoglycans on its surface to protect the transitional cells from the effect of urine, and this substance was absent from the mucosa of these patients. They administered sodium pentosanpolysulfate (Elmiron) orally, in doses of either 50 mg 4 times a day or 150 mg twice daily, for 4–8 weeks. Of 24 patients, 20 noted at least 80% relief of urgency, frequency, and nocturia; and 2 noted 50–80% relief. These 22 patients continue to improve. Two patients experienced no apparent relief.

Cortisone acetate, 100 mg, or prednisone (Meticorten), 10–20 mg/d, in divided doses orally for 21 days, followed by decreasing amounts for an additional 21 days, has also been found effective (Badenoch, 1971). Transcystoscopic injection of the lesions with prednisone has its proponents.

Antihistamines (eg, pyribenzamine, 50 mg 4 times a day) may also afford some relief. Heparin sodium (long-acting), 20,000 units intravenously daily, also blocks the action of histamine, and its use in the treatment of interstitial cystitis is encouraging.

Freiha, Faysal, and Stamey (1980) performed cystolysis in 5 patients who did not respond to oxychlorosene; all improved. If the bladder becomes fibrotic and the capacity small, ceco- or ileocystoplasty can be done to augment vesical capacity (Green, Mitcheson, and McGuire, 1983; Chang et al, 1980). Most patients are cured or greatly improved; those who are not may require urinary diversion.

Denervation by presacral and sacral neurectomy and perivesical procedures (cystolysis, cystoplasty, transvaginal neurotomy) is to be condemned, as it is rarely of lasting benefit. In severe contracture, augmentation cystoplasty is indicated.

B. General Measures: General or vesical sedatives may be prescribed but seldom afford relief. If urinary infection is found (usually following instrumentation), it should be treated by appropriate antibiotics. If senile urethritis is discovered, diethylstilbestrol vaginal suppositories may prove helpful.

C. Treatment of Complications: If progressive hydronephrosis develops secondary to ureteral stenosis, little will be gained by ureteral dilatations. Diversion of the urinary stream (eg, ureteroileocutaneous anastomosis) may therefore be necessary.

Prognosis

Most patients respond to one of the conservative measures mentioned above. Those who do not may require operation.

EXTERNAL VESICAL HERNIATION

The bladder of a young girl may protrude through a patulous urethra and present itself externally. Treatment requires gentle pressure upon the mass, with the patient in the Trendelenburg position. After reduction, a small urethral catheter should be left in the bladder for a few days. If herniation recurs, the bladder and urethra should be sutured to the linea alba.

INTERNAL VESICAL HERNIATION

One side of the bladder may become involved in an inguinal hernia (in men) or a femoral hernia (in women) (Fig 29–2). Such a mass may recede on urination. It is most often found as a previously unsuspected complication during surgical correction of a hernia (Bell and Witherington, 1980). Weitzenfeld et al (1980) reported a case in which the right kidney and ureter as well as the left ureter were in scrotal inguinal hernias.

URINARY STRESS INCONTINENCE

Stress incontinence, the loss of urine with physical strain (eg, coughing, sneezing), is a common complaint of older women. Although it usually occurs as an aftermath of childbirth, it has been observed in girls and nulliparous women also.

Normal urethral resistance is about 100 cm of water; this is the sum of the resistance of the smooth muscle urethral sphincter (50 cm of water) and the striated midurethral sphincter (50 cm of water). Normally, with strain or cough, intraperitoneal pressure rises sharply but the resistance in the mid urethra rises also, thus maintaining the relatively high urethra-to-detrusor pressure ratio. In patients with stress incontinence, the basic lesion is loss of normal midurethral resistance caused by a severe sagging of the vesical base and urethra due to poor support of these structures. The sphincter muscles are usually normal, but with the descent of the urethra and bladder, they cannot work efficiently. Normally, the length of the urethra is 4 cm. Urethral pressure studies show little closure pressure in the proximal half of the urethra. Thus, the functional length of such urethras is about 2 cm (Tanagho, 1979). In addition, the area of the posterior urethra and bladder neck has fallen out of the true pelvis, so that the strain which suddenly increases intravesical pressure is associated with decreased resistance in the proximal and mid urethra, thereby leading to incontinence.

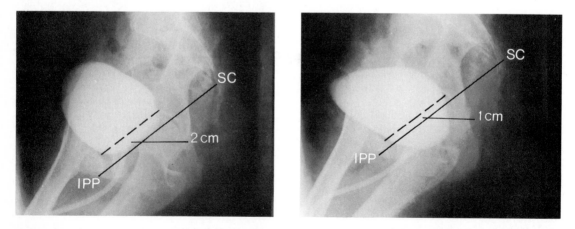

Figure 29–2. Internal vesical hernia; lateral cystograms in stress incontinence. *Above left:* Female, 6 months old. Cystogram of excretory urogram showing tongue of bladder in right femoral hernia (*see arrows*). In the 2 films shown below, the dashed line shows the normal position of the base of the normal bladder. Line SCIPP is a reference line drawn from the sacrococcygeal (SC) joint to the inferior point of the pubic bone (IPP). *Below left:* Resting cystogram in a stress incontinence. The bladder base lies 2 cm below the normal position. *Right:* Cystogram taken with straining in a patient with stress incontinence. The base of the bladder descends about 4 cm, revealing poor support of the urethrovesical junction. (Courtesy of John A Hutch.)

Susset et al (1976), Gershon and Diokno (1978), Faysal et al (1981), and Lockhart et al (*Urology*, 1982) have also published definitive studies on the urodynamics of urinary stress incontinence.

Clinical Findings

Patients complain of loss of urine only with straining in the upright position. They remain dry while in bed. Some degree of urethrocele is usually noted. Of some diagnostic value is the demonstration that support to the bladder neck will cause the patient to be continent with cough or strain. This test must be performed with the patient standing. The region of the bladder neck is lifted well up under the pubic symphysis with 2 fingers or 2 clamps. (If clamps are used, infiltration with a local anesthetic is required.) False-positive tests are sometimes elicited.

An important test in establishing the diagnosis of true stress incontinence is the lateral cystogram taken both with and without straining. A beaded chain or catheter should be placed in the bladder to delineate the urethrovesical junction (Fig 29–2). In the normal female, the base of the bladder lies about 2 cm above a line drawn from the inferior margin of the pubis to the sacrococcygeal joint (the SCIPP line). With straining, the vesical base should descend no more than 1.5 cm. With true stress incontinence, the static lateral cystogram may reveal some sagging of the bladder; this is markedly accentuated on the film taken when the patient strains to void (Noll and Hutch, 1969; Susset et al, 1976).

Differential Diagnosis

Careful history taking will usually differentiate between stress and urgency incontinence. The latter implies the presence of either local inflammatory disease or nervous tension. The following diseases must be differentiated from the lesion causing stress incontinence if good surgical results are to be obtained: ectopic ureteral orifice, neurogenic bladder, senile urethritis, urethral diverticulum, and local lesions of the urethra and bladder (eg, cystitis, urethritis). The history, physical examination, urinalysis, and renal function tests as well as cystoscopy, excretory urography, lateral cystography, and cystometry should make the differentiation. If urodynamic studies can be done, the diagnosis becomes highly accurate.

Treatment

If hypoestrogenism of the vagina and urethra is discovered, give estrogens locally or by mouth (see Chapter 31). If the degree of incontinence is mild, Stewart, Banowsky, and Montague (1976) recommend Ornade Spansules (a sustained-release preparation containing phenylpropanolamine, 50 mg; chlorpheniramine, 8 mg; and isopropamide iodide, 2.5 mg), 1 capsule daily. This treatment appears to be worth trying before surgery is recommended.

Although a vaginal approach designed to afford support to the bladder neck is most commonly employed, it appears that retropubic urethrovesical suspension (Marshall-Marchetti operation) affords a better result (Tanagho, 1976; Parnell, Marshall, and Vaughan, 1982). Stamey, Schaeffer, and Condy (1975) employ a similar procedure done through the endoscope with good results. Cobb and Ragde (1978) also report good results with this technique. Other operations largely based on the above principles include a modification of the Pereyra procedure (Roberts et al, 1981) and a modified Burch operation (Lockart, Maggiolo, and Politano, 1983).

Lockhart et al (*J Urol*, 1982) reviewed the causes of failure of these operations. They include improper surgical indications, suture misplacement, and failure to correct the urethrovesical angle.

Prognosis

If the proper diagnosis has been made, the cure rate approaches 85–90%. Unfortunately, stress incontinence recurs in a few cases after a year or so. Reoperation may therefore be necessary.

URINARY INCONTINENCE

Partial or complete urinary incontinence may develop after prostatectomy, particularly the transurethral type. Intrinsic damage to the smooth muscle urethral sphincter is implied. Though it is common to incriminate damage to or resection of the external voluntary sphincter, this is very rare. Such a patient can stop the voiding stream by contracture of the latter sphincter, but prolonged control is impossible because of fatigue of striated muscle. Only the smooth muscle with its constant tone can afford continence.

Scott, Bradley, and Timm (1974) and Light and Scott (1983) have described an ingenious method for affording urinary control. The entire silicone prosthesis is buried in the patient. It consists of a reservoir of fluid in a silastic bag placed deep to the abdominal wall near the bladder and a collar of silastic material that can encircle either the bladder neck or the bulbar urethra. The former is used in females, the latter in males. One silastic bulb is implanted in one scrotal (or labial) sac. This bulb has a special pressurized valve that will inflate or deflate the cuff around the urethra; compressed fluid will pass from the cuff to the reservoir, permitting free voiding. The cuff will refill spontaneously after a delay of 2 minutes. This device has been successful in affording control in most instances. Results are perfect in 75% or more of cases. Most failures follow technical difficulties with the prosthesis, eg, leakage, which requires reoperation.

Numerous other operations for cure of total incontinence have been designed. Kaufman has devised a number of procedures that apply pressure to the perineal urethra just distal to the prostate. These include apposition or transposition of the ischiocavernosus muscles and implantation of a plastic prosthesis. His most recent device (Kaufman and Raz, 1979) consists of a silastic container embedded in the perineum over the bulbous urethra. Silicon gel is instilled into the container until the desired occlusive pressure is reached. If leakage still occurs in the postoperative period, more silicon can be instilled percutaneously. Politano (1982) injects Polytef (Teflon) into the perineal periurethral tissues or submucosally at the bladder neck to afford suitable compression and claims excellent results.

Some of the mild cases may respond to ephedrine. Diokno and Taub (1975) prescribed up to 200 mg/d in 4 divided doses, with good response. Children were also benefited by the elixir, which contains 11 mg of ephedrine per 5 mL.

Tanagho and Smith (1972) have designed a procedure based upon sound anatomic principles that has been quite successful in restoring urinary continence. A rectangular flap of the heavy layer of the middle circular layer of the detrusor muscle, anteriorly, is formed into a tube, thus affording sphincteric action. This is anastomosed to the prostatic urethra. With this procedure, 44 of 50 patients suffering from postprostatectomy incontinence were cured. Williams and Snyder (1976) have successfully utilized this procedure in children.

ENURESIS

Enuresis originally meant incontinence of urine, but usage has caused the term to be restricted to bedwetting after age 3 years. Most children have achieved normal bladder control by that time, girls earlier than boys. At age 6 years, 10% have enuresis. Even at age 14 years, 5% still wet the bed (Simonds, 1977). It is difficult to be sure, but it seems that more than 50% of cases are caused by delayed maturation of the nervous system or an intrinsic myoneurogenic bladder dysfunction; 30% are of psychic origin; and 20% are secondary to more obvious organic disease. Most children with functional enuresis spontaneously gain nocturnal control by age 10 years.

Psychodynamics

Training in bladder control should begin after age 1½ years; attempts made before this are usually fruitless and may be harmful. If the parents fail in this teaching, the child may not develop cerebral inhibitory control over the infantile uninhibited bladder until much later in childhood. If the parents are emotionally unstable, their anxieties may be transmitted to the child, who may express tension through enuresis.

The birth of a sibling may cause loss of the child's paramount position in the family. The child may then regress to an infancy pattern in order to recapture the parents' affection. An acute illness may be accompanied or followed by recurrence of incomplete nocturnal control. Physiologic or psychologic stress (fear and anxiety) may reestablish an uninhibited bladder.

Possibly 40% of enuretic children have electroencephalograms that are borderline or compatible with epilepsy or delayed maturation of the central nervous system.

Clinical Findings

A. Symptoms: A child may wet the bed occasionally or regularly. Careful questioning of the parents or observation by the physician reveals that the patient voids a free stream of normal caliber. This tends to rule out obstruction of the lower tract as a cause of the enuresis. Children with daytime incontinence are apt to have more than psychogenic enuresis. Many void frequently and are found to have a diminished vesical capacity, although capacity is normal under anesthesia. This is probably a reflection of delayed maturation.

There is no burning, although frequency and urgency are common. The urine is clear.

Observation of the parents often reveals that they are anxious and tense, traits that can only be aggravated by the child's bedwetting.

B. Signs: General physical and urologic examinations are normal.

C. Laboratory Findings: In the emotional and delayed maturation group, all tests, including urinalysis, are normal. An electroencephalogram may be abnormal, however.

D. X-Ray Findings: Excretory urograms show no abnormality. The accompanying cystogram reveals no trabeculation; a film of the bladder taken immediately after voiding shows no residual urine.

E. Instrumental Examination: A catheter of suitable size passes readily to the bladder, thereby ruling out stricture. If the catheter is passed after urination, no residual urine is found. Urethrocystoscopy is normal. Cystometric studies are usually abnormal, and a curve typical of the "uninhibited" (hyperirritable) neuropathic bladder is often obtained. Unless infection or some more obvious organic disease is discovered, instrumentation, x-ray, and urodynamic studies are not necessary.

Differential Diagnosis

A. Obstruction: Lower tract obstruction (eg, posterior urethral valves, meatal stenosis) causes a urinary stream of decreased caliber. Painful, frequent urination during the day and night, pyuria, and fever (eg, pyelonephritis) are often present, and the bladder may be distended. Urinalysis usually reveals evidence of infection. Anemia and impairment of renal function may be demonstrated.

Excretory urograms may show dilatation of the bladder and the upper urinary tract. Incomplete vesical emptying may be seen on the postvoiding film. Cystography may demonstrate distal urethral stenosis or reflux. Urethrocystoscopy reveals the organic cause.

Severe obstruction from severe spasm of the entire pelvic floor musculature on a psychosomatic basis can cause damage to the bladder and kidneys; infection is the rule.

B. Infection: Chronic urinary tract infection not due to obstruction usually produces frequency both day and night and pain on urination, although such infections may occur without symptoms of vesical irritability. Recurrent fever with exacerbations is common.

General examination may be normal. Anemia may be noted. Urinalysis will show pus cells or bacteria, or both. Renal function may be deficient. Excretory urograms may be essentially normal, although changes compatible with healed pyelonephritis are often seen. Cystoscopy will show the changes caused by infection. Urine specimens obtained by ureteral catheter may reveal renal infection. Cystography may show vesicoureteral reflux.

C. Neurogenic Disease: Children suffering from sacral cord or root abnormality (eg, myelodysplasia) may have incomplete urinary control both day and night. Since they ordinarily have significant amounts of residual urine, infection is usually found on urinalysis. The passage of a catheter, or the postvoiding film taken in conjunction with excretory urograms, will demonstrate the presence of residual urine. A plain film of the abdomen may reveal spina bifida.

The cystometrogram is usually typical of a flaccid neurogenic bladder. Cystoscopy demonstrates an atonic bladder with moderate trabeculation and evidence of infection.

D. Distal Urethral Stenosis: This congenital anomaly is the cause of enuresis in many young girls, even in the absence of cystitis. Urethral calibration will establish this diagnosis.

Complications

The complications of functional enuresis are psychic, not organic. These children are particularly disturbed when they begin to attend school. Even more pressure is brought to bear by their parents; these children find it impossible to stay overnight at the homes of their playmates. Unhealthy introversion may be their lot. Enuresis may be prolonged because of undue emphasis on dryness or as a result of punitive or shaming measures.

Late Sequels

Occasionally an adult is seen who, under stress, develops nocturnal frequency without comparable diurnal frequency. Thorough urologic investigation proves to be negative. Many of these people will give histories of enuresis of long duration in childhood. It is suggested that their cerebrovesical pathways again break down under undue emotional tension; nocturnal frequency may be the adult expression of enuresis.

Treatment

Treatment should be considered if enuresis persists after age 3 years.

A. General Measures: Fluids should be limited after supper. The bladder should be completely emptied at bedtime, and the child should be completely awakened a little before the usual time of bedwetting and allowed to void.

Drug therapy has its proponents.

1. Imipramine has been reported to cure 50–70% of patients and is probably the drug of choice. Start with 25 mg before dinner. Increase the dose as needed to 50 mg. Usually, 25 mg is sufficient (Kass, Diokno, and Montealegre, 1979).

2. Parasympatholytic drugs such as atropine or belladonna, by decreasing the tone of the detrusor, may at times be of value. Methantheline bromide, 25–75 mg at bedtime, is more potent.

3. Sympathomimetic drugs, eg, dextroamphetamine sulfate, 5–10 mg at bedtime, may cause enough wakefulness so that the child perceives the urge to void.

4. Phenytoin has been found to control some of those children whose electroencephalograms are abnormal.

The use of mechanical devices such as metal-covered pads that when wet cause an alarm to ring may be of benefit in cases of delayed maturation by setting up a conditioned reflex (Close, 1980).

Urologic treatments (eg, urethral dilation, urethral instillations of silver nitrate), though often recommended, should be condemned in the absence of demonstrable local disease. They are physically and psychically traumatic and can only cause further apprehension and fear in an already disturbed child.

B. Psychotherapy: Analytic evaluation and treatment may be indicated for some enuretic children and their parents. Responsibility for correction of the patient's feelings of insecurity rests with the parents, who must be cautioned not to punish the child or in any way contribute further to existing feelings of guilt and insecurity. The handling of the parents may prove difficult, in which case psychiatric referral may be necessary.

Prognosis

Retraining the enuretic child and, above all, reeducating the parents is difficult and time-consuming. Psychiatric referral for the parents and, at times, for the child may be necessary. Most patients conquer their enuresis by age 10 years. A few, however, do not, and they may later develop vesical irritability of the psychogenic type in response to acute or chronic tension or anxiety.

FOREIGN BODIES INTRODUCED INTO THE BLADDER & URETHRA

Numerous objects have been found in the urethra and bladder of both men and women. Some of them find their way into the urethra in the course of inquisitive self-exploration. Others are introduced (in the male) as contraceptive devices in the hope that plugging the urethra will block emission of the ejaculate.

The presence of a foreign body causes cystitis. Hematuria is not uncommon. Embarrassment may cause the victim to delay medical consultation. A plain x-ray of the bladder area will disclose metal objects. Nonopaque objects sometimes become coated with calcium. Cystoscopy will visualize them all.

Cystoscopic or suprapubic removal of the foreign body is indicated. If not removed, the foreign body will lead to infection of the bladder. If the infecting organisms are urea-splitting, the alkaline urine (which causes increased insolubility of calcium salts) contributes to rapid formation of stone upon the foreign object (Fig 16–13).

VESICAL MANIFESTATIONS OF ALLERGY

So many mucous membranes are affected by allergens that the possibility of allergic manifestations involving the bladder must be considered. Hypersensitivity is occasionally suggested in cases of recurrent symptoms of acute "cystitis" in the absence of urinary infection or other demonstrable abnormality. During the attack, general erythema of the vesical mucosa may be seen and some edema of the ureteral orifices noted.

A careful history may reveal that these attacks follow the ingestion of a certain food not ordinarily eaten (eg, fresh lobster). Sensitivity to spermicidal creams is occasionally observed. If vesical allergy is suspected, it may be aborted by the subcutaneous injection of 0.5–1 mL of 1:1000 epinephrine. Control may also be afforded by the use of one of the antihistamines. Skin testing has not generally proved helpful in determining the source of allergy.

DIVERTICULUM

Most vesical diverticula are acquired and are secondary to either obstruction distal to the vesical neck or the upper motor neuron type of neurogenic bladder. Increased intravesical pressure causes vesical mucosa to insinuate itself between hypertrophied muscle bundles, so that a mucosal extravesical sac develops. Often this sac lies just superior to the ureter and causes vesicoureteral reflux (Hutch saccule; Fig 12–6). The diverticulum is devoid of muscle and therefore has no expulsive power; residual urine is the rule, and infection is perpetuated. If the diverticulum has a narrow opening that interferes with its emptying, transurethral resection of its neck will improve drainage (Vitale and Woodside, 1979). Reece et al (1974) suggest the use of a fiberoptic bronchoscope passed through a panendoscope sheath to inspect the wall of the diverticulum, because carcinoma occasionally develops on its wall. Mićić and Ilić (1983) discovered 13 diverticula harboring malignant tumors: 9 transitional cell tumors, 2 squamous cell tumors, and 2 adenocarcinomas. Gerridzen and Futter (1982) saw 48 cases of vesical diverticula. Transitional cell tumors were found in 5 of these patients, but almost all the rest had abnormal histopathology: chronic inflammation and metaplasia. These authors stress the need for visualizing the interior of diverticula during endoscopy. At the time of open prostatectomy, resection of a diverticulum should be considered.

VESICAL FISTULAS

Vesical fistulas are common. The bladder may communicate with the skin, intestinal tract, or female reproductive organs. The primary disease is usually not urologic. The causes are as follows: (1) primary intestinal disease—diverticulitis, 50–60%; cancer of the colon, 20–25%; and Crohn's disease, 10% (Badlani et al, 1980); (2) primary gynecologic disease—pressure necrosis during difficult labor; advanced cancer of the cervix; (3) treatment for gynecologic disease following hysterectomy, low cesarean section, or radiotherapy for tumor; (4) trauma.

Malignant tumors of the small or large bowel, uterus, or cervix may invade and perforate the bladder. Inflammations of adjacent organs may also erode through the vesical wall. Severe injuries involving the bladder may lead to perivesical abscess formation, and these abscesses may rupture through the skin of the perineum or abdomen. The bladder may be inadvertently injured during gynecologic or intestinal surgery; cystotomy for stone or prostatectomy may lead to a persistent cutaneous fistula.

Clinical Findings

A. Vesicointestinal Fistula: Symptoms arising from a vesicointestinal fistula include vesical irritability, the passage of feces and gas through the urethra, and usually a change in bowel habits (eg, constipation, abdominal distention, diarrhea) caused by the primary intestinal disease. Signs of bowel obstruction may be elicited; abdominal tenderness may be found if the cause is inflammatory. The urine is always infected.

A barium enema, upper gastrointestinal series, or sigmoidoscopic examination may demonstrate the communication. Following a barium enema, centrifuged urine should be placed on an x-ray cassette and an exposure made. The presence of radiopaque barium will establish the diagnosis of vesicocolonic fistula. Cystograms may reveal gas in the bladder or reflux of the opaque material into the bowel (Fig 29–3). Cystoscopic examination, the most useful diagnostic procedure, will show a severe localized inflammatory reaction from which bowel contents may exude. Catheterization of the fistulous tract may be feasible; the instillation of radiopaque fluid will often establish the diagnosis (Carson, Malek, and Remine, 1978).

B. Vesicovaginal Fistula: This relatively common fistula is secondary to obstetric, surgical, or radiation injury or to invasive cancer of the cervix. The constant leakage of urine is most distressing to the patient. Pelvic examination usually reveals the fistulous opening, which can also be visualized with the cystoscope. It may be possible to pass a ureteral catheter through the fistula into the vagina. Vaginography often successfully shows ureterovaginal, vesicovaginal, and rectovaginal fistulas. A 30-mL Foley catheter is inserted into the vagina and the balloon is distended. A

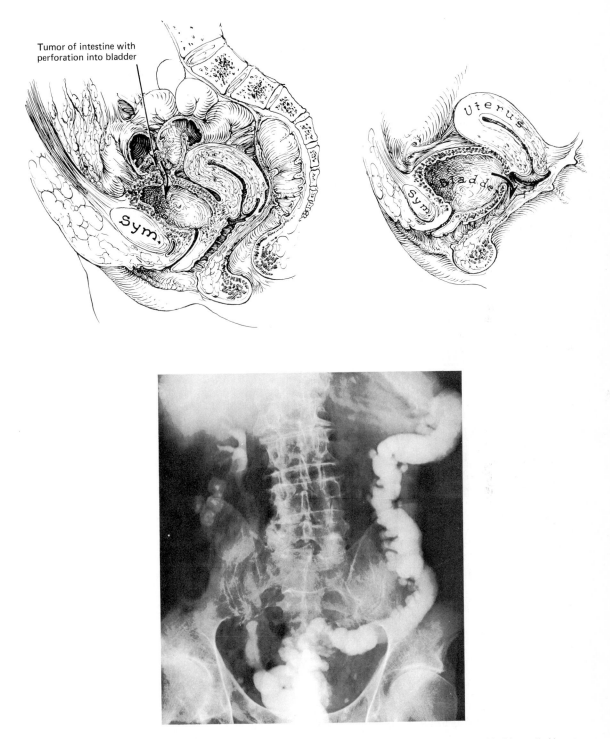

Figure 29–3. Vesical fistulas. *Above left:* Primary carcinoma of the sigmoid, with perforation through bladder wall. *Above right:* Injury to base of bladder following delivery by forceps. *Below:* Cystogram showing radiopaque fluid entering sigmoid containing multiple diverticula; right ureteral reflux, gallbladder calculi.

radiopaque solution is then instilled and appropriate x-rays are taken. Biopsy of the edges of the fistula may show carcinoma. Persky, Forsythe, and Herman (1980) describe vesicovaginal fistulas in 6 children; all occurred as a complication of surgery, 3 following transurethral resection of the bladder neck.

C. Vesicoadnexal Fistula: This rare fistula can be diagnosed by vaginal examination and by seeing the fistulous opening through the cystoscope.

Differential Diagnosis

It is necessary to differentiate ureterovaginal from vesicovaginal fistula.

Give pyridium by mouth to color the urine orange. One hour later, insert 3 cotton pledgets into the vagina and then instill methylene blue solution into the bladder. The patient should then walk around, after which the pledgets are examined. If the proximal cotton ball is wet and stained orange, the fistula is ureterovaginal. If the deep cotton pledget contains blue fluid, the diagnosis is vesicovaginal fistula. If only the distal pledget is blue, the patient probably has urinary incontinence (Raghavaiah, 1974).

Treatment

A. Vesicointestinal Fistula: If the lesion is in the rectosigmoid, treatment consists of proximal colostomy. When the inflammatory reaction has subsided, the involved bowel may be resected, with closure of the opening in the bladder. The colostomy can be closed later. Some authors recommend that the entire procedure be performed in one stage, thus avoiding the need for preliminary colostomy. Small bowel or appendiceal vesical fistulas require bowel or appendiceal resection and closure of the vesical defect (Goodwin and Scardino, 1980).

B. Vesicovaginal Fistula: Tiny fistulous openings may seal following the introduction of an electrode into the fistula. As the electrode is withdrawn, the fistula is coagulated with the electrosurgical unit to destroy the epithelium of the tract. An indwelling catheter should be left in place for 2 weeks or more. Aycinena (1977) reports good results in cases of small vesicovaginal fistulas treated by inserting a metal screw through the vaginal stoma. It is moved up and down to act as a curet. The vaginal mucosa is then closed and an indwelling catheter placed for 3 weeks.

Larger fistulas secondary to obstetric or surgical injuries respond readily to surgical repair, which may be done either through the vagina or transvesically (Goodwin and Scardino, 1980). Persky, Herman, and Guerrier (1979) advise repairing such fistulas immediately rather than waiting for 3–6 months as counseled by most surgeons. Fistulas that develop following radiation therapy for cancer of the cervix are much more difficult to close because of the avascularity of the tissues (Patil, Waterhouse, and Laungani, 1980). Surgical closure of fistulas that arise from direct invasion of the bladder by cervical carcinoma is impossible; diversion of the urinary stream above the level of the bladder (eg, ureterosigmoidostomy) is therefore necessary.

C. Vesicoadnexal Fistula: These fistulas are cured by removal of the involved female reproductive organs, with closure of the opening in the bladder (Henricksen, 1981).

Prognosis

The surgical repair of fistulas caused by benign disease or operative trauma is highly successful. Postirradiation necrosis offers a more guarded prognosis. Fistulas secondary to invading cancers present difficult problems.

PERIVESICAL LIPOMATOSIS

The cause of this lesion is not known. The disorder seems to affect principally black males in the 20- to 40-year age group. There are no pathognomonic symptoms. There may be some dysuria or mild urinary obstructive symptoms. Examination may demonstrate a distended or enlarged pear-shaped bladder. Excretory urograms and cystography may show dilatation of both upper tracts and an upward displacement and lateral compression of the bladder. In the perivesical area, x-ray reveals areas of radiolucency compatible with fatty tissue. A barium x-ray may show extrinsic pressure on the rectosigmoid. Angiography shows no evidence of neoplastic vessels.

CT scan in association with the above findings establishes the diagnosis by clearly demonstrating the fatty nature of the perivesical tissue (Levine, Farber, and Lee, 1978; Susmano and Dolin, 1979). Church and Kazam (1979) found sonography equally helpful.

On surgical exploration, lipomatous tissue is found surrounding the bladder and rectosigmoid. Though it is tempting to proceed with its resection, there are no cleavage planes. Such dissections have usually failed to relieve the ureteral obstruction. Sacks and Dresnick (1975) report that a low-calorie diet led to relief of ureteral obstruction in one case. Dilatation recurred when the patient again gained weight.

Ballesteros (1977) feels that surgical excision is feasible and reported excellent results in one such case. Crane and Smith (1977) found, after a 5-year follow-up, that hydronephrosis progressed in most. Many patients finally required urinary diversion.

RADIATION CYSTITIS

Many women receiving radiation treatment for carcinoma of the cervix develop some degree of vesical irritability. These symptoms may develop months after cessation of treatment. The urine may or may not be sterile. Vesical capacity is usually appreciably reduced. Cystoscopy will reveal a pale mucous membrane with multiple areas of telangiectatic blood vessels. Vesical ulceration may be noted, and vesicovaginal fistulas may develop. If symptoms are severe and prolonged, diversion of urine from the bladder may be necessary.

NONINFECTIOUS HEMORRHAGIC CYSTITIS

Some patients, following radiotherapy for carcinoma of the cervix or bladder, are prone to intermittent, often serious vesical hemorrhage. The same is true of those given cyclophosphamide.

In the case of the latter, the drug must be stopped. To control bleeding, cystoscopic fulguration can be tried, though it usually fails. The instillation of 3.9% formalin (prepared by diluting the standard 39% solution 10 times) is more efficacious. Clamp the catheter for 30 minutes and then lavage the bladder with 10% alcohol. A second or third instillation may be necessary on subsequent days. Holstein et al (1973) recommend the transurethral placement of a large balloon in the bladder. The balloon is filled to a pressure level equal to the systolic blood pressure and left in place for 6 hours. McGuire et al (1974) consider this the procedure of choice.

Pyeritz et al (1978) were unable to stop the hemorrhage with formalin or silver nitrate, but a continuous intravenous infusion of vasopressin caused it to cease. Giulani et al (1979) report success by selective transcatheter embolization of the internal iliac arteries. Ostroff and Chenault (1982) believe that the best and least harmful method of treatment is continuous irrigation with 1% alum solution (the ammonium or potassium salt) through a 3-way Foley catheter.

Despite these measures, the mortality rate is significant. Droller, Saral, and Santos (1982) have evolved a plan for reducing the incidence of cyclophosphamide-induced hemorrhagic cystitis: they produce diuresis and have the patient void frequently (or use open catheter drainage). This reduces the concentration of cyclophosphamide metabolites and the duration of their contact with bladder mucosa. Before the institution of this regimen, 8 of 97 such patients died; afterward, 1 of 198 patients died.

EMPYEMA OF THE BLADDER

If supravesical diversion of the urine is performed without cystectomy, severe infection of the bladder may develop because of lack of washout. In males, cystostomy or cutaneous vesicostomy may be necessary. In females, the formation of a vesicovaginal fistula will permit drainage (Spence and Allen, 1971). Occasionally, cystectomy may be necessary.

CONGENITAL ANOMALIES OF THE PROSTATE & SEMINAL VESICLES

Congenital anomalies of the prostate are rare. Cysts of the prostate and the seminal vesicles have been reported. Enlargements of the prostatic utricle are often found in association with penoscrotal or perineal hypospadias. They are usually small, lying in the midline posterior to the prostate and emptying through the verumontanum. These cysts represent embryologic remnants of the distal end of the müllerian ducts (see Chapter 2). Rarely, they become large enough to be easily palpable rectally or even abdominally. Through local pressure, they may cause symptoms of obstruction of the bladder neck.

BLOODY EJACULATION

Hemospermia is a not uncommon complaint of middle-aged men. It is the wife who usually recognizes the symptom. It is thought by some to be caused by hyperplasia of the mucosa of the seminal vesicles. For this reason, the use of diethylstilbestrol, 5 mg/d for 1 week, has been suggested. In the author's hands, it has worked well. Tolley and Castro (1975) stated that thorough urologic investigation of men without other symptoms never reveals a pathologic lesion. The cause is therefore not clear. Stein, Prioleau, and Catalona (1980) have observed this symptom to be caused by adenomatous polyps in 3 men and to accompany a prostatic intraductal carcinoma in another. Cattolica (1982) cured 3 patients by electrocoagulation of granulations of the posterior urethra. Van Poppel et al (1983) found the blood to emanate from a utricular cyst. Needle aspiration cured it.

REFERENCES

Exstrophy

Ansel JS: Surgical treatment of exstrophy of the bladder with emphasis on neonatal primary closure. Personal experience with 28 consecutive cases treated at the University of Washington hospitals from 1962 to 1977: Techniques and results. *J Urol* 1979;**121**:650.

Boyce WH: A new concept concerning treatment of exstrophy of the bladder: 20 years later. *J Urol* 1972;**107**:476.

DeMaria JE et al: Renal function in continent patients after surgical closure of bladder extrophy. *J Urol* 1980;**124**:85.

Gregoire W, Schulman CC: Exstrophy of the bladder. Treatment by trigonosigmoidostomy: Long-term results. *Br J Urol* 1978;**50**:90.

Ikeme AC: Pregnancy in women after repair of bladder exstrophy: Two case reports. *Br J Obstet Gynaecol* 1981;**88**:327.

Jeffs RD: Complications of exstrophy surgery. *Urol Clin North Am* 1983;**10**:509.

Johnston JH: The genital aspects of exstrophy. *J Urol* 1975;**113**:701.

Kandzari SJ et al: Exstrophy of urinary bladder complicated by adenocarcinoma. *Urology* 1974;**3**:496.

Lattimer JK et al: Long-term follow-up after exstrophy closure: Late improvement and good quality of life. *J Urol* 1978;**119**:664.

Light JK, Scott, FB: Treatment of the epispadias-exstrophy complex with the AS792 artificial urinary sphincter. *J Urol* 1983;**129**:738.

Lima SVC et al: Bladder exstrophy: Primary reconstruction with human dura mater. *Br J Urol* 1981;**53**:119.

Mollard P: Bladder reconstruction in exstrophy. *J Urol* 1980;**124**:525.

Rudin L, Tannenbaum M, Latimer JK: Histologic analysis of the exstrophied bladder after anatomical closure. *J Urol* 1972;**108**:802.

Spence HM, Hoffman WW, Pate VA: Exstrophy of the bladder. 1. Long-term results in a series of 37 cases treated by ureterosigmoidostomy. *J Urol* 1975;**114**:133.

Toguri AG et al: Continence in cases of bladder exstrophy. *J Urol* 1978;**119**:538.

Turner WR, Ransley PG, Williams DI: Patterns of renal damage in the management of vesical exstrophy. *J Urol* 1980;**124**:412.

Weed JC, McKee DM: Vulvoplasty in cases of exstrophy of the bladder. *Obstet Gynecol* 1974;**43**:512.

Persistent Urachus

Bauer SB, Retik AB: Urachal anomalies and related umbilical disorders. *Urol Clin North Am* 1978;**5**:195.

Blichert-Toft M, Kock F, Nielsen OV: Anatomic variants of the urachus related to clinical appearance and surgical treatment of urachal lesions. *Surg Gynecol Obstet* 1973;**137**:51.

Morin ME et al: Urachal cyst in the adult: Ultrasound diagnosis. *AJR* 1979;**132**:831.

Walden TB, Karafin L, Kendall AR: Urachal diverticulum in a 3-year-old boy. *J Urol* 1979;**122**:554.

Contracture of the Bladder Neck

Chang SL et al: Cecocystoplasty in the surgical management of the small contracted bladder. *J Urol* 1980;**124**:338.

Green D, Mitcheson HD, McGuire EJ: Management of the bladder by augmentation ileocecocystoplasty. *J Urol* 1983;**130**:133.

Grieve J: Bladder neck stenosis in children: Is it important? *Br J Urol* 1967;**39**:13.

Kaplan GW, King LR: An evaluation of Y-V vesicourethroplasty in children. *Surg Gynecol Obstet* 1970;**130**:1059.

Leadbetter GW Jr: Urinary tract infection and obstruction in children. *Clin Pediatr* 1966;**5**:377.

Moir JC: Vesicovaginal fistulae caused by wedge-resection of the bladder neck. *Br J Surg* 1966;**53**:102.

Nunn IN: Bladder neck obstruction in children. *J Urol* 1965;**93**:693.

Ochsner MG, Burns E, Henry HH Jr: Incidence of retrograde ejaculation following bladder neck revision in the child. *J Urol* 1970;**104**:596.

Shopfner CE: Roentgenologic evaluation of bladder neck obstruction. *Am J Roentgenol* 1967;**100**:162.

Smith DR: Critique on the concept of vesical neck obstruction in children. *JAMA* 1969;**207**:1686.

Interstital Cystitis

Badenoch AW: Chronic interstitial cystitis. *Br J Urol* 1971;**43**:718.

Fowler JE: Prospective study of intravesical dimethylsulfoxide in treatment of suspected early interstitial cystitis. *Urology* 1981;**18**:21.

Freiha FS, Faysal MH, Stamey TA: The surgical treatment of intractable interstitial cystitis. *J Urol* 1980;**123**:632.

Gordon HL et al: Immunologic aspects of interstitial cystitis. *J Urol* 1973;**109**:228.

Greenberg E et al: Transurethral resection of Hunner's ulcer. *J Urol* 1974;**111**:764.

Jacobo EJ, Stamler FW, Culp DA: Interstitial cystitis followed by total cystectomy. *Urology* 1974;**3**:481.

Jokinen EJ, Oravisto KJ, Alfthan OS: The effect of cystectomy on antitissue antibodies in interstitial cystitis. *Clin Exp Immunol* 1973;**15**:457.

Lapides J: Observations on interstitial cystitis. *Urology* 1975;**5**:610.

Messing EM, Freiha FS: Complications of clorpactin WCS-90 therapy for interstitial cystitis. *Urology* 1979;**13**:389.

Messing EM, Stamey TA: Interstitial cystitis: Early diagnosis, pathology and treatment. *Urology* 1978;**12**:381.

Oravisto KJ, Alfthan OS, Jokinen EJ: Interstitial cystitis: Clinical and immunological findings. *Scand J Urol Nephrol* 1970;**4**:37.

Parsons CL, Schmidt JD, Pollen JJ: Successful treatment of interstitial cystitis with sodium pentosanpolysulfate. *J Urol* 1983;**130**:51.

Rosin RD et al: Interstitial cystitis. *Br J Urol* 1979;**51**:524.

Stewart BH, Shirley SW: Further experience with intravesical dimethyl sulfoxide in the treatment of interstitial cystitis. *J Urol* 1976;**116**:36.

Utz DC, Zinke H: The masquerade of bladder cancer as interstitial cystitis. *J Urol* 1974;**111**:160.

Worth PHL, Turner-Warwick R: The treatment of interstitial cystitis by cystolysis with observations on cystoplasty. *Br J Urol* 1973;**45**:65.

External Vesical Herniation

Ray B et al: Massive inguinoscrotal bladder herniation. *J Urol* 1977;**118**:330.

Redman JF et al: The treatment of massive scrotal herniation of the bladder. *J Urol* 1973;**110**:59.

Internal Vesical Herniation

Bell ED, Witherington R: Bladder hernias. *Urology* 1980;**15**:127.

Liebeskind AL, Elkin M, Goldman SH: Herniation of the bladder. *Radiology* 1973;**106**:257.

McCarthy MP: Obturator hernia of urinary bladder. *Urology* 1976;**7**:312.

Weitzenfeld MB et al: Scrotal kidney and ureter: An unusual hernia. *J Urol* 1980;**123**:437.

Urinary Stress Incontinence

Beck RP et al: Recurrent urinary stress incontinence treated by the fascia lata sling procedure. *Am J Obstet Gynecol* 1974;**120**:613.

Biggers RD, Soderdahl DW: Per os pubis (POP) urethropexy. *Urology* 1980;**16**:36.

Cobb OE, Ragde H: Simplified correction of female stress incontinence. *J Urol* 1978;**120**:418.

Faysal MH et al: The impact of bladder neck suspension on the resting and stress urethral pressure profile: A prospective study comparing controls with incontinent patients preoperatively and postoperatively. *J Urol* 1981;**125**:55.

Gershon CR, Diokno AC: Urodynamic evaluation of female stress urinary incontinence. *J Urol* 1978;**119**:787.

Lockhart JL, Maggiolo LF, Politano VA: Modified Burch colposuspension in treatment of female urinary incontinence. *Urology* 1983;**21**:382.

Lockhart JL et al: Urodynamics in women with stress incontinence. *Urology* 1983;**20**:333.

Lockhart JL et al: Vesicourethral dysfunction following cystourethropexy. *J Urol* 1982;**128**:943.

Noll LE, Hutch JA: The SCIPP line: An aid in interpreting the voiding lateral cystourethrogram. *Obstet Gynecol* 1969;**33**:680.

Parnell JP, Marshall VF, Vaughan ED Jr: Primary management of urinary stress incontinence by the Marshall-Marchetti-Krantz vesicourethropexy. *J Urol* 1982;**127**:679.

Roberts JA et al: Modified Pereyra procedure for stress incontinence. *J Urol* 1981;**125**:787.

Stamey TA, Schaeffer AJ, Condy M: Clinical and roentgenographic evaluation of endoscopic suspension of the vesical neck for urinary incontinence. *Surg Gynecol Obstet* 1975;**14**:355.

Stewart BH, Banowsky HW, Montague DK: Stress incontinence: Conservative therapy with sympathomimetic drugs. *J Urol* 1976;**115**:558.

Susset JG et al: Urodynamic assessment of stress incontinence and its therapeutic implications. *Surg Gynecol Obstet* 1976;**142**:343.

Tanagho EA: Colpocystourethropexy: The way we do it. *J Urol* 1976;**116**:751.

Tanagho EA: Simplified cystography in stress urinary incontinence. *Br J Urol* 1974;**46**:295.

Tanagho EA: Urodynamics of female urinary incontinence with emphasis on stress incontinence. *J Urol* 1979;**122**:200.

Urinary Incontinence

Diokno AC, Taub M: Ephedrine in treatment of urinary incontinence. *Urology* 1975;**5**:624.

Farghaly SA, Hindmarsh JR: Changes in urethral function following hysterectomy. *Proc Int Continence Soc* 1985;**15**:195.

Furlow WL: Postprostatectomy urinary incontinence: Etiology, prevention, and selection of surgical treatment. *Urol Clin North Am* 1978;**5**:347.

Gleason DM, Bottaccini MR: The effect of a fine urethral pressure-measuring catheter on urinary flow in females. *Neurourol Urodynam* 1984;**3**:163.

Glen ES, Eadie A, Rowan D: Urethral closure pressure profile measurements in female urinary incontinence. *Acta Urol Belg* 1984;**52**:174.

Hertogs K, Stanton SL: Mechanism of urinary continence after colposuspension: Barrier studies. *Br J Obstet Gynaecol* 1985;**92**:1184.

Hetzenauer A, Bazzanella A, Reider W: Unstable female urethra: Incidence and significance. *Proc Int Continence Soc* 1985;**15**:111.

Kaufman JJ, Raz S: Urethral compression procedure for the treatment of male urinary incontinence. *J Urol* 1979;**121**:605.

Kramer AEJL, Venema PL: Dynamic urethral pressure measurements in the diagnosis of incontinence in women. *World J Urol* 1984;**2**:203.

Massey A, Abrams P: Urodynamics of the female lower urinary tract. *Urol Clin North Am* 1985;**12**:231.

McGuire EJ, Woodside JR: Suprapubic suspension of Kaufman urinary incontinence prosthesis. *Urology* 1980;**15**:256.

Pagani JJ et al: Radiographic evaluation of an artificial urinary sphincter. *Radiology* 1980;**134**:311.

Persky L, Forsythe WE, Herman G: Vesicovaginal fistulae in childhood. *Urology* 1980;**15**:36.

Politano VA: Periurethral polytetrafluoroethylene injection for urinary incontinence. *J Urol* 1982;**127**:439.

Raezer DM et al: A clinical experience with the Scott genitourinary sphincter in the management of urinary incontinence in the pediatric age group. *J Urol* 1980;**123**:546.

Raz S: Diagnosis of urinary incontinence in the male. *Urol Clin North Am* 1978;**5**:305.

Raz S: Pathophysiology of male incontinence. *Urol Clin North Am* 1978;**5**:295.

Scott FB, Bradley WE, Timm GW: Treatment of urinary incontinence by implantable prosthetic urinary sphincter. *J Urol* 1974;**112**:75.

Sørensen S et al: Urethral pressure variations in healthy females. *Proc Int Continence Soc* 1985;**15**:109.

Tanagho EA: Bladder neck reconstruction for total urinary incontinence: 10 years of experience. *J Urol* 1981;**125**:321.

Tanagho EA, Schmidt RA: Bladder pacemaker: Scientific basis and clinical features. *Urology* 1982;**20**:614.

Tanagho EA, Smith DR: Clinical evaluation of a surgical technique for the correction of complete urinary incontinence. *J Urol* 1972;**107**:402.

Westby M, Asmussen M: Anatomical and functional changes in the lower urinary tract after radical hysterectomy with lymph node dissection as studied by dynamic urethrocystography and simultaneous urethrocystometry. *Gynecol Oncol* 1985;**21**:261.

Williams DI, Snyder H: Anterior detrusor tube repair for urinary incontinence in children. *Br J Urol* 1976;**48**:671.

Winter CC: Peripubic urethropexy for urinary stress incontinence in women. *Urology* 1982;**20**:408.

Enuresis

Andersen OO, Petersen KE: Enuresis: An attempt at classification of genesis. *Acta Paediatr Scand* 1974;**63**:512.

Arnold ST, Ginsburg A: Enuresis: Incidence and pertinence of genitourinary disease in healthy enuretic children. *Urology* 1973;**2**:437.

Bradley WE, Anderson JT: Techniques for analysis of micturition reflex disturbances in childhood. *Pediatrics* 1977;**59**:546.

Butcher C, Donnai D: Vaginal reflux and enuresis. *Br J Radiol* 1972;**45**:501.

Buttarazzi PJ: Oxybutynin chloride (Ditropan) in enuresis. *J Urol* 1977;**118**:46.

Campbell EW, Young JD Jr: Enuresis and its relationship to electroencephalographic disturbances. *J Urol* 1966;**96**:947.

Close GC: Nocturnal enuresis and the buzzer alarm: Role of the general practitioner: *Br Med J* 1980;**281**:483.

Forsythe WI, Redmond A: Enuresis and spontaneous cure rate: Study of 1129 enuretics. *Arch Dis Child* 1974;**49**:259.

Fraser MS: Nocturnal enuresis. *Practitioner* 1972;**208**:203.

Gibbon NO et al: Transection of the bladder for adult enuresis and allied conditions. *Br J Urol* 1973;**45**:306.

Kass EJ, Diokno AC, Montealegre A: Enuresis: Principles of management and results of treatment. *J Urol* 1979;**121**:794.

Kolvin I: Enuresis in childhood. *Practitioner* 1975;**214**:33.

Linderholm BE: The cystometric findings in enuresis. *J Urol* 1966;**96**:718.

Marshall S, Marshall HH, Lyon RP: Enuresis: An analysis of various therapeutic approaches. *Pediatrics* 1973;**52**:813.

Martin GI: Imipramine pamoate in the treatment of childhood enuresis. *Am J Dis Child* 1971;**122**:42.

Murphy S et al: Adolescent enuresis: A multiple contingency hypothesis. *JAMA* 1971;**218**:1189.

Oppel WC, Harper PA, Rider RV: Social, psychological, and neurological factors associated with nocturnal enuresis. *Pediatrics* 1968;**42**:627.

Simonds JF: Enuresis: A brief survey of current thinking with respect to pathogenesis and management. *Clin Pediatr* 1977;**16**:79.

Foreign Bodies Introduced into the Bladder & Urethra

Najafi E, Maynard JF: Foreign body in lower urinary tract. *Urology* 1975;**5**:117.

Prasad S et al: Foreign bodies in urinary bladder. *Urology* 1973;**2**:258.

Vesical Manifestations of Allergy

Pastinszky I: The allergic diseases of the male genitourinary tract with special reference to allergic urethritis and cystitis. *Urol Int* 1960;**9**:288.

Rubin L, Pincus MD: Eosinophilic cystitis: The relationship of allergy in the urinary tract to eosinophilic cystitis and the pathophysiology of eosinophilia. *J Urol* 1974;**112**:457.

Diverticulum

Barrett DM, Malek RS, Kelalis PP: Observations on vesical diverticulum in childhood. *J Urol* 1976;**116**:234.

Bauer SB, Retik AB: Bladder diverticula in infants and children. *Urology* 1974;**3**:712.

Gerridzen R, Futter NG: Ten-year review of vesical diverticula. *Urology* 1982;**10**:33.

Mićić S, Ilić V: Incidence of neoplasm in vesical diverticula. *J Urol* 1983;**129**:734.

Reece RW et al: Evaluation of bladder diverticulum using fiberoptic bronchoscope. *Urology* 1974;**3**:790.

Vitale PJ, Woodside JR: Management of bladder diverticula by transurethral resection: Re-evaluation of an old technique. *J Urol* 1979;**122**:744.

Vesical Fistulas

Aycinena JF: Small vesicovaginal fistula. *Urology* 1977;**9**:543.

Badlani G et al: Enterovesical fistulas in Crohn disease. *Urology* 1980;**16**:599.

Birkhoff JD, Wechsler M, Romas NA: Urinary fistulas: Vaginal repair using labial fat pad. *J Urol* 1977;**177**:595.

Carson CC, Malek RS, Remine WH: Urologic aspects of vesicoenteric fistulas. *J Urol* 1978;**119**:744.

Goodwin WE, Scardino PT: Vesicovaginal and ureterovaginal fistulas: A summary of 25 years of experience. *J Urol* 1980;**123**:370.

Gross M, Peng B: Appendico-vesical fistula. *J Urol* 1969;**102**:697.

Henricksen HM: Vesicouterine fistula following cesarean section. *J Urol* 1981;**125**:884.

Krompier A et al: Vesicocolonic fistulas in diverticulitis. *J Urol* 1976;**115**:664.

Patil U, Waterhouse K, Laugani G: Management of 18 difficult vesicovaginal and urethrovaginal fistulas with modified Ingelman-Sundberg and Martius operations. *J Urol* 1980;**13**:653.

Persky L, Forsythe WE, Herman G: Vesicovaginal fistulas in childhood. *Urology* 1980;**15**:36.

Persky L, Herman G, Guerrier K: Nondelay in vesicovaginal fistula repair. *Urology* 1979;**13**:273.

Raghavaiah NV: Double-dye test to diagnose various types of vaginal fistulas. *J Urol* 1974;**112**:811.

Shield DE et al: Urologic complications of inflammatory bowel disease. *J Urol* 1976;**115**:701.

Wolfson JS: Vaginography for demonstration of ureterovaginal, vesicovaginal and rectovaginal fistulas, with case reports. *Radiology* 1964;**83**:438.

Perivesical Lipomatosis

Ambos MA et al: The pear-shaped bladder. *Radiology* 1977;**122**:85.

Ballesteros JJ: Surgical treatment of perivesical lipomatosis. *J Urol* 1977;**118**:329.

Church PA, Kazam E: Computed tomography and ultrasound in diagnosis of pelvic lipomatosis. *Urology* 1979;**14**:631.

Crane DB, Smith MJV: Pelvic lipomatosis: Five-year follow-up. *J Urol* 1977;**118**:547.

Joshi KK, Wise HA II: Pelvic lipomatosis: 9-year follow-up in a woman. *J Urol* 1983;**129**:1233.

Levine E, Farber B, Lee KR: Computed tomography in diagnosis of pelvic lipomatosis. *Urology* 1978;**12**:606.

Radinsky S, Cabal E, Shields J: Pelvic lipomatosis. *Urology* 1976;**7**:108.

Sacks SA, Dresnick EJ: Pelvic lipomatosis: Effect of diet. *Urology* 1975;**6**:609.

Susmano DE, Dolin EH: Computed tomography in diagnosis of pelvic lipomatosis. *Urology* 1979;**13**:215.

Yalla SV et al: Cystitis glandularis with perivesical lipomatosis: Frequent association of two unusual proliferative conditions. *Urology* 1975;**5**:383.

Radiation Cystitis

Maatman TJ et al: Radiation-induced cystitis following intracavitary irradiation for superficial bladder cancer. *J Urol* 1983;**130**:338.

Mallik MKB: Study of radiation necrosis of the urinary bladder following treatment of carcinoma of the cervix. *Am J Obstet Gynecol* 1962;**83**:393.

Noninfectious Hemorrhagic Cystitis

Bennett AH: Cyclophosphamide and hemorrhagic cystitis. *J Urol* 1974;**111**:603.

Droller MJ, Saral K, Santos G: Prevention of cyclophosphamide-induced hemorrhagic cystitis. *Urology* 1982;**20**:256.

Giulani L et al: Gelatin foam and isobutyl-2-cyanoacrylate in the treatment of life-threatening bladder haemorrhage by selective transcatheter embolisation of the internal iliac arteries. *Br J Urol* 1979;**51**:125.

Holstein P et al: Intravesical hydrostatic pressure treatment: New method for control of bleeding from bladder mucosa. *J Urol* 1973;**109**:234.

McGuire EJ et al: Hemorrhagic radiation cystitis: Treatment. *Urology* 1974;**3**:204.

Marshall FF, Klinefelter HF: Late hemorrhagic cystitis following low-dose cyclophosphamide therapy. *Urology* 1979;**14:**573.

Moinuddin SM, Upton DW: Urothelial carcinoma after cyclophosphamide therapy. *J Urol* 1983;**129:**143.

Ostroff EB, Chenault OW Jr: Alum irrigation for the control of massive bladder hemorrhage. *J Urol* 1982;**128:**929.

Pyeritz RE et al: An approach to the control of massive hemorrhage in cyclophosphamide-induced cystitis by intravenous vasopressin: A case report. *J Urol* 1978;**120:** 253.

Scott MP Jr, Marshall S, Lyon RP: Bladder rupture following formalin therapy for hemorrhage secondary to cyclophosphamide therapy. *Urology* 1974;**3:**364.

Spiro LH et al: Formalin treatment for massive bladder hemorrhage. *Urology* 1973;**2:**669.

Empyema of the Bladder

Dretler SP: The occurrence of empyema cystitis: Management of the bladder to be defunctionalized. *J Urol* 1972; **108:**82.

Spence HM, Allen TD: Vaginal vesicostomy for empyema of the defunctionalized bladder. *J Urol* 1971;**106:**862.

Congenital Anomalies of the Prostate & Seminal Vesicles

Donohue RE, Greenslade NF: Seminal vesical cyst and ipsilateral renal agenesis. *Urology* 1973;**2:**66.

Feldman RA, Weiss RM: Urinary retention secondary to Müllerian duct cyst in a child. *J Urol* 1972;**108:**647.

Rieser C, Griffin TL: Cysts of the prostate. *J Urol* 1964; **91:**282.

Warren MM, Greene LF: Calculus in the prostatic utricle. *J Urol* 1972;**107:**82.

Bloody Ejaculation

Cattolica EV: Massive hemospermia: A new etiology and simplified treatment. *J Urol* 1982;**128:**151.

Ross JC: Haemospermia. *Practitioner* 1969;**203:**59.

Stein AJ, Prioleau PG, Catalona WJ: Adenomatous polyps of the prostatic urethra: A cause of hematospermia. *J Urol* 1980;**124:**298.

Tolley DA, Castro JE: Hemospermia. *Urology* 1975;**6:**331.

Van Poppel R et al: Hemospermia owing to utricular cyst: Embryological summary and surgical review. *J Urol* 1983;**129:**608.

30 Disorders of the Penis & Male Urethra

Jack W. McAninch, MD

CONGENITAL ANOMALIES OF THE PENIS

APENIA

Congenital absence of the penis (apenia) is extremely rare. In this condition, the urethra generally opens on the perineum or inside the rectum.

Patients with apenia must be assigned the female gender. Castration should be done and vaginoplasty performed in combination with estrogen treatment as the child develops.

MEGALOPENIS

The penis enlarges rapidly in childhood (megalopenis) in boys with abnormalities that have increased production of testosterone, eg, interstitial cell tumors of the testicle or hyperplasia or tumors of the adrenal cortex. Management is by correction of the underlying endocrine problem.

MICROPENIS

Micropenis is a more common anomaly and has been attributed to a testosterone deficiency that results in poor growth of organs that are targets of this hormone. A penis smaller than 2 standard deviations from the norm is considered a micropenis (see Table 30–1). The testicles are small and frequently undescended. Other organs, including the scrotum, may be involved. Early evidence suggests that the ability of the hypothalamus to secrete luteinizing hormone-releasing hormone (LHRH) is decreased. The pituitary-gonadal axis appears to be intact, since the organs respond to testosterone, although this response may be sluggish at times. Studies have shown that topical application of 5% testosterone cream causes increased penile growth, but its effect is due to absorption of the hormone, which then systemically stimulates genital growth (Jacobs, Kaplan, and Gittes, 1975). Patients with micropenis must be carefully evaluated for other endocrine and central nervous system anomalies. Retarded bone growth, anosmia, learning disabilities, and deficiencies of adrenocorticotropic hormone (ACTH) and thyrotropin (TSH) have been associated with micropenis. In addition, the possibility of intersex problems must be carefully investigated before therapy is begun.

The approach to management of micropenis has undergone gradual change in recent years, but androgen replacement is the basic requirement. The objective is to provide sufficient testosterone to stimulate penile growth without altering growth and closure of the epiphyses. Allen (1980) recommends giving testosterone in doses of 25 mg orally every 3 weeks for no more than 4 doses. Penile growth is assessed by measuring the length of the stretched penis (pubis to glans) before and after treatment. Therapy should be started by age 1 year and aimed at maintaining genital growth commensurate with general body growth. Repeat courses of therapy may be required if the size of the penis falls behind as the child grows. For undescended testicles, orchiopexy should be done before the child is 2 years old. In the future, treatment with LHRH may correct micropenis as well as cause descent of the testicles, but at present, LHRH is not commercially available or approved for such use.

Table 30–1. Size of unstretched penis and testis from infancy to adulthood.*

Age (Years)	Length of Penis (cm ± SD)	Diameter of Testis (cm ± SD)
0.2–2	2.7 ± 0.5	1.4 ± 0.4
2.1–4	3.3 ± 0.4	1.2 ± 0.4
4.1–6	3.9 ± 0.9	1.5 ± 0.6
6.1–8	4.2 ± 0.8	1.8 ± 0.3
8.1–10	4.9 ± 1	2 ± 0.5
10.1–12	5.2 ± 1.3	2.7 ± 0.7
12.1–14	6.2 ± 2	3.4 ± 0.8
14.1–16	8.6 ± 2.4	4.1 ± 1
16.1–18	9.9 ± 1.7	5 ± 0.5
18.1–20	11 ± 1.1	5 ± 0.3
20.1–25	12.4 ± 1.6	5.2 ± 0.6

*Reproduced, with permission, from Winter JSD, Faiman C: Pituitary-gonadal relations in male children and adolescents. *Pediatr Res* 1972;**6**:126.

CONGENITAL ANOMALIES OF THE URETHRA

DUPLICATION OF THE URETHRA

Duplication of the urethra is rare. The structures may be complete or incomplete (Wirtshafter et al, 1980).

Resection of all but one complete urethra is recommended.

URETHRAL STRICTURE

Congenital urethral stricture is uncommon in infant boys. The fossa navicularis and membranous urethra are the 2 most common sites. Severe strictures may cause bladder damage and hydronephrosis (see pp 172–175), with symptoms of obstruction (urinary frequency and urgency) or urinary infection. A careful history and physical examination are indicated in patients with these complaints. Excretory urography and excretory voiding urethrography will often define the lesion and the extent of obstruction. Retrograde urethrography (Fig 30–1) may also be helpful. Cystoscopy and urethroscopy should be performed in all patients in whom urethral stricture is suspected.

Strictures can be treated at the time of endoscopy. Diaphragmatic strictures respond to dilation. Other strictures should be treated under direct vision by internal urethrotomy with the currently available pediatric urethrotome. It may be necessary to repeat these procedures in order to remove the stricture. Open surgical repair is desirable if the obstruction recurs.

POSTERIOR URETHRAL VALVES

Posterior urethral valves, the most common obstructive urethral lesions in infants and newborns, occur only in males and are found at the distal prostatic urethra. The valves are mucosal folds that look like thin membranes; they may cause varying degrees of obstruction when the child attempts to void (Fig 30–2).

Clinical Findings

A. Symptoms and Signs: Children with posterior urethral valves may present with mild, moderate, or severe symptoms of obstruction (Uehling, 1980). They often have a poor, intermittent, dribbling urinary stream. Urinary infection and sepsis occur frequently. Severe obstruction may cause hydronephrosis (see pp 172–175), which is apparent as a palpable abdominal mass. A palpable midline mass in the lower abdomen is typical of a distended bladder. Occasionally, palpable flank masses indicate hydronephrotic kidneys. In many patients, failure to thrive may be the only significant symptom, and examination may reveal nothing more than evidence of chronic illness.

B. Laboratory Findings: Azotemia and poor concentrating ability of the kidney are common findings. The urine is often infected, and anemia may be found if infection is chronic. Serum creatinine and blood urea nitrogen levels and creatinine clearance are the best indicators of the extent of renal failure.

C. X-Ray Findings: Voiding cystourethrography is the best radiographic study available to establish the diagnosis of posterior urethral valves. The presence of large amounts of residual urine will be apparent on initial catheterization done in conjunction with radiographic studies, and an uncontaminated urine specimen should be obtained via the catheter and sent for culture. The cystogram may show vesicoureteral reflux and the severe trabeculations of long-standing obstruction, and the voiding cystourethrogram often demonstrates elongation and dilatation of the posterior urethra, with a prominent bladder neck (Fig 30–1). Excretory urograms may reveal hydroureter and hydronephrosis when obstruction is severe and long-standing.

D. Ultrasonography: Ultrasonography can be used to detect hydronephrosis, hydroureter, and bladder distention in children with severe azotemia. It can also detect fetal hydronephrosis, which is typical of urethral valves, as early as 28 weeks' gestation; when the obstruction is from valves, an enlarged bladder with bilateral hydroureteronephrosis is usually present (Fig 30–3).

E. Instrumental Examination: Urethroscopy and cystoscopy, performed with the patient under general anesthesia, will show vesical trabeculation and cellules and, occasionally, vesical diverticula. The bladder neck and trigone may be hypertrophied. The diagnosis is confirmed by visual identification of the valves at the distal prostatic urethra. Supravesical compression will show that the valves cause obstruction.

Treatment

Treatment consists of destruction of the valves, but the approach will depend on the degree of obstruction and the general health of the child. In children with mild to moderate obstruction and minimal azotemia, transurethral fulguration of the valves is usually successful (Johnston and Kulatilake, 1971). Occasionally, catheterization, cystoscopy, or urethral dilation by perineal urethrostomy) destroys the valves.

The more severe degrees of obstruction create varying grades of hydronephrosis requiring individual variation in management. Treatment of children with urosepsis and azotemia associated with hydronephrosis includes use of antibiotics, catheter drainage of the bladder, and correction of the fluid and electrolyte imbalance. Vesicostomy may be of benefit in patients with reflux and renal dysplasia.

In the most severe causes of hydronephrosis, vesicostomy or removal of the valves may not be

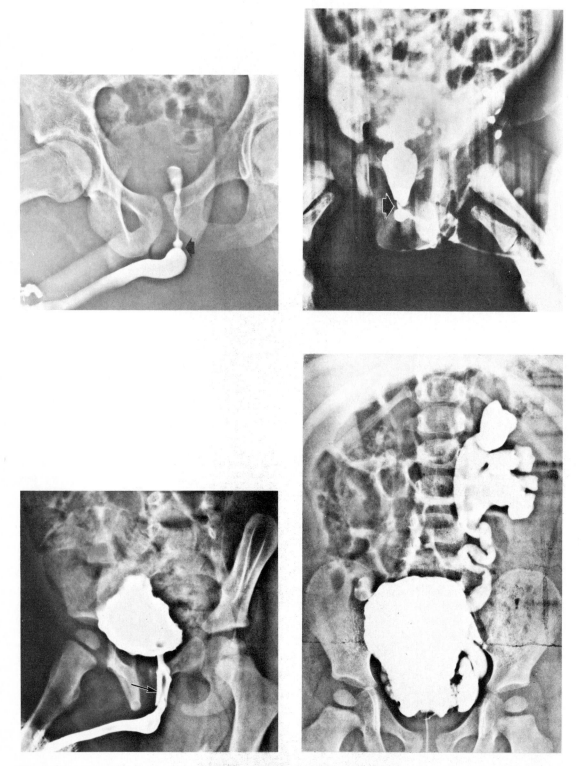

Figure 30–1. *Upper left:* Retrograde urethrogram showing congenital diaphragmatic stricture. *Upper right:* Posterior urethral valves revealed on voiding cystourethrography. Arrow points to area of severe stenosis at distal end of prostatic urethra. *Lower left:* Posterior urethral valves. Patient would not void with cystography. Retrograde urethrogram showing valves (*arrow*). *Lower right:* Cystogram, same patient. Free vesicoureteral reflux and vesical trabeculation with diverticula.

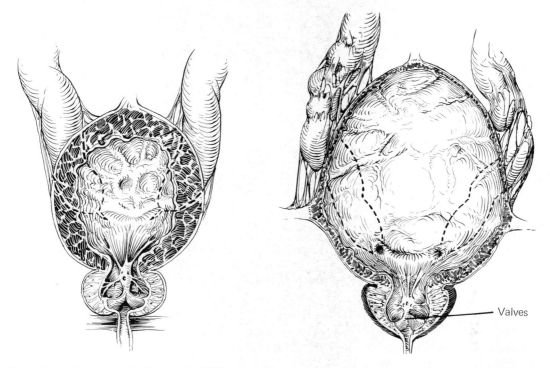

Figure 30–2. Posterior urethral valves. *Left:* Dilatation of the prostatic urethra, hypertrophy of vesical wall and trigone in stage of compensation; bilateral hydroureters secondary to trigonal hypertrophy. *Right:* Attenuation of bladder musculature in stage of decompensation; advanced ureteral dilatation and tortuosity, usually secondary to vesicoureteral reflux.

sufficient, because of ureteral atony, obstruction of the ureterovesical junction from trigonal hypertrophy, or both. In such cases, percutaneous loop ureterostomies may be done to preserve renal function and allow resolution of the hydronephrosis. After renal function is stabilized, valve ablation and reconstruction of the urinary tract can be done.

The period of proximal diversion should be as short as possible, since vesical contracture can be permanent after prolonged supravesical diversion (Tanagho, 1974).

Johnston (1979) found that approximately 50% of children with urethral valves had vesicoureteral reflux and that the prognosis is worse if the reflux is bilateral. After removal of the obstruction, reflux will cease spontaneously in about one-third of patients. In the remaining two-thirds of patients, the reflux should be corrected surgically.

Long-term use of antimicrobial drugs is often required to prevent recurrent urosepsis and urinary tract infection even though the obstruction has been relieved.

Prognosis

Early detection is the best way to preserve kidney and bladder function. This can be accomplished by ultrasonography in utero, by careful physical examination and observation of voiding in the newborn, and by thorough evaluation of children who have urinary tract infections. Children in whom azotemia and infection

persist after relief of obstruction have a poor prognosis.

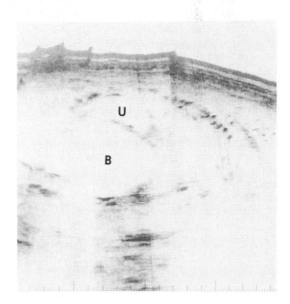

Figure 30–3. Intrauterine ultrasonogram demonstrating fetal hydronephrosis at 32 weeks' gestation. Massive enlarged bladder (B) and ureter (U) are typical of posterior urethral valves.

ANTERIOR URETHRAL VALVES

Signs of anterior urethral valves, a rare congenital anomaly, are urethral dilatation or diverticula proximal to the valve, bladder outlet obstruction, postvoiding incontinence, and infection. Enuresis may be present. Urethroscopy and voiding cystourethrography will demonstrate the lesion, and endoscopic electrofulguration will effectively correct the obstruction.

URETHRORECTAL & VESICORECTAL FISTULAS

Urethrorectal and vesicorectal fistulas are rare and are almost always associated with imperforate anus. Failure of the urorectal septum to develop completely and separate the rectum from the urogenital tract permits communication between the 2 systems (see Chapter 2). The child with such a fistula passes fecal material and gas through the urethra. If the anus has developed normally (ie, if it opens externally), urine may pass through the rectum.

Cystoscopy and panendoscopy usually show the fistulous opening. Radiographic contrast material given by mouth will reach the blind rectal pouch, and the distance between the end of the rectum and the perineum can be seen on appropriate radiograms.

Imperforate anus must be opened immediately and the fistula closed, or if the rectum lies quite high, temporary sigmoid colostomy should be performed. Definitive surgery, with repair of the urethral fistula, can be done later.

HYPOSPADIAS

In hypospadias, the urethral meatus opens on the ventral side of the penis proximal to the tip of the glans penis (Fig 30–4).

Sexual differentiation and urethral development begin in utero at approximately 8 weeks and are complete by 15 weeks. The urethra is formed by the fusion of the urethral folds along the ventral surface of the penis, which extends to the corona on the distal shaft. The glandular urethra is formed by canalization of an ectodermal cord that has grown through the glans to communicate with the fused urethral folds (see Chapter 2). Hypospadias results when fusion of the urethral folds is incomplete.

Hypospadias occurs in one in every 300 male children. Estrogens and progestins given during pregnancy are known to increase the incidence. Although a familial pattern of hypospadias has been recognized, no specific genetic traits have been established.

Classification

There are several forms of hypospadias, classified according to location: (1) glandular, ie, opening on the proximal glans penis; (2) coronal, ie, opening at the coronal sulcus; (3) penile shaft; (4) penoscrotal; and (5) perineal. About 70% of all cases of hypospadias are distal penile or coronal.

Hypospadias in the male is evidence of feminization: Patients with penoscrotal and perineal openings should be considered to have potential intersex problems requiring appropriate evaluation. Hypospadiac newborns should not be circumcised, because the preputial skin may be useful for future reconstruction.

Clinical Findings

A. Symptoms and Signs: Although newborns and young children seldom have symptoms related to hypospadias, older children and adults may complain of difficulty directing the urinary stream and stream spraying. Chordee (curvature of the penis) will cause ventral bending and bowing of the penile shaft, which can prevent sexual intercourse. Perineal or penoscrotal hypospadias will necessitate voiding in the sitting position, and these proximal forms of hypospadias in adults can be the cause of infertility. An additional complaint of almost all patients is the abnormal (hooded) appearance of the penis, caused by deficient or absent ventral foreskin. The hypospadiac meatus may be stenotic and should be carefully examined and calibrated. (A meatotomy should be done when stenosis exists.) There is an increased incidence of undescended testicles in children with hypospadias; scrotal examination is necessary to establish the position of the testicles.

B. Laboratory, X-Ray, and Endoscopic Findings: Since children with penoscrotal and perineal hypospadias often have a bifid scrotum and ambiguous genitalia, a buccal smear and karyotyping are indicated to help establish the genetic sex. Urethroscopy and cystoscopy are of value to determine whether internal male sexual organs are normally developed. Excretory urography is also indicated in these patients to detect additional congenital anomalies of the kidneys and ureters.

Some authors recommend routine use of excretory urography for all patients with hypospadias; however, this seems to be of little value in the more distal types of the disorder, because there appears to be no increased incidence of upper urinary tract anomalies.

Differential Diagnosis

Any degree of hypospadias is an expression of feminization. Perineal and scrotal urethral openings should be carefully evaluated to ascertain that the patient is not a female with androgenized adrenogenital syndrome. Urethroscopy and cystoscopy will aid in evaluating the development of internal reproductive organs.

Treatment

For psychologic reasons, hypospadias should be repaired before the patient reaches school age.

More than 150 methods of corrective surgery for hypospadias have been described. Currently, one-

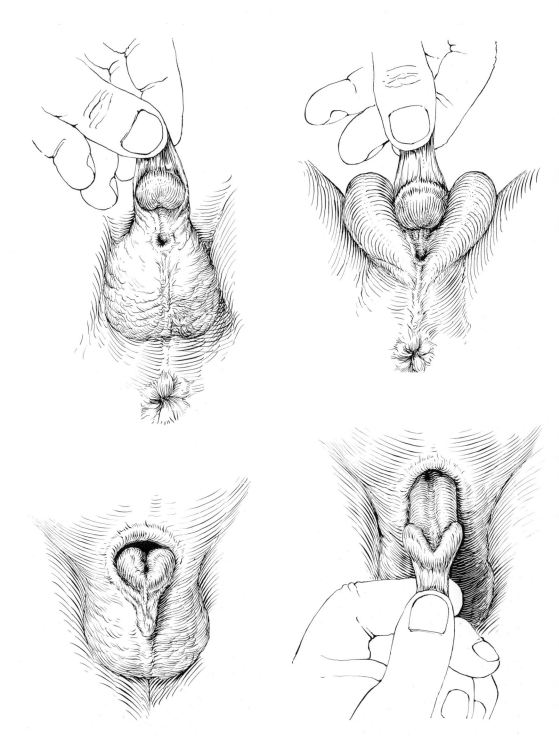

Figure 30–4. Hypospadias and epispadias. *Upper left:* Hypospadias, penoscrotal type. Redundant dorsal foreskin that is deficient ventrally; ventral chordee. *Upper right:* Hypospadias, midscrotal type. Chordee more marked. Penis often small. *Lower left:* Epispadias. Redundant ventral foreskin that is absent dorsally; severe dorsal chordee. *Lower right:* Traction on foreskin reveals dorsal defect.

stage repairs using island flap and free skin grafts are performed by more and more urologists. Fistulas occur in 15–30% of such cases, but the fistula repair is considered a small, second-stage reconstruction. Two-stage repairs have produced excellent results over the years and are the safest method for the surgeon who does occasional hypospadias repairs.

All types of repair involve straightening the penis by removal of the chordee. The chordee removal can be confirmed by producing an artificial erection in the operating room following urethral reconstruction and advancement. Most successful techniques for repair of hypospadias utilize local skin and foreskin in developing the neourethra. In recent years, advancement of the urethra on to the glans penis has become technically feasible and cosmetically acceptable.

Prognosis

After corrective surgery, most patients will be able to void in the standing position as well as to deposit semen into the vagina. The overall cosmetic appearance and the prevention of fistula formation remain the greatest challenges in these repairs.

CHORDEE WITHOUT HYPOSPADIAS

Congenital ventral chordee without hypospadias is seen occasionally and is caused by a short urethra, fibrous tissues surrounding the corpus spongiosum, or both. The urethral opening is in the normal position on the glans penis; only with erection does the penis bow, thus preventing satisfactory vaginal penetration. During examination, if the patient cannot achieve an erection naturally, erection can be induced by injecting saline solution into the corpus cavernosum after placing a tourniquet at the base of the penis. This technique should also be used during corrective surgery to be certain that the penis will be straight after operation.

If the penis is adequate in length, the dorsal surface can be shortened (1) by excising elliptical portions of the tunica albuginea on the dorsum of the penis on either side of the midline (Redman, 1978) or (2) by making transverse cuts in a similar position and then closing them longitudinally, thus shortening the dorsum (Udall, 1980). Fibrous tissue found in association with the urethra and corpus spongiosum should be totally excised.

EPISPADIAS

The incidence of complete epispadias is approximately 1 in 120,000 males and 1 in 450,000 females. The urethra is displaced dorsally, and classification is based on its position in males. In glandular epispadias, the urethra opens on the dorsal aspect of the glans, which is broad and flattened. In the penile type, the urethral meatus, which is often broad and gaping, is located between the pubic symphysis and the coronal sulcus. A distal groove usually extends from the meatus through the splayed glans. The penopubic type has the urethral opening at the penopubic junction, and the entire penis has a distal dorsal groove extending through the glans.

Patients with glandular epispadias seldom have urinary incontinence. However, with penopubic and penile epispadias, incontinence is present in 95% and 75% of cases, respectively (Kramer and Kelalis, 1982).

Females with epispadias have a bifid clitoris and separation of the labia. Most are incontinent.

Urinary incontinence is a common problem because of maldevelopment of the urinary sphincters. Dorsal curvature of the penis (dorsal chordee) is also present (Fig 30–4). The pubic bones are separated as in exstrophy of the bladder. Epispadias is a mild form of bladder exstrophy, and in severe cases, exstrophy and epispadias coexist.

Surgery is required to correct the incontinence, remove the chordee to straighten the penis, and extend the urethra out onto the glans penis. Repair of the urinary sphincter has not been very successful, but Tanagho and Smith (1972) obtained complete continence by interposing a tube graft of anterior bladder wall between the bladder and prostatic urethra. Chordee excision and urethroplasty with advancement of the meatus have been successful in achieving acceptable cosmetic and functional results (Kramer and Kelalis, 1982; Duckett, 1978; Hendren, 1979). Urinary diversion may be required in patients whose incontinence cannot be corrected.

ACQUIRED DISEASES & DISORDERS OF THE PENIS & MALE URETHRA

PRIAPISM

Priapism is an uncommon condition of prolonged erection. It is usually painful for the patient, and no sexual excitement or desire is present. The disorder is idiopathic in 60% of cases, while the remaining 40% of cases are associated with diseases (eg, leukemia, sickle cell disease, pelvic tumors, pelvic infections), penile trauma, spinal cord trauma, or use of medications. In Egypt, scorpion stings are a common cause of priapism in children. Although the idiopathic type often is initially associated with prolonged sexual stimulation, cases of priapism due to the other causes are unrelated to psychic sexual excitement.

The patient usually presents with a history of several hours of painful erection. The glans penis and corpus spongiosum are soft and uninvolved in the process. The corpora cavernosa are tense with congested blood and tender to palpation. The current theories regarding the mechanism of priapism remain in debate, but most authorities believe the major abnormality to be physiologic obstruction of the venous drainage

(Fitzpatrick, 1973). This obstruction causes buildup of highly viscous, poorly oxygenated blood within the corpora cavernosa. If the process continues for several days, interstitial edema and fibrosis of the corpora cavernosa will develop, causing impotence.

Priapism must be considered a urologic emergency. Sedation followed by enemas of ice-cold saline solution may induce subsidence of the erection. Ketamine hydrochloride given intravenously or intramuscularly has been reported to be effective in 50% of patients (Sagalowsky, 1982). Epidural or spinal anesthesia can also be used. The sludged blood can then be evacuated from the corpora cavernosa through a large needle placed through the glans. Multiple wedges of tissue can be removed via a Travenol biopsy needle to create a shunting fistula between the glans penis and corpora cavernosa (Winter, 1978). This technique, which has been very successful, provides an internal fistula to keep the corpora cavernosa decompressed. To maintain continuous fistula drainage, pressure should be exerted intermittently (every 15 minutes) on the body of the penis. The patient can do this manually after he has recovered from anesthesia.

If the shunt described above fails, another shunting technique may be utilized. Barry (1976) described an easy method of accomplishing shunting by anastomosing the superficial dorsal vein to the corpora cavernosa. Other effective shunting methods are corpora cavernosa to corpus spongiosum shunt by perineal anastomosis; saphenous vein to corpora cavernosa shunt; and pump decompression, as described by Gates and Middleton (1980).

Patients with sickle cell disease have benefited from massive blood transfusions, exchange transfusions, or both (Baron and Leiter, 1978). Hyperbaric oxygen also has been suggested for these patients. Patients with leukemia should receive prompt chemotherapy. Appropriate management of any underlying cause should be instituted without delay. Such treatment should not prevent aggressive management of the priapism if the erection persists for several hours.

Impotence is the worst sequel of priapism. It is more common after prolonged priapism (several days). Early recognition (within hours) and prompt treatment of priapism offer the best opportunity to avoid this major problem.

PEYRONIE'S DISEASE

Peyronie's disease (plastic induration of the penis) was first described in 1742 and is a well-recognized clinical problem affecting middle-aged and older men. Patients present with complaints of painful erection, curvature of the penis, and poor erection distal to the involved area. The penile deformity may be so severe that it prevents satisfactory vaginal penetration. The patient has no pain when the penis is in the nonerect state.

Examination of the penile shaft reveals a palpable dense, fibrous plaque of varying size involving the tu-

nica albuginea. The plaque is usually near the dorsal midline of the shaft. Multiple plaques are sometimes seen. In severe cases, calcification and ossification are noted and confirmed by radiography. Although the cause of Peyronie's disease remains obscure, the dense fibrous plaque is microscopically consistent with findings in severe vasculitis. The condition has been noted in association with Dupuytren's contracture of the tendons of the hand, in which the fibrosis resembles that of Peyronie's disease when examined microscopically.

There is no satisfactory treatment for this disease. However, spontaneous remission occurs in about 50% of cases. Initially, observation and emotional support are advised. If remission does not occur, *p*-aminobenzoic acid powder or tablets or vitamin E tablets may be tried for several months. However, these medications have limited success (Wild, Devine, and Horton, 1979). In recent years, a number of operative procedures have been used in refractory cases. Successful excision of the plaque and replacement with a dermal graft have been reported by several authors (Wild, Devine, and Horton, 1979). Das (1980) reported success with the use of tunica vaginalis grafts after plaque incision. Bruskewitz and Raz (1980) incised the plaque and inserted penile prostheses in the corpora cavernosa. Other methods used include radiation therapy and injection of steroids, dimethyl sulfoxide (DMSO), or parathyroid hormone into the plaque. The success of such treatments is poorly documented.

PHIMOSIS

Phimosis is a condition in which the contracted foreskin cannot be retracted over the glans. Chronic infection from poor local hygiene is its most common cause. Most cases occur in uncircumcised males, although excessive skin left after circumcision can become stenotic and cause phimosis. Calculi and squamous cell carcinoma may develop under the foreskin. Phimosis can occur at any age. In diabetic older men, chronic balanoposthitis may lead to phimosis and may be the initial presenting complaint. Children under 2 years of age seldom have true phimosis; their relatively narrow preputial opening gradually widens and allows for normal retraction of foreskin over the glans. Circumcision for phimosis should be avoided in children requiring general anesthesia; except in cases with recurrent infections, the procedure should be postponed until they reach an age when local anesthesia can be used.

Edema, erythema, and tenderness of the prepuce and the presence of purulent discharge usually cause the patient to seek medical attention. Inability to retract the foreskin is a less common complaint.

The initial infection should be treated with broad-spectrum antimicrobial drugs. The dorsal foreskin can be slit if improved drainage is necessary. Circumcision, if indicated, should be done after the infection is controlled.

PARAPHIMOSIS

Paraphimosis is the condition in which the foreskin, once retracted over the glans, cannot be replaced in its normal position. This is due to chronic inflammation under the redundant foreskin, which leads to contracture of the preputial opening (phimosis) and formation of a tight ring of skin when the foreskin is retracted behind the glans. The skin ring causes venous congestion leading to edema and enlargement of the glans, which make the condition worse. As the condition progresses, arterial occlusion and necrosis of the glans may occur.

Paraphimosis can usually be treated by firmly squeezing the glans for 5 minutes to reduce the tissue edema and decrease the size of the glans. The skin can then be drawn forward over the glans. Occasionally, the constricting ring will require incision under local anesthesia. Antibiotics should be administered and circumcision should be done after inflammation has subsided.

CIRCUMCISION

Although circumcision is routinely performed in some countries for religious or cultural reasons, it is usually not necessary if adequate penile cleanliness and good hygiene can be maintained. There is a higher incidence of penile carcinoma in uncircumcised males, but chronic infection and poor hygiene are usually underlying factors in such instances. Circumcision is indicated in patients with infection, phimosis, or paraphimosis (see above).

URETHRAL STRICTURE

Acquired urethral stricture is common in men but rare in women. (Congenital urethral stricture is discussed above.) Most acquired strictures are due to infection or trauma. Although gonococcal urethritis is seldom a cause of stricture today, infection remains a major cause—particularly infection from long-term use of indwelling urethral catheters. Large catheters and instruments are more likely than small ones to cause ischemia and internal trauma. External trauma, eg, pelvic fracture (see Chapter 17), can partially or completely sever the membranous urethra and cause severe and complex strictures. Straddle injuries can produce bulbar strictures.

Urethral strictures are fibrotic narrowings composed of dense collagen and fibroblasts. Fibrosis usually extends into the surrounding corpus spongiosum, causing spongiofibrosis. These narrowings restrict urine flow and cause dilation of the proximal urethra and prostatic ducts. Prostatitis is a common complication of urethral stricture. The bladder muscle may become hypertrophic, and increased residual urine may be noted. Severe, prolonged obstruction can result in decompensation of the ureterovesical junction, reflux, hydronephrosis, and renal failure. Chronic urinary stasis makes infection likely. Urethral fistulas and periurethral abscesses commonly develop in association with chronic, severe strictures.

Clinical Findings

A. Symptoms and Signs: A decrease in urinary stream is the most common complaint. Spraying or double stream is often noted, as is postvoiding dribbling. Chronic urethral discharge, occasionally a major complaint, is likely to be associated with chronic prostatitis. Acute cystitis or symptoms of infection are seen at times. Acute urinary retention seldom occurs unless infection or prostatic obstruction develops. Urinary frequency and mild dysuria may also be initial complaints.

Induration in the area of the stricture may be palpable. Tender enlarged masses along the urethra usually represent periurethral abscesses. Urethrocutaneous fistulas may be present. The bladder may be palpable if there is chronic retention of urine.

B. Laboratory Findings: If urethral stricture is suspected, urinary flow rates should be determined. The patient is instructed to accumulate urine until the bladder is full and then begin voiding; a 5-second collection of urine should be obtained during midstream maximal flow and its volume recorded. After the patient repeats this procedure 8–10 times over several days in a relaxed atmosphere, the mean peak flow can be calculated. With strictures creating significant problems, the flow rate will be less than 10 mL/s (normal, 20 mL/s).

Urine culture may be indicated. The midstream specimen is usually bacteria-free, with some pyuria (8–10 white blood cells per high power field) in a carefully obtained first aliquot of urine. If the prostate is infected, bacteria will be present in a specimen obtained after prostatic massage. In the presence of cystitis, the urine will be grossly infected.

C. X-Ray Findings: A urethrogram or voiding cystourethrogram (or both) will demonstrate the location and extent of the stricture. Urethral fistulas and diverticula are sometimes noted. Vesical stones, trabeculations, or diverticula may also be seen.

D. Instrumental Examination: Urethroscopy allows visualization of the stricture. Small-caliber strictures will prevent passage of the instrument through the area. Direct visualization aids in determining the extent, location, and degree of scarring. Additional areas of scar formation adjacent to the stricture may be detected by urethroscopy.

The stricture can be calibrated by passage of bougies à boule (see Chapter 10).

Differential Diagnosis

Benign or malignant prostatic obstruction can cause symptoms similar to those of stricture. After prostatic surgery, bladder neck contracture can develop and induce stricturelike symptoms. Rectal examination and panendoscopy will adequately define such abnormalities of the prostate. Urethral carcinoma is often associated with stricture; urethroscopy will demonstrate a definite irregular lesion, and biopsy will establish the diagnosis of carcinoma.

Complications

Complications include chronic prostatitis, cystitis, chronic urinary infection, diverticula, urethrocutaneous fistulas, periurethral abscesses, and urethral carcinoma. Vesical calculi may develop from chronic urinary stasis and infection.

Treatment

A. Specific Measures:

1. Dilation—Dilation of urethral strictures is not usually curative, but it fractures the scar tissue of the stricture and temporarily enlarges the lumen. As healing occurs, the scar tissue re-forms.

Dilation may initially be required because of severe symptoms of chronic retention of urine. The urethra should be liberally lubricated with a water-soluble medium before instrumentation. A filiform is passed down the urethra and gently manipulated through the narrow area into the bladder. A follower can then be attached (see Chapter 10) and the area gradually dilated (with successively larger sizes) to approximately 22F. A 16F silicone catheter can then be inserted. If difficulty arises in passing the filiform through the stricture, urethroscopy should be used to guide the filiform under direct vision.

An alternative method of urethral dilation employs Van Buren sounds. These instruments are best used by an experienced urologist familiar with the size and extent of the stricture involved. A 22F sound should first be passed down to the stricture site and gentle pressure applied. If this fails, a 20F sound should be used. Smaller sounds should not be used, because they can easily perforate the urethral wall and produce false passages. Bleeding and pain are major problems caused by dilation.

2. Urethrotomy under endoscopic direct vision—Lysis of urethral strictures can be accomplished using a sharp knife attached to an endoscope. The endoscope provides direct vision of the stricture during cutting. A filiform should be passed through the stricture and used as a guide during lysis. The stricture is usually incised dorsally, but multiple incisions in other areas may be required to open a narrow segment. A 22F instrument should pass with ease. A catheter is left in place for a short time to prevent bleeding and pain. Results of this procedure have been satisfactory in 70–80% of patients (Sacknoff and Kerr, 1980; Walther, Parsons, and Schmidt, 1980). The procedure has several advantages: (1) Minimal anesthesia is required—in some cases, only topical anesthesia combined with sedation; (2) it is easily repeated if the stricture recurs; and (3) it is very safe, with few complications.

3. Surgical reconstruction—If urethrotomy under direct vision fails, open surgical repair should be performed. Short strictures (≤ 1.5 cm) of the anterior urethra should be completely excised and primary anastomosis done. If possible, the segment to be excised should extend 1 cm beyond each end of the stricture to allow for removal of any existing spongiofibrosis and improve postoperative healing.

Strictures more than 2 cm in length can be managed by patch graft urethroplasty (Devine, Wendelken, and Devine, 1979). The urethra is incised in the midline for the full length of the stricture plus an additional 1.5 cm proximal and distal to its ends. A full-thickness skin graft is obtained—preferably from the penile skin—and all subcutaneous tissue is carefully removed. The graft is then tailored to cover the defect and meticulously sutured into place (Fig 30–5). If penile skin is not available, skin from the medial upper arm, abdomen, or neck (ie, areas without hair) should be used. The urethra should be approximately 30F in diameter at the completion of the procedure.

In cases of very narrow, long, densely fibrotic stricture, total excision of the stricture and placement of a full-thickness tube graft can be done successfully. Several studies have reported satisfactory results in about 85% of patients treated by procedures utilizing skin grafts.

Strictures involving the membranous urethra ordinarily result from external trauma (see Chapter 17) and present problems in reconstruction. The 2-stage scrotal inlay procedure described by Turner-Warwick (1977) has been well accepted. Other workers (Pierce, 1979; Tilak, Dhayagude, and Joshi, 1976) have successfully utilized a perineal approach. The author has found repair of such strictures easier when the perineal approach is combined with the transpubic approach popularized by Waterhouse, Laungani, and Patil (1980) and McAninch (1981) (Fig 30–6). Removal of the symphysis portion of the pubic bone provides excellent exposure for reconstruction and does not create postoperative problems involving the gait or the stability of the bony pelvis.

B. Treatment of Complications: Urinary tract infection in patients with strictures requires specific antimicrobial therapy, followed by long-term prophylactic therapy until the stricture has been corrected. Periurethral abscesses require drainage and use of antimicrobial drugs. Urethral fistulas usually require surgical repair.

Prognosis

A stricture should not be considered "cured" until it has been observed for at least 1 year after therapy, since it may recur at any time during that period. Urinary flow rate measurements and urethrograms are helpful to determine the extent of residual obstruction.

URETHRAL CONDYLOMATA ACUMINATA (Urethral Warts)

Condylomata acuminata are uncommon in the urethra and are almost always preceded by lesions on the skin (see p 600). They are wartlike papillomas caused by a papovavirus and are usually transmitted by direct

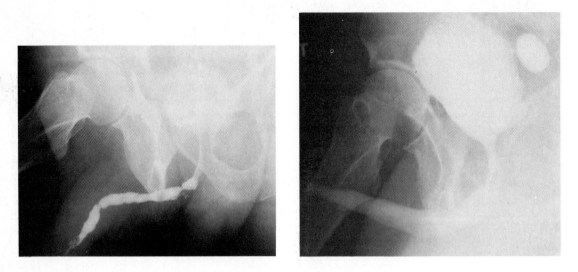

Figure 30–5. *Left:* Urethrogram demonstrating multiple anterior urethral strictures. *Right:* Voiding cystourethrogram following a patch skin graft of 14 cm in the same patient. There are no residual strictures.

sexual contact but may possibly be transmitted nonsexually.

Patients commonly complain of bloody spotting from the urethra and occasionally have dysuria and urethral discharge. Examination of the urethral meatus often reveals a small, protruding papilloma. If a lesion is not found in this location, the meatus should be separated with the examining fingers so that the distal urethra can be inspected. About 90% of such lesions are situated in the distal urethra. Complete urethroscopy must be done to be certain other lesions do not exist.

Lesions of the meatus can be treated by local excision. A local anesthetic is applied to the area at the base of the lesions, and the pedunculated lesions are sharply incised with small scissors. The area is then fulgurated by electrocautery. Meatotomy may be indicated for excision of lesions in the fossa navicularis and glandular urethra.

Deeper lesions may be fulgurated transurethrally with a resectoscope or Bugby electrode. Recently, lesions have been successfully destroyed using a carbon dioxide laser. Laser therapy does minimal damage to the urethral mucosa, and stricture formation seems less likely with its use (Fuselier et al, 1980).

Multiple lesions have also been treated with fluorouracil, 5% solution or cream. The drug is instilled in the urethra for 20 minutes twice a week for 5 weeks. Care must be taken to protect the penile skin and scrotum from coming in contact with the medication, since it may produce severe irritation (Weimer et al, 1978).

Lesions may become infected and ulcerated. This suggests carcinoma, and histopathologic confirmation of the diagnosis should be obtained. Rarely, giant condylomata (Buschke-Löwenstein tumors) involving the glans penis and often the urethra may be seen. Such lesions suggest carcinoma and must be biopsied. Surgical excision is the treatment of choice.

To prevent recurrence of condylomata acuminata, the sexual partner must also be examined and treated if necessary.

STENOSIS OF THE URETHRAL MEATUS

Newborns are often suspected of having meatal stenosis of some degree. This condition is thought to be secondary to ammonia dermatitis following circumcision and resulting in prolonged irritative meatitis.

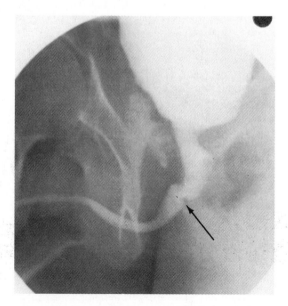

Figure 30–6. Voiding urethrogram following transpubic repair of traumatic posterior urethral stricture. Arrow indicates that area of repair is stricture-free.

Calibration is important, since the visual appearance of the meatus does not correlate well with its actual size. The urethra should easily accept the tip of an 8F pediatric feeding tube. The significance of meatal stenosis is debated, but a meatal caliber less than 8F in children under 10 years of age is an indication for meatotomy (Litvak, Morris, and McRoberts, 1976).

PENILE PHLEBOTHROMBOSIS & LYMPHATIC OCCLUSION

Superficial veins and lymphatic vessels of the dorsal penile shaft just proximal to the corona may become irritated and inflamed. A careful history usually indicates that minor trauma to the area (eg, from prolonged sexual intercourse) has occurred. Examination reveals a tender, indurated, cordlike structure on the distal penile shaft. Slight erythema may be present.

For clinical purposes, there is no need to distinguish lymphatic and venous causes, since both penile phlebothrombosis and lymphatic occlusion will resolve spontaneously. The patient must be reassured.

REFERENCES

CONGENITAL ANOMALIES

Penis & Urethra

Allen TD: Congenital microphallus. Page 327 in: *Current Urologic Therapy*. Kaufman JJ (editor). Saunders, 1980.

Hinman F Jr: Microphallus: Distinction between anomalous and endocrine types. *J Urol* 1980;**123:**412.

Jacobs SC, Kaplan GW, Gittes RF: Topical testosterone therapy for penile growth. *Urology* 1975;**6:**708.

Johnston WG Jr, Yeatman GW, Weigel JW: Congenital absence of the penis. *J Urol* 1977;**117:**508.

Jones HW Jr, Park IJ, Rock JA: Technique of surgical sex reassignment for micropenis and allied conditions. *Am J Obstet Gynecol* 1978;**132:**870.

Klugo RC, Cerny JC: Response of micropenis to topical testosterone and gonadotropin. *J Urol* 1978;**119:**667.

Kogan SJ, Williams DI: The micropenis syndrome: Clinical observations and expectations for growth. *J Urol* 1977;**118:**311.

Naparstek S et al: Complete duplication of male urethra in children. *Urology* 1980;**16:**391.

Wilson SA, Walker RD: Megalourethra and hypospadias. *J Urol* 1983;**129:**556.

Wirtshafter A et al: Complete trifurcation of the urethra. *J Urol* 1980;**123:**431.

Urethral Stricture

Kaplan GW, Brock WA: Urethral strictures in children. *J Urol* 1983;**129:**1200.

Kramer SA et al: Transpubic urethroplasty in children. *J Urol* 1981;**126:**767.

Redman JF, Fraiser LP: Apparent congenital anterior urethral strictures in brothers. *J Urol* 1979;**122:**707.

Posterior Urethral Valves

Egami K, Smith ED: A study of the sequelae of posterior urethral valves. *J Urol* 1982;**127:**84.

Friedland GW et al: Posterior urethral valves. *Clin Radiol* 1977;**27:**367.

Johnston JH: Vesicoureteric reflux with urethral valves. *Br J Urol* 1979;**51:**100.

Johnston JH, Kulatilake AE: The sequelae of posterior urethral valves. *Br J Urol* 1971;**43:**743.

Pinto MH, Markland C, Fraley EE: Posterior urethral valves managed by cutaneous ureterostomy with subsequent ureteral reconstruction. *J Urol* 1978;**119:**696.

Rabinowitz R et al: Upper tract management when posterior urethral valve ablation is insufficient. *J Urol* 1979;**122:**370.

Schoenberg HW, Miyai K, Gregory JG: Posterior urethral valves. *Urology* 1976;**7:**611.

Scott TW: Urinary ascites secondary to posterior urethral valves. *J Urol* 1976;**116:**87.

Tanagho EA: Congenitally obstructed bladder: Fate after prolonged defunctionalization. *J Urol* 1974;**111:**102.

Tank ES, Carey TC, Seifert AL: Management of neonatal urinary ascites. *Urology* 1980;**16:**270.

Uehling DT: Posterior urethral valves: Functional classification. *Urology* 1980;**15:**27.

Whitaker RH: The ureter in posterior urethral valves. *Br J Urol* 1973;**45:**395.

Anterior Urethral Valves

Firlit RS, Firlit CF, King LR: Obstructing anterior urethral valves in children. *J Urol* 1978;**119:**819.

Golimbu M et al: Anterior urethral valves. *Urology* 1978;**12:**343.

Urethrorectal & Vesicorectal Fistulas

Blandy JP, Singh M: Fistulae involving the adult male urethra. *Br J Urol* 1972;**44:**632.

Glenn JF: Eccentric flap repair of urethral fistulas. *J Urol* 1983;**129:**510.

Wesolowski S, Bulinski W: Vesico-intestinal fistulae and recto-urethral fistulae. *Br J Urol* 1973;**45:**34.

Hypospadias

Aarskog D: Current concepts in cancer: Maternal progestins as a possible cause of hypospadias. *N Engl J Med* 1979;**300:**75.

Bauer SB, Bull MJ, Retik AB: Hypospadias: A familial study. *J Urol* 1979;**121:**474.

Belman BA, Kass EJ: Hypospadias repair in children less than 1 year old. *J Urol* 1982;**128:**1273.

Devine CJ Jr, Franz JP, Horton CE: Evaluation and treatment of patients with failed hypospadias repair. *J Urol* 1978;**119:**223.

Devine CJ Jr, Horton CE: Hypospadias repair. *J Urol* 1977;**118:**188.

Duckett JW: Island flap technique for hypospadias repair. *Urol Clin North Am* 1981;**8:**503.

Duckett JW: MAGPI (meatoplasty and glanuloplasty): A procedure for subcoronal hypospadias. *Urol Clin North Am* 1981;**8:**513.

Genetics of hypospadias. *Br Med J* 1972;**4**:189.

Golimbu M, al-Askari S, Morales P: One-stage hypospadias repair. *Urology* 1977;**9**:672.

Gonzales ET et al: The management of distal hypospadias with meatal-based vascularized flaps. *J Urol* 1983; **129**:119.

Kelalis PP, Benson RC Jr, Culp OS: Complications of single and multistage operations for hypospadias: A comparative review. *J Urol* 1977;**118**:657.

Lutzker LG, Kogan SJ, Levitt SB: Is routine intravenous urography indicated in patients with hypospadias? *Pediatrics* 1977;**59**:630.

Shima H et al: Developmental anomalies associated with hypospadias. *J Urol* 1979;**122**:619.

Smith DR: Repair of hypospadias in the preschool child: A report of 150 cases. *J Urol* 1967;**97**:723.

Wettlaufer JN: Cutaneous chordee: Fact or fancy? *Urology* 1974;**4**:293.

Woodard JR, Cleveland R: Application of Horton-Devine principles to the repair of hypospadias. *J Urol* 1982; **127**:1155.

Chordee Without Hypospadias

Kaplan GW, Lamm DL: Embryogenesis of chordee. *J Urol* 1975;**114**:769.

Kramer SA et al: Chordee without hypospadias in children. *J Urol* 1982;**128**:559.

Perlmutter AD, Vatz AD: Meatal advancement for distal hypospadias without chordee. *J Urol* 1975;**113**:850.

Redman JF: Extended application of Nesbit ellipses in the correction of childhood penile curvature. *J Urol* 1978;**119**:122.

Udall DA: Correction of 3 types of congenital curvature of the penis, including the first reported case of dorsal curvature. *J Urol* 1980;**124**:50.

Epispadias

Ambrose SS, O'Brien DP III: Surgical embryology of the exstrophy-epispadias complex. *Surg Clin North Am* 1974;**54**:1379.

Duckett JW Jr: Epispadias. *Urol Clin North Am* 1978;**5**:107.

Hendren WH: Penile lengthening after previous repair of epispadias. *J Urol* 1979;**121**:527.

Kramer SA, Kelalis PP: Assessment of urinary continence in epispadias: Review of 94 patients. *J Urol* 1982;**128**:290.

Light JK, Scott FB: Treatment of the epispadias-exstrophy complex with the AS792 artificial urinary sphincter. *J Urol* 1983;**129**:738.

Tanagho EA, Smith DR: Clinical evaluation of a surgical technique for the correction of complete urinary incontinence. *J Urol* 1972;**107**:402.

ACQUIRED DISEASES & DISORDERS

Priapism

Baron M, Leiter E: The management of priapism in sickle cell anemia. *J Urol* 1978;**119**:610.

Barry JM: Priapism: Treatment with corpus cavernosum to dorsal vein of penis shunts. *J Urol* 1976;**116**:754.

Erocle CJ, Pierce JM Jr: Changing surgical concepts in the treatment of priapism. *J Urol* 1981;**125**:210.

Fitzpatrick TJ: Spongiograms and cavernosograms: A study of their value in priapism. *J Urol* 1973;**109**:843.

Gates CL Jr, Middleton RG: Extracorporeal corpus-venous shunting for priapism. *J Urol* 1980;**123**:595.

Goulding FJ: Modification of cavernoglandular shunt for priapism. *Urology* 1980;**15**:64.

Guerriero WG: Corpus cavernosum-corpus spongiosum shunts. *Surg Gynecol Obstet* 1978;**146**:792.

Kinney TR et al: Priapism in association with sickle hemoglobinopathies in children. *J Pediatr* 1975;**86**:241.

Lue TF et al: Priapism: Refined approach to diagnosis and treatment. *J Urol* 1986;**136**:104.

Persky L, Kursh E: Post-traumatic priapism. *J Urol* 1977; **118**:397.

Resnick MI et al: Priapism in boys: Management with cavernosaphenous shunt. *Urology* 1975;**5**:492.

Sagalowsky AI: Priapism. *Urol Clin North Am* 1982;**9**:255.

Schreibman SM, Gee TS, Grabstald H: Management of priapism in patients with chronic granulocytic leukemia. *J Urol* 1974;**111**:786.

Seeler RA: Intensive transfusion therapy for priapism in boys with sickle cell anemia. *J Urol* 1973;**110**:360.

Wear JB Jr, Crummy AB, Munson BO: A new approach to the treatment of priapism. *J Urol* 1977;**117**:252.

Winter CC: Priapism cured by creation of fistulas between glans penis and corpora cavernosa. *J Urol* 1978;**119**:227.

Peyronie's Disease

Bruskewitz R, Raz S: Surgical considerations in treatment of Peyronie disease. *Urology* 1980;**15**:134.

Das S: Peyronie's disease: Excision and autografting with tunica vaginalis. *J Urol* 1980;**124**:818.

Helvie WW, Ochsner SF: Radiation therapy in Peyronie's disease. *South Med J* 1972;**65**:1192.

Hicks CC et al: Experience with the Horton-Devine dermal graft in the treatment of Peyronie's disease. *J Urol* 1978; **119**:504.

Nyberg ML et al: Identification of an inherited form of Peyronie's disease with autosomal dominant inheritance and association with Dupuytren's contracture. *J Urol* 1982; **128**:48.

Poutasse EF: Peyronie's disease. *J Urol* 1972;**107**:419.

Pryor JP, Fitzpatrick JM: New approach to correction of penile deformity in Peyronie's disease. *J Urol* 1979; **122**:622.

Wild RM, Devine CJ Jr, Horton CE: Dermal graft repair of Peyronie's disease: Survey of 50 patients. *J Urol* 1979; **121**:47.

Phimosis

Redman AJ, Scribner LJ, Bissada NK: Postcircumcision of phimosis and its management. *Clin Pediatr* 1975;**14**:407.

Paraphimosis

Oster J: Further fate of the foreskin: Incidence of preputial adhesions, phimosis, and smegma among Danish boys. *Arch Dis Child* 1968;**43**:200.

Skoglund RW Jr, Chapman WH: Reduction of paraphimosis. *J Urol* 1970;**104**:137.

Circumcision

Dagher R, Selzer ML, Lapides J: Carcinoma of the penis and the anti-circumcision parade. *J Urol* 1973;**110**:79.

Fetus and Newborn Committee, Canadian Pediatric Society: Benefits and risks of circumcision: Another view. *Can Med Assoc J* 1982;**126**:1399.

Murdock MI, Selikowitz SM: Diabetes-related need for circumcision. *Urology* 1974;**4**:60.

Urethral Stricture

Azoury BS, Freiha FS: Excision of urethral stricture and end to end anastomosis. *Urology* 1976;**8**:138.

Bekirov HM et al: Internal urethrotomy under direct vision in men. *J Urol* 1982;**128**:37.

Betts JM, Texter JH Jr, Crane DB: Single stage urethroplasty as treatment for stricture disease. *J Urol* 1978;**120:**412.

Blandy JP et al: Urethroplasty in context. *Br J Urol* 1976;**48:**697.

Devine PC, Wendelken JR, Devine CJ Jr: Free full thickness skin graft urethroplasty: Current technique. *J Urol* 1979;**121:**282.

Madduri S, Kamat MH, Seebode J: Urethral stricture treated with soft catheter dilatation: Reappraisal of an old technique. *Urology* 1974;**4:**504.

Malek RS, O'Dea MJ, Kelalis PP: Management of ruptured posterior urethra in childhood. *J Urol* 1977;**117:**105.

McAninch JW: Traumatic injuries to the urethra. *J Trauma* 1981;**21:**291.

Oswalt GC Jr, Lloyd LK, Bueschen AJ: Full thickness skin graft urethroplasty for anterior urethral strictures. *Urology* 1979;**13:**45.

Pierce JM Jr: Posterior urethral stricture repair. *J Urol* 1979;**121:**739.

Quartey JKM: One-stage penile/preputial cutaneous island flap urethroplasty for urethral stricture. *J Urol* 1983;**129:**284.

Sacknoff EJ, Kerr WS Jr: Direct vision cold knife urethrotomy. *J Urol* 1980;**123:**492.

Schreiter F: Mesh-graft urethroplasty: Our experience with a new procedure. *Eur Urol* 1984;**10:**338.

Tilak GH, Dhayagude HC, Joshi SS: Badenoch's pull-through operation for urethral stricture. *Br J Urol* 1976; **48:**83.

Turner-Warwick R: Complex traumatic posterior urethral strictures. *J Urol* 1977;**118:**564.

Walther PC, Parsons CL, Schmidt JD: Direct vision internal urethrotomy in the management of urethral strictures. *J Urol* 1980;**123:**497.

Waterhouse K, Laungani G, Patil U: The surgical repair of membranous urethral strictures: Experience with 105 consecutive cases. *J Urol* 1980;**123:**500.

Urethral Condylomata Acuminata

Bissada NK, Redman JF, Sulieman JS: Condyloma-acuminatum of the male urethra: Successful management with 5-fluorouracil. *Urology* 1974;**3:**499.

Bruns TNC et al: Buschke-Lowenstein giant condylomas: Pitfalls in management. *Urology* 1975;**5:**773.

Dretler SP, Klein LA: The eradication of intraurethral condyloma acuminatum with 5 percent 5-fluorouracil cream. *J Urol* 1975;**113:**195.

Fuselier HA Jr et al: Treatment of condylomata acuminata with carbon dioxide laser. *Urology* 1980;**15:**265.

Pollack HM et al: Urethrographic manifestations of venereal warts (condyloma acuminata). *Radiology* 1978;**126:**643.

Rosenberg SK et al: Some guidelines in treatment of urethral condylomata with carbon dioxide laser. *J Urol* 1982; **127:**906.

Weimer GW et al: 5-Fluorouracil urethral suppositories for the eradication of condyloma acuminata. *J Urol* 1978; **120:**174.

Stenosis of the Urinary Meatus

Allen JS, Summers JL: Meatal stenosis in children. *J Urol* 1974;**112:**526.

Belman AB et al: Urethral meatal stenosis in males. *Pediatrics* 1978;**61:**778.

Litvak AS, Morris JA Jr, McRoberts JW: Normal size of the urethral meatus in boys. *J Urol* 1976;**115:**736.

Penile Thrombophlebitis & Lymphatic Occlusion

Harrow BR, Sloane JA: Thrombophlebitis of superficial penile and scrotal veins. *J Urol* 1963;**89:**841.

31

Disorders of the Female Urethra

Emil A. Tanagho, MD

CONGENITAL ANOMALIES OF THE FEMALE URETHRA

DISTAL URETHRAL STENOSIS IN INFANCY & CHILDHOOD
(Spasm of the External Urinary Sphincter)

There has been considerable confusion about the site of lower tract obstruction in little girls who suffer from enuresis, a slow and interrupted urinary stream, recurrent cystitis, and pyelonephritis and who, on thorough examination, often exhibit vesicoureteral reflux. Treatment has largely been directed to the bladder neck on rather empirical grounds. Most of these children, however, have congenital distal urethral stenosis with secondary spasm of the striated external sphincter rather than bladder neck obstruction due to functional or organic causes.

At birth, calibration of the urethra with bougies à boule reveals no evidence of a distal ring of urethral stenosis (Fisher et al, 1969). Within a few months, however, such a ring develops as a normal anatomic structure. After puberty, the ring disappears. The inference is that the absence of estrogens leads to the development of this lesion. Lyon and Tanagho (1965) found that the ring calibrates at 14F at age 2 and at 16F between the ages of 4 and 10. Even though from the hydrodynamic standpoint such a stenotic area should not be obstructive, almost all observers agree that dilatation of the ring does relieve symptoms in these children and that it results in cure or amelioration of persistent infection or vesical dysfunction in 80% of cases. Lyon and Tanagho thought it possible that the basic cause of these urinary difficulties might be reflex spasm of periurethral striated sphincter and noted that voiding cystourethrograms supported that view (Fig 31–1).

Tanagho et al (1971) measured pressures in the bladder and in the proximal and mid urethra simultaneously in symptomatic girls and found high resting pressures, some as high as 200 cm of water (normal, 100 cm of water) in the midurethral segment. Attempts at voiding caused intravesical pressures as high as 225 cm of water (normal, 30–40 cm of water) to develop. Under curare, the urethral closing pressures dropped to normal (40–50 cm of water), proving that these obstructing pressures were caused by spasm of the striated sphincter muscle. If the distal urethral ring was treated and symptoms abated, repeat pressure studies showed normal midurethral and intravesical voiding pressures. If, on the other hand, symptoms persisted, pressures were found to remain at extremely high levels.

It seems clear, therefore, that the major cause of urinary problems in little girls is spasm of the external sphincter and not vesical neck stenosis (Smith, 1969).

In addition to recurrent urinary tract infections, these patients have hesitancy in initiating micturition and a slow, hesitant, or interrupted urinary stream. Enuresis and involuntary loss of urine during the day are common complaints. Abdominal straining may be required in order to void. Small amounts of residual urine are found, which impair the vesical defense mechanism (Hinman, 1966). A voiding cystourethrogram may reveal an open bladder neck and ballooning of the proximal urethra secondary to spasm of the external sphincter (Fig 31–1).

The voiding cystourethrogram may reveal evidence of the distal ring, but typical findings are not always seen, particularly if the flow rate is slow. Definitive diagnosis is made by bougienage.

The simplest and least harmful treatment is overdilatation with sounds up to 32–36F or with the Kollmann dilator (Lyon and Tanagho, 1965; Lyon and Marshall, 1971; Hendry, Stanton, and Williams, 1973). With either method, the ring "cracks" anteriorly, with some bleeding. Recurrence of the ring is rare. Internal urethrotomy has its proponents (Immergut and Gilbert, 1973; Hradec et al, 1973), but Kaplan, Sammons, and King (1973) found that results with urethrotomy were poor, since incising the urethra along its entire length does not cut the external sphincter, whose abnormal tone is the cause of the obstruction, whereas "cracking" the ring by overdilatation accomplishes this purpose.

In 80% of affected children destruction of the ring of distal urethral stenosis will help to overcome enuresis and achieve a normal free voiding pattern and to cure recurrent cystitis or persistent bacteriuria (Lyon and Marshall, 1971). Spontaneous resolution of reflux is possible only in the case of "borderline" values that tend to give way in the presence of increased voiding pressure and infection.

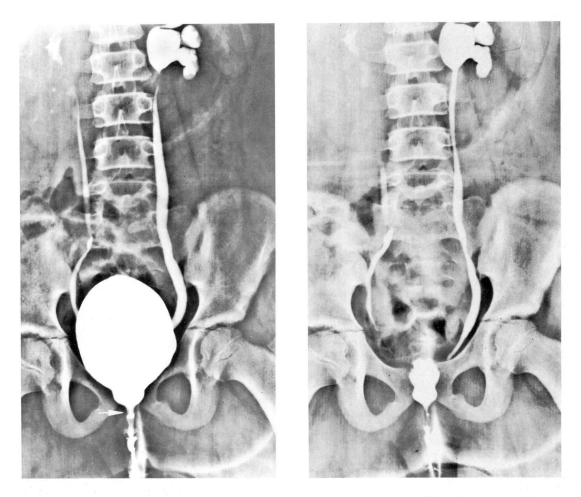

Figure 31–1. Distal urethral stenosis with reflux spasm of voluntary urethral sphincter. *Left:* Voilding cystourethrogram showing bilateral vesicoureteral reflux, a wide-open vesical neck, and severe spasm of the striated urethral sphincter in the mid portion of the urethra (*arrow*) secondary to distal urethral stenosis. *Right:* Postvoiding film. The bladder is empty and the vesical neck open, but the dilated urethra contains radiopaque fluid proximal to the stenotic zone. Bacteria in the urethra thus can flow back into the bladder. (Courtesy of AD Amar.)

Since the ring normally disappears at puberty, it is possible to await spontaneous cure; however, the ring should be broken if symptoms have been severe enough to bring the child to the attention of a urologist.

LABIAL FUSION
(Synechia Vulvae)

Some children with recurring urinary infection are found to have fused labia minora, which are apt to obstruct the flow of urine so that it tends to pool in the vagina. Local application of estrogen cream twice daily for 2–4 weeks usually causes spontaneous separation. Forceful separation or dissection has its advocates (Podolsky, 1973; Christensen and Oster, 1971).

ACQUIRED DISEASES
OF THE FEMALE URETHRA

ACUTE URETHRITIS

Acute urethritis frequently occurs with gonorrheal infection in women. Urinary symptoms are often present at the onset of the disease. Cultures and smears establish the diagnosis. Prompt cure can be achieved with antimicrobial drugs.

The detergents in bubble bath or certain spermicidal jellies may cause vaginitis and urethritis. Symptoms of vesical irritability may occur.

CHRONIC URETHRITIS

Chronic urethritis is one of the most common urologic problems of females. The distal urethra normally harbors pathogens, and the risk of infection may be increased by wearing contaminated diapers, by insertion of an indwelling catheter, by spread from cervical or vaginal infections, or by intercourse with an infected partner. Urethral inflammation may also occur from the trauma of intercourse or childbirth, particularly if urethral stenosis, either congenital or following childbirth, is present.

Clinical Findings

The urethral mucosa is reddened, quite sensitive, and often stenotic. Granular areas are often seen, and polypoid masses may be noted just distal to the bladder neck.

A. Symptoms: The symptoms resemble those of cystitis, although the urine may be clear. Complaints include burning on urination, frequency, and nocturia. Discomfort in the urethra may be felt, particularly when walking.

B. Signs: Examination may disclose redness of the meatus, hypersensitivity of the meatus and of the urethra on vaginal palpation, and evidence of cervicitis or vaginitis. There is no urethral discharge.

C. Laboratory Findings: When the initial and midstream urine are collected in separate containers, the first glass contains pus and the second does not (Marshall, Lyon, and Schieble, 1970). *Ureaplasma urealyticum* (formerly called T strains of mycoplasmas) is often identifiable in the first glass. These findings are similar to those of nongonococcal (chlamydial) urethritis in males. Clinically, the presence of white blood cells in the absence of bacteria on a routine stain or culture suggests nongonococcal urethritis. In other cases, various bacteria (eg, *Streptococcus faecalis, Escherichia coli*) may be cultured from both the urethral washings and a specimen taken from the introitus.

D. Instrumental Examination: A catheter, bougie à boule, or sound may meet resistance because of urethral stenosis. Panendoscopy reveals redness and a granular appearance of the mucosa. Inflammatory polyps may be seen in the proximal portion of the urethra. Cystoscopy may show increased injection of the trigone (trigonitis), which often accompanies urethritis.

Differential Diagnosis

Differentiation of urethritis from cystitis depends upon bacteriologic study of the urine; panendoscopy demonstrates the urethral lesion. Both urethritis and cystitis may be present.

Psychologic disorders may cause symptoms identical to those of chronic urethritis. A history of short bouts of frequency without nocturia is suggestive of functional illness. The neurotic makeup of the patient is usually obvious (Zufall, 1963).

Treatment & Prognosis

Gradual urethral dilatations (up to 36F in the adult) are indicated for urethral stenosis; this allows for some inevitable contracture. Immergut and Gilbert (1973) prefer internal urethrotomy. *U urealyticum* is fairly sensitive to tetracycline or erythromycin. Chlamydial urethritis usually responds to sulfonamides or tetracyclines. For ascending bacterial infections, Bruce et al (1973) recommend the regular local application of an antiseptic (eg, hexachlorophene, chlorhexidine cream) to the introitus in order to prevent bacteria from the area of the perineum, vagina, and vulva from reinfecting the urethra.

SENILE URETHRITIS

After physiologic (or surgical) menopause, hypoestrogenism occurs and retrogressive (senile) changes take place in the vaginal epithelium, so that it becomes rather dry and pale. Similar changes develop in the lower urinary tract, which arises from the same embryologic tissues as the female reproductive organs. Some eversion of the mucosa about the urethral orifice, from foreshortening of the vaginal canal, is usually seen. This is commonly misdiagnosed as caruncle.

Clinical Findings

A. Symptoms: Many postmenopausal women have symptoms of vesical irritability (burning, frequency, urgency) and stress incontinence. They may complain of vaginal and vulval itching and some discharge.

B. Signs: The vaginal epithelium is dry and pale. The mucosa at the urethral orifice is often reddened and hypersensitive; eversion of its posterior lip from foreshortening of the urethrovaginal wall is common.

C. Laboratory Findings: The urine is usually free of microorganisms. The diagnosis can be made by the following procedure: A dry smear of vaginal epithelial cells is stained with Lugol's solution. The slide is then washed with water and immediately examined microscopically while wet. In hypoestrogenism, the cells take up the iodine poorly and are therefore yellow. When the mucosa is normal, these cells stain deep brown because of their glycogen content. The diagnosis may also be confirmed by a Papanicolaou smear.

D. Instrumental Examination: Panendoscopy usually demonstrates a reddened and granular urethral mucosa. Some urethral stenosis may be noted.

Differential Diagnosis

Senile urethritis is often mistaken for urethral caruncle. Eversion of the posterior lip of the urinary meatus is evident in both conditions; however, a hypersensitive vascular tumor is not present in senile urethritis.

Before operations to relieve stress incontinence are performed, estrogen (or androgen) therapy should be tried.

Treatment

Senile urethritis responds well to diethylstilbestrol vaginal suppositories, 0.1 mg nightly for 3 weeks. Estrogen creams applied locally are also effective. Estrogen urethral suppositories have been recommended, but they offer no advantages and are difficult to insert. After 3 weeks of treatment, the drug is withheld for 1 week and the course is then repeated. Three or more courses are occasionally indicated, depending upon the symptoms and the appearance of the vaginal smear stained as outlined above.

If vaginal irritation or bleeding upon discontinuing estrogen suppositories is a problem, methyltestosterone buccal tablets can be used as vaginal suppositories. Insert one 5-mg tablet vaginally daily for 5–8 weeks. Diethylstilbestrol, 0.1 mg/d orally, is also effective.

Prognosis

Senile urethritis usually responds promptly to estrogen or androgen therapy.

URETHRAL CARUNCLE

Urethral caruncle is a benign, red, raspberrylike, friable vascular tumor involving the posterior lip of the external urinary meatus. It is rare before the menopause. Microscopically, it consists of connective tissue containing many inflammatory cells and blood vessels and is covered by an epithelial layer.

Clinical Findings

Symptoms include pain on urination, pain with intercourse, and bloody spotting from even mild trauma. A sessile or pedunculated red, friable, tender mass is seen at the posterior lip of the meatus.

Differential Diagnosis

Carcinoma of the urethra may involve the urethral meatus. Palpation reveals definite induration. Biopsy will establish the true diagnosis.

Senile urethritis is often associated with a polypoid reaction of the urinary meatus and in fact is the most common cause of masses in this region. The diagnosis can be made by verifying the patient's hypoestrogenic status and by demonstrating a favorable response to estrogen replacement therapy. Biopsy should be done if doubt exists.

Thrombosis of the urethral vein presents as a bluish, swollen, tender lesion involving the posterior lip of the urinary meatus. It has the appearance of the thrombosed hemorrhoid. It subsides without treatment.

Treatment

Local excision is indicated only if symptoms are troublesome.

Prognosis

True caruncle is usually cured by excision, but in a few instances it does recur.

THROMBOSIS OF THE URETHRAL VEIN

Spontaneous thrombosis of the urethral vein on the floor of the distal urethra occurs in older women, who complain of a sudden onset of local pain followed shortly thereafter by the appearance of a mass at the urethral orifice. Examination reveals a purple mass protruding from the posterior lip of the urethra; early, it is quite tender. The abrupt onset tends to rule out caruncle or cancer. If there is doubt about the true nature of the lesion, biopsy should be done.

No treatment is usually required, since the process gradually resolves. Evacuation of the clot has been recommended.

PROLAPSE OF THE URETHRA

Prolapse of the female urethra is not common. It usually occurs only in children or in paraplegics suffering from a lower motor neuron lesion. The protruding urethral mucosa presents as an angry red mass that may become gangrenous if it is not reduced promptly. When a little girl has a protruding mass, urethral prolapse must be differentiated from prolapse of a ureterocele.

After reduction, cystoscopy should be done to rule out ureterocele. Recurrences are rare following reduction; the accompanying inflammation probably "fixes" the tissue in place as healing progresses. If the prolapsed urethra cannot be reduced or if it recurs, an indwelling catheter should be inserted, traction placed upon it, and a heavy piece of suture material tightly tied over the tissue and catheter just proximal to the mass. The tissue later sloughs off. Using this same technique, the tissue can be resected, preferably with an electrosurgical cautery.

URETHROVAGINAL FISTULA

Urethrovaginal fistulas may follow local injury secondary to fracture of the pelvis or obstetric or surgical injury (see Chapter 16). A common cause is accidental trauma to the urethra or its blood supply in the course of surgical repair of a cystocele or excision of urethral diverticula. Vaginal urethroplasty is indicated.

URETHRAL DIVERTICULUM

Diverticulation of the urethral wall is not common. Diverticula are at times multiple. Most cases are probably secondary to obstetric urethral trauma or severe urethral infection. A few cases of carcinoma in such diverticula have been reported. Urethral diverticula are usually associated with recurrent attacks of cystitis. Purulent urethral discharge is sometimes noted as the infected diverticulum empties. Dyspareunia some-

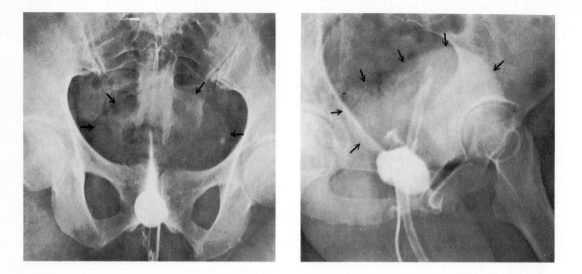

Figure 31–2. Urethral diverticulum containing stone. *Left:* Plain film showing stone. Arrows outline bladder. *Right:* Diverticulum filled with radiopaque fluid instilled through ureteral catheter. Bladder outlined by arrows.

times results. On occasion, the diverticulum may be large enough to be discovered by the patient.

The diagnosis is usually made on feeling a rounded cystic mass in the anterior wall of the vagina that leaks pus from the urethral orifice when pressure is applied. Endoscopy may reveal the urethral opening. The postvoiding film of an excretory urographic series may demonstrate the lesion. It may be possible to introduce a small catheter through which radiopaque fluid can be instilled. Appropriate x-ray films are then exposed (Fig 31–2). The plain film may show a stone in the diverticulum. If these methods fail, the following procedures can be used:

(1) Empty the diverticulum manually. Via a catheter, instill 5 mL of indigo carmine and 60 mL of contrast medium into the bladder. Remove the catheter and have the patient begin to void. Occlude the meatus with a finger. This maneuver usually causes the diverticulum to fill with the test solution. Take appropriate x-rays, and perform panendoscopy to look for leakage of blue dye from the mouth of the diverticulum (Borski and Stutzman, 1965).

(2) Insert a Davis-TeLinde catheter. This looks like a Foley catheter but is surrounded by a second movable balloon. Pass the catheter to the bladder and inflate the proximal balloon. While exerting tension on the catheter, slide the second balloon against the urinary meatus and inflate it. Then inject contrast medium into the catheter. The radiopaque fluid will escape from the catheter through a hole between the balloons and will fill the urethra and diverticulum, after which x-rays can be exposed.

Treatment consists of removal of the sac through an incision in the anterior vaginal wall, care being taken not to injure the urethral sphincteric musculature. Incision is carried down to the diverticular mucosa, and the plane of cleavage is then followed all around to the neck of the diverticulum. The diverticular sac is completely excised and the defect in the urethra repaired. Elik (1957) recommends that the diverticulum be opened, stuffed with Oxycel, and then closed; the resulting inflammatory reaction destroys the cyst. A suprapubic cystostomy should be left in place for 15 days following surgical excision of the diverticulum.

The outcome is usually good unless the diverticulum is so situated that its excision injures the external urinary sphincter mechanism. In a few cases, urethrovaginal fistula may develop. If the fistula does not close with adequate suprapubic drainage, surgical repair will be necessary 2–3 months later.

URETHRAL STRICTURE

True organic stricture of the adult female urethra is not common. (Functional urethral obstruction is more common.) It may be congenital or acquired. The trauma of intercourse and especially of childbirth may lead to periurethral fibrosis with contracture, or the stricture may be caused by the surgeon during vaginal repair. It may develop secondary to acute or chronic urethritis.

Persistent hesitancy in initiating urination and a slow urinary stream are the principal symptoms of stricture. Burning, frequency, nocturia, and urethral pain may occur from secondary urethritis or cystitis. If secondary infection of the bladder is present, pus and bacteria will be found in the urine. A fairly large catheter (22F) may pass to the bladder only with difficulty. Panendoscopy may demonstrate the point of narrowness and disclose evidence of urethritis. Cystoscopy often reveals trabeculation (hypertrophy) of the bladder wall.

Chronic cystitis may cause similar symptoms, but

urinalysis will reveal evidence of infection. Cancer of the urethra causes progressive narrowing of the urethra, but induration and infiltration of the urethra will be found on vaginal examination. Panendoscopy with biopsy establishes the diagnosis. Vesical tumor involving the bladder neck will cause hesitancy and impairment of the urinary stream. Cystoscopy is definitive. Chronic urethritis commonly accompanies urethral stenosis; either may be primary. Recurrent or chronic cystitis is often secondary to stenosis.

Treatment consists of gradual urethral dilatation (up to 36F) at weekly intervals. Slight overstretching is necessary, since some contracture will occur after therapy is discontinued. Measures to combat urethritis and cystitis must also be employed. Internal urethrotomy also has its proponents.

With proper overdilatation of the urethra and specific therapy of the urethritis that is usually present, the prognosis is good.

REFERENCES

Distal Urethral Stenosis

Farrar DJ, Green NA, Ashken MH: An evaluation of the Otis urethrotomy in female patients with recurrent urinary tract infections: A review after 6 years. *Br J Urol* 1980;**52**:68.

Firlit CF: Urethral anomalies. *Urol Clin North Am* 1978;**5**:31.

Fisher RE et al: Urethral calibration in newborn girls. *J Urol* 1969;**102**:67.

Hendry WF, Stanton SL, Williams DI: Recurrent urinary infections in girls: Effects of urethral dilatation. *Br J Urol* 1973;**45**:72.

Hinman F Jr: Mechanisms for the entry of bacteria and the establishment of urinary infection in female children. *J Urol* 1966;**96**:546.

Hojsgaard A: The urethral pressure profile in female patients with meatal stenosis. *Scand J Urol Nephrol* 1976;**10**:97.

Hradec E et al: Significance of urethral obstruction in girls. *Urol Int* 1973;**28**:440.

Immergut MA, Gilbert EC: Internal urethrotomy in recurring urinary infections in girls. *J Urol* 1973;**109**:126.

Kaplan GW, Sammons TA, King LR: A blind comparison of dilatation, urethrotomy and medication alone in the treatment of urinary tract infection in girls. *J Urol* 1973;**109**:917.

Kilner TP, Peet EW: *Urethra and Bladder: Congenital Malformations.* Butterworth, 1953.

Lyon RP, Marshall S: Urinary tract infections and difficult urination in girls: Long-term follow-up. *J Urol* 1971;**105**:314.

Lyon RP, Tanagho EA: Distal urethral stenosis in little girls. *J Urol* 1965;**93**:379.

Obrink A, Bunne G, Hedlund PO: Cultures from different parts of the urethra in female urethral syndrome. *Urol Int* 1979;**34**:70.

Smith DR: Critique on the concept of vesical neck obstruction in children. *JAMA* 1969;**207**:1686.

Tanagho EA, Lyon RP: Urethral dilatation versus internal urethrotomy. *J Urol* 1971;**105**:242.

Tanagho EA, Meyers FH, Smith DR: Urethral resistance: Its components and implications. 1. Smooth muscle component. 2. Striated muscle component. *Invest Urol* 1966;**7**:136,195.

Tanagho EA et al: Spastic external sphincter and urinary tract infection in girls. *Br J Urol* 1971;**43**:69.

Uehling DT: The normal caliber of the adult female urethra. *J Urol* 1978;**120**:176.

Van Gool J, Tanagho EA: External sphincter activity and recurrent urinary tract infection in girls. *Urology* 1977;**10**:348.

Vermillion CD, Halverstadt DB, Leadbetter GW Jr: Internal urethrotomy and recurrent urinary tract infection in female children. 2. Long-term results in the management of infection. *J Urol* 1971;**106**:154.

Walker D, Richard GA: A critical evaluation of urethral obstruction in female children. *Pediatrics* 1973;**51**:272.

Labial Fusion

Aribarg A: Topical oestrogen therapy for labial adhesions in children. *Br J Obstet Gynaecol* 1975;**82**:424.

Christensen EH, Oster J: Adhesions of labia minora (synechia vulvae) in childhood: A review and report of fourteen cases. *Acta Paediatr Scand* 1971;**60**:709.

Podolsky ML: Labial fusion: A cause of recurrent urinary tract infections. *Clin Pediatr* 1973;**12**:345.

Acute Urethritis

Bass HN: "Bubble bath" as an irritant to the urinary tract of children. *Clin Pediatr* 1968;**7**:174.

Marshall S: The effect of bubble bath on the urinary tract. *J Urol* 1965;**93**:112.

Chronic Urethritis

Batra SC, Iosif CS: Female urethra: Target for estrogen action. *J Urol* 1983;**129**:418.

Bruce AW et al: Recurrent urethritis in women. *Can Med Assoc J* 1973;**108**:973.

Farrar DJ, Green NA, Ashken MH: An evaluation of Otis urethrotomy in female patients with recurrent urinary tract infections: A review after 6 years. *Br J Urol* 1980;**52**:68.

Immergut MA, Gilbert EC: The clinical response of women to intestinal urethrotomy. *J Urol* 1973;**109**:90.

Marshall S, Lyon RP, Schieble J: Nonspecific urethritis in females. *Calif Med* (*June*) 1970;**112**:9.

Moore T, Hira NR, Stirland RM: Differential urethrovesical urinary cell-count. *Lancet* 1965;**1**:626.

Obrink A, Bunne G, Hedlund P-O: Cultures from different parts of the urethra in female urethral syndrome. *Urol Int* 1979;**34**:70.

O'Neil AGB: The bacterial content of the female urethra: A new method of study. *Br J Urol* 1981;**53**:368.

Pfau A, Sacks T: Bacterial flora of vaginal vestibule, urethra and vagina in normal premenopausal woman. *J Urol* 1977;**118**:292.

Zimskind PD, Mannes HA: Approach to bladder neck and urethral obstruction in women. *Surg Clin North Am* 1973;**53**:571.

Zufall R: Treatment of the urethral syndrome in women. *JAMA* 1963;**184**:894.

Senile Urethritis

Quinlivan LG: The treatment of senile vaginitis with low

doses of synthetic estrogens. *Am J Obstet Gynecol* 1965; **92:**172.

Smith P: Age changes in the female urethra. *Br J Urol* 1972;**44:**667.

Urethral Caruncle

Marshall FC, Uson AC, Melicow MM: Neoplasms and caruncles of the female urethra. *Surg Gynecol Obstet* 1960;**110:**723.

Thrombosis of the Urethral Vein

Falk HC: Treatment of urethral vein thrombosis. *Obstet Gynecol* 1964;**23:**85.

Harrow BR: The thrombosed urethral hemorrhoid: 3 case reports. *J Urol* 1967;**98:**482.

Prolapse of the Urethra

Capraro VJ, Bayonet-Rivera NP, Magoss I: Vulvar tumor in children due to prolapse of urethral mucosa. *Am J Obstet Gynecol* 1970;**108:**572.

Devine PC, Kessel HC: Surgical correction of urethral prolapse. *J Urol* 1980;**123:**856.

Klaus H, Stein, RT: Urethral prolapse in young girls. *Pediatrics* 1973;**52:**645.

Potter BM: Urethral prolapse in girls. *Radiology* 1971; **98:**287.

Smith HW Jr, Campbell EW Jr: Benign periurethral masses in women. *J Urol* 1976;**116:**451.

Turner RW: Urethral prolapse in female children. *Urology* 1973;**2:**530.

Urethrovaginal Fistula

Gray L: Urethrovaginal fistulas. *Am J Obstet Gynecol* 1968;**101:**28.

Hendren WH: Construction of female urethra from vaginal wall and perineal flap. *J Urol* 1980;**123:**657.

Tehan TJ, Nardi JA, Baker R: Complications associated with surgical repair of urethrovaginal fistula. *Urology* 1980; **15:**31.

Urethral Diverticulum

Benjamin J et al: Urethral diverticulum in adult female: Clinical aspects, operative procedure, and pathology. *Urology* 1974;**3:**1.

Borski AA, Stutzman RE: Diverticulum of female urethra: A simplified diagnostic aid. *J Urol* 1965;**93:**60.

Bracken RB et al: Primary carcinoma of the female urethra. *J Urol* 1976;**116:**188.

Dretler SP, Vermillion CD, McCullough DL: The roentgenographic diagnosis of female urethral diverticula. *J Urol* 1972;**107:**72.

Elik M: Diverticulum of the female urethra: A new method of ablation. *J Urol* 1957;**77:**243.

Glassman TA, Weinerth JL, Glenn JF: Neonatal female urethral diverticulum. *Urology* 1975;**5:**249.

Golimbu M, al-Askari S: High pressure voiding urethrography. *Urology* 1974;**3:**717.

Lapides J: Transurethral treatment of urethral diverticula in women. *J Urol* 1979;**121:**736.

Marshall S, Hirsch K: Carcinoma within urethral diverticula. *Urology* 1977;**10:**161.

Palagiri A: Urethral diverticulum with endometriosis. *Urology* 1978;**11:**271.

Presman D, Rolnick D, Zumerchek J: Calculus formation within a diverticulum of the female urethra. *J Urol* 1964;**91:**376.

Roberts TW, Melicow MM: Pathology and natural history of urethral tumors in females: Review of 65 cases. *Urology* 1977;**10:**583.

Sholem SL, Wechsler M, Roberts M: Management of the urethral diverticulum in women: A modified operative approach. *J Urol* 1974;**112:**485.

Spence, HM, Duckett JW Jr: Diverticulum of the female urethra: Clinical aspects and presentation of a simple operative technique for cure. *J Urol* 1970;**104:**432.

Torres SA, Quattlebaum RB: Carcinoma in a urethral diverticulum. *South Med J* 1972;**65:**1374.

Urethral Stricture

Essenhigh DM, Ardran GM, Cope V: A study of the bladder outlet in lower urinary tract infections in women. *Br J Urol* 1968;**40:**268.

Immergut MA, Gilbert EC: The clinical response of women to internal urethrotomy. *J Urol* 1973;**109:**90.

Surgical Repair

Hajj SN, Evans MI: Diverticula of the female urethra. *Am J Obstet Gynecol* 1980;**136:**335.

Hendren WH: Construction of female urethra from vaginal wall and perineal flap. *J Urol* 1980;**123:**657.

Steward M, Bretland PM, Stidolph NE: Urethral diverticula in the adult female. *Br J Urol* 1981;**53:**353.

Symmonds RE, Hill LM: Loss of the urethra: A report on 50 patients. *Am J Obstet Gynecol* 1978;**53:**130.

Woodhouse CRJ et al: Urethral diverticulum in females. *Br J Urol* 1980;**52:**305.

Disorders of the Testis, Scrotum, & Spermatic Cord

32

Jack W. McAninch, MD

DISORDERS OF THE SCROTUM

Hypoplasia of the scrotum accompanies cryptorchidism. Bifid scrotum is present with midscrotal or perineal hypospadias and in certain cases of intersexuality. In both instances, the 2 scrotal sacs simulate labia majora.

Idiopathic edema of the scrotum is occasionally seen in children. It may involve one or both sacs and also the penis, the perineum, or the inguinal region. The exact cause is not known; it may represent an allergic response or angioneurotic edema. Antihistamines may be of value, though the condition does resolve spontaneously.

Conn (1971) has observed scrotal edema caused by development of a fistula between the peritoneum and the subcutaneous tissue following paracentesis for cirrhosis of the liver. In women, the edema involves the labia. Three instances of scrotal emphysema were observed: (1) following treatment of rectal polyp, (2) following an open renal biopsy, and (3) in traumatic pneumothorax. It must be remembered, however, that torsion of the spermatic cord may affect the scrotal skin in a similar manner. Udall, Drake, and Rosenberg (1981) recognized acute scrotal swelling in an infant as a possible sign of acute peritonitis. Such a reaction requires a patent processus vaginalis.

In association with healed meconium peritonitis, masses may develop in the scrotum (or in the inguinal area) (Heydenrych and Marcus, 1976). Examination at birth may lead to the diagnosis of hydrocele, but a month later, the scrotal masses will have become firm. A plain film of the abdomen will reveal calcification in both the masses and the abdomen. This will differentiate the masses from teratoma.

CONGENITAL ANOMALIES OF THE TESTIS

ANOMALIES OF NUMBER

Absence of one or both testes is very rare. Broth-

ers, Weber, and Ball (1978) stress the need for a careful search for the absent organ. They cite 13 cases of testicular tumor in infra-abdominal cryptorchidism most of which were seminomas. Selective gonadal venography, sonography, CT scanning, and laparoscopy are useful in locating nonpalpable testes.

A review of the literature shows 53 instances of polyorchidism. A spermatocele or tumor of the spermatic cord is often mistaken for a third gonad.

HYPOGONADISM

Males suffering from either congenital or prepubertal primary testicular eunuchoidism or pituitary hypogonadism (congenital or secondary to a brain lesion) are tall and have disproportionately long extremities because of delay in fusion of the epiphyses. The testes are small, and there is lack of development of secondary sexual characteristics associated with some deficiency in libido and potency. These men are sterile. A somewhat feminine fat distribution may be noted, and there are wrinkles about the eyes. The primary gonadal defect is often associated with color blindness and mental retardation.

X-ray studies of the bones reveal delay in closure of the epiphyses. The differential diagnosis of these 2 disorders often depends upon determination of FSH and 17-ketosteroid (or serum testosterone) excretion in the urine. The pituitary type will excrete no FSH; the androgen level is very low. The gonadal eunuch excretes high levels of FSH (above 80 mouse units/24 h) but only moderately decreased amounts of urinary 17-ketosteroids or serum testosterone. The pituitary eunuchoid male may have an enlarged sella turcica or visual field defects secondary to tumor.

Both conditions are treated with long-acting esters of testosterone, 200 mg per month intramuscularly, or a comparable preparation by mouth daily.

Stearns et al (1974) have studied declining testicular function due to age. They found that serum testosterone levels remained normal to age 70 years. After age 40, however, a slight but steady increase in serum LH and FSH was observed.

For a discussion of Klinefelter's syndrome, see Chapter 34.

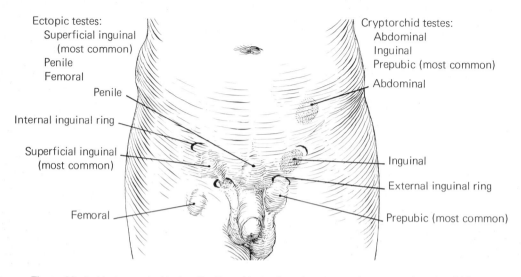

Figure 32–1. Undescended testes. Position of testes in various types of ectopy and cryptorchidism.

ECTOPY & CRYPTORCHIDISM

In ectopy, the testis has strayed from the path of normal descent; in cryptorchidism, it is arrested in the normal path of descent. Ectopy may be due to an abnormal connection of the distal end of the gubernaculum testis that leads the gonad to an abnormal position. The ectopic sites are as follows (Fig 32–1):

(1) Superficial inguinal (most common site): After passing through the external inguinal ring, the testis proceeds superolaterally to a position superficial to the aponeurosis of the external oblique muscle.

(2) Perineal (rare): The testis is found just in front of the anus and to one side of the midline (Middleton, Beamon, and Gillenwater, 1976).

(3) Femoral or crural (rare): The testis is found in Scarpa's triangle superficial to the femoral vessels. The cord passes under the inguinal ligament.

(4) Penile (rare): The testis is placed under the skin at the root of the dorsum of the penis.

(5) Transverse or paradoxic descent (rare): Both testes descend the same inguinal canal (Golladay and Redman, 1982). Some 85 examples have been collected from the literature.

(6) Pelvic (rare): The testis is found in the true pelvis (discovered only by surgical exploration).

Cryptorchidism is a condition in which a testicle is arrested at some point in its normal descent anywhere between the renal and scrotal areas. Unilateral arrest is more common than bilateral arrest. At the time of birth (9-month gestation), the incidence of maldescent is 3.4%; half of such testicles descend in the first month of life. The incidence of cryptorchidism in adults is 0.7–0.8%. In the premature infant, it is 30%. A few cryptorchid testes may descend at puberty.

Chromosomal studies in cases of cryptorchidism revealed no abnormalities. Bartone and Schmidt (1982) found normal chromosomes in 48 of 50 consecutive cases of cryptorchidism. One of the 2 patients with abnormal chromosomes was found to have Klinefelter's syndrome.

Etiology

The cause of maldescent is not clear. The following possibilities must be considered.

A. Abnormality of the Gubernaculum Testis: Differential growth of the embryo appears to cause descent of the gonad from its lumbar origin. Descent is guided by the gubernaculum, a cordlike structure that extends from the lower pole of the testis to the scrotum. In the embryo, of course, it is very short. Absence or abnormality of this structure may be a cause of maldescent.

B. Intrinsic Testicular Defect: Maldescent may be caused by a congenital gonadal (dysgenetic) defect that makes the testicle insensitive to gonadotropins. This theory is the best explanation for unilateral cryptorchidism. It would also explain why many patients with bilateral cryptorchidism are sterile, even when given definitive therapy at the optimum age.

C. Deficient Gonadotropic Hormonal Stimulation: Lack of adequate maternal gonadotropins may be a cause of incomplete descent. This seems to be the obvious explanation for bilateral cryptorchidism in the premature infant, since the elaboration of maternal gonadotropins remains at a low level until the last 2 weeks of gestation. It is difficult, however, to apply this theory to unilateral cryptorchidism.

Rajfer and Walsh (1977) have shown that testicular descent is an androgen-mediated event regulated by pituitary gonadotropin. This process leads to high levels of dihydrotestosterone. They point out that the testis must also have free access to the scrotum for normal descent.

Pathogenesis & Pathology

Moore clearly showed the efficacy of the scrotum as a temperature regulator for the tests, which are kept about 1 °C (1.8 °F) cooler than body temperature. The spermatogenic cells are sensitive to body temperature. Cooper demonstrated microscopic changes in the retained organ in boys at age 2. Mininberg, Rodger, and Bedford (1982) studied the ultrastructure of the cryptorchid testis and found deleterious changes in the first year of life. By age 4 years, massive collagen deposition was evident. They concluded that the testes had to be in the scrotum by age 1 year.

After age 6 years, changes become more obvious. The diameter of the tubules is smaller than normal. The number of spermatogonia decreases, and fibrosis between the tubules becomes marked. The cryptorchid testis after puberty may be fairly normal in size, but is markedly deficient in spermatogenic components; infertility is the rule.

It must be remembered that about 10% of these testes are congenitally defective (primary hypogonadism, hypogonadism secondary to hypopituitarism). These gonads will show subnormal spermatogenic activity in spite of treatment.

Fortunately, the Leydig cells are not affected by body temperature and are therefore usually found in normal numbers in the cryptorchid organ. An endocrinologic cause of impotence is rare in this group.

In a study employing the latest analytical methods, no chromosomal abnormalities could be found in biopsies of undescended testes. Maldescent and carcinomatous degeneration cannot be attributed to defects in chromosomes in the undescended organ.

Marshall and Shermeta (1979) point out that epididymal abnormalities are commonly found in these testes. The anomalies include agenesis, atresia, and elongated epididymides poorly connected to the gonad.

Clinical Findings

A. Symptoms: The cardinal symptom of ectopy or cryptorchidism is the absence of one or both testes from the scrotum. The patient may complain of pain from trauma to the testis, which may be situated in a vulnerable position (eg, over the public bone). The adult patient with bilateral cryptorchidism may present with a complaint of infertility.

B. Signs: In true maldescent, the scrotum on the affected side is atrophic. The testis either is not palpable (lying within or even proximal to the inguinal canal) or can be felt external to the inguinal ring. It cannot be manipulated into the scrotum. A common position for such a testis is in the region of the inguinal canal. A testis felt in this area would have to be a superficial inguinal ectopic testis (lying subcutaneously), for it is unlikely that a small testis could be palpated through the heavy external oblique aponeurosis. Inguinal hernia is often present on the affected side.

C. Laboratory Findings: Studies of the urinary 17-ketosteroids, gonadotropins, and serum testosterone may help in tracing the cause of cryptorchidism. In primary hypogonadism, the urinary gonadotropins (FSH) are markedly elevated, whereas the androgens are moderately reduced. In primary hypopituitarism, the androgens and pituitary gonadotropins are definitely depressed. In "primary" bilateral cryptochidism, the androgens and pituitary gonadotropins are often moderately diminished.

If neither testis can be demonstratred, Shapiro and Bodai (1978) suggest using herniography, venography, and arteriography. If these are unrevealing, they suggest using the human chorionic gonadotropin (hCG) test. This is done by establishing a baseline serum testosterone level and then giving hCG, 2000 units daily for 4 days. On the fifth day, the serum testosterone estimation should be repeated. If testes are present, this hormone will be elevated as much as 10-fold.

D. X-Ray Findings: Selective gonadal venography appears to be the most consistently useful test for proving the presence and position of a testis. Demonstration of a pampiniform plexus makes it almost certain that a testis is attached (Khan et al, 1982; Pommerville et al, 1982). However, Greenberg et al (1981) described 2 cases in which no testes were found although pampiniform plexuses were present.

E. Computed Tomography: Using CT scanning, Lee et al (1980) demonstrated 3 lower abdominal and 5 inguinal testes in the 8 patients they studied. CT scanning is more useful in postpubertal patients when the intra-abdominal testicle is sufficiently enlarged to be detected.

F. Ultrasonography: Using ultrasonography, Madrazo et al (1979) had no difficulty in identifying testes in the groin but were less successful if the organ was in the pelvis. Testes within the inguinal canal or positioned just inside the internal ring can easily be detected.

Differential Diagnosis

Physiologic cryptorchidism (retractile or migratory testis) is a common phenomenon requiring no treatment. Because of the small mass of the prepubertal testis and the strength of the cremaster muscle, which inserts upon the spermatic cord, the testes are apt to be involuntarily retracted out of the scrotum in cold weather or with excitement or physical activity. The diagnosis is made by noting that the scrotum on the suspected side is normally developed and that the "inguinal" testis can be pushed into and to the bottom of the scrotum. It may be necessary to place the child in a warm tub to afford maximum muscular relaxation, in which case the testis is found in the normal position. Such a testis descends at puberty and has been found to be normal (Puri and Nixon, 1977).

Complications

Associated inguinal hernia is found in 25% of patients with maldescent. At surgery, 95% of such patients are found to have a patent processus vaginalis.

Torsion of the spermatic cord is occasionally seen as a complication of cryptorchidism. Phillips and Holmes (1972) believe it is most commonly seen in spastic neurologic disease. Torsion of the cord must be differentiated from strangulated hernia, appendicitis, and diverticulitis.

Most authorities agree that cancer is 35 to 48 times more common in a misplaced testis than in the normally descended organ (Batata et al, 1980). This further substantiates the theory that many of these testes are dysgenetic. Martin (1979) collected 220 instances of cancer in undescended testes. Seminoma is the most common tumor. It is rare before age 10. Because of this evidence, he suggests that the undescended testis in a patient 10 years of age or older should be removed rather than treated by orchiopexy. Hinman (1979) recommends orchidectomy for the unilateral abdominal testis, because it is less likely to be fertile, more prone to cancer, and more difficult to place in the scrotum.

Treatment

Since definite histologic change can be demonstrated in the cryptorchid testis by age 1 year, placement of the testis in the scrotum should be accomplished by that age. Scorer (1967) recommends surgical correction at about age 1 year. He found that 83% of patients had an associated inguinal hernia. A successful operation will not ensure fertility if the testis is congenitally defective.

A. Hormone Therapy: Job et al (1982) suggest the use of hormone therapy before surgery is attempted. They find that although the optimal age for hormone therapy is 5 years of age, it can be effective at age 3 years. Give hCG, 1500 units/m² intramuscularly every other day or 3 times a week for a total of 9 injections. The inguinal testis responds best.

If physiologic cryptorchidism has been ruled out, hormone therapy will cause descent in about a month in 10–20% of cases, with more success in bilateral than unilateral cryptorchidism. Some of these cases may have been physiologic retractile testes that were misdiagnosed despite frequent examination. Descent with hormone therapy will save the child an operation and the surgeon embarrassment, although, if this treatment is successful, the testis would probably have descended spontaneously at puberty.

B. Surgical Treatment: If hormone therapy fails, or if inguinal hernia can be demonstrated, orchiopexy (and hernioplasty) should be done immediately. The testis must be placed at the bottom of the scrotum, without tension; the blood supply to the or-

gan must be meticulously preserved. Dissection of the inguinal area sometimes reveals that the vascular pedicle is too short to allow placement of the testis in the bottom of the scrotum. If so, the organ should be placed as low as possible, and 2 years later, the testicle should be advanced to the scrotum. In 62 cases, Zer, Wolloch, and Dintsman (1975) found that 17% of patients with atrophy of the testis required orchiectomy. In the past, a few authors have recommended division of the spermatic artery if the vascular pedicle was too short. This was originally described by Fowler and Stephens in 1959. They claimed that viability of the testis was preserved. Datta et al (1977) divided this artery at the internal ring, taking care to preserve collateral arteries to the vas deferens, cremaster muscle, and scrotum. They observed radionuclide evidence of normal vascular perfusion of the testicle. This is probably the procedure of choice for the short cord. Gibbons, Cromie, and Duckett Jr (1979) also recommend this procedure. However, Jones and Bagley (1979) used an extraperitoneal approach to place the testis in the scrotum in 85 of 86 subjects. Microsurgery has been used to place the abdominal testis in the scrotum by anastomosing the artery and vein of the testis to the inferior epigastric artery and vein (Martin and Salibian, 1980; Silber, 1981). If the testis is not discovered or is very atrophic and is therefore removed, a prosthesis can be placed in the scrotum. Orchiopexy can be done as an outpatient procedure (Caldamone and Rabinowitz, 1982).

Prognosis

The testicle that is properly placed in the scrotum provides adequate hormonal function and gives the scrotum a normal appearance. Approximately 20% of males with unilateral undescended testes will remain infertile even though orchiopexy is performed at an appropriate age (Gross and Replogle, 1963). A man with one untreated cryptorchid testis produces sperm of a lower concentration and poorer quality than a man with normally descended testes (Lipschultz et al, 1976). In bilateral undescended testes, treated or untreated, fertility rates are uniformly poor (Scheiber et al, 1981).

CONGENITAL ANOMALIES OF THE EPIDIDYMIS

Congenital absence of the epididymis is rare. At times the epididymis may be anterior rather than posterior to the testis. Fusion of the epididymis and testis may not occur.

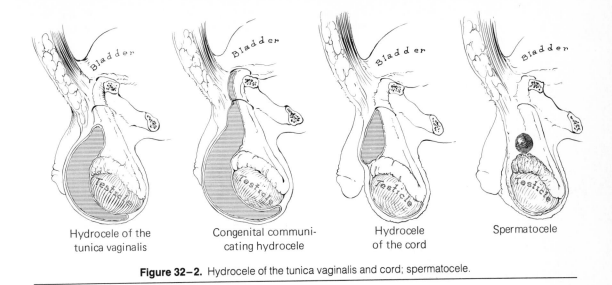

Hydrocele of the
tunica vaginalis

Congenital communi-
cating hydrocele

Hydrocele
of the cord

Spermatocele

Figure 32–2. Hydrocele of the tunica vaginalis and cord; spermatocele.

DISORDERS OF
THE SPERMATIC CORD*

SPERMATOCELE

A spermatocele is a painless cystic mass containing sperms. It lies just above and posterior to the testis but is separate from it (Fig 32–2). Most spermatoceles are less than 1 cm in diameter, although they are occasionally quite large and may be mistaken for hydroceles. They may be firm, simulating solid tumor. The cause is not entirely clear, although they probably arise from the tubules that connect the rete testis to the head of the epididymides (vasa efferentia) or from cystic structures on the upper pole of the testis or epididymis.

Since they are relatively small, spermatoceles are usually discovered by the physician during routine examination of the genitalia; at times they may be large enough to come to the attention of the patient. Examination reveals a freely movable transilluminating cystic mass lying above the testicle. Microscopic examination of aspirated contents reveals sperms, usually dead. Grossly, the fluid is thin, white, and cloudy.

Spermatocele is differentiated from hydrocele of the tunica vaginalis in that the latter covers the entire anterior surface of the testicle. Aspiration of hydrocele recovers yellow but clear fluid. A tumor of the coverings of the spermatic cord (eg, mesothelioma, fibroma) may feel like a tense spermatocele. It does not, however, contain fluid and will not transilluminate.

Spermatocele requires no therapy unless it is large enough to annoy the patient, in which case it should be excised.

VARICOCELE
(See also Male Infertility, pp 637–662.)

Varicocele is found in approximately 10% of young men and consists of dilatation of the pampiniform plexus above the testis, with the left side most commonly affected. These veins drain into the internal spermatic vein in the region of the internal inguinal ring. The internal spermatic vein passes lateral to the vas deferens at the internal inguinal ring and, on the left side, drains into the renal vein. On the right it empties into the vena cava.

Incompetent valves are more common in the left internal spermatic vein. This condition, combined with the effect of gravity, may lead to poor drainage of the pampiniform plexus, the veins of which gradually undergo dilation and elongation. The area may be painful, particularly in sexually continent men.

The sudden development of a varicocele in an older man is sometimes a late sign of renal tumor when tumor cells have invaded the renal vein, thereby occluding the spermatic vein.

Examination of a man with varicocele when he is upright reveals a mass of dilated, tortuous veins lying posterior to and above the testis. It may extend up to the external inguinal ring and is often tender. The degree of dilatation can be increased by the Valsalva maneuver. In the recumbent position, venous distention abates. Testicular atrophy from impaired circulation may be present.

Sperm concentration and motility are significantly decreased in 65–75% of subjects. Infertility is often observed and can be reversed in a high percentage of patients by correction of the varicocele. The most use-

---

* The primary congenital anomaly that affects the spermatic cord is absence of the vas deferens. If the vas is absent on both sides, infertility results.

ful surgical procedure is ligation of the internal spermatic veins at the internal inguinal ring. This can be done as an outpatient procedure. Recently, percutaneous methods, eg, balloon catheter, sclerosing fluids, have been used to occlude the veins. This is particularly useful when the infertile patient is undergoing percutaneous internal spermatic venography. One or both veins can be occluded as indicated (Formanek et al, 1981; Reidl, Lunglmayr, and Stacki, 1981; Walsh and White, 1981). A trial of scrotal support can be helpful in patients with chronic pain.

HYDROCELE

A hydrocele consists of a collection of fluid within the tunica or processus vaginalis. Although it may occur within the spermatic cord, it is most often seen surrounding the testis. A number of cases of hydrocele of the canal of Nuck have been reported. A hydrocele may develop rapidly secondary to local injury, radiotherapy, acute nonspecific or tuberculous epididymitis, or orchitis. It may complicate testicular neoplasm. Chronic hydrocele is more common. Its cause is usually unknown, and it usually afflicts men past age 40 years. Fluid collects about the testis, and the mass grows gradually (Fig 32–2). It may be soft and cystic or quite tense. The fluid is clear and yellow.

Communicating hydrocele of infancy and childhood is caused by a patent processus vaginalis, which is continuous with the peritoneal cavity. It is also a form of indirect inguinal hernia. If the hydrocele is large, bowel may be found within the contents. Most communicating hydroceles of infancy will close spontaneously before 1 year of age. If the presence of bowel in the sac is suspected, surgical correction should be done.

Clinical Findings

Young boys with hydrocele commonly have a history of a cystic mass that is small and soft in the morning but larger and more tense at night. This indicates that a small communication exists in the processus vaginalis (Fig 32–2). Hernia or communicating hydrocele is therefore the proper diagnosis. Hydrocele is usually painless unless it is accompanied by acute epididymal infection. The patient may, however, complain of its bulk or weight.

The diagnosis is made by finding a rounded cystic intrascrotal mass that is not tender unless underlying inflammatory disease is present. The mass transilluminates. If the hydrocele is enclosed within the spermatic cord, a cystic fusiform swelling is noted in the groin or in the upper scrotum. Sonography should be done if the diagnosis is in question.

A tense hydrocele must be differentiated from tumor of the testis, which does not transilluminate. However, if hydrocele develops in a young man without apparent cause, careful evaluation of the testicle and epididymis should be done in order to rule out cancer or tuberculosis.

Complications include compression of the blood supply of the testicle, which leads to atrophy, and hemorrhage into the hydrocele sac following trauma.

Treatment

Unless complications are present, active therapy is not required. The indications for treatment are a very tense hydrocele that might embarrass circulation to the testicle or a large, bulky mass that is cosmetically unsightly and perhaps uncomfortable for the patient.

Spontaneous closure and resolution of the hydrocele may occur in infancy. If it persists beyond 1 year of age, closure is unlikely. When treatment is necessary, surgical therapy is definitive. In children, high ligation of the patent processus vaginalis at the internal inguinal ring followed by excision of the distal sac corrects the problem. Inguinal incisions should be made in all children undergoing hydrocele repair, in order to correct the patent processus. In adults, Lord (1972) has described a simple operation wherein the hydrocele sac, after being opened, is merely stitched together to collapse the wall (Haas et al, 1978). The results of both procedures are good, though in a few cases the hydrocele recurs.

TORSION OF THE SPERMATIC CORD

Torsion of the spermatic cord (torsion of the testicle) is an uncommon affliction that is most commonly seen in adolescent males. It causes strangulation of the blood supply to the testis. Unless treatment is given within 3 or 4 hours, testicular atrophy may occur.

The cryptorchid testis is prone to undergo torsion. Many cases of torsion occur in the neonatal period (Guiney and McGlinchey, 1981; Jerkins et al, 1983). Lee, Wright, and McLoughlin (1983) found that 26% of their patients with torsion were over age 21. Shulka et at (1982) observed that most cases occurred in cold weather. Trauma may be an initiating factor. A few intra-abdominal cancerous testes have undergone torsion. In about half of patients, this disorder occurs during sleep. In most instances, congenital abnormality of the tunica vaginalis or spermatic cord is present. Torsion seems to be most often due to a voluminous tunica vaginalis that inserts well up on the cord. This allows the testis to rotate within the tunica. The initiating factor seems to be spasm of the cremaster muscle, which inserts obliquely on the cord. The contraction of this muscle causes the patient's left testis to rotate counterclockwise and his right testis clockwise (as the physician observes the patient from the foot of the bed). With vascular occlusion, there is edema of the testis and the cord up to the point of occlusion. This leads to gangrene of the testis and epididymis.

Clinical Findings

The diagnosis is suggested when a young boy suddenly develops severe pain in one testicle, followed by swelling of the organ, reddening of the scrotal skin, lower abdominal pain, and nausea and vomiting.

However, torsion of the cord may be accompanied only by moderate scrotal swelling and little or no pain.

Examination usually reveals a swollen, tender organ that is retracted upward as a result of shortening of the cord by volvulus. Testes that are apt to undergo torsion lie horizontally with the patient standing. He recognized this abnormality in a number of boys who had, in the past, suffered from transient testicular pain representing torsion with spontaneous detorsion. Pain may be increased by lifting the testicle up over the symphysis. (The pain from epididymitis is usually alleviated by this maneuver.) Within a few hours after onset leukocytosis may develop.

The diagnosis may be made in the early stages if the epididymis can be felt in an abnormal position (eg, anterior). After a few hours, however, the entire gonad becomes so swollen that the epididymis cannot be distinguished from the testis by palpation. Torsion can be differentiated from the epididymitis with limited success by using the Doppler stethoscope in conjunction with ultrasound (Rodriguez et al, 1981). The testis made ischemic by torsion will not echo sound; the hypervascularity of epididymitis will increase sound (Smith and King, 1979). The most definitive test appears to be the scintillation scan using ^{99m}Tc-pertechnetate. It is accurate in 90–100% of cases. The twisted testis is avascular, while epididymitis is "hot." Testicular tumors show increased vascularity; trauma shows decreased vascularity (Thomas et al, 1981).

Differential Diagnosis

The differential diagnosis includes acute epididymitis, acute orchitis, and trauma. Epididymitis is rare before puberty and is often accompanied by pyuria. Mumps orchitis, also rare before puberty, is usually accompanied by parotitis. Without a history or findings of injury, traumatic orchitis may be misdiagnosed as torsion of the cord.

Epididymitis is unusual before age 16. Differential diagnosis from tension may be difficult if epididymitis is not complicated by pyuria. In case of doubt, scintillation scanning is indicated (Valvo et al, 1982; Levy et al, 1983).

Treatment

If the patient is seen within a few hours of onset, manual detorsion may be attempted (King et al, 1974). Torsion causes the left testis to rotate conunterclockwise and the right one clockwise; therefore, one may twist a testis in the opposite direction. The right testis should be "unscrewed" and the left one "screwed up." This maneuver is facilitated by infiltration of the spermatic cord, near the external inguinal ring, with 10–20 mL of 1% xylocaine hydrochloride. Even if this is successful, surgical fixation of both testes should be done within the next few days. If manual detorsion fails, immediate surgical detorsion must be performed, although after 4–6 hours infarction usually will have occurred in those testes subjected to a 720-degree twist of the cord. Using early surgery, Cattolica et al (1982) obtained viable testes in 79% of their cases of torsion. Discounting those cases that they saw late, the salvage rate was 93%. Whether the testis appears to be viable or not, it should probably be sutured down to preclude subsequent torsion. Even though the seminiferous tubules may become necrotic, the more hardy interstitial cells may remain viable. Excision of the parietal tunica vaginalis will cause agglutination of the testicle to the scrotal wall. Because the opposite testicle usually is affected by the same abnormal attachments, prophylactic fixation of that organ is imperative.

Prognosis

Unfortunately, the diagnosis is usually made and treatment instituted too late, and atrophy is to be expected in these instances. Wright (1977) observed that detorsion within 12 hours of onset affords a good result; that recovery is possible if treatment is given 12–24 hours later; and that preservation is doubtful after 24 hours. If detorsion is delayed beyond 48 hours, orchiectomy is advised.

● ● ●

TORSION OF THE APPENDICES OF THE TESTIS & EPIDIDYMIS

On the upper poles of both the testis and epididymis, there are small vestigial appendages that may be sessile or pedunculated (Fig 1–8). The latter type may spontaneously undergo torsion, which leads to an inflammatory reaction followed by ischemic necrosis and absorption.

This phenomenon usually affects boys up to age 16 years, though Altaffer and Steele (1980) were able to find reports of 350 instances of torsion in adults. Sudden onset of testicular pain is noted. Shortly after onset, a small tender lump may be felt at the upper pole of the testis or epididymis; this sign is pathognomonic, particularly if the lump appears to be blue when the skin is held tight over the mass (Dresner, 1973; Puri and Boyd, 1976).

At later examination, the entire testicle is swollen and tender. The differential diagnosis is then between torsion of these appendages and torsion of the spermatic cord. Immediate surgical exploration is indicated, for time is a critical factor in the treatment of torsion of the cord. If an appendix is twisted, it should be excised. Holland, Graham, and Ignatoff (1981) feel that if the examination shows the problem to be torsion of an appendix of the testis or epididymis, no surgical intervention is necessary. The pain will slowly subside over 5–7 days and the scrotal swelling resolve.

REFERENCES

SCROTUM

Conn HO: Sudden scrotal edema in cirrhosis: A postparacentesis syndrome. *Ann Intern Med* 1971;**74:**943.

Heydenrych JJ, Marcus PB: Meconium granulomas of the tunica vaginalis. *J Urol* 1976;**115:**596.

Kaplan GW: Acute idiopathic scrotal edema. *J Pediatr Surg* 1977;**12:**647.

Malloy TR, Wein AJ, Gross P: Scrotal and penile lymphedema: Surgical considerations and management. *J Urol* 1983;**130:**263.

Udall DA, Drake DJ Jr, Rosenberg RS: Acute scrotal swelling: A physical sign of primary peritonitis. *J Urol* 1981;**125:**750.

TESTIS

Anomalies of Number

Brothers LR III, Weber CH Jr, Ball TP Jr: Anorchism versus cryptorchidism: The importance of a diligent search for intra-abdominal testes. *J Urol* 1978;**119:**707.

Goldberg LM, Skaist LB, Marrow JW: Congenital absence of the testes: Anorchism and monorchism. *J Urol* 1974;**111:**840.

Lazarus BA, Tessler AN: Polyorchidism with normal spermatogenesis. *Urology* 1974;**3:**615

Reckler JM, Rose LI, Harrison JH: Bilateral anorchism. *J Urol* 1975;**113:**869.

Hypogonadism

Clarke BF, Ewing DJ, Campbell IW: Clinical features of diabetic autonomic neuropathy. *Horn Metab Res (Suppl)* 1980;**9:**50.

Federman DD: The assessment of organ function: The testis. *N Engl J Med* 1971;**285:**901.

Handelsman DJ, Swerdloff RS: Male gonadal dysfunction. *Clin Endocrinol Metab* 1985;**14:**89.

Stearns EL et al: Declining testicular function with age. *Am J Med* 1974;**57:**761.

Ectopy & Cryptorchidism

Bartone FF, Schmidt MA: Cryptorchidism: Incidence of chromosomal anomalies in 50 cases. *J Urol* 1982; **127:**1105.

Batata MA et al: Cryptorchidism and testicular cancer. *J Urol* 1980;**124:**286.

Caldamone AA, Rabinowitz R: Outpatient orchiopexy. *J Urol* 1982;**127:**286.

Datta NS et al: Division of spermatic vessels in orchiopexy: Radionuclide evidence of preservation of testicular circulation. *J Urol* 1977;**118:**447.

Fowler R, Stephens FD: The role of testicular vascular anatomy in the salvage of the high undescended testes. *Aust NZ J Surg* 1959;**29:**92.

Gibbons MD, Cromie WJ, Duckett JW Jr: Management of the abdominal undescended testicle. *J Urol* 1979;**122:**76.

Giuliani L, Carmignani G: Microsurgical testis autotransplantation: A critical review. *Eur Urol* 1983;**9:**129.

Golladay ES, Redman JF: Transverse testicular ectopia. *Urology* 1982;**19:**181.

Greenberg SH et al: The falsely positive gonadal venogram: Presence of a pampiniform plexus without a gonad. *J Urol* 1981;**125:**887.

Gross RE, Replogle RL: Treatment of the undescended testis. *Postgrad Med* 1963;**34:**266.

Hinman F Jr: Unilateral abdominal crytorchidism. *J Urol* 1979;**122:**71.

Job JC et al: Hormonal therapy of cryptorchidism with human chorionic gonadotropin (HCG). *Urol Clin North Am* 1982;**9:**405.

Jones PF, Bagley FH: An abdominal extraperitoneal approach for the difficult orchidopexy. *Br J Surg* 1979; **66:**14.

Khan O et al: Testicular venography for the localization of the impalpable undescended testis. *Br J Surg* 1982; **69:**660.

Lee JKT, Glazer HS: Computed tomography in the localization of the non-palpable testis. *Urol Clin North Am* 1982; **9:**397.

Lee JKT et al: Utility of computed tomography in the localization of the undescended testis. *Radiology* 1980; **135:**121.

Lipshultz LI et al: Testicular function after orchiopexy for unilaterally undescended testis. *N Engl J Med* 1976; **295:**15.

Madrazo BL et al: Ultrasonographic demonstration of undescended testes. *Radiology* 1979;**133:**181.

Marshall FF, Shermeta DW: Epididymal abnormalities associated with undescended testis. *J Urol* 1979;**121:**341.

Martin DC: Germinal cell tumors of the testis after orchiopexy. *J Urol* 1979;**121:**422.

Martin DC, Salibian AH: Orchiopexy using microvascular surgical technique. *J Urol* 1980;**123:**435.

Middleton GW, Beamon CR, Gillenwater JV: Two rare cases of ectopic testis. *J Urol* 1976;**115:**455.

Miller HC: Transseptal orchiopexy for cryptorchism. *J Urol* 1967;**98:**503.

Mininberg DT, Rodger JC, Bedford JM: Ultrastructural evidence of the onset of testicular pathological conditions in the cryptorchid human testis within the first year of life. *J Urol* 1982;**128:**782.

Phillips NB, Holmes TW Jr: Torsion infarction in ectopic cryptorchidism: A rare entity occurring most commonly with spastic neuromuscular disease. *Surgery* 1972; **71:**335.

Pommerville P et al: The role of gonadal venography in the management of the adult with non-palpable undescended testis. *Br J Urol* 1982;**54:**408.

Puri P, Nixon HH: Bilateral retractile testes: Subsequent effects on fertility. *J Pediatr Surg* 1977;**12:**563.

Rajfer J, Walsh PC: Hormonal regulation of testicular descent: Experimental and clinical observations. *J Urol* 1977;**118:**985.

Rajfer J et al: The use of computerized tomography scanning to localize the impalpable testis. *J Urol* 1983;**129:**972.

Saha SK: Cordopexy: A new approach to the undescended testis: A review of 2- to 5-year follow-up. *J Urol* 1983; **129:**561.

Scheiber K et al: Late results after surgical treatment of maldescended testes with special regard to exocrine and endocrine testicular function. *Eur Urol* 1981;**7:**268.

Scorer CG: Early operation for the undescended testis. *Br J Surg* 1967;**54:**694.

Shapiro SR, Bodai BI: Current concepts of the undescended testis. *Surg Gynecol Obstet* 1978;**147:**617.

Sheldon CA: Undescended testis and testicular torsion. *Surg Clin North Am* 1985;**65:**1303.

Silber SJ: The intra-abdominal testes: Microvascular autotransplantation. *J Urol* 1981;**125**:329.

Smolko MJ, Kaplan GW, Brock WA: Location and fate of the nonpalpable testis in children. *J Urol* 1983;**129**:1204.

Weiss RM, Glickman MG: Venography of the undescended testis. *Urol Clin North Am* 1982;**9**:387.

Zer M, Wolloch Y, Dintsman M: Stage orchiorrhaphy: Therapeutic procedure in cryptorchic testicle with a short spermatic cord. *Arch Surg* 1975;**110**:387.

SPERMATIC CORD

Spermatocele

Clarke BG, Bamford SB, Gherardi GJ: Spermatocele: Pathologic and surgical anatomy. *Arch Surg* 1963;**86**:351.

Lord PH: A bloodless operation for spermatocele or cyst of the epididymis. *Br J Surg* 1970;**57**:641.

Schoenberg HW, Murphy JJ: The differential diagnosis of intrascrotal masses. *GP* (March) 1962;**25**:82.

Varicocele

Formanek A et al: Embolization of the spermatic vein for treatment of infertility: A new approach. *Radiology* 1981;**139**:315.

Reidl P, Lunglmayr G, Stacki W: A new method of transfemoral testicular vein obliteration for varicocele using a balloon catheter. *Radiology* 1981;**139**:323.

Ross LS, Lipson S, Dritz S: Surgical treatment of varicocele. *Urology* 1982;**19**:179.

Shafik A: Venous tension patterns in cord veins. 2. After varicocele correction. *J Urol* 1983;**129**:749.

Turner TT: Varicocele: Still an enigma. *J Urol* 1983;**129**:695.

Walsh PC, White RI: Balloon occlusion of the internal spermatic vein for the treatment of varicoceles. *JAMA* 1981;**246**:1701.

Hydrocele

Ariyan S: Hydrocele of the canal of Nuck. *J Urol* 1973;**110**:172.

Black RE et al: Abdominoscrotal hydrocele: Cause of abdominal mass in children. *Pediatrics* 1981;**67**:420.

Haas JA et al: Operative treatment of hydrocele: Another look at Lord's procedure. *Urology* 1978;**12**:578.

Kaye KW, Clayman RV, Lange PH: Outpatient hydrocele and spermatocele repair under local anesthesia. *J Urol* 1983;**130**:269.

Lord PH: Bloodless surgical procedures for the cure of idiopathic hydrocoele and epididymal cyst (spermatocoele). *Prog Surg* 1972;**10**:94.

Rifkin MD: Ultrasonography of the lower genitourinary tract. *Urol Clin North Am* 1985;**12**:645.

Rodriguez WC, Rodriguez DD, Fortuño RF: The operative treatment of hydrocele: A comparison of 4 basic techniques. *J Urol* 1981;**125**:804.

Torsion of the Spermatic Cord

Anderson PA, Giacomantonio JM: The acutely painful scrotum in children: Review of 113 consecutive cases. *Can Med Assoc J* 1985;**132**:1153.

Bartsch G et al: Testicular torsion: Late results with special regard to fertility and endocrine function. *J Urol* 1980;**124**:375.

Cattolica EV et al: High testicular salvage rate in torsion of the spermatic cord. *J Urol* 1982;**128**:66.

Cos LR et al: Torsion of intrascrotal malignant testis tumors. *J Urol* 1983;**130**:145.

Guiney EJ, McGlinchey J: Torsion of the testes and spermatic cord in the newborn. *Surg Gynecol Obstet* 1981;**152**:273.

Jerkins GR et al: Spermatic cord torsion in the neonate. *J Urol* 1983;**129**:121.

Kay R, Strong DW, Tank ES: Bilateral spermatic cord torsion in the neonate. *J Urol* 1980;**123**:293.

King LM et al: Untwisting in delayed treatment of torsion of the spermatic cord. *J Urol* 1974;**122**:217.

Knight PJ, Vassy LE: The diagnosis and treatment of the acute scrotum in children and adolescents. *Ann Surg* 1984;**200**:664.

Lee LM, Wright JE, McLoughlin MG: Testicular torsion in the adult. *J Urol* 1983;**130**:93.

Levy OM et al: Diagnosis of acute testicular torsion using radionuclide scanning. *J Urol* 1983;**129**:975.

Rodriguez DD et al: Doppler ultrasound vs testicular scanning in the evaluation of the acute scrotum. *J Urol* 1981;**125**:343.

Schneider RE, Laycob LM, Griffin WT: Testicular torsion in utero. *Am J Obstet Gynecol* 1973;**117**:1126.

Sellu DP, Lynn JA: Intermittent torsion of the testis. *J R Coll Surg Edinb* 1984;**29**:107.

Shulka RB et al: Association of cold weather with testicular torsion. *Br Med J* 1982;**285**:1459.

Smith SP, King LR: Torsion of the testis: Techniques of assessment. *Urol Clin North Am* 1979;**6**:429.

Stage KH, Schoenvogel R, Lewis S: Testicular scanning: Clinical experience with 72 patients. *J Urol* 1981;**125**:334.

Thomas WEG et al: Dynamic radionuclide scanning of the testis in acute scrotal conditions. *Br J Surg* 1981;**68**:621.

Valvo JR et al: Nuclear imaging in the pediatric acute scrotum. *Am J Dis Child* 1982;**136**:831.

Wright JE: Torsion of the testis. *Br J Surg* 1977;**64**:274.

Appendices of the Testis & Epididymis

Altaffer LF III, Steele SM Jr: Torsion of testicular appendages in men. *J Urol* 1980;**124**:56.

Dresner ML: Torsed appendage diagnosis and managment: Blue dot sign. *Urology* 1973;**1**:63.

Holland JM, Graham JB, Ignatoff JM: Conservative management of twisted testicular appendages. *J Urol* 1981;**125**:213.

Puri P, Boyd E: Torsion of the appendix testis: A survey of 22 cases. *Clin Pediatr* 1976;**15**:949.

33

Skin Diseases of the External Genitalia*

Timothy G. Berger, MD

INFLAMMATORY DERMATOSES

Almost any skin condition, including psoriasis, seborrheic dermatitis, lichen planus, eczema, etc, can affect the region of the external genitalia and perineum. The patient should be questioned and examined for other possible areas of involvement. In any case of itching or infected dermatitis in this area, it is important to rule out diabetes and pediculosis or scabies.

Associated vaginal and other urologic conditions should be corrected. Self-treatment and overtreatment may alter and complicate genital lesions. Emotional factors associated with repeated scratching and rubbing tend to prolong and complicate genital conditions.

Many individuals with involvement in this area have a fear of sexually transmitted disease; if there is no question of this, the fear should be dispelled.

CONTACT DERMATITIS

Contact dermatitis includes changes produced by both primary irritants and true allergic sensitizers. Possible causes are cosmetics, feminine deodorant sprays, douches, contraceptives, soaps, local medications ("overtreatment dermatitis"), wearing apparel, plants (poison oak and ivy), etc.

Treatment must include removal of the suspected agent, if possible. Cool wet dressings constitute excellent initial treatment, and corticosteroid creams may be used topically if infection is not present. The fluorinated corticosteroid creams are more likely to produce atrophic striae in the groin than is hydrocortisone.

CIRCUMSCRIBED NEURODERMATITIS
(Lichen Simplex Chronicus)

These thickened lesions are of great importance in the persistence of any vulval or scrotal skin condition regardless of the original cause. Rubbing and scratching can prolong any eruption indefinitely, and it is usually this problem that causes the patient to seek medical care. The rubbing or scratching may be done almost subconsciously. A continuing itch-scratch cycle is established that must be broken before healing can occur.

Treatment is as for contact dermatitis (above) plus stopping the rubbing or scratching.

ATOPIC DERMATITIS

This lesion presents as dry lichenified dermatitis on the penis and scrotum, in the groin, or on the vulva. Similar changes are usually present also on the face and neck and in the antecubital and popliteal spaces. Generalized dryness is present. There is usually a personal or family history of asthma or hay fever.

Treatment is as for contact dermatitis (see above) plus an oral antihistamine (hydroxyzine or diphenhydramine).

INTERTRIGO

Intertrigo (sodden, macerated dermatitis) is due to chafing and friction of contiguous surfaces. It occurs in the groins, inframammary areas, skin folds, etc, usually in obese individuals, and is more common in hot, humid weather. Superficial bacterial or candidal infection is often present. Treatment is cool soaks to dry the lesions, followed by application of a combination of a nonfluorinated topical steroid and an anticandidal cream (see Candidiasis, below).

DRUG ERUPTIONS

Most drug eruptions are widespread but may first appear in the genital area. A fixed drug eruption, due usually to laxatives (phenolphthalein), sulfonamides, or barbiturates, may present as a perfectly round,

---

* Sexually transmitted disease is discussed in Chapter 15; tumors in Chapter 19.

bright red to violaceous macule that quickly vesiculates and produces a superficial erosion. It occurs in the same site with reexposure to the drug. Lesions of erythema multiforme in the genital area have a similar clinical appearance.

PSORIASIS

Psoriasis may involve flexural surfaces (inverse psoriasis), such as the groin and the perianal cleft, and intermammary areas. It tends to be bright red and moist and is usually free of scales. Itching may be intense. Occasionally, the only involvement may be in the anogenital area. A solitary plaque may present on the penis, leading to confusion with Bowen's disease or some other more serious disorder. The diagnosis usually can be made by inspection and by noting other areas of involvement such as on the scalp, elbows, and knees. Pitting of the nails, when present, is almost pathognomonic of psoriasis. Treatment is with 0.1% anthralin ointment rubbed in sparingly morning and night for intertriginous lesions. Hydrocortisone cream, 1%, may be used concomitantly.

SEBORRHEIC DERMATITIS

Seborrheic dermatitis may appear as scaly erythematous patches and is easily confused with candidiasis, intertrigo, and psoriasis. Typical areas of involvement are usually present elsewhere, eg, on the scalp or brows, in creases of the cheeks and chin, in and around the ears, on the presternum, and in the axillas. Corticosteroid creams are very useful, especially in combination with an imidazole cream. Highly potent corticosteroid creams should not be used for prolonged periods, because temporary atrophy and atrophic striae will appear in susceptible individuals.

LICHEN PLANUS

Lichen planus may appear on the glans penis or on the labia and introitus. The lesions are small, polygonal, violet-hued papules about 1–2 cm in diameter, with milky striations over their shiny surfaces. They may become clustered together to form plaques. Itching is usually a problem. There may be generalized involvement or typical lesions in the buccal mucosa that look like spilled milk.

Corticosteroid creams may be helpful in relieving the pruritus. The disease usually disappears after a course of several months.

LICHEN SCLEROSUS ET ATROPHICUS

This is a distinct entity characterized by flat-topped white papules that coalesce to form white patches without infiltration. The surface shows comedolike plugs or dells. The end stages may resemble very thin parchment or tissue paper. It occurs most frequently in patches on the upper back, chest, and breasts, mostly in women. It almost inevitably involves the anogenital regions, where painful fissures may develop and severe itching may be a distressing symptom. On the penis, this condition occurs as balanitis xerotica obliterans, which may lead to urethral stenosis and atrophy with telangiectasia about the meatus and on the glans and may cause phimosis. There is a direct relationship between these conditions and carcinoma, although this is quite rare and should not call for prophylactic surgery of these genital lesions. Anogenital lichen sclerosus et atrophicus may be misdiagnosed as leukoplakia.

Lichen sclerosus et atrophicus may involute spontaneously, especially in young girls.

Circumcision for balanitis xerotica obliterans is not particularly helpful.

Testosterone propionate ointment, 2%, is of benefit in females. In males, and in females who do not respond to topical testosterone, bland ointment or mild topical steroids in combination with a topical anesthetic (pramoxine hydrochloride, 1%) may be of benefit.

COMMON SUPERFICIAL INFECTIONS

ARTHROPODS

Pediculosis Pubis (Pubic Lice, Crabs)

Pediculosis is a parasitic infestation of the skin of the scalp, trunk, or pubic area. Pediculosis pubis may be sexually or nonsexually transmitted.

Itching may be intense, leading to scratching. This may lead to pyoderma. The nits are found on the hair shafts. Treatment consists of application of lindane (gamma benzene hexachloride), 1% lotion or cream, which should remain in place for 8 hours and then be washed out. Pyrethrins in lotion form (Rid, Pyrinate) are equally effective. The sexual partner should also be examined and treated. All clothing, bedding, and towels should be washed in very hot water or drycleaned. If lice are found 1 week later, the treatment should be repeated.

Scabies

A severely pruritic, widespread dermatitis frequently involving the genital area is caused by the mite *Sarcoptes scabiei*. In males, very itchy papules or nodules with a central crust are common on the glans or shaft of the penis or on the scrotum. These nodules often persist for weeks to months after effective treatment. In adults, scabies is often a sexually transmitted disease. Treatment consists of application of lindane (gamma benzene hexachloride), 1% lotion or cream, to the entire body below the neck for 12–24 hours. All household members (> 6 years of age) and sexual contacts must be similarly treated. Crotamiton should be used to treat children age 6 years or younger. All clothing, bedding, and towels should be washed or drycleaned. Treatment may be repeated in 1 week. Topical steroids or tar gels may be used to treat persistent genital nodules.

FUNGAL INFECTIONS
(Tinea Cruris)

Heat, moisture, and darkness favor these infections. They are frequently aggravated by overtreatment.

Tinea cruris is characterized by marginated, slightly elevated, scaling patches on the inner thighs and in the groin. There may be an active vesicular border. Pruritus may be intense. Direct microscopic examination of skin scrapings in potassium hydroxide solution will reveal hyphae. The differential diagnosis includes seborrheic dermatitis, psoriasis, intertrigo, and localized neurodermatitis. Miconazole, 2% cream or lotion; clotrimazole, 1% cream or lotion; econazole, 1% cream; ciclopirox olamine, 1% cream; and haloprogin, 1% cream, applied twice daily, are good treatment alternatives. If they are irritating, 1% hydrocortisone cream may be used concomitantly. Griseofulvin (micronized), 500 mg orally, may be given twice daily for 4–6 weeks.

CANDIDIASIS

Infection with *Candida albicans* is characterized by erythematous, weeping, circumscribed lesions with peripheral satellite vesiculopustules. Lesions occur most commonly on the inner thighs, with a predilection for the creases. Scrotal involvement is common in candidiasis and rare in tinea cruris. "Pingpong" infections between sexual partners may occur. Pregnancy, diabetes, obesity, and immunosuppression are predisposing factors. Broad-spectrum antibiotic therapy or estrogen therapy may be followed by an overgrowth of *Candida*. The skin involvement may be secondary to vaginal involvement. Lesions occur under the prepuce. High-power microscopic examination of skin scrapings in potassium hydroxide solution shows clusters of tiny spores and fine mycelial filaments. Nystatin appears to be effective in most instances. It is available as dusting powder, cream, vaginal inserts, and oral tablets. Miconazole, 2% cream or lotion; clotrimazole, 1% cream or lotion; econozole, 1% cream; ciclopirox olamine, 1% cream; and haloprogin, 1% cream, applied twice daily, are good alternatives to nystatin. Ketoconazole, 200 mg orally daily for 10 days, will cure most cases of candidiasis.

BACTERIAL INFECTIONS
(Pyoderma)

Staphylococcus aureus is the most common cause of primary bacterial infections in the genital area. In addition, many inflammatory dermatoses may be secondarily infected by *S aureus* or other bacteria. A gram-stained smear will show clumps of cocci and many polymorphonuclear leukocytes. Culture is mandatory to confirm the diagnosis. *S aureus* produces 2 types of primary lesions, a follicular pustule (folliculitis) and a superficial blister (impetigo).

Staphylococcal folliculitis begins as a superficial infection of the follicle but may extend deeply (furunculosis). It is usually acute but may be chronic or recurrent. Chronic folliculitis is usually due to nasal carriage of *Staphylococcus*. Deep, draining abscesses are rarely due to bacteria alone and suggest the presence of secondary infection of a chronic suppurative disorder, eg, histiocytosis X, regional enteritis, lymphoma, hidradenitis suppurativa, schistosomiasis, or amebiasis. Recurrent folliculitis in the groin is common in acquired immunodeficiency syndrome (AIDS).

Topical treatment alone is often inadequate for bacterial folliculitis. A penicillinase-resistant penicillin (dicloxacillin) is the treatment of choice. Penicillin-allergic individuals may be treated with a cephalosporin or erythromycin. Treatment is continued until all lesions are healed. Adding rifampin to the above treatment is recommended for frequent recurrences. Washing the affected area with an antibacterial soap or a benzoyl peroxide wash may be useful adjunctively and may help to suppress recurrences.

Staphylococcal impetigo starts as a very superficial blister that quickly breaks, leaving a crusted, weeping erosion. Treatment is the same as for staphylococcal folliculitis but usually of shorter duration.

VIRAL INFECTIONS

Warts
Warts are common in the vulval region, under the prepuce, and on the shaft of the penis. If present on the mucous or mucocutaneous surfaces, they are called condylomata acuminata. Condylomata acuminata are wartlike anogenital papillomas caused by a sexually transmitted papovavirus. Although they tend to involve the external genitalia, anal or oral intercourse may lead to involvement of the anal canal or the mouth. They must be differentiated from condylomata lata, the lesions of syphilis. Condylomata acuminata are usually moist and macerated. They frequently respond to topical treatment with podophyllum resin, 25% in compound tincture of benzoin applied sparingly once a week. The resin should be washed off after several hours. Fulguration may be necessary if podophyllum is not successful. Liquid nitrogen can be used with a cotton-tipped applicator. Each lesion may

be frozen for 10–30 seconds. Urethral warts are discussed on p 577. To prevent recurrence of condylomata acuminata, the sexual partner must also be examined and treated if necessary.

Molluscum Contagiosum

Molluscum contagiosum is a common cutaneous infection that is sexually transmitted in adults. It is caused by a poxvirus that has not yet been successfully cultured. The characteristic lesion is a smooth-surfaced, firm, pearly papule 2–5 mm long, with a central umbilication. Most infected persons have 5–15 lesions located on the lower abdomen, upper thighs, or skin of the genitalia. Extensive molluscum contagiosum outside the genital area in adults is rare except in immunosuppressed patients. Treatment involves local destruction of the lesions by curettage, cryotherapy, or light electrodesiccation.

Herpes Simplex

Eighty-five percent of genital infections with herpes simplex virus are due to the type 2 virus. Initial or primary infection may present as a painful, widespread, symmetric, blistering eruption with moderate systemic symptoms and a duration averaging longer than 2 weeks. Dysuria is common, especially in females. Autoinoculation of other sites (fingers, eyes) may occur. Culture or a Tzanck preparation is necessary to confirm the diagnosis. Acyclovir (Zovirax), 200 mg orally 5 times daily, is recommended.

Herpes simplex virus type 2 frequently causes recurrent genital herpes. Recurrent herpes infection presents as localized, grouped blisters; there are few systemic symptoms and a course of about 1 week. Frequently, local pain or itching occurs as a prodrome to the blisters. Most patients with recurrent herpes infection should be given local drying treatment only (eg, benzoyl peroxide 5% gel). Individuals with frequent, disabling recurrences of infection that has been confirmed on culture may be treated with acyclovir, 200 mg orally 5 times daily for 5 days at the onset of symptoms or blisters. For the most severely affected patients, chronic suppressive therapy with acyclovir, 200 mg 3 times daily, may be considered. Persistent ulcerations in the genital or perianal area of an immunosuppressed person require culture for herpes simplex virus and intravenous acyclovir therapy if cultures are positive.

REFERENCES

General

Fitzpatrick TB et al: *Dermatology in General Medicine*. McGraw-Hill, 1986.

Holmes KK et al (editors): *Sexually Transmitted Diseases*. McGraw-Hill, 1984.

Moschella SL, Pillsbury DM, Hurley JF Jr: *Dermatology*. Saunders, 1985.

Rook A, Wilkinson DS, Ebling FJ: *Textbook of Dermatology*. Blackwell, 1985.

Inflammatory Dermatoses

Chalmers RJG et al: Lichen sclerosis et atrophicus: A common and distinctive cause of phimosis in boys. *Arch Dermatol* 1984;**120:**1025.

Farber EM, Abel EA, Charuworn A: Recent advances in the treatment of psoriasis. *J Am Acad Dermatol* 1983;**8:**311.

Fisher A: *Contact Dermatitis,* 3rd ed. Lea & Febiger, 1986.

Ford GP et al: The response of seborrhoeic dermatitis to ketoconazole. *Br J Dermatol* 1984;**111:**603.

Hanifin JM: Atopic dermatitis. *J Am Acad Dermatol* 1982;**6:**1.

Mahmood JM: Familial lichen planus: A report of 9 cases from 4 families with a brief review of the literature. *Arch Dermatol* 1983;**119:**292.

Wintroub BU, Stern R: Cutaneous drug reactions: Pathogenesis and clinical classification. *J Am Acad Dermatol* 1985;**13:**167.

Common Superficial Infections

Bunney MH: *Viral Warts: Their Biology and Treatment*. Oxford Univ Press, 1982.

Corey L et al: Genital herpes simplex virus infections: Clinical manifestations, course, and complications. *Ann Intern Med* 1983;**98:**958.

Feingold DS, Wagner RF Jr: Antibacterial therapy. *J Am Acad Dermatol* 1986;**14:**535.

Smith EB (editor): Superficial fungal infections. *Dermatol Clin* 1984;**2:**1. [Entire issue.]

34

Abnormalities of Sexual Differentiation*

Felix A. Conte, MD, & Melvin M. Grumbach, MD

Advances in cytogenetics, experimental embryology, steroid biochemistry, and methods of evaluation of the interaction between the hypothalamus, pituitary, and gonads have helped to clarify problems of sexual differentiation. Anomalies may occur at any stage of intrauterine maturation and can lead to gross ambisexual development or to subtle abnormalities that do not become manifest until sexual maturity is achieved.

Acronyms Used in This Chapter

ACTH	Adrenocorticotropic hormone
DHEA	Dehydroepiandrosterone
DHT	Dihydrotestosterone
DNA	Deoxyribonucleic acid
DOC	Deoxycorticosterone
DOCA	Deoxycorticosterone acetate
FSH	Follicle-stimulating hormone
GH	Growth hormone
GnRH	Gonadotropin-releasing hormone
hCG	Human chorionic gonadotropin
HLA	Human leukocyte antigen
LH	Luteinizing hormone
RNA	Ribonucleic acid
TSH	Thyroid-stimulating hormone; thyrotropin

NORMAL SEX DIFFERENTIATION

Chromosomal Sex

The normal human diploid cell contains 22 autosomal pairs of chromosomes and 2 sex chromosomes (two X or one X and one Y). Arranged serially and numbered according to size and centromeric position, they are known as a karyotype. Advances in the techniques of staining chromosomes (Fig 34–1) permit positive identification of each chromosome by its unique "banding" pattern. Bands can be produced with the fluorescent dye quinacrine (Q bands), in the region of the centromere (C bands), and with Giemsa's stain (G bands). Fluorescent banding (Fig 34–2) is particularly useful because the Y chromosome stains so brightly that it can be identified easily in both interphase and metaphase cells. The standard nomenclature for describing the human karyotype is shown in Table 34–1.

Studies in patients with abnormalities of sexual differentiation indicate that the sex chromosomes (the X and Y chromosomes) and quite likely the autosomes carry genes that influence sexual differentiation by causing the bipotential gonad to develop either as a testis or as an ovary. Two normally functioning X chromosomes, in the absence of a Y chromosome and the genes for testicular organogenesis, lead to the formation of an ovary.

---

*Figs 34–1 to 34–4, Figs 34–7 to 34–10, Fig 34–14, and Tables 34–1, 34–2, 34–4, and 34–5 are reproduced, with permission, from Grumbach MM, Van Wyk JJ: Disorders of sex differentiation. Chap 8, pp 423–501, in: *Textbook of Endocrinology,* 5th ed. Williams RH (editor). Saunders, 1974.

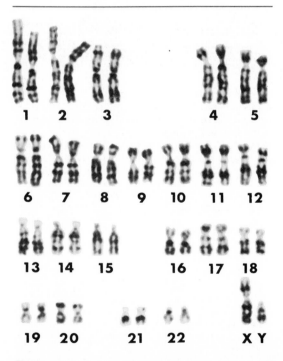

Figure 34–1. A normal 46,XY karyotype stained with Giemsa's stain to produce G bands. Note that each chromosome has a specific banding pattern.

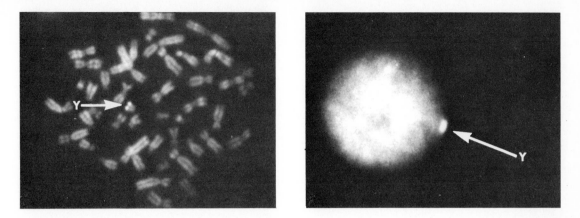

Figure 34–2. Metaphase chromosomes stained with quinacrine and examined through a fluorescence microscope. Note the bright fluorescence of the distal arms of the Y chromosome, which can also be seen in interphase cells (*"Y body"* at *right*).

Careful examination of the karyotype in humans reveals a marked discrepancy in size between the X and Y chromosomes. There is evidence that gene dosage compensation is achieved in all persons with 2 or more X chromosomes in their genetic constitution by inactivation of all X chromosomes except one. This phenomenon, the so-called Lyon hypothesis, is thought to be a random process that occurs in each cell in the late blastocyst stage of embryonic development. The result of this process is formation of one or more sex chromatin bodies (Barr bodies) in the interphase cells of persons having 2 or more X chromosomes (Fig 34–3).

Recent data indicate that the distal portion of the short arm of the X chromosome escapes inactivation. Several genes have been localized to this region, including steroid sulfatase, the XG^a red cell antigen, and the cell surface antigen MIC2, as well as a locus influencing the expression of H-Y antigen. Furthermore, it is this segment of the X chromosome which pairs with the short arm of the Y chromosome during meiosis, suggesting the possibility of homology between these pairing regions. In buccal mucosal smears of 46, XX females, a sex chromatin body is evident in 20–30% of the nuclei examined, whereas in normal

46, XY males, a comparable sex chromatin body is absent. In patients with more than two X chromosomes, the maximum number of sex chromatin bodies in any diploid nucleus is one less than the total number of X chromosomes. By utilizing sex chromatin and Y fluorescent staining (Fig 34–4), one can determine indirectly the sex chromosome complement of any individual (Table 34–2).

H-Y Antigen

In 1955, Eichwald and Silmser showed that among inbred strains of mice, most male-to-female skin grafts were rejected, whereas male-to-male and female-to-female grafts survived. This phenomenon was attributed to a specific Y-linked histocompatibility locus, the H-Y antigen.

Utilizing a sperm cytotoxicity assay to test for this antigen, Wachtel and his coworkers expanded the study of H-Y antigen from inbred mice to rats, guinea pigs, rabbits, and humans. They demonstrated the association of H-Y antigen with the heterogametic sex (usually the male) in a wide range of vertebrates. In mammals, H-Y antigen is expressed in the het-

Table 34–1. Nomenclature for describing the human karyotype pertinent to designating sex chromosome abnormalities.

Paris Conference	Description	Former Nomenclature
46,XX	Normal female karyotype	XX
46,XY	Normal male karyotype	XY
47,XXY	Karyotype with 47 chromosomes including an extra X chromosome	XXY
45,X	Monosomy X	XO
45,X/46,XY	Mosaic karyotype composed of 45,X and 46,XY cell lines	XO/XY
p	Short arm	p
q	Long arm	q
46,X,del (X) (qter→p21:)	Deletion of the short arm of the X distal to band Xp21	XXp–
46,X,del (X) (pter→q21:)	Deletion of the long arm of the X distal to band Xq21	XXq–
46,X,i (Xq)	Isochromosome of the long arm of X	XXqi
46,X,i (Xp)	Isochromosome of the short arm of X	XXpi
46,X,r (X)	Ring X chromosome	XXr
46,X,t (Y;7) (q11;q36)	Translocation of the distal fluorescent portion of the Y chromosome to the long arm of chromosome 7	46,XYt (Yq–7q+)

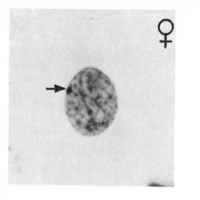

Figure 34–3. X chromatin body in the nucleus of a buccal mucosal cell from a normal female.

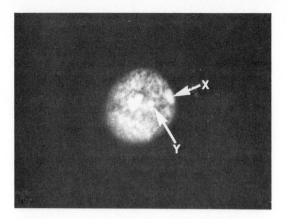

Figure 34–4. An interphase nucleus stained with quinacrine and examined by fluorescence microscopy. This cell reveals a "Y body" and an X chromatin body. The patient has a 47,XXY karyotype.

erogametic male but not usually in the homogametic XX female.

Wachtel and Ohno and their associates noted the striking conservation throughout evolution of this ubiquitous minor cross-reacting plasma membrane histocompatibility antigen, its appearance early in embryonic development (in the 8-cell male mouse embryo), and its association with heterogametic sex. These observations led them to suggest that this phylogenetically conserved antigen is the factor responsible for inducing testicular organogenesis of the bipotential fetal gonads. They examined their hypothesis by testing patients with testicular tissue who had XX karyotypes, eg, XX males and XX true hermaphrodites. Despite the absence of a Y chromosome in these patients, H-Y antigen was detected in all patients tested (although it is usually at lower levels than those observed in control 46, XY males). In addition, the gonad of the bovine freemartin (the intersex XX twin of a male fetus) is positive for H-Y antigen. Further evidence indicates that even in the absence of a discrete Y chromosome, or karyotypic evidence of a Y-to-X chromo-

some, or Y-to-autosome translocation or insertion, the presence of testicular tissue is invariably associated with a positive test for H-Y antigen. The chromosome sites of the structural and regulatory genes for the expression of H-Y antigen are uncertain. Evidence suggests that there are sites in the pericentromeric region of the Y chromosome, on the short arm of the X chromosome, and possibly on autosomes that affect the synthesis and action of H-Y antigen.

According to Ohno, biologically active H-Y antigen is a protein (MW 16,000–18,000) composed of hydrophobic peptide units that are linked by intersubunit disulfide bonds. The only cell known to disseminate H-Y antigen is the primitive Sertoli cell. H-Y antigen has been detected on all cell membranes from "normal" XY males except those of immature germ cells. Apparently, there are 2 receptors for H-Y antigen. Ohno has proposed that one receptor is nonspecific and ubiquitous and represents the stable cell membrane anchorage sites for H-Y antigen on all male cells; this anchorage site has been conceived as an association of "major histocompatibility complex" cell surface antigens (HLA) with β_2-microglobulin. The second receptor is found only on gonadal cells, both male and female, and binds free H-Y antigen with a greater affinity than do nonspecific anchorage sites.

A hypothesis for the organogenesis of the indifferent embryonic gonad as testis can be summarized as follows: The pericentromeric region of the Y chromosome contains a locus (or loci) that either codes for H-Y antigen or regulates its expression. H-Y antigen is disseminated by cells in the gonadal blastema, binds to gonad-specific H-Y receptors, and induces differentiation of the primitive gonad as a testis by the seventh week of gestation (Fig 34–5). In the absence of critical levels of H-Y antigen and in the presence of 2 structurally normal X chromosomes, a functional ovary will develop. Indirect evidence suggests the presence of a specific ovarian organizing antigen.

Table 34–2. Sex chromosome complement correlated with X chromatin and Y bodies in somatic interphase nuclei.*

Sex Chromosomes	Maximum Number in Diploid Somatic Nuclei	
	X Bodies	Y Bodies
45,XO	0	0
46,XX	1	0
46,XY	0	1
47,XXX	2	0
47,XXY	1	1
47,XYY	0	2
48,XXXX	3	0
48,XXXY	2	1
48,XXYY	1	2
49,XXXXX	4	0
49,XXXXY	3	1
49,XXXYY	2	2

*The maximum number of X chromatin bodies in diploid somatic nuclei is one less than the number of Xs, whereas the maximum number of Y fluorescent bodies is equivalent to the number of Ys in the chromosome constitution.

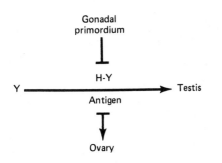

Figure 34–5. Interaction of H-Y antigen, germ cells, and somatic elements of the primordial gonad in testicular differentiation.

All of the evidence discussed previously in support of the testis-organizing function of H-Y antigen is indirect and circumstantial. However, in vitro experimental data provide more direct evidence for this hypothesis. In a series of experiments, Ohno and Zenzius and their coworkers have reported cell dissociation and reaggregation experiments on newborn rat and mouse gonads (Fig 34–6). The Moscona technique was used to obtain a suspension of single cells from newborn mouse or rat testes. The free cell suspension was exposed to excess anti-H-Y serum and incubated in rotation culture. The H-Y antibody-treated dissociated testicular cells reaggregated to form ovarian "primordiumlike follicles," whereas untreated testicular cells reorganized as "seminiferous tubule-like structures." In a subsequent experiment (Fig 34–6), Ohno and his coworkers purified H-Y antigen from culture media of a ("Daudi") human male, Burkitt lymphoma cell line, which lacks the putative β_2-microglobulin H-Y anchorage site. Bovine fetal XX indifferent gonads exhibited testicular organization in the presence of purified H-Y antigen. Thus, these experiments directly demonstrate the capacity of H-Y antigen to induce differentiation of the indifferent fetal gonad into a testis.

Recently, several groups have reported the detection of H-Y antigen in unexpected circumstances, ie, in patients with Turner's syndrome (XO and XXqi). Questions of the specificity, reproducibility, and quantification of these technically difficult serologic assays for H-Y antigen must be addressed before one can interpret these discrepancies between a putative immunoreactive H-Y antigen and gonadal and chromosomal sex (see Ohno, 1986).

TESTICULAR & OVARIAN DIFFERENTIATION

Until the 12-mm stage (approximately 42 days of gestation), the embryonic gonads of males and females are indistinguishable. By 42 days, 300–1300 primordial germ cells have seeded the undifferentiated gonad. These large cells later become oogonia and spermatogonia, and lack of these cells is incompatible with further ovarian differentiation. Under the influence of the genes that code for the H-Y antigen, the gonad will begin testicular differentiation by 43–50 days of gestation. The appearance of Sertoli cells is the earliest recognizable event in testicular organogenesis. This is correlated with the development of seminiferous cords. Thereafter, Leydig cells are apparent by about 60 days, the tunica albuginea develops, and differentiation of male external genitalia occurs by 65–77 days of gestation.

In the gonad destined to be an ovary, the lack of differentiation persists. At 77–84 days, long after differentiation of the testis in the male fetus, a significant number of germ cells enter meiotic prophase to characterize the transition of oogonia into oocytes, which marks the onset of ovarian differentiation from the undifferentiated gonads (Fig 34–7).

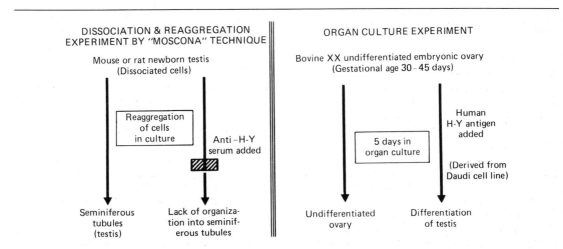

Figure 34–6. Diagrammatic scheme summarizing experimental evidence supporting H-Y antigen as the inducer of the testis in gonadal organogenesis. (Reproduced, with permission, from Grumbach MM, Conte FA: Disorders of sex differentiation. Chapter 9 in: *Textbook of Endocrinology,* 6th ed. Williams RH [editor]. Saunders, 1981.)

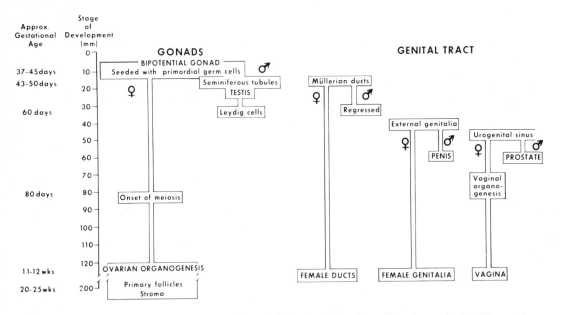

Figure 34-7. Schematic sequence of sexual differentiation in the human fetus. Note that testicular differentiation precedes all other forms of differentiation.

Differentiation of Genital Ducts
(Fig 34-8)

By the seventh week of intrauterine life, the fetus is equipped with the primordia of both male and female genital ducts. The müllerian ducts, if allowed to persist, form the uterine tubes, the uterus, the cervix, and the upper third of the vagina. The wolffian ducts, on the other hand, have the potential for differentiating into the epididymis, vas deferens, seminal vesicles, and ejaculatory ducts of the male. In the presence of a functional testis, the müllerian ducts involute under the influence of "müllerian duct inhibitory factor," a nonsteroid macromolecule secreted by Sertoli cells. This substance acts "locally" to cause müllerian duct repression ipsilaterally. The differentiation of the wolffian duct is stimulated by testosterone secretion from the testis. In the presence of an ovary or in the absence of a functional fetal testis, müllerian duct differentiation occurs, and the wolffian ducts involute.

Differentiation of External Genitalia
(Fig 34-9)

Up to the eighth week of fetal life, the external genitalia of both sexes are identical and have the capacity to differentiate into the genitalia of either sex. Female sex differentiation will occur in the presence of an ovary or streak gonads or if no gonad is present (Fig 34-10). Differentiation of the external genitalia along male lines depends on the action of testosterone and particularly dihydrotestosterone, the 5α-reduced metabolite of testosterone. In the male fetus, testosterone is secreted by the Leydig cells, possibly autonomously at first, and thereafter under the influence of hCG, and then by stimulation from fetal pituitary

LH and FSH. Masculinization of the external genitalia and urogenital sinus of the fetus results from the action of dihydrotestosterone, which is converted from testosterone in the target cells by the enzyme 5α-reductase. Dihydrotestosterone is bound to a cytosol receptor (binding protein) in the target cell. It is then translocated to the nucleus of the cell, where chromatin binding occurs, which initiates DNA-directed, RNA-mediated transcription and results in androgen-induced differentiation and growth of the cell. The gene that codes for the cytosol androgen-binding protein is located on the X-chromosome. Thus, an X-linked gene controls the androgen response of all somatic cell types by specifying the cytosol androgen receptor protein.

As in the case of the genital ducts, there is an inherent tendency for the external genitalia and urogenital sinus to develop along female lines. Differentiation of the external genitalia along male lines requires androgenic stimulation early in fetal life. The testosterone metabolite dihydrotestosterone and its specific cytosol receptor must be present to effect masculinization. Dihydrotestosterone stimulates growth of the genital tubercle, fusion of the urethral folds, and descent of the labioscrotal swellings to form the penis and scrotum. Androgens also inhibit descent and growth of the vesicovaginal septum and differentiation of the vagina. There is a critical period for action of the androgen. After about the 12th week of gestation, fusion of the labioscrotal folds will not occur even under intense androgen stimulation, although phallic growth can be induced. Impairment in the synthesis or secretion of fetal testosterone or in its conversion to dihydrotestosterone, deficient or defective androgen receptor activity, or defective production and local action of

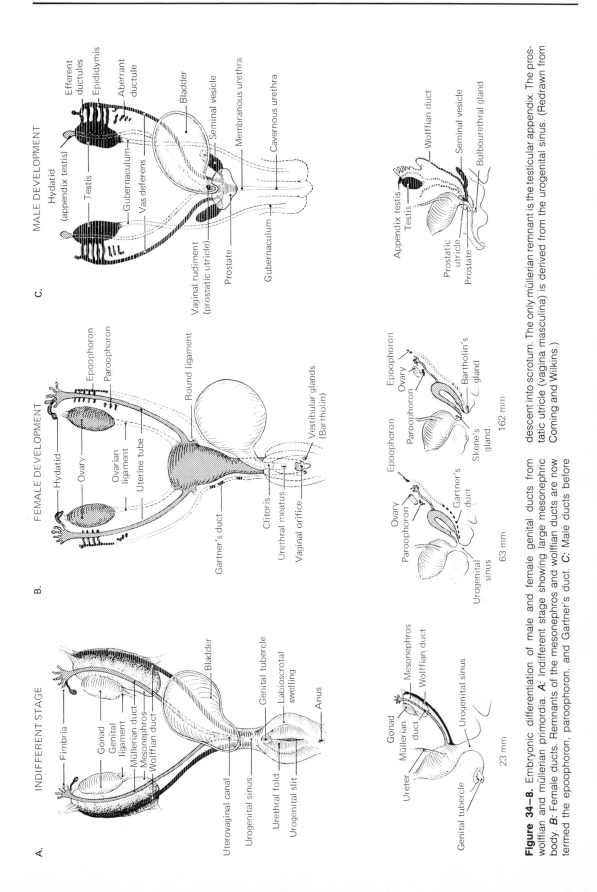

Figure 34–8. Embryonic differentiation of male and female genital ducts from wolffian and müllerian primordia. **A:** Indifferent stage showing large mesonephric body. **B:** Female ducts. Remnants of the mesonephros and wolffian ducts are now termed the epoophoron, paroophoron, and Gartner's duct. **C:** Male ducts before descent into scrotum. The only müllerian remnant is the testicular appendix. The prostatic utricle (vagina masculina) is derived from the urogenital sinus. (Redrawn from Corning and Wilkins.)

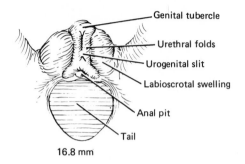

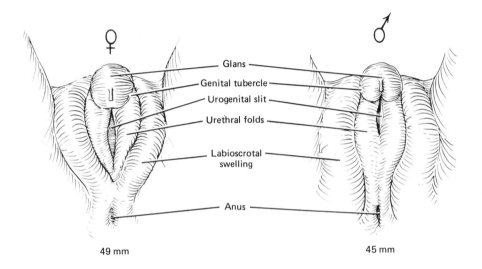

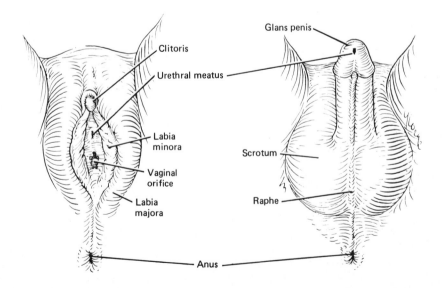

Figure 34–9. Differentiation of male and female external genitalia from bipotential primordia.

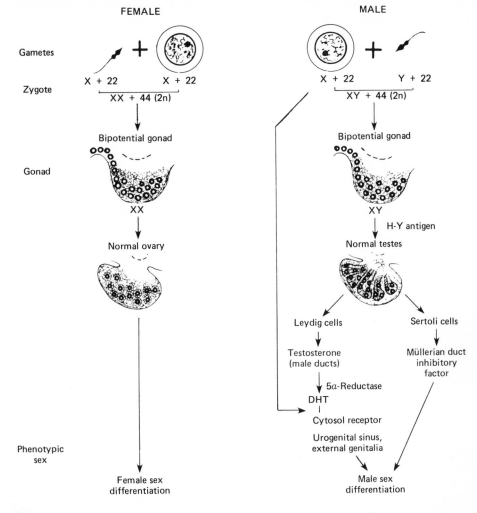

Figure 34–10. Diagrammatic summation of human sexual differentiation. DHT, dihydrotestosterone.

müllerian duct inhibitory factor leads to incomplete masculinization of the male fetus (Fig 34–10). Exposure of the female fetus to abnormal amounts of androgens from either endogenous or exogenous sources, especially before the 12th week of gestation, can result in virilization of the external genitalia.

PSYCHOSEXUAL DIFFERENTIATION

Psychosexual differentiation may be classified into 4 broad categories: (1) gender identity, defined as the identification of self as either male or female; (2) gender role, ie, those aspects of behavior in which males and females differ from one another in our culture at this time; (3) gender orientation, which is the choice of erotic partner; and (4) cognitive differences.

Studies of individuals who have been reared in the sex opposite to their chromosomal or gonadal sex—as well as prenatally androgenized females with virilizing adrenal hyperplasia—provide strong evidence that gender identity is not coded for primarily by sex chromosomes or prenatal sex steroid exposure. Rather, it appears to be "imprinted" postnatally by words, attitudes, and comparison of one's body with those of others. Generally, gender identity agrees with the sex of assignment in the intersex patient, provided that the child is reared *unambiguously* and appropriate surgical and hormonal therapy is instituted, so that the child has an unambiguously male or female phenotype. Under these circumstances, gender identity is usually established by 18–30 months of age. If, at puberty, discordant secondary sexual characteristics are allowed to develop and persist, some intersex patients develop doubts about their gender identity and request a change of sex. Thus, it appears that gender identity may be more plastic than previously thought and that at puberty, sex steroids as well as socialization reinforce gender identity. However, the weight of evidence still strongly supports environmental factors as the principal determinant of gender identity in our society.

ABNORMAL SEX DIFFERENTIATION

Classification of Errors in Sex Differentiation
(Table 34–3)

Disorders of sexual differentiation are the result of abnormalities in the complex processes of sexual differentiation, which originate in genetic information on the X and Y chromosomes as well as on the autosomes. A true hermaphrodite is defined as a person who possesses both ovarian and testicular tissue. A male pseudohermaphrodite is one whose gonads are exclusively testes but whose genital ducts or external genitalia, or both exhibit incomplete masculinization. A female pseudohermaphrodite is a person whose gonadal tissue is exclusively ovarian but whose genital development exhibits an ambiguous or male appearance.

SEMINIFEROUS TUBULE DYSGENESIS: CHROMATIN-POSITIVE KLINEFELTER'S SYNDROME & ITS VARIANTS

Klinefelter's syndrome is one of the most common forms of primary hypogonadism and infertility in males. These patients usually have an XXY sex chromosome constitution and an X chromatin-positive buccal smear, although patients with a variety of sex chromosome constitutions, including mosaicism, have been described. Virtually all of these variants have in common the presence of at least two X chromosomes and a Y chromosome, except for the rare group in which only an XX sex chromosome complement is found.

Surveys of the prevalence of XXY fetuses by karyotype analysis of unselected newborn infants indicate an incidence of one per 1000 newborn males. The invariable clinical features of Klinefelter's syndrome in adults are a male phenotype; small, firm testes less than 3 cm in length; and azoospermia. Prepubertally, the disorder is characterized by disproportionately long legs, small testes, personality and behavioral dis-

Table 34–3. Classification of anomalous sexual development.

Disorders of Gonadal Differentiation
  A. Seminiferous tubular dysgenesis (Klinefelter's syndrome).
  B. Syndrome of gonadal dysgenesis and its variants (Turner's syndrome).
  C. Complete and incomplete forms of XX and XY gonadal dysgenesis.
  D. True hermaphroditism.

Female Pseudohermaphroditism
  A. Congenital virilizing adrenal hyperplasia.
  B. Androgens and synthetic progestins transferred from maternal circulation.
  C. Malformations of intestine and urinary tract (nonadrenal female pseudohermaphroditism).
  D. Other teratologic factors.

Male Pseudohermaphroditism
  A. Testicular unresponsiveness to hCG and LH (Leydig cell agenesis or hypoplasia).
  B. Inborn errors of testosterone biosynthesis:
    1. Enzyme defects affecting synthesis of both corticosteroids and testosterone (variants of congenital adrenal hyperplasia).
      a. Cholesterol side-chain cleavage deficiency, P-450$_{scc}$ deficiency (congenital lipoid adrenal hyperplasia).
      b. 3β-Hydroxysteroid dehydrogenase deficiency.
      c. 17α-Hydroxylase deficiency.
    2. Enzyme defects primarily affecting testosterone biosynthesis by the testes.
      a. 17,20-Lyase deficiency.
      b. 17β-Hydroxysteroid oxidoreductase deficiency.
  C. Defects in androgen-dependent target tissues:
    1. End organ resistance to androgenic hormones (androgen receptor and postreceptor defects):
      a. Complete syndrome and androgen resistance and its variants (testicular feminization and its variant forms).
      b. Incomplete syndrome of androgen resistance and its variants (Reifenstein's syndrome).
      c. Androgen resistance in infertile men.
    2. Defects in testosterone metabolism by peripheral tissues: 5α-Reductase deficiency–pseudovaginal perineoscrotal hypospadias.
  D. Dysgenetic male pseudohermaphroditism:
    1. X chromatin–negative variants of the syndrome of gonadal dysgenesis (eg, XO/XY,XYp–).
    2. Incomplete form of XY gonadal dysgenesis.
    3. Associated with degenerative renal disease.
    4. "Vanishing testes" (embryonic testicular regression; XY agonadism→XY gonadal agenesis→rudimentary testes→anorchia).
  E. Defects in synthesis, secretion, or response to müllerian duct inhibitory factor: Female genital ducts in otherwise normal men–"uteri herniae inguinale"; persistent müllerian duct syndrome.
  F. Maternal ingestion of estrogens and progestins.

Unclassified Forms of Abnormal Sexual Development
  A. In males:
    1. Hypospadias.
    2. Ambiguous external genitalia in XY males with multiple congenital anomalies.
  B. In females: Absence or anomalous development of the vagina, uterus, and uterine tubes (Rokitansky-Küster syndrome).

orders, and a lower verbal IQ score when compared with controls, but no significant difference in overall IQ. Gynecomastia and other signs of androgen deficiency such as diminished facial and body hair, a small phallus, poor muscular development, and a eunuchoid body habitus occur postpubertally in affected patients. Adult males with an XXY karyotype tend to be taller than average, mainly because of the disproportionate length of their legs. They also have an increased incidence of mild diabetes mellitus, varicose veins, chronic pulmonary disease, and carcinoma of the breast. Sexual precocity due to an hCG-secreting polyembryoma has been described in six XXY males.

The testicular lesion appears to be progressive and gonadotropin-dependent. It is characterized in the adult by extensive seminiferous tubular hyalinization and fibrosis, absent or severely deficient spermatogenesis, and pseudoadenomatous clumping of the Leydig cells. Although hyalinization of the tubules is usually extensive, it varies considerably from patient to patient and even between testes in the same patient. Spermatogenesis is rarely found, and patients who have been reported to be fertile have been XY/XXY mosaics.

Advanced maternal age and meiotic nondisjunction have been found to play a role in the genesis of the XXY karyotype. Pedigree studies indicate that both X chromosomes are of maternal origin in 67% of XXY patients.

The diagnosis of Klinefelter's syndrome is suggested by the classic phenotype and hormonal changes. It is confirmed by the finding of an X chromatin-positive buccal smear and demonstration of an XXY karyotype in blood, skin, or gonads. After puberty, serum and urinary gonadotropins, especially FSH, are elevated, whereas plasma testosterone levels can be low or normal. Testicular biopsy reveals the classic findings of hyalinization of the seminiferous tubules, severe deficiency of spermatogonia, and pseudoadenomatous clumping of Leydig cells.

Treatment of patients with Klinefelter's syndrome is directed toward androgen replacement, if necessary. Testosterone enanthate in oil, 200 mg intramuscularly every 2 weeks, is recommended as a replacement dose in adults. Gynecomastia is not amenable to hormone therapy but can be surgically corrected if it is severe or psychologically disturbing to the patient.

Variants of Chromatin-Positive Seminiferous Tubule Dysgenesis

A. XY/XXY Mosaicism: This is the second most common chromosome complement associated with the Klinefelter phenotype. Mosaicism with any XY cell line may modify the clinical syndrome and result in less severe gynecomastia, as well as a lesser degree of testicular pathology. Some of these patients are fertile. Mean testosterone levels tend to be higher in XY/XXY patients than in XXY patients. In order to rule out XY/XXY mosaicism, cultures for karyotype analysis should be obtained from 2 or more tissues, and a

sufficient number of cells (50 or more) should be examined from each tissue. Therapy depends on the severity of the clinical and gonadal aberrations associated with the XXY cell line.

B. XXYY: These patients comprise 3% of chromatin-positive males. In addition to exhibiting the usual characteristics of Klinefelter's syndrome, they tend to be tall, and almost all reported patients have been mentally retarded. Therapy with testosterone is similar to that in patients with XXY Klinefelter's syndrome.

C. XXXY and XXXYY: All of these patients have had significant mental retardation; developmental anomalies (short neck, epicanthal folds, radioulnar synostosis, and clinodactyly) are present in half of patients.

D. XXXXY: These patients are more severely affected than those with a lesser number of X chromosomes. In addition to severe mental retardation, they exhibit radioulnar synostosis, hypoplastic external genitalia, and cryptorchid testes. Other anomalies such as congenital heart disease, cleft palate, strabismus, and microcephaly may be present. The facies is characteristic, with prognathism, hypertelorism, and myopia.

E. XX Males: Over 100 phenotypic males with a 46, XX karyotype have been described since 1964. In general, they have a male phenotype, male psychosocial gender identity, and testes with histologic features similar to those observed in patients with an XXY karyotype. At least 10% of patients have had hypospadias or ambiguous external genitalia. XX males have normal body proportions and a mean final height that is shorter than patients with an XXY karyotype or normal males but taller than normal females. As in XXY males, testosterone levels are low or low normal, gonadotropins are elevated, and spermatogenesis is impaired. Gynecomastia is present in approximately one-third of the patients.

The presence of testes and male sexual differentiation in 46,XX individuals has been a perplexing problem. However, the paradox has been clarified by the discovery that XX males are H-Y antigen-positive.

Three theories have been advanced to explain this rare example of sex reversal: (1) the presence of hidden sex chromosome mosaicism in an XX male with an undetected cell line containing a Y chromosome; (2) interchange or translocation between a Y and an X chromosome or an autosome that results in relocation of masculinizing genes from the Y chromosome onto an X chromosome (as has been described in the sex-reversed mouse) or an autosome; and (3) a putative mutant autosomal gene that leads to the differentiation of testes in an XX embryo, as in the "Saanen" goat. Recent evidence indicates that two-thirds of XX males tested have inherited Y-chromosome-derived sequences, presumably by Y-to-X translocation during male meiosis. Of note is an increased incidence of ambiguous genitalia in XX males without detectable Y chromosome sequences. The presence of XX males and XX true hermaphrodites in the same family in mammals suggests that the pathogenesis of these conditions is related.

SYNDROME OF GONADAL DYSGENESIS: TURNER'S SYNDROME & ITS VARIANTS

Turner's Syndrome: XO Gonadal Dysgenesis

One in 10,000 newborn females has an XO sex chromosome constitution. The cardinal features of XO gonadal dysgenesis are a variety of somatic anomalies, sexual infantilism at puberty secondary to gonadal dysgenesis, and short stature. Patients with an XO karyotype can be recognized in infancy usually because of lymphedema of the extremities and loose skin folds over the nape of the neck. In later life, the typical patient is often recognizable by her distinctive facies, in which micrognathia, epicanthal folds, prominent low-set ears, a fishlike mouth, and ptosis are present to varying degrees. The chest is shieldlike and the neck short, broad, and webbed (40% of patients). Additional anomalies associated with Turner's syndrome include coarctation of the aorta (10%), bicuspid aortic valve, hypertension, renal abnormalities (50%), pigmented nevi, cubitus valgus, a tendency to keloid formation, puffiness of the dorsum of the hands, short fourth metacarpals, and recurrent otitis media. Routine intravenous urography or ultrasonography is indicated for all patients to rule out a surgically correctable renal abnormality. The internal ducts as well as the external genitalia of these patients are female.

Short stature is an invariable feature of the syndrome of gonadal dysgenesis. Mean final height in XO patients is 142 cm, with a range of 133–153 cm. Current data suggest that the short stature found in patients with the syndrome of gonadal dysgenesis is not due to a deficiency of growth hormone, somatomedin, sex steroids, or thyroid hormone. No significant increase in final height has been documented in these patients after therapy with anabolic steroids or estrogens. Short-term linear growth data on treatment with pharmacologic doses of growth hormone alone or together with oxandrolone appear promising, but no final heights are yet available.

Gonadal dysgenesis is another feature of patients with an XO sex chromosome constitution. The gonads are typically streaklike and usually contain only fibrous stroma arranged in whorls. Longitudinal studies of both basal and GnRH-evoked gonadotropin secretion in patients with gonadal dysgenesis indicate a lack of feedback inhibition of the hypothalamic-pituitary axis by the dysgenetic gonads in affected infants and children (Fig 34–11). Thus, plasma and urinary gonadotropin levels, particularly FSH levels, are high, especially during early infancy and after 10 years of age. Since ovarian function is impaired, puberty does not usually ensue spontaneously; thus, sexual infantilism is a hallmark of this syndrome.

A variety of disorders are associated with this syndrome, including obesity, diabetes mellitus, Hashimoto's thyroiditis, rheumatoid arthritis, aortic rupture, and inflammatory bowel disease.

Phenotypic females with the following features should have a buccal smear for sex chromatin and a karyotype analysis: (1) short stature (> 2.5 SD below the mean value per age); (2) somatic anomalies associated with the syndrome of gonadal dysgenesis; and (3) delayed adolescence and increased concentration of plasma gonadotropins. In normal XX females, 20–30% of the nuclei are sex chromatin-positive. Although a buccal smear for sex chromatin is useful, karyotype analysis should be performed for definitive diagnosis.

Therapy is directed toward the institution of estrogen therapy in order to produce secondary sexual characteristics and menarche at an age commensurate with normal peers. A successful regimen is to initiate therapy at age 12–13 years with either 0.3 mg of conjugated estrogens, or ethinyl estradiol, 5 μg by mouth for the first 21 days of the calendar month. Thereafter, the dose of estrogen is gradually increased over the next 2–3 years to 0.6–1.25 mg of conjugated estrogens daily or 10 μg of ethinyl estradiol daily. The patient is maintained on the minimum dose of estrogen necessary to maintain secondary sexual characteristics and menses. Medroxyprogesterone acetate, 5 mg daily, is given on the 12th–21st days of the cycle to ensure physiologic menses and to try to reduce the risk of endometrial carcinoma from sustained estrogen stimulation.

In vitro fertilization with donor oocytes has been reported recently and affords the possibility of a normal pregnancy in selected patients with the syndrome of gonadal dysgenesis.

X Chromatin-Positive Variants of the Syndrome of Gonadal Dysgenesis

Patients with structural abnormalities of the X chromosome (deletions and additions) and mosaicism with XX cell lines may manifest the somatic as well as the gonadal features of the syndrome of gonadal dysgenesis (Table 34–4). Evidence suggests that genes on both the long and short arms of the X chromosome control gonadal differentiation, whereas genes on the proximal short arms of the X prevent the short stature and somatic anomalies that are seen in XO patients. In general, mosaicism with an XX cell line in association with an XO cell line will modify the phenotype toward normal and can even result in normal gonadal function.

X Chromatin-Negative Variants of the Syndrome of Gonadal Dysgenesis

These patients usually have mosaicism with an XO- and a Y-bearing cell line—XO/XY, XO/XXY, XO/XY/XYY—or perhaps a structurally abnormal Y chromosome. They range from phenotypic females with the features of Turner's syndrome through pa-

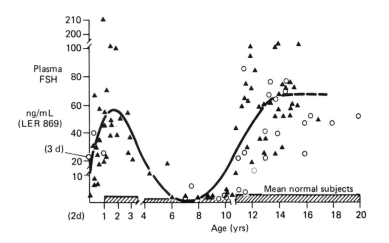

Figure 34–11. Diphasic variation in basal levels of plasma FSH (ng/mL-LER 869) in patients with an XO karyotype (solid triangles) and patients with structural abnormalities of the X chromosome, and mosaics (open circles). Note that mean basal levels of plasma FSH in patients with gonadal dysgenesis are in the castrate range before 4 years and after 10 years of age. (Reproduced, with permission, from Conte FA, Grumbach MM, Kaplan SL: A diphasic pattern of gonadotropin secretion in patients with the syndrome of gonadal dysgenesis. *J Clin Endocrinol Metab* 1975;**40**:670.)

tients with ambiguous genitalia to (rarely) completely virilized males with a few stigmas of Turner's syndrome. The gonadal differentiation varies from bilateral streaks to bilateral dysgenetic testes, along with asymmetric development, ie, a streak on one side and a dysgenetic testicle (or, rarely, a nearly normal testis) on the other side, sometimes called "mixed gonadal dysgenesis." The development of the external genitalia as well as the internal ducts correlates well with the degree of testicular differentiation and, presumably, the capacity of the fetal testes to secrete müllerian duct inhibitory factor and testosterone.

The risk of development of gonadal tumors is greatly increased in patients with XO/XY mosaicism, and prophylactic removal of streak gonads or dysgenetic undescended testes in this syndrome is indicated. Breast development at or after the age of puberty in these patients is associated with a gonadal neoplasm, usually a gonadoblastoma. Pelvic sonography, CT scanning, and MRI are all useful in screening for neoplasms in these patients. Gonadoblastomas are fre-

quently calcified, so that they may be visible even on a plain film of the abdomen.

The diagnosis of XO/XY mosaicism can be established by the demonstration of both XO and XY cells in blood, skin, or gonadal tissue. The decision as to the sex of rearing of the child should be based on the age at diagnosis and the potential for normal function of the external genitalia. In patients assigned a female gender role, the gonads should be removed and the external genitalia repaired. Estrogen therapy should be initiated at the age of puberty, as in patients with an XO karyotype (see above). In affected infants who are assigned a male gender role, all gonadal tissue except that which appears histologically normal and is in the scrotum should be removed. Removal of the müllerian structures and repair of hypospadias are also indicated. At puberty, depending on the functional integrity of the retained gonad, androgen replacement therapy may be indicated in doses similar to those for patients with XY gonadal dysgenesis (see below).

Table 34–4. Relationship of structural abnormalities of the X and Y chromosomes to clinical manifestations of the syndrome of gonadal dysgenesis.[*]

Type of Sex Chromosome Abnormality	Karyotypes[†]	Phenotype	Sexual Infantilism	Shortness of Stature	Somatic Anomalies of Turner's Syndrome
Loss of an X or Y	XO	Female	+	+	+
‡Deletion of short arm of an X	XXqi	Female	+ (occ. ±)	+	+
	XXp–	Female	+ , ± , or –	+ (–)	+ (–)
‡Deletion of long arm of an X	XXpi	Female	+	–	– or (±)
	XXq–	Female	+	– (+)	– or (±)
Deletion of ends of both arms of an X	XXr	Female	– or +	+	+ or (±)
Loss of short arm of Y	XYp–	Ambiguous	+	+	+

*Modified and reproduced, with permission, from Grumbach MM, Conte FA, in: *Textbook of Endorcrinology,* 5th ed. Williams RH (editor). Saunders, 1974.
†See Table 34–1 for newer nomenclature (Paris Conference).
‡In XXp– and XXq–, the extent and site of the deleted segment are variable.
XXqi = isochromosome for long arm of an X; XXp– = deletion of short arm of an X; XXpi = isochromosome for short arm of an X; XXq– = deletion of long arm of an X; XXr = ring chromosome derived from an X; XYp– = deletion of short arm of Y.

XX & XY GONADAL DYSGENESIS

The terms XX and XY gonadal dysgenesis have been applied to XX or XY patients who have bilateral streak gonads, a female phenotype, and no stigmas of Turner's syndrome. After puberty, they exhibit sexual infantilism, castrate levels of plasma and urinary gonadotropins, normal or tall stature, and eunuchoid proportions.

XX Gonadal Dysgenesis

Familial and sporadic cases of XX gonadal dysgenesis have been reported. Pedigree analysis of familial cases is consistent with autosomal recessive inheritance. In 3 families, XX gonadal dysgenesis was associated with deafness of the sensorineural type. In several affected groups of siblings, a spectrum of clinical findings occurred, eg, varying degrees of ovarian function, including breast development and menses followed by secondary amenorrhea. The diagnosis of XX gonadal dysgenesis should be suspected in phenotypic females with sexual infantilism and normal müllerian structures who lack the somatic stigmas of the syndrome of gonadal dysgenesis (Turner's syndrome). Karyotype analysis reveals only 46,XX cells. As in Turner's syndrome, gonadotropin levels are high, estrogen levels are low, and treatment consists of cyclic estrogen replacement.

Sporadic cases of XX gonadal dysgenesis may represent a heterogeneous group of patients from a pathogenetic point of view. XX gonadal dysgenesis should be distinguished from ovarian failure due to infections such as mumps, antibodies to gonadotropin receptors, biologically inactive FSH, and gonadotropin-insensitive ovaries as well as errors in estrogen biosynthesis.

XY Gonadal Dysgenesis

XY gonadal dysgenesis occurs both sporadically and in familial aggregates. Patients with this syndrome have female external genitalia, normal or tall stature, bilateral streak gonads, müllerian duct development, sexual infantilism, eunuchoid habitus, and a 46,XY karyotype. Clitorimegaly is common, and in familial cases, a continuum of involvement ranging from the complete syndrome to ambiguity of the external genitalia has been described. The phenotypic difference between the complete form of XY gonadal dysgenesis and the incomplete form is due to the degree of differentiation of the testicular tissue and its functional capacity to produce testosterone and müllerian duct inhibitory factor.

Analysis of familial cases suggests that XY gonadal dysgenesis is transmitted as an X-linked recessive or sex-limited autosomal dominant trait. Both H-Y antigen-positive and H-Y antigen-negative forms of this syndrome have been described and reflect the genetic heterogeneity of this syndrome. XY gonadal dysgenesis may result from a mutant gene that affects the expression of H-Y antigen (H-Y negative); from a defect in the gonad-specific H-Y antigen receptor (H-Y positive); or possibly from the production of a serologically reactive but abnormal H-Y antigen that lacks affinity for H-Y antigen receptors on gonadal cells (H-Y antigen-positive). Sporadic cases may represent teratologic defects in gonadal morphogenesis.

Therapy for patients with XY gondadal dysgenesis who have female external genitalia involves prophylactic gonadectomy and estrogen substitution at puberty. In the incomplete form of XY gonadal dysgenesis, assignment of a male gender role may be possible. It depends upon the degree of ambiguity of the genitalia and the potential for normal function. Prophylactic gonadectomy must be considered, since fertility is unlikely and there is an increased risk of malignant gonadal transformation in these patients. Recent studies have suggested a relationship between the development of gonadal neoplasms and H-Y antigen serotype; 95% of patients who had a gonadal tumor were H-Y antigen-positive. Prosthetic testes should be implanted at the time of gonadectomy, and androgen substitution therapy is instituted at the age of puberty. Testosterone enanthate in oil is utilized, beginning with 50 mg intramuscularly monthly and gradually increasing the dose over 3–4 years to a full replacement dose of 200 mg intramuscularly every 2 weeks.

TRUE HERMAPHRODITISM

True hermaphrodites have both ovarian and testicular tissue present in either the same or opposite gonads. Differentiation of the internal and external genitalia is highly variable. The external genitalia may simulate those of a male or female, but most often they are ambiguous. Cryptorchidism and hypospadias are common. In all cases, a uterus is present. The differentiation of the genital ducts usually follows that of the ipsilateral gonad. The ovotestis is the most common gonad found in true hermaphrodites, followed by the ovary and, least commonly, the testis. At puberty, breast development is usual in untreated patients, and menses occur in over 50% of cases. Whereas the ovary or the ovarian portion of an ovotestis may function normally, the testis or testicular portion of an ovotestis is almost always dysgenetic.

Sixty percent of true hermaphrodites have a 46,XX karyotype; 20% have 46,XY; and about 20% have mosaicism or XX/XY chimerism. True hermaphroditism may result from (1) sex chromosome mosaicism or chimerism, (2) Y-to-autosome or Y-to-X chromosome translocation or interchange, or (3) an autosomal mutant gene. There is evidence to support each of these possibilities in the pathogenesis of this clinically and anatomically heterogeneous syndrome, and all could lead to the serologic expression of H-Y antigen.

The diagnosis of true hermaphroditism should be considered in all patients with ambiguous genitalia. The finding of an XX/XY karyotype or a bilobed gonad compatible with an ovotestis in the inguinal region or labioscrotal folds suggests the diagnosis. If all other forms of male and female pseudohermaphroditism have been excluded, laparotomy and histologic confirmation of both ovarian and testicular tissue establish the diagnosis. The management of true hermaphroditism is contingent upon the age at diagnosis and a careful assessment of the functional capacity of the gonads, genital ducts, and external genitalia.

Gonadal Neoplasms in Dysgenetic Gonads

While gonadal tumors are rare in patients with Klinefelter's syndrome and XO gonadal dysgenesis, the incidence of gonadal neoplasms is greatly increased in patients with certain types of dysgenetic gonads. Gonadoblastomas, dysgerminomas, seminomas, and teratomas are found most frequently. The frequency is increased (1) in XO/XY mosaicism and in patients with a structurally abnormal Y chromosome and (2) in XY gonadal dysgenesis, either with a female phenotype or with ambiguous genitalia. Prophylactic gonadectomy is advised in these 2 categories as well as in individuals with gonadal dysgenesis who manifest signs of virilization, regardless of karyotype.

The gonad should be preserved in patients who are being raised as males only if it is a relatively normal testicle that can be relocated in the scrotum. The fact that a gonad is palpable in the scrotum does not preclude malignant degeneration and spread, since seminomas tend to metastasize at an early stage before a local mass is obvious.

FEMALE PSEUDOHERMAPHRODITISM

These individuals have normal ovaries and müllerian derivatives associated with ambiguous external genitalia. In the absence of testes, a female fetus will be masculinized if subjected to increased circulating levels of androgens derived from an extragonadal source. The degree of masculinization depends upon the stage of differentiation at the time of exposure (Fig 34–12). After 12 weeks of gestation, androgens will produce only clitoral hypertrophy. Rarely, ambiguous genitalia that superficially resemble those produced by androgens are the result of teratogenic malformations.

Congenital Adrenal Hyperplasia (Fig 34–13)

There are 6 major types of adrenal hyperplasia, all transmitted as autosomal recessive disorders. The common denominator of all 6 types is a defect in the synthesis of cortisol that results in an increase in ACTH and then in adrenal hyperplasia. Both males and females can be affected, but males are rarely diagnosed at birth unless they have ambiguous genitalia or are salt losers and manifest adrenal crises. Types I–III are defects confined to the adrenal gland that produce virilization. Types IV–VI have in common blocks in cortisol and sex steroid synthesis, in both the adrenals and the gonads. The latter 3 types produce primarily incomplete masculinization in the male and little (type IV) or no virilization in the female (Table 34–5). Consequently, these will be discussed primarily as forms of male pseudohermaphroditism.

A. Type I–C21 Hydroxylase Deficiency Primarily Affecting C21 Hydroxylation in the Zona Fasciculata (Simple Virilization): This is the most common type of congenital adrenal hyperplasia, with a prevalence of 1:5000 to 1:15,000 live births in Caucasians. It is inherited in an autosomal recessive manner. Recent data indicate that the locus for the gene which codes for 21-hydroxylation is on the short arm of chromosome 6 in close proximity to the locus for C4 (complement) between HLA-B and HLA-D. Thus, the gene for 21-hydroxylase deficiency is closely linked to the HLA gene complex. In addition, certain specific HLA subtypes are found to be statistically increased in patients with 21-hydroxylase deficiency. These include B5 in the simple virilizing form and Bw47 in the salt-losing form.

A defect in 21-hydroxylase activity of the adrenal cortex results in impaired cortisol synthesis, increased ACTH levels, and increased adrenal androgen and androgen precursor production. Prior to 12 weeks of gestation, high fetal androgen levels lead to a varying degree of labioscrotal fusion and clitoral enlargement in the female fetus; exposure to androgen after 12 weeks induces clitorimegaly alone. In the male fetus, no structural abnormalities in the external genitalia are

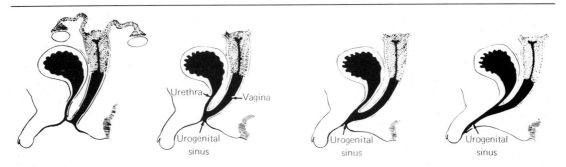

Figure 34–12. Female pseudohermaphroditism induced by prenatal exposure to androgens. Exposure after the 12th fetal week leads only to clitoral hypertrophy (*diagram on left*). Exposure at progressively earlier stages of differentiation (depicted from left to right in drawings) leads to retention of the urogenital sinus and labioscrotal fusion. If exposure occurs sufficiently early, the labia will fuse to form a penile urethra. (Reproduced, with permission, from Grumbach MM, Ducharme J: *Fertil Steril* 1960;11:757.)

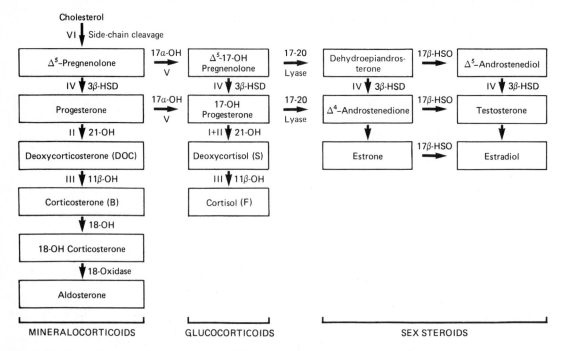

Figure 34–13. A diagrammatic representation of the steroid biosynthetic pathways in the adrenal and gonads. I to VI correspond to enzymes whose deficiency results in congenital adrenal hyperplasia. Enzyme abbreviations on arrows: OH, hydroxy; 3β-HSD, 3β-hydroxysteroid dehydrogenase; 17β-HSO, 17β-hydroxysteroid oxidoreductase. (Reproduced, with permission, from Conte FA, Grumbach MM: Pathogenesis, classification, diagnosis, and treatment of anomalies of sex. Chapter 106 in: *Endocrinology.* DeGroot L [editor]. Grune & Stratton, 1979.)

evident at birth, but the phallus may be enlarged. These patients produce sufficient amounts of aldosterone to prevent the signs and symptoms of mineralocorticoid deficiency. Recently, the heterogeneity of 21-hydroxylase deficiency has been demonstrated by the finding that "classical," acquired (late onset), and cryptic 21-hydroxylase deficiency are all HLA-linked and thus represent forms of 21-hydroxylase deficiency with a wide range of clinical and biochemical severity. The "nonclassical" variants of 21-hydroxylase deficiency have been postulated to be due to allelic variants of the 21-hydroxylase gene on chromosome 6 (New, 1986).

B. Type II–C21 Hydroxylase Deficiency Affecting C21 Hydroxylation in the Zona Fasciculata and Glomerulosa (Virilization With Salt Wasting): The salt-losing variant of 21-hydroxylase deficiency involves a more severe deficit of 21-hydroxylase in the zona fasciculata and zona glomerulosa of the adrenal cortex, which leads to impaired secretion of both cortisol (fasciculata) and aldosterone (glomerulosa). This results in electrolyte and fluid losses which usually manifest after the fifth day of life as hyponatremia, hyperkalemia, acidosis, dehydration, and vascular collapse. Masculinization of the external genitalia of affected females tends to be more

Table 34–5. Clinical manifestations of the various types of congenital adrenal hyperplasia.

Enzymatic Defect	Cholesterol Side-Chain Cleavage (P-450scc)		3β-Hydroxysteroid Dehydrogenase		17α-Hydroxylase		11β-Hydroxylase		21α-Hydroxylase	
Type	VI		IV		V		III		II and I	
Chromosomal	XX	XY	XX	XY	XX	XY	XX	XY	XX	XY
External genitalia	Female	Female	Female (clitorimegaly)	Ambiguous	Female	Female or ambiguous	Ambiguous	Male	Ambiguous	Male
Postnatal virilization	– (Sexual infantilism at puberty)		±	Mild to moderate	– (Sexual infantilism at puberty)		+		+	
Addisonian crises	+		+		–		–		+ in 66% (type II)	
Hypertension	–		–		+		(±)		–	

severe than that found in patients with simple 21-hydroxylase deficiency.

The diagnosis of 21-hydroxylase deficiency should always be considered (1) in patients with ambiguous genitalia who have an XX karyotype and are thus female pseudohermaphrodites; (2) in apparent cryptorchid males; (3) in any infant who presents with shock, hypoglycemia, and chemical findings compatible with adrenal insufficiency; and (4) in males and females with signs of virilization prior to puberty. In the past, the diagnosis of 21-hydroxylase deficiency was based on the finding of elevated levels of 17-ketosteroids and pregnanetriol in the urine. Although still valid and useful, urinary steroid determinations have been replaced by the measurement of plasma 17-hydroxyprogesterone. The concentration of plasma 17-hydroxyprogesterone is normally elevated in umbilical cord blood but rapidly decreases into the range of 100–200 ng/dL by 24 hours after delivery. In patients affected with 21-hydroxylase deficiency, the 17-hydroxyprogesterone values usually range from 3000 to 40,000 ng/dL, depending on the age of the patient and the severity of 21-hydroxylase deficiency. Patients with mild 21-hydroxylase deficiency, ie, late-onset and cryptic forms, may have borderline basal 17-hydroxyprogesterone values, but they can be distinguished from heterozygotes on the basis of an augmented 17-hydroxyprogesterone response to the administration of ACTH. Salt losers can be ascertained clinically, usually by chemical evidence of hyponatremia and hyperkalemia on a regular or low-salt diet. In these patients, aldosterone levels in both plasma and urine are low in relation to the serum electrolyte pattern, while plasma renin activity is elevated. HLA typing as well as amniotic fluid 17-hydroxyprogesterone levels have been utilized in the prenatal diagnosis of affected infants. Heterozygosity has been ascertained by HLA typing in informative families and by the use of ACTH-induced rises in plasma 17-hydroxyprogesterone levels.

C. Type III–C11 Hydroxylase Deficiency (Virilization With Hypertension): A defect in hydroxylation at C11 leads to the hypersecretion of 11-deoxycorticosterone and 11-deoxycortisol in addition to adrenal androgens. Patients with this form of adrenal hyperplasia exhibit virilization secondary to increased androgen production and hypertension caused by increased 11-deoxycorticosterone secretion. Recent data suggest that the defect in 11β-hydroxylation may be primarily in the zona fasciculata. The 11β-hydroxylase gene is not linked to the HLA complex. As in other forms of congenital adrenal hyperplasia, mild forms of 11β-hydroxylase deficiency may not become manifest until adolescence or early adulthood.

The diagnosis of 11β-hydroxylase deficiency can be confirmed by demonstration of elevated plasma levels of 11-deoxycortisol and 11-deoxycorticosterone and increased excretion of their metabolites in urine (mainly tetrahydro 11-deoxycortisol).

D. Type IV–3β-Hydroxysteroid Dehydrogenase Deficiency (Male or Female Pseudo-

hermaphroditism and Adrenal Insufficiency): See p 618.

E. Type V–17α-Hydroxylase Deficiency (Male Pseudohermaphroditism, Sexual Infantilism, Hypertension, and Hypokalemic Alkalosis): See p 619.

F. Type VI–Cholesterol Side-Chain Cleavage Deficiency, p-450 Side-Chain Cleavage Deficiency, Congenital Lipoid Adrenal Hyperplasia (Male Pseudohermaphroditism, Sexual Infantilism, and Adrenal Insufficiency): See p 618.

Treatment

Treatment of patients with adrenal hyperplasia may be divided into acute and chronic phases. In acute adrenal crises, a deficiency of both cortisol and aldosterone results in hypoglycemia, hyponatremia, hyperkalemia, hypovolemia, and shock. An infusion of 5% glucose in isotonic saline should be started immediately. In the first hour, if the patient is in shock, 20 mL/kg of saline may be given; thereafter, fluid and electrolyte replacement is calculated on the basis of deficits and standard maintenance requirements. Hydrocortisone sodium succinate, 50 mg/m^2, should be given as a bolus and another 50–100 mg/m^2 added to the infusion fluid over the first 24 hours of therapy. If profound hyponatremia and hyperkalemia are present, deoxycorticosterone acetate (DOCA), 1–2 mg, may be given every 12–24 hours intramuscularly. The amount of DOCA and the concentration and amount of saline solution must be adjusted according to the results of frequent electrolyte determinations, assessments of the state of hydration, and blood pressure measurements. Excess DOCA and salt can result in hypokalemia, hypertension, congestive heart failure, and hypertensive encephalopathy, whereas too little salt and DOCA will fail to correct the electrolyte imbalance.

Once the patient is stabilized and a definitive diagnosis with appropriate steroid studies has been made, the patient should receive maintenance doses of glucocorticoids to permit normal growth, development, and bone maturation (hydrocortisone, approximately 18 mg/m^2/d by mouth in 3 divided doses). Salt losers need treatment with mineralocorticoids (fludrocortisone 0.50–0.1 mg/d orally) and added dietary salt. The dose of mineralocorticoid should be adjusted so that plasma renin activity is maintained in the normal range for age.

Patients with ambiguous external genitalia should have plastic repair of the external genitalia before age 1 year. Clitoral recession or clitoroplasty rather than clitoridectomy is preferred. Of major importance to the family with an affected child is the assurance that their child will grow and develop into a normal functional adult. In patients with the most common form of adrenal hyperplasia—21-hydroxylase deficiency—fertility in males and feminization, menstruation, and fertility in females can be expected with adequate treatment. Long-term psychologic guidance and support for the patient and family by the physician is essential.

Aberrant adrenal rests are common in males with adrenal hyperplasia who are undertreated; these may be mistaken for either adult testicular maturation or testicular neoplasms. These adrenal rests are often bilateral and are made up of cells that appear indistinguishable from Leydig cells histologically except for the fact that they lack Reinke crystalloids. It is strongly recommended that for all patients with adrenal hyperplasia a lifelong regimen of replacement glucocorticoid therapy—and, if necessary, mineralocorticoid therapy—be continued in order to mitigate the risks of adrenal insufficiency, adrenal carcinoma, pituitary hyperplasia, and hyperplasia of aberrant adrenal rests in the testes.

MATERNAL ANDROGENS & PROGESTINS

Masculinization of the external genitalia of a female infant can occur if the mother ingested testosterone or androgen derivatives (ie, danazol) during the first trimester of pregnancy. After the 12th week of gestation, exposure results in clitorimegaly only. Synthetic progestational agents such as norethindrone, ethisterone, norethynodrel, and medroxyprogesterone acetate have been implicated in masculinization. In rare instances, masculinization of a female fetus may be secondary to an ovarian or adrenal tumor, adrenal hyperplasia, or luteoma of pregnancy.

The diagnosis of female pseudohermaphroditism arising from transplacental passage of androgenic steroids is based on exclusion of other forms of female pseudohermaphroditism and a history of drug exposure. Surgical correction of the genitalia, if needed, is the only therapy necessary. Nonadrenal female pseudohermaphroditism can be associated with imperforate anus, renal anomalies, and other congenital anomalies of the lower intestine and urinary tract. Sporadic as well as familial cases have been reported.

MALE PSEUDOHERMAPHRODITISM

Male pseudohermaphrodites have gonads that are testes, but the genital ducts or external genitalia are not completely masculinized. Male pseudohermaphroditism can result from deficient testosterone secretion as a consequence of (1) failure of testicular differentiation, (2) failure of secretion of testosterone or müllerian duct inhibitory factor, (3) failure of target tissue response to testosterone or dihydrotestosterone, and (4) failure of conversion of testosterone to dihydrotestosterone.

Testicular Unresponsiveness to hCG & LH

Male sexual differentiation is dependent upon the production of testosterone by fetal Leydig cells. Data indicate that Leydig cell testosterone secretion is under the influence of placental hCG during the critical period of male sexual differentiation, and, thereafter, fe-

tal pituitary LH and FSH during gestation.

The finding of normal male sexual differentiation in XY males with anencephaly, apituitarism, and congenital hypothalamic hypopituitarism suggests that male sex differentiation can occur independently of the secretion of fetal pituitary gonadotropins.

Absence, hypoplasia, or unresponsiveness of Leydig cells to hCG-LH would result in deficient testosterone production and, consequently, male pseudohermaphroditism. The extent of the genital ambiguity is a function of the degree of testosterone deficiency. A small number of patients with absent, hypoplastic, or unresponsive Leydig cells (attributed to a lack of receptor activity for hCG-LH) have been reported, as well as an animal model—the "vet" rat. In most of the patients thus far reported, the defect resulted in female-appearing external genitalia. Müllerian duct regression was complete. Basal gonadotropin levels, as well as GnRH-evoked responses, were elevated in postpubertal patients. Basal plasma 17α-hydroxyprogesterone, androstenedione, and testosterone levels were low, and hCG elicited little or no rise in these steroids.

Inborn Errors of Testosterone Biosynthesis

Fig 34–14 demonstrates the major pathways in testosterone biosynthesis in the gonads; each step is associated with an inherited defect that results in testosterone deficiency and, consequently, male pseudohermaphroditism. Steps 1, 2, and 3 are enzymatic deficiencies that occur in both the adrenals and gonads and result in defective synthesis of both corticosteroids and testosterone. Thus, they represent forms of congenital adrenal hyperplasia.

(1) Cholesterol side-chain cleavage deficiency, P-450 side-chain cleavage deficiency, type VI adrenal hyperplasia, congenital lipoid adrenal hyperplasia (male pseudohermaphroditism, sexual infantilism, and adrenal insufficiency): This is a very early defect in the synthesis of all steroids and results in severe adrenal and gonadal insufficiency. Affected males have female (or rarely, ambiguous) external genitalia with a blind vaginal pouch and hypoplastic male genital ducts but no müllerian derivatives; the genitalia of affected females are normal. Large lipid-laden adrenals that displace the kidneys downward may be demonstrated on intravenous urography, sonography, or CT scan. Death in early infancy from adrenal insufficiency is not uncommon. Affected males have female-appearing external genitalia. The diagnosis is confirmed by the lack of or low levels of all steroids in plasma and urine and an absent response to ACTH stimulation.

(2) 3β-Hydroxysteroid dehydrogenase deficiency, type IV congenital adrenal hyperplasia (male or female pseudohermaphroditism and adrenal insufficiency): 3β-Hydroxysteroid dehydrogenase defi-ciency is an early defect in steroid synthesis that results in inability of the adrenals and gonads to convert 3β-hydroxy-Δ⁵-steroids to 3-keto-Δ⁴-ste-

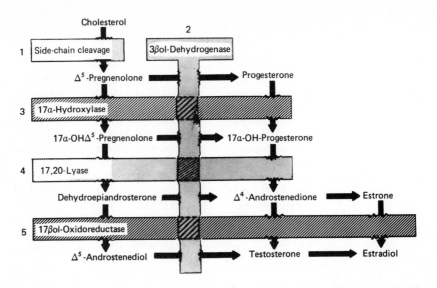

Figure 34–14. Enzymatic defects in the biosynthetic pathway for testosterone. All 5 of the enzymatic defects cause male pseudohermaphroditism in affected males. Although all of the blocks affect gonadal steroidogenesis, those at steps 1, 2, and 3 are associated with major abnormalities in the biosynthesis of glucocorticoids and mineralocorticoids in the adrenal.

roids. This defect in its complete form results in a deficiency of aldosterone, cortisol, testosterone, and estradiol. Mild forms of this defect may not be manifested clinically until adolescence and are not associated with severe salt loss. Males with this defect are incompletely masculinized, and females have mild clitorimegaly. Salt loss and adrenal crises usually occur in early infancy in affected patients.

As in other forms of congenital adrenal hyperplasia, mild or "nonclassical" cases with normal genitalia (or mild hypospadias in males) and normal mineralocorticoid activity have been described. These patients usually present with premature pubarche or hirsutism.

The diagnosis of 3β-hydroxysteroid dehydrogenase deficiency is based on finding elevated concentrations of 17α-hydroxypregnenolone, dehydroepiandrosterone (DHEA) and its sulfate, and other 3β-hydroxy-Δ⁵-steroids in the plasma and urine of patients with a consistent clinical picture. Suppression of the increased plasma and urinary 3β-hydroxy-Δ⁵-steroids by the administration of dexamethasone distinguishes 3β-hydroxysteroid dehydrogenase deficiency from a virilizing adrenal tumor.

(3) 17α-Hydroxylase deficiency, type V congenital adrenal hyperplasia (male pseudohermaphroditism, sexual infantilism, hypertension, and hypokalemic alkalosis): A defect in 17α-hydroxylation in the zona fasciculata of the adrenal and in the gonads results in impaired synthesis of 17α-hydroxyprogesterone and 17α-hydroxypregnenolone and, consequently, cortisol and sex steroids. The secretion of large amounts of corticosterone and deoxycorticosterone (DOC) leads to hypertension, hypokalemia, and alkalosis. Increased DOC secretion with resultant hypertension produces suppression of renin and consequently aldosterone secretion.

The clinical manifestations results from the adrenal and gonadal defect. XX females have normal development of the internal ducts and external genitalia but manifest sexual infantilism with elevated gonadotropin concentrations at puberty. XY males have impaired testosterone synthesis by the fetal testes, which results in female or ambiguous genitalia. At adolescence, sexual infantilism and hypertension are the hallmarks of this defect.

The diagnosis of 17α-hydroxylase deficiency should be suspected in XY males with female or ambiguous genitalia or XX females with sexual infantilism, who also manifest hypertension associated with hypokalemic alkalosis. High levels of progesterone, Δ⁵-pregnenolone, DOC, and corticosterone in plasma and increased excretion of their urinary metabolites establish the diagnosis. Plasma renin activity and aldosterone secretion are markedly diminished in these patients.

The following errors affect testosterone and estrogen biosynthesis in the gonads primarily:

(4) 17,20-Lyase deficiency: This is a rare defect in testosterone synthesis that affects the conversion of the C21 steroids 17α-hydroxyprogesterone and 17α-hydroxy-Δ⁵-pregnenolone to the C19 steroids androstenedione and DHEA. Patients described with 17,20-desmolase deficiency have been male pseudohermaphrodites with either female or ambiguous genitalia and inguinal or intra-abdominal testes. Müllerian derivatives are absent, presumably as a result of the secretion of müllerian duct inhibitory factor. At puberty, incomplete virilization without gynecomastia may occur.

Patients with 17,20-desmolase deficiency have low circulating levels of testosterone, androstenedione, DHEA, and estradiol. The diagnosis can be confirmed by demonstration of an increased ratio of 17α-hydroxy

C21 steroids to C19 steroids (testosterone, DHEA, Δ^5-androstenediol, and androstenedione) after stimulation with ACTH or chorionic gonadotropin.

(5) 17β-Hydroxysteroid oxidoreductase deficiency: The last step in testosterone and estradiol biosynthesis by the gonads involves the reduction of androstenedione to testosterone and estrone to estradiol. At birth, males with a deficiency of the enzyme 17β-hydroxysteroid oxidoreductase have female or mildly ambiguous external genitalia resulting from testosterone deficiency during male differentiation. They have male duct development, absent müllerian structures with a blind vaginal pouch, and inguinal or intra-abdominal testes. At puberty, progressive virilization with clitoral hypertrophy occurs, often associated with the concurrent development of gynecomastia. Plasma gonadotropin, androstenedione, and estrone levels are high, whereas testosterone and estradiol concentrations are low.

17β-Hydroxysteroid oxidoreductase deficiency should be included in the differential diagnosis of (1) male pseudohermaphrodites with absent müllerian derivatives who have no abnormality in glucocorticoid or mineralocorticoid synthesis and (2) male pseudohermaphrodites who virilize at puberty, especially if gynecomastia is present. The diagnosis of 17β-hydroxysteroid oxidoreductase deficency can be confirmed by the demonstration of inappropriately high plasma levels of estrone and androstenedione and decreased ratios of plasma testosterone to androstenedione and estradiol to estrone before and after stimulation with hCG.

Management of the patients, as with other forms of male pseudohermaphroditism, depends on the age at diagnosis and the degree of ambiguity of the external genitalia. In the patient assigned a male gender identity, plastic repair of the genitalia and testosterone replacement therapy at puberty will be necessary. In patients reared as females (the usual case), the appropriate treatment is castration, followed by estrogen replacement therapy at puberty.

Defects in Androgen-Dependent Target Tissues

The complex mechanism of action of steroid hormones at the cellular level has been clarified (Fig 34–15). Free testosterone enters the target cells and undergoes 5α reduction to dihydrotestosterone, which in turn is bound to a receptor protein; the receptor protein complex is translocated into the nucleus of the target cell. In the nucleus, the receptor-dihydrotestosterone complex binds to chromatin and initiates transcription. Messenger RNA is synthesized, modified, and exported to the cytoplasm of the cell, where ribosomes translate mRNA into new proteins that have an androgen effect on the cell. A lack of androgen effect at the end organ and consequently male pseudohermaphroditism may result from abnormalities in 5α-reductase activity, dihydrotestosterone receptor activity, translocation of the steroid-receptor complex, nuclear binding, transcription, or translation.

End Organ Insensitivity to Androgenic Hormones (Androgen Receptor & Postreceptor Defects)

A. Complete Syndrome of Androgen Resistance and Its Variants (Testicular Feminization): The complete syndrome of androgen resistance (testicular feminization) is characterized by a 46,XY karyotype, bilateral testes, female-appearing external genitalia, a blind vaginal pouch, and absent müllerian derivatives. At puberty, female secondary sexual characteristics develop, but menarche does not ensue. Pubic and axillary hair are usually sparse and in one-third of patients totally absent. Some patients have a variant form of this syndrome and exhibit slight clitoral enlargement. At puberty, these patients may exhibit mild virilization in addition to the development of breasts and a female habitus.

Androgen resistance during embryogenesis prevents masculinization of the external genitalia and differentiation of the wolffian ducts. Secretion of müllerian duct inhibitory factor by the fetal Sertoli cells leads to regression of the müllerian ducts. Thus, affected patients are born with female external genitalia and a blind vaginal pouch. At puberty, androgen resistance results in augmented LH secretion with subsequent increases in testosterone and estradiol. Estradiol arises from conversion of testosterone and androstenedione as well as from direct secretion by the testes. Androgen resistance coupled with increased estradiol secretion results in the development of female secondary sexual characteristics at puberty.

Data on rodents as well as other mammals indicate that androgen resistance is modulated, at least in part, by abnormalities in androgen receptor activity in androgen-sensitive tissues. Studies utilizing fibroblasts cultured from genital skin indicate that patients with complete androgen insensitivity are genetically heterogeneous. Patients have been described who have (1) an undetectable or low amount of androgen receptor activity, (2) a qualitatively abnormal (thermolabile, unstable, or both) androgen receptor, and (3) a normal amount of androgen receptor activity (a presumed postreceptor defect). Inheritance in all forms appears to be X-linked.

The diagnosis of complete androgen insensitivity can be suspected from the clinical features. Prepubertally, testislike masses in the inguinal canal or labia in a phenotypic female suggest the diagnosis. Postpubertally, the patients present with primary amenorrhea, normal breast development, and absent or sparse sexual hair. Characteristically, the concentrations of LH and testosterone are markedly elevated. This latter finding is an important hormonal feature of androgen resistance. The family history, phenotype, endocrine evaluation, androgen receptor studies, and, if necessary, the metabolic response to testosterone will help confirm the diagnosis.

Therapy of patients with complete androgen resistance involves affirmation and reinforcement of their female gender identity. Castration, either prior to or

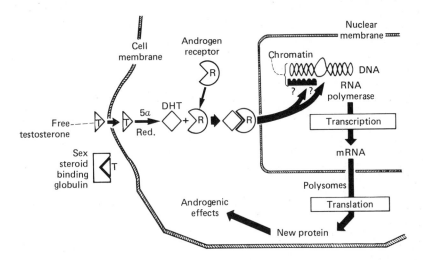

Figure 34–15. A simplified diagrammatic representation of the mechanism of action of testosterone at the target organ. 5α-Red., 5α-reductase; DHT, dihydrotestosterone. (Reproduced, with permission, from Conte FA, Grumbach MM: Pathogenesis, classification, diagnosis, and treatment of anomalies of sex. Chapter 106 in: *Endocrinology.* DeGroot L [editor]. Grune & Stratton, 1979.)

after puberty, is indicated because of the increased risk of gonadal neoplasms with age. Thereafter, estrogen replacement therapy must be instituted.

B. Incomplete Syndrome of Androgen Resistance and Its Variants (Reifenstein's Syndrome): Patients with incomplete androgen resistance manifest a wide spectrum of phenotypes as far as masculinization is concerned. The external genitalia at birth can range from ambiguous, with a blind vaginal pouch, to hypoplastic male genitalia. Müllerian duct derivatives are absent and wolffian duct derivatives present, but they are usually hypoplastic. At puberty, virilization is poor; pubic and axillary hair as well as gynecomastia are usually present. The testes remain small and exhibit azoospermia as a consequence of germinal cell arrest. As in the case of patients with complete androgen resistance, there are high levels of plasma LH, testosterone, and estradiol. However, the degree of feminization in these patients despite high estradiol levels is less than that found in the complete syndrome of androgen resistance.

Androgen receptor studies in these patients have revealed (1) a partial deficiency of androgen receptor activity and (2) a qualitatively abnormal androgen receptor. As in the complete syndrome of androgen insensitivity, inheritance appears to be X-linked.

Androgen Resistance in Infertile Men

Partial androgen resistance has been described in a group of infertile men who have normal male genitalia and may exhibit gynecomastia. Unlike other patients with androgen resistance, some of these patients have normal LH and testosterone levels. Thus, infertility in otherwise normal men may be the only clinical manifestation of androgen resistance. Infertility represents one extreme of the highly variable phenotypic expression of androgen resistance in patients with a comparable deficiency of androgen receptor activity as determined by in vitro studies.

Defects in Testosterone Metabolism by Peripheral Tissues; 5α-Reductase Deficiency (Male Pseudohermaphroditism with Masculinization at Puberty, Pseudovaginal Perineoscrotal Hypospadias)

The defective conversion of testosterone to dihydrotestosterone produces a unique form of male pseudohermaphroditism (Fig 34–16). At birth, ambiguous external genitalia are manifested by a small hypospadiac phallus bound down in chordee, a bifid scrotum, and a urogenital sinus that opens onto the perineum. A blind vaginal pouch is present. The testes are either inguinal or labial. The müllerian structures are absent, and the wolffian structures are well differentiated. At puberty, affected males virilize; the voice deepens, muscle mass increases, and the phallus enlarges to 4–8 cm in length. The bifid scrotum becomes rugate and pigmented. The testes enlarge and descend into the labioscrotal folds, and spermatogenesis may ensue. Gynecomastia is notably absent in these patients. Of note also is the absence of acne, temporal hair recession, and hirsutism. A remarkable feature of this form of male pseudohermaphroditism has been the reported change in gender identity from female to male at puberty, primarily in affected individuals living in rural communities in the Dominican Republic.

After the onset of puberty, patients with 5α-reductase deficiency have normal to elevated testosterone levels and elevated plasma concentrations of LH. As expected, plasma dihydrotestosterone is low and the testosterone/dihydrotestosterone ratio is abnormally

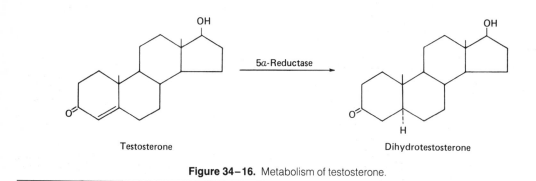

Figure 34–16. Metabolism of testosterone.

high. Apparently, lack of 5α reduction of testosterone to dihydrotestosterone in utero during the critical phases of male sex differentiation results in incomplete masculinization of the external genitalia, while testosterone-dependent wolffian structures are normally developed. The marked virilization that occurs at puberty in these patients is in sharp contrast to that which occurs in utero and is as yet not well explained. Since the androgen receptor binds both dihydrotestosterone and testosterone (but with a lower affinity), the sustained high levels of circulating testosterone attained at puberty may be a factor in the virilization achieved. In addition, the enzyme defect is incomplete, and at puberty the plasma concentration of dihydrotestosterone, while low, is detectable. Also, the hormonal environment is markedly different at puberty in that large quantities of competitive steroids (estrogens and progestins) are not present as they are in utero. In particular, high concentrations of progesterone may have a marked effect on 5α-reductase activity in utero, whereas at puberty progesterone levels are low in males. 5α-Reductase deficiency is inherited as an autosomal recessive trait, and the enzymatic defect exhibits genetic heterogeneity.

5α-Reductase deficiency should be suspected in male pseudohermaphrodites with a blind vaginal pouch. The diagnosis can be confirmed by demonstration of an abnormally high plasma testosterone/dihydrotestosterone ratio, either under basal conditions or after hCG stimulation. Other confirmatory findings include an increased 5β:5α ratio of urinary C19 steroid metabolites of testosterone, a decreased level of 5α-reductase activity in genital skin in vitro, and decreased conversion of infused testosterone to dihydrotestosterone in vivo.

The early diagnosis of this condition is particularly critical. In view of the natural history of this disorder, affected males might be assigned a male gender identity, treated with dihydrotestosterone, and have appropriate plastic repair of their external genitalia. In patients who are diagnosed after infancy, in whom gender identity is unequivocally female, prophylactic orchiectomy and estrogen substitution therapy is still considered the treatment of choice until further experience with this biochemical entity and sex reversal in our culture is available.

Dysgenetic Male Pseudohermaphroditism (Ambiguous Genitalia Due to Dysgenetic Gonads)

Defective gonadogenesis results in ambiguous development of the genital ducts, urogenital sinus, and external genitalia. Patients with XO/XY mosaicism, structural abnormalities of the Y chromosome, and forms of XY gonadal dysgenesis manifest defective gonadogenesis and thus defective virilization. These disorders are classified under disorders of gonadal differentiation but also are included as a subgroup of male pseudohermaphroditism.

A. Ambiguous Genitalia Associated With Degenerative Renal Disease: Several cases are recorded of male pseudohermaphroditism associated with degenerative renal disease and hypertension as well as with Wilms' tumor. In this syndrome, both the kidneys and the testes are dysgenetic, and a predisposition for renal neoplasms exists.

B. Vanishing Testes Syndrome (Embryonic Testicular Regression Syndrome; XY Agonadism; Rudimentary Testes Syndrome; Congenital Anorchia): Cessation of testicular function during the critical phases of male sex differentiation can lead to varying clinical syndromes depending on when testicular function ceases. At one end of the clinical spectrum of these heterogeneous conditions are the XY patients in whom testicular functional deficiency occurred prior to 8 weeks of gestation, which results in female differentiation of the internal and external genitalia. At the other end of the spectrum are the patients with "anorchia" or "vanishing testes." These patients have perfectly normal male differentiation of their internal and external structures, but gonadal tissue is absent. The diagnosis of anorchia should be considered in all cryptorchid males. Administration of hCG, 1000–2000 units intramuscularly every other day for 7 doses, is a useful test of Leydig cell function. In the presence of normal Leydig cell function, there will be a rise in plasma testosterone from concentrations of less than 20 ng/dL to over 200 ng/dL in prepubertal males. In infants under 4 years of age and children over 10 years of age, plasma FSH levels are a sensitive index of gonadal integrity. The gonadotropin response to a 100-μg bolus injection of

GnRH can also be utilized to diagnose the absence of gonadal feedback on the hypothalamus and pituitary. In gonadal children, GnRH will elicit a rise in LH and FSH levels that is greater than that achieved in prepubertal children with normal gonadal function. Patients with high gonadotropin levels and no testosterone response to hCG are invariably found to lack recognizable gonadal tissue at laparotomy (Lustig, 1987).

Defects in the Synthesis, Structure, or Response to Müllerian Duct Inhibitory Factor

A small number of patients have been described in whom normal male development of the external genitalia has occurred but in whom the müllerian ducts persist. The retention of müllerian structures can be ascribed to failure of the Sertoli cells to synthesize müllerian duct inhibitory factor or to a defect in the response of the duct to that factor. This condition appears to be transmitted as an autosomal recessive trait. Therapy involves removal of the müllerian structures.

UNCLASSIFIED FORMS OF ABNORMAL SEXUAL DEVELOPMENT IN MALES

Hypospadias

Hypospadias is a common urogenital anomaly occurring in 1–8 per 1000 newborn males. On an embryologic basis, deficient virilization of the external genitalia implies subnormal Leydig cell functions in utero, end organ resistance, or disjointed chronologic correlation between hormone level and the critical time for tissue response. Although in most patients there is little reason to suspect these mechanisms, recent reports in a small number of patients have suggested that simple hypospadias may be associated with an abnormality in androgen receptor activity, nuclear localization of the androgen receptor, or an aberration in the maturation of the hypothalamic-pituitary-gonadal axis. Further studies are necessary to determine the role of these factors in the pathogenesis of this condition.

In one prospective study of 100 patients with hypospadias, one patient was found to be a genetic female with congenital adrenal hyperplasia, 5 with sex chromosome abnormalities, and one with the incomplete form of XY gonadal dysgenesis. Nine patients were from pregnancies in which the mother had taken progestational compounds during the first trimester. Thus, a pathogenetic mechanism was found in only 15% of these patients. Hypospadias has been described in association with chromosomal abnormalities and with generalized dysmorphic syndromes, eg, as Smith-Lemli-Opitz syndrome.

Microphallus

Microphallus can result from a heterogeneous group of disorders, but by far the most common is fetal testosterone deficiency. In the human male fetus, testosterone synthesis by the fetal Leydig cell during the critical period of male differentiation (8–12

weeks) is under the influence of placental hCG. After midgestation, fetal pituitary LH as well as placental hCG seems to modulate fetal testosterone synthesis by the Leydig cell and, consequently, growth of the phallus. GH also appears to play a role in growth of the phallus. Thus, males with congenital hypopituitarism as well as isolated gonadotropin deficiency and "late" testicular failure can present with normal male differentiation and microphallus at birth (phallus less than 2.5 cm in length in a full-term infant). Patients with hypothalamic hypopituitarism or pituitary aplasia may also have midline defects, hypoglycemia, and giant cell hepatitis. After appropriate evaluation of anterior pituitary function (ie, GH, ACTH, cortisol, TSH, and gonadotropins) and stabilization of the patient with hormone replacement, if necessary, an hCG stimulation test should be performed. Thereafter, a trial of testosterone therapy should be administered to all patients with microphallus before definitive gender assignment is made. Patients with fetal testosterone deficiency as a cause of their microphallus respond to 25–50 mg of testosterone enanthate intramuscularly monthly for 3 months with a mean increase of 2 cm in phallic length (Fig 34–17). If a trial of testosterone therapy does not result in a reasonable increase in phallic size, castration and assignment of a female gender may then be a prudent course to follow in the management of patients with microphallus.

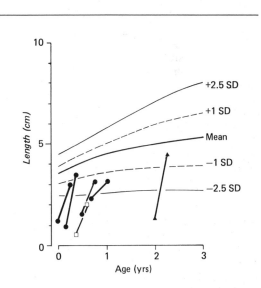

Figure 34–17. The response in phallic length to a 3-month course of testosterone in 6 patients with microphallus under 2 years of age. Each patient was given 25 mg of testosterone enanthate in oil intramuscularly monthly for 3 months. ▲, □ indicate 2 patients who subsequently underwent a second course of testosterone therapy. (Reproduced, with permission, from Burstein S, Grumbach MM, Kaplan SL: Early determination of androgen-responsiveness is important in the management of microphallus. *Lancet* 1979;2:983.)

UNCLASSIFIED FORMS OF ABNORMAL SEXUAL DEVELOPMENT IN FEMALES

Congenital absence of the vagina occurs in one in 5000 female births. It can be associated with müllerian derivatives that vary from normal to absent. Ovarian function is usually normal. Therapy involves plastic repair of the vagina, if indicated.

MANAGEMENT OF PATIENTS WITH INTERSEX PROBLEMS

Choice of Sex

The goal of the physician in the management of patients with ambiguous genitalia is to establish a diagnosis and to assign a sex for rearing that is most compatible with a well-adjusted life and sexual adequacy. Once the sex for rearing is assigned, the gender role is reinforced by the use of appropriate surgical, hormonal, or psychologic measures. Except in female pseudohermaphrodites, ambiguities of the genitalia are caused by lesions that almost always make the patient infertile. In recommending male sex assignment, the adequacy of the size of the phallus should be the most important consideration.

Differential Diagnosis

The steps in the diagnosis of intersexuality are delineated in Fig 34–18.

Reassignment of Sex

Reassignment of sex in infancy and childhood is always a difficult psychosocial problem for the patient, the parents, and the physicians involved. While easier in infancy than after 2 years of age, it should always be undertaken with much deliberation and with provision for long-term medical and psychiatric supervision and counseling.

Reconstructive Surgery

It is desirable to initiate plastic repair of the external genitalia prior to 6–12 months of age. In children raised as females, the clitoris should be salvaged, if possible, by clitoroplasty or clitoral recession. Reconstruction of a vagina, if necessary, can be deferred until adolescence.

Removal of the gonads in children with the variant forms of gonadal dysgenesis should be performed at the time of initial repair of the external genitalia, because gonadoblastomas, seminomas, and dysgerminomas have been reported to occur during the first decade of life.

In a patient with testicular feminization, the gonads may be left in situ (provided they are not situated in the labia majora) to provide estrogen until late adolescence. The patient may then undergo prophylactic castration, having had her female identity reinforced by normal feminization at puberty.

In patients with incomplete testicular feminization reared as females or in patients with errors of testosterone biosynthesis in whom some degree of masculinization occurs at puberty, gonadectomy should be performed prior to puberty.

Hormonal Substitution Therapy

Cyclic estrogen and progestin are used in individuals reared as females in whom a uterus is present (see p 612). In males, virilization is achieved by the administration of repository testosterone (see p 614).

Psychologic Management

Sex is not a single biologic entity but the summation of many morphogenetic, functional, and psychologic potentialities. There must never be any doubt in the mind of the parent or child as to the child's true sex. Chromosomal and gonadal sex are secondary matters; the sex of rearing is paramount. With proper surgical reconstruction and hormone substitution, the individual whose psychosexual gender is discordant with chromosomal gender need not have any psychologic catastrophes as long as the sex of rearing is accepted with conviction by the family and others during the critical early years. These individuals should reach adulthood as well-adjusted men or women capable of normal sexual interaction, albeit usually not of procreation.

REFERENCES

Austin CR, Edwards RB (editors): *Mechanisms of Sex Differentiation in Animals and Man.* Academic Press, 1981.

Bandmann JH, Breit R (editors): *Klinefelter's Syndrome.* Springer-Verlag, 1984.

Conte FA, Grumbach MM: Pathogenesis, classification, diagnosis, and treatment of anomalies of sex. In: *Endocrinology,* 2nd ed. DeGroot L (editor). Grune & Stratton, 1987.

George FW, Wilson JD: Embryology of the genital tract. In: *Campbell's Urology,* 5th ed. Walsh PC et al (editors). Saunders, 1986.

Goodfellow PN: The case of the missing H-Y antigen. *Trends Genet* 1986;**2:**87.

Griffin JE, Wilson JD: Disorders of sexual differentiation. In: *Campbell's Urology,* 5th ed. Walsh PG et al (editors). Saunders, 1986.

Griffin JE, Wilson JD: The syndromes of androgen resistance. *N Engl J Med* 1980;**302:**198.

Grumbach MM, Conte FA: Disorders of sex differentiation. In: *Williams Textbook of Endocrinology,* 7th ed. Wilson JD, Foster DW (editors). Saunders, 1985.

Hamerton JL: *Human Cytogenetics.* Vols 1 and 2. Academic Press, 1971.

Imperato-McGinley JL et al: Androgens and the evolution of

Diagnosis of Intersexuality

1. History: Family, pregnancy.
2. Physical examination: Palpation of inguinal region, labioscrotal folds, and rectal examination.
3. Initial studies: X chromatin pattern, karyotype analysis, serum electrolytes. 17-hydroxyprogesterone, androstenedione, dehydro-epiandrosterone, testosterone, and dihydrotestosterone. Sonogram of kidneys, ureters, and pelvic contents.
4. Provisional diagnosis: "Abnormal" external genitalia—proceed as shown below.

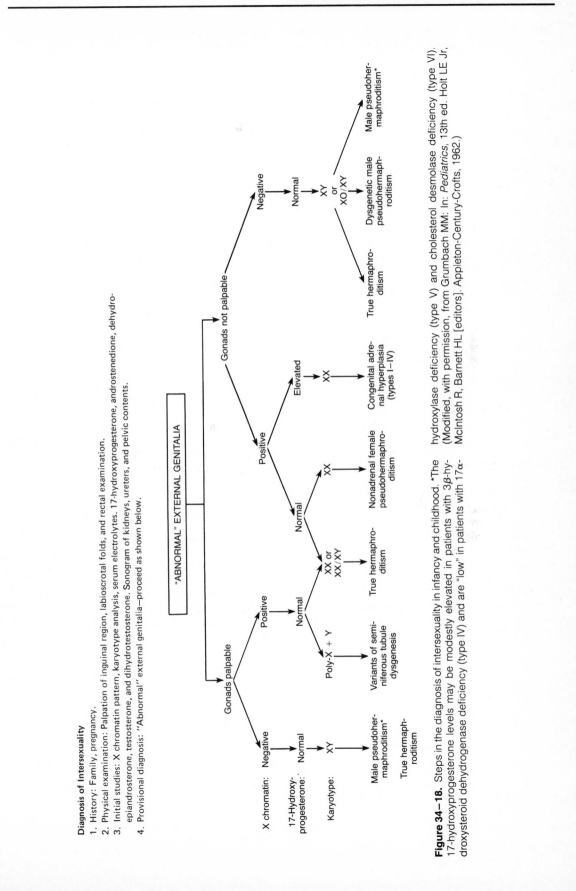

Figure 34–18. Steps in the diagnosis of intersexuality in infancy and childhood. *The 17-hydroxyprogesterone levels may be modestly elevated in patients with 3β-hy-droxysteroid dehydrogenase deficiency (type IV) and are "low" in patients with 17α-hydroxylase deficiency (type V) and cholesterol desmolase deficiency (type VI). (Modified, with permission, from Grumbach MM: In: *Pediatrics*, 13th ed. Holt LE Jr, McIntosh R, Barnett HL [editors]. Appleton-Century-Crofts, 1962.)

male-gender identity among male pseudohermaphrodites with 5α-reductase deficiency. *N Engl J Med* 1979;**300:**1233.

Lee PA et al (editors): *Congenital Adrenal Hyperplasia.* University Park Press, 1977.

Lustig RH et al: Ontogeny of gonadotropin secretion in congenital anorchia: Sexual dimorphism versus syndrome of gonadal dysgenesis and diagnostic considerations. *J Urol* 1987; **138:**587.

McKusick VA: *Mendelian Inheritance in Man,* 6th ed. Johns Hopkins Univ Press, 1983.

Money J, Ehrhardt AA: *Man and Woman, Boy and Girl: The Differentiation and Dimorphism of Gender Identity From Conception to Maturity.* Johns Hopkins Univ Press, 1972.

New MI, Levine LS: Steroid 21-hydroxylase deficiency. Pages 83–94 in: *Adrenal Diseases in Childhood.* New MI, Levine LS (editors). Karger, 1984.

New MI, Speiser PW: Genetics of adrenal steroid 21-hydroxylase deficiency. *Endocr Rev* 1986;**7:**331.

Ohno S: *Major Sex Determining Genes.* Springer-Verlag, 1979.

Ohno S: The Y-linked testis determining gene and H-Y plasma membrane antigen gene: Are they one and the same? *Endocr Rev* 1986;**6:**421.

Peters H, McNulty KP: *The Ovary.* Univ of California Press, 1980.

Peterson RE et al: Male pseudohermaphroditism due to steroid 5α-reductase deficiency. *Am J Med* 1977;**62:**170.

Rosenfield RL, Lucky AW, Allen TD: The diagnosis and management of intersex. *Curr Probl Pediatr* 1980;**10:**1. [Entire issue.]

Serio M et al (editors): *Sexual Differentiation: Basic and Clinical Aspects.* Vol 11 of: *Serono Symposia.* Raven Press, 1984.

Simpson JL, Photopulos G: The relationship of neoplasia to disorders of abnormal sexual differentiation. *Birth Defects* 1976;**12(Suppl 1):**15.

Singh L, Jones KW: Sex reversal in the mouse (*Mus musculus*) is caused by a recurrent nonreciprocal crossover involving the X and an aberrant Y chromosome. *Cell* 1982;**28:**205.

Vallet HL, Porter IH (editors): *Symposium on Genetic Mechanisms of Sexual Development.* Academic Press, 1979.

Van Niekerk WA: *True Hermaphroditism: Clinical, Morphological and Cytogenetic Aspects.* Harper & Row, 1974.

Wachtel SS: *H-Y Antigen and the Biology of Sex Determination.* Grune & Stratton, 1983.

Wilson JD et al: The androgen resistance syndromes: 5α-Reductase deficiency, testicular feminization, and related disorders. Chap 48, pp 1001–1026, in: *The Metabolic Basis of Inherited Disease,* 5th ed. Stanbury JB et al (editors). McGraw-Hill, 1983.

Renovascular Hypertension

35

R. Ernest Sosa, MD, & E. Darracott Vaughan, Jr., MD

Hypertension affects about 50 million Americans. In most patients, the cause is unknown, and the disease is termed **essential hypertension.** Renal disease is found to be the cause in 5–15% of patients with hypertension, who are said to have **renal hypertension.** Renal hypertension may be vascular in nature (ie, secondary to renal artery disease [Table 35–1]); may be related to renal parenchymal disease (Table 35–2); or may result from a combination of these 2 processes. Many cases of renal hypertension are reversible if hypertension is properly diagnosed and treated.

Etiology

Renal disease in association with hypertension has been recognized since the early 19th century. In 1898, Tigerstadt and Bergman demonstrated that a water-soluble substance—extracted from the renal cortex of a healthy rabbit and termed **renin**—produced marked and sustained hypertension when injected intravenously into a second healthy rabbit.

In 1934, Goldblatt's classic experiments with dogs demonstrated that reversible elevation in systemic blood pressure could be produced by clamping the main renal artery of one of 2 healthy kidneys. Blood pressure returned to normal on removal of the clamp or the involved kidney. In this model, excessive secretion of renin from the ischemic kidney was implicated as the underlying pathogenetic abnormality in renovascular hypertension (Fig 35–1). In humans, as in the Goldblatt 2-kidney, 1-clip model of hypertension, unilateral renal ischemia has been shown to produce high-renin, angiotension-dependent hypertension that can be cured by reconstruction of the renal artery, per-

Table 35–1. Causes of renovascular hypertension.

Common causes
  Atherosclerosis (66%)
  Fibromuscular dysplasia (33%)
    Intimal fibroplasia (about 5%)
    Fibromuscular hyperplasia (about 2%)
    Medial fibroplasia (about 80%)
    Perimedial fibroplasia (about 15%)
Rare causes (≤ 1%)
  Polyarteritis nodosa
  Takayasu's arteritis
  Arteriovenous fistula
  Aortic aneurysm
  Coarctation of the aorta
  Middle aortic syndrome
  Radiation arteritis

Table 35–2. Nonvascular causes of renal hypertension in unilateral renal parenchymal disease.

Surgery indicated
  Renal cell carcinoma
  Wilms' tumor
  Reninoma
  Obstructive uropathy
  Nonfunctioning atrophic kidney
Surgery only upon proved indications
  Chronic pyelonephritis associated with vesicoureteral reflux
  Polycystic kidney
  Radiation nephritis
  Perinephric scarring (Page kidney)
  Segmental hypoplasia (Ask-Upmark kidney)
  Renal tuberculosis

cutaneous balloon catheter dilation of the stenosed arterial segment, or nephrectomy.

Pathogenesis

The renin-angiotension-aldosterone system (Fig 35–2) is an integrated hormonal cascade that simultaneously controls blood pressure and sodium and potassium balance and influences regional blood flow. Renin is a proteolytic enzyme produced in the juxtaglomerular cells of the afferent arterioles. It acts on renin substrate (angiotensinogen), an α-2 globulin produced in the liver, to form the decapeptide angiotensin I. Converting enzyme, found in the lung and kidney, cleaves 2 amino acids from angiotensin I to form the octapeptide angiotensin II, a potent arterial vasoconstrictor. Angiotensin II also stimulates the zona glomerulosa of the adrenal gland to secrete aldosterone. Elevation of blood pressure and restoration of sodium balance inhibit further renin secretion.

The mechanisms responsible for renin secretion include an afferent arteriolar baroreceptor responding to decreased renal perfusion pressure, a sensor at the macula densa responding to decreased delivery of sodium and chloride to the distal tubule, and increased activity of the sympathetic nervous system, mediated by β_1-adrenergic receptors. Frequent causes of hypersecretion of renin include sodium depletion, hemorrhage, shock, congestive heart failure, and renal artery stenosis.

Plasma renin activity is closely related to the patient's sodium intake and urinary sodium excretion, ie, sodium balance. The renin-angiotensin-aldosterone system is activated in response to sodium restriction and suppressed by sodium loading. Plasma renin activity must therefore be correlated with the sodium

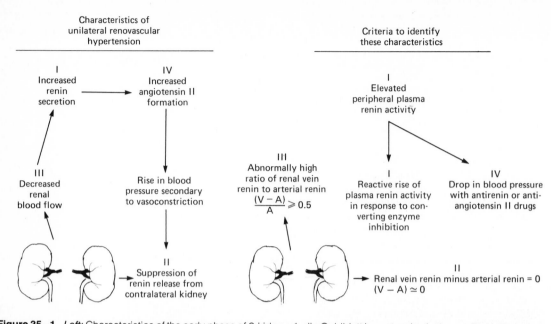

Figure 35–1. *Left:* Characteristics of the early phase of 2-kidney, 1-clip Goldblatt hypertension in the rat. *Right:* The criteria derived from the animal model that serve to identify patients with correctable renal hypertension. Roman numerals relate left and right parts of figure. (Modified and reproduced, with permission, from Vaughan ED Jr et al: Clinical evaluation of renovascular hypertension and therapeutic decisions. *Urol Clin North Am* 1984;11:393.)

balance in order to be meaningful. Fig 35–3 illustrates how the plasma renin activity varies with the sodium balance, which is determined in normal subjects by measuring the urinary excretion of sodium in a 24-hour specimen.

Pathology

Stenosis of the renal artery (and, therefore, renovascular hypertension) is most commonly caused by arteriosclerotic plaques and fibromuscular dysplasia (Table 35–1). Not all renal artery stenoses are physiologically significant and cause hypertension, however. A lesion must produce a reduction in luminal diameter of at least 70% before renal plasma flow is reduced to the point that clinically significant ischemia results. The clinical significance of an anatomic stenosis noted on angiography (Fig 35–4) is assessed by renin assays, as discussed below.

Other urologic lesions that may cause renin-dependent hypertension include obstructive uropathy, benign and malignant renal masses, and chronic pyelonephritis, the latter most commonly associated with vesicoureteral reflux (Table 35–2). In some patients, elevated levels of plasma renin activity returned to normal and hypertension was alleviated after appropriate surgical treatment of the underlying urologic disorder. However, hypertension due to renal parenchymal disease is not usually curable by surgical means. Most patients require medical management to control blood pressure.

History & Physical Examination

A. History: A complete and thorough medical history and physical examination provide important information about the patient's current general health, past medical history, and family medical history. Clinical clues and other factors suggestive of renovascular hypertension are set forth in Table 35–3. The patient's age and circumstances at onset of hypertension, recorded blood pressure ranges, previous treatment, results of therapy, and history of end organ damage are noted. The past history is investigated for evidence of diseases (eg, glomerulonephritis, chronic pyelonephritis with or without vesicoureteral reflux, hydronephrosis, urolithiasis) or other factors (eg, renal trauma, radiation therapy to the abdomen) that could contribute to the development of hypertension.

Hypertension may have an abrupt onset and progress rapidly in children with Wilms' tumor, in young adults with fibromuscular dysplasia, and in older patients with arteriosclerotic occlusion of the renal artery. Anorexia, weight loss, and malaise may be signs of malignant disease leading to elevated blood pressure. However, the absence of symptoms is not sufficient to rule out a diagnosis of curable hypertension.

B. Physical Examination: Physical examination should include serial measurements of the patient's blood pressure to establish the degree of hypertension. Measurements are taken in each arm with an appropriate-sized cuff while the patient is standing, sitting, and lying down. If 3 measurements are higher than 140/90 mm Hg in an adult, further evaluation is warranted. The physician should palpate all peripheral pulses. Diminution of pulses and decreased blood pressure in the lower extremities in a young patient

Angiotensinogen (α_2-globulin)

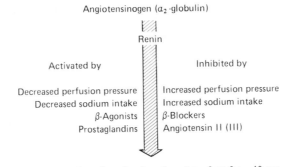

Renin

Activated by | Inhibited by

Decreased perfusion pressure | Increased perfusion pressure
Decreased sodium intake | Increased sodium intake
β-Agonists | β-Blockers
Prostaglandins | Angiotensin II (III)

$H_2N\text{-}Asp^1\text{-}Arg^2\text{-}Val^3\text{-}Tyr^4\text{-}Ile^5\text{-}His^6\text{-}Pro^7\text{-}Phe^8\text{-}His^9\text{-}Leu^{10}\text{-}OH$

Angiotensin I

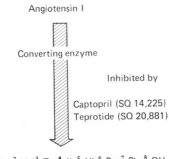

Converting enzyme

Inhibited by

Captopril (SQ 14,225)
Teprotide (SQ 20,881)

$H_2N\text{-}Asp^1\text{-}Arg^2\text{-}Val^3\text{-}Tyr^4\text{-}Ile^5\text{-}His^6\text{-}Pro^7\text{-}Phe^8\text{-}OH$

Angiotensin II

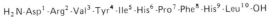

Angiotensin II receptor

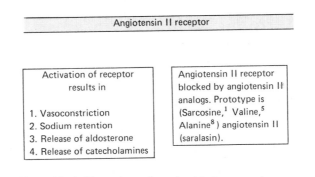

Activation of receptor results in	Angiotensin II receptor blocked by angiotensin II analogs. Prototype is (Sarcosine,^{1} Valine,^{5} Alanine^8) angiotensin II (saralasin).
1. Vasoconstriction 2. Sodium retention 3. Release of aldosterone 4. Release of catecholamines	

Figure 35–2. The renin-angiotensin-aldosterone system.

may signify coarctation of the aorta; an intrascapular murmur is another characteristic sign. In patients with renal artery stenosis, a continuous abdominal bruit may be heard on either side of the midline immediately above the umbilicus.

Laboratory Evaluation

A. Renovascular Hypertension:

1. Basic tests–Laboratory examination of the patient with suspected renovascular hypertension (Fig 35–5) should begin with basic tests that assess the patient's general health: complete blood count, serum electrolyte and fasting blood glucose determinations, blood urea nitrogen and serum creatinine measurements, urinalysis and urine culture, and an ECG.

2. Plasma renin activity profile–In patients in whom the diagnosis of hypertension has been definitively established, evaluation should start with a plasma renin activity profile (plasma renin activity must be plotted against 24-hour urinary sodium excretion). These measurements should be obtained while the patient is on a diet containing normal amounts of sodium; antihypertensive medication must be withheld for 2 weeks prior to sampling. The blood sample for the renin determination is drawn at the end of the 24-hour period in which the urine is collected and after 4 hours of ambulatory activity. This test will reveal elevated plasma renin activity levels in about 80% of patients with renovascular hypertension (Fig 35–6, left).

3. Captopril challenge test–Peripheral plasma renin activity is measured before and 60 minutes after administration of captopril (a converting enzyme inhibitor), 25 mg orally. In renin-dependent hypertension, inhibition of the converting enzyme occurs as shown in Table 35–4. If the 3 criteria shown in Table 35–4 are present in a patient with normal renal func-

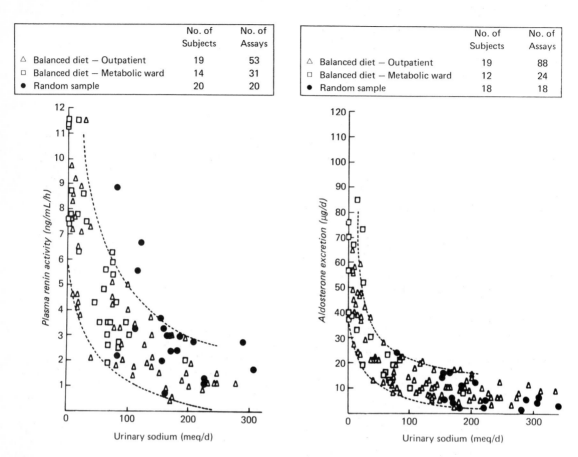

	No. of Subjects	No. of Assays
△ Balanced diet — Outpatient	19	53
□ Balanced diet — Metabolic ward	14	31
● Random sample	20	20

	No. of Subjects	No. of Assays
△ Balanced diet — Outpatient	19	88
□ Balanced diet — Metabolic ward	12	24
● Random sample	18	18

Figure 35–3. Plasma renin activity levels obtained at noon (*left*) and 24-hour urinary aldosterone excretion levels (*right*) in relation to daily urinary sodium excretion levels in normal subjects. In such subjects, plasma renin activity and excretion of aldosterone describe similar hyperbolic curves in relation to sodium excretion. The fact that a random sampling of nonhospitalized subjects consuming uncontrolled diets yielded similar results enhances the validity of this nomogram for use in studies of outpatients or subjects not consuming a constant diet. (Reproduced, with permission, from Laragh JH: *Hypertension Manual.* York Medical Books, 1973.)

tion who is not taking diuretics, renovascular hypertension can be distinguished from essential hypertension with a specificity of 100% and a sensitivity of 95% (Muller et al, 1986). Prior sodium depletion due to use of diuretics or dietary restrictions increases plasma renin activity and causes the captopril challenge test to be nonspecific. Patients taking beta-blockers remain responsive to the test as described above, unless the baseline plasma renin activity is less than 2.5 ng/mL/h, in which case the test may be unreliable.

4. Renal vein renin sampling—Patients with high peripheral plasma renin activity levels or those in whom the captopril challenge test is positive should undergo further evaluation with renal vein sampling for renin. Samples are collected from each renal vein (V1 and V2) and from the distal inferior vena cava before and after administration of captopril, 25 mg orally (Table 35–5).

According to criteria established by Vaughan et al (1973), potentially reversible hypertension is charac-

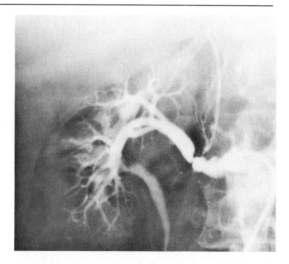

Figure 35–4. Selective renal arteriogram showing severe renal artery stenosis in a 65-year-old patient with normal blood pressure. (Reproduced, with permission, from Vaughan ED Jr: Laboratory tests in the evaluation of renal hypertension. *Urol Clin North Am* 1979;6:485.)

Table 35–3. Clinical clues suggestive of renovascular hypertension.

	Comment
Clues from history	
Hypertension in the absence of any family history of hypertensive disease	Suspect renovascular hypertension if the family history is negative; however, about one-third of patients with renovascular hypertension have a positive family history.
Age of onset of hypertension is under 25 years or over 45 years	Average age of onset of essential hypertension is 31 ± 10 (SD) years. Children and young adults usually have fibromuscular disease, whereas adults over age 45 years are more likely to have atherosclerotic narrowing of the arteries.
Abrupt onset of moderate to severe hypertension	Essential hypertension usually begins with a labile phase before mild hypertension becomes established, whereas the natural history in renovascular hypertension is usually more compressed, with the disease often appearing initially as moderate hypertension of recent onset.
Development of severe or malignant hypertension	Renovascular hypertension often becomes moderately severe and may cause accelarated or malignant hypertension; both forms of hypertension involve markedly increased secretion of renin.
Headaches	Essential hypertension is usually asymptomatic; headaches occur more commonly with renovascular hypertension and may be related to its greater severity or the high levels of angiotensin II (a potent cerebrovascular vasoconstrictor) associated with this disease.
Cigarette smoking	A recent survey showed that 74% of patients with fibromuscular renal artery stenosis are smokers; 88% of those with atherosclerotic disease smoke.
White race	Renovascular hypertension is uncommon in blacks.
Resistance to or escape from adequate control of blood pressure with standard diuretic or antiadrenergic therapy	Renovascular hypertension typically responds poorly to diuretics and often responds only transiently to antiadrenergic drugs.
Excellent antihypertensive response to converting enzyme inhibitors, eg, captopril	Converting enzyme inhibitors block the renin-angiotensin-aldosterone system most effectively and are highly specific agents.
Clues from physical examination and routine laboratory studies	
Retinopathy	Hemorrhage, exudates, or papilledema indicates accelerated or malignant hypertension.
Abdominal or flank bruit	Bruits are not pathognomonic of renovascular hypertension, since they are common in elderly persons and occasionally occur in younger patients who have no apparent vascular stenosis.
Carotid bruits or other evidence of large-vessel disease	Vascular pathologic processes are not limited to the renal bed.
Hypokalemia exists in the untreated state or persists even after administration of a thiazide diuretic	Increased aldosterone secretion by the renin-angiotensin-aldosterone system reduces serum potassium level. This does not occur in untreated *essential* hypertension. Thiazide diuretics accentuate this phenomenon in *renovascular* hypertension.

terized by ipsilateral hypersecretion of renin ($[V1 - A] \div A \geq 0.50$), contralateral suppression of renin secretion ($[V2 - A] \div A \cong 0$), and an increase in the peripheral plasma renin activity level (Table 35–5). Because interventional treatment such as transluminal angioplasty (see Chapter 7) is likely to be of benefit to patients who meet these criteria, further anatomic avaluation should be performed. Renin secretion returns to normal levels after successful angioplasty (Figs 35–6 and 35–7).

B. Other Tests: Excretory urography is not generally recommended as an initial screening test for renovascular hypertension because it has a sensitivity of only 75% and a specificity of 86% (Harvey et al, 1985). It is nonetheless useful in patients with a history of verified or suspected urologic disease and in the localization of anatomic defects before surgery.

Arteriography or digital intravenous subtraction angiography (see Chapter 6) is preferred in screening for hypertension and evaluating anatomic abnormalities. These methods involve intravenous injection of contrast material to delineate the anatomy of the renal arteries and urinary tract. However, arteriographic or angiographic demonstration of an arterial lesion must be supplemented by evidence of abnormal levels of renin secretion in order to prove that unilateral ischemia is the cause of renovascular hypertension.

C. Renal Parenchymal Disease: In patients with suspected renal parenchymal disease, preoperative evaluation of plasma renin activity is similar to that described for patients with renovascular hypertension. It should be noted that peripheral plasma renin levels are normal in many such patients who are later shown to have lateralizing renal vein renin ratios. The captopril challenge test is therefore recommended in these patients in order to elicit evidence of a reactive rise in plasma renin activity and a fall in blood pressure. Hypertension due to renal parenchymal disease

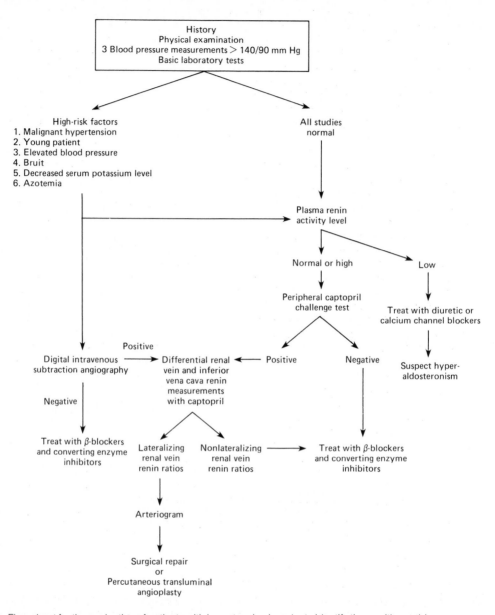

Figure 35–5. Flow sheet for the evaluation of patients with hypertension in order to identify those with curable renovascular disease. (Modified and reproduced, with permission, from Sosa RE: Vol 2, No. 31 of: *AVA Update Series.* Office of Education, American Urological Association, Houston, Texas, 1982.)

is less frequently curable by surgical treatment than is renovascular hypertension. Nephrectomy should be avoided if the blood pressure can be controlled with antihypertensive medication and if the glomerular filtration rate in the involved kidney is sufficient to ensure the patient's survival if removal of the contralateral kidney is ever necessary.

Treatment

Patients with known or suspected hypertension must be methodically evaluated in order to identify those with renin-dependent hypertension and plan individualized treatment.

A. Medical Measures: Management of patients with renovascular hypertension using conventional antihypertensive drugs has been difficult. In a prospective study of 214 patients with renovascular hypertension, 100 patients underwent surgical repair of renal artery stenosis and 114 patients were medically treated (Hunt, 1975). After 7–14 years of follow-up, morbidity and mortality rates were shown to be significantly greater in the medically treated group. Cure or improvement of hypertension was achieved in 90% of the surgically treated patients, whereas adequate control was attained in fewer than 50% of patients in the medically treated group. This study sug-

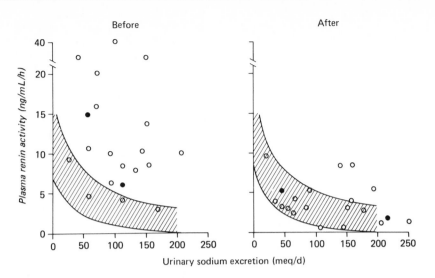

Figure 35–6: Effect of angioplasty on peripheral plasma renin activity level plotted against 24-hour urinary sodium excretion. *Left:* Before angioplasty. *Right:* Six months after angioplasty. Hatched area shows normal range. ○ = Cured or improved, ● = Failed to improve. (Reproduced, with permission, from Pickering TG et al: Predictive value and changes of renin secretion in hypertensive patients with unilateral renovascular disease undergoing successful renal angioplasty. *Am J Med* 1984;76:398.)

gested the efficacy of surgery for renovascular hypertension, but subsequent studies have revealed that the operative mortality rate for such patients is significant—in the range of 2–9%.

Recently, the development of drugs such as captopril and beta-blockers has made medical management of renovascular hypertension more effective. Renal artery lesions are progressive, however, and total occlusion of the renal artery may occur even in patients successfully treated with these drugs. Therefore, interventional uroradiologic procedures are the initial treatment of choice in selected cases.

Medical treatment with converting enzyme inhibitors and beta-blockers should be reserved for higher-risk patients who are not good candidates for

Table 35–4. Single-dose captopril test. Criteria distinguishing patients with renovascular hypertension from those with essential hypertension.*

Stimulated plasma renin activity of 12 ng/mL/h or more **and**
Absolute increase in plasma renin activity of 10 ng/mL/h or more **and**
Percent increase in plasma renin activity of 150% or more **or** of 400% if the baseline plasma renin activity is less than 3 ng/mL/h.

*Reproduced, with permission, from Muller FB et al: The captopril test for identifying renovascular disease in hypertensive patients. *Am J Med* 1986;**80**:633.

Table 35–5. Renin values for predicting reversibility of renovascular hypertension.*

Collection of samples (Patient should have moderate sodium intake, ie, 40–100 meq/d.)
1. With patient ambulatory, measure peripheral plasma renin level and 24-hour urinary excretion of sodium under steady-state conditions (ie, not on the day of arteriography).
2. Before and after blockade with converting enzyme inhibitor, collect blood for measurement of plasma renin levels.
3. With patient supine, collect blood samples for measurement of renin levels†: sample from renal vein of kidney thought to be affected (V1), matching sample from aorta (A1) or inferior vena cava (IVC1), sample from renal vein of contralateral kidney (V2), and second matching sample from aorta (A2) or inferior vena cava (IVC2).
4. If results of initial renin determinations are inconclusive, enhance renin secretion by using converting enzyme inhibitor blockade.

Criteria for predicting reversibility
High plasma renin level in relation to urinary sodium level. Indicates hypersecretion of renin.
Marked reactive rise in plasma renin level and fall in blood pressure in response to converting enzyme inhibitor.
In contralateral kidney, $V2 - A2 \approx 0$. Indicates suppression of renin secretion in this kidney.
In affected kidney, $(V1 - A1) \div A1 > 0.5$. Indicates unilateral renin secretion and reduced renal blood flow.
In patients with high plasma renin levels, low ratios of renal vein renin to aorta renin ($[V1 - A1] \div A1 + [V2 - A2] \div A2 \leq 0.5$) indicate incorrect sampling or segmental disease. Repeat measurements with segmental sampling.

*Modified and reproduced, with permission, from Vaughan ED Jr: Renal artery stenosis. Chapter 10 in: *Hypertension.* Vol 8 of: *Contemporary Issues in Nephrology.* Brenner BM, Stein JH (editors). Churchill Livingstone, 1981.
†Renin levels in inferior vena cava (IVC) can be substituted for those in aorta (A); values are identical (Sealey, 1973).

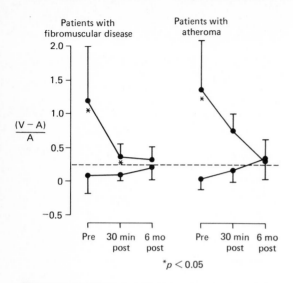

Patients with fibromuscular disease

Patients with atheroma

$\dfrac{(V - A)}{A}$

Pre / 30 min post / 6 mo post

Pre / 30 min post / 6 mo post

*$p < 0.05$

Figure 35–7. Effect of angioplasty on renal vein renin levels. Blood samples were drawn immediately before, 30 minutes after, and 6 months after angioplasty. The higher values are for the ischemic kidney; the lower ones, for the contralateral kidney. The asterisks indicate a significant difference between the 2 kidneys, and the dashed line represents the normal level of $(V - A) \div A$ (0.24). (Reproduced, with permission, from Pickering TG et al: Predictive value and changes of renin secretion in hypertensive patients with unilateral renovascular disease undergoing successful renal angioplasty. *Am J Med* 1984;**76**:398.)

surgery and for those patients in whom revascularization procedures have failed. Medical management of patients with correctable renal artery lesions requires close monitoring of both blood pressure control and renal function.

B. Transluminal Angioplasty (Angiodilation): Patients who meet the criteria for reversible renovascular hypertension can now be treated with percutaneous transluminal balloon dilation of the stenotic renal artery (transluminal angioplasty; see Chapter 7). Preliminary results have been encouraging. In successful cases, angiograms obtained after transluminal angioplasty show enlargement of the diameter of the renal artery (Fig 35–8), and measurements show that the renin activity returns to normal levels and the blood pressure likewise returns to normal or near normal levels. In a series of 89 patients with atheromatous and fibromuscular stenoses (Sos et al, 1983), angiodilation was technically successful in 87% of patients with fibromuscular stenoses and 47% of those with unilateral atheromatous stenoses. Technical difficulties were encountered in patients with bilateral atheromatous stenosis, total occlusion, or ostial stenosis, in whom only 10% of lesions could be completely dilated. Following successful angiodilation, blood pressure returned to normal levels or was lowered in 93% of patients with fibromuscular dysplasia and 84% of patients with unilateral atheromatous disease. Although the long-term stability of the blood

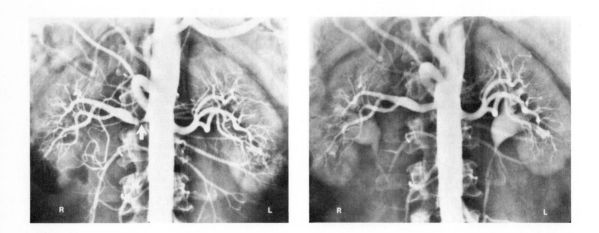

Figure 35–8. Aortograms showing unilateral right renal artery stenosis before (*left*) and after (*right*) successful percutaneous transluminal angioplasty. (Reproduced, with permission, from Vaughan ED Jr: Renal artery stenosis. Chapter 10 in: *Hypertension.* Brenner BM, Stein JH [editors]. Vol 8 of: *Contemporary Issues in Nephrology.* Churchill Livingstone, 1981.)

pressure after it decreases in response to angiodilation is not known, transluminal angioplasty is an acceptable alternative to surgical correction, especially in patients with diffuse atherosclerotic disease who are poor surgical risks. Successful dilation precludes the need for major surgery and can lower blood pressure while preserving or improving renal function.

C. Surgical Measures: Surgery is reserved for patients in whom percutaneous transluminal dilation is not successful. The first surgical cure of hypertension was achieved by unilateral nephrectomy. However, unilateral nephrectomy has benefited only 26–37% of the large group of unselected patients with hypertension who have been so treated. Unilateral nephrectomy is now reserved for treatment of 2 groups of patients with hypertension: (1) those who have poor or absent renal function in the involved kidney but normal function in the contralateral kidney and in whom attempts at revascularizaton have failed, and (2) those

at such high risk that the loss of functioning nephrons is offset by the elimination of the cause of significant excess renin secretion. Partial nephrectomy may be performed if the kidney has multiple renal arteries and only one is stenotic.

Today, surgical treatment emphasizes preservation of renal function. Accordingly, various methods may be used to attempt to revascularize an ischemic kidney; these include endarterectomy, aortorenal bypass graft utilizing the saphenous vein or hypogastric artery, and hepatorenal and splenorenal bypass procedures for patients with severely diseased aortas. Hypertension has been cured or improved in over 90% of the carefully selected patients treated surgically by experienced operating teams; the mortality rate has been about 2%. More favorable results have been achieved in patients with fibromuscular disease, who tend to be younger and healthier than the more elderly patients presenting with atheromatous disease.

REFERENCES

Ayers CR, Harris RH, Lefer LG: Control of renin release in experimental hypertension. *Circ Res* 1969;**24/25(Suppl 1):**103.

Blake WD et al: Effect of renal arterial constriction on excretion of sodium and water. *Am J Physiol* 1950;**163:**422.

Brenner BM, Stenin JH (editors): *Hypertension.* Vol 8 of: *Contemporary Issues in Nephrology.* Churchill Livingstone, 1981.

Brunner HR et al: Angiotensin II blockade in man by sar1-ala8-angiotensin II for understanding and treatment of high blood pressure. *Lancet* 1973;**2:**1045.

Brunner HR et al: Essential hypertension: Renin and aldosterone, heart attack, and stroke. *N Engl J Med* 1972;**286:**441.

Brunner HR et al: Hypertension of renal origin: Evidence for two different mechanisms. *Science* 1971;**174:**1344.

Case DB, Atlas SA, Laragh JH: Physiologic effects and blockade. Pages 541–550 in: *Frontiers in Hypertension Research.* Laragh JH, Buhler FR, Seldin DW (editors). Springer-Verlag,1982.

Case DB, Atlas SA, Laragh JH: Reactive hyperreninemia to angiotensin blockade-identified renovascular hypertension. *Clin Sci* 1979;**57(Suppl 5):**313S.

Case DB et al: Possible role of renin in hypertension as suggested by renin-sodium profiling and inhibition of converting enzyme. *N Engl J Med* 1977;**296:**641.

Eyler WR et al: Angiography of the renal areas, including a comparative study of renal arterial stenosis in patients with and without hypertension. *Radiology* 1962;**78:**879.

Foster JH et al: Renovascular occlusive disease: Results of operative treatment. *JAMA* 1975;**231:**1043.

Goldblatt H, Lynch J, Hangel R: Studies on experimental hypertension. *J Exp Med* 1934;**59:**347.

Harvey RJ et al: Screening for renovascular hypertension. *JAMA* 1985;**254:**388.

Holley KE et al: Renal artery stenosis: A clinical-pathologic study in normotensive patients. *Am J Med* 1964;**37:**14.

Howard JE et al: Hypertension resulting from unilateral renovascular disease and its relief by nephrectomy. *Bull Johns Hopkins Hosp* 1954;**94:**51.

Hunt JC et al: Renal and renovascular hypertension: A reasoned approach to diagnosis and management. *Arch Intern Med* 1975;**133:**988.

Judson WE, Helmer OM: Diagnostic and prognostic values of renin activity in renal venous plasma in renovascular hypertension. *Hypertension* 1965;**13:**79.

Kaufman JJ: Renovascular hypertension: The UCLA experience *J Urol* 1979;**121:**139.

Laragh JH (editor): *Hypertension Manual.* York Medical Books, 1973.

Liard JF et al: Renin, aldosterone, body fluid volumes, and the baroreceptor reflex in the development and reversal of Goldblatt hypertension in conscious dogs. *Circ Res* 1974;**34:**549.

Libertino JA et al: Renal artery revascularization: Restoration of renal function. *JAMA* 1980;**244:**1340.

Lyons DF et al: Captopril stimulation of differential renins in renovascular hypertension. *Hypertension* 1983;**5:**615.

Marks LS, Maxwell MH: Renal vein renin value and limitations in the prediction of operative results. *Urol Clin North Am* 1975;**2:**311.

Maxwell MH, Lupu AN: Excretory urogram in renal arterial hypertension. *J Urol* 1968;**100:**395.

Maxwell MH, Lupu AN, Kaufman JJ: Individual kidney function tests in renal arterial hypertension. *J Urol* 1968;**100:**384.

Maxwell MH, Lupu AN, Taplin GV: Radioisotope renogram in renal arterial hypertension. *J Urol* 1968;**100:**376.

Miller ED Jr, Samuels AI, Haber E: Inhibition of angiotensin conversion in experimental renovascular hypertension. *Science* 1972;**177:**1108.

Muller FB et al: The captopril test for identifying renovascular disease in hypertensive patients. *Am J Med* 1986;**80:**633.

Nicholson JP et al: Cigarette smoking in renovascular hypertension. *Lancet* 1983;**2:**765.

Novick AC Et al: Diminished operative morbidity and mortality following revascularization for atherosclerotic renovascular disease. *JAMA* 1981;**246:**749.

Osborne RW et al: Digital video subtraction angiography: Screening technique for renovascular hypertension. *Surgery* 1981;**90:**932.

Pickering TG et al: Predictive value and changes of renin secretion in hypertensive patients with unilateral renovascular disease undergoing successful renal angioplasty. *Am J Med* 1984;**76**:398.

Sealey JE et al: The physiology of renin secretion in essential hypertension: Estimation of renin secretion rate and renal plasma flow from peripheral and renal vein renin levels. *Am J Med* 1973;**55**:391.

Simon N et al: Clinical characteristics of renovascular hypertension. *JAMA* 1972;**220**:1209.

Sos TA et al: Percutaneous transluminal renal angioplasty in renovascular hypertension due to atheroma or fibromuscular dysplasia. *N Engl J Med* 1983;**309**:274.

Stockigt JR et al: Renal-vein renin in various forms of renal hypertension. *Lancet* 1972;**1**:1194.

Thibonnier M et al: Improved diagnosis of unilateral renal artery lesions after captopril administration. *JAMA* 1984;**25**:56.

Vaughan ED Jr: Laboratory tests in the evaluation of renal hypertension. *Urol Clin North Am* 1979;**6**:485.

Vaughan ED Jr et al: Clinical evaluation of renovascular hypertension and therapeutic decisions. *Urol Clin North Am* 1984;**11**:393.

Vaughan ED Jr et al: Hypertension and unilateral parenchymal renal disease: Evidence for abnormal vasoconstriction-volume interaction. *JAMA* 1975;**233**:1177.

Vaughan ED Jr et al: Renovascular hypertension: Renin measurements to indicate hypersecretion and contralateral suppression, estimate renal plasma flow, and score for surgical curability. *Am J Med* 1973;**55**:402.

Male Infertility

36

R. Dale McClure, MD, FRCS(C)

MALE REPRODUCTIVE PHYSIOLOGY

Understanding reproductive physiology is pivotal in the evaluation and therapy of male infertility. The human testis is an organ of dual function: spermatogenesis, which occurs in the seminiferous tubules; and secretion of steroid hormones (androgens) by the Leydig cells, which are present in the interstitial tissue. These testicular functions are intimately related, as testosterone synthesis is required not only for sperm production but also for the development of secondary sexual characteristics and normal sexual behavior. The anterior pituitary controls both these functions through secretion of gonadotropins, luteinizing hormone (LH), and follicle-stimulating hormone (FSH). In turn, the anterior pituitary is regulated by many parts of the brain via hypothalamic secretion of gonadotropin-releasing hormone (GnRH), also known as luteinizing hormone-releasing hormone (LHRH). This hypothalamic-pituitary-gonadal axis consists of a closed-loop feedback control mechanism directed at maintaining normal reproductive function.

HYPOTHALAMIC-PITUITARY-GONADAL AXIS

The hypothalamus, the integrative center of the reproductive axis, receives messages from both the central nervous system and the testis to regulate the synthesis and secretion of GnRH. Neurotransmitters (norepinephrine, dopamine, serotonin, acetylcholine) and neuropeptides (endogenous opioid peptides) have both inhibitory and stimulatory influence on the hypothalamus. The hypothalamus releases the single decapeptide GnRH episodically. This pulsatile nature of GnRH secretion appears to be essential for stimulating the synthesis and release of both LH and FSH. Paradoxically, after the initial stimulation of these gonadotropins, the exposure to constant GnRH results in inhibition of their release.

LH and FSH are glycoproteins synthesized in the anterior pituitary and are secreted episodically in response to the pulsatile release of GnRH. The lower plasma concentration and longer circulating half-life of FSH as compared to LH results in less obvious pulsatile changes. LH and FSH bind to specific receptors on the membrane of the Leydig cells and Sertoli cells, respectively, to stimulate cellular metabolism.

The hypothalamic-pituitary-gonadal axis consists of a closed-loop feedback control mechanism. The rise in both serum FSH and LH that occurs after orchidectomy demonstrates that gonadal hormones have an inhibitory effect on the secretion of LH and FSH. Testosterone, the major secretory product of the testes, is a primary inhibitor of LH secretion in males. Testosterone may be metabolized in peripheral tissue to the potent androgen dihydrotestosterone or the potent estrogen estradiol. These androgens and estrogens act independently to modulate LH secretion. The rise in LH levels after endogenous GnRH administration is lessened during estradiol administration but is normal during testosterone infusion. This suggests that estradiol acts at the pituitary level, while testosterone acts at the hypothalamic level. Although a positive feedback mechanism of estrogen is clearly demonstrated in females (a rise in LH secretion in response to prolonged estrogen exposure), it is still controversial in males. However, this mechanism has been demonstrated in individuals with primary testicular failure (ie, hypergonadotropic hypergonadism, Klinefelter's syndrome, Sertoli cell-only syndrome).

The mechanism for feedback control of FSH secretion is more controversial than that of LH. After castration, FSH increases, indicating negative feedback from the testes. Numerous animal and human studies have demonstrated that a nonsteroidal Sertoli cell factor, inhibin, is extremely important in the feedback regulation of FSH. Decreases in spermatogenesis are accompanied by decreased production of inhibin, and this reduction in negative feedback is associated with reciprocal elevation of FSH levels. Isolated increased levels of FSH constitute an important, sensitive marker of the state of the germinal epithelium.

Evidence also exists to support negative feedback of FSH from the sex steroid testosterone. Several animal studies have demonstrated that if testosterone is replaced in physiologic doses after castration, levels of both LH and FSH can be maintained within the normal range. Serum FSH levels in males with seminiferous tubule damage consequent to chemotherapy are only 50% of those of castrated individuals; this supports the theory that sex steroids play a role in mediating FSH secretion in humans. Both gonadal steroids and inhibin are important in maintaining normal FSH concentrations (Fig 36–1).

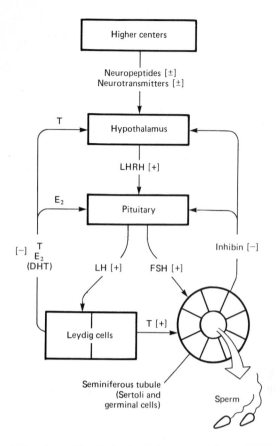

Figure 36–1. Hypothalamic-pituitary-gonadal axis. (DHT = dihydrotestosterone; E$_2$ = estradiol; FSH = follicle-stimulating hormone; LH = luteinizing hormone; LHRH = luteinizing hormone-releasing hormone; T = testosterone; + = positive influence; − = negative influence.) (Reproduced, with permission, from McClure RD: Endocrine investigation and therapy. Urol Clin North Am 1987;**14**:471.)

Prolactin also has a complex interrelationship with gonadotropins. In males with hyperprolactinemia and testosterone deficiency, serum LH levels are inappropriately low, indicating that in such patients, the hypothalamic-pituitary axis fails to respond to the reduced levels of testosterone. Prolactin also inhibits production of GnRH; individuals with prolactin-secreting tumors respond to an infusion of GnRH with an increase in LH. Besides inhibiting androgen secretion, elevated prolactin levels may have a direct effect on the central nervous system. In individuals with elevated prolactin levels who are given androgen, libido and sexual function do not return to normal as long as prolactin levels are elevated.

THE TESTES

Leydig Cells

Testosterone is secreted episodically from the Ley-

dig cells in response to LH pulses and has a diurnal pattern, with the peak level in the early morning and the nadir in the evening. Several mechanisms alter the ability of the Leydig cells to produce testosterone in response to LH and constitute an intratesticular control system for regulating testosterone production. In intact testes, LH receptors decrease (down-regulation) after exogenous LH administration. Large doses of GnRH or its analogs also reduce the numbers of LH receptors and inhibit LH secretion. (This has been applied clinically to cause medical castration in men with prostate cancer.) Estrogen inhibits enzymes in the testosterone synthetic pathways and therefore directly affects production. In the animal model, prolactin increases the number of receptors. There also appears to be an intratesticular ultrashort loop feedback such that exogenous testosterone will override the effect of LH and inhibit testosterone production.

In normal males, 2% of testosterone is free (unbound); 44% is bound to testosterone-estradiol-binding globulin (TeBG; also called sex hormone-binding globulin); and 54% is bound to albumin and other proteins. In the seminiferous tubules, testosterone is bound to androgen-binding protein (ABP), a Sertoli cell product. These steroid-binding proteins modulate androgen action. It was formerly believed that the physiologically active androgen moiety was the non-protein-bound "free" testosterone. It now appears that transport of steroid hormone into cells is more complicated and that enhanced rates of hormone dissociation from the binding proteins may occur in the microcirculation. Pardridge (1981) has demonstrated that albumin-bound testosterone is also available for transport into target tissues such as the brain and the liver. TeBG has a higher affinity for testosterone than for estradiol, and changes in TeBG alter or amplify the hormonal milieu.

TeBG levels are increased by estrogens, thyroid administration, and cirrhosis of the liver and may be decreased by androgens, growth hormone (GH), and obesity.

The biologic effects of androgens are exerted on target organs that contain a specific androgen receptor protein in the cell cytosol. Testosterone leaves the circulation and enters the target cells, where it may be converted to the more potent androgen dihydrotestosterone by 5-alpha-reductase, and either testosterone or DHT binds to a receptor protein. This androgen receptor complex is translocated into the nucleus, where it binds to nuclear chromatin and results in the synthesis of messenger RNA (mRNA). mRNA causes protein synthesis and other expressions of androgen action (Fig 36–2).

The major functions of androgen in target tissue include (1) regulation of gonadotropin secretion by the hypothalamic-pituitary axis, (2) initiation and maintenance of spermatogenesis, (3) differentiation of the internal and external male genital system during fetal development, and (4) promotion of sexual maturation at puberty.

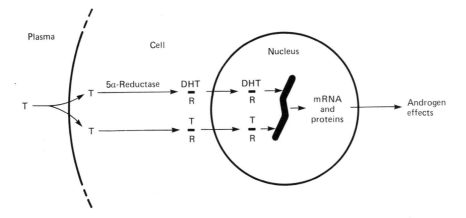

Figure 36–2. Mechanism of androgen action. Action of testosterone (T) on target cells includes conversion of testosterone to dihydrotestosterone (DHT) by 5-alpha reductase; binding of T/DHT to cytoplasmic androgen receptors (R); translocation of the receptor complex into the nucleus with binding to the chromosome; and stimulation of the synthesis of messenger RNA (mRNA) and proteins. (Reproduced, with permission, from McClure RD: Endocrine investigation and therapy. *Urol Clin North Am* 1987;**14**:471.)

Seminiferous Tubules

Seminiferous tubules contain germ cells at various stages of maturation and Sertoli cells; these account for 85–90% of testicular volume.

A. Sertoli Cells: Sertoli cells are fixed-population or nondividing support cells. They rest on the basement membrane of the seminiferous tubules and extend filamentous cytoplasmic ramifications toward the lumen of the tubule. Sertoli cells are linked by tight junctions that divide the seminiferous tubule into a basal and adluminal compartment. These junctional complexes, coupled with the close approximation of the myoid cells of the peritubular contractile cell layer, serve to form the blood-testis barrier. This barrier provides a unique microenvironment that facilitates spermatogenesis and maintains these germ cells in an immunologically privileged location. This isolation is important because spermatozoa are produced during puberty, long after the period of self-recognition by the immune system. If these developing spermatozoa were not immunologically protected, they would be recognized as foreign and attacked by the body's immune system.

Sertoli cells appear to be involved in the nourishment of developing germ cells as well as phagocytosis of damaged cells. Spermatogonia and young spermatocytes are in the basal compartment, whereas mature spermatocytes and spermatids are sequestered behind the permeability barrier in the adluminal compartment.

Although our knowledge is incomplete, it is apparent that multiple spermatogenic control sites must exist between Sertoli cells and germ cells. This relationship probably has the following components: (1) the presence of specific high-affinity membrane-bound receptors for FSH on Sertoli cells; (2) the production or concentration by Sertoli cells of a soluble high-affinity androgen-binding protein found in the seminiferous tubule fluid, which serves as a reservoir of androgen hormone within the seminiferous tubule; (3) the production of a macromolecule by the seminiferous tubule that preferentially inhibits FSH secretion (inhibin); and (4) the (probable) metabolism of certain steroids by Sertoli cells to 5-alpha-reduced androgens and estrogens. The ascribed functional role of androgen-binding protein is that of concentrating androgens in the adluminal region of the tubule, thus facilitating spermatogenesis as well as concentrating testosterone in the epididymal tubule.

B. Germinal Cells: The spermatogenic cells are arranged in an orderly manner from the basement membrane to the lumen. Spermatogonia lie directly on the basement membrane, and next in order, progressing centrally, are found primary spermatocytes, secondary spermatocytes, and spermatids. Heller and Clermont (1964) revealed 13 different germ cells thought to represent different stages in the developmental process. Proceeding from the least to the most differentiated, they are named dark type A spermatogonia (Ad); pale type A spermatogonia (Ap); type B spermatogonia (B); preleptotene primary spermatocytes (R); leptotene primary spermatocytes (L); zygotene primary spermatocytes (Z); pachytene primary spermatocytes (P); secondary spermatocytes (II); and Sa, Sb, Sc, Sd_1, and Sd_2 spermatids.

Spermatogenesis

Spermatogenesis is a complex process whereby primitive stem cells, spermatogonia, either divide to reproduce their number (stem cell renewal) or produce daughter cells that will later become spermatocytes. The most primitive undifferentiated spermatogonia are the stem cells. To provide for constant renewal of stem cells, following mitotic division, the primitive stem cells, dark type A spermatogonia (Ad), produce a fresh stock of Ad cells as well as pale type A spermatogonia (Ap). The pale type A spermatogonia undergo mitotic divisions into preleptotene primary spermatocytes via type B spermatogonia. The primary spermatocytes undergo the first maturation division by a process of meiosis, reducing the number of chromosomes from 46 to 23. Each primary spermatocyte gives rise to 2 secondary spermatocytes, and each of these divides into 2 spermatids. The spermatids then undergo a transformation into spermatozoa, a process termed spermiogenesis. This transformation includes nuclear condensation, acrosome formation, loss of most of the cytoplasm, development of a tail, and arrangement of mitochondria into the middle piece of the sperm.

In the human testes, groups of germ cells connected by intercellular bridges in the same stages of development pass through spermatogenesis together. This sequence phase of developing germ cells is called a generation. These generations of germ cells are not mixed at random but form a limited number of cell associations (stages). Histologically on cross-section, many germ cells are repeatedly seen only in association with certain other cells. These specific cellular associations are known as stages of the seminiferous epithelium, of which there are 6 in human males (Heller and Clermont, 1964) (Fig 36–3). The process of spermatogenesis progressively involves the cell association of each stage sequentially. The progression from stage I through stage VI in any one segment of the seminiferous tubule constitutes one cycle. In humans, the duration of each cycle is approximately 16 days, and 4.6 cycles are required for a mature sperm to develop from an early spermatogonium. Therefore, the duration of the entire spermatogenic cycle in humans is 74 days (4.6 × 16).

HORMONAL CONTROL OF SPERMATOGENESIS

There is an intimate structural and functional relationship between the 2 separate compartments of the testes. LH affects spermatogenesis only indirectly in that it stimulates endogenous testosterone production. Sertoli cells are the target for FSH, as they possess specific high-affinity FSH receptors. Therefore, testosterone and FSH are the hormones that are directed at the seminiferous tubule epithelium. Androgen-binding protein, a Sertoli cell product, carries androgens intracellularly and may serve as an androgen reservoir within the seminiferous tubule in addition to transporting testosterone from the testes into the epididymal tubule. The physical proximity of the Leydig cells to the seminiferous tubule and elaboration by the Sertoli cells of androgen-binding protein cause a high level of androgen to be maintained in the microenvironment of the developing spermatozoa (Fig 36–4).

The hormonal requirements for *initiation* of spermatogenesis appear to be independent of the *maintenance* of this process. For spermatogenesis to be maintained immediately after hypophysectomy (pituitary

obliteration), testosterone alone is required; however, if it is to be reinitiated after the germinal epithelium has been allowed to regress completely, both FSH and testosterone are required. The amount of hormone needed depends on whether the goal is qualitative restoration of spermatogenesis (production of a few advance spermatids) or quantitative restoration (complete restoration of spermatid numbers). For qualitative restoration, testosterone will initiate and maintain spermatogenesis in humans, but because of the difficulty of restoring high enough blood levels of testosterone, quantitative maintenance in human males has not been achieved. In humans, FSH probably has little impact on the maintenance of spermatogenesis but is necessary for production of quantitatively normal sperm. FSH is important for initiating spermatogenesis in pubertal males and for reinitiating spermatogenesis in adult males in whom the germinal epithelium has been allowed to regress after hypophysectomy.

TRANSPORT-MATURATION-STORAGE OF SPERM

Although the testis is responsible for sperm production, the epididymis is intimately involved with the maturation, storage, and transport of spermatozoa. Testicular spermatozoa are nonmotile and incapable of fertilizing ova. Spermatozoa gain progressive motility and fertilizing ability after passing through the epididymis.

The tunica albuginea, or the testicular capsule, extends fibrosepta into the testicle, resulting in formation of approximately 250 pyramidal lobules each of which contains coiled seminiferous tubules. These tubules terminate in the rete testis, which in turn coalesces to form the ductuli efferentes, which conduct testicular fluid and spermatozoa into the caput epididymidis. The epididymis consists of a single convoluted tubule, 5–6 m in length. The epididymis is divided into the caput, corpus, and cauda epididymidis. Sperm are immotile in the male reproductive tract but are transported by a hydrostatic pressure difference, ciliary propulsion, and peristaltic contraction of myoid cells along the epididymis. Although epididymal transit time varies with age (testicular sperm production rate) and sexual activity, the estimated transit time of spermatozoa through the caput, corpus, and cauda epididymidis in healthy males is 0.7, 0.7, and 1.8 days, respectively. It is during the period of maturation in the caput and corpus (< 2 days) that sperm develop the increased capacity for progressive motility characterized by high-frequency, low-amplitude beats and also acquire the ability to penetrate oocytes during fertilization. Human spermatozoa are able to bind to zona-free hamster eggs (human surrogate egg system), but only spermatozoa from the cauda epididymidis are able to bind and penetrate eggs. This implies that the fertilizing capability of human sperm is completed at the level of the cauda epididymidis. The epididymis

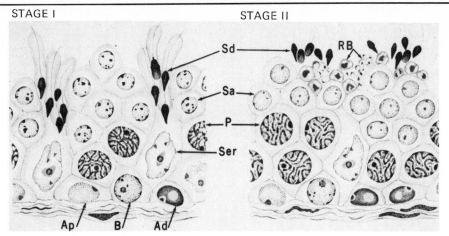

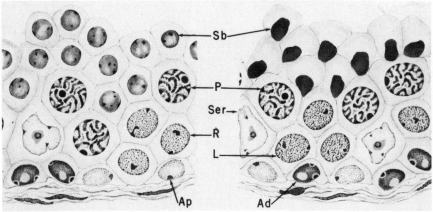

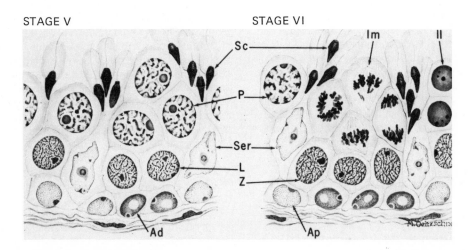

Figure 36–3. Diagrammatic representation of the 6 recognizable cell associations corresponding to the stages of the cycle of the human seminiferous epithelium. Ser = Sertoli cell; Ad and Ap = dark and pale type A spermatogonia; B = type B spermatogonia; R = resting primary spermatocyte; L = leptotene spermatocyte; Z = zygotene spermatocyte; P = pachytene spermatocyte; Im = primary spermatocyte in division; II = secondary spermatocyte in interphase; Sa, Sb, Sc, Sd = spermatids in various stages of differentiation; RB = residual bodies of Regnaud. (Reproduced, with permission, from Clermont Y: *Am J Anat* 1963;**112**:35.)

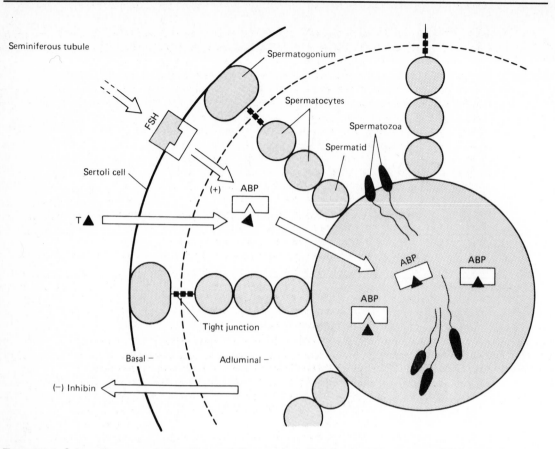

Figure 36–4. Schematic representation of the seminiferous tubule. Follicle-stimulating hormone (FSH) and testosterone (T) act on the Sertoli cells, which produce both androgen-binding protein (ABP) and inhibin. (Reproduced, with permission, from McClure RD: Endocrine investigation and therapy. *Urol Clin North Am* 1987;**14**:471.)

also serves as a reservoir or storage area for sperm; it is estimated that the extragonadal sperm reserve is 440×10^6 spermatozoa and that more than 50% of these are located in the cauda epididymidis.

These spermatozoa stored in the cauda epididymidis enter the vas deferens, a muscular duct 30–35 cm long, which propels its contents by peristaltic motion into the ejaculatory duct. Sperm are transported to the outside of the male reproductive tract by emission and ejaculation. During emission, secretions from the seminal vesicles and prostate are deposited into the posterior urethra. Prior to ejaculation, peristalsis of the vas deferens and bladder neck occurs under sympathetic nervous control. During ejaculation, the external sphincter relaxes and the semen is propelled through the urethra by rhythmic contractions of the perineal and bulbourethral muscles, both under somatic control.

The first portion of the ejaculate contains a small volume of fluid from the vas deferens, which is rich in sperm. The major volume of the seminal plasma comes from the seminal vesicles (60%) and prostate (20%). The seminal vesicles provide the nourishing substrate fructose as well as prostaglandins, phosphorylcholine, and coagulating substrates. A recognized function of the seminal plasma is its buffering effect

on the acidic vaginal environment. The coagulum formed by the ejaculated semen liquefies within 20 minutes as a result of prostatic proteolytic enzymes. The prostate adds zinc, phospholipids, spermine, and phosphatase to the seminal fluid. Additional fluid may be added by the bulbourethral glands (Cowper's glands) and urethral glands (Littre's glands) during transport of the fluid through the penile urethra. The first portion of the ejaculate characteristically contains most of the spermatozoa and most of the prostatic secretions, while the second portion is composed primarily of seminal vesical secretions and contains only a few spermatozoa.

FERTILIZATION

Fertilization normally takes place within the uterine tubes after ovulation has occurred. During the menstrual mid cycle, the cervical mucus changes to become more abundant, thinner, and more watery. These changes serve to facilitate entry of the sperm into the uterus and to protect the sperm from the highly acidic vaginal secretions. Physiologic changes in the spermatozoa ("capacitation") must occur within the female reproductive tract in order for fertilization to occur. As the sperm cell interacts with the egg, there is initiation of new flagellar movement ("hyperactive motility") and morphologic changes in the sperm that result in the release of lytic enzymes and exposure of parts of the sperm's structure ("acrosome reaction"). As a result of these changes, the fertilizing sperm cell is able to reach the oocyte, traverse its various layers, and become incorporated into the ooplasm.

MALE INFERTILITY

Approximately 15% of all married couples will experience reproductive difficulty. Conception normally is achieved within 12 months in 80% of couples who use no contraceptive measures, and persons presenting after this time should therefore be regarded as possibly infertile and should be evaluated.

About a third of cases of infertility result from pathologic factors in the man, a third from factors in the woman, and a third from contributing factors in both parties. Therefore, the male factor is at least partly responsible in about 50% of infertile couples. It is extremely important in the evaluation of infertility to consider the couple as a unit in evaluation and treatment and to proceed in a parallel investigative manner until a significant problem is uncovered. The simultaneous evaluation of the female is strongly recommended, since subtle abnormalities are frequently found. Pregnancy rates of up to 50% have been reported when only the woman has been investigated and treated even when the man was found to have moderately severe abnormalities of semen quality.

CLINICAL FINDINGS

History

The cornerstone of the evaluation of the infertile man is a careful history and physical examination. Specific childhood illnesses should be sought, including cryptorchidism, postpubertal mumps orchitis, and testicular trauma or pain (torsion). Timing of puberty is important, as precocious puberty may indicate the presence of adrenal-genital syndrome, whereas delayed puberty may indicate Klinefelter's syndrome or idiopathic hypogonadism. Prenatal exposure to diethylstilbestrol should be ascertained because this may cause an increased incidence of epididymal cysts and a slightly increased frequency of cryptorchidism. A detailed history of exposure to occupational and environmental toxins (eg, dibromochloropropane [DBCP]), excessive heat, or radiation should be elicited. Cancer chemotherapy has a dose-dependent, potentially devastating effect on the testicular germinal epithelium. The drug history should be reviewed; anabolic steroids, cimetidine, and spironolactone may affect the reproductive cycle. Medications such as sul-fasalazine and nitrofurantoin may affect sperm motility. Illicit drugs and excessive alcohol consumption are associated with a decrease in sperm count and hormonal abnormalities.

Previous medical and surgical diseases and their treatment may occasionally compromise reproductive function. Men with unilateral undescended testes will have overall semen quality of considerably less than normal, even after therapy. Previous surgical procedures such as a bladder neck operation (Y-V-plasty) or retroperitoneal lymph node dissection for testicular cancer may cause retrograde ejaculation or absent emission. Diabetic neuropathy may result in either retrograde ejaculation or impotence. Both the vas deferens and the testicular blood supply can easily be injured during hernia repair. In cystic fibrosis, the vas deferens or epididymis and seminal vesicles may be absent.

Any generalized fever or illness can impair spermatogenesis. The ejaculate may not be affected for 3 months after the event, as spermatogenesis takes about 74 days from initiation to the appearance of mature spermatozoa, and there is also a variable transport time in the ducts. Therefore, events that have occurred in the previous 3–6 months are extremely important.

Sexual habits, including frequency of intercourse, type of ejaculation, use of coital lubricants (spermicides), and the patient's understanding of the ovulatory cycle should be discussed. Previous infertility evaluation and treament and the reproductive history from previous marriages should be ascertained.

Recurrent respiratory infections and infertility may be associated with the immotile cilia syndrome, in which the sperm count is normal but spermatozoa are completely nonmotile due to ultrastructural defects. Kartagener's syndrome, a variant of immotile cilia syndrome, consists of chronic bronchiectasis, sinusitis, situs inversus, and immotile spermatozoa. In Young's syndrome, also associated with pulmonary disease, the cilia ultrastructure is normal but the epididymis is obstructed due to inspissated material, and these patients present with azoospermia.

Loss of libido associated with headaches, visual abnormalities, and galactorrhea may suggest a pituitary tumor. Other medical problems that have been associated with infertility include thyroid disease, seizure disorders (phenytoin decreases FSH), and liver disease. Chronic systemic diseases such as renal disease and sickle cell disease are associated with abnormal reproductive hormonal parameters.

Physical Examination

During the examination, particular attention should be paid to discerning features of hypogonadism, if present: poorly developed secondary sexual characteristics, eunuchoidal skeletal proportions (arm span 2 inches greater than height); ratio of upper body segment (crown to pubis) to lower body segment (pubis to floor) less than one; and lack of normal male hair distribution (sparse axillary, pubic, facial, and body hair; lack of temporal hair recession) (Table 36–1).

Table 36–1. Features of eunuchoidism.*

Eunuchoid skeletal proportions
  Upper-body: lower-body ratio below 1; arm span more than 2
  in greater than height
Lack of adult male hair distribution
  Sparse axillary, pubic, facial, and body hair; lack of temporal
  lobe hair recession
Infantile genitalia
  Small penis, testes, and prostate; underdeveloped scrotum
Diminished muscular development and mass

*Reproduced, with permission, from McClure RD: Endocrine
investigation and therapy. *Urol Clin North Am* 1987;**14**:471.

A careful examination of the testes is an essential part of the examination. The seminiferous tubules account for approximately 95% of testicular volume. Normal adult testes are an average of 4.6 cm long (range 3.6–5.5 cm) and 2.6 cm wide (range 2.1–3.2 cm), with a mean volume of 18.6 ± 4.8 (SD) mL (Figs 36–5 and 36–6). A ruler, caliper, or Prader orchidometer may be used to measure testicular size. If the seminiferous tubules were damaged before puberty, the testes are small and firm; with postpubertal damage, they are usually small and soft.

Gynecomastia is a consistent feature of a feminizing state. Men with congenital hypogonadism may have associated midline defects such as anosmia, color blindness, cerebellar ataxia, harelip, and cleft palate. Hepatomegaly may be associated with problems of hormonal metabolism. Proper neck examination may help rule out thyromegaly, a bruit or nodularity associated with thyroid disease. Neurologic examination should test the visual fields and reflexes.

Irregularities in the epididymis suggest a previous infection and possible obstruction. Examination may reveal a small prostate with androgen deficiency or slight tenderness (bogginess) in men with prostatic infection. Any penile abnormalities (hypospadias, abnormal curvature, phimosis) should be looked for. The scrotal contents should be carefully palpated with the patient in both the supine and standing positions. Many varicoceles are not visible and may only be discernible when the patient stands or performs the Valsalva maneuver. Varicoceles often result in smaller left testes, and a discrepancy in size between the 2 testes should arouse suspicion. Both vasa should be palpated, as 2% of infertile men have congenital absence of the vasa and seminal vesicles.

Laboratory Findings

A. Semen Analysis: A carefully performed semen analysis provides important information concerning the male reproductive hormonal cycle, spermatogenesis, and the patency of the reproductive tract. The World Health Organization laboratory manual for examination of human semen and semen-cervical mucus interactions is highly recommended for technical details. The standard techniques of analysis allow variations of up to 20% between laboratories. Besides laboratory error, there are marked variations in sperm density, motility, and morphology among multiple samples from a given man. Abstinence intervals give a large source of variability. With each day of abstinence (up to one week), semen volume increases by 0.4 mL, sperm concentration by 10–15 million/mL, and total sperm count by 50–90 million. Sperm motility and morphology appear to be unaffected by 5–7 days of abstinence, but longer periods lead to impaired motility.

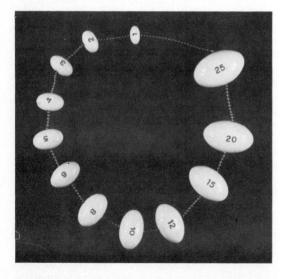

Figure 36–5. Prader orchidometer for measuring testicular volume. (Reproduced, with permission, from McClure RD: Endocrine investigation and therapy. *Urol Clin North Am* 1987;14:471.)

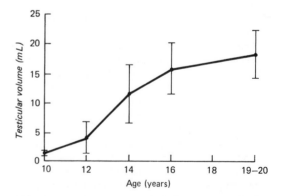

Figure 36–6. Normal values for testicular volume in relation to age. (Redrawn and reproduced, with permission, from Zachman M et al: Testicular volume during adolescence: Cross-sectional and longitudinal studies. *Helv Paediatr Acta* 1974;**29**:61 and McClure RD: Endocrine investigation and therapy. *Urol Clin North Am* 1987;14:471.)

Interpretation of semen analysis must take into consideration the variations between samples that exist in individuals. The minimum number of specimens to define good or poor quality of semen is 3 samples over a 2-month interval with a consistent period of abstinence (48–72 hours). In a longitudinal analysis of semen from both fertile and infertile men, Sherins, Brightwell, and Sternthal (1977) found that 97% of men with initial good sperm concentration would continue to show good density after as many as 3–6 specimens. Those rated poor at the first visit also remained poor at the third and sixth visits. For those rated equivocal, the first visit was of little value, and at least 3 visits were needed to obtain stability. In this longitudinal study, there were only minor changes in semen volume and the percentage of sperm with normal morphology remained stable.

Conventional semen analysis is an indirect assessment of fertility potential. Pregnancy is the only irrefutable proof of the sperm's capability to fertilize. Prediction by semen analysis of an individual's fertility can be markedly improved by proper collection and interpretation of the data obtained.

1. Collection of semen–After 48–72 hours' abstinence, the specimen should be collected by masturbation into a wide-necked clear glass or plastic container. (Alternatively, coitus interruptus may be used, but the first part of the ejaculate, which is rich in sperm, may be lost.) Because assessment of motility is extremely important, the specimen should be analyzed within one hour of collection and kept at body temperature. Therefore, collection at the site of analysis is ideal. If the patient must transport the sample from home, he should keep it close to his body (for example, in his jacket pocket).

2. Sperm concentration–Clinical studies of infertile patients have established the limits of adequacy of semen quality below which the initiation of a pregnancy is increasingly improbable. For most clinicians, 20×10^6 per milliliter is the lower limit of normal. MacLeod and Gold (1951), in their classic study, found little difference in the distribution of sperm counts of 1000 fertile men and 1000 infertile men until the count fell below 20×10^6 per milliliter.

Semen volume must be taken into consideration in assessing total sperm production by the testes. Semen volume per se, however, affects fertility only when it falls below 1.5 mL (inadequate buffering of vaginal acidity) or is more than 5 mL. Low volumes may be associated with retrograde ejaculation, incomplete collection, or androgen deficiency.

3. Sperm motility–Adequate motor activity of the sperm cell is required for normal transport through the female reproductive tract and for penetrating the ovum. Sperm motility is the single most important measure of semen quality and can be a compensatory factor in men with low sperm counts. Sperm motility is usually rated in 2 ways: the number of motile sperm as a percentage of the total, and the quality of sperm movement (how fast and how straight the sperm swim). The degree of forward progression is a classification based on the pattern displayed by the majority of motile spermatozoa and ranges from 0 (no movement) to 4 (excellent forward progression). A normal value for sperm motility in the semen is at least 50–60% motile cells and a quality greater than 2. The subjectivity of this assessment may limit its usefulness and has led to the use of more sophisticated methods (lasers, computers, video cameras).

4. Sperm morphology–Human sperm morphology is subject to great variation, and it is unusual to see specimens that contain more than 80% normal sperm heads. Morphology is assessed on stained seminal smears and is usually scored as a percentage of normal cells. To be classified as normal, a sperm cell must have an oval head and a normal midpiece and tail. In fertile semen, the percentage is usually 60% or more. MacLeod and Gold showed that cytologic study is a sensitive index of the state of the germinal epithelium and is remarkably constant, with variations reflecting testicular insult.

Although the "stress" pattern of cytology (increased number of tapered, amorphous, and immature cells) was thought to be pathognomonic of varicocele, Rodriquez-Rigau et al found this pattern to be equally common in oligospermic men with and without varicocele. They showed that the percentage of tapered and amorphous spermatozoa was inversely correlated with sperm counts and was not related to the presence of varicocele. Semen with particularly tapered forms are not pathognomonic of varicocele but represent altered testicular function.

5. Fructose–Fructose is androgen-dependent and is produced in the seminal vesicles. Fructose levels should be determined in any patient with azoospermia and especially in those whose ejaculate volume is less than 1 mL, suggesting seminal vesicle obstruction or atresia. The usual test for fructose is a qualitative test that uses resorcinol and hydrochloric acid (50 mg powdered resorcinol and 33 mg concentrated hydrochloric acid diluted to 100 mL with water). The semen is mixed with these reagents in a 1:10 ratio and boiled. The presence of fructose within 60 seconds of boiling is shown by a change in the sample to an orange-red color. Absence of fructose, low semen volume, and failure of the semen to coagulate indicate either congenital absence of the vas deferens and seminal vesicles or obstruction of the ejaculatory duct.

6. Additional criteria–Semen from normal men coagulates and then, over the next 5–20 minutes, liquefies. Delayed liquefaction of semen (> 60 minutes) may indicate disorders of accessory gland function. Diagnosis of a liquefaction problem should be made if there is absence of sperm in the postcoital tests. If spermatozoa are capable of reaching the cervical mucus, problems of semen liquefaction are not clinically relevant.

Increased semen viscosity, which is unrelated to the coagulation-liquefaction phenomenon, signifies a disorder of accessory gland function and may affect the accuracy of assessment of both sperm density and motility. It is only clinically relevant when there are very few sperm in the postcoital tests. Occasional clumps of agglutinated sperm are not infrequently seen in semen samples, but increasing clumping suggests an inflammatory or immunologic process.

7. Normal values—Semen specimens should be regarded as abnormal if the following values for these different characteristics persist: volume of less than 1.5 mL or more than 5 mL; sperm concentration of less than 20×10^6 per mL; total sperm number of fewer than 50×10^6; sperm motility of less than 60% of cells with forward progression and quality graded below 2; and sperm morphology of less than 60% oval forms.

8. Newer techniques for semen analysis—The Coulter Counter is a rapid technique for determining sperm density, but the accuracy of this technique is reduced with sperm densities of less than 10 million/mL. The Makler Chamber Device, similar to a hemocytometer, determines sperm density and motility simultaneously.

Until recently, sperm density was the only characteristic of human semen that could be measured objectively and quantitatively. Sophisticated computers, lasers, and video cameras now allow simultaneous assessment of sperm density and motility parameters, including the percentage of motile sperm, directional velocity, and forward progression. Further comparative work with all these new techniques and standard tests of sperm function need to be carried out to allow a more meaningful inference about these new tests.

B. Hormone Evaluation: Most cases of male infertility are nonendocrine in origin. Routine evaluation of hormonal parameters is not warranted unless sperm density is extremely low or there is clinical suspicion of an endocrinopathy. The incidence of primary endocrine defects in infertile men is less than 3%. Such defects are rare in men with a sperm concentration of greater than 5×10^6 per milliliter. When an endocrinopathy is discovered, however, specific hormonal therapy is often successful.

1. Baseline hormone evaluation—Because of the episodic nature of LH secretion and its short half-life, a single LH determination has an accuracy of plus or minus 50%. Similarly, testosterone is secreted episodically in response to LH pulses and has a diurnal pattern with an early morning peak. To overcome these sampling inaccuracies, 3 blood samples should be drawn at least 15–20 minutes apart and an equal volume of semen from each pooled for a single determination. Since LH should be interpreted in light of serum testosterone, levels of both should be assessed from the pooled samples. Serum FSH has a longer half-life, and these fluctuations are less obvious.

A low serum testosterone level is one of the best indicators of hypogonadism of hypothalamic or pituitary origin. Mean serum LH and FSH concentrations are significantly lower in hypogonadotropic patients than in normal men, although in some individuals they can overlap with the lower limits of normal. Low LH and FSH values concurrent with low serum testosterone levels indicate hypogonadotropic hypogonadism, which may also be apparent clinically.

Elevated serum FSH and LH values help to distinguish primary testicular failure (hypergonadotropic hypogonadism) from secondary testicular failure (hypogonadotropic hypogonadism). Most patients with primary hypogonadism have severe, irreversible testicular defects. On the other hand, secondary hypogonadism has a hypothalamic or pituitary origin, and in these patients, infertility may be correctable.

Decreases in spermatogenesis are generally accompanied by decreased "inhibin" production, and these reductions in negative feedback are associated with reciprocal elevation of FSH levels. Elevated FSH levels are usually a reliable indicator of germinal epithelial damage and are usually associated with azoospermia or severe oligospermia ($< 5 \times 10^6$ sperm per milliliter), depicting significant and usually irreversible germ cell damage. In azoospermic and severely oligospermic patients with normal FSH levels, primary spermatogenic defects cannot be distinguished from obstructive lesions by hormonal investigation alone; scrotal exploration, testicular biopsy, and vasography should be considered. An elevated serum FSH level associated with small, atrophic testes implies irreversible infertility, and biopsy is not warranted.

Hyperprolactinemia has been reported to cause oligospermia, but the diagnostic value of prolactin measurements is extremely low in men with semen abnormalities unless these are associated with decreased libido, impotence, and evidence of hypogonadism. Prolactin measurement is warranted in patients with low serum testosterone levels without an associated increase in serum LH levels.

Individuals with gynecomastia or suspected androgen resistance (elevated serum testosterone and LH levels with undermasculinization) should have a serum estradiol determination. Individuals with a rapid loss of secondary sex characteristics implying both testicular and adrenal failure (deficiency of adrenal androgens) should undergo investigation of adrenal function. In men with a history of precocious puberty, one should consider congenital adrenal hyperplasia. In the common variant (21-hydroxylase deficiency), serum levels of 17-hydroxyprogesterone are elevated, as is urinary pregnanetriol. In 11-hydroxylase deficiency, serum 11-deoxycortisol levels are elevated.

In patients with hypogonadotropic hypogonadism, the pituitary hormones other than LH and FSH should also be assessed (adrenal corticotropic hormone [ACTH], thyroid-stimulating hormone [TSH], and growth hormone [GH]). Thyroid dysfunction is such a rare cause of infertility that routine screening for a thyroid abnormality should be discouraged.

In addition to the standard radioimmunoassay for LH, bioassays have been developed to measure the response of mouse Leydig cells to LH in serum. Rarely, a patient may be infertile due to immunologically active but biologically inactive LH.

2. Dynamic hormonal testing—These tests are rarely required in an infertility workup.

a. hCG test—Human chorionic gonadotropin (hCG), which has a biologic action similar to that of LH, is used to establish the presence of testicular tissue or Leydig cell reserve in patients with testicular disorders or hypogonadotropic states, particularly if therapeutic use of hCG is anticipated. Administration of 4000 IU for 4 days produces a doubling of serum testosterone levels in 3–4 days. However, depending on the degree of testicular failure and the previous stimulation by endogenous gonadotropins, responses can be poor.

b. GnRH test—Because GnRH should have a direct effect on the pituitary gland, it was hoped that its injection would differentiate hypogonadotropic hypogonadism of pituitary or hypothalamic origin. Theoretically, patients with pituitary disease would not respond, whereas those with hypothalamic disease would secrete LH and FSH after injection of GnRH. Often, a single injection of GnRH is inadequate to produce the response, and multiple-dose priming injections must be given. If the pituitary gland has been chronically understimulated, it may not have the reserves or the biosynthetic machinery to respond normally to a single challenge. Hypogonadal individuals with pituitary tumors often have a normal response, which reflects the amount of stored hormone in the pituitary related to endogenous production of GnRH. Therefore, a normal response is of no diagnostic value, either in determining the presence or absence of disease or in distinguishing hypothalamic from pituitary disease.

C. Chromosomal Studies: Analysis of the buccal smear provides evidence of the number of X chromosomes, as in general, there is one chromatid, or Barr body, for every X chromosome in excess of one. For difficult diagnostic problems or when chromosomal mosaicism or structural alteration is suspected (especially when serum gonadotropin levels are elevated), peripheral blood leukocytes, fibroblasts, or gonadal tissue should be submitted for tissue culture and karyotyping.

Only in isolated cases has infertility been documented in association with a specific chromosomal abnormality, but subtle genetic studies should be considered in men with severe oligospermia and azoospermia to look for both autosomal and sex chromosomal abnormalities. The diagnostic yield is greatest in men with small testes, azoospermia, and elevated FSH levels.

D. Immunologic Studies: Sperm antibodies have been reported in 3–7% of infertile men and may be a relative cause of infertility. Physicians should be aware of clinical parameters that may correlate with antibody-mediated infertility in men. A history of orchitis; inflammation of the genitourinary tract; or testicular injury, torsion, atrophy, or obstruction may lead to the development of sperm antibodies.

Although most infertile men with sperm immunity have normal findings on semen analysis, the presence of spontaneous agglutination or severe abnormalities in motility should alert the clinician to the possibility of antibodies. Often, sperm agglutination is nonspecific and may relate to the presence of bacteria, viruses, or cellular debris and may not reflect an immunologic problem. Serial postcoital testings provide an excellent means of screening for antisperm antibodies (postcoital testing involves microscopic examination of cervical mucus after intercourse). If fewer than 5 motile sperm per field are seen in a well-estrogenized mucus sample or if the sperm are seen to shake or vibrate, sperm antibody testing should be performed.

Circulating antisperm antibodies belong to the IgG and IgM classes, while seminal plasma antibodies are predominantly IgG and IgA. IgG in semen is largely the result of prostatic transudation of serum IgG, while IgA is largely the product of local secretion. The 3 main sites of sperm antigen activity include (1) the tail end-piece, which is probably of no clinical significance; (2) the main tail portion, which reacts to IgG or IgM antibodies and produces decreased motility; and (3) the head portion. Antibodies against the head portion have no effect on motility but will decrease the ability of sperm to attach on the zona pellucida. It appears that not only the site of antigen activity but the type and number of antibodies present affect fertility impairment.

Functional tests such as sperm agglutination or immobilizing assays were the first to identify antisperm antibodies. Sperm agglutination tests (Franklin-Dukes test, Kibrick test, Tray agglutination test, microagglutination test) are indirect assays that rely on agglutination of sperm by the binding of antibodies to antigenic sites. The number of binding sites on the immunoglobulin surface determines the degree of agglutination. These agglutination studies are confounded by nonimmunoglobulin-mediated factors such as bacterial contamination as well as by nonimmunoglobulin proteins in serum. These lead to false-positive reactions. The sperm immobilization test (Isojima test) involves complement-dependent IgG and IgM antibodies, which result in loss of motility, usually accompanied by cytotoxicity. This is a highly reliable, reproducible test with essentially no false-positive results.

Newer techniques have been devised to detect the presence and type of immunoglobulins on the surface of the sperm. This technique appears to be more direct, with greater clinical relevance. The immunobead-binding (IBB) technique uses polyacrylamide spheres (Immunobeads [produced by Bio-Red]) to which isotype-specific rabbit antihuman antibodies are linked. It detects the presence of antibodies, the site on the sperm's surface to which the antibodies are attached, and the isotype of the antibody (IgG, IgM, IgA). A recent comparative study shows that the immunobead-binding technique correlated well with tray and gelatin agglutination testing, as well as with sperm immobilization testing. It is a quick, simple test, provided that sufficient motile sperm are present for study. With poor sperm motility, indirect im-

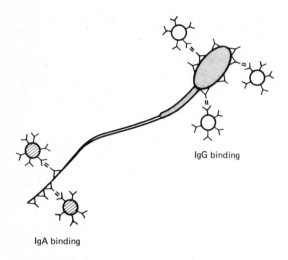

IgG binding

IgA binding

Figure 36–7. Immunobead reaction. The antibody to human IgG and IgA (immunobead) attached to sperm-bound antibody.

munobead-binding testing may be used with serum or seminal plasma and donor sperm (Fig 36–7).

E. Testicular Biopsy; Seminal Vesiculography and Vasography: The use of testicular biopsy has declined in recent years. Histologic study of the biopsy specimen does not indicate the degree of testicular function present or the cause of testicular damage. However, in azoospermic patients with normal FSH levels, primary spermatogenic defects cannot be differentiated from obstructive lesions by hormonal investigation alone, and testicular biopsy and vasography should be considered. When patients have azoospermia or severe oligospermia and markedly shrunken testes, serum FSH levels should be determined; if they are elevated (> twice normal), testicular biopsy can be avoided. Such a patient almost always has irreversible germ cell damage. The exception is the patient who has undergone chemotherapy, in whom the elevated FSH level may normalize with return of spermatogenesis.

Rarely, testicular biopsy is warranted in men with severe oligospemia to rule out partial obstruction. However, this is so uncommon that routine biopsy for severe oligospermia is not indicated. Before biopsy, obvious causes of azoospermia should be eliminated, and at least 2 semen analyses should reveal azoospermia. Retrograde ejaculation should be ruled out by examining the postejaculatory urine. In men with acidic semen (pH < 7.0) and a volume of less than 1 mL, suspect ejaculatory obstruction or congenital absence of the seminal vesicles and vas deferens. For confirmation, seminal fructose levels should be determined. The presence of fructose rules out obstruction or atresia of the ejaculatory ducts but does not verify total ductal patency. Vasography must be done to verify the point of obstruction.

Only when there is clinical suggestion of different pathologic conditions on each side are bilateral biop-

sies indicated. The sample of testicular tissue should be placed atraumatically into a container with Bouin's, Zenker's, or Conroy's solution. Formalin should be avoided, as it distorts the testicular architecture.

When vasography is performed, the dye should be injected in a distal direction (toward the penis). If the dye is injected in a proximal direction (toward the testis), it is extremely difficult to interpret the images of the epididymal anatomy, and there is a significant risk of rupturing the delicate epididymal tubule. Injection of 3–5 mL of diatrizoate sodium 50% (Hypaque) or diatrizoate meglumine 52% plus diatrizoate sodium 8% (Renografin-60) will provide adequate films of the vas, seminal vesicles, and ejaculatory duct (Fig 36–8).

F. Sperm Function Tests:

1. Sperm-cervical mucus interaction– Aspects of sperm function related to transport in the female may be assessed by evaluation of sperm with cervical mucus. The postcoital test involves microscopic examination of the cervical mucus 2–8 hours after intercourse at the time of expected ovulation. A positive result implies normal semen and mucus, while a poor result in an individual with normal semen parameters implies either cervical abnormality or the presence of sperm antibodies. The postcoital test is subject to several variables, including the timing of ovulation. At times other than the mid cycle, cervical mucus is extremely hostile to spermatozoa.

The interaction of sperm and cervical mucus may also be evaluated on a microscope slide or in a capillary tube. Several in vitro sperm-mucus tests are now available that use bovine mucus or mucus from a proved fertile donor. The rate of sperm movement can be objectively compared as a mucus-filled chamber is incubated in a pool of test semen. This allows for evaluation of sperm-mucus interaction under defined conditions with known normal standards. Unfortunately, none of these tests directly evaluate fertility.

If the postcoital test appears abnormal, a semen-mucus cross-penetration test may be performed with the patients and fertile donors in a 4-way comparison to pinpoint the abnormality.

2. Sperm penetration assay (zona-free hamster egg penetration test)– The zona pellucida is the principal barrier to interspecies fertilization between human spermatozoa and oocytes of the golden hamster. When hamster eggs are rendered zona-free and penetrated by human spermatozoa in vitro, they serve as a substitute for human ova in a preliminary assessment of fertilizing capacity. Because both capacitation and the acrosome reaction are required before sperm fusion with (and penetration of) the hamster ovum, this test evaluates the fertilizing capacity of human spermatozoa directly. A positive result occurs when the ova have been penetrated and the sperm head is identified inside the oocyte (Fig 36–9).

Many investigators have shown that fertile and subfertile populations can be differentiated by the sperm penetration assay. Sperm from fertile men will pene-

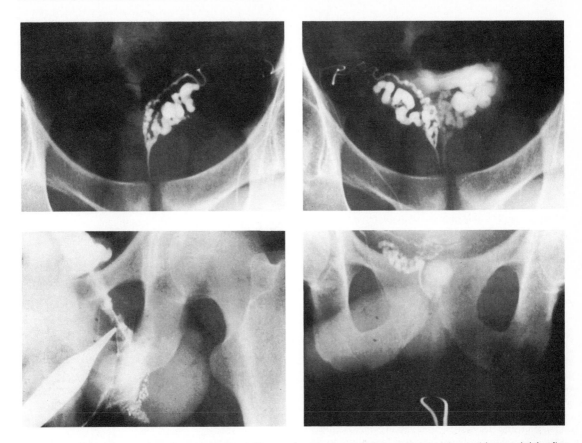

Figure 36–8. Vasography demonstrating (*upper left*) normal-appearing vas and seminal vesicles and (*upper right*) reflux into the bladder, verifying distal patency. Epididymal imaging showing extravasation (*lower left*) and demonstrating the difficulty of determining the point of epididymal obstruction with proximal vasography. *Lower right:* Azoospermia is shown to be the result of a cyst of the ejaculatory duct (*arrow*). (Reproduced, with permission, from McClure RD: Evaluation of the infertile male. In: *Problems in Urology.* DeVere White R [editor]. Lippincott, 1987. [In press.])

trate between 14 and 100% of ova; sperm from infertile men will penetrate less than 10%. Although variations still exist between laboratories, there appears to be general agreement that less than 10% penetration is evidence of sperm dysfunction and male infertility.

The principal advantage of the sperm penetration assay is its ability to detect defects in sperm function that are not assessable by conventional semen analysis. In a series of 62 fertile men, the false-negative rate (sensitivity) was 32% with conventional analysis and 18% with the sperm penetration assay (Rogers, 1985). Excluding individuals with very low sperm counts (who may not be able to impregnate their partners) and those with large numbers of white blood cells in their semen (this causes false-negative findings on sperm penetration assay), the false-negative rate could be lowered to 6.5%. In the same report, the false-positive rate (specificity) in 53 infertile men was 30% for routine semen analysis and only 2% for the sperm penetration assay. Of 143 men whose sperm showed no evidence of penetration on the sperm penetration assay, 16.3% had no readily detectable abnormality on routine semen analysis.

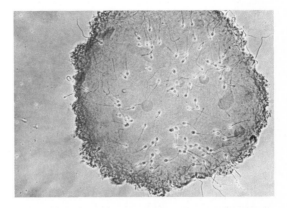

Figure 36–9. Sperm penetration assay. Note the swollen sperm head with tail attached, indicating that the hamster egg has been penetrated. (Reproduced, with permission, from McClure RD: Evaluation of the infertile male. In: *Problems in Urology.* DeVere White R [editor]. Lippincott, 1987. [In press.])

Although the sperm penetration assay is a reliable indicator of the fertilizing capacity of human spermatozoa, it does not predict the ability of sperm to penetrate the zona pellucida or the sperm's motility and progression in the female reproductive tract. Now available clinically, it may be particularly useful in unraveling the causes of unexplained infertility.

G. Bacteriologic Investigation: During the first visit, all individuals should undergo urinalysis to rule out pyuria or bacteriuria. If bacterial prostatitis is implicated by either the history or physical examination, a "3-glass" urinalysis and appropriate cultures are indicated. The common sexually transmitted organisms such as *Chlamydia trachomatis, Mycoplasma hominis,* and *Ureaplasma urealyticum* have been implicated in reproductive failure in animals and humans. On the basis of this supposition, physicians have instituted antibiotic therapy without obtaining evidence of infection in the hope of improving fertility. We recently could find no evidence for the role of current asymptomatic infection due to *Mycoplasma* or *Chlamydia* in male infertility. Without evidence of inflammation (> 5 white blood cells on VB_1), there is no indication for routine culture or antibiotic treatment of infertile men.

H. Androgen-Receptor Abnormalities: Because diagnosis of androgen-receptor abnormalities is extremely difficult and, in these patients, infertility is not treatable, few physicians investigate the possibility of such an abnormality. In several research centers, genital skin fibroblasts are obtained for culture to determine the number of androgen receptors.

I. Radiologic Investigation: Both clinical and laboratory investigations have provided convincing evidence that varicoceles are detrimental to spermatogenesis in some men. Dubin and Amelar (1970) reported that improvement in semen quality after varicocelectomy bears no relation to the palpable size of the varicocele. Because small but clinically significant varicoceles may be missed, even on careful physical examination, several diagnostic techniques have been tried. The Doppler pencil-probe stethoscope is one of the earliest techniques. Questionable regurgitant sounds are a drawback with the Doppler stethoscope, and unequivocal answers cannot be obtained in cases of questionable varicoceles. A polygraph recording helps remove reliance on the physician's ability to recognize auditory venous pulse waves. Another diagnostic technique is scrotal thermography; however, in patients with a single or atrophic testicle or bilateral varicoceles, this test is inadequate, since diagnosis relies on temperature differences between the 2 sides of the scrotum.

Scrotal ultrasonography is a readily available noninvasive method that can detect many intrascrotal abnormalities and has a unique ability to visualize both the testicle and the surrounding structures (Fig 36–10).

Venography appears to be the most specific method of identification, but it is invasive and associated with some morbidity, requires specialized skills and equip-

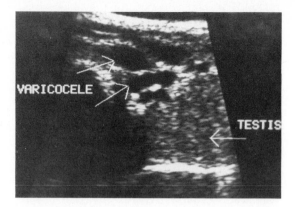

Figure 36–10. Scrotal ultrasound. Varicoceles (*arrow*) are imaged as tubular echo-free structures. (Reproduced, with permission, from McClure RD, Hricak H: Scrotal ultrasound in the infertile male: Detection of subclinical unilateral and bilateral varicoceles. *J Urol* 1986;135:711. ©Williams & Wilkins, 1986.)

ment, and is expensive. It should be reserved for use in recurrent varicoceles for postoperative detection of aberrant veins.

CAUSES

1. PRETESTICULAR CAUSES (Table 36–2)

Hypothalamic Disease

A. Isolated Gonadotropin Deficiency (Kallmann's Syndrome): Isolated gonadotropin deficiency occurs in both the sporadic and familiar form, and although uncommon (1:10,000 men), it is second to Klinefelter's syndrome as a cause of hypogonadism. The original report described the familiar form associated with anosmia, but the eponym now refers to both variants, with and without anosmia. This syndrome may also be associated with other congenital anomalies (eg, congenital deafness, harelip, cleft palate, craniofacial asymmetry, renal abnormalities, color blindness). The hypothalamic hormone GnRH appears to be absent, as exogenous GnRH administra-

Table 36–2. Pretesticular causes of infertility.

Hypothalamic disease
  Isolated gonadotropin deficiency (Kallmann's syndrome)
  Isolated LH deficiency ("fertile eunuch")
  Isolated FSH deficiency
  Congenital hypogonadotropic syndromes
Pituitary disease
  Pituitary insufficiency (tumors, infiltrative processes, operation, radiation)
  Hyperprolactinemia
  Hemochromatosis
  Exogenous hormones (estrogen-androgen excess, glucocorticoid excess, hyper- and hypothyroidism)

tion stimulates the release of both LH and FSH from the pituitary. Except for the gonadotropin deficiency, anterior pituitary function is intact. The syndrome appears to be inherited either as an autosomal recessive trait or an autosomal dominant trait with incomplete penetrance.

The differential diagnosis includes constitutionally delayed puberty, but the presence of anosmia, somatic midline defects, or a positive family history is a clinical clue. Another distinguishing feature of Kallmann's syndrome is testes less than 2 cm in diameter.

B. Isolated LH Deficiency ("Fertile Eunuch"): Individuals with isolated LH deficiency have eunuchoid proportions with variable degrees of virilization and, often, gynecomastia. They characteristically have large testes and ejaculate containing a few sperm. Plasma FSH levels are normal, but both serum LH and serum testosterone concentrations are low normal. The cause appears to be partial gonadotropin deficiency, in which there is adequate LH to stimulate high intratesticular testosterone with resultant spermatogenesis but insufficient testosterone to promote virilization.

C. Isolated FSH Deficiency: In isolated FSH deficiency (rare), patients are normally virilized and have normal testicular size and baseline levels of LH and testosterone. Sperm counts range from nil (azoospermia) to a few (severe oligospermia). Serum FSH levels are low and do not respond to GnRH stimulation.

D. Congenital Hypogonadotropic Syndromes: These are congenital syndromes associated with secondary hypogonadism and a multitude of other somatic findings. Prader-Willi syndrome is characterized by hypogonadism, hypomentia, hypotonia at birth, and obesity. Serum testosterone levels increase after hCG stimulation, and LH and FSH levels respond to chronic GnRH therapy. These findings suggest that the basic defect is a hypothalamic deficiency of GnRH. Laurence-Moon-Bardet-Biedl syndrome, an autosomal recessive trait, is characterized by mental retardation, retinitis pigmentosa, polydactyly, and hypogonadism. As in Prader-Willi syndrome, the hypogonadism is thought to be of hypothalamic origin.

Pituitary Disease

Pituitary insufficiency may result from tumors, infarctions, iatrogenic causes (surgery, irradiation), or one of several infiltrative and granulomatous processes. If pituitary insufficiency occurs prior to puberty, growth retardation associated with adrenal and thyroid deficiency is the major clinical presentation.

Hypogonadism that occurs in a sexually mature male usually has its origin in a pituitary tumor. Decreasing libido, impotence, and infertility may occur years before other symptoms of an expanding tumor, such as headaches, visual abnormalities, and deficiency of thyroid or adrenal hormones. Once an individual has passed through normal puberty, it takes a long time for the secondary sexual characteristics to disappear unless adrenal insufficiency is present. The testes become small and soft. The diagnosis is made by low serum testosterone levels with low or low normal plasma gonadotropin concentrations. Depending upon the degree of panhypopituitarism, plasma corticosteroids will be reduced, as will plasma TSH and growth hormone levels.

A. Hyperprolactinemia: Excessive serum prolactin levels cause both reproductive and sexual dysfunction. Prolactin-secreting tumors of the pituitary gland, whether from a microadenoma (< 10 mm) or macroadenoma, result in loss of libido, impotence, galactorrhea, gynecomastia, and altered spermatogenesis. Patients with a macroadenoma first present with visual field abnormalities and headaches. They should undergo CT scanning of the pituitary and laboratory testing of anterior pituitary, thyroid, and adrenal function. These patients have low serum testosterone levels, but basal serum levels of LH and FSH are either low or low normal and reflect an inadequate pituitary response to depressed testosterone, implicating impaired GnRH secretion. Particularly in individuals with macroadenoma, signs and symptoms of other hormonal derangements (hypothyroidism and hypoadrenalism) should be sought.

B. Hemochromatosis: Approximately 80% of men with this disease have testicular dysfunction. Their hypogonadism may be secondary to iron deposition in the liver or may be primarily testicular, as the result of iron deposition in the testes. Recently, however, iron deposits have been found in the pituitary, implicating this gland as the major site of abnormality.

Exogenous or Endogenous Hormones

A. Estrogen/Androgen Excess: Adrenocortical tumors, Sertoli cell tumors, and interstitial cell tumors of the testes may all at times be estrogen-producing. Similarly, hepatic cirrhosis is often associated with increased endogenous estrogens. Estrogens act primarily by suppressing pituitary gonadotropin secretion, resulting in secondary testicular failure.

Androgens also suppress pituitary gonadotropins to lead to secondary testicular failure. The current use of exogenous androgens (anabolic steroids) by professional athletes may result in temporary sterility. Endogenous excess may be due to an androgen-producing adrenocortical tumor or testicular tumor but more likely congenital adrenal hyperplasia. In this disorder, the enzyme 21-hydroxylase is commonly deficient, resulting in defective cortisol synthesis and excessive production of ACTH. As a consequence, the production of androgenic steroids by the adrenal cortex is increased, resulting in premature development of secondary sexual characteristics and abnormal phallic enlargement. The testes fail to mature because of gonadotropin inhibition and are characteristically small. In the absence of precocious puberty, the diagnosis is extremely difficult, since excessive virilization is difficult to detect in an otherwise normal sexually mature man. Careful laboratory evaluation is essential, particularly in patients with a mild enzyme deficiency. When 21-hydroxylase is deficient, serum levels of 17-hydroxyprogesterone and adrostenedione and urinary pregnanetriol levels should be evaluated.

In the case of classic disease that has been recognized in childhood in patients with precocious puberty and short stature, follow-up has shown that some achieve a normal sperm count and fertility, even when not treated with glucocorticoids. When 21-hydroxylase deficiency is complicated by testicular adrenal rest tumors, oligospermia may develop from mechanical obstruction, destruction of seminiferous tubules, or changes in the testicular or hormonal milieu. Adrenal rest tumors must be differentiated from Leydig cell tumors, as the former are treated by steroids and the latter by orchiectomy.

Infertility caused by documented congenital adrenal hyperplasia is treatable with corticosteroids. However, physicians have used corticosteroids in individuals with idiopathic infertility with a presumptive diagnosis of an attenuated form of congenital adrenal hyperplasia. Unless these abnormalities can be documented, steroid therapy has no place.

B. Glucocorticoid Excess: Whether glucocorticoid excess is exogenous (eg, therapy of ulcerative colitis, asthma, rheumatoid arthritis) or endogenous (Cushing's syndrome), the result is decreased spermatogenesis. The elevated plasma cortisone levels depress LH secretion and cause secondary testicular dysfunction. Correction of the glucocorticoid excess results in improvement of spermatogenesis.

C. Hyper- and Hypothyroidism: Elevated or depressed levels of serum thyroid hormone alter spermatogenesis. Hyperthyroidism affects both pituitary and testicular function, with alterations in the secretion of releasing hormones and increased conversion of androgens to estrogens.

2. TESTICULAR CAUSES
(Table 36–3)

Chromosomal Abnormalities

Several somatic chromosomal abnormalities are associated with male infertility, the incidence increasing as the sperm count decreases. In a study of 1263 barren couples, Kjessler (1974) found the overall incidence of male chromosomal abnormalities to be 6.2%.

Table 36–3. Testicular cause of infertility.

Chromosomal anomalies (Klinefelter's syndrome, XX disorder [sex reversal syndrome], XYY syndrome)
Noonan's syndrome (male Turner's syndrome)
Myotonic dystrophy
Bilateral anorchia (vanishing testes syndrome)
Sertoli-cell-only syndrome (germinal cell aplasia)
Gonadotoxins (drugs, radiation)
Orchitis
Trauma
Systemic disease (renal failure, hepatic disease, sickle cell disease)
Defective androgen synthesis or action
Cryptorchidism
Varicocele

In a subgroup in which the male partner's sperm count was less than 10 million, the incidence rose to 11%. In azoospermic subjects, 21% had significant chromosomal abnormalities. Only in isolated cases, however, has infertility been documented in association with a specific chromosomal abnormality, including D–D translocations, ring abnormalities, reciprocal translocation, and Robertsonian aberrations, but cytogenic studies should be considered in men with severe oligospermia or azoospermia to look for autosomal and sex chromosomal abnormalities.

A. Klinefelter's Syndrome: This genetic disorder is due to the presence of an extra X chromosome in the male, the common karyotype being either 47,XXY (the classic form) or 46,XY/47,XXY (the mosaic form). The incidence is approximately 1:500 males.

Characteristically, these individuals have small, firm testes, decreased androgenicity (delayed sexual maturation), azoospermia, and gynecomastia (Fig 36–11). Because features of hypogonadism are not evident until puberty, the diagnosis is usually delayed. The decrease in testicular mass is usually due to sclerosis and hyalinization of the seminiferous tubules; although the Leydig cells may appear hyperplastic, their total number per testis is normal. The testes characteristically have a length of less than 2 cm and always less than 3.5 cm (corresponding to 2- and 12-mL volumes, respectively).

Gonadotropin levels are characteristically elevated, particularly FSH. Plasma testosterone levels can range from normal to low but decrease with age. Serum estradiol levels are often increased, with a resultant increase in TeBG. The elevated TeBG, resulting in higher levels of bound than free testosterone, explains the difference between the total serum testosterone levels and the degree of androgenicity. The higher estrogen levels relative to testosterone cause the feminized appearance and gynecomastia.

Approximately 10% of these patients have chromosomal mosaicism. They have less severe features of Klinefelter's syndrome and may be fertile, as there may be a normal clone of cells within the testes.

Klinefelter's syndrome may be associated with other endocrine disorders such as thyroiditis and diabetes. Mild mental deficiency and restrictive pulmonary disease occur more frequently in these patients than in the general population.

Infertility is reversible. Later in life, most men will require androgen replacement therapy for optimal virilization and normal sexual function.

B. XX Disorder (Sex Reversal Syndrome): This sex reversal syndrome is a variant of Klinefelter's syndrome. The signs are similar, except that the average height is less than normal, hypospadias is common, and the incidence of mental deficiency is not increased. These patients have a 46,XX chromosome complement. This paradox is explained by the fact that their cells express H-Y antigen, which is coded for by genetic material normally located on the Y chromosome and presumably present somewhere in the genomes of these patients.

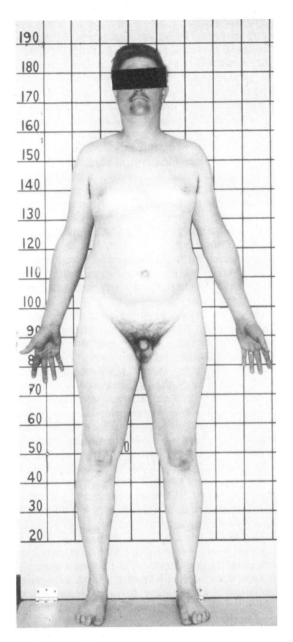
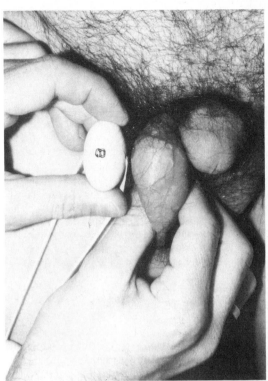

Figure 36–11. Klinefelter's syndrome. *Left:* Note the eunuchoid habitus, female escutcheon, gynecomastia, lack of temporal blading. *Right:* Characteristic firm, small testes. Growth of bones in the lower extremities may be increased, altering the usual upper segment : lower segment ratio seen in hypogonadism. (Reproduced, with permission, from McClure RD: Endocrine investigation and therapy. *Urol Clin North Am* 1987;14:471.)

C. XYY Syndrome: The incidence of XYY syndrome is the same as that of Klinefelter's syndrome, but its phenotypic expression is much more variable. Ejaculates from these subjects may vary from azoospermic to normal. These patients are excessively tall and have had pustular acne. A percentage have antisocial behavior. Most have normal plasma LH and testosterone levels, and the plasma FSH levels depend on the extent of germ cell damage. There is no therapy for individuals with impaired spermatogenesis.

Noonan's Syndrome (Male Turner's Syndrome)

Noonan's syndrome is the male counterpart of Turner's syndrome (XO), and these individuals typically have similar features (short stature, webbed neck, low-set ears, cubitus valgus, ocular abnormalities [ptosis]) and cardiovascular abnormalities. Most males with Noonan's syndrome have cryptorchidism and diminished spermatogenesis and are infertile. Those with diminished testicular function will have elevated serum FSH and LH levels. They demonstrate on karyotype analysis a sex chromosome abnormality such as XO/XY mosaicism and represent a partial sex chromosome monosomy variant of Turner's syndrome. There is no treatment for their impaired spermatogenesis.

Myotonic Dystrophy

In addition to myotonia (delayed relaxation after initial contraction), the major clinical features of myotonic dystrophy include lenticular opacities, frontal baldness, and testicular atrophy. Inheritance is autosomal dominant, and expression is variable (ie, 80% will develop testicular atrophy). Pubertal development is usually normal, and testicular damage occurs later in adult life. Leydig cell function remains normal, and there is no gynecomastia. The serum FSH level is elevated proportionate to the degree of testicular atrophy. There is no therapy for the infertility, and as testosterone levels are normal, no androgen therapy is required.

Bilateral Anorchia
(Vanishing Testes Syndrome)

Bilateral anorchia is an extremely rare disorder (1:20,000 males). Patients present with nonpalpable testes and sexual immaturity because of the absence of testicular androgens. The karyotype is normal, but serum LH and FSH levels are elevated, and serum levels of testosterone are extremely low. The testes may have been lost due to testicular torsion, trauma, vascular injury, or infection. However, functioning testicular tissue must have been present during the first 14–16 weeks of fetal life in order for wolffian duct growth and müllerian duct regression to occur (no uterine remnants) and for the external genitalia to differentiate along male lines. Testosterone does not increase in response to hCG stimulation, in contrast to the increase seen in other patients with bilateral nonpalpable testes. These patients have eunuchoid proportions but no gynecomastia. Therapy is directed at the androgen deficiency.

Sertoli-Cell-Only Syndrome
(Germinal Cell Aplasia)

Sertoli-cell-only syndrome may have several causes, including congenital absence of germ cells, genetic defects, or androgen resistance. Testicular biopsy will reveal complete absence of germinal elements. Clinical findings include azoospermia in association with normal virilization, testes of normal consistency but slightly smaller size, and no gynecomastia. Plasma testosterone and serum LH levels are normal, but plasma FSH levels are usually elevated. With other testicular disorders (mumps, cryptorchidism, damage due to irradiation or toxins, adult seminiferous tubule failure), the seminiferous tubules may also contain only Sertoli cells, but in these men the testes are small, the histologic pattern is not as uniform, and severe sclerosis and hyalinization are prominent features. The prognosis is poor.

Gonadotoxins

A. Drugs: The germinal epithelium, a rapidly dividing tissue, is susceptible to interference of cell division. Cancer chemotherapy has a dose-dependent, potentially devastating effect on the testicular germinal epithelium and may also damage the Leydig cells. The effect also varies with drug class and the age of the patient. The germinal epithelium appears to be more resistant to toxic drugs before puberty than in adulthood. The alkylating agents (chlorambucil, cyclophosphamide, nitrogen mustard) are particularly toxic to the testes. Prevention of chemotherapeutic toxicity to the testes is still under investigation. In several animal studies, the testes were successfully protected during chemotherapy by suppression of testicular activity, but definitive results in humans have yet to be determined. In some patients, cryopreservation of semen can be performed before cancer chemotherapy is begun; however, many untreated patients will have testicular defects and decreased sperm counts caused by the malignant disease.

Drugs may cause infertility by inhibiting testosterone synthesis directly, blocking peripheral androgen action, inhibiting pituitary gonadotropin secretion, or enhancing estrogen levels. Cyproterone, ketoconazole, spironolactone, and alcohol all interfere with testosterone synthesis. The most commonly administered drug known to be an androgen antagonist is cimetidine. Men treated with cimetidine present with gynecomastia and may have decreased sperm counts. Recreational drugs (eg, marihuana, heroin, methadone) are associated with lower serum testosterone levels without a concomitant elevation in plasma LH levels, suggesting a central abnormality as well as a testicular defect. Certain pesticides (eg, dibromochloropropane [DBCP]) have been found to impair testicular function in men.

B. Radiation: Germ cells are particularly sensitive to radiation, while Leydig cells are relatively resistant. At single exposures below 600 rads, germ cell damage is reversible, but above this level of exposure, permanent damage is likely. In patients receiving irradiation for Hodgkin's disease, the testes receive approximately 200 rads. Spermatogenesis may be recovered in these men, but it may take 2–3 years. Elevated serum FSH levels reflect impaired spermatogenesis; once the testes recover, with normalization of spermatogenesis, FSH levels may return to normal.

Orchitis

Approximately 15–25% of adult men who contract mumps (epidemic parotitis) develop orchitis, which is commonly unilateral (bilateral involvement occurs in only 10% of affected men). Testicular atrophy can develop within 1–6 months or may take years. With the advent of the mumps vaccine, the incidence of mumps and associated orchitis is becoming increasingly rare. Fewer than one-third of men with bilateral orchitis recover normal semen parameters.

Syphilis may involve the testicle, producing orchitis with diffuse interstitial edema, gumma formation, and endarteritis.

Trauma

The exposed position of the testicles makes them susceptible to injury and subsequent atrophy. Iatrogenic injury may occur during inguinal surgery and may interfere with testicular blood supply or the ductal system (vas deferens).

Systemic Disease

A. Renal Failure: Uremia in males is associated with decreased libido, impotence, altered spermatogenesis, and gynecomastia. Plasma testosterone levels are decreased, and plasma LH and FSH levels are increased. The rise in serum testosterone to exogenous gonadotropin is blunted, suggesting a primary defect at the testicular level.

The cause of hypogonadism in uremia is still controversial and is probably multifactorial. Serum prolactin levels are elevated in one-fourth of patients. Another theory proposes that the impotence is due to a direct neurotoxic effect of high serum parathyroid hormone levels, and a third theory implicates zinc deficiency. An excess of estrogen may be paramount in the derangement of the hypothalamic-pituitary-gonadal axis. Other nonhormonal factors such as antihypertensive drugs or uremic neuropathy may also play a role in uremic impotence and hypogonadism. In patients who have undergone successful renal transplantation, uremic hypogonadism improves.

B. Cirrhosis of the Liver: A large percentage of males with cirrhosis of the liver have testicular atrophy, impotence, and gynecomastia. Plasma testosterone levels and metabolic clearance rates are decreased. Plasma estradiol is increased as the result of decreased hepatic extraction of androgens with increased conversion to estrogen peripherally. The response of plasma testosterone to hCG stimulation is diminished, suggesting a defect at the testicular level. Basal serum LH and FSH levels are only moderately elevated relative to the low serum testosterone levels; coupled with the lack of hyperresponsiveness to GnRH, this also suggests diminished function at the level of the hypothalamic-pituitary axis. Independent of its effect on the liver, ethanol also acutely reduces testosterone levels by inhibiting testicular testosterone synthesis.

C. Sickle Cell Disease: Many men with sickle cell disease have evidence of hypogonadism (delayed sexual maturation, impaired skeletal growth, reduced testicular size, and, in some, reduced sperm count). Serum testosterone levels are low, but studies have shown basal serum LH and FSH levels to be normal, elevated, or reduced. These discrepancies make it impossible to state definitely that the hypogonadism of sickle cell disease is primary (testicular), secondary (pituitary-hypothalamic), or a mixture of both.

Defective Androgen Synthesis or Action

High intratesticular levels of testosterone are required for spermatogenesis, which thus will be markedly inhibited by any defect in testosterone synthesis or action. Several rare hereditary disorders due to enzymatic defects result in defective testosterone synthesis and are associated with inadequate virilization that is evident at birth as ambiguous genitalia. Enzymatic defects in their mildest form could cause infertility, but at the present time this has not been reported.

Several forms of androgen resistance result in undermasculinization and infertility in males with normally developed external genitalia. Diagnosis is made by the finding of abnormal androgen receptors in a culture of genital skin fibroblasts. Characteristically, there is elevation of serum testosterone and serum LH levels, but these findings are not reliable predictors of which men have a receptor defect. Aimann and Griffin (1982) found that in a group of men with idiopathic infertility (azoospermia), 40% had androgen-receptor deficiency. More recent studies have not verified androgen resistance as a common cause of male infertility.

Cryptorchidism

Crytorchidism is a common developmental defect with an incidence of 0.8% in adult males. The undescended testes start to become morphologically abnormal after age 2. In spite of prophylactic orchidopexy, unilateral cryptorchid patients have reduced fertility potential. It appears that in the cryptorchid individual, there is dysgenesis of both the normally and abnormally descended testes. Semen quality is particularly poor in most patients with bilateral cryptorchidism. Although baseline serum gonadotropin and testosterone levels are normal, there is a supranormal response of both LH and FSH to GnRH stimulation, reflecting compromised testicular function. Although early morphologic alterations in the cryptorchid testes may or may not be reversed by orchidopexy, surgery is recommended at 24 months of age.

Varicocele

Varicocele, or dilation of the veins of the pampiniform plexus, is the most common causative finding in infertile men. It results from backflow of blood secondary to incompetent or absent valves in the spermatic veins. This valvular deficiency, combined with the long vertical course of the internal spermatic vein on the left side, leads to the formation of most varicoceles on the left side (90%). Varicoceles are not commonly seen on the right side, because of the oblique course of the right internal spermatic vein from the vena cava. A unilateral right-sided varicocele suggests venous thrombosis (tumor) or situs inversus. Although it was formerly thought that bilateral varicoceles were rare, newer diagnostic tests have shown the incidence of bilateral varicoceles to be greater than 40%.

The incidence of varicoceles in the adult male population is between 10 and 15% and in individuals evaluated for infertility, between 21 and 41%. Fifty percent of men with varicoceles will have impaired semen quality, but many men with varicoceles are fertile.

To explain the abnormalities in spermatogenesis with varicocele, the following theories have been proposed, though none have been proved: (1) elevation of testicular temperature due to venous stasis; (2) retrograde flow of toxic metabolites from the adrenal or kidney; (3) blood stagnation, with germinal epithelial hypoxia; and (4) alterations in the hypothalamic-pituitary-gonadal axis. Recent experimental models have demonstrated bilateral increase in both testicular blood flow and temperature with altered spermatogenesis.

Idiopathic Infertility

At least 40% of infertile men have idiopathic infertility for which no cause can be identified. As knowledge of male reproductive physiology expands, more unknown causes will be elucidated.

3. POSTTESTICULAR CAUSES
(Table 36–4)

Disorders of Sperm Transport

A. Congenital Disorders: Rarely, portions of the male ductal system are absent or atretic. Absence of the vas deferens can occur on either or both sides and is usually accompanied by absence of the seminal vesicles, ampulla, and a major portion of the epididymis. Males with cystic fibrosis have a high incidence of congenital hypoplasia or absence of these reproductive ducts. Absence of the seminal vesicles is always associated with azoospermia, semen that does not coagulate at ejaculation, and absence of fructose. In Young's syndrome, which is associated with pulmonary disease, the ultrastructure of the cilia is normal but the epididymis is obstructed owing to inspissated material, and these patients are azoospermic.

B. Acquired Disorders: Today, bacterial infection *(Escherichia coli)* in older individuals (> 35 years of age) or *C trachomatis* in younger males may acutely or chronically involve the epididymis, with subsequent scarring and obstruction. Apart from voluntary sterilization, the vas may be accidentally ligated during herniorrhaphy, orchiopexy, and even varicocelectomy.

Table 36–4. Posttesticular causes of infertility.

Disorders of sperm transport
Congenital disorders
Acquired disorders
Functional disorders
Disorders of sperm motility or function
Congenital defects of the sperm tail
Maturation defects
Immunologic disorders
Sexual dysfunction
Infection

C. Functional Obstruction: Injuries to the sympathetic nerves during retroperitoneal lymphadenectomy or extensive pelvic surgery may cause aperistalsis of the vas deferens, resulting in retrograde ejaculation due to failure of bladder neck closure or of emission. Diabetic males with autonomic neuropathy frequently present with both impotence and retrograde ejaculation. Various pharmacologic agents such as phenoxybenzamine, guanethidine, and methyldopa may interfere with the sympathetic nervous system as well.

Spinal cord lesions resulting in quadriplegia or paraplegia will affect spermatozoa transport. There is also impaired spermatogenesis that increases the longer the time from injury and may be related to altered testicular temperature regulation.

Disorders of Sperm Motility or Function

A. Congenital Defects of the Sperm Tail: Immotile cilia syndrome is a group of disorders characterized by immotility or poor motility of spermatozoa. Kartagener's syndrome, a variant of immotile cilia syndrome, consists of chronic sinusitis, bronchiectasis, situs inversus, and immotile sperm. In all these disorders, testicular biopsy is normal and the sperm count adequate, but sperm motility is either markedly reduced or absent. The defective structural abnormality leading to impairment of both the cilia and spermatozoa is seen only with the electron microscope. The defects known to cause immotile cilia syndrome include absent dynein arms, short or absent spokes with no central sheath, and missing central microtubules.

Motility problems may also be associated with a deficiency of the protein carboxylmethylase in the tail of the sperm. This enzyme is required for sperm movement.

B. Maturation Defects: Normal sperm counts but poor motility following vasectomy reversal may be a result of epididymal dysfunction. Chronic intratubular pressure following vasectomy may have a deleterious effect on the epididymis such that spermatozoa may not gain their usual maturation and capacity for motility as they pass through the epididymis following reversal.

C. Immunologic Defects: Breakdown of the blood-testis barrier by infection, trauma, or operation allows sensitization of spermatozoa antigens. Sperm antibodies may be a relative cause of infertility in 3–7% of infertile males. Immunity does not appear to be an all-or-none phenomenon but may contribute to reduced fertility potential. It appears that the number of sperm, the site of antigen activity, and the type of antibody are important.

D. Sexual Dysfunction: Decreased sexual drive, impotence, premature ejaculation, and failure of intromission are all potentially correctable causes of reproductive failure. Decreasing libido and impotence may reflect low serum testosterone levels with an organic cause. Orthodox Jewish couples may, for religious reasons, practice abstinence for one week following the last menstrual flow; this obviously may interfere with the proper coital timing for pregnancy to occur.

E. Infection: High concentrations of gram-negative bacteria (*E coli*) in the semen impair sperm motility. Sexually transmitted organisms such as *C trachomatis, M hominis,* and *U urealyticum* have rarely been implicated in reproductive failure. In both animals and humans, there is no convincing evidence to support the use of routine cultures or empiric therapy in asymptomatic infertile males.

TREATMENT

Surgical Measures

A. Varicocelectomy: The relationship between varicocele, altered spermatogenesis, and infertility is now so widely accepted that varicocelectomy is the most common surgical procedure for infertility in males. This operation improves semen quality in about two-thirds of men and doubles the chance of conception. Ligation of varicoceles eliminates testicular venous reflux by interruption of the internal spermatic veins. Operation may involve a scrotal, inguinal, or retroperitoneal approach. The scrotal approach is the least popular because of the numerous veins encountered as well as the possibility of arterial injury. More recently, percutaneous venographic oc-

clusion has become a popular alternative to surgery. Morbidity rates for this procedure range from 0.5 to 9%, compared with 1–3% with surgical treatment. Risks include peripheral migration of a balloon with lung embolization as well as increased radiation to the gonads. Even surgery is not without the complications of recurrent varicoceles or hydroceles.

B. Vasovasostomy: The popularity of vasectomy as a form of male contraception combined with high rates of divorce and remarriage has led to an increasing number of vasectomy reversals (Fig 36–12). Microscopic techniques have resulted in accurate reapproximation of these fine ductal structures. The success of vasovasostomy appears to be influenced by the length of time that has passed since the vasectomy was performed. Up to 7–8 years postvasectomy, the rate of successful reapproximation (sperm present in the ejaculate) is 80–90%, with a functional success rate (pregnancy rate) of 50–60%. Failures of vasovasostomy may be attributed to anastomotic stenosis, sperm antibodies, epididymal dysfunction, or an unrecognized epididymal tubule blowout with subsequent obstruction. The latter condition should be suspected when, at the time of the initial vasovasostomy, there is lack of fluid containing spermatozoa in the cut end of the testicular portion of the vas. Chronic intratubular pressure may cause an epididymal blowout, with subsequent spermatic granuloma and obstruction in the epididymal tubule.

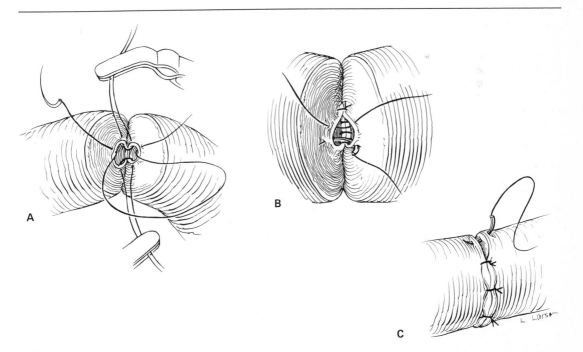

Figure 36–12. Two-layer microsurgical vasovasostomy. *A:* The first 2 mucosal sutures of 10–0 nylon are placed anteriorly 180 degrees apart and held in neurosurgical Heifetz microclips. Suture includes the elastic layer next to the mucosa. The third stitch is placed between these sutures and tied. The clips are removed and the first 2 sutures tied. *B:* The muscularis layer of the anterior layer is completed with 9–0 nylon sutures. The clamp is then flipped 180 degrees, and the posterior layer of the vas is sewn. *C:* Placement of sutures in the posterior muscularis layer. (Reproduced, with permission, from McClure RD: Microsurgery of the male reproductive system. *World J Urol* 1986;4:105.)

C. Epididymovasostomy: The solitary epididymal tubule may be obstructed due to a granuloma as described above. This may be a congenital disorder or due to an inflammatory condition. Spermatozoa gain maturation and the capacity for motility as they move from the caput to the cauda of the epididymis. The bypass anastomosis should therefore be placed as low on the epididymis as possible. Microsurgery allows direct microtubular anastomosis between the epididymal tubule and the cut end of the vas. This operation is much more difficult than vasovasostomy, and success rates are usually less than 30%.

D. Transurethral Resection of Ejaculatory Duct: Patients present with azoospermia, normal-sized testes, normal testicular biopsy, and vasography demonstrating ejaculatory duct obstruction. Before transurethral resection of the orifice of the ejaculatory duct, the posterior urethra and bladder neck are inspected endoscopically. The distal ends of the ducts must be incised or unroofed as they lie within the posterior floor of the prostatic urethra, lateral to the verumontanum but proximal to the external sphincter.

E. Artificial Spermatocele: Surgeons have devised reservoirs (artificial spermatoceles) to collect spermatozoa from individuals with irreparable reproductive ducts (congenital aplasia of the vas deferens, extensive vasal scarring, obstruction of the ejaculatory duct). The spermatozoa collected from these devices have been used for artificial insemination. The resultant low pregnancy rate (nil in the USA) is due to failure to maintain the patency of the epididymal tubule and the extremely poor motility of the collected spermatozoa. A recent review of European literature shows that of a total of 130 spermatoceles placed in 91 patients, there were only 5 live births. Individuals with less than 20% motile sperm interoperatively should not undergo implantation of the device. A viable alternative treatment of obstructive azoospermia is to collect spermatozoa by microaspiration and perform in vitro fertilization.

F. Ablation of Pituitary Adenoma: Therapeutic use of the dopamine agonist bromocriptine or, in selected cases, transphenoidal surgical ablation of a pituitary micro- or macroadenoma may be required in individuals with impotence and a spermatogenic defect associated with elevated prolactin levels (hyperprolactinemia).

G. Prophylactic Surgical Measures:

1. Orchidopexy–Few testes descend spontaneously after 9 months of age. Histologic data show a progressive decrease in the numbers of spermatogonia per tubule beginning before age 2, and orchidopexy is therefore recommended prior to this age. The variable success of medical therapy with hCG has led to the recent use of intranasal GnRH. A number of studies have suggested that it is effective in causing the testicles to descend, while others have not demonstrated any effect. The difference may be related to timing and dosage of the drug.

2. Operation for testicular torsion–A great deal of animal data but few human studies have shown a deleterious effect of an infarcted testis (posttorsion testis) on the contralateral testicle. This effect was thought to be mediated through an autoimmune process resulting from breakdown of the intact blood-testis barrier. It is therefore recommended that the nonviable testicle be removed at the time of diagnosis of torsion.

Medical Measures

A. Endocrine Therapy: Infertile men with hypogonadotropic hypogonadism (secondary hypogonadism) are the only appropriate candidates for exogenous gonadotropin therapy. Previous androgen therapy during puberty will not affect the later responsiveness of the testes.

For initiation of spermatogenesis, LH must be given to stimulate the Leydig cells to produce high intratesticular testosterone levels. hCG (Pregnyl, Profasi HP, APL), 2000 IU intramuscularly 3 times a week, is usually effective in stimulating adequate production of testosterone for full androgenization. Once the patient is fully androgenized and 8–12 months of hCG therapy have not led to production of sperm, FSH therapy should be initiated. FSH is available as human menopausal gonadotropin (hMG). The commercial preparation Pergonal contains 75 IU of FSH and 75 IU of LH per vial. The usual dosage is one-half to one vial intramuscularly 3 times weekly. As hCG and hMG are compatible in solution, the same syringe may be used. It takes months for sperm to appear in the ejaculate after initiation of FSH therapy, and therefore it is important to perform a monthly semen analysis. With a normal response, most patients achieve a sperm count of between 2 and 5 million per ejaculate. In spite of these low counts, impregnation is possible.

Once pregnancy has occurred, FSH therapy can be stopped, and in many individuals, spermatogenesis will be maintained with hCG alone.

An alternative to exogenous gonadotropins is the use of GnRH to stimulate LH and FSH endogenously. GnRH must be given in a pulsatile manner, as continuous administration down-regulates the pituitary. The initial dosage is 25–50 ng/kg every 2 hours by a small infusion pump. Therapy is monitored by its effect on levels of gonadotropins and testosterone, and, eventually, on spermatogenesis. Pituitary disease is not amenable to GnRH therapy, and combined treatment with hCG and hMG will be necessary. Both the gonadotropins and GnRH are expensive, and although GnRH achieves a more physiologic pattern of gonadotropin stimulation, its superiority has yet to be proved.

Individuals with the fertile eunuch syndrome (partial LH deficiency) may respond to hCG therapy alone.

B. Therapy for Immunologic Infertility: Although sperm washing has been used for immunologic infertility, once antibodies are attached, simple washing is unlikely to be effective. One of the oldest methods is the use of condoms for a 6- to 7-month period to decrease the levels of sperm antibodies in the female. There have been no studies to document a decrease in antibody levels or the efficacy of this method.

The optimal form of therapy appears to be corticosteroids. Low doses of 15 mg of prednisone daily for 3–12 months have resulted in normalization of sperm counts in two-thirds of oligospermic patients and pregnancy in the partners of one-third of oligospermic males (Hendry, 1979). Better results have been obtained using short-term, high-dose steroids (pregnancy rate of 44%). Methylprednisolone, 96 mg/d for 7 days starting at day 21 of the woman's cycle for 3 consecutive cycles, is recommended. Side effects of these large doses include gastrointestinal distress, hypertension, personality changes, and, rarely, aseptic necrosis of the hip. A more moderate approach is prednisone, 40 mg twice a day for 10 days, with tapering of dosages on days 11 and 12 (20 mg twice a day for 1 day, and 10 mg twice a day for 1 day) (Lipshultz, personal communication).

C. Therapy for Retrograde Ejaculation: Alkylation of the bladder urine with oral sodium bicarbonate and retrieval of sperm from the bladder after ejaculation have been used successfully for artificial insemination. The addition of 4% human albumin to the retrieved sperm may increase their fertility potential.

Antegrade ejaculation may be induced by treatment with alpha-adrenergic stimulation using sympathomimetic agents. Phenylpropanolamine (Ornade), 1 capsule twice a day, and pseudoephedrine are commonly used agents. Others have had equal success with the antidepressant imipramine (Tofranil), 25–50 mg/d.

D. Treatment of Infection: Individuals with symptomatic genitourinary tract infection should be treated with the appropriate antibiotics. Tetracycline is the drug of choice for both *Chlamydia* and *Mycoplasma*.

E. Empiric Therapy: A large percentage of infertile men (40%) fall into the category of idiopathic or unexplained infertility. Many are treated empirically. The great number of these therapeutic modalities attests to the inability to find one or 2 that really work. Most of these drug trials have not been controlled, blind, or cross-over in nature. Although there are few scientific data on which to base therapy, almost all patients wish to be treated even though the only available therapy is nonspecific.

1. Antiestrogens–Antiestrogens interfere with the normal feedback of circulating estrogens and result in an increase in GnRH that stimulates endogenous gonadotropin secretion. The resulting testicular stimulation increases intratesticular testosterone levels and, in theory, should improve spermatogenesis.

Clomiphene (Clomid), one of the most widely used drugs in male infertility, acts as a competitive inhibitor of estrogen action. Clomiphene is given in a dose of 25–50 mg/d for 3–6 months. Although there are multiple studies that show a positive effect of the drug on semen parameters, there is no absolute evidence that clomiphene will substantially improve pregnancy

rates. Recent studies (Wang, 1985) have shown an increase in sperm counts in some individuals but without concomitant changes in sperm function on sperm penetration assay.

Tamoxifen (Nolvadex), similar in action to clomiphene, is a popular drug for male infertility in Europe. It is given in a dose of 20 mg/d. As with clomiphene, there is no evidence to show overall effectiveness in infertile men with normal levels of gonadotropins.

Testolactone (Teslac), an aromatase inhibitor, prevents the conversion of testosterone to estradiol. Because estrogen has a detrimental effect on spermatogenesis and interferes with the reproductive axis, it was thought that testolactone might improve spermatogenesis. The initial study of 10 individuals treated for 6–12 months with 1 g/d showed a significant increase in sperm counts, no change in sperm motility, and 3 pregnancies. Unfortunately, a subsequent study with a control group showed no significant improvement.

2. Androgens–Testosterone rebound was at one time a popular form of therapy. Parenteral testosterone suppressed the gonadotropins, resulting in inhibition of spermatogenesis. After testicular function was suppressed temporarily for 3–4 months, the therapy was stopped, and it was hoped that spermatogenesis would rebound, producing sperm of better quality and number than before therapy. The enthusiastic report by Rowley and Heller (1972) of 157 men with a subsequent 41% pregnancy rate has not been equaled by other investigators. The inconvenience of parenteral injections as well as the occasional failure of sperm counts to return to normal after suppression has led to its disuse.

Low-dose oral androgens at therapeutic levels not thought to suppress gonadotropins have been used to directly stimulate the germinal epithelium and epididymis. Methyltestosterone, 10–15 mg/d, fluoxymesterone, 15–20 mg/d, or mesterolone, 50–75 mg/d, may not suppress spermatogenesis, although there is no convincing evidence that sperm motility improves. Although Brown (1975) reported increased motility in 30–58% of asthenospermic men, others have had variable success with androgen therapy.

3. hMG and hCG–Based on the stimulation of spermatogenesis by gonadotropins in hypogonadotropic individuals, clinicians have used hMG and hCG in an attempt to stimulate spermatogenesis. Administration of hMG alone has increased sperm density, but the conception rate has been less than 20%, and several reports have not been sufficiently favorable to encourage its use. Sherins (1974) treated 11 males with idiopathic infertility with hCG and found a doubling of serum testosterone levels, but semen quality did not improve and there were no pregnancies. Subsequent therapy with combined hCG and hMG produced no improvement in either sperm quality or the pregnancy rate. hCG has been used in individuals with sperm density of less than 10 million who were undergoing varicocelectomies. This has improved the fertility rate with operation alone from 22 to 44%.

4. GnRH— Trials of GnRH as a therapeutic agent for infertility are still in their infancy. Several trials in Europe have shown an increase in sperm count and motility (67 and 71%, respectively), with a pregnancy rate of 24–49%. This drug has a short biologic half-life and must be administered in a pulsatile fashion with the use of a portable pump or frequent nasal sprays.

5. Kallikrein— Kallikrein is a tissue hormone-releasing polypeptide that releases kinins in both male and female genital secretions. These kinins are reported to enhance sperm motility, and in European studies there has been a 67% increase in sperm motility, with a pregnancy rate of 17–38%. Epididymal or prostatic inflammation is a side effect of this drug.

6. Historical therapies— Arginine, bromocriptine, corticosteroids, and thyroid should be relegated to the shelf, as they have not had any effect on infertility when used empirically.

Artificial Insemination (AIH)

By definition, artificial insemination involves use of the husband's sperm for insemination. AIH is particularly useful with low semen volumes or in cases where repeated postcoital tests have shown cervical hostility. There is no documented advantage in individuals with oligospermia or asthenospermia. The technique of AIH may vary; semen can be placed in the vagina, on the cervix, or within the uterine cavity.

Use of ultrasound to document enlarging follicles and urine testing to predict the timing of the LH surge (ovulation) will increase the success rate.

New Therapies

A. Semen Processing: Various attempts at in vitro manipulation by enhancing spermatic function by removing adverse seminal fluid factors or by extracting a more normal and motile sperm population have potential usefulness. Percoll gradients or albumin gradients have been used for selection of motile spermatozoa (sperm enhancement). The swim-up technique allows the more motile spermatozoa to swim up to a capacitating solution (Ham's F-10 or Bigger's-Whitten-Whittingham [BWW] solution). There appears to be significant increase in the number of progressively motile sperm selected by these techniques. These techniques hold promise for use in intrauterine or in vitro fertilization settings.

B. In Vitro Fertilization (IVF): Originally intended for individuals with female factor or unexplained infertility, use of in vitro fertilization has been expanded to include couples with male factor infertility. Presently, human ova can be fertilized using this technique, with concentrations of 20,000–100,000 motile sperm. IVF eliminates many of the formidable obstacles to human spermatozoa in the female reproductive tract. Proper screening methods are being devised to select which oligoasthenospermic individuals may benefit from IVF.

REFERENCES

Male Reproductive Physiology

Amann RP, Howards SS: Daily spermatozoal production and epididymal spermatozoal reserves of the human male. *J Urol* 1980;**124**:211.

Bardin CW, Paulson CA: The testes. In: *Textbook of Endocrinology,* 6th ed. Williams RH (editor). Saunders, 1981.

Clermont Y: The cycle of the seminiferous epithelium in man. *Am J Anat* 1963;**112**:35.

Ewing LL, Chang TSK: The testis, epididymis, and ductus deferens. In: *Campbell's Urology,* 5th ed. Walsh PC et al (editors). Saunders, 1986.

Griffin JE, Wilson JD: Disorders of the testes and male reproductive tract. In: *Williams Textbook of Endocrinology,* 7th ed. Wilson JD, Foster DW (editors). Saunders, 1985.

Heller CG, Clermont Y: Kinetics of the germinal epithelium. *Recent Prog Horm Res* 1964;**20**:545.

Hinrichsen MJ, Blaquier JA: Evidence supporting the existence of sperm maturation in the human epididymis. *J Reprod Fertil* 1980;**60**:291.

Howards SS: The epididymis, sperm maturation and capacitation. In: *Infertility in the Male.* Lipshultz LI, Howards SS (editors). Churchill Livingstone, 1983.

Matsumoto AM, Karpas AE, Bremner WJ: Chronic human chorionic gonadotropin administration in normal men: Evidence that follicle-stimulating hormone is necessary for the maintenance of quantitatively normal spermato-

genesis in man. *J Clin Endocrinol Metab* 1986;**62**:1184.

Pardridge WM: Transport of protein-bound hormones into tissues in vivo. *Endocr Rev* 1981;**2**:103.

Steinberger E: Hormonal control of mammalian spermatogenesis. *Physiol Rev* 1971;**51**:1.

Vigersky RA: Normal testicular physiology. In: *Urologic Endocrinology.* Rajfer J (editor). Saunders, 1986.

Evaluation of Male Infertility

Aitken RJ: Use of sperm-ova penetration tests to evaluate the infertile couple. In: *Male Reproductive Dysfunction.* Santen RJ, Swerdloff RS (editors). Marcel Dekker, 1986.

Baker HWG et al: Relative incidence of etiological disorders in male infertility. In: *Male Reproductive Dysfunction.* Santen RJ, Swerdloff RS (editors). Marcel Dekker, 1986.

Beitins IZ et al: Hypogonadism in a male with an immunologically active, biologically inactive luteinizing hormone: Characterization of the abnormal hormone. *J Clin Endocrinol Metab* 1981;**52**:1143.

Boreau J: *Images of the Seminal Tracts.* Karger, 1974.

Bronson R et al: Anti-sperm antibodies, detected by agglutination, immobilization, microcytoxicity and immunobead-binding assays. *J Reprod Immunol* 1985;**8**:279.

Dubin L, Amelar RD: Varicocele size and results of varicocelectomy in selected subfertile men with varicocele. *Fertil Steril* 1970;**21**:606.

Eil C et al: Whole cell and nuclear androgen uptake in skin

fibroblasts from infertile men. *J Androl* 1985;**6**:365.

Eliasson R et al: The immotile-cilia syndrome: A congenital ciliary abnormality as an etiologic factor in chronic airway infections and male sterility. *N Engl J Med* 1977;**297**:1.

Goldzieher JW et al: Improving the diagnostic reliability of rapidly fluctuating plasma hormone levels by optimized multiple-sampling techniques. *J Clin Endocrinol Metab* 1976;**43**:824.

Hellström WJG et al: Is there a role for *Chlamydia trachomatis* and genital mycoplasma in male infertility? *Fertil Steril* 1987;**48**:337.

Katz DF et al: Real-time analysis of sperm motion using automatic video image digitization. *Comput Methods Programs Biomed* 1985;**21**:173.

Kidd GS, Glass AR, Vigersky RA: The hypothalamic-pituitary-testicular axis in thyrotoxicosis. *J Clin Endocrinol Metab* 1979;**48**:798.

Kjessler B: Facteurs genetiques dans la subfertile male humaine. In: *Fécondité et Stérilité du Male: Acquisitions récentes*. Masson, 1972.

Lipshultz LI, Howards SS: Evaluation of the subfertile male. In: *Infertility in the Male*. Lipshultz LI, Howards SS (editors). Churchill Livingstone, 1983.

MacLeod J, Gold RZ: The male factor in fertility and infertility. 2. Spermatozoan counts in 1000 men of known fertility and in 1000 cases of infertile marriage. *J Urol* 1951;**66**:436.

Marshall JC: Investigative procedures. *Clin Endocrinol Metab* 1975;**4**:545.

McClure RD: Endocrine investigation and therapy. *Urol Clin North Am* 1987;**14**:471.

McClure RD: Evaluation of the infertile male. In: *Problems in Urology*. DeVere White R (editor). Lippincott, 1987. [In press.]

McClure RD, Hricak H: Scrotal ultrasound in the infertile man: Detection of subclinical unilateral and bilateral varicoceles. *J Urol* 1986;**135**:711.

Overstreet JW: Sperm penetration of cervical mucus. *Fertil Steril* 1986;**45**:324.

Rajfer J (editor): Cryptorchidism. *Urol Clin North Am* 1982;**9**:315.

Rodriguez-Rigau LJ, Smith KD, Steinberger E: Varicocele and the morphology of spermatozoa. *Fertil Steril* 1981;**35**:54.

Rogers BJ: The sperm penetration assay: Its usefulness reevaluated. *Fertil Steril* 1985;**43**:821.

Santen RJ, Bardin CW: Episodic luteinizing hormone secretion in man: Pulse analysis, clinical interpretation, physiologic mechanisms. *J Clin Invest* 1973;**52**:2617.

Saypol DC: Varicocele. *J Androl* 1981;**2**:61.

Sherins RJ, Brightwell D, Sternthal PM: Longitudinal analysis of semen of fertile and infertile men. In: *The Testis in Normal and Infertile Men*. Troen P, Nankin HR (editors). Raven Press, 1977.

Smith KD, Rodriguez-Rigau LJ, Steinberger E: Relation between indices of semen analysis and pregnancy rate in infertile couple. *Fertil Steril* 1977;**28**:1314.

Snyder PJ et al: Repetitive infusion of gonadotropin-releasing hormone distinguishes hypothalamic from pituitary hypogonadism. *J Clin Endocrinol Metab* 1979;**48**:864.

Swerdloff RS, Boyers SP: Evaluation of the male partner of an infertile couple: An algorithmic approach. *JAMA* 1982;**247**:2418.

World Health Organization: *Laboratory Manual for the Examination of Human Semen and Semen-Cervical Mucus Interaction*. Belsey MA et al (editors). Press Concern, 1980.

Zachmann M et al: Testicular volume during adolescence: Cross-sectional and longitudinal studies. *Helv Paediatr Acta* 1974;**29**:61.

Causes of Male Infertility—Pretesticular

Bray GA et al: The Prader-Willi syndrome: A study of 40 patients and a review of the literature. *Medicine* 1983;**62**:59.

Carter JN et al: Prolactin-secreting tumors and hypogonadism in 22 men. *N Engl J Med* 1978;**299**:847.

Charbonnel B et al: Pituitary function in idiopathic haemochromatosis: Hormonal study in 36 male patients. *Acta Endocrinol* 1981;**98**:178.

Cutfield RG, Bateman JM, Odell WD: Infertility caused by bilateral testicular masses secondary to congenital adrenal hyperplasia (21-hydroxylase deficiency). *Fertil Steril* 1983;**40**:809.

Danish RK et al: Micropenis. 2. Hypogonadotropic hypogonadism. *Johns Hopkins Med J* 1980;**146**:177.

Fairman C et al: The "fertile eunuch" syndrome: Demonstration of isolated luteinizing hormone deficiency by radioimmunoassay technique. *Mayo Clin Proc* 1968;**43**:661.

Lieblich JM et al: Syndrome of anosmia with hypogonadotropic hypogonadism (Kallmann syndrome): Clinical and laboratory studies in 23 cases. *Am J Med* 1982;**73**:506.

Mozaffarian GA, Higley M, Paulsen CA: Clinical studies in an adult male patient with "isolated follicle stimulating hormone (FSH) deficiency." *J Androl* 1983;**4**:393.

Segal S, Polishuk WZ, Ben-David M: Hyperprolactinemic male infertility. *Fertil Steril* 1976;**27**:1425.

Urban MD, Lee PA, Migeon CJ: Adult height and fertility in men with congenital virilizing adrenal hyperplasia. *N Engl J Med* 1978;**299**:1392.

Causes of Male Infertility—Testicular

Abbasi AA et al: Gonadal function abnormalities in sickle cell anemia: Studies in adult male patients. *Ann Intern Med* 1976;**85**:601.

Aiman J, Griffin JE: The frequency of androgen receptor deficiency in infertile men. *J Clin Endocrinol Metab* 1982;**54**:725.

Aynsley-Green A et al: Congenital bilateral anorchia in childhood: A clinical, endocrine and therapeutic evaluation of twenty-one cases. *Clin Endocrinol* 1976;**5**:381.

Beard CM et al: The incidence and outcome of mumps orchitis in Rochester, Minnesota, 1935 to 1974. *Mayo Clin Proc* 1977;**52**:3.

Collins E, Turner G: The Noonan syndrome: A review of the clinical and genetic features of 27 cases. *J Pediatr* 1973;**83**:941.

Damewood MD, Grochow LB: Prospects for fertility after chemotherapy or radiation for neoplastic disease. *Fertil Steril* 1986;**45**:443.

De Kretser DM et al: Hormonal, histological and chromosomal studies in adult males with testicular disorders. *J Clin Endocrinol Metab* 1972;**35**:392.

Fowler JE Jr: Infections of the male reproductive tract and infertility: A selected review. *J Androl* 1981;**3**:121.

Griffin JE, Wilson JD: The syndromes of androgen resistance. *N Engl J Med* 1980;**302**:198.

Handelsman DJ: Hypothalamic-pituitary gonadal dysfunction in renal failure, dialysis and renal transplantation. *Endocr Rev* 1985;**6**:151.

Kjessler B: Chromosomal constitution and male reproductive failure. In: *Male Fertility and Sterility*. Mancini RE, Martini L (editors). Academic Press, 1974.

Lipshultz LI et al: Testicular function after orchiopexy for unilaterally undescended testis. *N Engl J Med* 1976;**295**:15.

Paulsen CA et al: Klinefelter's syndrome and its variants: A hormonal and chromosomal study. *Recent Prog Horm Res* 1968;**24**:321.

Saypol DC: Varicocele. *J Androl* 1981;**2**:61.

Schilsky RL, Sherins RJ: Gonadal dysfunction. In: *Cancer: Principles and Practice of Oncology.* DeVita VT Jr, Hellman S, Rosenberg S (editors). Lippincott, 1985.

Takeda R, Ueda M: Pituitary-gonadal function in male patients with myotonic dystrophy: Serum luteinizing hormone, follicle stimulating hormone and testosterone levels and histological damage of the testis. *Acta Endocrinol* 1977;**84**:382.

Toth A et al: Subsequent pregnancies among 161 couples treated for T-mycoplasma genital-tract infection. *N Engl J Med* 1983;**308**:505.

Van Thiel DH, Lester R, Sherins RJ: Evidence for a defect in pituitary secretions of luteinizing hormone in chronic alcoholic men. *J Clin Endocrinol Metab* 1978;**47**:499.

Whorton MD: Male occupational reproductive hazards. *West J Med* 1982;**137**:521.

Wong TW et al: Pathological aspects of the infertile testis. *Urol Clin North Am* 1978;**5**:503.

Causes of Male Infertility–Posttesticular

Afzelius BA, Mossberg B: The immotile-cilia syndrome including Kartagener's syndrome. Chap 91, pp 1986–1994, in: *The Metabolic Basis of Inherited Disease,* 5th ed. Stanbury JB et al (editors). McGraw-Hill, 1983.

Bronson R, Cooper G, Rosenfeld D: Sperm antibodies: Their role in infertility. *Fertil Steril* 1984;**42**:171.

Gagnon C et al: Deficiency of protein-carboxyl methylase in immotile spermatozoa of infertile men. *N Engl J Med* 1982;**306**:821.

Handelsman DJ et al: Young's syndrome: Obstructive azoospermia and chronic sinopulmonary infections. *N Engl J Med* 1984;**310**:3.

Nagler HM, Deitch AD, deVere White R: Testicular torsion: Temporal considerations. *Fertil Steril* 1984;**42**:257.

Treatment

Acosta AA et al: In vitro fertilization and the male factor. *Urology* 1986;**28**:1.

Al-Ansari AA et al: Isolated follicle-stimulating hormone deficiency in men: Successful long-term gonadotropin therapy. *Fertil Steril* 1984;**42**:618.

Aparicio NJ et al: Treatment of idiopathic normogonadotropic oligoasthenospermia with synthetic luteinizing hormone-releasing hormone. *Fertile Steril* 1976;**27**:549.

Belker AM et al: Absence of motile epididymal sperm contraindicates implantation of alloplastic spermatocele. *J Androl* 1985;**6**:26.

Brown JS: The effect of orally administered androgens on sperm motility. *Fertil Steril* 1975;**26**:305.

Buvat J et al: Increased sperm count in 25 cases of idiopathic normogonadotropic oligospermia following treatment with tamoxifen. *Fertil Steril* 1983;**39**:700.

Clark RV, Sherins RJ: Clinical trial of testolactone for treatment of idiopathic male infertility. (Abstract.) *J Androl* 1983;**4**:31.

Dubin L, Amelar RD: Varicocelectomy as therapy in male infertility: A study of 504 cases. *Fertil Steril* 1975;**26**:217.

Finkel DM, Phillips JL, Snyder PJ: Stimulation of spermatogenesis by gonadotropins in men with hypogonadotropic hypogonadism. *N Engl J Med* 1985;**313**:651.

Hendry WF et al: Cyclic prednisolone therapy for male infertility associated with autoantibodies to spermatozoa. *Fertil Steril* 1986;**45**:249.

Hendry WF et al: The results of intermittent high dose steroid therapy for male infertility due to antisperm antibodies. *Fertil Steril* 1981;**36**:351.

Hendry WF et al: Steroid treatment of male subfertility caused by antisperm antibodies. *Lancet* 1979;**2**:498.

Homonnai ZT, Shilon M, Paz G: Evaluation of semen quality following kallikrein treatment. *Gynecol Obstet Invest* 1978;**9**:132.

Lee HY: Observations of the results of 300 vasovasostomies. *J Androl* 1980;**1**:11.

McClure RD: Microsurgery of the male reproductive system. *World J Urol* 1986;**4**:105.

Rajfer J et al: Hormonal therapy of cryptorchidism: A randomized, double-blind study comparing human chorionic gonadotropin and gonadotropin-releasing hormone. *N Engl J Med* 1986;**314**:466.

Ronnberg L: The effect of clomiphene treatment on different sperm parameters in men with idiopathic oligozoospermia. *Andrologia* 1980;**12**:261.

Rowley MJ, Heller CG: The testosterone rebound phenomenon in the treatment of male infertility. *Fertil Steril* 1972;**23**:498.

Schill WB: Treatment of idiopathic oligozoospermia by kallikrein: Results of a double-blind study. *Arch Androl* 1979;**2**:163.

Sherins RJ: Clinical aspects of treatment of male infertility with gonadotropins: Testicular response of some men given HCG with and without pergonal. Page 545 in: *Male Infertility and Sterility.* Mancini RE, Martini L (editors). Academic Press, 1974.

Sherins RJ: Hypogonadotropic hypogonadism. In: *Current Therapy of Infertility,* 2nd ed. Garcia CR et al (editors). Mosby, 1984.

Shulman JF, Shulman S: Methylprednisolone treatment of immunologic infertility in the male. *Fertil Steril* 1982;**38**:591.

Silber SJ: Vasectomy and its microsurgical reversal. *Urol Clin North Am* 1978;**5**:573.

Spratt DI, Hoffman AR, Crowley WF: Hypogonadotropic hypogonadism and its treatment. In: *Male Reproductive Dysfunction.* Santen RJ, Swerdloff RS (editors). Marcel Dekker, 1986.

Vance ML, Thorner MO: Medical treatment of male infertility. *Semin Urol* 1984;**2**:115.

Vigersky RA, Glass AR: Effects of delta 1-testolactone on the pituitary-testicular axis in oligospermic men. *J Clin Endocrinol Metab* 1981;**52**:897.

Vigersky RA, Glass AR: Treatment of idiopathic oligospermia with testolactone plus tamoxifen. Page 262 in: *Proceedings of the Endocrine Society 65th Annual Meeting, San Antonio, 1983.*

Wang C et al: Clomiphene citrate does not improve spermatozoal fertilizing capacity in idiopathic oligospermia. *Fertil Steril* 1985;**44**:102.

Male Sexual Dysfunction

37

Tom F. Lue, MD

A better understanding of male sexual dysfunction has recently been made possible by innovative laboratory and clinical research in the hemodynamics, neurophysiology, and pharmacology of penile erection. Erectile function can now be evaluated in the office setting by intracavernous injection of vasoactive agents. Improved diagnostic tests can differentiate among types of impotence. More treatment options are being developed, and the latest generation of penile prostheses is more sophisticated and durable than earlier ones. Continuing research offers the possibility of a more physiologic solution to erectile dysfunction.

PHYSIOLOGY OF PENILE ERECTION

Innervation of the Penis

The spinal centers controlling erection were recently demonstrated by a nerve tracing technique that uses horseradish peroxidase (Lue et al, 1984B). The autonomic erection center is located in the intermediolateral nucleus of the spinal cord at levels S_2-S_4 and $T_{12}-L_2$. Branches of the thoracolumbar segments join the inferior hypogastric plexus, which sends branches to the pelvic plexus, which is formed by contributions from sacral nerves. Bundles from these plexuses radiate to the pelvic organs. The fibers innervating the penis (the cavernous nerves) travel along the posterolateral aspect of the seminal vesicles and prostate and then accompany the membranous urethra through the genitourinary diaphragm (Walsh and Donker, 1982). At the prostatic urethra, these fibers are located at the 5 and 7 o'clock positions, and at the membranous urethra, they are at the 3 and 9 o'clock positions; they ascend gradually to the 1 and 11 o'clock positions (at the level of the mid-urethral bulb) and finally enter the hilum of the penis at the level of the distal urethral bulb (Fig 37–1). Some fibers enter the corpora cavernosa and corpus spongiosum with the cavernous and urethral arteries. Others travel farther distally and penetrate the tunica albuginea at mid shaft. The terminal branches of the cavernous nerves innervate the helicine arteries and the trabecular smooth muscle and are responsible for the vascular events during tumescence and detumescence.

The center for somatic motor nerves is located at the Onuf nucleus of the ventral horn of the S_2-S_4 segment (Gomes de Araujo, Schmidt, and Tanagho, 1982). The motor fibers join the pudendal nerve to innervate the bulbocavernosus and ischiocavernosus muscles. The somatic sensory nerves originate at the receptors in the penile skin and glans. Sensations of pain and temperature ascend via the spinothalamic tract; vibratory stimuli are carried in the dorsal column; touch and pressure sensations are transmitted via both pathways to the thalamus. The perception of pleasant or unpleasant emotions probably involves past experience and cortical interpretation.

Three types of erection can be identified: reflexogenic, psychogenic, and nocturnal. Reflexogenic erection is induced by genital stimulation. Afferent fibers controlling this type of erection are in the pudendal nerve and efferent fibers in the sacral parasympathetic nerves. This can be preserved in patients with cervical or thoracic spinal cord lesions. Psychogenic erection, resulting from visual or auditory stimuli or fantasy, is more complex. Cerebral im-

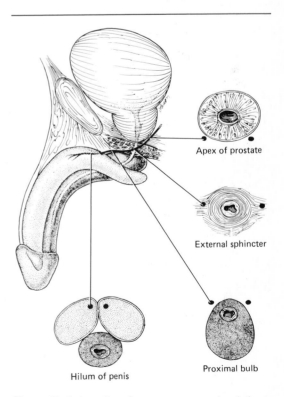

Figure 37–1. Location of cavernous nerves in relation to urethra.

Apex of prostate

External sphincter

Proximal bulb

Hilum of penis

pulses probably pass through the thoracolumbar and sacral centers to the cavernous nerves. The fact that only a small percentage of patients with complete sacral cord lesions can achieve erection suggests that the sacral center exerts major control. Nocturnal (subconscious) erection usually occurs during REM (rapid eye movement) sleep and can be monitored by nocturnal penile tumescence (NPT) testing. This function is quite separate from erection induced by visual or genital stimulation and is retained in psychogenic (Karacan et al, 1975; Fisher et al, 1975) and hormonal impotence (Bancroft and Wu, 1983; Kwan et al, 1983) and in some patients with neurogenic impotence.

Hemodynamics of Penile Erection

The paired internal pudendal artery is the major carrier of the blood supply to the penis. The terminal portion of this artery divides into 4 branches: the artery to the urethral bulb, the urethral artery, the dorsal artery, and the cavernosal artery (deep artery). The cavernosal artery supplies the corpora cavernosa; the dorsal artery, the glans penis; and the bulbar and urethral arteries supply the corpus spongiosum during erection. The venous drainage of the glans is mainly through the deep dorsal vein. The corpus spongiosum is drained via the circumflex and bulbar veins, but the drainage of the corpora cavernosa is more complex: the mid and distal shaft are drained by the deep dorsal vein to the preprostatic plexus; the proximal corpora by the cavernous veins to the preprostatic plexus and internal pudendal vein. The drainage of all 3 corpora originates in the subtunical venules, which unite to form emissary veins that pierce the tunica albuginea. The emissary veins may empty directly or through the circumflex veins into the deep dorsal vein. The glans penis possesses numerous large and small veins that communicate freely with the dorsal veins. The penile skin and subcutaneous tissue are drained by superficial dorsal veins, which then empty into the saphenous veins.

Investigations of human penile blood flow have included Newman's infusion study in cadavers (Newman, Northrup, and Devlin, 1964) and the radioactive xenon washout studies of Wagner and Uhrenholdt (1980) and Shirai et al (1978) in volunteers during visual erotic stimulation. Although the contribution of increased arterial flow has been well established, the role of the venous system has remained controversial. However, studies in dogs and monkeys after electrical stimulation of the cavernous and pudendal nerves and in humans during papaverine-induced erection have finally clarified the role of the arterial, venous, and sinusoidal systems.

The erection process can be divided into phases as shown in Table 37–1 and Fig 37–2.

Studies of erection during visual sexual stimulation (Wagner, 1986 [personal communication]) and REM sleep (Karacan, Aslan, and Hirschkowitz, 1983) have shown synergistic activity of the bulbocavernosus and ischiocavernosus muscles during the erectile process.

Table 37–1. Phases of the erection process.*

Flaccid phase (1)
Minimal arterial and venous flow; blood gas values equal those of venous blood. Flow rate: 2.5–8 mL/100 g/min (Wagner and Uhrenholdt, 1980); 0.5–6.5 mL/100 g/min (Shirai et al, 1978).

Latent (filling) phase (2)
Increased flow in the internal pudendal artery during both systolic and diastolic phases. Decreased pressure in the internal pudendal artery; unchanged intracavernous pressure. Some elongation of the penis.

Tumescent phase (3)
Rising intracavernous pressure until full erection is achieved. Penis shows more expansion and elongation with pulsation. The arterial flow rate decreases as the pressure rises. When intracavernous pressure rises above diastolic pressure, flow occurs only in the systolic phases.

Full erection phase (4)
Intracavernous pressure can rise to as much as 80–90% of the systolic pressure. Pressure in the internal pudendal artery increases but remains slightly below systemic pressure. Arterial flow is much less than in the initial filling phase but is still higher than in the flaccid phase. Although the venous channels are mostly compressed, the venous flow rate is slightly higher than during the flaccid phase. Blood gas values are similar to those of arterial blood.

Skeletal or rigid erection phase (5)
As a result of contraction of the ischiocavernous muscle, the intracavernous pressure rises well above the systolic pressure, resulting in rigid erection. During this phase, almost no blood flows through the cavernous artery; however, the short duration prevents the development of ischemia or tissue damage.

Detumescent phase (6)
After ejaculation or cessation of erotic stimuli, sympathetic tonic discharge resumes, resulting in contraction of the smooth muscles around the sinusoids and arterioles. This effectively diminishes the arterial flow to flaccid levels, expels a large portion of blood from the sinusoidal spaces, and reopens the venous channels. The penis returns to its flaccid length and girth.

*Numbers 1–6 correspond to phases shown in Fig 37–2.

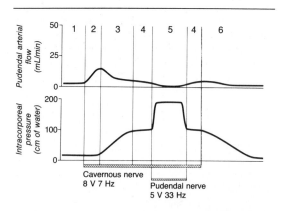
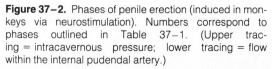

Figure 37–2. Phases of penile erection (induced in monkeys via neurostimulation). Numbers correspond to phases outlined in Table 37–1. (Upper tracing = intracavernous pressure; lower tracing = flow within the internal pudendal artery.)

Separate electrode implantation on the cavernous and pudendal nerves in the animal model as well as papaverine injection in humans and animals has made it possible to study the relative contribution of the autonomic and somatic nerves in the erectile process. Autonomic neural stimulation is responsible for the **vascular stage of erection,** ie, filling and trapping of blood in the cavernous bodies. After full erection is achieved, contraction of the ischiocavernosus muscle compresses the proximal corpora and raises the pressure in the entire corpora well above the systolic blood pressure, resulting in rigid erection (Table 37–1) **(skeletal muscle stage of erection).** This rigid phase occurs naturally during masturbation or sexual intercourse but can also occur from slight bending of the penis, without muscular action. Studies in the animal models (Lue, 1986B) have shown almost no flow in the internal pudendal artery during the rigid erection phase; however, bcause this phase usually lasts only a short period of time, ischemia or tissue damage does not occur.

The hemodynamics of the glans penis are somewhat different. Arterial flow increases in a similar manner in the glans as in the shaft. However, because it lacks the tunica albuginea, the glans functions as an arteriovenous fistula during the full erection phase. Partial compression of the deep dorsal vein within Buck's fascia by the expanded corpora does contribute to the pressure increase in the glans and dorsal vein. Nevertheless, during rigid erection, most of the venous channels are temporarily compressed, and further engorgement of the glans can be observed.

Mechanism of Penile Erection

Based on human cadaveric dissections, Conti (1952) proposed the theory that penile erection is regulated by polsters in the penile arteries and veins. Synergistic contraction or relaxation of these polsters would control the arteriovenous shunting of blood and result in erection or detumescence. This theory was recently challenged by Newman and Tchertkoff (1980), who could not find polsters in newborns, and by Benson et al (1980), who believe that what Conti described were not polsters but atherosclerotic lesions.

By fixing the corpus cavernosum in the erect and flaccid states, anatomic changes can be examined in the dog and monkey (Lue, 1986A). In these models, dilatation of the arterial tree, expansion of the sinusoids, and compression of the subtunical and emissary veins were clearly seen on the erect side in both histologic studies and scanning electron microscopic examination of corrosion casts. The flaccid corpus cavernosum showed contracted sinusoids and tortuous and constricted arteries and arterioles; the subtunical venules and emissary veins were wide open. Histologic examinations and scanning electron microscopic study of human penile tissue and corrosion casts revealed findings similar to those in the flaccid animal corpus. From these studies and observation of papaverine-induced erections, it appears that the smooth muscles in the arteriolar tree and the trabeculae are the key mechanisms in the erectile process. The intrinsic smooth muscle tone and, possibly, the adrenergic tonic discharge maintain contraction of the smooth muscles in the flaccid state. This high peripheral resistance distributed throughout the contracted sinusoids and tortuous and constricted arteriolar and arterial tree allows only a minimal amount of flow to enter the sinusoidal spaces. When the smooth muscles relax due to release of neurotransmitters or injection of alpha-adrenergics or a smooth-muscle relaxant, the compliance of the sinusoidal spaces and the arterial tree increases and the resistance to incoming flow drops to a minimum. This allows arterial and arteriolar vasodilatation and easy expansion of the sinusoids to receive a large increase of flow. Trapping of blood due to increased compliance of the entire sinusoidal system causes the penis to lengthen and widen rapidly until the capacity of the tunica albuginea is reached. Meanwhile, expansion of the sinusoidal walls against one another and against the tunica albuginea results in compression of the subtunical venular plexus. Further expansion will stretch the tunica albuginea and effectively reduce the flow in the emissary veins to a minimum (Fig 37–3A and B). Because flow to the penis is not constant (as evidenced by the tremendous flow increase in the internal pudendal artery during erection), there is no need to have an arteriovenous shunt to divert excess blood from the penis. Thus, polsters, if they do exist, serve no necessary function. Furthermore, it becomes obvious that contraction and relaxation of the smooth muscles of the trabeculae and the arteriolar tree are the mechanisms that control erection.

Hormones & Sexual Function

Androgens are essential for male sexual maturity. Testosterone regulates gonadotropin secretion and muscle development; dihydrotestosterone mediates all other aspects of male sexual maturation, including hair growth, acne, male-pattern baldness, and spermatogenesis. In adults, androgen deficiency results in loss of sexual interest and impaired seminal emission. The frequency, magnitude, and latency of nocturnal penile erections are reduced. However, studies have shown that erection in response to visual sexual stimulation is not affected by androgen withdrawal in hypogonadal men, suggesting that androgen enhances but is not essential for erection (Bancroft and Wu, 1983; Kwan et al, 1983).

A progressive decline in testosterone occurs after the seventh decade. Studies suggest that this may be partly of testicular origin and partly due to hypothalamic-pituitary dysfunction (Deslypere and Vermeulen, 1984). It is not known whether there is a threshold level of androgen above which a further increase will have no effect on sexual interest. However, it has been shown that exogenous testosterone does increase sexual interest in some men with levels in the "laboratory normal" range. Further studies are needed to determine if there is such a threshold and whether it changes with age (O'Carroll and Bancroft, 1984).

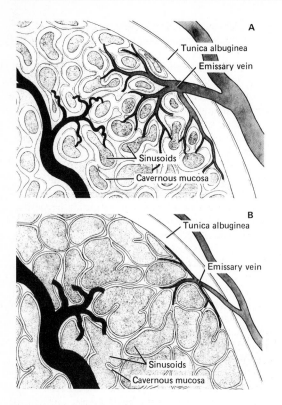

Figure 37–3. The mechanism of penile erection. In the flaccid state *(A)*, the arteries, arterioles, and sinusoids are contracted. The intersinusoidal and subtunical venular plexuses are wide open, with free flow to the emissary veins. In the erect state *(B)*, the muscles of the sinusoidal wall and the arterioles relax, allowing maximal flow to the compliant sinusoidal spaces. Most of the venules are compressed between the expanding sinusoids. Even the larger intermediary venules are sandwiched and flattened by distended sinusoids and the noncompliant tunica albuginea. This effectively reduces the venous capacity to a minimum.

Neurotransmitters & the Pharmacology of Erection

The neurotransmitters controlling penile erection are still under investigation, but several have been shown to be present in the penile tissue and around the helicine arteries: vasoactive intestinal polypeptide (VIP) (Polack et al, 1981); acetylcholine (Saenz de Tejada et al, 1985); and norepinephrine (Levin and Wein, 1980; McConnell, Benson, and Wood, 1979). Others that have been proposed are serotonin, histamine, prostaglandins, and endothelium-derived relaxation factor (EDRF). The tumescence process probably involves multiple transmitters. One possibility is that the release of VIP and acetylcholine acts synergistically to relax arteriolar and trabecular smooth muscles. Inhibition of alpha-adrenergic tonic discharge could also play a role. Detumescence is probably due to recovery of intrinsic muscle tone and reactivation of norepinephrine release, which contracts the muscles of the trabeculae and the arteriolar system to decrease inflow and facilitate outflow.

Table 37–2. Agents that induce or inhibit penile erection in human males.

Inducers	Inhibitors
Vasoactive intestinal polypeptide (VIP)	Metaraminol
Phentolamine*	Epinephrine
Papaverine*	Norepinephrine
Nitroglycerin	Ephedrine
Thymoxamine	Dopamine
Imipramine	Phenylephrine
Verapamil	Guanethidine
Phenoxybenzamine	

*Alone and in combination.

Direct injection of vasoactive agents, on the other hand, has helped in the understanding of the pharmacology of the penis and changed diagnosis and treatment strategies. The agents capable of inducing erection and causing detumescence are summarized in Tables 37–2 and 37–3. Although the actions of different agents vary, when given in large doses, all erection-inducing agents cause the smooth muscles to relax and all detumescence-inducing agents cause them to contract.

MALE SEXUAL DYSFUNCTION

Male sexual dysfunction, denoting the inability to achieve a satisfactory sexual relationship, may involve inadequacy of erection or problems with emission, ejaculation, or orgasm.

Erectile impotence is the inability to achieve and maintain a firm erection. Patients should seek medical advice if this occurs consistently over a 6-month period and in more than 50% of attempts.

Premature ejaculation refers to uncontrolled ejaculation before or shortly after entering the vagina.

Retarded ejaculation is unusually delayed ejaculation.

Retrograde ejaculation denotes backflow of semen into the bladder during ejaculation due to an incompetent bladder neck mechanism.

Table 37–3. Agents known to contract or relax human cavernous smooth muscles in vitro.

Contracting Agents	Relaxing Agents
Norepinephrine	Vasoactive intestinal polypeptide (VIP)
Epinephrine	Carbachol
Substance P	PGE_1
$PGF_2\alpha$	PGE_2
PGI_2	Papaverine
Acetylcholine	Phentolamine
	Phenoxybenzamine
	Acetylcholine

PATHOGENESIS

Erection involves psychologic, neurologic, hormonal, arterial, venous, and sinusoidal factors (Fig 37–4). Impotence of clearly defined origin is discussed below under the appropriate heading. Cases resulting from more than one factor or from causes that cannot be precisely determined are discussed under Other Causes, below.

Psychologic Disorders

Early theories attributed erectile failure to anxiety (Wolpe, 1958; Ellis, 1962). Masters and Johnson (1970) introduced the concept of performance anxiety and the spectator role. Recently, LoPiccolo (1986) refined the differentiation of various psychologic causes as religious orthodoxy, obsessive-compulsive or anhedonic personality, sexual phobias or deviation, widower's syndrome, depression, lack of physical attraction or poor body image, the "madonna-prostitute" syndrome, concern over aging, or lack of knowledge of physiologic changes with age. In the 1950s, 90% of cases of impotence were believed to be psychogenic. Most authors now believe that more than 50% have an organic cause, and in the older population, the percentage is probably higher (Collins et al, 1983; Legros, Mormont, and Servais, 1978; Montague et al, 1979; Spark, White, and Connolly, 1980). The pathogenesis of psychogenic impotence is unknown. Sympathetic overactivity and inhibition of neurotransmitter release are some of the proposed causes.

Neurogenic Disorders

Erectile impotence can be caused by disease or dysfunction of the brain, spinal cord, cavernous and pudendal nerves, and terminal nerve endings and receptors. Among these, spinal cord injury is particularly intriguing. Bors and Comarr (1971) found that about 95% of patients with complete upper motor neuron lesions are capable of erection (reflexogenic), while only about 25% of those with complete lower motor

neuron lesions can have erections (psychogenic). With incomplete lesions, however, more than 90% of patients in both groups retain erectile ability. It is suggested that diseases at the level of the brain (eg, tumors, epilepsy, cerebrovascular accidents, and Parkinson's or Alzheimer's disease) probably cause erectile failure through decreased sexual interest or overinhibition of the spinal erection centers (Weiss, 1972). Diseases at the spinal level (eg, spina bifida, disk herniation, syringomyelia, cord tumor, tabes dorsalis, and multiple sclerosis) may affect either the afferent or efferent nerve pathway to the penis. Peripheral neuropathy as seen in diabetes mellitus, chronic alcohol consumption, or vitamin deficiency may affect the nerve endings and result in a deficiency of neurotransmitters. Direct injury to the cavernous or pudendal nerves from trauma or radical prostatic or rectal surgery can also cause disruption of the neural pathway and result in impotence.

Hormonal Disorders

Diabetes mellitus is the most common hormonal disease associated with erectile failure. However, impotence in diabetics is due mostly to vascular, neurogenic, or psychologic factors (or a combination of these) rather than to the hormonal aberration per se. Hypogonadism due to hypothalamic or pituitary tumors, estrogen or antiandrogen therapy, or orchiectomy for prostatic cancer can suppress sexual interest and nocturnal erections. However, these patients can achieve normal erection during visual sexual stimulation (Bancroft and Wu, 1983), and, thus, the erectile ability is intact. Similarly, impotence resulting from hyperprolactinemia is probably caused by suppressed sexual interest. Hyperthyroidism, hypothyroidism, Cushing's syndrome, and Addison's disease are all reported to cause decreased libido and impotence. Whether the hormonal disturbance or other factors are responsible for the impotence needs further investigation.

Arterial Disorders

When the penis is in the flaccid state, a minimal amount of blood enters the corpora cavernosa to meet the metabolic needs and the corporeal blood gas levels are the same as in venous blood. After sexual stimulation, a large amount of arterial flow instantaneously passes through the dilated arterioles to expand the entire sinusoidal system (tumescence), until a new equilibrium is established at around 100 mm Hg (full erection), when only threshold amounts of flow enter and leave the corpora to maintain the erection.

In animal experiments, the time required to achieve full erection gradually increases with increasing arterial insufficiency. Narrowing of the arterial lumen (or hardening of the arterial wall in humans) results in low pressure in the cavernous arteries and poor arterial flow that can only partially fill the sinusoidal system and is not adequate to expand the sinusoidal wall fully to compress most of the venules. This insufficiency results in partial erection, difficulty in maintaining erec-

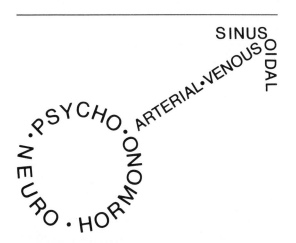

Figure 37–4. Erection involves psychologic, neurologic, hormonal, arterial, venous, and sinusoidal factors.

tion, or early detumescence—the most frequent complaints.

Michal, Kovac, and Belan (1984) found that the incidence and age at onset of coronary disease and impotence are parallel. Except when arteriogenic impotence is due to trauma or is congenital, most often it is probably a component of generalized systemic arterial disease. The distribution and severity of the disease, however, differ from person to person. Some patients with severe arterial disease may still be potent as long as the arterial flow exceeds the venous flow; conversely, some patients with minimal arterial disease may be partially or completely impotent because of relatively large venous outflow, cavernous smooth muscle dysfunction, or inadequate neurotransmitter release. Therefore, in evaluating the arterial system, other contributing factors must also be taken into consideration.

Arterial disease can be classified as extra- or intrapenile arterial insufficiency. Extrapenile arterial disease is amenable to surgical repair and comprises diseases of the internal pudendal, internal and common iliac arteries, and aorta (Leriche syndrome [Leriche and Morel, 1968]), the pelvic steal syndrome (Michal and Pospichal, 1978), and pelvic trauma. Intrapenile arterial disease such as that resulting from aging, arteriosclerosis, or diabetes mellitus does not respond well to present surgical techniques.

Venous & Sinusoidal Disorders

The relationship between aberrant venous flow and erectile dysfunction was confirmed by Ebbehoj and Wagner (1979), who used cavernosography during visual erotic stimulation. Animal experiments have shown that venous compression by the expanding sinusoidal wall and tunica albuginea depends on trabecular smooth muscle relaxation and a compliant sinusoidal system. Currently, 3 types of venous flow abnormalities are identifiable: (1) a defect of the tunica albuginea or excessive number or increased size of veins; (2) insufficient neurotransmitter release; and (3) fibrous replacement of cavernous smooth muscles. Examples of the first abnormality have been described by Tudoriu and Bourmer (1983) in young patients with primary impotence and in old patients with a thin, "worn" tunica albuginea or after a shunt operation for priapism. Insufficient neurotransmitter release can be due to a neurogenic disorder, psychogenic inhibition, or even to cigarette smoking. Patients with diabetes mellitus or severe arterial disease or those who have experienced priapism can develop fibrosis of the corpora cavernosa.

With an insufficient venous occlusion mechanism, erection will be only partial or short-lived. Patients may have primary impotence or may become impotent at a young age, in their early thirties or forties. Local disease such as Peyronie's disease, penile tumor, or penile fracture may involve the sinusoids and prevent erection. Impotence occurs in more than 50% of patients after priapism due to fibrosis of the corpora (Winter, 1978).

Other Causes

Other causes may affect one or more of the factors controlling the erectile mechanism. However, because of the lack of scientific studies, their precise pathogenetic relationship remains speculative.

A. Drugs: In older patients taking several medications for different diseases, it is often difficult to distinguish whether sexual dysfunction results from a specific drug, from interactions among several drugs, from underlying diseases, or from associated psychologic factors (Van Arsdalen, Malloy, and Wein, 1983).

Almost all antihypertensive drugs have been implicated in impotence, especially the central-acting sympatholytics such as methyldopa, clonidine, and reserpine. Their major effect is probably through central nervous system depression, elevated prolactin levels, and decreased libido (Reichgott, 1979). The peripheral alpha-adrenergic blockers such as phenoxybenzamine or prazosin rarely affect erection, although retrograde ejaculation is a known side effect. The beta blockers such as propranolol reportedly decrease libido, as does spironolactone, which causes gynecomastia in some patients. Theoretically, diuretics and vasodilators should not cause erectile dysfunction; however, patients with severe atherosclerosis may require higher blood pressure to deliver sufficient flow to the penis, and the lowering of blood pressure by these agents may result in partial erection.

Antidepressants such as tricyclics and monoamine-oxidase inhibitors depress the libido, probably through their sedative and anticholinergic effects. The major and minor tranquilizers and hypnotics have also been reported to cause decreased libido. Suggested mechanisms are sedation, an anticholinergic effect, and prolactin release through the inhibition of dopamine receptors. These 2 groups of medications include phenothiazines, benzodiazepines, meprobamate, and barbiturates.

Other drugs or chemicals known to cause impotence include estrogen and antiandrogens (cimetidine, ketoconazole, cyproterone acetate). Marihuana depresses the testosterone level; alcohol may induce alcoholic neuropathy or increase estrogen due to hepatic dysfunction; narcotics decrease the libido; and cigarette smoking contributes to vasoconstriction and venous leakage.

B. Systemic Disease and Other Disorders:

1. Diabetes mellitus—Impotence reportedly occurs in 25% of young diabetics and in almost 75% of older patients (Rubin and Babbott, 1958). However, insulin dosage and duration and adequacy of control appear unrelated to sexual dysfunction. Although diabetes is an endocrine disorder, most studies reveal no other hormonal dysfunction or androgen deficiency that might be contributory to impotence (Jensen et al, 1979; Kolodny et al, 1974B). Psychogenic impotence is probably rare; however, secondary psychologic factors compounding organic impotence are common.

The major impact of diabetes is on the nervous and vascular systems. After 10–15 years, a functional abnormality of the somatic and autonomic nervous system can often be found on neurologic testing. Faerman et al (1974) showed a good correlation between sexual dysfunction and the presence of peripheral neuropathy but not retinopathy or arrhythmia. The pathogenesis of neurogenic impotence in diabetes is still under investigation. Recently, decreased levels of vasoactive intestinal polypeptide (Crowe et al, 1983) and norepinephrine (Melman and Henry, 1979) have been reported. Diabetes is also known to affect both large and small vessels. Ružbarský and Michal (1977) have reported fibrotic lesions of the cavernous arteries with intimal proliferation, calcification, and stenosis of the lumen in 15 men with diabetes of an average of 13 years' duration. Jevtich et al (1982) reported a high incidence of abnormal results on Doppler examination of the penile arteries. Although a neurologic deficit or arterial disease alone may not cause impotence if adequate compensation can be recruited, the presence of both simultaneously will certainly aggravate the disability.

2. Renal disease–Impotence occurs in about 50% of patients undergoing dialysis (Sherman, 1975; Thurm, 1975). Multiple factors are involved, including decreased testosterone levels; autonomic neuropathy; accelerated vascular disease; multiple medications; worsening of the primary disease; and psychologic stress. In a series of patients who underwent successul renal transplantation, potency was restored in 75% (Salvatierra, Fortmann, and Belzer, 1975). Bilateral renal transplantation with end-to-end anastomosis to internal iliac arteries can result in postoperative impotence due to compromised internal pudendal arterial flow.

3. Other diseases–Patients who have recently recovered from myocardial infarction and those with angina or heart failure can develop impotence due to anxiety, arterial insufficiency, or the effects of drugs. Patients with severe pulmonary emphysema with dyspnea often develop impotence because of anxiety, which may exacerbate the dyspnea and cause interpersonal conflicts with the sexual partner. In patients who have colostomies, ileostomies, or ileal conduits, problems may also occur due to depression and loss of self-esteem. Cirrhosis of the liver, scleroderma, chronic debilitation, and cachexia are also known to cause impotence.

Although hypertension is common among impotent patients, Newman and Marcus (1985) found that the frequency of erectile failure was little different from that in a control group of similar age. They also found that aging has a negative impact in all groups, with or without hypertension or diabetes.

DIAGNOSIS & TREATMENT

A detailed medical and sexual history and a thorough physical examination are the most important steps in the differential diagnosis of sexual dysfunction. Interviewing the partner, if available, is indispensable in eliciting a reliable history, planning treatment, and obtaining a successful outcome. Because multiple contributing factors may exist, a routine noninvasive workup aimed at determining the major cause should be performed in all patients. This should include basic laboratory tests such as a complete blood count, urinalysis, fasting and 2-hour postprandial blood glucose determinations, serum creatinine levels, morning serum testosterone and prolactin levels, and serologic test for syphilis. In patients with symptoms of prostatic disease, expressed prostatic secretions should be examined.

Psychogenic Impotence

In the past, impotence was arbitrarily classified as either organic or psychogenic. When it was associated with a disease known to cause erectile failure, impotence was classified as organic; all other cases were labeled psychogenic. In fact, the pattern of sexual dysfunction, rather than the presence or absence of an organic factor, is probably the most important factor in making a diagnosis. Because psychogenic impotence is the result of changes in affect and mood, it usually occurs in a specific pattern. A suggestive history includes sudden onset, selective dysfunction (eg, rigid erection with one partner and poor erection with others, or normal erection during masturbation or fantasy but not during intercourse), and normal pattern of nocturnal erections but abnormal pattern during waking hours. This is often associated with anxiety, guilt, fear, emotional stress, and religious or parental inhibition.

Complementary psychometric testing (eg, Minnesota Multiphasic Personality Inventory, Walker Sex Form, and Derogatis Sexual Function Inventory) is reported to be helpful in assessing psychologic status. However, some researchers find that these tests do not provide much information. The recently developed papaverine test can be used to help establish the diagnosis. When a neurologic deficit and hormonal disease are absent, the positive result (full erection after papaverine injection) strongly suggests a psychogenic cause.

Theoretically, the preferred treatment of psychogenic impotence should be psychotherapy. Several techniques have been developed. Individual therapy using the psychoanalytic method is based on Freud's theory that erectile failure is the result of unconscious fears centering on the Oedipus complex. Subsequently, Masters and Johnson (1976) developed individual and couple counseling based on the concept of performance anxiety. This was followed by psychodynamically oriented couple therapy developed by Kaplan (1979). Other techniques include behaviorist therapy, feedback training, and hypnotherapy. Because of the urologist's limited knowledge of psychotherapy, referral to a sex therapist or psychotherapist is recommended. If the patient refuses to undergo psychotherapy or fails to improve after a reasonable number of sessions, an alternative treatment can be recommended. This includes a penile prosthesis and pharmacotherapy with agents such as yohimbine or intracavernous injection of vasoactive drugs. (Pharmacotherapy is still in an early stage of development.)

Neurogenic Impotence

Ideally, neurologic examination should assess the integrity of the entire nervous system, including the afferent and efferent components of the central and peripheral and the autonomic and somatic functions. However, such a thorough examination is time-consuming and unrewarding in most cases. Furthermore, since erectile capability can be retained in the presence of neuropathy (eg, in some diabetics), an abnormal neurologic finding may not be the cause of impotence. Correlation with the history and other test results is essential before neurogenic impotence can be diagnosed.

A practical approach should begin with a detailed medical history. Particular attention should be directed to the autonomic and somatic functions of the sacral nerves (urinary, bowel, and sphincter control; sensation of the external genitalia, including the experience of pleasure or pain with penile stimulation; and direction and force of ejaculation). A history of diabetes, alcoholism, trauma or lesion of the head and spinal cord, or multiple sclerosis should also be sought. If the medical history reveals no neurologic disease or deficit, a simple neurologic examination, including pinprick, touch, and vibratory stimulation of the external genitalia, perineum, and lower extremities and evaluation of the bulbocavernous reflex, is probably sufficient. When responses are normal, the chance of finding a neurologic lesion is rare.

In patients with a history of neurologic disease or deficit or abnormal findings on testing, more sophisticated testing is warranted. The patient should be referred to a neurologist if the urologist does not have the equipment for the following tests.

A. Somatosensory and Motor Function: Biothesiometry (Newman, 1970; Padma-Nathan, Goldstein, and Krane, 1986A) can be used to quantify dorsal nerve dysfunction because loss of vibratory sense is one of the early signs of diabetic peripheral neuropathy. Evoked potential techniques are useful to determine dorsal nerve conduction velocity (Gerstenberg and Bradley, 1983), sacral evoked potential (Ertekin and Reel, 1976; Krane and Siroky, 1980) and genitocerebral responses (Haldeman et al, 1982).

B. Autonomic Afferent and Efferent Components: There are several procedures for assessing autonomic neuropathy: (1) heart rate variations during deep breathing (Watkins and MacKay, 1980), which indicate abnormal cardiac reflex—an early sign of autonomic neuropathy; (2) pupillary response to light; (3) crystometry with or without bethanechol testing and urethral pressure profile; and (4) bulbocavernous reflex to stimulation of the prostatic urethra. However, all these tests are indirect, and direct testing of erectile function is not presently available. Ideally, this should include evaluation of the genital stimulation reflex, which involves the dorsal nerve (somatic) and the cavernous nerve (autonomic), and of the visual sexual stimulation reflex, which involves the optic nerves, cerebral and spinal centers, and cavernous nerves.

C. Central Nervous System: Nocturnal penile tumescence testing (NPT) represents the standard evaluation of nocturnal erections. Karacan and Moore (1982) have perfected this technique by adding electroencephalography (EEG), electromyography (EMG), and electrocardiography (ECG). Irregularities revealed by these tests combined with abnormal NPT results may suggest a central nervous system abnormality.

Because dissociation between penile tumescence and rigidity has been noted in some patients during nocturnal testing, several techniques have been introduced to measure rigidity, such as the stamp test (Barry, Blank, and Boileau, 1980), SnapGauge test (Ek, Bradley, and Krane, 1983), and the newly developed Rigiscan continuous testing technique (Kaneko and Bradley, 1986).

Recently, Spark, Wills, and Royal (1984) identified a group of men with sexual dysfunction and temporal lobe epilepsy. They suggested that sleep-deprived EEG or single photon emission computerized tomography (SPECT) be used to locate lesions causing the sexual dysfunction.

Treatment of neurogenic impotence depends on the severity of the disease and associated factors. Patients with purely neurogenic disease may be treated with intracavernous injection of vasoactive drugs or a penile prosthesis. Implantation of electrodes on the erectile nerves is currently under investigation. In patients whose neuropathy is due to alcoholism or nutritional deficiency, vitamin supplements and a decrease in alcohol consumption may be helpful.

Hormonal Impotence

Evaluation of endocrine function should begin with a thorough medical history and systemic review. The hypothalamic-pituitary-gonadal axis should be assessed, as should thyroid and adrenal function. Diabetes mellitus is the most common endocrine disorder, although its effect is mainly on vascular and neurologic functions. A history of chemotherapy; irradiation; exposure to toxins, alcohol, and drugs; or chronic renal failure should be elicited. Most patients with endocrine abnormalities report decreased sexual interest rather than erectile failure, and a detailed sexual history is helpful in differential diagnosis.

During physical examination, particular attention should be directed toward signs of hypogonadism (small atrophic testes, loss of beard and body hair, and gynecomastia). If Leydig cell failure occurs before puberty, signs of eunuchoidism will be apparent (sparse facial, pubic, and axillary hair, infantile genitalia, and a high-pitched voice). Laboratory tests should include testosterone and prolactin levels. Because 97% of the testosterone in plasma is bound to protein, a free testosterone determination may be necessary if a protein-binding problem is suspected.

Patients with an elevated prolactin level should undergo repeat testing; if the result is still abnormal, they should be referred to an endocrinologist for suspicion of a pituitary tumor. Patients with low morning testosterone levels should also have repeat studies and determination of luteinizing hormone (LH) and follicle-stimulating hormone (FSH) levels. When testosterone levels are low but LH and FSH levels are not elevated, endocrine consultation should be requested for investigation of pituitary or hypothalamic dysfunction. When LH and FSH levels are appropriately elevated in the presence of low testosterone levels, primary testicular failure is the cause of impotence.

Patients with diseases of the thyroid, adrenal, or pituitary glands should be referred to an endocrinologist for treatment. Diseases of the testicle such as primary testicular failure can be treated with intramuscular or oral testosterone preparations. Luteinizing hormone-releasing hormone (LHRH) has also been reported to be useful in patients with hypothalamic-pituitary-gonadal axis abnormalities. In patients with hypopituitarism, human chorionic gonadotropin (hCG) can be used to stimulate the production of testosterone from the testicle. In patients with hyperprolactinemia, treatment with a dopaminergic drug, bromocriptine, has been reported to improve sexual function. In patients with a pituitary tumor secreting excessive prolactin, treatment with bromocriptine or surgery also restores potency.

Arteriogenic Impotence

Except in traumatic cases, arterial disease is a generalized systemic disorder and usually involves multiple organ systems. A history of peripheral vascular disease, intermittent claudication, and atrophic change of the extremities will provide clues to the possible involvement of the penile arteries. Patients with coronary or peripheral vascular bypass have a high incidence of impotence due to arterial disease. The physical examination should include palpation of the carotid, brachial, femoral, and dorsal penile arteries.

Measurement of the penile blood pressure has been advocated as a screening test for penile arterial disease. The ratio of penile systolic blood pressure to brachial systolic pressure, expressed as the penile brachial pressure index (PBI), is reportedly a good indicator of arterial disease. A ratio below 0.6 is strongly indicative of arteriogenic impotence. Continuous-wave Doppler analysis is used for the PBI. This technique measures a mixture of signals from all the penile arteries rather than signals from a single artery, and, thus, a low value (eg, 0.6) correlates well with arteriography showing severe arterial disease. However, a normal PBI does not indicate normal penile blood flow. Pressure is measured in the flaccid penis and is not predictive of erectile function. Nevertheless, if this test is combined with pelvic exercise, the pelvic steal syndrome may be unmasked (Goldstein et al, 1982). Some authors report a better correlation between penile arteriography and other techniques (eg, determining the difference between mean arterial pressure and penile blood pressure [Montague, James,

and deWolfe, 1980]; pulse wave from analysis [Velcek et al, 1980]; and pulse volume recording [Merchant and DePalma, 1981]).

A. Functional Evaluation of Penile Arteries: The xenon washout technique performed during visual erotic stimulation provides an excellent functional test of psychogenic erection (Wagner, 1981). Different washout curves can be demonstrated in patients with abnormal venous leakage or arterial disease. However, this technique requires a radioisotope, and the individual response to erotic videotapes varies greatly.

The introduction of intracavernous injection of vasoactive agents opened a new era in the functional study of penile vasculature. Although in rare situations psychologic apprehension can affect the patient's response (Buvat et al, 1986), in most situations intracavernous injection can reliably assess penile vascular status (Abber et al, 1986). A negative response (no erection or partial erection) is not diagnostic; however, if the patient develops full erection within 12 minutes of injection of 60 mg of papaverine, adequate arterial flow and an intact venous mechanism can be assumed. Patients with less than full erection after papaverine injection can be further evaluated with high-resolution ultrasonography combined with pulsed Doppler analysis of the penile arteries during papaverine-induced erection (Lue et al, 1986A). This technique can scan the architecture of the penis, define the thickness of Peyronie's plaque, measure changes in the diameter of the cavernous arteries before and after papaverine injection, and visually assess the pulsation of the penile arteries. Pulsed Doppler wave analysis can also measure the velocity of the flow through individual vessels in the penis. Sonography combined with Doppler analysis is a noninvasive way of assessing the individual penile arteries and is much more accurate than the penile brachial pressure index (Fig 37–5).

Internal iliac or pudendal arteriography is indicated in selected cases of pelvic injury or in young healthy patients suspected of having isolated arterial disease. In most instances, the cavernous arteries are poorly visualized if arteriography is performed under local anesthesia due to high resistance and minimal flow in the flaccid state. Intracavernous or intra-arterial injection of a vasodilator before imaging will aid in assessment of the functional capacity of the penile arteries (Fig 37–6) (Virag et al, 1984; Zorgniotti and Lefleur, 1985).

B. Treatment of Arteriogenic Impotence: Isolated stenosis or occlusion of the extrapenile arteries is amenable to surgical repair. Restoration of potency has been reported after surgery of the internal iliac, internal pudendal, and dorsal arteries. Michal et al (1977) pioneered the use of extrapenile vessels to revascularize the corpora cavernosa (epigastric-corporeal anastomosis). Subsequent modifications include using a venous graft for femorocorporeal anastomosis and direct anastomosis of the epigastric artery to the cavernous artery (Crespo et al, 1982). Although short-

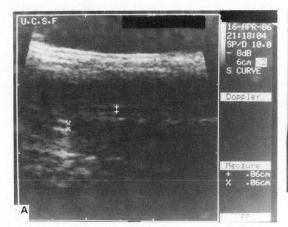

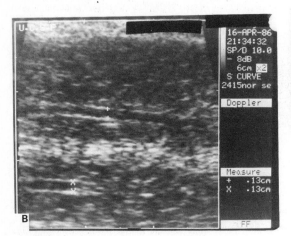

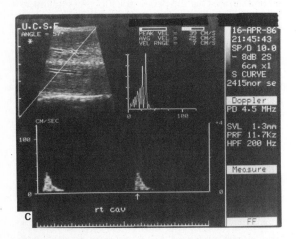

Figure 37–5. Duplex ultrasonography and Doppler analysis of the arterial response to intracavernous papaverine injection. In the flaccid state (*A*), the luminal diameter of the cavernous artery is 0.06 cm; after papaverine injection (*B*), this increases to 0.13 cm. Wave analysis (*C*) shows normal flow in the cavernous artery (peak velocity, 39 cm/ ⟨ sec).

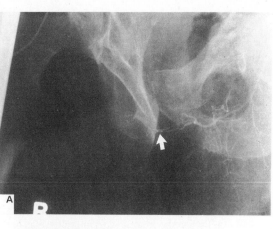

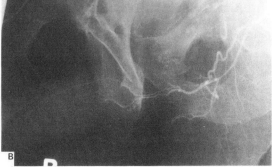

Figure 37–6. Internal iliac arteriogram in the flaccid penis (*A*) shows poor visualization of penile arteries, simulating occlusion (arrow). After intracavernous injection of 60 mg of papaverine (*B*), all the branches of the penile artery are well visualized.

term results for all 3 techniques are good, long-term results of the epigastric-corporeal and femorocorporeal anastomoses have been poor (they are not yet available for the epigastric-cavernous arterial bypass). Anastomosis of the epigastric artery to the deep dorsal vein was first described by Virag (1982C), the intention being to divert blood from the dorsal vein back to the cavernous spaces. Further modification by anastomosing a branch of the dorsal vein to the corpora cavernosa after anastomosing the epigastric artery to the deep dorsal vein reportedly achieves better results, although the follow-up period has been short.

Penile prostheses continue to be refined (Table 37–4). In addition to the improved durability of the semirigid prostheses (Small-Carrion, Jonas, Flexirod, AMS, and Mentor malleable), the mechanics and strength of the inflatable prosthesis (eg, AMS inflatable, Mentor inflatable) have also been upgraded. Two newly designed prostheses are now available. One is the single-component inflatable prosthesis (Flexi-Flate and Hydroflex) with inflating and deflating mechanisms contained within a single cylinder for easier implantation. The other (OmniPhase) consists of a segmented hinge and a cable that runs

Table 37–4. Types of penile prostheses.

Semirigid
Small-Carrion
Flexirod
Jonas
AMS 600 (malleable)
Mentor malleable
Inflatable (multicomponent)
AMS 700
Mentor
Inflatable (single-component)
Hydroflex
Flexi-Flate
Segmented, hinged
OmniPhase

through the center of each segment with a mechanical activator on one end. Gratifying results have been achieved in more than 95% of cases after penile prosthesis insertion, especially if preoperative counseling is given to both the patient and the partner (Kaufman, Lindner, and Raz, 1982; Montague, 1983). The major complications are infection, prolonged pain, tenderness, and problems resulting from inadequate length (SST syndrome).

Intracavernous injection of vasoactive agents provides an attractive alternative to surgery. The reported agents are papaverine alone (Virag, 1982B) or with phentolamine (Zorgniotti and Lefleur, 1985; Sidi et al, 1986), phenoxybenzamine (Brindley, 1983), and prostaglandin E_1 (Ishii et al, 1986). These cause prolonged arterial dilatation and venous compression, and a large number of patients have been able to achieve and maintain erections better than their own. Repeated injection can improve penile hemodynamics; after short-term treatment, some patients have achieved good erections without injection. Several complications have been reported: ecchymosis at the injection site; transient dizziness or a drop in blood pressure; paresthesia; failure of ejaculation; infection; and priapism. Priapism of less than 24 hours' duration may be treated by aspiration or instillation of alpha-adrenergic agents such as epinephrine, norepinephrine, metaraminol, phenylephrine, or ephedrine (Lue et al, 1986B). In priapism of longer duration, a shunting procedure may be required, and several patients have reportedly become completely impotent due to fibrosis of the corpora after prolonged priapism (Halsted et al, 1986). Reports from 3 years' follow-up in some large series also noted several cases of fibrosis of the cavernous tissue (Zorgniotti, 1986) and elevated liver enzymes (Goldstein, I: personal communication) after frequent and repeated injections. Monkeys receiving 100 papaverine injections over a one-year period showed some fibrosis near the injection site and smooth muscle hypertrophy in the other portion of the corpus. The significance of these findings needs further study.

Another alternative is the use of a vacuum suction device with a constrictive band placed at the base of the penis. With proper use, a number of patients have been able to achieve and maintain erections adequate for sexual intercourse. Ecchymosis and petechiae developed in about 40%, and some reported transient numbness of the penis (Nadig, Ware, and Blumoff, 1986). The long-term results of this modality are not available.

Venogenic Impotence & Diseases of the Cavernous Smooth Muscles

A. Diagnosis: Detection of penile venous incompetence was pioneered by Wagner's group, who used cavernosography during visual erotic stimulation (Wagner, 1981). Virag (1982A) and Wespes et al (1984) modified this approach and introduced the technique of cavernosometry (ie, measuring the rate of saline perfusion required to achieve and maintain erection) before cavernosography. A further refinement with the addition of intracavernous papaverine injection is probably a better way to study the functional status of the penile venous occlusion mechanism. Wespes' group (1986) has determined that in potent volunteers, the maintenance rate after papaverine is less than 5 mL/min. Visualization of the penile veins depends on the amount of contrast medium present in the venous system. Therefore, a high maintenance rate results in visualization of abnormal venous systems and a low rate will show minimal or no venous drainage outside the corpora cavernosa (Fig 37–7). An abnormal communication between the corpora cavernosa and the corpus spongiosum or the glans penis can sometimes be demonstrated. However, cavernosography without cavernosometry is not adequate in the diagnosis of venous leakage.

A history of rapid detumescence or partial erection, especially in young men, is strongly suggestive of venous incompetence, although arterial insufficiency can produce the same symptoms. Dizziness, facial flushing, or even a drop in systemic blood pressure after papaverine injection can be due to autonomic neuropathy or a large venous leak. Confirmation with cavernosometry is necessary.

The most widely recognized disease of the cavernous muscle is fibrosis after priapism and local replacement with fibrotic plaque in Peyronie's disease. Diseases of the cavernous muscles due to severe arterial disease, diabetic angiopathy, and aging are not well defined. In these cases, history, physical examination, penile ultrasound, and cavernosography may not be diagnostic. Biopsy of the cavernous tissue and special staining may be necessary.

B. Treatment: Although improvement of potency after ligation of the penile veins was described in the early 20th century, urologists were skeptical until cavernosography and cavernosometry provided a scientific demonstration of venous leakage. Ligation and stripping of the superficial and deep dorsal veins and repair of a fistula between the glans and the cavernous bodies are the procedures reported. Virag's technique of anastomosis of the epigastric artery to the deep dorsal vein probably also decreases venous outflow because of higher venous resistance. Although this technique appears promising, only a few series have been

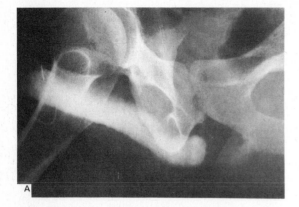

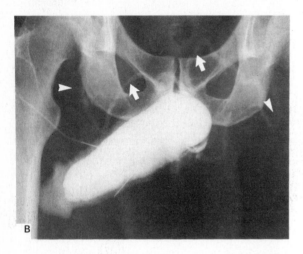

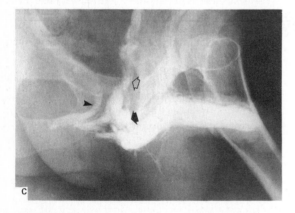

Figure 37–7. Cavernosography after intracavernous injection of papaverine. In a normal man (**A**), the cavernosogram shows opacification of the erect corpora cavernosa and nonvisualization of penile veins. In (**B**), the patient has a large leak through both superficial dorsal veins (**arrows**) to the saphenous veins (**arrowheads**). Film (**C**) shows abnormal venous drainage via the cavernous veins (**solid arrow**) into the preprostatic plexus (**open arrow**) and the internal pudendal veins (**arrowhead**). (Reproduced, with permission, from Lue TF, Tanagho EA: Physiology of erection and pharmacological management of impotence. *J Urol* 1987;**137**:829. © by Williams & Wilkins, 1987.)

reported, and long-term results are not available (Wespes and Schulman, 1985; Lewis and Puyau, 1986).

When impotence is due to disease of the cavernous tissue, treatment is generally surgical. If only a limited amount of cavernous tissue is involved, such as in Peyronie's plaque, injection of collagenase may decrease the plaque and improve the penile curvature (Gelbard, Lindner, and Kaufman, 1985). A prosthesis is required in the majority of patients when fibrosis involves most of the corpora cavernosa.

Impotence Due to Other Causes

The medical history, systemic review, laboratory examination, and drug history cannot always reveal the precise cause of erectile dysfunction. Evaluation of potency after systemic disease has been adequately treated or a medication discontinued or changed sometimes may be the only way of diagnosing the cause of impotence. Conservative management should always be tried first, with surgery to be considered a last resort.

MALE SEXUAL DYSFUNCTION INVOLVING EMISSION, EJACULATION, & ORGASM

Physiology of Emission, Ejaculation, & Orgasm

Different mechanisms are involved in erection, emission, ejaculation, and orgasm, and these events can be dissociated from one another (eg, a frequent complaint of impotent patients is ejaculating through a "limp penis"). Except for nocturnal emissions or "wet dreams," emission and ejaculation require stimulation of the external genitalia. Impulses traveling from the pudendal nerves reach the upper lumbar spinal sympathetic nuclei. Efferent signals traveling in the hypogastric nerve activate secretions and transport sperm from the distal epididymis, vasa deferentia, seminal vesicles, and prostate to the prostatic urethra. Coordinated closing of the internal urethral sphincter and relaxation of the external sphincter direct the semen into the bulbous urethra (emission). Subsequent rhythmic contractions of the bulbocavernous muscles force the semen through a pressurized conduit—the much narrowed urethral lumen compressed by the engorged corpora cavernosa and corpus spongiosum within Buck's fascia—to produce the 2- to 5-mL ejaculate. The external ejaculation process involves the somatomotor efferent of the pudendal nerve to contract the bulbocavernous muscle. However, since this action is involuntary, integrated autonomic and somatic action is required.

The mechanism of orgasm is the least understood of the sexual processes. It probably involves cerebral interpretation and response to sexual stimulation. Along with emission and ejaculation, several nongenital responses also occur. These include involuntary rhythmic contractions of the anal sphincter, hyperventilation, tachycardia, and elevation of blood pressure.

Disorders Affecting Emission, Ejaculation, & Orgasm

Bilateral sympathectomy at the L2 level has resulted in ejaculatory dysfunction in about 40% of patients. High bilateral retroperitoneal lymphadenectomy causes an even higher percentage of emission failure.

Retrograde ejaculation is usually the result of dysfunction of the internal sphincter or the bladder neck, as seen after prostatectomy, with alpha-blocker therapy, and in autonomic neuropathy due to diabetes.

Successful emission and ejaculation without orgasm occur in some patients with spinal cord injury. Phantom orgasm in a paraplegic man also has been described. A history of disease or surgery is helpful in differentiating emission failure from retrograde ejaculation. If microscopic examination confirms the presence of sperm in bladder urine after a dry ejaculation, retrograde ejaculation can be diagnosed. If no sperm is found, emission failure is the cause.

Treatment

Elimination of alpha blockers will cure some patients with emission failure or retrograde ejaculation. Alpha sympathomimetics such as ephedrine or a combination of chlorpheniramine maleate and phenylpropanolamine hydrochloride (Ornade) have been used successfully in patients with retrograde ejaculation. Electroejaculation via a rectal probe has been applied in patients suffering from spinal cord injury with some success (Brindley, 1981; Perkash et al, 1985). Patients who have normal "wet dreams" but cannot achieve orgasm and ejaculation may benefit from psychosexual counseling. Premature ejaculation can be treated by desensitization (Semans, 1956), the squeezing technique (Masters and Johnsons, 1976), or application of a local anesthetic or a condom to reduce the sensitivity of the glans and frenulum.

REFERENCES

Physiology of Penile Erection

Adaikan PG, Kottegoda SR, Ratnam SS: Is vasoactive intestinal polypeptide the principal transmitter involved in human penile erection? *J Urol* 1986;**135**:638.

Adaikan PG et al: Cholinoreceptors in the corpus cavernosum muscle of the human penis. *J Auton Pharmacol* 1983;**3**:107.

Bancroft J, Wu FCW: Changes in erectile responsiveness during androgen replacement therapy. *Arch Sex Behav* 1983;**12**:59.

Benson GS: Penile erection: In search of a neurotransmitter. *World J Urol* 1983;**1**:209.

Benson GS et al: Neuromorphology and neuropharmacology of the human penis: An in vitro study. *J Clin Invest* 1980;**65**:506.

Brindley GS: Pilot experiments on the actions of drugs injected into the human corpus cavernosum penis. *Br J Pharmacol* 1986;**87**:495.

Carati CJ et al: Pharmacology of the erectile tissue of the canine penis. *Pharmacol Res Commun* 1985;**3**:951.

Conti G: L'erection du penis humain et ses bases morphologico-vasculaires. *Acta Anat* 1952;**14**:217.

Deslypere JP, Vermeulen A: Leydig cell function in normal men: Effect of age, life-style, residence, diet, and activity. *J Clin Endocrinol Metab* 1984;**59**:955.

Fisher C et al: The assessment of nocturnal REM erection in the differential diagnosis of sexual impotence. *J Sex Marital Ther* 1975;**1**:277.

Fournier GR Jr et al: Mechanism of venous occlusion during canine penile erection: Anatomic demonstration. *J Urol* 1987;**137**:163.

Gomes de Araujo C, Schmidt RA, Tanagho EA: Neural pathways to lower urinary tract identified by retrograde axonal transport of horseradish peroxidase. *Invest Urol* 1982;**19**:290.

Hedlund H, Andersson KE: Contraction and relaxation induced by some prostanoids in isolated human penile erectile tissue and cavernous artery. *J Urol* 1985;**134**:1245.

Juenemann KP et al: Hemodynamics of papaverine- and phentolamine-induced penile erection. *J Urol* 1986;**136**:158.

Karacan I, Aslan C, Hirshkowitz M: Erectile mechanisms in man. *Science* 1983;**220**:1080.

Karacan I et al: Sleep-related penile tumescence as a function of age. *Am J Psychiatry* 1975;**132**:932.

Kawatani M, Nagel J, de Groat WC: Identification of neuropeptides in pelvic and pudendal nerve afferent pathways to the sacral spinal cord of the cat. *J Comp Neurol* 1986;**249**:117.

Klinge E, Sjöstrand NO: Comparative study of some isolated mammalian smooth muscle effectors of penile erection. *Acta Physiol Scand* 1977;**100**:354.

Kwan M et al: The nature of androgen action on male sexuality: A combined laboratory/self-report study on hypogonadal men. *J Clin Endocrinol Metab* 1983;**57**:557.

Levin RM, Wein AJ: Adrenergic alpha receptors outnumber beta receptors in human corpus cavernosum. *Invest Urol* 1980;**18**:225.

Lue TF: The erectile mechanism. Pages 7–9 in: *The Scientific Basis of Sexual Dysfunction.* US Government Printing Office Publication No. 491–292:41090, 1986A.

Lue TF: The mechanism of penile erection in the monkey. *Semin Urol* 1986B;**4**:217.

Lue TF et al: Hemodynamics of canine corpora cavernosa during erection. *Urology* 1984A;**24**:347.

Lue TF et al: Hemodynamics of erection in the monkey. *J Urol* 1983;**130**:1237.

Lue TF et al: Neuroanatomy of penile erection: Its relevance to iatrogenic impotence. *J Urol* 1984B;**131**:273.

Marberger H: The mechanisms of ejaculation. In: *Physiology and Genetics of Reproduction.* Coutinho E, Fuchs F (editors). Plenum Press, 1974.

McConnell J, Benson GS, Wood J: Autonomic innervation of the mammalian penis: A histochemical and physiological study. *J Neural Transm* 1979;**45**:227.

Michal V et al: Haemodynamics of erection in man. *Physiol Bohemoslov* 1983;**32**:497.

Newman HF, Northup JP, Devlin J: Mechanism of human penile erection. *Invest Urol* 1964;**1**:350.

Newman HF, Tchertkoff V: Penile vascular cushions and erection. *Invest Urol* 1980;**18**:43.

O'Carroll R, Bancroft J: Testosterone therapy for low sexual interest and erectile dysfunction in men: A controlled study. *Br J Psychiatry* 1984;**145**:146.

Padma-Nathan H et al: In vivo and in vitro studies on the physiology of penile erection. *Semin Urol* 1986;**4**:209.

Polack JM et al: VIP-ergic nerves in the penis. *Lancet* 1981;**2**:217.

Saenz de Tejada I et al: Cholinergic neurotransmission in human penile corpus cavernosum smooth muscle. *Fed Proc* 1985;**256**:454.

Shirai M et al: Hemodynamic mechanism of erection in the human penis. *Arch Androl* 1978;**1**:345.

Virag R: Intracavernous injection of papaverine for erectile failure. *Lancet* 1982;**2**:938.

Wagner G, Uhrenholdt A: Blood flow measurement by the clearance method in the human corpus cavernosum in the flaccid and erect states. Pages 41–46 in: *Vasculogenic Impotence*. (Proceedings of the First International Conference on Corpus Cavernosum Revascularization.) Zorgniotti AW, Rossi G (editors). Thomas, 1980.

Wagner G et al: New theory on the mechanism of erection involving hitherto undescribed vessels. *Lancet* 1982;**1**:416.

Walsh PC, Donker PJ: Impotence following radical prostatectomy: Insight into etiology and prevention. *J Urol* 1982;**128**:492.

Willis E et al: Vasoactive intestinal polypeptide (VIP) as a possible neurotransmitter involved in penile erection. *Acta Physiol Scand* 1981;**113**:545.

Male Sexual Dysfunction

Abber JC et al: Diagnostic tests for impotence: Comparison of papaverine injection with penile-brachial index and nocturnal penile tumescence monitoring. *J Urol* 1986;**135**:923.

Abelson D: Diagnostic value of the penile pulse and blood pressure: A Doppler study of impotence in diabetics. *J Urol* 1975;**113**:636.

Adlercreutz H: Hepatic metabolism of estrogens in health and disease. *N Engl J Med* 1974;**290**:1081.

Antoniou LD et al: Reversal of uraemic impotence by zinc. *Lancet* 1977;**2**:895.

Bancroft J, Wu FCW: Changes in erectile responsiveness during androgen therapy. *Arch Sex Behav* 1983;**12**:59.

Barry JM, Blank B, Boileau M: Nocturnal penile tumescence monitoring with stamps. *Urology* 1980;**15**:171.

Bennett AH: Revascularization using the dorsal vein of the penis in vasculogenic impotence. *Semin Urol* 1986;**4**:259.

Bors E, Comarr AE: *Neurological Urology*. University Park Press, 1971.

Bradley WE et al: New method for continuous measurement of nocturnal penile tumescence and rigidity. *Urology* 1985;**26**:4.

Brindley GS: Cavernosal alpha-blockade: A new technique for investigating and treating erectile impotence. *Br J Psychiatry* 1983;**143**:332.

Brindley GS: Electroejaculation: Its technique, neurological implication and uses. *J Neurol Neurosurg Psychiatry* 1981;**44**:9.

Brindley GS: Pilot experiments on the actions of drugs injected into the human corpus cavernosum penis. *Br J Pharmacol* 1986;**87**:495.

Britt DB, Kemmerer WT, Robison JR: Penile blood flow determination by mercury strain gauge plethysmography. *Invest Urol* 1971;**8**:673.

Buvat J et al: Is intracavernous injection of papaverine a reliable screening test for vascular impotence? *J Urol* 1986;**135**:476.

Collins WE et al: Multidisciplinary survey of erectile impotence. *Can Med Assoc J* 1983;**128**:1393.

Crespo E et al: Treatment of vasculogenic sexual impotence by revascularizing of cavernous and/or dorsal arteries using microvascular techniques. *Urology* 1982;**20**:271.

Crowe R et al: Vasoactive intestinal polypeptide-like immunoreactive nerves in diabetic penis: A comparison between streptozotocin-treated rats and man. *Diabetes* 1983;**32**:1075.

DePalma RG, Levine SB, Feldman S: Preservation of erectile function after aortoiliac reconstruction. *Arch Surg* 1978;**113**:958.

Ebbehoj J, Wagner G: Insufficient penile erection due to abnormal drainage of cavernous bodies. *Urology* 1979;**13**:507.

Ek A, Bradley WE, Krane RJ: Nocturnal penile rigidity measured by the snap gauge band. *J Urol* 1983;**129**:964.

Ellenberg M: Impotence in diabetes: The neurologic factor. *Ann Intern Med* 1971;**75**:213.

Ellis A: *Reason and Emotion in Psychotherapy*. Lyle Stuart, 1962.

Engel G, Burnham SJ, Carter MF: Penile blood pressure in the evaluation of erectile impotence. *Fertil Steril* 1978;**30**:687.

Ertekin C, Reel F: Bulbocavernosus reflex in normal men and in patients with neurogenic bladder and/or impotence. *J Neurol Sci* 1976;**28**:1.

Faerman J et al: Impotence and diabetes: Histological studies of the autonomic nervous fibers of the corpora cavernosa in impotent diabetic males. *Diabetes* 1974;**23**:971.

Finkle A, Prian D: Sexual potency in elderly men before and after prostatectomy. *JAMA* 1966;**196**:125.

Finney RP: Finney flexirod prosthesis. *Urology* 1984;**23(5 Spec No)**:79.

Finney RP: Flexi-flate penile prosthesis. *Semin Urol* 1986;**4**:244.

Fishman IJ: Experience with the Hydroflex penile prosthesis. *Semin Urol* 1986;**4**:239.

Fishman IJ, Shabsign R, Scott FB: A comparison of the hydroflex and inflatable penile prostheis. *J Urol* 1986;**135**:358.

Flanigan DP et al: Elimination of iatrogenic impotence and improvement of sexual function after aortoiliac revascularization. *Arch Surg* 1982;**117**:544.

Flanigan DP et al: Internal iliac artery revascularization in the treatment of vasculogenic impotence. *Arch Surg* 1985;**120**:271.

Forsberg L, Olsson AM, Neglen P: Erectile function before and after aortoiliac reconstruction: A comparison between measurements of Doppler acceleration ratio, blood pressure and angiography. *J Urol* 1982;**127**:379.

Gaskell P: The importance of penile blood pressure in cases of impotence. *Can Med Assoc J* 1971;**105**:1047.

Gelbard MK, Lindner A, Kaufman JJ: The use of collagenase in the treatment of Peyronie's disease. *J Urol* 1985;**134**:280.

Gerstenberg TC, Bradley WE: Nerve conduction velocity measurement of dorsal nerve of the penis in normal and impotent males. *Urology* 1983;**21**:90.

Gerstenberger DL, Osborne D, Furlow WL: Inflatable penile prosthesis: Follow-up study of patient-partner satisfaction. *Urology* 1979;**14**:583.

Ginestie J, Romieu A: *Radiologic Exploration of Impotence*. Martinus Nijhoff, 1978.

Goldstein I: Arterial revascularization procedures. *Semin Urol* 1986;**4**:252.

Goldstein I: Neurologic impotence. In: *Male Sexual Dysfunction*. Krane RJ, Siroky MB, Goldstein I (editors). Little, Brown, 1983.

Goldstein I et al: Vasculogenic impotence: Role of the pelvic steal test. *J Urol* 1982;**128**:300.

Gordon GG et al: Effect of alcohol (ethanol) administration on sex-hormone metabolism in normal men. *N Engl J Med* 1976;**295**:793.

Haldeman S, Bradley WE, Bhatia N: Evoked responses from the pudendal nerve. *J Urol* 1982;**128**:974.

Haldeman S et al: Pudendal evoked responses. *Arch Neurol* 1982;**39**:280.

Halsted DS et al: Papaverine-induced priapism. *J Urol* 1986;**136**:109.

Ishii N et al: Therapeutic trial with prostaglandin E_1 for organic impotence. *Jpn J Urol* 1986;**77**:954.

Jensen SB et al: Sexual function and pituitary axis in insulin treated diabetic men. *Acta Med Scand* 1979;**624 (Suppl)**:65.

Jevtich MJ: Importance of penile arterial pulse sound examination in impotence. *J Urol* 1980;**124**:820.

Jevtich MJ et al: Vascular factor in erectile failure among diabetics. *Urology* 1982;**19**:163.

Kaneko S, Bradley WE: Evaluation of erectile dysfunction with continuous monitoring of penile rigidity. *J Urol* 1986;**136**:1026.

Kaplan HS: *Disorders of Sexual Desire*. Brunner/Mazel, 1979.

Karacan I, Moore CA: Nocturnal penile tumescence: An objective diagnostic aid for erectile dysfunction. Pages 62–72 in: *Management of Male Impotence*. Bennett AH (editor). Williams & Wilkins, 1982.

Karacan I et al: Sleep-related penile tumescence as a function of age. *Am J Psychiatry* 1975;**132**:932.

Kaufman JJ, Lindner A, Raz S: Complications of penile prosthesis surgery for impotence. *J Urol* 1982;**128**:1192.

Kedia KR, Markland C: The effect of pharmacologic agents on ejaculation. *J Urol* 1975;**114**:237.

Kedia KR, Markland C, Fraley EE: Sexual function following high retroperitoneal lymphadenectomy. *J Urol* 1975;**114**:237.

Kolodny RC et al: Depression of plasma testosterone levels after chronic intensive marihuana use. *N Engl J Med* 1974A;**290**:872.

Kolodny RC et al: Sexual dysfunction in diabetic men. *Diabetes* 1974B;**23**:306.

Krane RJ: Omniphase penile prosthesis. *Semin Urol* 1986;**4**:247.

Krane RJ, Siroky MB: Studies on sacral-evoked potentials. *J Urol* 1980;**124**:872.

Legros JJ, Mormont C, Servais J: Psychoneuroendocrinological study of erectile "psychogenic impotence": A comparison between normal patients and patients with abnormal reaction to glucose tolerance test. Pages 301–319 in: *Clinical Psychoneuroendocrinology in Reproduction*. Carenza L, Pancheri P, Zichella L (editors). Academic Press, 1978.

Leriche A, Morel A: The syndrome of thrombotic obliteration of aortic bifurcation. *Ann Surg* 1968;**127**:193.

Lewis RW, Puyau FA: Procedures for decreasing venous drainage. *Semin Urol* 1986;**4**:263.

LoPiccolo J: Diagnosis and treatment of male sexual dysfunction. *J Sex Marital Ther* 1986;**11**:215.

Lowsley OS, Bray JL: The surgical relief of impotence: Further experiences with a new operative procedure. *JAMA* 1936;**107**:2029.

Lue TF et al: Functional evaluation of penile veins by cavernosography in papaverine-induced erection. *J Urol* 1986A;**135**:479.

Lue TF et al: Priapism: A refined approach to diagnosis and treatment. *J Urol* 1986B;**136**:104.

Lue TF et al: Vasculogenic impotence evaluated by high-resolution ultrasonography and pulsed Doppler spectrum analysis. *Radiology* 1985;**155**:777.

MacGregor RJ, Konnak JW: Treatment of vasculogenic erectile dysfunction by direct anastamosis of the inferior epigastric artery to the central artery to the corpus cavernosum. *J Urol* 1982;**127**:136.

Mackay JD et al: Diabetic autonomic neuropathy: The diagnostic value of heart rate monitoring. *Diabetologia* 1980;**18**:471.

Masters WH, Johnson VE: *Human Sexual Inadequacy*. Little, Brown, 1970.

Masters WH, Johnson VE: Principles of the new sex therapy. *Am J Psychol* 1976;**133**:548.

Melman A, Henry D: The possible role of the catecholamines of the corpora in penile erection. *J Urol* 1979;**121**:419.

Merchant RF Jr, DePalma RG: Effects of femorofemoral grafts on postoperative sexual function: Correlation with penile pulse volume recordings. *Surgery* 1981;**90**:962.

Merrill DC: Clinical experience with Mentor inflatable penile prosthesis in 206 patients. *Urology* 1986;**28**:185.

Michal V, Kovac J, Belan A: Arterial lesions in impotence: Phalloarteriography. *Int Angiol* 1984;**3**:247.

Michal V, Kramar R, Pospichal J: External iliac "steal syndrome." *J Cardiovasc Surg* 1978;**19**:355.

Michal V, Pospichal J: Phalloarteriography in the diagnosis of erectile impotence. *World J Surg* 1978;**2**:239.

Michal V et al: Aortoiliac occlusive disease. Chapter 24 in: *Vasculogenic Impotence*. Zorgniotti AW, Rossi G (editors). Thomas, 1980.

Michal V et al: Arterial epigastricocavernous anastomosis for the treatment of sexual impotence. *World J Surg* 1977;**1**:515.

Money J: Phantom orgasm in the dreams of paraplegic men and women. *Arch Gen Psychiatry* 1960;**3**:373.

Montague DK: Experience with semirigid rod and inflatable penile prostheses. *J Urol* 1983;**129**:967.

Montague DK, James RE, deWolfe V: Diagnostic screening for vasculogenic impotence. In: *Vasculogenic Impotence*. Zorgniotti AW, Rossi G (editors). Thomas, 1980.

Montague DK et al: Diagnostic evaluation, classification, and treatment of men with sexual dysfunction. *Urology* 1979;**14**:545.

Morales A et al: Nonhormonal pharmacological treatment of organic impotence. *J Urol* 1982;**128**:45.

Morley JE, Melmed S: Gonadal dysfunction in systemic disorders. *Metabolism* 1979;**28**:1051.

Moul JW, McLeod DG: Experience with the AMS 600 malleable penile prosthesis. *J Urol* 1986;**135**:929.

Nadig PW, Ware JC, Blumoff R: A noninvasive device to produce and maintain an erection-like state. *Urology* 1986;**27**:126.

Newman HF: Vibratory sensitivity of the penis. *Fertil Steril* 1970;**21**:791.

Newman HF, Marcus H: Erectile dysfunction in diabetes and hypertension. *Urology* 1985;**26**:135.

Padma-Nathan H, Goldstein I, Krane RJ: Evaluation of the impotent patient. *Semin Urol* 1986A;**4**:225.

Padma-Nathan H, Goldstein I, Krane RJ: Treatment of prolonged or priapistic erections following intracavernosal papaverine therapy. *Semin Urol* 1986B;**4:**236.

Papadopoulos C: Cardiovascular drugs and sexuality: A cardiologist's review. *Arch Intern Med* 1980;**140:**1341.

Perkash I et al: Reproductive biology of paraplegics: Results of semen collection, testicular biopsy and serum hormone evaluation. *J Urol* 1985;**134:**284.

Reichgott MJ: Problems of sexual function in patients with hypertension. *Cardiovasc Med* 1979;**4:**149.

Rubin A, Babbott D: Impotence and diabetes mellitus. *J Am Med Assoc* 1958;**168:**498.

Ružbarský V, Michal V: Morphologic changes in the arterial bed of the penis with aging: Relationship to the pathogenesis of impotence. *Invest Urol* 1977;**15:**194.

Rydin E, Lundberg PO, Brattberg A: Cystometry and micrometry as tools in diagnosing neurogenic impotence. *Acta Neurol Scand* 1981;**63:**181.

Salvatierra O, Fortmann JL, Belzer FO: Sexual function of males before and after renal transplantation. *Urology* 1975;**5:**64.

Semans JH: Premature ejaculation: A new approach. *South Med J* 1956;**49:**353.

Sharlip ID: Penile arteriography in impotence after pelvic trauma. *J Urol* 1981A;**126:**477.

Sharlip ID: Penile revascularization in the treatment of impotence. *West J Med* 1981B;**134:**206.

Sherman FP: Impotence in patients with chronic renal failure on dialysis: Its frequency and etiology. *Fertil Steril* 1975;**26:**221.

Sidi AA et al: Intracavernous drug-induced erections in the management of male erectile dysfunction: Experience with 100 patients. *J Urol* 1986;**135:**704.

Siroky MB, Krane RJ: Physiology of sexual function. Chapter 3 in: *Clinical Neuro-Urology.* Krane RJ, Siroky MB (editors). Little, Brown, 1979.

Small MP: Surgical treatment of impotence with Small-Carrion prosthesis: Preoperative, intraoperative, and postoperative considerations. *J Urol* 1984;**23(5 Spec No):**93.

Spark RF, White RA, Connolly PB: Impotence is not always psychogenic: Newer insights into hypothalamic-pituitary-gonadal dysfunction. *JAMA* 1980;**243:**750.

Spark RF, Wills CA, Royal H: Hypogonadism, hyperprolactinaemia, and temporal lobe epilepsy in hyposexual men. *Lancet* 1984;**1:**413.

Thurm J: Sexual potency of patients on chronic hemodialysis. *Urology* 1975;**5:**60.

Tudoriu T, Bourmer H: The hemodynamics of erection at the level of the penis and its local deterioration. *J Urol* 1983;**129:**741.

Van Arsdalen KN, Malloy TR, Wein AJ: Erectile physiology, dysfunction and evaluation. 2. Etiology and evaluation of erectile dysfunction. *Monogr Urol* 1983;**4:**165.

Van Thiel DH et al: Hypothalamic-pituitary-gonadal dysfunction in men using cimetidine. *N Engl J Med* 1979;**300:**1012.

Velcek D et al: Penile flow index utilizing a Doppler pulse wave analysis to identify penile vascular insufficiency. *J Urol* 1980;**123:**669.

Virag R: Arterial and venous hemodynamics in male impotence. Chap 7, pp 108–126, in: *Management of Male Impotence.* Bennett AH (editor). Williams & Wilkins, 1982A.

Virag R: Intracavernous injection of papaverine for erectile failure. (Letter.) *Lancet* 1982B;**2:**938.

Virag R: Revascularization of the penis. Chap 17, pp 219–233, in: *Management of Male Impotence.* Bennett AH (editor). Williams & Wilkins, 1982C.

Virag R et al: Intracavernous injection of papaverine as a diagnostic and therapeutic method in erectile failure. *Angiology* 1984;**35:**79.

Wagner G: Methods for differential diagnosis of psychogenic and organic erectile failure. Chap 8, pp 89–130, in: *Impotence: Physiological, Psychological, Surgical Diagnosis and Treatment.* Wagner G, Green R (editors). Plenum Press, 1981.

Wagner G, Uhrenholdt A: Blood flow measurement by the clearance method in the human corpus cavernosum in the flaccid and erect status. Chapter 6 in: *Vasculogenic Impotence.* Zorgniotti AW, Rossi G (editors). Thomas, 1980.

Walsh PC, Donker PJ: Impotence following radical prostatectomy: Insight into etiology and preservation. *J Urol* 1982;**128:**492.

Waltzer WC: Sexual and reproductive function in men treated with hemodialysis and renal transplantation. *J Urol* 1981;**126:**713.

Watkins PJ, Mackay JD: Assessment of diabetic autonomic neuropathy using heart rate monitoring. *Horm Metab Res* 1980;**9(Suppl):**69.

Weinstein MH, Machleder HI: Sexual function after aortoiliac surgery. *Ann Surg* 1975;**181:**787.

Weinstein MH, Roberts M: Sexual potency following surgery for rectal carcinoma: A follow-up of 44 patients. *Ann Surg* 1977;**185:**295.

Weiss HD: The physiology of human penile erection. *Ann Intern Med* 1972;**76:**793.

Wespes E, Schulman CC: Parameters of erection. *Br J Urol* 1984;**56:**416.

Wespes E, Schulman CC: Venous leakage: Surgical treatment of a curable cause of impotence. *J Urol* 1985;**133:**796.

Wespes E et al: Cavernometry-cavernography: Its role in organic impotence. *Eur Urol* 1984;**10:**229.

Wespes E et al: Pharmacocavernometry-cavernography in impotence. *Br J Urol* 1986;**58:**429.

Whitelaw GP, Smithwick RA: Some secondary effects of sympathectomy with particular reference to sexual function. *N Engl J Med* 1951;**245:**121.

Winter CC: Priapism. *Urol Surv* 1978;**28:**163.

Winter CC: Priapism treated by modification of creation of fistulas between glans penis and corpora cavernosa. *J Urol* 1979;**121:**743.

Wolpe J: *Psychotherapy by Reciprocal Inhibition.* Stanford Univ Press, 1958.

Wooten JS: Ligation of the dorsal vein of the penis as a cure for atonic impotence. *Tex Med J* 1902–1903;**18:**325.

Zorgniotti AW: Corpus cavernosum blockade for impotence: Practical aspects and results in 250 cases. *J Urol* 1986;**135:**306.

Zorgniotti AW, Lefleur RS: Auto-injection of the corpus cavernosum with a vasoactive drug combination for vasculogenic impotence. *J Urol* 1985;**133:**39.

Appendix:
Normal Laboratory Values*

Marcus A. Krupp, MD

HEMATOLOGY

Bleeding time: Ivy method, 1–7 minutes (60–420 seconds). Template method, 3–9 minutes (180–540 seconds).

Cellular measurements of red cells: Average diameter = 7.3 μm (5.5–8.8 μm).
Mean corpuscular volume (MCV): Men, 80–94 fL; women, 81–99 fL (by Coulter counter).
Mean corpuscular hemoglobin (MCH): 27–32 pg.
Mean corpuscular hemoglobin concentration (MCHC): 32–36 g/dL red blood cells (32–36%).
Color, saturation, and volume indices: 1 (0.9–1.1).

Clot retraction: Begins in 1–3 hours; complete in 6–24 hours. No clot lysis in 24 hours.

Coagulation time (Lee-White): At 37 °C, 6–12 minutes; at room temperature, 10–18 minutes.

Fibrinogen split products: Negative > 1:4 dilution.

Fragility of red cells: Begins at 0.45–0.38% NaCl; complete at 0.36–0.3% NaCl.

Hematocrit (PCV): Men, 40–52%; women, 37–47%.

Hemoglobin: [B] Men, 14–18 g/dL (2.09–2.79 mmol/L as Hb tetramer); women, 12–16 g/dL (1.86–2.48 mmol/L). [S] 2–3 mg/dL.

Partial thromboplastin time: Activated, 25–37 seconds.

Platelets: 150,000–400,000/μL (0.15–0.4 × 10^{12}/L). ·

Prothrombin: [P] 75–125%. Less than 2 seconds deviation from control.

Red blood count (RBC): Men, 4.5–6.2 million/μL (4.5–6.2 × 10^{12}/L); women, 4–5.5 million/μL (4–5.5 × 10^{12}/L).

Reticulocytes: 0.2–2% of red cells.

Sedimentation rate: Less than 20 mm/h (Westergren); 0–10 mm/h (Wintrobe).

White blood count (WBC) and differential: 5000–10,000/μL (5–10 × 10^9/L).

Myelocytes	0 %
Juvenile neutrophils	0 %
Band neutrophils	0–5 %
Segmented neutrophils	40–60%
Lymphocytes	20–40%
Eosinophils	1–3 %
Basophils	0–1 %
Monocytes	4–8 %

Lymphocytes: Total, 1500–4000/μL	
B cell	5–25%
T cell	60–88%
Suppressor	10–43%
Helper	32–66%
H:S	> 1

BLOOD, PLASMA, OR SERUM CHEMICAL CONSTITUENTS
(Values vary with method used.)

Acetone and acetoacetate: [S] 0.3–2 mg/dL (3–20 mg/L).

Aldolase: [S] Values vary with method used.

α-Amino acid nitrogen: [S, fasting] 3–5.5 mg/dL (2.2–3.9 mmol/L).

Aminotransferases:
Aspartate aminotransferase (AST; SGOT): [S] 6–25 IU/L at 30 °C; SMA, 10–40 IU/L at 37 °C; SMAC, 0–41 IU/L at 37 °C.
Alanine aminotransferase (ALT; SGPT): [S] 3–26 IU/L at 30 °C; SMAC, 0–45 IU/L at 37 °C. Values vary with method used.

Ammonia: [B] 80–110 μg/dL (47–65 μmol/L) (diffusion method). Do not use anticoagulant containing ammonium oxalate.

---

* Blood [B], Plasma [P], Serum [S], Urine [U].

Amylase: [S] 80–180 units/dL (Somogyi). Values vary with method used.

α_1-Antitrypsin: [S] > 180 mg/dL.

Ascorbic acid: [P] 0.4–1.5 mg/dL (23–85 μmol/L).

Base, total serum: [S] 145–160 meq/L (145–160 mmol/L).

Bicarbonate: [S] 24–28 meq/L (24–28 mmol/L).

Bilirubin: [S] Total, 0.2–1.2 mg/dL (3.5–20.5 μmol/L). Direct conjugated, 0.1–0.4 mg/dL (< 7 μmol/L). Indirect, 0.2–0.7 mg/dL (< 12 μmol/L).

Calcium: [S] 8.5–10.3 mg/dL (2.1–2.6 mmol/L). Values vary with albumin concentration.

Calcium, ionized: [S] 4.25–5.25 mg/dL; 2.1–2.6 meq/L (1.05–1.3 mmol/L).

β-Carotene: [S, fasting] 50–300 μg/dL (0.9–5.58 μmol/L).

Ceruloplasmin: [S] 25–43 mg/dL (1.7–2.9 μmol/L).

Chloride: [S or P] 96–106 meq/L (96–106 mmol/L).

Cholesterol: [S or P] 150–265 mg/dL (3.9–6.85 mmol/L). (See Lipid fractions.) Values vary with age.

Cholesteryl esters: [S] 65–75% of total cholesterol.

CO_2 content: [S or P] 24–29 meq/L (24–29 mmol/L).

Complement: [S] C3 (β_{1C}), 90–250 mg/dL. C4 (β_{1E}), 10–60 mg/dL. Total (CH_{50}), 75–160 mg/dL.

Copper: [S or P] 100–200 μg/dL (16–31 μmol/L).

Cortisol: [P] 8:00 AM, 5–25 μg/dL (138–690 nmol/L); 8:00 PM. < 10 μg/dL (275 nmol/L).

Creatine kinase (CK): [S] 10–50 IU/L at 30 °C. Values vary with method used.

Creatinine: [S or P] 0.7–1.5 mg/dL (62–132 μmol/L).

Cyanocobalamin: [S] 200 pg/mL (148 pmol/L).

Epinephrine: [P] Supine, < 0.1 μg/L (< 0.55 nmol/L).

Ferritin: [S] Adult women, 20–120 ng/mL; men, 30–300 ng/mL. Child to 15 years, 7–140 ng/mL.

Folic acid: [S] 2–20 ng/mL (4.5–45 nmol/L). [RBC] > 140 ng/mL (> 318 nmol/L).

Glucose: [S or P] 65–110 mg/dL (3.6–6.1 mmol/L).

Haptoglobin: [S] 40–170 mg of hemoglobin-binding capacity.

Iron: [S] 50–175 μg/dL (9–31.3 μg/dL).

Iron-binding capacity: [S] Total, 250–410 μg/dL (44.7–73.4 μmol/L). Percent saturation, 20–55%.

Lactate: [B, special handling] Venous, 4–16 mg/dL (0.44–1.8 mmol/L).

Lactate dehydrogenase (LDH): [S] 55–140 IU/L at 30 °C; SMA, 100–225 IU/L at 37 °C; SMAC, 60–200 IU/L at 37 °C. Values vary with method used.

Lipase: [S] 0.2–1.5 units.

Lipid fractions: [S or P] Desirable levels: HDL cholesterol, > 40 mg/dL; LDL cholesterol, < 180 mg/dL; VLDL cholesterol, < 40 mg/dL. (To convert to mmol/L, multiply by 0.026.)

Lipids, total: [S] 450–1000 mg/dL (4.5–10 g/L).

Magnesium: [S or P] 1.8–3 mg/dL (0.75–1.25 mmol/L).

Norepinephrine: [P] Supine, < 0.5 μg/L (< 3 nmol/L).

Osmolality: [S] 280–296 mosm/kg water (280–296 mmol/kg water).

Oxygen:
 Capacity: [B] 16–24 vol%. Values vary with hemoglobin concentration.
 Arterial content: [B] 15–23 vol%. Values vary with hemoglobin concentration.
 Arterial % saturation: 94–100% of capacity.
 Arterial P_{O_2} (P_{aO_2}): 80–100 mm Hg (10.67–13.33 kPa) (sea level). Values vary with age.

P_{aCO_2}: [B, arterial] 35–45 mm Hg (4.7–6 kPa).

pH (reaction): [B, arterial] 7.35–7.45 (H^+ 44.7–45.5 nmol/L).

Phosphatase, acid: [S] 1–5 units (King-Armstrong), 0.1–0.63 units (Bessey-Lowry).

Phosphatase, alkaline: [S] Adults, 5–13 units (King-Armstrong). 0.8–2.3 (Bessey-Lowry); SMA, 30–85 IU/L at 37 °C; SMAC, 30–115 IU/L at 37 °C.

Phospholipid: [S] 145–200 mg/dL (1.45–2 g/L).

Phosphorus, inorganic: [S, fasting] 3–4.5 mg/dL (1–1.5 mmol/L).

Potassium: [S or P] 3.5–5 meq/L (3.5–5 mmol/L).

Protein:
Total: [S] 6–8 g/dL (60–80 g/L).
Albumin: [S] 3.5–5.5 g/dL (35–55 g/L).
Globulin: [S] 2–3.6 g/dL (20–36 g/L).
Fibrinogen: [P] 0.2–0.6 g/dL (2–6 g/L).

Prothrombin clotting time: [P] By control.

Pyruvate: [B] 0.6–1 mg/dL (70–114 μmol/L).

Serotonin: [B] 0.05–0.2 μg/mL (0.28–1.14 μmol/L).

Sodium: [S or P] 136–145 meq/L (136–145 mmol/L).

Specific gravity: [B] 1.056 (varies with hemoglobin and protein concentration). [S] 1.0254–1.0288 (varies with protein concentration).

Sulfate: [S or P] As sulfur, 0.5–1.5 mg/dL (156–468 μmol/L).

Transferrin: [S] 200–400 mg/dL (23–45 μmol/L).

Triglycerides: [S] < 165 mg/dL (1.9 mmol/L). (See Lipid fractions.)

Urea nitrogen: [S or P] 8–25 mg/dL (2.9–8.9 mmol/L). Do not use anticoagulant containing ammonium oxalate.

Uric acid: [S or P] Men, 3–9 mg/dL (0.18–0.54 mmol/L); women, 2.5–7.5 mg/dL (0.15–0.45 mmol/L).

Vitamin A: [S] 15–60 μg/dL (0.53–2.1 μmol/L).

Vitamin B$_{12}$: [S] > 200 pg/mL (> 148 pmol/L).

Vitamin D: [S] Cholecalciferol (D$_3$): 25-Hydroxy-cholecalciferol, 8–55 ng/mL (19.4–137 nmol/L); 1,25-dihydroxycholecalciferol, 26–65 pg/mL (62–155 pmol/L); 24,25-dihydroxycholecalciferol, 1–5 ng/mL (2.4–12 nmol/L).

Volume, blood (Evans blue dye method): Adults, 2990–6980 mL. Women, 46.3–85.5 mL/kg; men, 66.2–97.7 mL/kg.

Zinc: [S] 50–150 μg/dL (7.65–22.95 μmol/L).

HORMONES, SERUM OR PLASMA

Pituitary:
Growth hormone (GH): [S] Adults, 1–10 ng/mL (46–465 pmol/L) (by RIA).
Thyroid-stimulating hormone (TSH): [S] < 10 μU/mL.
Follicle-stimulating hormone (FSH): [S] Prepubertal, 2–12 mIU/mL; adult men, 1–15 mIU/mL; adult women, 1–30 mIU/mL; castrate or postmenopausal, 30–200 mIU/mL (by RIA).
Luteinizing hormone (LH): [S] Prepubertal, 2–12 mIU/mL; adult men, 1–15 mIU/mL; adult women, < 30 mIU/mL; castrate or postmenopausal, > 30 mIU/mL.
Corticotropin (ACTH): [P] 8:00–10:00 AM, up to 100 pg/mL (22 pmol/L).
Prolactin: [S] 1–25 ng/mL (0.4–10 nmol/L).
Somatomedin C: [P] 0.4–2 U/mL.
Antidiuretic hormone (ADH; vasopressin): [P] Serum osmolality 285 mosm/kg, 0–2 pg/mL; > 290 mosm/kg, 2–12 + pg/mL.

Adrenal:
Aldosterone: [P] Supine, normal salt intake, 2–9 ng/dL (56–250 pmol/L); increased when upright.
Cortisol: [S] 8:00 AM, 5–20 μg/dL (0.14–0.55 μmol/L); 8:00 PM, < 10μg/dL (0.28 μmol/L).
Deoxycortisol: [S] After metyrapone, > 7 μg/dL (> 0.2 μmol/L).
Dopamine: [P] < 135 pg/mL.
Epinephrine: [P] < 0.1 ng/mL (< 0.55 nmol/L).
Norepinephrine: [P] < 0.5 μg/L (< 3 nmol/L).
See also Miscellaneous Normal Values.

Thyroid:
Thyroxine, free (FT$_4$): [S] 0.8–2.4 ng/dL (10–30 pmol/L).
Thyroxine, total (TT$_4$): [S] 5–12 μg/dL (65–156 nmol/L) (by RIA).
Thyroxine-binding globulin capacity (T$_4$): [S] 12–28 μg/dL (150–360 nmol/L).
Triiodothyronine (T$_3$): [S] 80–220 ng/dL (1.2–3.3 nmol/L).
Reverse triiodothyronine (rT$_3$): [S] 30–80 ng/dL (0.45–1.2 nmol/L).
Triiodothyronine uptake (RT$_3$U): [S] 25–36%; as TBG assessment (RT$_3$U ratio), 0.85–1.15.
Calcitonin: [S] < 100 pg/mL (< 29.2 pmol/L).

Parathyroid: Parathyroid hormone levels vary with method and antibody. Correlate with serum calcium.

Islets:
Insulin: [S] 4–25 μU/mL (29–181 pmol/L).
C-peptide: [S] 0.9–4.2 ng/mL.
Glucagon: [S, fasting] 20–100 pg/mL.

Stomach:

Gastrin: [S, special handling] Up to 100 pg/mL (47 pmol/L). Elevated, > 200 pg/mL.

Pepsinogen I: [S] 25–100 ng/mL.

Kidney:

Renin activity: [P, special handling] Normal sodium intake: Supine, 1–3 ng/mL/h; standing, 3–6 ng/mL/h. Sodium depleted: Supine, 2–6 ng/mL/h; standing, 3–20 ng/mL/h.

Gonad:

Testosterone, free: [S] Men, 10–30 ng/dL; women, 0.3–2 ng/dL. (1 ng/dL = 0.035 nmol/L.)

Testosterone, total: [S] Prepubertal, < 100 ng/dL; adult men, 300–1000 ng/dL; adult women, 20–80 ng/dL; luteal phase, up to 120 ng/dL.

Estradiol (E_2): [S, special handling] Men, 12–34 pg/mL; women, menstrual cycle 1–10 days, 24–68 pg/mL; 11–20 days, 50–300 pg/mL; 21–30 days, 73–149 pg/mL (by RIA). (1 pg/mL = 3.6 pmol/L.)

Progesterone: [S] Follicular phase, 0.2–1.5 ng/mL; luteal phase, 6–32 ng/mL; pregnancy, > 24 ng/mL; men, < 1 ng/mL (by RIA). (1 ng/mL = 3.2 nmol/L.)

Placenta:

Estriol (E_3): [S] Men and nonpregnant women, < 0.2 μg/dL (< 7 nmol/L) (by RIA).

Chorionic gonadotropin: [S] Beta subunit: Men, < 9 mIU/mL; pregnant women after implantation, > 10 mIU/mL.

NORMAL CEREBROSPINAL FLUID VALUES

Appearance: Clear and colorless.

Cells: Adults, 0–5 mononuclears/μL; infants, 0–20 mononuclears/μL.

Glucose: 50–85 mg/dL (2.8–4.7 mmol/L). (Draw serum glucose at same time.)

Pressure (reclining): Newborns, 30–80 mm water; children, 50–100 mm water; adults, 70–200 mm water (avg = 125).

Proteins: Total, 20–45 mg/dL (200–450 mg/L) in lumbar cerebrospinal fluid. IgG, 2–6 mg/dL (0.02–0.06 g/L).

Specific gravity: 1.003–1.008.

RENAL FUNCTION TESTS

p-**Aminohippurate (PAH) clearance (RPF):** Men, 560–830 mL/min; women, 490–700 mL/min.

Creatinine clearance, endogenous (GFR): Approximates inulin clearance (see below).

Filtration fraction (FF): Men, 17–21%; women, 17–23%. (FF = GFR/RPF.)

Inulin clearance (GFR): Men, 110–150 mL/min; women, 105–132 mL/min (corrected to 1.73 m^2 surface area).

Maximal glucose reabsorptive capacity (Tm_G): Men, 300–450 mg/min; women, 250–350 mg/min.

Maximal PAH excretory capacity (Tm_{PAH}): 80–90 mg/min.

Osmolality: On normal diet and fluid intake: Range 500–850 mosm/kg water. Achievable range, normal kidney: Dilution 40–80 mosm; concentration (dehydration) up to 1400 mosm/kg water (at least 3–4 times plasma osmolality).

Specific gravity of urine: 1.003–1.030.

MISCELLANEOUS NORMAL VALUES

Adrenal hormones and metabolites:

Aldosterone: [U] 2–26 μg/24 h (5.5–72 nmol). Values vary with sodium and potassium intake.

Catecholamines: [U] Total, < 100 μg/24 h. Epinephrine, < 10 μg/24 h (< 55 nmol); norepinephrine, < 100 μg/24 h (< 591 nmol). Values vary with method used.

Cortisol, free: [U] 20–100 μg/24 h (0.55–2.76 μmol).

11,17-Hydroxycorticoids: [U] Men, 4–12 mg/24 h; women, 4–8 mg/24 h. Values vary with method used.

17-Ketosteroids: [U] Under 8 years, 0–2 mg/24 h; adolescents, 2–20 mg/24 h. Men, 10–20 mg/24 h; women, 5–15 mg/24 h. Values vary with method used. 1 mg = 3.5 μmol.

Metanephrine: [U] < 1.3 mg/24 h(< 6.6 μmol) or < 2.2 μg/mg creatinine. Values vary with method used.

Vanillylmandelic acid (VMA): [U] Up to 7 mg/24 h (< 35 μmol).

Fecal fat: Less than 30% dry weight.

Lead: [U] < 80 μg/24 h (< 0.4 μmol/d).

Porphyrins:
　Delta-aminolevulinic acid: [U] 1.5–7.5 mg/24 h
　　(11.4–57.2 μmol).
　Coproporphyrin: [U] < 230 μg/24 h (<345 nmol).
　Uroporphyrin: [U] < 50 μg/24 h (< 60 nmol).
　Porphobilinogen: [U] < 2 mg/24 h (< 8.8 μmol).

Urobilinogen: [U] 0–2.5 mg/24 h (< 4.23 μmol).

Urobilinogen, fecal: 40–280 mg/24 h (68–474 μmol).

Index

Oxygen, blood, normal values, 680
Oxytetracycline, 237

P pili, in urinary tract infection, 200
Pacemaker, bladder, 447
Pa$_{CO2}$, normal values, 680
PAH, 143
clearance of, normal values, 682
Pain
back, 30, 33
bladder, 33
in cancer, palliation of, 417
colicky, 30
epididymal, 33
flank, 39
kidney, 29, 39
local and referred, in genitourinary tract disorders, 29
prostatic, 33
pseudorenal, 29
radicular, 39
renal, 29
mimicry in, 33
with stones, 276, 277
suprapubic, 33
testicular, 33
ureteral, 30
in urogenital tract neoplasms, 330
Palpation
of female genital tract, 42
of kidney, 38
of penis, 40
Pampiniform plexus, venous, 11
Pancreas, cysts or tumors of, 495
Pa$_{O2}$, normal values, 680
Papaverine, in treatment of impotence, 673
Papaverine test, 669
Papillary necrosis, 212
renal, 521
Paquin operation, 193
Para-aminohippuric acid, 143
Paradidymis, 24
Paradoxic incontinence, 35, 175
Paraneoplastic syndromes, 414
Paraphimosis, 40
Parasympatholytic drugs, in spastic neuropathic bladder, 447
Parasympathomimetic drugs, in flaccid neuropathic bladder, 448
Paratesticular tissues, tumors of, 384
Parathyroid hormone, normal values, 681
PBI, 671
PCV, normal values, 679
Peakometer, 453
Pediculosis pubis, 599
Pelvic inflammatory disease, acute, defined, 198
Pelvic steal syndrome, 671
Pelvis
hematoma of, 312
renal, 5
anatomy of, 4

Penicillin, 236
Penicillin G, 236, 237, 238
in renal failure, 234
Penile brachial pressure index, 671
Penile prostheses, 672, 673
Penile urethra, 26
Penis
absence or duplication of, 26, 568
anatomy of, 10, 13
angiography of, 76
arteries of, 664
carcinoma of, chemotherapy for, 417
congenital anomalies of, **568–574**
deep artery of, 13
diseases of, acquired, **574–579**
disorders of, **568–581**
erection of
agents inducing or inhibiting, 666
hemodynamics of, 664
mechanism of, 665, 666
nocturnal, 664
pharmacology of, 666
phases of, 664
physiology of, 663
psychogenic, 663
reflexogenic, 663
examination of, 40
fracture of, 316
injuries to, 316
innervation of, 663
inspection of, 40
lymphatic occlusion of, 579
nerves of, 663
phlebothrombosis of, 579
plastic induration of, 575
size of
from infancy to adulthood, 568
in infant or child, 36
suspensory ligament of, 10
transverse section of, 10
tumors of, **395–398**
staging of, 396
Pepsinogen I, serum, normal values, 682
Peptostreptococci, in urinary tract infection, 196
Percussion, of kidneys, 39
Percutaneous antegrade endourology, **125–141**
puncture in, 125
Percutaneous nephrolithotomy, 125, 132, 133
Percutaneous nephrostomy, 114, 125
Perfusion profilometry, 461
Perfusion-chemolysis, of renal stones, 131
Perfusion/pressure studies, 128
Pericardial effusions, in cancer, palliation of, 419
Perinephric abscess, 38, 215, 218, 219
Perirenal fascia, 1
Peritoneal dialysis, chronic, 531
Peritoneal irritation, 33

Peritonitis, meconium, 589
Periurethral glands, 8
of Skene, 14
Perivesical cysts, 259
Perivesical lipomatosis, 562
Peyronie's disease, 40, 575
Pflüger's tubes, 22
pH, blood, normal values, 680
Phallus, 26
Pharmaceutical(s), in biotherapy, 325
Pharyngitis, 516
Phenacetin
abuse of, and renal tumors, 348
and necrotizing papillitis, 521
Phenoxybenzamine
in treatment of impotence, 673
and urethral pressure, 464
Phenylalanine mustard, in cancer chemotherapy, 404, 407, 409
Pheochromocytoma, 485
Phimosis, 40, 575
Phlebothrombosis, penile, 579
Phosphatase
acid, serum, normal values, 680
alkaline, serum, normal values, 680
Phosphates, and glucose, absorption of, defects of, 523
Phospholipids, serum, normal values, 681
Phosphorus
absorption of, defects of, 523
inorganic, serum, normal values, 681
Physiologic retractile testis, 41
Pili
bacterial, 200
in urinary tract infection, 200
Piperacillin, 237
Pituitary gland
adenoma of, ablation of, 658
disease of, in infertility, 651
hormones of, normal values, 682
microadenoma of, transsphenoidal resection of, 478
Pituitary hypogonadism, 589
Pituitary-adrenal interrelationship, 478
Placenta, hormones of, normal values, 682
Plain film of abdomen, 59
Plasma, chemical constituents of, 679
Plasmodium malariae, 516
Platelets, normal values, 679
Platinol, in cancer chemotherapy, 404, 408, 411
Pleural effusions, in cancer, palliation of, 419
Plexus, medullary, 5
Pneumaturia, 35, 222
Pneumocystis carinii, pneumonia due to, 272
PNL, 125, 132, 133
Politano-Leadbetter operation, 193

Lange Medical Books are available at medical bookstores within the United States. To order directly from the publisher, complete and mail the postage-paid card below.

BASIC SCIENCE TEXTBOOKS

1. **Correlative Neuroanatomy, 20th Ed.,** *deGroot and Chusid,* A1340-7, $22.50
2. **Biochemistry: A Synopsis,** *Colby,* A0033-9, $14.00
3. **Review of Medical Physiology, 13th Ed.,** *Ganong,* A8435-8, $24.00
4. **Physiology: A Study Guide,** *Ganong,* 2nd Ed., A7864-0, $16.50
5. **Review of Medical Microbiology, 17th Ed.,** *Jawetz et al.,* A8432-5, $22.00
6. **Basic Histology, 5th Ed.,** *Junqueira et al.,* A0570-0, $24.00
7. **Basic & Clinical Pharmacology, 3rd Ed.,** *Katzung,* A0553-6, $29.50
8. **Pharmacology: A Review,** *Katzung and Trevor,* A0031-3, $14.00
9. **Harper's Review of Biochemistry, 21st Ed.,** *Murray et al.,* A3648-1, $29.00
10. **Basic & Clinical Immunology, 6th Ed.,** *Stites et al.,* A0548-6, $29.00

CLINICAL SCIENCE TEXTBOOKS

11. **Principles of Clinical Electrocardiography, 12th Ed.,** *Goldman,* A0008-1, $22.00
12. **Review of General Psychiatry, 2nd Ed.** *Goldman,* A8420-0, $25.00
13. **Electrocardiography: Essentials of Interpretation,** *Goldschlager and Goldman,* A0029-7, $16.50
14. **Basic & Clinical Endocrinology, 2nd Ed.,** *Greenspan and Forsham,* A0547-8, $27.00
15. **Smith's General Urology, 12th Ed.,** *Tanagho,* A8605-6, $29.95
16. **Clinical Cardiology, 4th Ed.,** *Sokolow and McIlroy,* A0023-0, $26.50
17. **General Ophthalmology, 11th Ed.,** *Vaughan and Asbury,* A3108-6, $23.50

CURRENT CLINICAL REFERENCES

18. **Current Obstetric & Gynecologic Diagnosis & Treatment, 6th Ed.,** *Pernoll and Benson,* A1412-4, $34.50
19. **Current Pediatric Diagnosis & Treatment, 9th Ed.,** *Kempe et al.,* A1414-0, $31.50
20. **Current Medical Diagnosis & Treatment 1988, 27th Ed.,** *Schroeder et al.,* A1344-9, $32.50
21. **Current Emergency Diagnosis & Treatment, 2nd Ed.,** *Mills et al.,* A0027-1, $29.50
22. **Current Surgical Diagnosis & Treatment, 8th Ed.,** *Way,* A1415-7, $34.50

HANDBOOKS

23. **Handbook of Obstetrics & Gynecology, 8th Ed.,** *Benson,* A0014-9, $13.00
24. **Handbook of Poisoning, 12th Ed.,** *Dreisbach and Robertson,* A3643-2, $16.50
25. **Physician's Handbook, 21st Ed.,** *Krupp et al.,* A0002-4, $16.50
26. **Handbook of Pediatrics, 15th Ed.,** *Silver et al.,* A3635-8, $16.50

NEW LANGE TITLES

27. **Clinical Anatomy,** *Lindner,* A1259-9, $25.00 (approx.)
28. **Clinical Thinking in Surgery,** *Sterns,* A5686-9, $24.00 (approx.)

LANGE CLINICAL MANUALS

29. **Psychiatry: Diagnosis & Therapy, '88-'89,** *Flaherty et al.,* A1277-1, $19.95
30. **Neonatology: Basic Management, On-Call Problems, Diseases, Drugs, '88-'89,** *Gomella,* A1280-5, $19.95
31. **Clinical Pharmacology, '88-'89,** *Katzung,* A1281-3, $19.95
32. **Internal Medicine: Diagnosis and Therapy, '88-'89,** *Stein,* A1275-5, $19.95

ORDER CARD

Please send the books I've circled below on 30-day approval:

1. deGroot, A1340-7, $22.50
2. Colby, A0033-9, $14.00
3. Ganong, A8435-8, $24.00
4. Ganong, A7864-0, $16.50
5. Jawetz, A8432-5, $22.00
6. Junqueira, A0570-0, $24.00
7. Katzung, A0553-6, $29.50
8. Katzung, A0031-3, $14.00
9. Murray, A3648-1, $29.00
10. Stites, A0548-6, $29.00
11. Goldman, A0008-1, $22.00
12. Goldman, A8420-0, $25.00
13. Goldschlager, A0029-7, $16.50
14. Greenspan, A0547-8, $27.00
15. Tanagho, A8605-6, $29.95
16. Sokolow, A0023-0, $26.50
17. Vaughan, A3108-6, $23.50
18. Pernoll, A1412-4, $34.50
19. Kempe, A1414-0, $31.50
20. Schroeder, A1344-9, $32.50
21. Mills, A0027-1, $29.50
22. Way, A1415-7, $34.50
23. Benson, A0014-9, $13.00
24. Dreisbach, A3643-2, $16.50
25. Krupp, A0002-4, $16.50
26. Silver, A3635-8, $16.50
27. Lindner, A1259-9, $25.00 (approx.)
28. Sterns, A5686-9, $24.00 (approx.)
29. Flaherty, A1277-1, $19.95
30. Gomella, A1280-5, $19.95
31. Katzung, A1281-3, $19.95
32. Stein, A1275-5, $19.95

☐ Payment enclosed. (Publisher pays postage & handling.) Please include your state sales tax.
☐ Bill me later.
Charge to: ☐ VISA ☐ Mastercard

Card # _____ Exp. Date _____

Signature _____

APPLETON & LANGE
25 Van Zant St.
E. Norwalk, CT 06855
Simon & Schuster Higher Education Group

NAME _____

ADDRESS _____

CITY/STATE/ZIP _____

Prices advertised are in U.S. dollars and applicable in the U.S. only. All prices are subject to change without notice.

In Canada, contact Prentice-Hall Canada, 1870 Birchmount Rd., Scarborough, Ontario M1P 2J7.

Outside the U.S. and Canada, contact Simon & Schuster Intl., Englewood Cliffs, NJ 07632.